FOURTEEN PAIRS OF DRUGS WHICH CAN CAUSE LIFE-THREATENING REACTIONS IF USED TOGETHER:

Propulsid with Biaxin

insulin with Inderal

warfarin (Coumadin) with Tagamet

Sporanox with Propulsid

Prozac with Desyrel

Lanoxin with Calan SR

Tagamet with Dilantin

Zocor with Posicor

Hismanal with Paxil

Mevacor with Lopid

Tegretol with erythromycin

Calan SR with quinidine

theophylline with Tagamet

Demerol with Nardil

Hundreds of other pairs of dangerously interacting drugs discussed inside!

WORST PILLS, BEST PILLS

A Consumer's Guide to Avoiding Drug-Induced Death or Illness

Sidney M. Wolfe, M.D.;

Larry D. Sasich, Pharm.D., M.P.H.; Rose-Ellen Hope, R.Ph.;

and Public Citizen's Health Research Group

POCKET BOOKS

New York   London   Toronto   Sydney   Tokyo   Singapore

Publisher's Note

The drug information contained in this book is based on product labeling published in the 1997 edition of *Physicians' Desk Reference*®, supplemented with facts from other sources the publisher believes reliable. While diligent efforts have been made to assure the accuracy of this information, the book does not list every possible adverse reaction, interaction, precaution, and effect of a drug; and all information is presented without guarantees by the authors, consultants, and publisher, who disclaim all liability in connection with its use.

This book is intended only as a reference for use in an ongoing partnership between doctor and patient in the vigilant management of the patient's health. It is not a substitute for a doctor's professional judgment, and serves only as a reminder of concerns that may need discussion. All readers are urged to consult with a physician before beginning or discontinuing use of any prescription drug or undertaking any form of self-treatment.

Brand names listed in this book are intended to represent only the more commonly used products. Inclusion of a brand name does not signify endorsement of the product; absence of a name does not imply a criticism or rejection of the product. The publisher is not advocating the use of any product described in this book, does not warrant or guarantee any of these products, and has not performed any independent analysis in connection with the product information contained herein.

 POCKET BOOKS, a division of Simon & Schuster Inc.
1230 Avenue of the Americas, New York, NY 10020

Copyright © 1990, 1993 by Public Citizen's Health Research Group
Copyright © 1999 by Public Citizen Foundation, Inc., Sidney M. Wolfe, M.D., and Public Citizen's Health Research Group

All rights reserved, including the right to reproduce this book or portions thereof in any form whatsoever. For information address Pocket Books, 1230 Avenue of the Americas, New York, NY 10020

ISBN: 0-671-01918-X

First Pocket Books trade paperback printing February 1999

10 9 8 7 6 5 4 3 2 1

POCKET and colophon are registered trademarks of Simon & Schuster Inc.

Cover design by Matt Galemmo
Front cover photo by Jonathan Kirn/Liaison Agency

Printed in the U.S.A.

This book is dedicated to all those people who need to intervene, armed with as much information as possible, to stop preventable drug-induced injuries or deaths from occurring to ourselves, our families, or our friends. There are tens of millions of us.

PREFACE

The latest edition of this extraordinarily useful reference book arrives at a critical time for both young and older Americans. During the past several years there have been many "recalls" of drugs with their licenses withdrawn by the Food and Drug Administration (FDA). This unhappy situation has been attributed to the pressure for speedy approval of new drugs exerted on the FDA by the drug industry and their supporters in Congress and the Senate. For example, fenfluramine, a purported appetite suppressant, was withdrawn after possibly as many as five million Americans had taken it. It seems this drug can, in rare cases, cause a potentially fatal lung disease called primary pulmonary hypertension and can commonly cause damage to the heart valves. Initial estimates are that perhaps as many as 10,000 or more fenfluramine users may have sustained valve damage from this drug. Other recently approved drugs listed as **Do Not Use** in this book may also end up being recalled.

Another baleful development is the passage of changes in the FDA regulations to allow "off-label" promotion of drugs by pharmaceutical industry salespersons in doctors' offices. Off-label use is the prescribing of an approved drug for an *unapproved* indication—one that has not been adequately tested nor approved by the FDA as the data submitted is inadequate to support the therapeutic claim.

I believe the increasing trend toward the use of so-called "alternative" therapy is dangerous, although at first glance it might seem empowering to the consumer. However, this sense of empowerment is illusory. The consumer has only gained the "right" to self-medicate with untested drugs, herbs, homeopathic concoctions and the like, without the protection of the FDA testing and evaluation. Such testing, while flawed, is still usually done quite well when the FDA is not pressured to speed up approval without adequate time for careful scrutiny.

Worst Pills, Best Pills is perhaps the best defense the health consumer can rely on for objective and evidence-based information and advice about drugs. Previous editions have sold many copies, attesting to its usefulness. This latest edition is updated in the continuing tradition of careful science merged with common sense advice. I urge you to keep this book handy to consult as your doctor prescribes for you and as you read about the claims made by manufacturers for their drugs. However, do not make the error of becoming nihilistic and cynical about drugs. We have an array of powerful and life-saving drugs which, when used properly, can make your life more comfortable and often cure previously dreaded illnesses. This book will help you distinguish those useful and reasonably safe drugs from those best avoided.

Paul D. Stolley, M.D.
Professor of Medicine and Preventive Medicine
University of Maryland School of Medicine
Baltimore, Maryland

ACKNOWLEDGMENTS

Worst Pills, Best Pills is the result of the talent, time, labor, and dedication of many people, including past and present members of the staff of Public Citizen's Health Research Group as well as many others outside the group.

The Authors
- Sidney M. Wolfe, M.D., Director, Public Citizen's Health Research Group
- Larry D. Sasich, pharmacist and researcher, Public Citizen's Health Research Group
- Rose-Ellen Hope, pharmacist, Silverton, Oregon

The Editorial and Production Staff
Thank you to:
- *Phyllis M. McCarthy* for her exceptional organizational skills, limitless know-how, attention to important details, preparation of the manuscript, proofreading, editing suggestions and her profound caring for those who will use and benefit from this book.

- *Alana Bame,* for editing, proofreading, fact checking and helping out in 100 other ways.
- *Benita Marcus Adler,* for proofreading and offering helpful design suggestions.
- *David Vladeck,* Director, Public Citizen's Litigation Group for a review of the manuscript as well as other helpful suggestions.

We also wish to acknowledge the additional authors of the 1988 edition of this report: Lisa Fugate, Elizabeth P. Hulstrand, and Laurie E. Kamimoto.

We would also like to thank our editor, Nancy Miller, and all of our friends at Pocket Books: Donna O'Neill, Donna Ruvituso, Erin Galligan, Kim Kanner, Lisa Feuer, Joann Foster, Emily Bestler, Gina Centrello, and finally, our copy editors, Miriam Varian and Jill Parsons.

CONTENTS

Introduction   xv

How This Book Was Compiled   xxi

Medical Advisers   xxiii

Index of Drugs   xxv

1: Misprescribing and Overprescribing of Drugs   1
    Evidence of Misprescribing and Overprescribing   2
    The Causes of Misprescribing and Overprescribing   4

2: Adverse Drug Reactions   9
    How Extensive Is the Problem of Specific
      Adverse Drug Reactions?   10
    Specific Patient Examples   12
    Nine Reasons Why Older Adults Are More Likely
      Than Younger Adults to Have Adverse
      Drug Reactions   15
    Which Adverse Effects Can Be Caused by
      Which Drugs?   18

        Summary of Adverse Reactions and the Drugs
          That Cause Them   18

        Drugs That Can Affect the Mind (Such as Those
          Causing Depression or Psychoses)   19

        Drugs That Can Cause Abnormal, Involuntary
          Movements   25

        Drugs That Can Disturb Balance   26

        Drugs That Can Cause Sexual Dysfunction   28

        Drugs That Can Affect the Gastrointestinal
          (GI) Tract   30

            Drugs That Can Cause Lung Toxicity   33
            Drugs That Can Affect the Urinary Tract   34

3: 456 Drugs Commonly Used by Consumers   39
    How to Use This Chapter   39
    Drugs for Heart Conditions   41
            Drug Listings   41
            High Blood Pressure   44
            Potassium Supplementation   49
            Beta-blockers   52
            Calcium Channel Blockers   53
            Cholesterol-lowering Drugs   54
            Drug Profiles   56

    Mind Drugs   177
            Drug Listings   177
            Tranquilizers and Sleeping Pills   178
            Antipsychotic Drugs   187
            Depression   196
            Drug Profiles   201

    Painkillers and Arthritis Drugs   259
            Drug Listings   259
            Salicylates   261
            Narcotics   264
            Arthritis and Inflammation   265
            Drug Profiles   270

    Gastrointestinal Drugs   351
            Drug Listings   351
            Diarrhea   352
            Constipation   354
            Gas   354
            Drug Profiles   354

    Cold, Cough, Allergy, and Asthma Drugs   400
            Drug Listings   400
            Cold   402
            Allergy and Hay Fever   405
            Asthma, Chronic Bronchitis, and Emphysema   408
            Drug Profiles   410

Drugs for Infections   466
        Drug Listings   466
        Antibiotics   468
        Penicillins and Cephalosporins   470
        Fluoroquinolones   472
        Tetracyclines   474
        Drug Profiles   475

Drugs for Diabetes   550
        Drug Listings   550
        Diabetes and Its Treatment   550
        Drug Profiles   555

Drugs for Neurological Disorders   569
        Drug Listings   569
        Drug Profiles   569

Nutritional Supplements   592
        Supplement Listings   592
        Nutritional Supplements   592
        Supplement Profiles   600

Eye Drugs   621
        Drug Listings   621
        General Instructions for Application of
                Eye Drops and Ointment   622
        Glaucoma   623
        Drug Profiles   624

Drugs for Other Conditions   649
        Drug Listings   649
        Corticosteroids   651
        Drug Profiles   654

4: Protecting Yourself and Your Family
    from Preventable Drug-induced Injury   745
    Sample Drug Worksheet   747

5: Saving Money While Avoiding Injury
    When Buying Prescription Drugs   756

Glossary   768

Drug Worksheet

INTRODUCTION

- A 40-year-old woman who dies from a heart arrhythmia
- A 58-year-old man who has just developed parkinsonism
- A 68-year-old woman with a hip fracture
- A 63-year-old woman whose memory and ability to think clearly are slipping, according to her daughter
- A 62-year-old man with recent onset of extreme dizziness and occasional fainting when he first gets up
- A 52-year-old woman who suddenly dies while having some dental work done

What Do These People Have In Common?

They are all tragic victims of serious but entirely preventable adverse reactions to prescription drugs. In each case, the drug was too dangerous to be used at all or was misprescribed. (See Chapter 2, "Adverse Drug Reactions," (p. 9.) In fact, a study in *The Journal of the American Medical Association* found that adverse drug reactions are responsible for 100,000 fatalities a year and afflicting 2.2 million people with serious drug-induced diseases.[1] Drug-induced illness is one of the leading causes of preventable disease and death in the United States. By reading and using *Worst Pills, Best Pills,* you can help protect yourself and your family from the dangers of misprescribed drugs. But first, you may have some questions. Here are the answers to some frequently asked ones.

Question: **Sure, once in a while prescription drugs, whether prescribed properly or not, can cause adverse drug reactions. But the six cases above are unusual, aren't they?**

Answer: Unfortunately, they are all too common. In addition to the fact that there are 100,000 deaths a year from adverse drug reactions, each year approximately 1.5 million people in the United States are injured so seriously by adverse drug reactions that they require hospitalization. Seven hundred thousand people a year develop adverse drug reactions *after* they have been hospitalized for other reasons. Also, there are *61,000 people with drug-induced parkinsonism; 32,000 with hip fractures, including 1,500 deaths attributable to drug-induced falls; 16,000 with injuries from car crashes caused by adverse drug reactions; 163,000 with drug-induced or drug-worsened memory loss; 41,000 with hospitalizations—3,300 of whom died—from ulcers caused by nonsteroidal anti-inflammatory drugs, usually for arthritis; and hundreds of thousands of people with drug-induced dizziness or fainting.*

Other drug reactions can also lead to death. Older drugs such as *digoxin* (see p. 113), a heart medicine, cause 28,000 cases of life-threatening or fatal adverse reactions each year in hospitals alone, often because the prescribed dose is too high or the drug is given to people who do not need to be taking it in the first place. Newer drugs, such as the powerful sedative/tranquilizer *Versed,* can also be extremely dangerous if not used carefully. Used for so-called conscious sedation during oral surgery or during diagnostic procedures such as gastroscopy, this drug has caused dozens of preventable deaths when the dose was needlessly high.

Question: **But why are so many people getting adverse drug reactions and how can they be prevented?**

Answer: First: Often, the "disease" for which a drug is prescribed is actually an adverse reaction to another drug, masquerading as a disease. Second: Many times a drug is used to treat a problem which, although susceptible in some cases to a pharmaceutical solution, should first be treated with common sense lifestyle changes. Third: The medical problem—as with viral infections such as colds and bronchitis in otherwise healthy children or adults—is both self-limited and completely unresponsive to treatments such as antibiotics or does not merit treatment with certain drugs. Fourth: A drug *is* the preferred treatment for the medical problem, but instead of using the safest, most effective—and often least expensive—treatment, one of the 160 **Do Not Use** drugs listed in this book—or another much less preferable alternative—is prescribed. Fifth: Different prescription drugs, each of which on its own may be safe and effective, together can interact to cause serious injury or death. Sixth: Adverse reactions can occur when two or more drugs in the same therapeutic category are used, even though the additional ones do not add to the effectiveness of the first but clearly increase the risk to the patient. Seventh: Many times the right drug is prescribed, but the dose is dangerously high.

Question: **Why do older adults suffer more, and more serious, adverse drug reactions than younger people?**

Answer: In Chapter 2, "Adverse Drug Reactions," p. 9, we discuss nine reasons, including both physical differences and differences and deficiencies in doctors' prescribing habits.

DRUGS THAT CAN CAUSE LIFE-THREATENING REACTIONS IF USED TOGETHER

Propulsid with Biaxin	Hismanal with Paxil
insulin with Inderal	Mevacor with Lopid
warfarin (Coumadin) with Tagamet	Tegretol with erythromycin
Sporanox with Propulsid	Calan SR with quinidine
Prozac with Desyrel	theophylline with Tagamet
Lanoxin with Calan SR	
Tagamet with Dilantin	
Zocor with Posicor	Demerol with Nardil

Recent studies have found that:

• Seventy percent of doctors treating Medicare patients flunked an exam concerning their knowledge of prescribing to older adults.

• Between 40% and 50% of drugs prescribed for older adults outside the hospital were overused.

• Among older patients being given three or more prescriptions upon leaving the hospital, 88% had prescriptions with one or more problems and 22% had prescription errors that were potentially serious or life-threatening. A closer look at these frequent, often-serious prescribing mistakes showed that:

• Fifty-nine percent of patients were prescribed a less-than-optimal drug or one not effective for their disease.

• Twenty-eight percent of patients were given doses that were too high.

• Forty-eight percent of patients were given drugs with one or more potential harmful interactions with other drugs.

But, according to the World Health Organization, *"quite often, the history and clinical examination of patients with side effects reveal that no valid indication [purpose] for the drug has been present."*[2]

Question: **Are you and the World Health Organization saying that if older people used fewer drugs, more selectively, most adverse reactions would be prevented?**

Answer: Yes, that is exactly what we are saying. Most older people and many younger people are using too many drugs, often for problems that are better treated with nondrug therapy. (See sections on sleeping pills and tranquilizers, p. 178, diabetes, p. 550, and hypertension, p. 44.)

Question: **Since more of these problems occur in older people, if I am not 60 or over, do I really need to worry about them?**

Answer: You certainly do, for two reasons. First, serious problems with prescription drugs do not suddenly start at age 60. Beginning in our thirties, the output of the heart and the ability of the liver to metabolize drugs and, even more importantly, of the kidney to clear drugs out of the body, begin to decrease. Since most people in their thirties or forties are not given many prescription drugs, these changes alone do not usually lead to a large number of drug-induced medical problems. **Most of the adverse reactions discussed in this book, however, can occur in anyone at any age. They just occur more often in older adults.**

However, as people enter their fifties, the amount of prescription drug use starts increasing significantly, and the odds of getting an adverse drug reaction also increase. The risk of an adverse drug reaction is about 33% higher in people aged 50 to 59 than in people aged 40 to 49.[3] It becomes two to three times higher as people get even older.[4]

For most of the categories of problems that can be caused by drugs, such as depression, sexual dysfunction, memory loss, hallucinations, insomnia, parkinsonism, constipation, and many others, we include lists of frequently prescribed drugs that can cause these problems in

people of any age (see Chapter 2). Only for the categories of drug-induced automobile crashes resulting in injuries, and hip fractures do the drug lists apply mainly to people 60 and older.

If you do not learn how to reduce (or keep low, if not at zero) the number of prescription drugs you are taking when you are in your thirties, forties, and fifties, you will be in great danger of becoming another overmedicated person at unnecessary risk of adverse drug reactions.

The second reason for concern, even though you may be less than 60 years old, is that all people under 60 have parents, grandparents, brothers, sisters, or friends who are over 60 and who could use some of your help in better coping with the onslaught of drugs and other treatments that most doctors are inclined to prescribe. (See Chapter 4, "Protecting Yourself and Your Family from Preventable Drug-Induced Injury," p. 745, for specific ways you can help others with the information in this book.)

Question: **How many of the drugs in this book should not be used?**

Answer: According to published studies and/or the Public Citizen's Health Research Group or its medical consultants, 160 of the 456 commonly prescribed drugs—one out of every three drugs—should not be used because safer alternative drugs are available. (See Chapter 3, p. 39, for the 160 **"Do Not Use"** drugs and their safer alternatives.)

*This list of **Do Not Use** drugs includes widely used sleeping pills and tranquilizers such as Valium, Restoril, Ativan, and Tranxene; antidepressants such as Elavil; painkillers or arthritis drugs such as Darvocet-N and Darvon, Ultram and Feldene; heart drugs such as Persantine, Lopid, Aldomet, Dyrenium, and Catapres; gastrointestinal drugs such as Bentyl, Donnatal, Librax, Lomotil, and Tigan; the widely used diabetes drugs Diabinese and Glucophage; and birth control pills such as Desogen and Ortho-Cept.*

These 23 Do Not Use drugs alone account for more than 100 million prescriptions filled a year, at a cost of well in excess of $2 billion a year.

When you look at the 160 **Do Not Use** drugs you will find 137 other drugs in addition to these 23. In three of the major categories of drugs, a large proportion are categorized as **Do Not Use** by our medical experts. They include:

- 20 of 46, or 43%, of the mind drugs (tranquilizers, sleeping pills, etc.)
- 43 of 110, or 39%, of the heart/blood pressure drugs
- 13 of 35, or 37%, of the gastrointestinal drugs.

Even for the 152 drugs that we categorize as **Limited Use** or the other drugs discussed in the book, the number of serious, life-threatening adverse reactions can be significantly reduced by using lower doses and avoiding the harmful interactions with other drugs or foods that we list.

Question: **What can be done about this serious epidemic of preventable drug-induced illness?**
Answer: The solution to this problem, a difficult one, will have to involve you, your doctor(s), and your pharmacist.

A good way to start is by being aware of the extraordinary variety of "illnesses" that are often written off to old age or to nervous problems but can be drug-induced. For example, all of the following medical problems have been found, in a significant number of instances, to occur as adverse drug reactions. The number of different drugs listed by name in the tables in Chapter 2 that can cause each type of adverse reaction is included:

- 148 drugs can cause depression
- 133 drugs can cause hallucinations or psychoses
- 128 drugs can cause sexual dysfunction

- 76 drugs can cause dementia
- 52 drugs can cause falls and hip fractures
- 20 drugs can cause auto accidents resulting in injuries
- 27 drugs can cause insomnia
- 105 drugs can cause constipation
- 36 drugs can cause parkinsonism

This list does not include those kinds of adverse reactions that are more difficult for patients or their friends to detect, such as early evidence of liver or lung damage, nor does it contain every drug, no matter how few prescriptions there are, which can cause the adverse effects listed here.

Further specific details of how to significantly reduce the risks of drug-induced death and injury are discussed in Chapter 4, including *Ten Rules for Safer Drug Use.*

The first step is to take an inventory of all the drugs you or your parents or other loved one have used in the last month, including over-the-counter and prescription drugs. The most accurate way to do this is **to put all the drugs in a brown bag** and, the next time you or your parents go to the doctor, bring all of them along and **get the doctor to help you fill out the Drug Worksheet for Patients, Family, Doctor and Pharmacist**, sample on p. 747. For each drug you or your parents are using, you will need to list the doses, how often the drug is taken and for how long, the medical conditions for which the doctor says each drug is being used, the adverse effects you or your parents are having from any of these drugs, and other information shown on the drug worksheet. Then you, your parents, and the doctor can begin the process of reducing the number of drugs being taken by eliminating the ones that are not absolutely necessary or are unnecessarily dangerous. At the same time, the dosage of drugs that are thought to be necessary can be reduced, if possible, to further decrease the risk of adverse drug reactions.

Question: **When I finally get down to the smallest number of drugs I really need to be taking and the lowest dose of each, is there any way that I can further cut down on the $1,200 a year I am now spending on prescription drugs?**

Answer: As discussed in much more detail in Chapter 5, *"Saving Money While Avoiding Injury When Buying Prescription Drugs"* (p. 756), each year a larger percentage of the drugs most commonly used by older adults is available in generic form—which is usually much less expensive—as the brand name versions come off patent. In this chapter, we also discuss and rebut the myths that brand name companies are using to frighten doctors and patients from using these much less expensive drugs.

In addition, many times you'll find that more expensive, but not safer or more effective drugs, are prescribed because they are heavily promoted to doctors.

A typical older adult might be prescribed Feldene for arthritis and Calan SR for high blood pressure. At costs of $1,200 per year for the Feldene and about $680 a year for Calan SR, the total would be $1,880. But Feldene is a **Do Not Use** drug, and both of the preferred *Worst Pills, Best Pills* alternatives for arthritis, generic enteric-coated aspirin and ibuprofen, cost about $280 a year. Similarly, Calan SR

costs about $680 a year, but the first choice drug for hypertension, generic hydrochlorothiazide, can be obtained for only $72 a year. Thus, the yearly drug bill for this typical person would be $352 a year instead of $1,880, or about one-fifth as much.

In the drug profiles in Chapter 3, the availability of a generic version of each drug is listed at the top (except for those in the **Do Not Use** category).

One last thought: When we hear the phrase *drug abuse* these days, the first thing that comes to mind is heroin, cocaine, smack, crack, or whatever drug is currently in the headlines. But what about drug abuse in older people? Well, older people do not use *those* kinds of drugs. *That* problem mainly has to do with younger people. But that is taking the narrow view that drug abuse means the drug-abusing person "chooses" to take drugs such as heroin and cocaine. If instead, we broaden the definition of drug abuse to include older or younger victims of the drug choices of others— such as patients of doctors—then **the greatest epidemic of drug abuse in American society is among those patients who are the victims of misprescribing or overprescribing.** Like other epidemics, it is preventable. This book will help you start that process.

1. Lazarou J, Pomeranz BH, Corey PN. Incidence of adverse drug reactions in hospitalized patients: a meta-analysis of prospective studies. *Journal of the American Medical Association* 1998; 279: 1200–5.

2. *Drugs for the Elderly*. 2nd ed. Copenhagen, Denmark: World Health Organization, 1997.

3. Vestal RE, ed. *Drug Treatment in the Elderly*. Sydney, Australia: ADIS Health Science Press, 1984. Calculation of 33% increase in risk of adverse reaction (age 50–59 vs. 40–49) is based on an average of all three studies listed on page 32.

4. Avorn JL, Lamy PP, Vestal RE. Prescribing for the elderly safely. *Patient Care* June 30, 1982:14–62.

HOW THIS BOOK WAS COMPILED

Which Drugs Are Included in the Book?

The decision as to which drugs were to be included in the book was based in part on data from the *American Druggist* list of the 200 most commonly prescribed drugs in the U.S. in 1997, all of which are included in the book. We also added a number of drugs that have only recently come on the market but which are likely to soon become among the most often prescribed drugs. In addition, we included many drugs which, although not in the top 200, are often used by older adults, and were in earlier editions of *Worst Pills, Best Pills*. We did not include in the book any drug if more than 50% of its use was in the hospital, such as a number of antibiotics, drugs for general anesthesia, and other drugs. Nor did we include most drugs used primarily for the treatment of cancer.

The total number of drugs listed in the book is 456; the names appear in the Index and the Table of Contents for each section in Chapter 3. The generic names are in lower-case letters, and the brand names are in capital letters.

What Information Goes Into the Discussions of Specific Drugs?

In addition to information that is referenced in the listed medical journal articles and books, much of the other information comes from the *Physicians' Desk Reference*® and the *USP DI* (the United States Pharmacopeia Drug Information), 1998 editions.

On What Basis Is a Drug Listed as "Do Not Use"?

For each of the 160 drugs listed as **"Do Not Use,"** at least one or more of the following reasons was used as the basis for the decision:

1. Published references explicitly stating not to use the drug in older adults and other information advising against use in younger people.

2. Single-ingredient drugs that, in the opinion of Public Citizen's Health Research Group and its consultants,* are not as safe as the alternative drug or other treatment that is always listed on the page to the right of the **"Do Not Use."**

3. Lack of evidence of effectiveness of the drug in the opinion of Public Citizen's Health Research Group and its consultants.* This was most commonly seen in combination drugs in which at least one ingredient has not been proven to be effective or the second ingredient has not been proven to significantly add to the effectiveness of the first. Therefore the combination drug is more dangerous than an alternative without the unproven ingredient because it has increased risks posed by the extra ingredient without any increased benefit.

4. Fixed-combination drugs that do not, in the opinion of Public Citizen's Health Research Group and its consultants* meet the criteria for justifying their use. Use fixed combinations of drugs only when they are logical and well studied and they either aid compliance or improve tolerance or efficacy obtained with a single ingredient. **Few fixed combinations meet this standard.**

On What Basis Is a Drug Listed as "Limited Use"?

Drugs were designated for "Limited Use" on the basis of one or more of the following criteria:

1. Published studies stating that the drug should only be used as a second-line drug if another drug does not work.

2. Published studies showing that the drug is more dangerous than another, preferable drug but not so much so that it merits being listed as **"Do Not Use."**

3. Published evidence that the drug, although effective and safe enough for the treatment of certain conditions, is widely used for inappropriate and therefore unnecessarily unsafe purposes. The widespread use of antipsychotic drugs for treating older adults who are not psychotic (see p. 187) is an example of this serious problem.

4. Combination drugs that should be reserved for second-choice use. (Most are **Do Not Use**.) Examples are many combination high blood pressure drugs which are required to carry a warning label. The label states that, because it is a fixed-combination drug, the drug is not indicated for initial treatment of high blood pressure.

On What Basis Is a Drug Listed as "Do Not Use Until Five Years After Release"?

Safety dictates the designation of a new drug as "Do Not Use Until Five Years After Release." The exception to this rule is a rare "breakthrough" drug that offers a documented therapeutic benefit over older proven drugs. The "Do Not Use Until Five Years After Release" designation is made for the following reasons:

1. New drugs are the most dangerous because we know the least about their safety.

2. New drugs are tested in a relatively small number of people before they are approved and much more is known about their effectiveness than their safety.

3. Though more is known about the effectiveness of new drugs, it is rarely known if they are more or less effective than older drugs.

4. Serious adverse effects or life-threatening drug interactions may not be detected until a new drug has been taken by hundreds of thousands of people.

5. A number of new drugs have been withdrawn from the market, or serious new adverse reaction warnings have been added to their labeling, usually within five years after they have been released.

The problem has become more serious in recent years because of the record numbers of new drugs that have been approved in the U.S. due to intense political pressure exerted by the pharmaceutical industry through Congress on a weakened Food and Drug Administration (FDA). In a period of only nine months, between September 1997 and June 1998, three new drugs with known safety problems were withdrawn, all on the market for less than five years. They should not have been approved but were approved by the FDA. Tragically, in each of these cases, there were multiple other older proven drugs available for treating the same conditions that these drugs were approved for and hundreds of people were needlessly killed or injured.

---

* All drugs were initially reviewed by Public Citizen's Health Research Group staff to decide which ones should be listed as **"Do Not Use."** Subsequently, most drugs were also reviewed, depending on their therapeutic category, by at least one specialist in areas including cardiology, diabetology, gastroenterology, infectious diseases, neurology, and psychiatry. Each drug met at least one of the criteria listed above for **"Do Not Use"** and/or was thought by Public Citizen's Health Research Group staff and at least one of the above consultants to merit a **"Do Not Use"** designation. (The names and affiliations of these consultants are listed on p. xxiii.)

MEDICAL ADVISERS

The following physicians, with expertise in various medical subspecialties, gave generously of their time to read and make helpful suggestions about the parts of the book that fell into their area of expertise.

Frank Calia, M.D., Chief of Infectious Diseases, University of Maryland and Chief of Medicine, Baltimore Veterans Administration Hospital (Drugs for Infections for all three editions)

Charles Gerson, M.D., physician in private practice of gastroenterology, New York City, and attending physician, Mount Sinai School of Medicine, New York (Gastrointestinal Drugs for all three editions)

Joseph Lowenstein, M.D., Professor of Internal Medicine, Texas Tech University Health Sciences Center, Odessa, Texas (Drugs for Diabetes for third edition)

Louis Rakita, M.D., Department of Cardiology, Cleveland Metropolitan General Hospital and Professor of Medicine, Case Western Reserve University School of Medicine, Cleveland, Ohio (Drugs for Heart Conditions for all three editions)

Fredric Solomon, M.D., Director, Division of Mental Health and Behavioral Medicine of the Institute of Medicine of the National Academy of Sciences, Washington, D.C., and Study Director of the Institute of Medicine study *Sleeping Pills, Insomnia, and Medical Practice.* (Sleeping Pills, Minor Tranquilizers, Antidepressants, and Antipsychotic Drugs for all three editions)

E. Fuller Torrey, M.D., practicing psychiatrist, author of *Surviving Schizophrenia,* former director of schizophrenic wards, St. Elizabeth's Hospital, Washington, D.C., and staff member, Public Citizen's Health Research Group (Antipsychotic Drugs and Antidepressants for first and third editions)

Maurice Victor, M.D., Distinguished Scholar, Veterans Administration, V.A. Hospital, White River Junction, Vermont, Professor Emeritus, Neurology, Case Western Reserve University School of Medicine, Cleveland, Ohio, and coauthor, *Principles of Neurology* (Neurological Drugs for all three editions)

INDEX OF DRUGS

You can use this index to look up any drug profiled in Chapter 3 of this book by either its generic name (lowercase letters) or its brand name (CAPITAL LETTERS). This index lists the limited number of brand names that are included in Chapter 3. There may be additional brand names for a listed generic drug. Always know both the brand and generic names of any drug you are taking.

> Talk to your doctor before deciding to make any changes in your prescription drugs based on information in this book.

acarbose	564	aluminum hydroxide	358
ACCOLATE	410	aluminum hydroxide and magnesium carbonate	373
ACCUPRIL	123	aluminum hydroxide and magnesium hydroxide	378
acebutolol	153	amantadine	536
acetaminophen	338	AMARYL	555
acetaminophen and codeine	340	AMBIEN	201
acetaminophen and hydrocodone	274	AMEN	723
acetaminophen and oxycodone	323	amiloride and hydrochlorothiazide	138
acetazolamide	632	aminophylline	417
acetohexamide	555	amiodarone	83
ACHROMYCIN	475	amitriptyline	216
ACTHAR	654	amitriptyline and chlordiazepoxide	224
ACTIFED	412	amitriptyline and perphenazine	250
acyclovir	544	amlodipine	142
ADALAT	56	amlodipine and benazepril	129
ADALAT CC	142	AMOLINE	417
ADSORBOCARPINE	624	amoxapine	203
ADVIL	311	amoxicillin	476
AEROBID	703	amoxicillin and clavulanate	476
AK-PENTOLATE	625	AMOXIL	476
albuterol	449	AMPHOJEL	358
ALDACTAZIDE	57	ampicillin	522
ALDACTONE	58	ANAPROX	317
ALDOMET	61	ANDROID	709
ALDORIL	61	ANSAID (oral tablets)	270
alendronate	687	antibiotic treatment for ulcer disease	354
ALERMINE	413	ANTIVERT	359
ALLEGRA	415	APRESAZIDE	63
allopurinol	347	APRESOLINE	64
alprazolam	222	AQUASOL A	611
ALTACE	123	ARISTOCORT	656

ARCO-CEE 614
ARICEPT 571
ARTANE 569
ARTHROPAN 336
artificial tears 642
ASCRIPTIN 280
ASCRIPTIN A/D 280
ASENDIN 203
aspirin 275
aspirin with codeine 273
aspirin and oxycodone 324
astemizole 439
ATARAX 420
atenolol 153
atenolol and chlorthalidone 161
ATIVAN 222
atorvastatin 130
atropine 361
atropine, hyoscyamine, methenamine, methylene
    blue, phenyl salicylate, and benzoic acid 538
atropine, hyoscyamine, scopolamine, and
    phenobarbital 372
ATROVENT 422
AUGMENTIN 476
aurothioglucose 329
AVAPRO 90
AVAPRO HCT 90
AVENTYL 230
AXID 383
AYGESTIN 723
azatadine and pseudoephedrine 458
azathioprine 299
azithromycin 543
AZULFIDINE 361
BACTRIM 478
BACTROBAN 480
BANCAP-HC 274
BAYCOL 130
BAYER ASPIRIN (GENUINE) 275
beclomethasone 736
BECLOVENT 736
BENADRYL 424
benazepril 123
benazepril and hydrochlorothiazide 127
BENEMID 278
BENTYL 363
benzonatate 457
benztropine 570
BETAGAN 626
betamethasone 675
BETA-2 426

betaxolol 154
betaxolol (eye drops) 629
bethanechol 735
BETOPTIC 629
BETOPTIC S 629
BIAXIN 481
bisacodyl 373
bismuth subsalicylate 354
bismuth subsalicylate/metronidazole/tetracycline 354
bisoprolol 154
bisoprolol and hydrochlorothiazide 169
BLEPHAMIDE 632
BLOCADREN 66
BRETHAIRE 449
BRETHINE 449
BRICANYL 449
bromfenac 292
bromocriptine 586
brompheniramine and phenylpropanolamine 433
BRONKODYL 426
BRONKOMETER 426
BRONKOSOL 426
buffered aspirin 280
BUFFERIN 280
bumetanide 70
BUMEX 70
bupropion (mind) 251
bupropion (smoking) 739
BUSPAR 206
buspirone 206
butabarbital 208
butalbital, acetaminophen, and caffeine 297
butalbital, caffeine, and aspirin 299
butalbital, caffeine, aspirin, and codeine 299
BUTAZOLIDIN 281
BUTISOL 208
butorphanol 331
CALAN 73
CALAN SR 73
CALCIFEROL 616
CALCIMAR 659
calcitonin 659
calcium carbonate 600
calcium citrate 600
calcium gluconate 600
calcium lactate 600
CALTRATE 600
CAPOTEN 123
CAPOZIDE 127
captopril 123
captopril and hydrochlorothiazide 127

CARAFATE	363
carbamazepine	588
CARDENE	142
CARDENE SR	142
CARDIZEM	76
CARDIZEM CD	76
carisoprodol	730
carteolol	154
CARTROL	154
carvedilol	85
CATAPRES	80
CECLOR	482
cefaclor	482
cefadroxil	496
cefixime	534
cefprozil	484
CEFTIN	484
cefuroxime axetil	484
CEFZIL	484
CENTRAX	222
CENTRUM	606
cephalexin	510
cephradine	486
CERESPAN	81
cerivastatin	130
certirizine	462
CEVI-BID	614
CHIBROXIN (eye drops)	519
chloramphenicol	488
chlordiazepoxide	222
chlordiazepoxide and clidinium	377
CHLOROMYCETIN	488
CHLOROSERPINE	93
chlorothiazide	100
chlorpheniramine	413
chlorpheniramine and phenylpropanolamine	446
chlorpheniramine, phenyltoloxamine, phenylpropanolamine, and phenylephrine	443
chlorpheniramine and pseudoephedrine	429
chlorpromazine	247
chlorpropamide	555
chlorthalidone	105
CHLOR-TRIMETON	413
CHLOR-TRIMETON 12 HOUR	429
chlorzoxazone	711
CHOLEDYL	430
cholestyramine	119
choline and magnesium salicylates	336
choline salicylate	336
CILOXAN EYE DROPS	489
cimetidine	395
CIPRO	489
ciprofloxacin	489
cisapride	392
CITRACAL	600
clarithromycin	481
CLARITIN	431
clemastine	454
clemastine and phenylpropanolamine	456
CLEOCIN	491
clindamycin	491
CLINORIL	281
clonazepam	579
clonidine	80
clonidine and chlorthalidone	81
clorazepate	222
clotrimazole	515
cloxacillin	493
clozapine	209
CLOZARIL	209
codeine	284
codeine and pseudoephedrine	444
codeine, pseudoephedrine, guaifenesin, and alcohol	444
COGENTIN	570
COGNEX	571
COLACE	365
colchicine	286
COMBIPRES	81
COMPAZINE	366
conjugated estrogens	714
CONSTANT-T	426
CORDARONE	83
COREG	85
CORGARD	154
CORTEF	660
corticotropin/adrenocorticotropic hormone (ACTH)	654
CORTISPORIN EAR DROPS (otic)	494
CORTROPHIN-ZINC	654
CORZIDE	169
COTRIM	478
COUMADIN	87
COVERA-HS	73
COZAAR	90
cromolyn	437
cyclandelate	93
cyclobenzaprine	686
CYCLOGYL	625
cyclopentolate	625
cyclophosphamide	663
CYCLOSPASMOL	93

cyproheptadine	447	DIPROSONE	675
CYTOTEC	369	dipyridamole	146
CYTOXAN	663	DISALCID	291
DALMANE	222	disopyramide	139
DARVOCET-N	288	DITROPAN	677
DARVON	288	DIULO	101
DARVON COMPOUND	288	DIUPRES	93
DARVON COMPOUND-65	288	DIURIL	100
DARVON-N	288	divalproex	572
DAYPRO	314	DOAN'S PILLS	336
DECADRON	665	docusate	365
DELTASONE	668	docusate and casanthranol	371
DEMEROL	289	DOLOBID	291
DEMI-REGROTON	150	donepezil	571
DEMULEN	670	DONNATAL	372
DEPAKENE	572	DORAL	222
DEPAKOTE	572	dorzolamide	645
DEPONIT	108	doxepin	203
deprenyl	576	doxycycline	541
DES	714	DULCOLAX	373
deserpidine and methyclothiazide	99	DURACT	292
desipramine	230	DURAGESIC	293
DESOGEN	673	DURAQUIN	94
desogestrel/ethinyl estradiol	673	DURICEF	496
desoximetasone	733	DYAZIDE	97
DESYREL	211	DYCILL	493
dexamethasone	665	DYMELOR	555
DIABETA	555	DYNACIRC	142
DIABINESE	555	DYNACIRC CR	142
DIALOSE PLUS	371	DYNAPEN	493
DIAMOX	632	DYRENIUM	99
diazepam	222	EASPRIN	275
diclofenac	343	ECOTRIN	275
dicloxacillin	493	EES	498
dicyclomine	363	EFFEXOR	213
diethylstilbestrol	714	EFUDEX	679
DIFLUCAN	495	ELAVIL	216
diflunisal	291	ELDEPRYL	576
digoxin	113	ELIXOPHYLLIN	426
dihydrocodeine, aspirin, and caffeine	331	enalapril	123
DILACOR XR	76	enalapril and hydrochlorothiazide	127
DILANTIN	574	ENDURON	101
DILAUDID	289	ENDURONYL	99
diltiazem	76	enoxacin	523
diltiazem and enalapril	129	ENTEX	434
DIMETAPP	433	ENTEX LA	436
DIOVAN	90	EQUANIL	216
diphenhydramine	424	ergoloid mesylates	578
diphenoxylate and atropine	378	ERYTHROCIN	498
dipivefrin	640	erythromycin	498
DIPROLENE	675	erythromycin estolate	507

ESGIC	297	fosinopril	123
ESIDRIX	100	FURADANTIN	513
ESKALITH	217	furosemide	116
estazolam	222	GANTRISIN	505
ESTRACE	714	GARAMYCIN	635
ESTRADERM	680	GASTROCOM	437
estradiol (cream)	714	GAVISCON	373
estradiol (patch)	680	GAVISCON-2	373
estropipate	714	gemfibrozil	121
ethynodiol diacetate/ethinyl estradiol	670	GENORA 1/35	689
etodolac	303	gentamicin	635
EUTHROID	732	glimepiride	555
EVISTA	683	glipizide	555
famotidine	383	GLUCOPHAGE	558
FELDENE	298	GLUCOTROL	555
felodipine	142	glyburide	555
felodipine and enalapril	129	gold sodium thiomalate	329
fenoprofen	314	grepafloxacin	523
fentanyl patches	293	guaifenesin	452
FEOSOL	604	guaifenesin and dextromethorphan	453
FEOSTAT	604	guaifenesin and phenylpropanolamine	436
FERGON	604	guaifenesin, phenylpropanolamine, and	
ferrous fumarate (iron)	604	phenylephrine	434
ferrous gluconate (iron)	604	guaifenesin and theophylline	451
ferrous sulfate (iron)	604	guanabenz	168
fexofenadine	415	guanfacine	158
finasteride	721	GYNE-LOTRIMIN	515
FIORICET	297	HABITROL	692
FIORINAL	299	halazepam	222
FIORINAL WITH CODEINE	299	HALCION	222
FLAGYL	500	HALDOL	219
FLEXERIL	686	haloperidol	219
FLOXIN	502	HALOTESTIN	709
fluconazole	495	HELIDAC	354
flunisolide	703	HEXADROL	665
fluocinolone	730	HISMANAL	439
fluocinonide	698	HUMALOG	559
fluorometholone	634	HUMULIN	559
FLUOROPLEX	679	HYDERGINE	578
fluorouracil	679	HYDERGINE LC	578
fluoxetine	233	hydralazine	64
fluoxymesterone	709	hydralazine and hydrochlorothiazide	63
fluphenazine	247	hydrochlorothiazide	100
flurazepam	222	hydrocodone and phenyltoloxamine	460
flurbiprofen	270	hydrocortisone	660
fluvastatin	130	HYDRODIURIL	100
fluvoxamine	233	hydromorphone	289
FML	634	HYDROPRES	103
folic acid (folate)	602	HYDROSERPINE	103
FOLVITE	602	hydroxychloroquine	325
FOSAMAX	687	hydroxyzine	420

HYGROTON	105	KLOTRIX	111
HY-PAM	420	KWELL	512
HYPOTEARS	642	labetalol	154
HYTRIN	105	LAMISIL	533
HYZAAR	90	LANOXICAPS	113
ibuprofen	311	LANOXIN	113
ILETIN	559	lansoprazole	389
ILOSONE	507	LARODOPA	582
IMDUR	108	LASIX	116
imipramine	203	LESCOL	130
IMITREX	695	LEVAQUIN	523
IMODIUM	375	LEVATOL	154
IMURAN	299	levobunolol	626
indapamide	101	levodopa	582
INDERAL	154	levodopa and carbidopa	582
INDERAL LA	154	levofloxacin	523
INDERIDE LA	169	LEVOTHROID	732
INDOCIN	302	levothyroxine	732
indomethacin	302	LEXXEL	129
INH	507	LIBRAX	377
INSULATARD	559	LIBRIUM	222
insulin (beef, pork)	559	LIDEX	698
insulin (human)	559	LIDEX-E	698
INTAL	437	lidocaine	346
ipratropium	422	LIMBITROL	224
irbesartan	90	LINCOCIN	513
irbesartan and hydrochlorothiazide	90	lincomycin	513
ISMO	108	lindane	512
isoetharine	426	liotrix	732
isoniazid	507	LIPITOR	130
ISOPTIN	73	lisinopril	123
ISOPTIN SR	73	lisinopril and hydrochlorothiazide	127
ISOPTO CARPINE	624	lithium	217
ISORDIL	108	LITHOBID	217
isosorbide dinitrate	108	LITHONATE	217
isosorbide-5-mononitrate	108	LOCHOLEST	119
isoxsuprine	167	LODINE	303
isradipine	142	LOESTRIN-FE 1.5/30	689
itraconazole	533	lomefloxacin	523
K-LOR	111	LOMOTIL	378
K-LYTE TABLETS	111	loperamide	375
KAOCHLOR	111	LO/OVRAL	689
KAON-CL	111	LOPID	121
KATO	111	LOPRESSOR	154
KAY CIEL	111	LOPRESSOR HCT	169
KEFLEX	510	LORABID	484
KENALOG	656	loracarbef	484
KERLONE	154	loratadine	431
ketoprofen	320	lorazepam	222
ketorolac	335	LORELCO	122
KLONOPIN	579	losartan	90

losartan and hydrochlorothiazide 90
LOTENSIN 123
LOTENSIN HCT 127
LOTREL 129
LOTRIMIN 515
lovastatin 130
LOZOL 101
LUDIOMIL 225
LUMINAL 584
LUVOX 233
MAALOX 378
MAALOX TC 378
MACROBID 513
MACRODANTIN 513
magaldrate 378
magnesium hydroxide 388
magnesium hydroxide, aluminum hydroxide, and simethicone 381
magnesium salicylate 336
maprotiline 225
MAVIK 123
MAXAIR 440
MAXAQUIN 523
MAXITROL 636
MAXZIDE 97
mebendazole 539
meclizine 359
meclofenamate 306
MECLOMEN 306
MEDIPREN 311
MEDROL 700
medroxyprogesterone 723
MELLARIL 247
meperidine 289
meprobamate 216
MERIDIA 702
METAHYDRIN 101
METAMUCIL 380
metformin 558
methazolamide 638
methocarbamol 728
methotrexate 327
methyclothiazide 101
methyldopa 61
methyldopa and hydrochlorothiazide 61
methylphenidate 726
methylprednisolone 700
methyltestosterone 709
METICORTEN 668
metoclopramide 393
metolazone 101

metoprolol 154
metoprolol and hydrochlorothiazide 169
metronidazole 500
MEVACOR 130
mexiletine 133
MEXITIL 133
MIACALCIN INJECTION 659
MIACALCIN NASAL SPRAY 659
mibefradil 146
miconazole 513
MICRO-K 111
MICRONASE 555
MILTOWN 216
MINIPRESS 136
MINITRAN 108
MINOCIN 309
minocycline 309
minoxidil 729
mirtazapine 237
misoprostol 369
MIXTARD 559
MODURETIC 138
moexipril 123
M.O.M. 388
MONISTAT 7 513
MONISTAT-DERM 513
MONOPRIL 123
MOTRIN 311
multivitamins 606
mupirocin 480
MYCELEX 515
MYCITRACIN 518
MYCOBIOTIC II 516
MYCOLOG II 516
MYCOSTATIN 517
MYDRIACYL 637
MYLANTA 381
MYLANTA-II 381
MYLICON 382
MYOCHRYSINE 329
nabumetone 303
nadolol 154
nadolol and bendroflumethiazide 169
NALDECON 443
NALFON 314
NAPROSYN 317
naproxen 317
NAQUA 101
NASALCROM 437
NASALIDE 703

NAVANE	227	OCUFLOX EYE DROPS	502
nefazodone	245	ofloxacin	502
NEMBUTAL	208	OGEN	714
NEODECADRON	638	olanzapine	253
neomycin and dexamethasone	638	omeprazole	389
neomycin, polymyxin B, and bacitracin	518	OMNIPEN	522
neomycin, polymyxin B, and dexamethasone	636	ORETON METHYL	709
neomycin, polymyxin B, and hydrocortisone	494	ORINASE	555
NEOSAR	663	ORNADE	446
NEOSPORIN MAXIMUM STRENGTH OINTMENT	518	orphenadrine	711
NEPTAZANE	638	orphenadrine, aspirin, and caffeine	319
niacin (nicotinic acid, vitamin B$_3$)	607	ORTHO-CEPT	673
niacin (sustained-release dosage)	609	ORTHO-CYCLEN	689
nicardipine	142	ORTHO-NOVUM 1/35	689
NICOBID	609	ORTHO-NOVUM 7/7/7	689
NICODERM	692	ORTHOTRI-CYCLEN	689
NICOLAR	607	ORUDIS	320
NICORETTE	692	OS-CAL 500	600
nicotine	692	oxaprozin	314
NICOTROL	692	oxazepam	242
nifedipine	142	oxtriphylline	430
nifedipine, short-acting forms	56	oxybutynin	677
nisoldipine	142	PAMELOR	230
NITRO-BID	108	PANMYCIN	475
NITRODISC	108	papaverine	81
NITRO-DUR	108	PARAFON FORTE DSC	711
nitrofurantoin	513	PARLODEL	586
nitroglycerin	108	paroxetine	233
NITROSTAT	108	PAVABID	81
nizatidine	383	PAXIL	233
NOLVADEX	706	PAXIPAM	222
norethindrone acetate	723	penbutolol	154
norethindrone/ethinyl estradiol	689	PENETREX	523
NORFLEX	708	penicillin G	527
norfloxacin	519	penicillin V	527
NORGESIC FORTE	319	pentazocine	332
norgestimate/ethinyl estradiol	689	pentazocine and naloxone	332
norgestrel/ethinyl estradiol	689	pentobarbital	208
NORMODYNE	154	pentoxifylline	166
NOROXIN (tablets)	519	PEN VEE K	527
NORPACE	139	PEPCID	383
NORPRAMIN	230	PEPTO-BISMOL	354
nortriptyline	230	PERCOCET	323
NORVASC	142	PERCODAN	324
NOVOLIN	559	PERCODAN-DEMI	324
NUCOFED (capsules and syrup)	444	PERDIEM	380
NUCOFED (expectorant syrup)	444	PERIACTIN	447
NUPRIN	311	PERI-COLACE	371
nystatin	517	PERSANTINE	146
nystatin and triamcinolone	516	PHAZYME	382
OCUFEN (eye solution)	270	phenazopyridine	725

PHENERGAN	385	PYRIDIUM	725
phenobarbital	584	quazepam	222
phenylbutazone	281	QUESTRAN	119
phenytoin	574	QUESTRAN LIGHT	119
PHILLIPS' MILK OF MAGNESIA	388	QUIBRON	451
pilocarpine	624	QUIBRON-T-SR	426
pindolol	154	QUINAGLUTE DURA-TABS	94
pirbuterol	440	quinapril	123
piroxicam	298	QUINIDEX	94
PLAQUENIL	325	quinidine	94
PLENDIL	142	quinine	150
POLYCILLIN	522	raloxifene	683
POSICOR	146	ramipril	123
potassium supplements	111	ranitidine	383
PRAVACHOL	130	ranitidine bismuth citrate	354
pravastatin	130	RAXAR	523
prazepam	222	REGLAN	393
prazosin	136	REGROTON	150
PRECOSE	564	RELAFEN	303
PRED FORTE	711	REMERON	237
prednisolone	711	RENOVA	726
prednisone	668	reserpine	152
PREMARIN	714	reserpine and chlorothiazide	93
PREVACID	389	reserpine and chlorthalidone	150
PRILOSEC	389	reserpine, hydralazine, and hydrochlorothiazide	157
PRINIVIL	123	reserpine and hydrochlorothiazide	103
PRINZIDE	127	reserpine and hydroflumethiazide	152
probenecid	278	RESTORIL	222
probucol	122	RETIN-A	726
procainamide	148	REZULIN	565
PROCANBID	148	RHEUMATREX DOSE PACK	327
PROCARDIA	56	RIFADIN	530
PROCARDIA XL	142	rifampin	530
prochlorperazine	366	RIMACTANE	530
PROLIXIN	247	RIOPAN	378
PROLOPRIM	528	RISPERDAL	239
promethazine	385	risperidone	239
PROPINE	640	RITALIN	726
propoxyphene	288	ROBAXIN	728
propoxyphene and acetaminophen	288	ROBITUSSIN	452
propoxyphene, aspirin, and caffeine	288	ROBITUSSIN DAC	444
propranolol	154	ROBITUSSIN-DM	453
propranolol and hydrochlorothiazide	169	ROGAINE	729
PROPULSID	392	salsalate	291
PROSCAR	721	SALUTENSIN	152
PROSOM	222	SECTRAL	153
PROSTEP	692	SELDANE	453
PROVENTIL	449	SELDANE-D	453
PROVERA	723	selegiline	576
PROZAC	233	SEPTRA	478
psyllium	380	SER-AP-ES	157

SERAX	242	TALWIN-NX	332
sertraline	233	tamoxifen	706
SERZONE	245	TARKA	129
sibutramine	702	TAVIST	454
SILVADENE	532	TAVIST-1	454
silver sulfadiazine	532	TAVIST-D	456
simethicone	382	TEARISOL	642
simvastatin	130	TEARS NATURALE	642
SINEMET	582	TECZEM	129
SINEQUAN	203	TEGRETOL	588
SLO-BID	426	temazepam	222
SLO-NIACIN	609	TENEX	158
SLO-PHYLLIN	426	TENORETIC	161
SLOW FE	604	TENORMIN	153
SLOW-K	111	TERAZOL 3 (cream or suppositories)	537
SOLFOTON	584	TERAZOL 7 (cream)	537
SOLGANAL	329	terazosin	105
SOMA	730	terbinafine	533
SOMINEX FORMULA	424	terbutaline	449
SOMOPHYLLIN	417	terconazole	537
SOMOPHYLLIN-CRT	426	terfenadine	453
SOMOPHYLLIN-DF	417	terfenadine and pseudoephedrine	453
SOMOPHYLLIN-T	426	TESSALON	457
SORBITRATE	108	tetracycline	475
sparfloxacin	523	THEO-24	426
spironolactone	58	THEO-DUR	426
spironolactone and hydrochlorothiazide	57	THEOLAIR	426
SPORANOX	533	theophylline	426
STADOL	331	THERAGRAN-M	606
STADOL NS	331	thiamine (vitamin B_1)	610
STELAZINE	247	thioridazine	247
sucralfate	363	thiothixene	227
SULAMYD	641	THORAZINE	247
SULAR	142	thyroid	732
sulfacetamide	641	THYROLAR	732
sulfacetamide and prednisolone	632	TIAZAC	76
sulfasalazine	361	TICLID	162
sulfisoxazole	505	ticlopidine	162
sulindac	281	TIGAN	397
sumatriptan	695	TIMOLIDE	169
SUPRAX	534	timolol	66
SURFAK	365	timolol (eye drops)	643
SUSTAIRE	426	timolol and hydrochlorothiazide	169
SYMMETREL	536	TIMOPTIC	643
SYNALAR	730	tobramycin	635
SYNALGOS-DC	331	TOBREX	635
SYNEMOL	730	tocainide	164
SYNTHROID	732	TOFRANIL	203
tacrine	571	tolazamide	555
TAGAMET	395	tolbutamide	555
TALWIN	332	TOLECTIN	332

TOLINASE	555	VANCENASE	736
tolmetin	332	VANCERIL	736
TONOCARD	164	VASERETIC	127
TOPICORT	733	VASOCIDIN	632
TOPROL XL	154	VASODILAN	167
TORADOL	335	VASOTEC	123
TORVAN	523	VELOSULIN	559
tramadol	342	venlafaxine	213
TRANDATE	154	VENTOLIN	449
trandolapril	123	verapamil	73
TRANSDERM-NITRO	108	verapamil and trandolapril	129
TRANXENE	222	VERELAN	73
trazodone	211	VERMOX	539
TRENTAL	166	VIBRAMYCIN	541
tretinoin	726	VICODIN	274
triamcinolone	656	VISKEN	154
triamterene	99	VISTARIL	420
triamterene and hydrochlorothiazide	97	vitamin A	611
TRIAVIL	250	vitamin B_{12} (cyanocobalamin)	613
triazolam	222	vitamin C (ascorbic acid)	614
trichlormethiazide	101	vitamin D	616
trifluoperazine	247	vitamin E (alpha tocopherol)	618
trihexyphenidyl	569	VOLTAREN	343
TRI-LEVLEN	689	warfarin	87
TRILISATE	336	WELLBUTRIN	251
trimethobenzamide	397	WYGESIC	288
trimethoprim	528	WYTENSIN	168
trimethoprim and sulfamethoxazole	478	XANAX	222
TRIMPEX	528	XYLOCAINE	346
TRINALIN	458	zafirlukast	410
TRIPHASIL	689	ZAGAM	523
triprolidine and pseudoephedrine	412	ZANTAC	383
TRITEC	354	ZAROXOLYN	101
troglitazone	565	ZEBETA	154
tropicamide	637	ZESTORETIC	127
trovafloxacin	523	ZESTRIL	123
TRUSOPT	645	ZIAC	169
TUSSIONEX	460	zileuton	461
TYLENOL	338	ZITHROMAX	543
TYLENOL NO. 3	340	ZOCOR	130
TYLOX	323	zolmitriptan	695
ULTRAM	342	ZOLOFT	233
UNIVASC	123	zolpidem	201
URECHOLINE	735	ZOMIG	695
URISED	538	ZOVIRAX	544
VALISONE	675	ZYBAN	739
VALIUM	222	ZYFLO	461
valproate	572	ZYLOPRIM	347
valproic acid	572	ZYPREXA	253
valsartan	90	ZYRTEC	462

1

MISPRESCRIBING AND OVERPRESCRIBING OF DRUGS: Evidence and Causes

The numbers are staggering: in 1997, an estimated 2.35 billion prescriptions were filled in retail drugstores in the United States. For those people who got at least one prescription filled, this amounts to an average of 11.6 prescriptions per person that year.[1]

There is no dispute that for many people, prescriptions are beneficial, even lifesaving in many instances. But hundreds of millions of these prescriptions are wrong, either entirely unnecessary or unnecessarily dangerous. At the very least, misprescribing wastes tens of billions of dollars, barely affordable by many people who pay for their own prescriptions. But there are much more serious consequences. As discussed in Chapter 2, p. 9, more than 1.5 million people are hospitalized and more than 100,000 die each year from largely preventable adverse reactions to drugs that should not have been prescribed as they were in the first place.[2] What follows is a summary of the **seven all-too-often-deadly sins of prescribing.**

First: The "disease" for which a drug is prescribed is actually an adverse reaction to another drug, masquerading as a disease but unfortunately not recognized by doctor and patient as such. Instead of lowering the dose of the offending drug or replacing it with a safer alternative, the physician adds a second drug to the regimen to "treat" the adverse drug reaction caused by the first drug. Examples discussed in this book (see later in this chapter and in Chapter 2) include drug-induced parkinsonism, depression, sexual dysfunction, insomnia, psychoses, constipation, and many other problems.

Second: A drug is used to treat a problem which, although in some cases susceptible to a pharmaceutical solution, should first be treated with common sense lifestyle changes. Problems such as insomnia and abdominal pain often have causes that respond very well to nondrug treatment, and often the physician can uncover these causes by taking a careful history. Other examples include medical problems such as high blood pressure, mild adult-onset diabetes, obesity, anxiety, and situational depression. Doctors should recommend lifestyle changes as the first approach for these conditions, rather than automatically reach for the prescription pad.

Third: The medical problem is both self-limited and completely unresponsive to treatments such as antibiotics or does not merit treatment with certain drugs. This is seen most clearly with viral infections such as colds and bronchitis in otherwise healthy children or adults.

Fourth: A drug *is* the preferred treatment for the medical problem, but instead of the safest, most effective—and often least expensive—treatment, the physician prescribes one of the 160 Do Not Use drugs listed in this book or another, much less preferable alternative. An example of a less preferable alternative would be a drug to

1

which the patient has a known allergy that the physician did not ask about.

Fifth: Two drugs interact. Each on its own may be safe and effective, but together they can cause serious injury or death.

Sixth: Two or more drugs in the same therapeutic category are used, the additional one(s) not adding to the effectiveness of the first but clearly increasing the risk to the patient. Sometimes the drugs come in a fixed combination pill, sometimes as two different pills. Often heart drugs or mind-affecting drugs are prescribed in this manner.

Seventh: The right drug is prescribed, but the dose is dangerously high. This problem is seen most often in older adults, who cannot metabolize or excrete drugs as rapidly as younger people. This problem is also seen in small people who are usually prescribed the same dose as that prescribed to people weighing two to three times as much as they do. Thus, per pound, they are getting two to three times as much medicine as the larger person.

Evidence of Misprescribing and Overprescribing

Here are some examples from recent studies by a growing number of medical researchers documenting misprescribing and overprescribing of drugs:

Treating Adverse Drug Reactions—as Diseases—with Other Drugs

Researchers at the University of Toronto and at Harvard have clearly documented and articulated what they call the *prescribing cascade*. It begins when an adverse drug reaction is misinterpreted as a new medical condition. Another drug is then prescribed, and the patient is placed at risk of developing additional adverse effects relating to this potentially unnecessary treatment.[3] To prevent this prescribing cascade, doctors—and patients—should follow what we

call Rule 3 of the Ten Rules for Safer Drug Use (see p. 746): **Assume that any new symptom you develop after starting a new drug might be caused by the drug. If you have a new symptom, report it to your doctor.**

Some of the instances of the prescribing cascade that these and other researchers have documented include:

• The increased use of anti-Parkinson's drugs to treat drug-induced parkinsonism caused by the heartburn drug metoclopramide[4] (REGLAN) or by some of the older antipsychotic drugs.

• A sharply increased use of laxatives in people with decreased bowel activity that has been caused by antihistamines such as diphenhydramine (BENADRYL), antidepressants such as amitriptyline (ELAVIL)—a **Do Not Use** drug—or some antipsychotic drugs such as thioridazine (MELLARIL).[5]

• An increased use of antihypertensive drugs in people with high blood pressure that was caused or increased by very high doses of nonsteroidal anti-inflammatory drugs (NSAIDs), used as painkillers or for arthritis).[6]

Failing to Treat Certain Problems with Nondrug Treatments

Research has shown that many doctors are too quick to pull the prescription trigger. In one study, in which doctors and nurse practitioners were presented with part of a clinical scenario—as would occur when first seeing a patient with a medical problem—and then encouraged to ask to find out more about the source of the problem, 65% of doctors recommended that a patient complaining of insomnia be treated with sleeping pills even though, had they asked more questions about the patient, they would have found that the patient was not exercising, was drinking coffee in the evening, and, although awakening at 4 A.M., was actually getting seven hours of sleep by then.[7]

In a similar study, doctors were presented with a patient who complained of abdominal pain and whose endoscopy showed diffuse irritation in the stomach. Sixty-five percent of the doctors recommended treating the problem with a drug—a histamine antagonist (such as Zantac, Pepcid, or Tagamet). Had they asked more questions they would have discovered that the patient was using aspirin, drinking a lot of coffee, smoking cigarettes, and was under considerable emotional stress—all potential contributing factors to abdominal pain and stomach irritation.

In summarizing the origin of this overprescribing problem, the authors stated: "Apparently quite early in the formulation of the problem, the conceptual focus [of the doctor] appears to shift from broader questions like 'What is wrong with this patient?' or 'What can I do to help?' to the much narrower concern, 'Which prescription shall I write?'" They argued that this approach was supported by the "barrage" of promotional materials that only address drug treatment, not the more sensible lifestyle changes to prevent the problem.[8]

In both of the above scenarios, nurse practitioners were much more likely than doctors to take an adequate history that elicited the causes of the problems and, not surprisingly, were only one-third as likely as the doctors to decide on a prescription as the remedy instead of suggesting changes in the patient's habits.

In Chapter 3, p. 39, in the discussions about insomnia, high blood pressure, situational depression, mild adult-onset diabetes, and other problems, you will find out about the proven-effective nondrug remedies that should first be pursued before yielding to the riskier pharmaceutical solutions.

Treating Viral Infections with Antibiotics or Treating Other Diseases with Drugs That Are Not Effective for Those Problems

Two recently published studies, based on nationwide data from office visits for children and adults, have decisively documented the expensive and dangerous massive overprescribing of antibiotics for conditions which, because of their viral origin, do not respond to these drugs. Forty-four percent of children under 18 years old were given antibiotics for treatment of a cold and 75% for treatment of bronchitis. Similarly, 51% of people 18 or older were treated with antibiotics for colds and 66% for bronchitis. Despite the lack of evidence of any benefit for most people from these treatments, more than 23 million prescriptions a year were written for colds, bronchitis, and upper respiratory infections. This accounted for approximately one-fifth of all prescriptions for antibiotics written for children or adults.[9,10] An accompanying editorial warned of "increased costs from unnecessary prescriptions, adverse drug reactions, and [subsequent] treatment failures in patients with antibiotic-resistant infections" as the reasons to try to reduce this epidemic of unnecessary antibiotic prescribing.[11]

Similar misprescribing of a drug useful and important for certain problems, but not necessary or effective—and often—dangerous for other problems can be seen in another recent study. In this case, 47% of the people admitted to a nursing home who were taking digoxin, an important drug for treating an abnormal heart rhythm called atrial fibrillation or for treating severe congestive heart failure, did not have either of these medical problems and were thereby being put at risk for life-threatening digitalis toxicity without the possibility of any benefit.[12]

A final example in this category involves the overuse of a certain class of drugs, in this case calcium channel blockers, which have not been established as effective for treating people who have had a recent heart attack. The study shows that this prescribing pattern actually did indirect damage to patients because their use was replacing the use of beta-blockers, drugs shown to be very effective for reducing the subsequent risk of death or hospitalization following a heart attack. Use of a calcium channel blocker instead of a beta-blocker was associated with a doubled risk of death, and beta-blocker recipients were hospitalized 22% less often than nonrecipients.[13]

The Prescribing of More Dangerous and/or Less Effective Do Not Use Drugs Instead of Safer Alternatives

There are 160 drugs listed in this book for which we recommend safer alternatives. Forty-three of these **Do Not Use** drugs are for heart disease or high blood pressure and make up 39% of all the drugs in the book for these problems. Twenty of the **Do Not Use** drugs are for treating insomnia, anxiety, depression, or other mental problems, and make up 43% of the drugs in the book for these problems. Another 20 of the **Do Not Use** drugs are for treating pain, and make up 36% of the drugs in the book for these problems. Thirteen of the **Do Not Use** drugs are for treating gastrointestinal problems and make up 37% of the drugs in the book for these problems. Twenty-four of the **Do Not Use** drugs are for treating coughs, colds, allergies, or asthma, and make up 63% of the drugs in the book for these problems. Sixteen of the **Do Not Use** drugs are for treating infections and make up 28% of the drugs in the book for these problems. Although the original determinations for these **Do Not Use** drugs were based on their use by older adults, we have concluded that the same warnings apply to use by any adults.

Included in this list of 160 are drugs we label **Do Not Use Until Five Years After Release.** We have applied this warning to drugs that have only recently appeared on the market, for which there is no evidence of their superiority over older drugs about which we have much more information as to long-term safety and effectiveness. Because of incomplete and worrisome safety information, there is a risk that some of these newer drugs will have to be banned. But by the time they have been on the market for five years, it is much less likely that they will be banned, and it is much more likely that, if they are still being used, there will be much better information about their safety and effectiveness.

Another category of drugs that is misprescribed even though there are safer alternatives, are drugs to which patients are known to be allergic, but which their physicians have not taken a careful medical history about.

The Causes of Misprescribing and Overprescribing: Drug Companies, the FDA, Doctors, Pharmacists, and Inadequately Informed or Not-Vigilant-Enough Patients

The Drug Industry

The primary culprit in promoting the misprescribing and overprescribing of drugs is the pharmaceutical industry, which now sells about $80 billion worth of drugs in the United States alone.[14] By intimidating the Food and Drug Administration (FDA) into approving record numbers of me-too drugs (drugs that offer no significant benefit over drugs already on the market) that often have dangerous adverse effects and by spending well in excess of $12 billion a year to promote drugs,[15] using advertising and promotional tricks that push at or through the envelope of being false and misleading, this industry has been extremely successful in distorting, in a profitable but dangerous way, the rational processes for approving and prescribing drugs. Two studies of the accuracy of ads for prescription drugs widely circulated to doctors both concluded that a substantial proportion of these ads contained information that was false or misleading and violated FDA laws and regulations concerning advertising.[16,17]

The fastest-growing segment of drug advertising is directed not at doctors but at patients. It has been estimated that from 1991 to 1998, DTC (direct-to-consumer) advertising expenditures in the United States grew from about $60 million a year to $1.5 billion a year, an increase of 25-fold in just seven years, employing misleading advertising campaigns similar to those used for doctors. A recent study by *Consumer Reports* of 28 such ads found that "only half were judged to convey important information on side effects in the main promotional text," only 40% were "honest about efficacy and fairly described the benefits and risks in the main text," and 39% of the ads were considered "more harmful than helpful" by at least one reviewer.[18] This campaign has been extremely successful. According to a drug industry spokesman, "There's a strong correlation between the amount of money pharmaceutical companies spend on DTC advertising and what drugs patients are most often requesting from physicians." The advertising "is definitely driving patients to the doctor's office, and in many cases, leading patients to request the drugs by name."[19] The problems with DTC advertising are best summed up in an article written by a physician ten years ago in *The New England Journal of Medicine,* before the current binge had really begun: "If direct [to consumer] advertising should prevail, the use of prescription medication would be warped by misleading commercials and hucksterism. The choice of a patient's medication, even of his or her physician, could then come to depend more on the attractiveness of a full-page spread or prime-time commercial than on medical merit . . . such advertising would serve only the ad-makers and the media, and might well harm our patients."[20]

The Food and Drug Administration (FDA)

Attempting to fend off FDA-weakening legislation even worse than that which was signed into law in 1997, the FDA has bent over backwards to approve more drugs, culminating in 1996 and 1997 when the agency approved a larger number than had ever been approved in

any two-year period. Thousands of people were injured or killed after taking one of three such recently approved drugs (which have subsequently been recalled from the market). These drugs were the weight loss drug dexfenfluramine (REDUX), a heart drug mibefradil (POSICOR), and the painkiller bromfenac (DURACT). Other drugs that would not have gotten approved in a more cautious era at the FDA have also been approved, but are likely either to be banned or to be forced to carry severe warnings that will substantially reduce their use. Many of these are included in this book and listed as **Do Not Use** drugs.

In the 27 years since the Public Citizen's Health Research Group started monitoring the FDA and the drug industry, the current pro-industry attitude at the FDA is as bad and dangerous as it has ever been. In addition to record numbers of approvals of questionable drugs, FDA enforcement over advertising has fallen behind. The division at FDA responsible for policing prescription drug advertising has not been given adequate resources to keep up with the torrent of newly approved drugs. As a result, the drug industry correctly believes it can get away with more violative advertising than in the past. The role of the U.S. Congress in pushing the FDA into approving more drugs, and passing, with the FDA's reluctant approval, legislation to further weaken the FDA's ability to protect the public, cannot be overlooked.

Physicians

The well-financed promotional campaigns by drug companies would not have as much of an impact as they do were there not such an educational vacuum about proper prescribing of drugs, a serious problem that must be laid at the feet of medical school and residency training. The varieties of overprescribing and misprescribing of drugs by doctors—**the seven all-too-often-deadly sins of prescribing** referred to on p. 1—are all strongly enhanced by the mind-altering properties of drug promotion. The best doctors, of whom there are many, do not waste their time talking to drug sales people, toss promotional materials away, and ignore drug ads in medical journals. Too many other doctors, however, are heavily influenced by drug companies, accepting free meals, free drinks, and free medical books in exchange for letting the drug companies "educate" them at symposia in which the virtues of certain drugs are extolled. Unfortunately, many of these doctors are too arrogant to realize that there is no such thing as a free lunch. The majority of doctors attending such functions have been found to increase their prescriptions for the targeted drugs following attendance at the "teach-in."[21]

Beyond traditional advertising and promotion and their influence, bias of drug-company-sponsored research, as published in medical journals, also can sway doctors toward more favorable impressions about drugs. An analysis was done of 56 trials that were paid for by drug companies and reported in 52 medical journals about drugs for arthritis and pain—nonsteroidal anti-inflammatory drugs (NSAIDs). (These drug-company-sponsored studies represented 85% of those that the researchers originally looked at.) In studies identifying the company's drug as less toxic than another drug, in barely one-half of the studies was there justification for the finding of less toxicity. This certainly explains why, contrary to fact, newer arthritis drugs almost always "seem" safer than older, usually much less expensive ones.[22]

A final example demonstrates the ignorance of many physicians, especially in dealing with prescribing drugs to older adults. A study of physicians who treat Medicare patients found that 70% of the doctors who took an examination concerning their knowledge of prescribing for older adults failed to pass the test. The majority of physicians who were contacted for participation in the study refused to take the test, often giving as their reason that they had

a "lack of interest in the subject." The authors concluded "many of these physicians [who failed the exam] had . . . not made good use of the best information on prescribing for the elderly."[23]

Pharmacists

A small fraction of pharmacists have, in our view, betrayed their professional ethics and are working for drug companies, engaging in such activities as calling doctors to get them to switch patients from drugs made by a company other than the one the pharmacist works for to the pharmacist's employer's drugs. In addition, pharmacy organizations such as the American Pharmaceutical Association and others have fought hard to prevent the FDA from requiring accurate patient package information to be dispensed with each prescription filled.

Too many pharmacists, despite having computers to aid them, have been willing to fill prescriptions for pairs of drugs which, because of life-threatening adverse drug interactions if used at the same time, should never be dispensed to the same person.

- Sixteen (32%) of 50 pharmacies in Washington, D.C., filled prescriptions for erythromycin and terfenadine (SELDANE) without comment.[24] These two drugs, if used in combination, can cause fatal heart arrhythmias.

- In another study, of 245 pharmacists in seven cities, about one-third of pharmacists, did not alert consumers to the potentially fatal and widely publicized interaction between Hismanal, a common antihistamine, and Nizoral, an often-prescribed antifungal drug. Only 4 out of 17 pharmacists warned of the interaction between oral contraceptives and Rimactane, an antibiotic that could decrease the effectiveness of the oral contraceptive. Only 3 out of 61 pharmacists issued any verbal warnings about the interaction between Vasotec and Dyazide—two drugs for treating hypertension—which may lead to dangerously high levels of potassium in the blood.[25]

• In yet another study, concurrent use of terfenadine (SELDANE) and contraindicated drugs declined over time. The rate of same-day dispensing declined by 84%, from an average of 2.5 per 100 persons receiving terfenadine in 1990 to 0.4 per 100 persons during the first six months of 1994, while the rate of overlapping use declined by 57% (from 5.4 to 2.3 per 100 persons). Most cases involved erythromycin. Despite substantial declines following reports of serious drug-drug interactions and changes in product labeling, concurrent use of terfenadine and contraindicated antibiotics such as erythromycin and clarithromycin (BIAXIN) and antifungals such as ketoconazole (NIZORAL) continued to occur.[26]

Patients

For too many patients, the system is stacked against you—drug companies, doctors, and pharmacists are too often making decisions that ultimately derive from what is best for the drug companies, doctors, and pharmacists, and not necessarily from what is best for you. This book has been researched and written to help you come out ahead in the struggle with our health care industry.

In Chapter 2, concerning adverse drug reactions, you can learn which common medical problems—depression, insomnia, sexual disorders, parkinsonism, falls and hip fractures, constipation, and many others—can actually be caused by drugs. Once you recognize these problems, you can take care of yourself and your family and bring the problems to an end by discussing safer alternatives with your physician.

Chapter 3, the largest section of the book, discusses 456 drugs, including 160 that we and our consultants think you should not use. For each of these, we recommend safer alternatives. In addition, Chapter 3 lists hundreds of drug combinations that should not be used because of serious interactions.

Chapter 4 presents a detailed strategy, beyond information on specific adverse effects and drugs, to help you to use drugs more safely, including Ten Rules for Safer Drug Use and how to use and maintain your own Drug Worksheet for Patient, Family, Doctor and Pharmacist. This is your personalized plan for avoiding becoming a victim of overprescribing or misprescribing.

Chapter 5 discusses the latest information about generic drugs and shows you how and why you can and should save hundreds of dollars a year or more.

In short, this book is intended to help you and your family to improve your health by using drugs, if necessary, more carefully and recognizing those you should avoid.

NOTES

1. According to data from the National Center for Health Statistics' National Health Information Survey of 1996, 79.1% of the civilian non-institutionalized population of the United States had contact with a physician at least once during the year. If we assume that at least one prescription was generated and filled for each of these people, this number, 210,055,000, can be used as the denominator of the fraction of total prescriptions divided by people getting one or more prescriptions filled. This will actually tend to underestimate the number of prescriptions filled per person since not all people having contact with a physician actually are prescribed a drug.

2. Lazarou J, Pomeranz BH, Corey PN. Incidence of adverse drug reactions in hospitalized patients: A meta-analysis of prospective studies. *Journal of the American Medical Association* 1998; 279:1200–5.

3. Rochon PA, Gurwitz JH. Optimising drug treatment for elderly people: The prescribing cascade. *British Medical Journal* 1997; 315:1096–9.

4. Ibid.

5. Monane M, Avorn J, Beers MH, Everitt DE. Anticholinergic drug use and bowel function in nursing home patients. *Archives of Internal Medicine* 1993; 153:633–8.

6. Rochon PA, Gurwitz JH. Drug therapy. *Lancet* 1995; 346:32–6.

7. Everitt DE, Avorn J. Clinical decision-making in the evaluation and treatment of insomnia. *The American Journal of Medicine* 1990; 89:357–62.

8. Avorn J, Everitt DE, Baker MW. The neglected medical history and therapeutic choices for abdominal pain. *Archives of Internal Medicine* 1991; 151:694–8.

9. Nyquist AC, Gonzales R, Steiner JF, Sande MA. Antibiotic prescribing for children with colds, upper respiratory tract infections, and bronchitis. *Journal of the American Medical Association* 1998; 279:875–7.

10. Gonzales R, Steiner JF, Sande MA. Antibiotic prescribing for adults with colds, upper respiratory tract infections, and bronchitis by ambulatory care physicians. *Journal of the American Medical Association* 1997; 278:901–4.

11. Schwartz B, Mainous AG, Marcy SM. Why do physicians prescribe antibiotics for children with upper respiratory tract infections? *Journal of the American Medical Association* 1998; 279:881–2.

12. Aronow WS. Prevalence of appropriate and inappropriate indications for use of digoxin in older patients at the time of admission to a nursing home. *Journal of the American Geriatric Society* 1996; 44:588–90.

13. Soumerai SB, McLaughlin TJ, Spiegelman D, Hertzmark E, Thibault G, Goldman L. Adverse outcomes of underuse of beta-blockers in elderly survivors of acute myocardial infarction. *Journal of the American Medical Association* 1997; 277:115–21.

14. Post-1990 launches represent 43% of RX Market, IMS says. *The Pink Sheet* 1998; 60(10):9–10.

15. Wolfe SM. Why do American drug companies spend more than $12 billion a year pushing drugs? Is it education or promotion? *Journal of General Internal Medicine* 1996; 11:637–9.

16. Wilkes MS, Doblin BH, Shapiro MF. Pharmaceutical advertisements in leading medical journals: Experts' assessments. *Annals of Internal Medicine* 1992; 116:912–9.

17. Stryer D, Bero LA. Characteristics of materials distributed by drug companies: An evaluation of appropriateness. *Journal of General Internal Medicine* 1996; 11:575–83.

18. Drug advertising. Is this good medicine? *Consumer Reports* June 1996:62–3.

19. The top 200 drugs. *American Druggist* February 1998:46–53.

20. Cohen EP. Direct-to-the-public advertisement of prescription drugs. *New England Journal of Medicine* 1988; 318:373–6.

21. *Medical Marketing and Media*, October 20, 1990.

22. Rochon PA, Gurwitz JH, Simms RW, Fortin PR, Felson DT, Minaker KL, et al. A study of manufacturer-supported trials of nonsteroidal anti-inflammatory drugs in the treatment of arthritis. *Archives of Internal Medicine* 1994; 154:157–63.

23. Ferry ME, Lamy P, Becker L. Physicians' knowledge of prescribing for the elderly. *Journal of the American Geriatrics Society* 1985; 33:616–25.

24. Cavuto NJ, Woosley RL, Sale M. Pharmacies and prevention of potentially fatal drug interactions. *Journal of the American Medical Association* 1996; 275:1086 [letter].

25. Headden S. Danger at the drugstore. *U.S. News & World Report* August 26, 1996:46–53.

26. Thompson D, Oster G. Use of terfenadine and contraindicated drugs. *Journal of the American Medical Association* 1996; 275:1339–41.

2

ADVERSE DRUG REACTIONS: How Serious Is the Problem and How Often and Why Does It Occur?

Although some adverse drug reactions are not very serious, others cause the death, hospitalization, or serious injury of more than 2 million people in the United States each year, including more than 100,000 fatalities. In fact, adverse drug reactions are one of the leading causes of death in the United States.[1] Most of the time, these dangerous events could and should have been avoided. Even the less drastic reactions, such as change in mood, loss of appetite, and nausea, may seriously diminish the quality of life.

Despite the fact that more adverse reactions occur in patients 60 or older, the odds of suffering an adverse drug reaction really begin to increase even before age 50. Almost half (49.5%) of Food and Drug Administration (FDA) reports of deaths from adverse drug reactions and 61% of hospitalizations from adverse drug reactions were in people younger than 60.[2] Many physical changes that affect the way the body can handle drugs actually begin in people in their thirties, but the increased prescribing of drugs does not begin for most people until they enter their fifties. By then, the amount of prescription drug use starts increasing significantly, and therefore the odds of having an adverse drug reaction also increase. **The risk of an adverse drug reaction is about 33% higher in people aged 50 to 59 than it is in people aged 40 to 49.**[3]

Adverse Reactions to Drugs Cause Hospitalization of 1.5 Million Americans Each Year

An analysis of numerous studies in which the cause of hospitalization was determined found that approximately 1.5 million hospitalizations a year were caused by adverse drug reactions.[4] This means that every day more than 4,000 patients have adverse drug reactions so serious that they need to be admitted to American hospitals. Although the rate of drug-induced hospitalization is higher in older adults (an average of about 10% of all hospitalizations for older adults are caused by adverse drug reactions) because they use more drugs, a significant proportion of hospitalizations for children is also caused by adverse drug reactions. In a review of more than 6,500 admissions of children to five different hospitals, 2.0% were prompted by adverse drug reactions.[5]

Adverse Reactions Occur to 770,000 People a Year During Hospitalization

In addition to the 1.5 million people a year who are admitted to the hospital *because* of adverse drug reactions, an additional three quarters of a million people a year develop an adverse reaction after they are hospitalized. According to national projections based on a study involving adverse drug reactions developing in patients in the hospital, 770,000 additional patients a year, more than 2,000 patients a day, suffer an adverse event caused by drugs once they are admitted. Many of the reactions in the patients studied were serious, even life-threatening, and included cardiac arrhythmias, kidney failure, bleeding, and dangerously low blood pressure. People with these adverse reactions had an almost two-fold higher risk of death compared to other otherwise comparable hospitalized patients who did not have a drug reaction. Most importantly, according to the researchers, almost 50% of these adverse reactions were preventable. Among the kinds of preventable problems were adverse interactions between drugs that should not have been prescribed together (hundreds of these are listed in Chapter 3 of this book), known allergies to drugs that had not been asked about before the patients got a prescription, and excessively high doses of drugs prescribed without considering the patient's weight and kidney function.[6]

Thus, adding the number of people with adverse drug reactions so serious that they require hospitalization to those in which the adverse reaction was "caused" by the hospitalization, more than 2.2 million people a year, or 6,000 patients a day, suffer these adverse reactions. In both situations, many of these drug-induced problems should have been prevented.

Dangerous Prescribing Outside the Hospital for 6.6 Million Older Adults a Year

Based on the **Do Not Use** principle we have advocated concerning certain drugs for more than ten years in our *Worst Pills, Best Pills* books and monthly newsletter, several published studies have examined the extent to which people are prescribed drugs that are contraindicated because there are safer alternatives. One study, whose authors stated that *"Worst Pills, Best Pills* stimulated this research," found that almost one out of four older adults living at home—6.6 million people a year—were prescribed a "potentially inappropriate" drug or drugs, placing them at risk of such adverse drug effects as mental impairment and sedation, even though the study only examined the use of a relatively short list of needlessly dangerous drugs (fewer than the number listed as **Do Not Use** drugs in this book).[7]

Other researchers looked not only at people for whom a contraindicated drug was prescribed, but also at prescriptions for older people involving two other categories: questionable combinations of drugs and excessive treatment duration. The authors categorized all of this as "high-risk prescribing" and limited their analysis to just the three classes of drugs most commonly causing drug-related illness: cardiovascular drugs, psychotropic drugs (ones that act on the mind) such as tranquilizers and antidepressants, and anti-inflammatory drugs. They found that 52.6% of all people 65 or older were given one or more prescriptions for a high-risk drug.[8] Thus, more than twice as many older adults were the victims of high-risk prescribing when these two additional categories were added.

How Extensive Is the Problem of Specific Adverse Drug Reactions?

The following national estimates are based on well-conducted studies, mainly in the United States:

• *Each year, in hospitals alone, there are 28,000 cases of life-threatening heart toxicity from adverse reactions to digoxin,* the most commonly used form of digitalis in older adults.[9] Since as many as 40% or more of these people are using this drug unnecessarily (see discussion on p. 113), many of these injuries are preventable.

- *Each year 41,000 older adults are hospitalized—and 3,300 of these die from ulcers caused by NSAIDs* (nonsteroidal anti-inflammatory drugs, usually for treatment of arthritis).[10] Thousands of younger adults are hospitalized.

- *Each year, more than 9.6 million adverse drug reactions occur in older Americans.* The referenced study found that 37% of these adverse reactions were not reported to the doctor, presumably because patients did not realize they were due to the drug. This is not too surprising considering that most doctors admitted they did not explain possible adverse effects to their patients.[11]

- *At least 16,000 injuries from auto crashes each year involving older drivers are attributable to the use of psychoactive drugs,* specifically benzodiazepines and tricyclic antidepressants.[12] (Psychoactive drugs are those that affect the mind or behavior.)

- *Each year 32,000 older adults suffer from hip fractures—contributing to more than 1,500 deaths—attributable to drug-induced falls.*[13] In one study, the main categories of drugs responsible for the falls leading to hip fractures were sleeping pills and minor tranquilizers (30%), antipsychotic drugs (52%), and antidepressants (17%). All of these categories of drugs are often prescribed unnecessarily, especially in older adults. (See section on minor tranquilizers and sleeping pills, antipsychotic drugs, and antidepressants, p. 178.) The in-hospital death rate for hip fractures in older adults is 4.9%.[14] Multiplying this times the 32,000 hip fractures a year in older adults attributable to drug-induced falls shows that 1,568 older adults die each year from adverse drug reactions that cause hip fractures.

- *Approximately 163,000 older Americans suffer from serious mental impairment (memory loss, dementia) either caused or worsened by drugs.*[15] In a study in the state of Washington, in 46% of the patients with drug-induced mental impairment, the problem was caused by minor tranquilizers or sleeping pills; in 14%, by high blood pressure drugs; and in 11%, by antipsychotic drugs.

- *Two million older Americans are addicted or at risk of addiction to minor tranquilizers or sleeping pills because they have used them daily for at least one year*, even though there is no acceptable evidence that the tranquilizers are effective for more than four months and the sleeping pills for more than 30 days.[16]

- *Drug-induced tardive dyskinesia has developed in 73,000 older adults; this condition is the most serious and common adverse reaction to antipsychotic drugs, and it is often irreversible.* Tardive dyskinesia is characterized by involuntary movements of the lips, tongue, and sometimes the fingers, toes, and trunk. Since most of the older people taking these drugs were not actually psychotic, they have a serious side effect from antipsychotic drugs prescribed without justification.[17]

- *Drug-induced parkinsonism has developed in 61,000 older adults due to the use of antipsychotic drugs such as Haldol, Thorazine, Mellaril, Stelazine, and Prolixin.* There are also other parkinsonism-inducing drugs, such as Reglan, Compazine, and Phenergan, prescribed for gastrointestinal problems.[18] As mentioned above, most (about 80%) of older adults receiving antipsychotic drugs do not have schizophrenia or other conditions that justify the use of such powerful drugs.

A serious problem exists because doctors and patients do not realize that **practically any symptom in older adults and in many younger adults can be caused or worsened by drugs.**[19] Some doctors and patients assume that what are actually adverse drug reactions are simply signs of aging. As a result, many serious adverse reactions are entirely overlooked or not recognized until they have caused significant harm.

Later in this chapter we will list the most common drug-induced adverse effects along with the drugs that can cause them. In the box below are some of the symptoms which, although they are frequently caused by drugs, are the kinds of problems that you or many doctors might first attribute simply to "growing old," or "getting nervous" instead of to a drug.

Mental Adverse Drug Reactions: depression, hallucinations, confusion, delirium, memory loss, impaired thinking

Nervous System Adverse Drug Reactions: parkinsonism, involuntary movements of the face, arms, legs (tardive dyskinesia), sexual dysfunction

Dizziness on Standing, Falls Sometimes Resulting in Hip Fractures, Automobile Accidents Resulting in Injury

Gastrointestinal Adverse Drug Reactions: loss of appetite, constipation

Urinary Problems: difficulty urinating, leaking of urine

The drugs responsible for the most serious adverse reactions in older adults are tranquilizers, sleeping pills, and other mind-affecting drugs; cardiovascular drugs such as high blood pressure drugs, digoxin, and drugs for abnormal heart rhythms;[20] and drugs for treating intestinal problems.

Specific Patient Examples

Forty-Year-Old Woman Dies from Dangerous Drug Interaction

Louise went to her family doctor for allergies and was prescribed Seldane, the nonsedating antihistamine that was widely promoted and prescribed (until it was recently taken off the market). When she later got a fungal infection of her toenails, she went to a dermatologist who prescribed an antifungal drug, ketoconazole (NIZORAL). The dermatologist did not question her about which other drugs she was taking and also did not know that the combination of the two drugs could, by preventing the body from getting rid of Seldane, cause toxic levels of Seldane to accumulate, levels that cause life-threatening heart arrhythmias. Louise died of such an arrhythmia not long after she started taking Nizoral.

Fifty-eight-Year-Old Man Develops Parkinsonism from Antipsychotic Drug Being Used to Treat His "Irritable Bowel" Problem

Larry, an otherwise healthy 58-year-old man with diarrhea believed to be due to "irritable bowel syndrome," was given Stelazine, a powerful antipsychotic tranquilizer to "calm down" his intestinal tract. Stelazine is not even approved for treating such medical problems. Six months after starting Stelazine, Larry developed severe parkinsonism and was started on L-dopa, a drug for treating Parkinson's disease. Presumably, the doctor did not realize the parkinsonism was drug-induced, and the Stelazine was continued. For seven years, Larry took both drugs. Then a neurologist specializing in Parkinson's disease saw Larry, recognized the real cause of his problem, stopped the Stelazine, and slowly withdrew the L-dopa over a six-month period. Larry's severe, disabling parkinsonism cleared completely.

As mentioned above, 61,000 older adults develop drug-induced parkinsonism each year. At least 80% of them, like Larry, should never have been put on the drugs causing the parkinsonism in the first place. Also, as in Larry's situation, a large proportion of these people have doctors who think that their parkinsonism developed spontaneously.

The doctors not only fail to suspect that it is caused by a drug such as Stelazine, or other

antipsychotic drugs (Reglan, Compazine, or Phenergan), but they add a second drug to treat the disease that has been caused by the first drug.

The same neurologist who "cured" Larry of his drug-induced parkinsonism saw, in just three years, 38 other patients with drug-induced parkinsonism and 28 with drug-induced tardive dyskinesia.

None of these people were psychotic, the one justification for antipsychotic medications. Rather, the most common reasons for using the parkinsonism-inducing drugs were chronic anxiety and gastrointestinal complaints. The most frequent culprit (in 19 of these 39 patients) was metoclopramide (REGLAN), usually prescribed for heartburn or for nausea and vomiting. Doctors often prescribe Reglan before trying other more conservative and safer methods. (See alternative treatment of nausea and vomiting, p. 366). Other drugs that brought on parkinsonism included Compazine, Haldol and Thorazine.[21]

Sarah's 80-Year-Old Father's Confusion and Hallucinations Were Induced by His Ulcer Drugs

Sarah wrote us about her father, saying that she had to repeatedly nag his doctor about the possible role of her dad's ulcer drugs in causing confusion and hallucinations before the doctor listened. Three different drugs—Tagamet, Zantac, and Pepcid—had been tried for her father's ulcers, and each had caused these adverse reactions. When the doctor finally switched Sarah's father to an antacid, Maalox, his mind completely cleared and he was his old self, no longer confused or hallucinating.

Seventy-nine-Year-Old Woman Has Reversible Mental Impairment

Sally, the mother-in-law of a physician, was noted by her son-in-law, who had not seen her for several months, to have suffered severe impairment of her otherwise sharp mind. She was acting confused and, for the first time in her life, was unable to balance her checkbook. When questioned by her son-in-law, she was able to remember that her problem had started around the time she was put on a tranquilizer, Ativan. After this link was discovered, the drug was slowly discontinued and all of the mental impairment that had begun when the drug was started disappeared.

Sixty-four-Year-Old Man Has Auto Accident After One Dose of Tranquilizer

Ben, the 64-year-old uncle of a physician, was scheduled to have a biopsy done at a local hospital at eight in the morning. So that he would be relaxed for the biopsy, four days before it was to be done the doctor gave him a free sample of a tranquilizer, Xanax, to take an hour or so before the procedure. Ben was not told that he should not use drugs like this if he was going to drive and, while driving to the hospital for the biopsy, he blacked out. The car went over a fence and sustained $6,000 worth of damage, but fortunately Ben was unhurt. (See Drugs That Can Cause Auto Accidents, p. 28.)

Sixty-three-Year-Old Gets into "Drug-Illness" Cycle

Nancy, a healthy 63-year-old woman, complained about difficulty going to sleep. Instead of taking a careful history and finding out that she had recently started drinking several cups of coffee at dinner, her doctor prescribed a sleeping pill. A subsequent referral was also made to a psychiatrist because of depression (possibly partly induced by the sleeping pill), and an antidepressant drug was also prescribed. If this patient also took an antihistamine-containing drug for a cold (not an effective treatment), she would be using three drugs, all of which have powerful sedative effects, which could make her so groggy that standing would be difficult, and falling would be easy.

Sixty-Year-Old Woman Given "Overdose" of Propranolol

Elsie, a 60-year-old woman who worked as an assistant at a senior citizens' center, was started on propranolol to treat her high blood pressure. Unfortunately, her doctor did not realize that the dose of this sometimes useful drug (see p. 154) must be reduced in older adults, and she was prescribed 80 milligrams twice a day. Two days after she started taking the drug, she began feeling very weak, so much so that by the third day, she went to a hospital emergency room, where her pulse rate was found to be thirty-six beats per minute. This dangerously low rate fully explained her weakness. The drug was stopped and Elsie's heart rate returned to normal. Later a low dose of a different drug was prescribed and had no adverse effects.

Seven-Year-Old Boy Dies from Drug Prescribed for Attention Deficit Hyperactivity Disorder

Bernie, a bright 7-year-old, was prescribed an antidepressant, imipramine (TOFRANIL), to treat attention deficit hyperactivity disorder. Because his parents were not provided with accurate, complete information about the drug, they were unaware that the drug could cause life-threatening heart arrhythmias, that the dose prescribed was too high, and that the tremor and convulsions that Bernie began to have were actually adverse drug reactions to imipramine. Treatment with the drug was continued, and one day, while at school, he collapsed and died of a heart arrhythmia. If his parents had been adequately warned about this drug, Bernie would be alive today.

In discussing the problem of adverse drug reactions in the elderly, the World Health Organization has stated some principles applicable to people of all ages: "*Quite often, the history and clinical examination of patients with side effects reveal that no valid indication [purpose]* *for the offending drug has been present. . . . Adverse reactions can to a large extent be avoided in the elderly by choosing safe and effective drugs and applying sound therapeutic principles in prescribing, such as starting with a small dose, observing the patient frequently, and avoiding excessive polypharmacy [the use of multiple drugs at the same time].*"[22]

In other words, according to the World Health Organization, patients who suffer adverse drug reactions are very often victims of drugs that there is no valid reason for them to take.

A carefully controlled study examined the details of prescriptions of people being discharged from a community hospital with three or more prescriptions to treat chronic illnesses.[23] The results of this study are quite disturbing, both in what they say about the doctors' prescribing practices and in the evidence as to the potential damage that could be done to older adults as a result of these practices. Of the 236 people intensively studied:

• Eighty-eight percent of the people had one or more prescribing problems with the prescriptions they were given. At least one potentially serious, life-threatening problem occurred which could have been as a result of the prescriptions written for 22% of these patients.

When the specific problems with the prescriptions were examined, the results were as follows:

• Fifty-nine percent of the patients had been given one or more prescriptions for a drug that was an inappropriate choice of therapy because it was either "less than optimal medication given the patient's diagnosis" or there was no established indication for it;
• Twenty-eight percent of the patients were given too high a dose of the drug, an "overdose";
• Forty-eight percent of the patients were given a combination of drugs that can result in one or more harmful drug interactions;

• Twenty percent of the patients were given drugs that unnecessarily duplicated the therapeutic effect of another drug they were taking.

The good news from this study, however, was that a consultant pharmacist, involved in the care of more than 50% of these patients, was able to reduce the risks by making recommendations to the prescribing physicians.

Nine Reasons Why Older Adults Are More Likely Than Younger Adults to Have Adverse Drug Reactions (Unless They Are Given Fewer Drugs and Smaller Doses)

Many of the studies and much of the information concerning the epidemic of drug-induced disease focuses on people 60 and over. As we have mentioned previously, some of the changes that eventually lead to great numbers of adverse reactions in older adults (in combination with increased drug use) really begin to occur in the mid-thirties. In connection with the idea that drug-induced disease begins to get more common before age 60, it is interesting to note that in a number of studies comparing the way "older" people clear drugs out of the body with the way younger people do, the definition of older is above 50, and younger is below 50.[24]

1. Smaller Bodies and Different Body Composition: Older adults generally weigh less and have a smaller amount of water and a larger proportion of fat than younger adults. Body weight increases from age 40 to 60, mainly due to increased fat, then decreases from age 60 to 70, with even sharper declines from 70 on. Therefore, the amount of a drug per pound of body weight or per pound of body water will often be much higher in an older adult than it would be if the same amount of the drug were given to a younger person. In addition, drugs that concentrate in fat tissue may stay in the body longer because there is more fat for them to accumulate in.

2. Decreased Ability of the Liver to Process Drugs: Because the liver does not work as well in older adults, they are less able than younger people to process certain drugs so that they can be excreted from the body. This has important consequences for a large proportion of the drugs used to treat heart conditions and high blood pressure, as well as many other drugs processed by the liver. The ability of the body to rid itself of drugs such as Valium, Librium, and many others is affected by this decrease in liver function.

3. Decreased Ability of the Kidneys to Clear Drugs Out of the Body: The ability of the kidneys to clear many drugs out of the body decreases steadily from age 35 to 40 on. By age 65, the filtering ability of the kidneys has already decreased by 30%. Other aspects of kidney function also decline progressively as people age. This has an effect on the safety of a large number of drugs.

4. Increased Sensitivity to Many Drugs: The problems of decreased body size, altered body composition (more fat, less water), and decreased liver and kidney function cause many drugs to accumulate in older people's bodies at dangerously higher levels and for longer times than in younger people. These age-related problems are further worsened by the fact that even at "normal" blood levels of many drugs, older adults have an increased sensitivity to their effects, often resulting in harm. This is seen most clearly with drugs that act on the central nervous system such as many **sleeping pills, alcohol, tranquilizers, strong painkillers such as morphine or pentazocine (TALWIN), and most drugs that have anticholinergic effects (see *Anticholinergic* in the Glossary, p. 768). This latter group includes antidepressants, antipsychotic drugs, antihistamines, drugs used to calm the intestinal tract (for treating ulcers or some kinds of colitis) such as Donnatal, atropine, and Librax, antiparkinsonian drugs, and other drugs such as Norpace.**

For all of the drugs in the above-mentioned groups that are listed in this book, we include an "anticholinergic" warning as follows:

WARNING: SPECIAL MENTAL AND PHYSICAL ADVERSE EFFECTS

Older adults are especially sensitive to the harmful anticholinergic (see Glossary, p. 768) effects of [name of drug class]. These drugs should not be used unless absolutely necessary.

Mental effects: confusion, delirium, short-term memory problems, disorientation, and impaired attention

Physical effects: dry mouth, constipation, difficulty urinating (especially for a man with an enlarged prostate), blurred vision, decreased sweating with increased body temperature, sexual dysfunction, and worsening of glaucoma.

Yet another example of the marked increase in the sensitivity of older adults to drugs has to do with stimulant drugs that are in the same family as amphetamines or "speed." Despite the dangers of these drugs for anyone, especially older adults, they are widely promoted and prescribed, including Ornade, Tavist-D, Entex LA, and Actifed. All of these contain amphetamine-like drugs such as PPA (phenylpropanolamine) or pseudoephedrine. For any of these drugs discussed in this book, most of which are listed as **Do Not Use** drugs, the following warning is given:

WARNING

[Name of drug] can cause or worsen high blood pressure. It is especially dangerous for people who have high blood pressure, heart disease, diabetes, or thyroid disease. People over 60 are more likely than younger people to experience effects on the heart and blood pressure, restlessness, nervousness, and confusion.

---

5. Decreased Blood-Pressure-Maintaining Ability: Because older adults are less able to compensate for some of the effects of drugs, there is yet another reason why they are more vulnerable to adverse effects of drugs and more sensitive to the intended effects. The most widespread example of older adults' decreased ability to compensate is seen when they get out of bed and/or suddenly rise from a seated position. As you rise, your blood pressure normally falls, decreasing the blood flow to your head, resulting in less blood flow to the brain. Younger people's bodies can compensate for this: receptors in the neck, sensing that the blood pressure is falling as the person rises, tighten up the blood vessels in other parts of the body, thus keeping the overall blood pressure high enough. In older adults, these receptors do not work as well. Often, upon standing, older adults feel giddy, lightheaded, and dizzy. They may even faint because the blood pressure in the head falls too rapidly.

The ability to maintain a proper blood pressure is further weakened when you use any of a very long list of drugs, **the most common examples being high blood pressure drugs. Other categories of drugs that cause an exaggerated blood pressure drop include sleeping pills, tranquilizers, antidepressants, antipsychotic drugs, antihistamines, drugs for heart pain (angina), and antiarrhythmics.** (See p. 26 for a full list of drugs that can cause this difficulty.)

This problem of so-called postural hypotension—the sudden fall in blood pressure on standing, brought about by a combination of aging and drugs—can be catastrophic, and the falls that often result can end in hip fractures, a leading cause of death in older adults, or other serious injuries.

6. Decreased Temperature Compensation: Younger adults are more easily able than older people to withstand very high or very low temperatures. They sweat and dilate (widen) blood vessels to get rid of excess heat when it is hot, and constrict (narrow) blood vessels to conserve heat when it is cold. Older adults' bodies are less able to do this. As in the case of blood pressure compensation, this "normal" temperature-regulating problem of older adults can be significantly worsened by any of a large number of prescription and over-the-counter drugs, resulting in fatal or life-threatening changes in body temperature. **Many older adults' deaths during heat waves or prolonged cold spells can be attributed to drugs that interfere with temperature regulation. Most of these people did not know they were at increased risk.** All drugs in this book that contain a warning about anticholinergic effects can have this harmful effect on withstanding heat waves.

7. More Diseases That Affect the Response to Drugs: Older adults are much more likely than younger adults to have at least one disease—such as liver or kidney damage (not just the decreased function of older age), poor circulation, and other chronic conditions—that alters their response to drugs. Little is known about the influence of multiple diseases on drug effects in the elderly.

One well-understood example, however, is the effect of heart failure on the way people can handle drugs. When the heart is not able to pump as much blood as it used to, the change that occurs in heart failure, there is also a decrease in the flow of blood to the kidneys. For the same reasons discussed in reason number 3, the reduced flow of blood to the kidneys decreases the kidneys' ability to rid drugs from the blood and excrete them in the urine.

8. More Drugs and, Therefore, More Adverse Drug Reactions and Interactions: Since older adults use significantly more prescription drugs than younger people, they have greatly increased odds of having a drug reaction caused by the dangerous interaction between two drugs. Often, older adults take one or more over-the-counter drugs in addition to their prescription drugs. This further increases the likelihood of

adverse drug interactions. One of the more common kinds of adverse drug interactions is the ability of some drug to cause a second drug to accumulate to dangerous levels in the body. At the end of the discussion of each drug in Chapter 3, except for the 160 **Do Not Use** drugs, there is a list of other drugs that can cause serious adverse interactions.

PARTIAL LIST OF DRUG INTERACTIONS

Some of these interactions are life-threatening or of great potential harm to patients. (See individual drug profiles for complete lists of interactions.)

Propulsid	with	Biaxin
Zocor	with	Posicor
Hismanal	with	Paxil
Sporanox	with	Propulsid
Mevacor	with	Lopid
Seldane	with	erythromycin
Aldactone	with	potassium
Prozac	with	Desyrel
Butazolidin	with	Orinase
insulin	with	Inderal
Tegretol	with	erythromycin
Tagamet	with	Dilantin
Nardil	with	Larodopa
Inderal	with	Tagamet
Demerol	with	Nardil
Calan SR	with	quinidine
theophylline	with	Tagamet
warfarin (Coumadin)	with	Tagamet
Lanoxin	with	Calan SR

---

9. Inadequate Testing of Drugs in Older Adults Before Approval: Although older adults use a disproportionate share of prescription drugs, few of these drugs are adequately tested in older adults before being approved by the FDA.

Dr. Peter Lamy of the University of Maryland School of Pharmacy has stated, "We test drugs in young people for three months; we give them to old people for 15 years." The FDA is slowly remedying this serious problem by requiring that the people on whom a drug is tested be representative of those who will use the drug if it is approved. Nonetheless, most drugs on the market today, which are heavily used by older adults, were not adequately tested in this age group.

In summary, there are significant differences between younger and older patients, often not realized by doctors or patients. Increasing awareness of these differences will result in the prescription of far fewer drugs to older adults, and those that are prescribed will be given at lower doses in most instances.

Which Adverse Effects Can Be Caused by Which Drugs?

The following charts are to be used by patients who have any of a variety of medical problems (or by doctors) to find out which drugs, especially ones they are using or are considering using, can cause specific adverse reactions. The lists are compiled from a variety of sources.[25,26,27,28,29,30]

Although some of these adverse effects occur most commonly in older adults, all of them have also been documented in younger people, although not as often in some instances.

SUMMARY OF ADVERSE REACTIONS AND THE DRUGS THAT CAUSE THEM

Only the most easily detectable problems are considered, and only the most common drugs causing each problem are listed.

Adverse Drug Reaction	(Number of Drugs)	Examples of Brand Names
Depression	(148)	Accutane, Cipro, Valium, Dalmane, Xanax, Catapres, Inderal, Reglan, Advil, Naprosyn, Tagamet, Talwin, Zantac, Pepcid, Norpace
Psychoses/ hallucinations	(133)	Lanoxin, Procanbid, Aldomet, Catapres, Inderal, Elavil, Valium, Halcion, Benadryl, Hismanal, Cipro, Tagamet, Dexatrim
Confusion/ delirium	(140)	Compazine, Mellaril, Elavil, Cipro, Amaryl, Valium, Xanax, Benadryl, Sinemet, Catapres, Tagamet, Zantac, DiaBeta, Diabinese, Dymelor

Adverse Drug Reaction	(Number of Drugs)	Examples of Brand Names
Dementia	(76)	Mellaril, Valium, Xanax, Restoril, Aldomet, Ser-Ap-Es, Regroton, Inderal, Tagamet, Zantac, Maxzide
Insomnia	(27)	Sudafed, Inderal, Lasix, Mevacor, Nicorette, Theo-24, Synthroid
Parkinsonism	(36)	Haldol, Mellaril, Thorazine, Elavil, Asendin, Aldomet, Prozac, Regroton, Compazine, Reglan
Tardive dyskinesia	(17)	Compazine, Haldol, Mellaril, Thorazine, Asendin, BuSpar, Wellbutrin, Risperdal, Zyprexa, Zyban
Dizziness on standing	(148)	Nitro-Bid, Isordil, Lasix, Hytrin, Cardura, Calan SR, Cardizem CD, Catapres, Minipress, Procardia, Inderal, Tenormin, Valium, Xanax, Prinivil, Elavil, Compazine, Haldol
Falls/hip fracture	(52)	Valium, Xanax, Restoril, Prozac, Nembutal, Elavil, Sinequan, Haldol, Compazine, Navane, Isordil, Dalmane
Auto accidents	(20)	Valium, Xanax, Ativan, Elavil, Tofranil, Asendin, Norpramin, Pamelor, Sinequan
Sexual dysfunction	(128)	Transderm-Scop, Proscar, Pepcid, Tagamet, Zantac, Calan SR, Norpace, Tegretol, Lopid, Prozac, Lopressor
Loss of appetite, nausea, vomiting	(58)	K-Lor, Lanoxin, Advil, Feldene, Demerol, EES, Sumycin, Feosol, Ultram, Theo-24, Daypro, Relafen
Abdominal pain, ulcers, GI bleeding	(40)	Advil, Motrin, Feldene, Indocin, Anaprox, Somophyllin, Theo-24, Cortone, Decadron, Relafen, Daypro
Constipation	(105)	Dilaudid, Ultram, Talwin, Tylenol No. 3, Tylox, Benadryl, Cogentin, Urised, Maalox, Inderal, Amphojel, Caltrate
Diarrhea	(46)	Aldomet, Precose, Maalox, Phillips' Milk of Magnesia, Dulcolax, Peri-Colace, Sumycin, Cipro
Lung toxicity	(60)	Tegretol, Inderal, Visken, Prinivil, Vasotec, Feldene
Blocked urination	(55)	Sinequan, Ultram, Elavil, Compazine, Haldol, Antivert, Bentyl, Benadryl, Tavist, Artane, Zyban
Urine leakage	(74)	Lasix, Esidrix, Zaroxolyn, Inderal, Tenormin, Minipress, Valium, Restoril, Xanax, Lithobid, Ziac, Hytrin

Drugs That Can Affect the Mind

Drugs That Can Cause Depression

BRAND NAME	GENERIC NAME

Acne drugs

Accutane	isotretinoin ·

Antibiotics and other anti-infective agents

	dapsone
	sulfonamides
Chibroxin, Noroxin	norfloxacin
Ciloxan, Cipro	ciprofloxacin
Flagyl	metronidazole
Floxin, Ocuflox	ofloxacin
INH	isoniazid
Lariam	mefloquine
Levaquin	levofloxacin
Maxaquin	lomefloxacin
Penetrex	enoxacin
Raxar	grepafloxacin
Seromycin	cycloserine
Trecator-SC	ethionamide
Zagam	sparfloxacin
Zovirax	acyclovir

Corticosteroids, systemic

Acthar	corticotropin (ACTH)
Azmacort	triamcinolone
Cortef	hydrocortisone
Cortone	cortisone
Decadron, Hexadrol	dexamethasone
Deltasone, Meticorten	prednisone
Diprolene, Valisone	betamethasone
Medrol	methylprednisolone
Metreton, Pred Forte	prednisolone

Eye drugs

Betagan	levobunolol
Cartrol	carteolol
OptiPranolol	metipranolol
Timoptic	timolol

Gastrointestinal drugs

Axid	nizatidine
Pepcid	famotidine
Reglan	metoclopramide
Tagamet	cimetidine
Zantac	ranitidine

Heart and blood vessel drugs
Antiarrhythmics

Norpace	disopyramide
Procanbid	procainamide

Cholesterol-lowering drugs

Baycol	cerivastatin
Lescol	fluvastatin
Lipitor	atorvastatin
Mevacor	lovastatin

BRAND NAME	GENERIC NAME
Pravachol	pravastatin
Zocor	simvastatin

High blood pressure drugs (beta-blockers)

Blocadren	timolol
Cartrol	carteolol
Coreg	carvedilol
Corgard	nadolol
Corzide	nadolol/bendroflumethiazide
Inderal, Inderal LA	propranolol
Inderide LA	propranolol/hydrochlorothiazide
Kerlone	betaxolol
Levatol	penbutolol
Lopressor, Toprol XL	metoprolol
Lopressor HCT	metoprolol/hydrochlorothiazide
Normodyne, Trandate	labetalol
Sectral	acebutolol
Tenoretic	atenolol/chlorthalidone
Tenormin	atenolol
Timolide	timolol/hydrochlorothiazide
Visken	pindolol
Zebeta	bisoprolol
Ziac	bisoprolol/hydrochlorothiazide

High blood pressure drugs (calcium channel blockers)

Adalat, Procardia, Adalat CC, Procardia XL	nifedipine
Calan SR, Covera-HS, Isoptin SR, Verelan	verapamil
Cardene, Cardene SR	nicardipine
Cardizem CD, Dilacor XR, Tiazac	diltiazem
DynaCirc, DynaCirc CR	isradipine
Lexxel	felodipine/enalapril
Lotrel	amlodipine/benazepril
Norvasc	amlodipine
Plendil	felodipine
Posicor	mibefradil
Sular	nisoldipine
Tarka	verapamil/trandolapril
Teczem	diltiazem/enalapril

High blood pressure drugs (diuretics)

Diupres	reserpine/chlorothiazide
Enduronyl	deserpidine/methyclothiazide
Hydropres	reserpine/hydrochlorothiazide
Regroton, Demi-Regroton	reserpine/chlorthalidone
Salutensin	reserpine/hydroflumethiazide
Ser-Ap-Es	reserpine/hydralazine/hydrochlorothiazide

High blood pressure drugs (other)

	reserpine
Aldomet	methyldopa
Catapres	clonidine
Hytrin	terazosin
Minipress	prazosin
Tenex	guanfacine

BRAND NAME	GENERIC NAME

Mind-affecting drugs
Antidepressants
Wellbutrin	bupropion

Barbiturates
Butisol	butabarbital
Luminal, Solfoton	phenobarbital
Nembutal	pentobarbital
Seconal	secobarbital

Tranquilizers or sleeping pills
Ativan	lorazepam
BuSpar	buspirone
Centrax	prazepam
Dalmane	flurazepam
Halcion	triazolam
Librium	chlordiazepoxide
Limbitrol	amitriptyline/chlordiazepoxide
Noludar	methyprylon
Restoril	temazepam
Serax	oxazepam
Tranxene	clorazepate
Valium	diazepam
Xanax	alprazolam

Neurological drugs
Anticonvulsants
Depakene/Depakote	divalproex, valproate, valproic acid
Dilantin	phenytoin
Klonopin	clonazepam
Luminal, Solfoton	phenobarbital
Mysoline	primidone
Tegretol	carbamazepine
Zarontin	ethosuximide

Antiparkinsonians
Eldepryl	selegiline, deprenyl
Larodopa	levodopa
Parlodel	bromocriptine
Permax	pergolide
Sinemet	levodopa/carbidopa

Painkillers/narcotics
Advil, Motrin	ibuprofen
Aleve, Anaprox, Naprosyn	naproxen
Ansaid, Ocufen	flurbiprofen
Butazolidin	phenylbutazone
Clinoril	sulindac
Daypro	oxaprozin
Demerol	meperidine
Dolobid	diflunisal
Duract	bromfenac
Feldene	piroxicam
Indocin	indomethacin
Lodine	etodolac
Meclomen	meclofenamate
MS Contin, Roxanol	morphine
Nalfon	fenoprofen

BRAND NAME	GENERIC NAME
Orudis	ketoprofen
Relafen	nabumetone
Talwin	pentazocine
Talwin-NX	pentazocine/naloxone
Tolectin	tolmetin
Ultram	tramadol
Voltaren	diclofenac

Other drugs
	amphetamines (during withdrawal)
	progestins
Amipaque	metrizamide
Antabuse	disulfiram
Dexatrim	phenylpropanolamine
Elspar	asparaginase
Lioresal	baclofen
Roferon-A, Intron A	interferon alfa
Seromycin	cycloserine
Velban	vinblastine
Zyban	bupropion

Drugs That Can Cause Psychoses, Such as Hallucinations

BRAND NAME	GENERIC NAME

Antibiotics and other anti-infective agents
	dapsone
	sulfonamides
Aralen	chloroquine
Atabrine	quinacrine
Chibroxin, Noroxin	norfloxacin
Ciloxan, Cipro	ciprofloxacin
Floxin, Ocuflox	ofloxacin
Fungizone	amphotericin B
INH	isoniazid
Lariam	mefloquine
Levaquin	levofloxacin
Maxaquin	lomefloxacin
Mintezol	thiabendazole
NegGram	nalidixic acid
Off	deet
Penetrex	enoxacin
Podofin	podophyllum
Raxar	grepafloxacin
Seromycin	cycloserine
Symmetrel	amantadine
Trecator-SC	ethionamide
Wycillin	penicillin G procaine
Zagam	sparfloxacin
Zovirax	acyclovir

Cold, cough, allergy and asthma drugs
Antihistamines
Alermine, Chlor-Trimeton	chlorpheniramine
Atarax, Vistaril	hydroxyzine

BRAND NAME	GENERIC NAME
Benadryl, Sominex Formula	diphenhydramine
Dimetane	brompheniramine
Hismanal	astemizole
Myidil	tripolidine
Optimine	azatadine
Periactin	cyproheptadine
Seldane	terfenadine
Tavist, Tavist-1	clemastine

Asthma drugs

Maxair	pirbuterol
Proventil, Ventolin	albuterol

Nasal decongestants

	ephedrine
Afrin	oxymetazoline
Naldecon	phenylephrine
Sudafed	pseudoephedrine

Corticosteroids, systemic

Acthar	corticotropin (ACTH)
Azmacort	triamcinolone
Cortef	hydrocortisone
Cortone	cortisone
Decadron, Hexadrol	dexamethasone
Deltasone, Meticorten	prednisone
Diprolene, Valisone	betamethasone
Medrol	methylprednisolone
Metreton, Pred Forte	prednisolone

Eye drugs

Betagan	levobunolol
Timoptic	timolol

Gastrointestinal drugs

Tagamet	cimetidine

Heart and blood vessel drugs

Lanoxicaps, Lanoxin	digoxin

Antiarrhythmics

Mexitil	mexiletine
Procanbid	procainamide
Tonocard	tocainide
Xylocaine	lidocaine

High blood pressure drugs

Aldomet	methyldopa
Capoten	captopril
Cartrol	carteolol
Catapres	clonidine
Coreg	carvedilol
Corgard	nadolol
Hytrin	terazosin
Inderal, Inderal LA	propranolol
Kerlone	betaxolol
Levatol	penbutolol
Lopressor, Toprol XL	metoprolol
Minipress	prazosin
Normodyne, Trandate	labetalol
Sectral	acebutolol
Tenex	guanfacine

BRAND NAME	GENERIC NAME
Tenormin	atenolol
Visken	pindolol
Zebeta	bisoprolol

Mind-affecting drugs

Antidepressants

Asendin	amoxapine
Aventyl, Pamelor	nortriptyline
Desyrel	trazodone
Elavil	amitriptyline
Limbitrol	amitriptyline/chlordiazepoxide
Ludiomil	maprotiline
Norpramin	desipramine
Sinequan	doxepin
Tofranil	imipramine
Triavil	amitriptyline/perphenazine
Wellbutrin	bupropion

Tranquilizers or sleeping pills

Ambien	zolpidem
BuSpar	buspirone
Halcion	triazolam
Noludar	methyprylon
Placidyl	ethchlorvynol
Valium	diazepam

Neurological drugs

Anticonvulsants

Dilantin	phenytoin
Klonopin	clonazepam
Mysoline	primidone
Tegretol	carbamazepine
Zarontin	ethosuximide

Antiparkinsonians

Eldepryl	selegiline, deprenyl
Larodopa	levodopa
Parlodel	bromocriptine
Permax	pergolide
Sinemet	levodopa/carbidopa

Painkillers/narcotics

Arthropan*	choline salicylate*
Ascriptin*, Bufferin*	buffered aspirin*
Genuine Bayer Aspirin*, Ecotrin*	aspirin*
Darvon, Darvon–N	propoxyphene
Disalcid*	salsalate*
Doan's Pills*	magnesium salicylate*
Indocin	indomethacin
Ketalar	ketamine
MS Contin, Roxanol	morphine
Orudis	ketoprofen
Talwin	pentazocine
Talwin-NX	pentazocine/naloxone
Trilisate*	choline and magnesium salicylates*

---

*Salicylates can cause psychoses when they are used in high doses.

Other drugs

BRAND NAME	GENERIC NAME
	amphetamines
	atropine
	barbiturates
	cocaine
Amicar	aminocaproic acid
Amipaque	metrizamide
Antabuse	disulfiram
Dexatrim	phenylpropanolamine
Epogen	erythropoietin
Ifex	ifosfamide
Levothroid, Synthroid	levothyroxine
Lioresal	baclofen
Nardil	phenelzine
Oncovin	vincristine
Ritalin	methylphenidate
Sansert	methysergide
Zanaflex	tizanidine
Zyban	bupropion

Drugs That Can Cause Sudden Onset of Confusion or Delirium

Antibiotics and other anti-infective agents

BRAND NAME	GENERIC NAME
Chibroxin, Noroxin	norfloxacin
Ciloxan, Cipro	ciprofloxacin
Cytovene	ganciclovir
Floxin, Ocuflox	ofloxacin
Levaquin	levofloxacin
Maxaquin	lomefloxacin
Penetrex	enoxacin
Raxar	grepafloxacin
Symmetrel	amantadine
Urised	atropine/hyoscyamine/methenamine/methylene blue/phenyl salicylate/benzoic acid
Zagam	sparfloxacin
Zovirax	acyclovir

Cold, cough, allergy, and asthma drugs

BRAND NAME	GENERIC NAME
Alermine, Chlor-Trimeton	chlorpheniramine
Atarax, Vistaril	hydroxyzine
Benadryl, Sominex Formula	diphenhydramine
Dimetane	brompheniramine
Hismanal	astemizole
Myidil	triprolidine
Optimine	azatadine
Periactin	cyproheptadine
Seldane	terfenadine
Tavist, Tavist-1	clemastine

Corticosteroids, systemic

BRAND NAME	GENERIC NAME
Acthar	corticotropin (ACTH)
Azmacort	triamcinolone
Cortef	hydrocortisone
Cortone	cortisone
Decadron, Hexadrol	dexamethasone
Deltasone, Meticorten	prednisone
Diprolene, Valisone	betamethasone
Medrol	methylprednisolone
Metreton, Pred Forte	prednisolone

Diabetes drugs

BRAND NAME	GENERIC NAME
Amaryl	glimepiride
DiaBeta, Micronase	glyburide
Diabinese	chlorpropamide
Dymelor	acetohexamide
Glucotrol	glipizide
Humalog, Humulin	insulin
Orinase	tolbutamide
Tolinase	tolazamide

Gastrointestinal drugs

BRAND NAME	GENERIC NAME
	atropine
Antivert	meclizine
Axid	nizatidine
Bentyl	dicyclomine
Compazine	prochlorperazine
Ditropan	oxybutynin
Donnatal	atropine/hyoscyamine/scopolamine/phenobarbital
Librax	chlordiazepoxide/clidinium
Lomotil	diphenoxylate/atropine
Pepcid	famotidine
Phenergan	promethazine
Tagamet	cimetidine
Tigan	trimethobenzamide
Zantac	ranitidine

Heart and blood vessel drugs

BRAND NAME	GENERIC NAME
Catapres	clonidine
Duraquin, Quinaglute Dura–tabs, Quinidex	quinidine
Lanoxicaps, Lanoxin	digoxin
Norpace	disopyramide
Tenex	guanfacine

Mind-affecting drugs
Antidepressants

BRAND NAME	GENERIC NAME
Asendin	amoxapine
Aventyl, Pamelor	nortriptyline
Desyrel	trazodone
Elavil	amitriptyline
Lithobid, Lithonate	lithium
Limbitrol	amitriptyline/chlordiazepoxide
Ludiomil	maprotiline
Norpramin	desipramine
Prozac	fluoxetine
Sinequan	doxepin
Tofranil	imipramine

BRAND NAME	GENERIC NAME
Triavil	amitriptyline/perphenazine
Wellbutrin	bupropion

Antipsychotics

Clozaril	clozapine
Compazine	prochlorperazine
Haldol	haloperidol
Mellaril	thioridazine
Navane	thiothixene
Prolixin	fluphenazine
Reglan	metoclopramide
Stelazine	trifluoperazine
Thorazine	chlorpromazine
Triavil	amitriptyline/perphenazine

Barbiturates

Butisol	butabarbital
Luminal, Solfoton	phenobarbital
Nembutal	pentobarbital

Tranquilizers or sleeping pills

Atarax, Vistaril	hydroxyzine
Ativan	lorazepam
BuSpar	buspirone
Centrax	prazepam
Dalmane	flurazepam
Doriden	glutethimide
Halcion	triazolam
Librium	chlordiazepoxide
Miltown, Equanil	meprobamate
Noctec	chloral hydrate
Noludar	methyprylon
Restoril	temazepam
Serax	oxazepam
Tranxene	clorazepate
Valium	diazepam
Xanax	alprazolam

Neurological drugs
Anticonvulsants

Dilantin	phenytoin
Klonopin	clonazepam

Antiparkinsonians

Artane	trihexyphenidyl
Cogentin	benztropine
Larodopa	levodopa
Parlodel	bromocriptine
Permax	pergolide
Sinemet	levodopa/carbidopa

Painkillers/narcotics

Advil, Motrin	ibuprofen
Aleve, Anaprox, Naprosyn	naproxen
Ansaid, Ocufen	flurbiprofen

BRAND NAME	GENERIC NAME
Arthropan*	choline salicylate*
Ascriptin*, Bufferin*	buffered aspirin*
Genuine Bayer Aspirin*, Ecotrin*	aspirin*
Butazolidin	phenylbutazone
Clinoril	sulindac
Daypro	oxaprozin
Disalcid*	salsalate*
Doan's Pills*	magnesium salicylate*
Dolobid	diflunisal
Duract	bromfenac
Feldene	piroxicam
Indocin	indomethacin
Lodine	etodolac
Meclomen	meclofenamate
Nalfon	fenoprofen
Orudis	ketoprofen
Relafen	nabumetone
Talwin	pentazocine
Talwin-NX	pentazocine/naloxone
Tolectin	tolmetin
Toradol	ketorolac
Trilisate*	choline and magnesium salicylates*
Voltaren	diclofenac

Other drugs

Adsorbocarpine, Isopto Carpine	pilocarpine
Amipaque	metrizamide
Cytosar-U	cytarabine
Elspar	asparaginase
Lioresal	baclofen
Zyban	bupropion

Drugs That Can Cause or Worsen Dementia (Mental Impairment—Forgetfulness, Slow Thinking, Inability to Care for Oneself, Confusion)

Unlike the drugs listed on p. 22, which cause sudden confusion and/or delirium, these drugs cause mental impairment that is much slower and more subtle in onset.[31] **The categories of drugs with the biggest risk for mental impairment are the sleeping pills and so-called minor tranquilizers.**

BRAND NAME	GENERIC NAME

Gastrointestinal drugs

Axid	nizatidine
Pepcid	famotidine
Tagamet	cimetidine
Zantac	ranitidine

*Salicylates can cause psychoses when they are used in high doses.

Heart and blood vessel drugs
High blood pressure drugs (beta-blockers)

Blocadren	timolol
Cartrol	carteolol
Coreg	carvedilol
Corgard	nadolol
Corzide	nadolol/ bendroflumethiazide
Inderal, Inderal LA	propranolol
Inderide LA	propranolol/ hydrochlorothiazide
Kerlone	betaxolol
Levatol	penbutolol
Lopressor, Toprol XL	metoprolol
Lopressor HCT	metoprolol/ hydrochlorothiazide
Normodyne, Trandate	labetalol
Sectral	acebutolol
Tenoretic	atenolol/chlorthalidone
Tenormin	atenolol
Visken	pindolol
Zebeta	bisoprolol
Ziac	bisoprolol/ hydrochlorothiazide

High blood pressure drugs (diuretics)

Aldactazide	spironolactone/ hydrochlorothiazide
Aldoril	methyldopa/ hydrochlorothiazide
Apresazide	hydralazine/ hydrochlorothiazide
Bumex	bumetanide
Combipres	clonidine/chlorthalidone
Demadex	torsemide
Diupres	reserpine/chlorothiazide
Diuril	chlorothiazide
Dyazide, Maxzide	triamterene/hydrochlorothiazide
Enduron	methyclothiazide
Enduronyl	deserpidine/methyclothiazide
Esidrix, HydroDiuril	hydrochlorothiazide
Hydropres	reserpine/hydrochlorothiazide
Hygroton	chlorthalidone
Inderide LA	propranolol/hydrochlorothiazide
Lozol	indapamide
Metahydrin, Naqua	trichlormethiazide
Moduretic	amiloride/hydrochlorothiazide
Regroton, Demi-Regroton	reserpine/chlorthalidone
Salutensin	reserpine/hydroflumethiazide
Ser-Ap-Es	reserpine/hydralazine/ hydrochlorothiazide
Tenoretic	atenolol/chlorthalidone
Zaroxolyn, Diulo	metolazone

High blood pressure drugs (other)

	reserpine
Aldomet	methyldopa

BRAND NAME	GENERIC NAME

Mind-affecting drugs
Antidepressants

Prozac	fluoxetine

Antipsychotics

Compazine	prochlorperazine
Haldol	haloperidol
Mellaril	thioridazine
Navane	thiothixene
Prolixin	fluphenazine
Stelazine	trifluoperazine
Thorazine	chlorpromazine
Triavil	amitriptyline/ perphenazine

Barbiturates

Butisol	butabarbital
Luminal, Solfoton	phenobarbital
Nembutal	pentobarbital

Tranquilizers or sleeping pills

Atarax, Vistaril	hydroxyzine
Ativan	lorazepam
BuSpar	buspirone
Centrax	prazepam
Dalmane	flurazepam
Doriden	glutethimide
Halcion	triazolam
Librium	chlordiazepoxide
Miltown, Equanil	meprobamate
Noctec	chloral hydrate
Noludar	methyprylon
Restoril	temazepam
Serax	oxazepam
Tranxene	clorazepate
Valium	diazepam
Xanax	alprazolam

Neurological drugs

Klonopin	clonazepam

Drugs That Can Cause Insomnia

BRAND NAME	GENERIC NAME

Antibiotics and other anti-infective agents

	dapsone
Flumadine	rimantadine
Symmetrel	amantadine
Zovirax	acyclovir

Cold, cough, allergy, and asthma drugs

Elixophyllin, Slo-Bid, Theo-24	theophylline
Sudafed	pseudoephedrine

Gastrointestinal drugs

Tagamet	cimetidine

Heart and blood vessel drugs

Aldomet	methyldopa

BRAND NAME	GENERIC NAME
Duraquin, Quinaglute Dura-tabs, Quinidex	quinidine
Esidrix, HydroDiuril	hydrochlorothiazide
Inderal, Inderal LA	propranolol
Lasix	furosemide
Mevacor	lovastatin

Mind-affecting drugs
  Tranquilizers or sleeping pills
  (Note: These drugs may cause rebound insomnia.)

Dalmane	flurazepam
Halcion	triazolam

Antidepressants

BuSpar	buspirone
Effexor	venlafaxine

Antipsychotics

Risperdal	risperidone

Neurological drugs

Dilantin	phenytoin
Larodopa	levodopa
Neurontin	gabapentin

Other drugs

	alcohol
	caffeine
	interferons
Levothroid, Synthroid	levothyroxine
Nicorette, Nicoderm	nicotine
Ritalin	methylphenidate

Drugs That Can Cause Abnormal, Involuntary Movements

Drugs That Can Induce Parkinsonism

The following drugs can cause a tremor often indistinguishable from Parkinson's disease. If signs of the disease develop after one begins to use one of these drugs, discontinuing the drug will often result in the disappearance of the parkinsonism. Unfortunately, doctors often do not recognize the drug-induced nature of this problem, and instead of discontinuing the drug that caused the problem, they add another drug to treat the parkinsonism.

BRAND NAME	GENERIC NAME

Heart and blood vessel drugs
  High blood pressure drugs (diuretics)

Diupres	reserpine/chlorothiazide
Enduronyl	deserpidine/methyclothiazide
Hydropres	reserpine/hydrochlorothiazide

BRAND NAME	GENERIC NAME
Regroton, Demi-Regroton	reserpine/chlorthalidone
Salutensin	reserpine/hydroflumethiazide
Ser-Ap-Es	reserpine/hydralazine/hydrochlorothiazide

High blood pressure drugs (other)

	reserpine
Aldomet	methyldopa

Mind-affecting drugs
  Antidepressants

Asendin	amoxapine
Aventyl, Pamelor	nortriptyline
Desyrel	trazodone
Elavil	amitriptyline
Limbitrol	amitriptyline/chlordiazepoxide
Ludiomil	maprotiline
Luvox	fluvoxamine
Norpramin	desipramine
Paxil	paroxetine
Prozac	fluoxetine
Sinequan	doxepin
Tofranil	imipramine
Triavil	amitriptyline/perphenazine
Wellbutrin	bupropion
Zoloft	sertraline

Antipsychotics

Compazine	prochlorperazine
Haldol	haloperidol
Mellaril	thioridazine
Navane	thiothixene
Prolixin	fluphenazine
Risperdal	risperidone
Stelazine	trifluoperazine
Thorazine	chlorpromazine
Triavil	amitriptyline/perphenazine
Zyprexa	olanzapine

Tranquilizers

BuSpar	buspirone

Other drugs

Reglan	metoclopramide
Zyban	bupropion

Drugs That Can Induce Tardive Dyskinesia

Tardive dyskinesia is the most common and serious adverse effect of antipsychotic drugs and is often irreversible. It is characterized by involuntary movements of the lips, tongue, and sometimes the fingers, toes, and trunk. It may occur in as many as 40% of people over the age of 60 taking antipsychotic drugs. **Tardive dyskinesia is more common and more severe in older adults, and antipsychotic** drugs are quite often prescribed unnecessarily in this age group. (See discussion of this in *Antipsychotic Drugs*, p. 187.)

BRAND NAME	GENERIC NAME
Mind-affecting drugs	
Antidepressants	
Asendin	amoxapine
Prozac	fluoxetine
Wellbutrin	bupropion
Antipsychotics	
Compazine	prochlorperazine
Haldol	haloperidol
Mellaril	thioridazine
Navane	thiothixene
Phenergan	promethazine
Prolixin	fluphenazine
Risperdal	risperidone
Stelazine	trifluoperazine
Thorazine	chlorpromazine
Triavil	amitriptyline/perphenazine
Zyprexa	olanzapine
Tranquilizers	
BuSpar	buspirone
Neurological drugs	
Eldepryl	selegiline, deprenyl
Other drugs	
Zyban	bupropion

Drugs That Can Disturb Balance

Drugs That Can Cause Dizziness on Standing (Postural Hypotension)

BRAND NAME	GENERIC NAME
Antibiotics and other anti-infective agents	
Chibroxin, Noroxin	norfloxacin
Ciloxan, Cipro	ciprofloxacin
Floxin, Ocuflox	ofloxacin
Levaquin	levofloxacin
Maxaquin	lomefloxacin
Penetrex	enoxacin
Raxar	grepafloxacin
Vermox	mebendazole
Zagam	sparfloxacin
Cold, cough, allergy, and asthma drugs	
Alermine, Chlor-Trimeton	chlorpheniramine
Atarax, Vistaril	hydroxyzine
Benadryl, Sominex Formula	diphenhydramine
Dimetane	brompheniramine
Hismanal	astemizole
Myidil	triprolidine
Optimine	azatadine

BRAND NAME	GENERIC NAME
Periactin	cyproheptadine
Seldane	terfenadine
Tavist, Tavist-1	clemastine
Eye drugs	
Betagan	levobunolol
Cartrol	carteolol
Neptazane	methazolamide
OptiPranolol	metipranolol
Timoptic	timolol
Heart and blood vessel drugs	
Antianginal drugs	
Ismo, Imdur	isosorbide-5-mononitrate
Isordil, Sorbitrate	isosorbide dinitrate
Nitro-Bid, Nitrostat, Transderm-Nitro	nitroglycerin
High blood pressure drugs (beta-blockers)	
Blocadren	timolol
Cartrol	carteolol
Coreg	carvedilol
Corgard	nadolol
Corzide	nadolol/bendroflumethiazide
Inderal, Inderal LA	propranolol
Inderide LA	propranolol/hydrochlorothiazide
Kerlone	betaxolol
Levatol	penbutolol
Lopressor, Toprol XL	metoprolol
Lopressor HCT	metoprolol/hydrochlorothiazide
Normodyne, Trandate	labetalol
Sectral	acebutolol
Tenoretic	atenolol/chlorthalidone
Tenormin	atenolol
Visken	pindolol
Zebeta	bisoprolol
Ziac	bisoprolol/hydrochlorothiazide
High blood pressure drugs (diuretics)	
Aldactazide	spironolactone/hydrochlorothiazide
Aldoril	methyldopa/hydrochlorothiazide
Apresazide	hydralazine/hydrochlorothiazide
Bumex	bumetanide
Combipres	clonidine/chlorthalidone
Demadex	torsemide
Diupres	reserpine/chlorothiazide
Diuril	chlorothiazide
Dyazide, Maxzide	triamterene/hydrochlorothiazide
Enduron	methyclothiazide
Enduronyl	deserpidine/methyclothiazide
Esidrix, HydroDiuril	hydrochlorothiazide
Hydropres	reserpine/hydrochlorothiazide
Hygroton	chlorthalidone
Inderide LA	propranolol/hydrochlorothiazide
Lasix	furosemide
Lozol	indapamide

BRAND NAME	GENERIC NAME
Metahydrin, Naqua	trichlormethiazide
Moduretic	amiloride/hydrochlorothiazide
Regroton, Demi-Regroton	reserpine/chlorthalidone
Salutensin	reserpine/hydroflumethiazide
Ser-Ap-Es	reserpine/hydralazine/hydrochlorothiazide
Tenoretic	atenolol/chlorthalidone
Zaroxolyn, Diulo	metolazone

High blood pressure drugs (other)

BRAND NAME	GENERIC NAME
	reserpine
Accupril	quinapril
Adalat, Adalat CC Procardia, Procardia XL	nifedipine
Aldactone	spironolactone
Aldomet	methyldopa
Altace	ramipril
Apresoline	hydralazine
Calan SR, Covera–HS, Isoptin SR, Verelan	verapamil
Capoten	captopril
Cardene, Cardene SR	nicardipine
Cardizem CD, Dilacor XR, Tiazac	diltiazem
Cardura	doxazosin
Catapres	clonidine
DynaCirc, DynaCirc CR	isradipine
Hytrin	terazosin
Ismelin	guanethidine
Lexxel	felodipine/enalapril
Lotensin	benazepril
Lotrel	amlodipine/benazepril
Mavik	trandolapril
Minipress	prazosin
Monopril	fosinopril
Norvasc	amlodipine
Plendil	felodipine
Posicor	mibefradil
Prinivil, Zestril	lisinopril
Sular	nisoldipine
Tarka	verapamil/trandolapril
Tenex	guanfacine
Univasc	moexipril
Vasotec	enalapril
Wytensin	guanabenz

Mind-affecting drugs
Antidepressants

BRAND NAME	GENERIC NAME
Asendin	amoxapine
Aventyl, Pamelor	nortriptyline
Desyrel	trazodone
Effexor	venlafaxine
Elavil	amitriptyline
Limbitrol	amitriptyline/chlordiazepoxide
Ludiomil	maprotiline

BRAND NAME	GENERIC NAME
Luvox	fluvoxamine
Norpramin	desipramine
Paxil	paroxetine
Prozac	fluoxetine
Serzone	nefazodone
Sinequan	doxepin
Tofranil	imipramine
Triavil	amitriptyline/perphenazine
Zoloft	sertraline

Antipsychotics

BRAND NAME	GENERIC NAME
Clozaril	clozapine
Compazine	prochlorperazine
Haldol	haloperidol
Mellaril	thioridazine
Navane	thiothixene
Prolixin	fluphenazine
Risperdal	risperidone
Stelazine	trifluoperazine
Thorazine	chlorpromazine
Triavil	amitriptyline/perphenazine
Zyprexa	olanzapine

Tranquilizers or sleeping pills

BRAND NAME	GENERIC NAME
Ambien	zolpidem
Atarax, Vistaril	hydroxyzine
Ativan	lorazepam
Centrax	prazepam
Dalmane	flurazepam
Doriden	glutethimide
Halcion	triazolam
Librium	chlordiazepoxide
Miltown, Equanil	meprobamate
Noctec	chloral hydrate
Noludar	methyprylon
Placidyl	ethchlorvynol
Restoril	temazepam
Serax	oxazepam
Tranxene	clorazepate
Valium	diazepam
Xanax	alprazolam

Neurological drugs
Anticonvulsants

BRAND NAME	GENERIC NAME
Klonopin	clonazepam

Antiparkinsonians

BRAND NAME	GENERIC NAME
Eldepryl	selegiline, deprenyl
Larodopa	levodopa
Parlodel	bromocriptine
Sinemet	levodopa/carbidopa

Drugs That Can Cause Falls/Hip Fractures

A study found that a significant proportion of hip fractures in older adults could be attributed to the use of four classes of drugs: sleeping pills, tranquilizers, antipsychotics, and antidepressant drugs. The following are examples of such drugs as well as others that have been associated with falls, which could also increase the risk of hip fractures. In addition to these drugs, all of the drugs listed above as causing dizziness on standing can also cause falls.

BRAND NAME	GENERIC NAME

Heart and blood vessel drugs
Ismo, Imdur	isosorbide-5-mononitrate
Isordil, Sorbitrate	isosorbide dinitrate
Nitro-Bid, Nitrostat, Transderm-Nitro	nitroglycerin

Mind-affecting drugs
Antidepressants
Asendin	amoxapine
Aventyl, Pamelor	nortriptyline
Desyrel	trazodone
Elavil	amitriptyline
Limbitrol	amitriptyline/ chlordiazepoxide
Ludiomil	maprotiline
Luvox	fluvoxamine
Norpramin	desipramine
Paxil	paroxetine
Prozac	fluoxetine
Sinequan	doxepin
Tofranil	imipramine
Triavil	amitriptyline/perphenazine
Wellbutrin	bupropion
Zoloft	sertraline

Antipsychotics
Compazine	prochlorperazine
Haldol	haloperidol
Mellaril	thioridazine
Navane	thiothixene
Prolixin	fluphenazine
Risperdal	risperidone
Stelazine	trifluoperazine
Thorazine	chlorpromazine
Triavil	amitriptyline/perphenazine
Zyprexa	olanzapine

Barbiturates
Butisol	butabarbital
Luminal, Solfoton	phenobarbital
Nembutal	pentobarbital

Tranquilizers or sleeping pills
Atarax, Vistaril	hydroxyzine
Ativan	lorazepam
BuSpar	buspirone
Centrax	prazepam
Dalmane	flurazepam
Doriden	glutethimide
Halcion	triazolam
Librium	chlordiazepoxide
Miltown, Equanil	meprobamate
Noctec	chloral hydrate

BRAND NAME	GENERIC NAME
Noludar	methyprylon
Placidyl	ethchlorvynol
Restoril	temazepam
Serax	oxazepam
Tranxene	clorazepate
Valium	diazepam
Xanax	alprazolam

Neurological drugs
Dilantin	phenytoin
Klonopin	clonazepam
Luminal, Solfoton	phenobarbital
Tegretol	carbamazepine

Other drugs
Zyban	bupropion

Drugs That Can Cause Automobile Accidents

BRAND NAME	GENERIC NAME

Mind-affecting drugs
Antidepressants
Anafranil	clomipramine
Asendin	amoxapine
Aventyl, Pamelor	nortriptyline
Elavil	amitriptyline
Limbitrol	amitriptyline/chlordiazepoxide
Ludiomil	maprotiline
Norpramin	desipramine
Sinequan	doxepin
Surmontil	trimipramine
Tofranil	imipramine
Triavil	amitriptyline/perphenazine
Vivactil	protriptyline

Tranquilizers and sleeping pills
Ativan	lorazepam
Centrax	prazepam
Librium	chlordiazepoxide
Paxipam	halazepam
Serax	oxazepam
Tranxene	clorazepate
Valium	diazepam
Xanax	alprazolam

Drugs That Can Cause Sexual Dysfunction

BRAND NAME	GENERIC NAME

Antibiotics and other anti-infective agents
Nizoral	ketoconazole
Tegison	etretinate

Anticholinergics
Banthine	methantheline
Bentyl	dicyclomine
Cantil	mepenzolate
Darbid	isopropamide

BRAND NAME	GENERIC NAME
Ditropan	oxybutynin
Homapin	homatropine
Pamine	methscopolamine
Pathilon	tridihexethyl
Pro-Banthine	propantheline
Quarzan	clidinium
Robinul	glycopyrrolate
Tral	hexocyclium
Transderm-Scop	scopolamine
Valpin	anisotropine

Cancer drugs

Intron A, Roferon-A	interferon alfa
Lupron	leuprolide
Nolvadex	tamoxifen
Rheumatrex Dose Pack	methotrexate

Eye drugs

Daranide	dichlorphenamide
Diamox	acetazolamide
Neptazane	methazolamide

Gastrointestinal drugs

Axid	nizatidine
Azulfidine	sulfasalazine
Pepcid	famotidine
Prilosec	omeprazole
Reglan	metoclopramide
Tagamet	cimetidine
Zantac	ranitidine

Heart and blood vessel drugs

Antianginal drugs

Adalat, Adalat CC Procardia, Procardia XL	nifedipine
Calan SR, Covera-HS, Isoptin SR, Verelan	verapamil
Lanoxicaps, Lanoxin	digoxin

Antiarrhythmics

Cordarone	amiodarone
Mexitil	mexiletine
Norpace	disopyramide

Blood vessel dilators

Cerespan, Pavabid	papaverine

Cholesterol-lowering drugs

Atromid-S	clofibrate
Lopid	gemfibrozil

High blood pressure drugs (beta-blockers)

Blocadren	timolol
Cartrol	carteolol
Coreg	carvedilol
Inderal, Inderal LA	propranolol
Kerlone	betaxolol
Levatol	penbutolol
Lopressor, Toprol XL	metoprolol
Normodyne, Trandate	labetalol
Tenormin	atenolol
Zebeta	bisoprolol

BRAND NAME	GENERIC NAME

High blood pressure drugs (diuretics)

Esidrix, HydroDiuril	hydrochlorothiazide
Hygroton	chlorthalidone
Lozol	indapamide
Midamor	amiloride

High blood pressure drugs (other)

	reserpine
Aldactone	spironolactone
Aldomet	methyldopa
Apresoline	hydralazine
Catapres	clonidine
Demser	metyrosine
Hylorel	guanadrel
Inversine	mecamylamine
Ismelin	guanethidine
Minipress	prazosin
Tenex	guanfacine
Wytensin	guanabenz

Mind-affecting drugs

Antidepressants

Asendin	amoxapine
Aventyl, Pamelor	nortriptyline
Desyrel	trazodone
Effexor	venlafaxine
Elavil	amitriptyline
Lithobid, Lithonate	lithium
Ludiomil	maprotiline
Luvox	fluvoxamine
Marplan	isocarboxazid
Nardil	phenelzine
Norpramin	desipramine
Parnate	tranylcypromine
Paxil	paroxetine
Prozac	fluoxetine
Serzone	nefazodone
Sinequan	doxepin
Tofranil	imipramine
Vivactil	protriptyline
Zoloft	sertraline

Antipsychotics

Clozaril	clozapine
Haldol	haloperidol
Mellaril	thioridazine
Moban	molindone
Navane	thiothixene
Orap	pimozide
Prolixin	fluphenazine
Risperdal	risperidone
Serentil	mesoridazine
Stelazine	trifluoperazine
Taractan	chlorprothixene
Thorazine	chlorpromazine
Trilafon	perphenazine
Zyprexa	olanzapine

BRAND NAME	GENERIC NAME
Barbiturates	
Nembutal	pentobarbital
Tranquilizers	
BuSpar	buspirone
Valium	diazepam
Xanax	alprazolam
Neurological drugs	
Anticonvulsants	
Dilantin	phenytoin
Tegretol	carbamazepine
Zarontin	ethosuximide
Antiparkinsonians	
Larodopa	levodopa
Parlodel	bromocriptine
Permax	pergolide
Painkillers/narcotics	
Aleve, Anaprox, Naprosyn	naproxen
Dolophine, Methadose	methadone
Indocin	indomethacin
Revia, Trexan	naltrexone
Other drugs	
	alcohol
	amphetamines
	cocaine
Antabuse	disulfiram
Danocrine	danazol
Depo-Testosterone	testosterone
Diprivan	propofol
Fastin	phentermine
Intralipid	fat emulsion
Lioresal	baclofen
Mazanor, Sanorex	mazindol
Plegine	phendimetrazine
Pondimin	fenfluramine
Proscar	finasteride
Synarel	nafarelin
Tenuate, Tepanil	diethylpropion

Drugs That Can Affect the Gastrointestinal (GI) Tract

Drugs That Can Cause Loss of Appetite, Nausea, or Vomiting

BRAND NAME	GENERIC NAME
Antibiotics and other anti-infective agents	
Achromycin, Panmycin, Sumycin	tetracycline
Biaxin	clarithromycin
Chibroxin, Noroxin	norfloxacin
Diflucan	fluconazole

BRAND NAME	GENERIC NAME
Erythrocin, EES	erythromycin
Flagyl	metronidazole
Floxin, Ocuflox	ofloxacin
Zithromax	azithromycin
Cancer drugs	
Many anticancer drugs affect the gastrointestinal tract. They are not listed in this book.	
Cold, cough, allergy, and asthma drugs	
Choledyl	oxtriphylline
Elixophyllin, Slo-Bid, Theo-24	theophylline
Somophyllin, Somophyllin-DF	aminophylline
Heart and blood vessel drugs	
Kato, K-Lor, Slow-K	potassium supplements
Lanoxicaps, Lanoxin	digoxin
Locholest, Questran	cholestyramine
Mevacor	lovastatin
Mind-affecting drugs	
BuSpar	buspirone
Effexor	venlafaxine
Luvox	fluvoxamine
Paxil	paroxetine
Prozac	fluoxetine
Risperdal	risperidone
Serzone	nefazodone
Wellbutrin	bupropion
Zoloft	sertraline
Neurological drugs	
Eldepryl	selegiline, deprenyl
Larodopa	levodopa
Sinemet	levodopa/carbidopa
Painkillers/narcotics	
	codeine
Advil, Motrin	ibuprofen
Aleve, Anaprox, Naprosyn	naproxen
Ansaid, Ocufen	flurbiprofen
Butazolidin	phenylbutazone
Clinoril	sulindac
Daypro	oxaprozin
Demerol	meperidine
Dolobid	diflunisal
Duract	bromfenac
Duragesic	fentanyl
Feldene	piroxicam
Imuran	azathioprine
Indocin	indomethacin
Lodine	etodolac
Meclomen	meclofenamate
Nalfon	fenoprofen
Orudis	ketoprofen
Relafen	nabumetone
Roxanol, MS Contin	morphine

BRAND NAME	GENERIC NAME
Stadol, Stadol NS	butorphanol
Talwin	pentazocine
Talwin-NX	pentazocine/naloxone
Tolectin	tolmetin
Ultram	tramadol
Voltaren	diclofenac

Other drugs

	estrogens
Estraderm, Estrace	estradiol
Feosol, Slow Fe	ferrous sulfate
Feostat	ferrous fumarate
Fergon	ferrous gluconate
Zyban	bupropion

Drugs That Can Cause Abdominal Pain, Ulcers, or Gastrointestinal Bleeding

Although all of these drugs can cause abdominal pain, bleeding, and ulcers, **piroxicam (FELDENE), indomethacin (INDOCIN), and phenylbutazone (BUTAZOLIDIN) are more dangerous than the others and should not be used by older adults.**

BRAND NAME	GENERIC NAME

Antibiotics and other anti-infective agents

Diflucan	fluconazole

Cold, cough, allergy, and asthma drugs

Choledyl	oxtriphylline
Elixophyllin, Slo-Bid, Theo-24	theophylline
Somophyllin, Somophyllin-DF	aminophylline

Corticosteroids, systemic

Acthar	corticotropin (ACTH)
Azmacort	triamcinolone
Cortef	hydrocortisone
Cortone	cortisone
Decadron, Hexadrol	dexamethasone
Deltasone, Meticorten	prednisone
Diprolene, Valisone	betamethasone
Medrol	methylprednisolone
Metreton, Pred Forte	prednisolone

Mind-affecting drugs

BuSpar	buspirone
Wellbutrin	bupropion

Neurological drugs

Eldepryl	selegiline, deprenyl

Painkillers/narcotics

Advil, Motrin	ibuprofen
Aleve, Anaprox, Naprosyn	naproxen
Ansaid, Ocufen	flurbiprofen
Arthropan	choline salicylate

BRAND NAME	GENERIC NAME
Ascriptin, Bufferin	buffered aspirin
Genuine Bayer Aspirin, Ecotrin	aspirin
Butazolidin	phenylbutazone
Clinoril	sulindac
Daypro	oxaprozin
Disalcid	salsalate
Doan's Pills	magnesium salicylate
Dolobid	diflunisal
Duract	bromfenac
Feldene	piroxicam
Indocin	indomethacin
Lodine	etodolac
Meclomen	meclofenamate
Nalfon	fenoprofen
Orudis	ketoprofen
Relafen	nabumetone
Tolectin	tolmetin
Toradol	ketorolac
Trilisate	choline and magnesium salicylates
Voltaren	diclofenac

Other drugs

Zyban	bupropion

Drugs That Can Cause Constipation

BRAND NAME	GENERIC NAME

Antibiotics and anti-infective agents

Urised	atropine/hyoscyamine/ methenamine/methylene blue/phenyl salicylate/ benzoic acid

Cold, cough, allergy, and asthma drugs

Alermine, Chlor-Trimeton	chlorpheniramine
Atarax, Vistaril	hydroxyzine
Benadryl, Sominex Formula	diphenhydramine
Dimetane	brompheniramine
Hismanal	astemizole
Myidil	triprolidine
Optimine	azatadine
Periactin	cyproheptadine
Seldane	terfenadine
Tavist, Tavist-1	clemastine

Eye drugs

Betagan	levobunolol

Gastrointestinal drugs

	atropine
Amphojel	aluminum hydroxide
Antivert	meclizine
Bentyl	dicyclomine
Caltrate, Os-Cal 500	calcium carbonate

BRAND NAME	GENERIC NAME
Compazine	prochlorperazine
Donnatal	atropine/hyoscyamine/ scopolamine/phenobarbital
Dulcolax*	bisacodyl*
Gaviscon, Gaviscon-2	aluminum hydroxide and magnesium carbonate
Librax	chlordiazepoxide/clidinium
Lomotil	diphenoxylate/atropine
Maalox, Maalox TC	aluminum and magnesium hydroxide
Mylanta, Mylanta II	magnesium hydroxide/ aluminum hydroxide/ simethicone
Phenergan	promethazine
Reglan	metoclopramide
Tigan	trimethobenzamide

Heart and blood vessel drugs
Antiarrhythmics

Mexitil	mexiletine
Norpace	disopyramide

Cholesterol-lowering drugs

Locholest, Questran	cholestyramine
Mevacor	lovastatin

High blood pressure drugs (beta-blockers)

Blocadren	timolol
Cartrol	carteolol
Coreg	carvedilol
Corgard	nadolol
Corzide	nadolol/bendroflumethiazide
Inderal, Inderal LA	propranolol
Inderide LA	propranolol/hydrochlorothiazide
Kerlone	betaxolol
Levatol	penbutolol
Lopressor, Toprol XL	metoprolol
Lopressor HCT	metoprolol/hydrochlorothiazide
Normodyne, Trandate	labetalol
Sectral	acebutolol
Tenoretic	atenolol/chlorthalidone
Tenormin	atenolol
Visken	pindolol
Zebeta	bisoprolol
Ziac	bisoprolol/hydrochlorothiazide

High blood pressure drugs (other)

Adalat, Adalat CC, Procardia, Procardia XL	nifedipine
Calan SR, Covera-HS, Isoptin SR, Verelan	verapamil
Cardene, Cardene SR	nicardipine
DynaCirc, DynaCirc CR	isradipine
Lexxel	felodipine/enalapril
Lotrel	amlodipine/benazepril
Norvasc	amlodipine
Plendil	felodipine

* Constipation can occur with prolonged use.

BRAND NAME	GENERIC NAME
Posicor	mibefradil
Sular	nisoldipine
Tarka	verapamil/trandolapril
Teczem	diltiazem/enalapril

Mind-affecting drugs
Antidepressants

Asendin	amoxapine
Aventyl, Pamelor	nortriptyline
Desyrel	trazodone
Elavil	amitriptyline
Limbitrol	amitriptyline/chlordiazepoxide
Ludiomil	maprotiline
Norpramin	desipramine
Sinequan	doxepin
Tofranil	imipramine
Triavil	perphenazine/amitriptyline
Wellbutrin	bupropion

Antipsychotics

Clozaril	clozapine
Compazine	prochlorperazine
Haldol	haloperidol
Mellaril	thioridazine
Navane	thiothixene
Prolixin	fluphenazine
Reglan	metoclopramide
Risperdal	risperidone
Stelazine	trifluoperazine
Thorazine	chlorpromazine
Triavil	amitriptyline/perphenazine

Tranquilizers and sleeping pills

BuSpar	buspirone
Doriden	glutethimide

Neurological drugs
Anticonvulsants

Klonopin	clonazepam

Antiparkinsonians

Artane	trihexyphenidyl
Cogentin	benztropine

Painkillers/narcotics

Darvocet-N, Wygesic	propoxyphene/ acetaminophen
Darvon, Darvon-N	propoxyphene
Darvon Compound, Darvon Compound-65	propoxyphene/aspirin/caffeine
Demerol	meperidine
Dilaudid	hydromorphone
Empirin with Codeine	aspirin/codeine
Percodan, Percodan-Demi	aspirin/oxycodone
Roxanol, MS Contin	morphine
Synalgos-DC	dihydrocodeine/aspirin/caffeine
Talwin	pentazocine
Talwin-NX	pentazocine/naloxone
Tylenol No. 3	acetaminophen/codeine
Tylox, Percocet	acetaminophen/oxycodone

BRAND NAME	GENERIC NAME
Ultram	tramadol
Vicodin	acetaminophen/hydrocodone

Other drugs

Ditropan	oxybutynin

Drugs That Can Cause Diarrhea

BRAND NAME	GENERIC NAME

Antibiotics and other anti-infective agents

Achromycin, Panmycin, Sumycin	tetracycline
Biaxin	clarithromycin
Ceftin	cefuroxime axetil
Cefzil	cefprozil
Chibroxin, Noroxin	norfloxacin
Ciloxan, Cipro	ciprofloxacin
Cleocin	clindamycin
Floxin, Ocuflox	ofloxacin
Ilosone	erythromycin estolate
Levaquin	levofloxacin
Lincocin	lincomycin
Lorabid	loracarbef
Maxaquin	lomefloxacin
Omnipen	ampicillin
Penetrex	enoxacin
Raxar	grepafloxacin
Suprax	cefixime
Vermox	mebendazole
Zagam	sparfloxacin
Zithromax	azithromycin

Gastrointestinal drugs

Cytotec	misoprostol
Dialose Plus, Peri-Colace	docusate/casanthranol
Dulcolax	bisacodyl
Maalox, Maalox TC	aluminum hydroxide and magnesium hydroxide
Mylanta, Mylanta-II	magnesium hydroxide/ aluminum hydroxide/ simethicone
Phillips' Milk of Magnesia	magnesium hydroxide

Heart and blood vessel drugs
Antianginal drugs

Lanoxicaps, Lanoxin	digoxin

Antiarrhythmics

Mexitil	mexiletine

High blood pressure drugs (diuretics)

Diupres	reserpine/chlorothiazide
Enduronyl	deserpidine/methyclothiazide
Hydropres	reserpine/hydrochlorothiazide
Regroton, Demi-Regroton	reserpine/chlorthalidone
Salutensin	reserpine/hydroflumethiazide

BRAND NAME	GENERIC NAME
Ser-Ap-Es	reserpine/hydralazine/ hydrochlorothiazide

High blood pressure drugs (other)

	reserpine
Aldomet	methyldopa
Ismelin	guanethidine

Mind-affecting drugs

BuSpar	buspirone
Luvox	fluvoxamine
Paxil	paroxetine
Prozac	fluoxetine
Wellbutrin	bupropion
Zoloft	sertraline

Painkillers/narcotics

Imuran	azathioprine

Other drugs

Nicorette, Nicoderm	nicotine
Precose	acarbose
Zyban	bupropion

Drugs That Can Cause Lung Toxicity

BRAND NAME	GENERIC NAME

Antibiotics and other anti-infective agents

Fansidar	pyrimethamine-sulfadoxine
Furadantin, Macrobid, Macrodantin	nitrofurantoin

Cancer drugs

Alkeran	melphalan
BiCNU	carmustine
Blenoxane	bleomycin
CeeNU	lomustine
Cytosar-U	cytarabine
Cytoxan	cyclophosphamide
Eldisine	vindesine
Leukeran	chlorambucil
Matulane	procarbazine
Mutamycin	mitomycin
Myleran	busulfan
Proleukin	aldesleukin/interleukin-2
Rheumatrex Dose Pack	methotrexate
Velban	vinblastine

Cold, cough, allergy, and asthma drugs

Brethaire, Brethine, Bricanyl	terbutaline

Eye drugs

Adsorbocarpine, Isopto Carpine	pilocarpine

Gastrointestinal drugs

Azulfidine	sulfasalazine

Heart and blood vessel drugs
Antiarrhythmics

Cordarone	amiodarone

BRAND NAME	GENERIC NAME
Rythmol	propafenone
Tonocard	tocainide
Xylocaine	lidocaine

High blood pressure drugs (beta-blockers)

Blocadren	timolol
Inderal, Inderal LA	propranolol
Visken	pindolol

High blood pressure drugs (diuretics)

Esidrix, HydroDiuril	hydrochlorothiazide

High blood pressure drugs (other)

Capoten	captopril
Prinivil, Zestril	lisinopril
Vasotec	enalapril

Mind-affecting drugs

Placidyl	ethchlorvynol

Neurological drugs
Anticonvulsants

Dilantin	phenytoin

Antiparkinsonians

Parlodel	bromocriptine
Tegretol	carbamazepine

Painkillers/narcotics

Advil, Motrin	ibuprofen
Aleve, Anaprox, Naprosyn	naproxen
Genuine Bayer Aspirin, Ecotrin	aspirin
Butazolidin	phenylbutazone
Clinoril	sulindac
Cuprimine, Depen	penicillamine
Darvon, Darvon-N	propoxyphene
Dolophine, Methadose	methadone
Feldene	piroxicam
Imuran	azathioprine
Indocin	indomethacin
Myochrysine	gold sodium thiomalate
Narcan	naloxone
Sansert	methysergide
Solganal	aurothioglucose
Voltaren	diclofenac

Other drugs

	cocaine
	protamine
	tryptophan
Anectine	succinylcholine
Dantrium	dantrolene
Norcuron	vercuronium
Pavulon	pancuronium
Tracrium	atracurium
Tubarine	tubocurarine
Yutopar	ritodrine

Drugs That Can Affect the Urinary Tract

Drugs That Can Block Urination

All of the following drugs can cause urinary retention, the inability to urinate or difficulty in urinating, particularly in men with enlarged prostate glands.

BRAND NAME	GENERIC NAME

Antibiotics and other anti-infective agents

Urised	atropine/hyoscyamine/ methenamine/methylene blue/phenyl salicylate/ benzoic acid

Cold, cough, allergy, and asthma drugs

Alermine, Chlor-Trimeton	chlorpheniramine
Atarax, Vistaril	hydroxyzine
Atrovent	ipratropium
Benadryl, Sominex Formula	diphenhydramine
Dimetane	brompheniramine
Hismanal	astemizole
Myidil	triprolidine
Optimine	azatadine
Periactin	cyproheptadine
Seldane	terfenadine
Tavist, Tavist-1	clemastine

Eye drugs

Neptazane	methazolamide

Gastrointestinal drugs

	atropine
Antivert	meclizine
Bentyl	dicyclomine
Compazine	prochlorperazine
Donnatal	atropine/hyoscyamine/ scopolamine/ phenobarbital
Librax	chlordiazepoxide/ clidinium
Lomotil	diphenoxylate/atropine
Phenergan	promethazine
Reglan	metoclopramide
Tigan	trimethobenzamide

Heart and blood vessel drugs
Antiarrhythmics

Norpace	disopyramide

High blood pressure drugs

Adalat, Adalat CC, Procardia, Procardia XL	nifedipine

BRAND NAME	GENERIC NAME
Cardene, Cardene SR	nicardipine
DynaCirc, DynaCirc CR	isradipine

Mind-affecting drugs

Antidepressants

Asendin	amoxapine
Aventyl, Pamelor	nortriptyline
Desyrel	trazodone
Elavil	amitriptyline
Limbitrol	amitriptyline/chlordiazepoxide
Ludiomil	maprotiline
Norpramin	desipramine
Prozac	fluoxetine
Sinequan	doxepin
Tofranil	imipramine
Triavil	amitriptyline/perphenazine
Wellbutrin	bupropion

Antipsychotics

Compazine	prochlorperazine
Haldol	haloperidol
Mellaril	thioridazine
Navane	thiothixene
Prolixin	fluphenazine
Reglan	metoclopramide
Stelazine	trifluoperazine
Thorazine	chlorpromazine
Triavil	amitriptyline/perphenazine

Tranquilizers

BuSpar	buspirone

Neurological drugs

Artane	trihexyphenidyl
Cogentin	benztropine
Eldepryl	selegiline, deprenyl

Other drugs

Ditropan	oxybutynin
Ultram	tramadol
Zyban	bupropion

Drugs That Can Cause Loss of Bladder Control (Incontinence)

All of the drugs listed above that may block urination can, when the bladder gets too full, cause "overflow" leakage. In addition, the following drugs can also cause urine to leak:

BRAND NAME	GENERIC NAME

Antibiotics and other anti-infective agents

Urised	atropine/hyoscyamine/ methenamine/methylene blue/phenyl salicylate/ benzoic acid

BRAND NAME	GENERIC NAME

Eye drugs

Betagan	levobunolol

Gastrointestinal drugs

Cytotec	misoprostol

Heart and blood vessel drugs

High blood pressure drugs (beta-blockers)

Blocadren	timolol
Cartrol	carteolol
Coreg	carvedilol
Corgard	nadolol
Corzide	nadolol/bendroflumethiazide
Inderal, Inderal LA	propranolol
Inderide LA	propranolol/hydrochlorothiazide
Kerlone	betaxolol
Levatol	penbutolol
Lopressor, Toprol XL	metoprolol
Lopressor HCT	metoprolol/hydrochlorothiazide
Normodyne, Trandate	labetalol
Sectral	acebutolol
Tenoretic	atenolol/chlorthalidone
Tenormin	atenolol
Visken	pindolol
Zebeta	bisoprolol
Ziac	bisoprolol/hydrochlorothiazide

High blood pressure drugs (diuretics)

Aldactazide	spironolactone/ hydrochlorothiazide
Aldoril	methyldopa/hydrochlorothiazide
Apresazide	hydralazine/hydrochlorothiazide
Bumex	bumetanide
Combipres	clonidine/chlorthalidone
Demadex	torsemide
Diupres	reserpine/chlorothiazide
Diuril	chlorothiazide
Dyazide, Maxzide	triamterene/hydrochlorothiazide
Enduron	methyclothiazide
Enduronyl	deserpidine/methyclothiazide
Esidrix, HydroDiuril	hydrochlorothiazide
Hydropres	reserpine/hydrochlorothiazide
Hygroton	chlorthalidone
Inderide LA	propranolol/hydrochlorothiazide
Lasix	furosemide
Lozol	indapamide
Metahydrin, Naqua	trichlormethiazide
Moduretic	amiloride/hydrochlorothiazide
Regroton, Demi-Regroton	reserpine/chlorthalidone
Salutensin	reserpine/hydroflumethiazide
Ser-Ap-Es	reserpine/hydralazine/ hydrochlorothiazide
Tenoretic	atenolol/chlorthalidone
Zaroxolyn, Diulo	metolazone

BRAND NAME	GENERIC NAME

High blood pressure drugs (other)
Adalat, Adalat CC Procardia, Procardia XL	nifedipine
Aldactone	spironolactone
Cardene, Cardene SR	nicardipine
Cardura	doxazosin
DynaCirc, DynaCirc CR	isradipine
Hytrin	terazosin
Minipress	prazosin

Mind-affecting drugs
Antidepressants
Lithobid, Lithonate	lithium
Prozac	fluoxetine
Wellbutrin	bupropion

Antipsychotics
| Zyprexa | olanzapine |

Tranquilizers or sleeping pills
Atarax, Vistaril	hydroxyzine
Ativan	lorazepam
BuSpar	buspirone
Centrax	prazepam
Dalmane	flurazepam
Doriden	glutethimide
Halcion	triazolam
Librium	chlordiazepoxide
Miltown, Equanil	meprobamate
Noctec	chloral hydrate
Noludar	methyprylon
Placidyl	ethchlorvynol
Restoril	temazepam
Serax	oxazepam
Tranxene	clorazepate
Valium	diazepam
Xanax	alprazolam

Neurological drugs
| Klonopin | clonazepam |

Other drugs
| Zyban | bupropion |

NOTES

1. Lazarou J, Pomeranz BH, Corey PN. Incidence of adverse drug reactions in hospitalized patients: A meta-analysis of prospective studies. *Journal of the American Medical Association* 1998; 279:1200–5.

2. *Second Annual Adverse Drug/Biologic Reaction Report: 1986.* Food and Drug Administration, 1987.

3. Vestal RE, ed. *Drug Treatment in the Elderly.* Sydney, Australia: ADIS Health Science Press, 1984. Calculation of 33% increase in risk of adverse reaction (age 50–59 vs 40–49) is based on an average of all three studies listed on page 32.

4. Lazarou, op. cit.

5. Mitchell AA, Lacouture PG, Sheehan JE, Kauffman RE, Shapiro S. Adverse drug reactions in children leading to hospital admission. *Pediatrics* 1988; 82:24–9.

6. Classen DC, Pestotnik SL, Evans RS, Lloyd JF, Burke JP. Adverse drug events in hospitalized patients: Excess length of stay, extra costs, and attributable mortality. *Journal of the American Medical Association* 1997; 277:301–6.

7. Willcox SM, Himmelstein DU, Woolhandler S. Inappropriate drug prescribing for the community-dwelling elderly. *Journal of the American Medical Association* 1994; 272:292–6.

8. Tamblyn RM, McLeod PJ, Abrahamowicz M, Monette J, Gayton DC, Berkson L, et al. Questionable prescribing for elderly patients in Quebec. *Canadian Medical Association Journal* 1994; 150:1801–9.

9. Using the same basis for estimating the number of admissions to medical wards of hospitals as used in reference 4 (above) of 6.05 million in 1990, and the estimate that in 22.4% of medical admissions the patients are using digoxin and that 2.06% of these suffer life-threatening heart toxicity from digoxin (both are from Miller RR, Greenblatt DJ. *Drug Effects in Hospitalized Patients.* New York: John Wiley and Sons, 1976), this amounts to 6.05 million times 22.4% times 2.06% or 27,917 older adults in hospitals who suffer from life-threatening heart toxicity from digoxin. This estimate understates the magnitude of the problem because the proportion of patients in the Miller/Greenblatt book using digoxin and experiencing life-threatening heart toxicity is based on all patients of all ages, whereas the rate of digoxin use and therefore the rate of life-threatening reactions is higher in older adults. The estimate is also lower because it does not include cases of digoxin toxicity that occur in surgical patients.

10. Ray WA, Griffin MR, Shorr RI. Adverse drug reactions and the elderly. *Health Affairs* Fall 1990:114–22.

11. Of the 42.34 million Americans 60 and older (*Statistical Abstracts of the United States 1992,* 1991 population data) approximately 90% are taking one or more medications for a total of 37.83 million older people. According to a study of verified adverse drug reactions (German PS, Klein LE. Adverse drug experience among the elderly. In *Pharmaceuticals for the Elderly.* Pharmaceutical Manufacturers Association, November 1986), 25.4% of the elderly patients 60 and older had at least one adverse drug reaction during the six-month interval that the study encompassed. Twenty-five and four-tenths percent of 37.83 million people is 9.61 million adverse reactions for the six-month period. The number of adverse reactions in a year would certainly be higher. The actual number of adverse reactions is also much higher since this calculation assumes all patients were being seen outside of the hospital or nursing home. Because the use of drugs in nursing homes and hospitals is much higher than in clinics, the number of adverse reactions is also higher.

12. Ray WA, Fought RL, Decker MD. Psychoactive drugs and the risk of injurious motor vehicle crashes in elderly drivers. *American Journal of Epidemiology* 1992; 136:873–83.

13. Ray WA, Griffin MR, Schaffner W, Baugh DK, Menton J. Psychotropic drug use and the risk of hip fracture. *New England Journal of Medicine* 1987; 316:363–9. The estimate of 32,000 hip fractures in older adults is based on projecting the findings of this study of drug-induced hip fractures in older Michigan Medicaid patients to the entire country.

14. Myers AP, Robinson EG, Van Natta ML, Michelson JD, Collins K, Baker SP. Hip fractures among the elderly: Factors associated with in-hospital mortality. *American Journal of Epidemiology* 1991; 134:1128–37.

15. Larson EB, Kukull WA, Buchner D, Reifler BV. Adverse drug reactions associated with global cognitive impairment in elderly persons. *Annals of Internal Medicine* 1987; 107:169–73. This estimate is based on projecting the findings of the Larson study on the 1.43 million Americans 65 and older who have dementia. See discussion on sleeping pills and tranquilizers (p. 178) for more details about this serious problem.

16. See discussion on sleeping pills and tranquilizers (p. 178) for more details on this estimate.

17. See discussion on antipsychotic drugs (p. 187) for more details about drug-induced tardive dyskinesia and misprescribing of antipsychotic drugs.

18. The estimate of 61,000 older adults suffering from drug-induced parkinsonism is derived as follows: As described in detail in the chapter on antipsychotic drugs (see p. 187), there are an estimated 750,000 people 65 and older in nursing homes or living in the community who are regularly (for three or four months or longer) being prescribed antipsychotic drugs. According to a survey in 1981 of 5,000 patients being treated with antipsychotic drugs, 13.2% had parkinsonism (see reference 65, p. 256 in the Mind Drugs section). Another study by the same researchers found that 62% became better (no longer had parkinsonism) within 30 days of discontinuing the drug. Thus, at least 62% of the 13.2% of patients getting antipsychotic drugs or 7.92% of all patients getting these drugs suffer from drug-induced parkinsonism. Calculating 7.92% of 750,000 patients getting these drugs for at least several months yields 61,380 patients with drug-induced parkinsonism. This is a very conservative estimate because it does not include either those patients using antipsychotic drugs for less than three to four months (an additional 1.16 million people) who are also at risk for drug-induced parkinsonism (because 90% of the cases occur within 72 hours after beginning the drug) or those who get drug-induced parkinsonism from the related drugs Reglan (metoclopramide), Compazine (prochlorperazine) and Phenergan (promethazine) usually prescribed for nausea.

19. Vestal, op. cit.

20. Ouslander JG. Drug therapy in the elderly. *Annals of Internal Medicine* 1981; 95:711–22.

21. Grimes JD. Drug-induced parkinsonism and tardive dyskinesia in non-psychiatric patients. *Canadian Medical Association Journal* 1982; 126:468.

22. *Drugs for the Elderly.* 2nd edition. Copenhagen, Denmark: World Health Organization, 1997: 28.

23. Lipton HL, Bero LA, Bird JA, McPhee SJ. The impact of clinical pharmacists' consultations on physicians' geriatric drug prescribing. *Medical Care* 1992; 30:646–58.

24. Vestal, op. cit., p. 364.

25. *Drugs for the Elderly,* op. cit.

26. *The Medical Letter on Drugs and Therapeutics.* New York: The Medical Letter, 1998; 40:21–4.

27. Davies DM, ed. *Textbook of Adverse Drug Reactions.* New York: Oxford University Press, 1977.

28. Aronson JK, Van Boxtel CJ, eds. *Side Effects of Drugs Annual* 18. Amsterdam: Elsevier, 1995.

29. Aronson JK. *Side Effects of Drugs Annual* 20. Amsterdam: Elsevier, 1997.

30. Aronson JK, Van Boxtel CJ. *Side Effects of Drugs Annual* 19. Amsterdam: Elsevier, 1996. Other sources included the *Physicians' Desk Reference* and outside consultants.

31. Larson, op. cit. Although this study found specific drugs in certain therapeutic classes to cause an increased risk of mental impairment, we list all of the drugs in that class here, since for benzodiazepines, beta-blockers, and major tranquilizers (antipsychotic drugs), for example, there is no reason to believe that the whole class would not have this adverse effect.

3

456 DRUGS COMMONLY USED BY CONSUMERS

How to Use This Chapter

This chapter gives a profile of 456 drugs commonly used by consumers. The profiles are divided into 11 sections based on the type of problem treated: Drugs for Heart Conditions, Mind Drugs, Painkillers and Arthritis Drugs, etc.

Each of these sections has (1) a Drug Listing of the brand and generic names of all drugs profiled in it and the page on which each profile begins, (2) discussions of the most important medical problems (for example, high blood pressure) and the types of treatment available, and (3) the drug profiles.

Before looking up any of the drugs in this chapter, please read the following guide to the format of the drug profiles.

GUIDE TO THE DRUG PROFILES

This page, showing the format of our drug profiles, will help you understand the information provided about each of the 456 drugs in this chapter. If a drug profile lacks any of the sections described below, it means there is no relevant information.

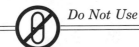 *Do Not Use*

We recommend that these drugs not be used and we suggest an alternative treatment. Listings for these drugs do not include information on whether or not a generic version is available, or sections titled Before You Use This Drug, When You Use This Drug, How to Use This Drug, Interactions with Other Drugs, Adverse Effects, or Periodic Tests.

Do Not Use Until Five Years After Release

We recommend that these drugs not be used for at least five years from date of release unless it is one of those rare "breakthrough" drugs that offers you a documented therapeutic advantage over older, proven drugs. (The year in which the drug will have been on the market for five years is given in the profile of each drug with this designation.)

Last Choice Drug

We believe that these drugs should be used only if other drugs are ineffective or cannot be used to treat your medical condition.

Limited Use

We believe that these drugs offer limited benefit or benefit only certain people or conditions.

Generic Name

This is the chemical name of the active ingredient(s).

BRAND NAME (Manufacturer)

These are the brand names used by the manufacturers. The names are those of the most frequently prescribed drugs. In most cases, no more than five brand names appear because of space limitations. You always should learn both the brand and the generic name of your drug.

GENERIC: Tells if a generic product is available that is sold under the chemical name of the drug.

FAMILY: This is the class of similar drugs.

The text section describes the drug's actions and effects, in older adults in particular, and the conditions for which the drug is prescribed. It explains how and why the drug should or should not be used.

Before You Use This Drug

• Presents information that your doctor should know before you start to use the drug, such as your past and present health conditions and prescription and nonprescription drugs that you use.

When You Use This Drug

• Presents information that will ensure your safety and maximum benefit while using the drug.

How to Use This Drug

• Tells you what to do about a missed dose and how to take the drug.

Interactions with Other Drugs

Alphabetically lists the names of the drugs that may interact most harmfully with the drug profiled if they are used at the same time. The generic drugs are in lower-case letters and the brand names are in CAPITAL LETTERS. Make sure you know the generic name of your drugs since only one or two brand names are listed for each generic drug.

Adverse Effects

• Presents the unwanted adverse effects that may occur while you use the drug (and sometimes after you stop). There are two categories of adverse effects: (1) those that require immediate medical attention, including signs of overdose for many drugs, and (2) signs that do not require immediate attention but should be brought to your doctor's attention if they persist.

Periodic Tests

• Names the medical tests that should or might need to be done during the time that you use this drug, such as complete blood count, complete urine test, electrocardiogram (ECG, EKG), or eye pressure exam. You should ask your doctor which of these tests you need.

Talk to your doctor before deciding to make any changes in your prescription drugs based on the information in this book.

Drugs for Heart Conditions

High Blood Pressure	**44**
Potassium Supplementation	**49**
Beta-blockers	**52**
Calcium Channel Blockers	**53**
Cholesterol-lowering Drugs	**54**

DRUG LISTINGS

DRUGS FOR HIGH BLOOD PRESSURE

Beta-blockers

acebutolol		153
atenolol		153
betaxolol		154
bisoprolol		154
BLOCADREN		66
carteolol		154
CARTROL		154
carvedilol	Do Not Use Until Five Years After Release	85
COREG	Do Not Use Until Five Years After Release	85
CORGARD		154
INDERAL		154
INDERAL LA		154
KERLONE		154
labetalol	Limited Use	154
LEVATOL		154
LOPRESSOR		154
metoprolol		154
nadolol		154
NORMODYNE	Limited Use	154
penbutolol		154
pindolol		154
propranolol		154
SECTRAL		153
TENORMIN		153
timolol		66
TOPROL XL		154
TRANDATE	Limited Use	154
VISKEN		154
ZEBETA		154

Calcium Channel Blockers

ADALAT	Ⓧ Do Not Use	56
ADALAT CC	Limited Use	142
amlodipine	Limited Use	142
amlodipine and benazepril	Ⓧ Do Not Use	129
CALAN	Limited Use	73
CALAN SR	Limited Use	73
CARDENE	Limited Use	142
CARDENE SR	Limited Use	142
CARDIZEM	Limited Use	76
CARDIZEM CD	Limited Use	76
COVERA-HS	Limited Use	73
DILACOR XR	Limited Use	76
diltiazem	Limited Use	76
diltiazem and enalapril	Ⓧ Do Not Use	129
DYNACIRC	Limited Use	142
DYNACIRC CR	Limited Use	142
felodipine	Limited Use	142
felodipine and enalapril	Ⓧ Do Not Use	129
ISOPTIN	Limited Use	73
ISOPTIN SR	Limited Use	73
isradipine	Limited Use	142
LEXXEL	Ⓧ Do Not Use	129
LOTREL	Ⓧ Do Not Use	129
mibefradil	Ⓧ Do Not Use	146
nicardipine	Limited Use	142
nifedipine	Limited Use	142
nifedipine, short-acting forms	Ⓧ Do Not Use	56
nisoldipine	Do Not Use Until Five Years After Release	142
NORVASC	Limited Use	142

Drug	Recommendation	Page
PLENDIL	Limited Use	142
POSICOR	⊘ Do Not Use	146
PROCARDIA	⊘ Do Not Use	56
PROCARDIA XL	Limited Use	142
SULAR	Do Not Use Until Five Years After Release	142
TARKA	⊘ Do Not Use	129
TECZEM	⊘ Do Not Use	129
TIAZAC	Limited Use	76
verapamil	Limited Use	73
verapamil and trandolopril	⊘ Do Not Use	129
VERELAN	Limited Use	73

Diuretics (water pills)/Antihypertensives

Drug	Recommendation	Page
ALDACTAZIDE	⊘ Do Not Use	57
ALDACTONE	Limited Use	58
ALDORIL	⊘ Do Not Use	61
amiloride and hydrochlorothiazide	⊘ Do Not Use	138
APRESAZIDE	Limited Use	63
atenolol and chlorthalidone	⊘ Do Not Use	161
AVAPRO HCT	Do Not Use Until Five Years After Release	90
benazepril and hydrochlorothiazide	Limited Use	127
bisoprolol and hydrochlorothiazide	Limited Use	169
bumetanide	Limited Use	70
BUMEX	Limited Use	70
CAPOZIDE	Limited Use	127
captopril and hydrochlorothiazide	Limited Use	127
CHLOROSERPINE	Do Not Use	93
chlorothiazide	Limited Use	100
chlorthalidone	⊘ Do Not Use	105
clonidine and chlorthalidone	⊘ Do Not Use	81
COMBIPRES	⊘ Do Not Use	81
CORZIDE	Limited Use	169
DEMI-REGROTON	⊘ Do Not Use	150
deserpidine and methyclothiazide	⊘ Do Not Use	99
DIULO	Limited Use	101
DIUPRES	⊘ Do Not Use	93
DIURIL	Limited Use	100
DYAZIDE	Limited Use	97
DYRENIUM	⊘ Do Not Use	99
enalapril and hydrochlorothiazide	Limited Use	127

Drug	Recommendation	Page
ENDURON	Limited Use	101
ENDURONYL	⊘ Do Not Use	99
ESIDRIX		100
furosemide	Limited Use	116
hydralazine and hydrochlorothiazide	Limited Use	63
hydrochlorothiazide		100
HYDRODIURIL		100
HYDROPRES	⊘ Do Not Use	103
HYDROSERPINE	⊘ Do Not Use	103
HYGROTON	⊘ Do Not Use	105
HYZAAR	Do Not Use Until Five Years After Release	90
indapamide	Limited Use	101
INDERIDE LA	Limited Use	169
irbesartan and hydrochlorothiazide	Do Not Use Until Five Years After Release	90
LASIX	Limited Use	116
lisinopril and hydrochlorothiazide	Limited Use	127
LOPRESSOR HCT	Limited Use	169
losartan and hydrochlorothiazide	Do Not Use Until Five Years After Release	90
LOTENSIN HCT	Limited Use	127
LOZOL	Limited Use	101
MAXZIDE	Limited Use	97
METAHYDRIN	Limited Use	101
methyclothiazide	Limited Use	101
methyldopa and hydrochlorothiazide	⊘ Do Not Use	61
metolazone	Limited Use	101
metoprolol and hydrochlorothiazide	Limited Use	169
MODURETIC	⊘ Do Not Use	138
nadolol and bendroflumethiazide	Limited Use	169
NAQUA	Limited Use	101
PRINZIDE	Limited Use	127
propranolol and hydrochlorothiazide	Limited Use	169
REGROTON	⊘ Do Not Use	150
reserpine and chlorothiazide	⊘ Do Not Use	93
reserpine and chlorthalidone	⊘ Do Not Use	150
reserpine, hydralazine and hydrochlorothiazide	⊘ Do Not Use	157
reserpine and hydrochlorothiazide	⊘ Do Not Use	103

reserpine and hydroflumethiazide	⊘ Do Not Use	152
SALUTENSIN	⊘ Do Not Use	152
SER-AP-ES	⊘ Do Not Use	157
spironolactone	Limited Use	58
spironolactone and hydrochlorothiazide	⊘ Do Not Use	57
TENORETIC	⊘ Do Not Use	161
TIMOLIDE	Limited Use	169
timolol and hydrochlorothiazide	Limited Use	169
triamterene	⊘ Do Not Use	99
triamterene and hydrochlorothiazide	Limited Use	97
trichlormethiazide	Limited Use	101
VASERETIC	Limited Use	127
ZAROXOLYN	Limited Use	101
ZESTORETIC	Limited Use	127
ZIAC	Limited Use	169

Other Drugs for High Blood Pressure

ACCUPRIL	Limited Use	123
ALDOMET	⊘ Do Not Use	61
ALTACE	Limited Use	123
APRESOLINE		64
AVAPRO	Do Not Use Until Five Years After Release	90
benazepril	Limited Use	123
CAPOTEN	Limited Use	123
captopril	Limited Use	123
CATAPRES	⊘ Do Not Use	80
clonidine	⊘ Do Not Use	80
COZAAR	Do Not Use Until Five Years After Release	90
DIOVAN	Do Not Use Until Five Years After Release	90
enalapril	Limited Use	123
fosinopril	Limited Use	123
guanabenz	⊘ Do Not Use	168
guanfacine	Limited Use	158
hydralazine		64
HYTRIN	Limited Use	105
irbesartan	Do Not Use Until Five Years After Release	90
lisinopril	Limited Use	123
losartan	Do Not Use Until Five Years After Release	90
LOTENSIN	Limited Use	123
MAVIK	Do Not Use Until Five Years After Release	123
methyldopa	⊘ Do Not Use	61

MINIPRESS	Limited Use	136
moexipril	Do Not Use Until Five Years After Release	123
MONOPRIL	Limited Use	123
prazosin	Limited Use	136
PRINIVIL	Limited Use	123
quinapril	Limited Use	123
ramipril	Limited Use	123
reserpine	⊘ Do Not Use	152
TENEX	Limited Use	158
terazosin	Limited Use	105
trandolapril	Do Not Use Until Five Years After Release	123
UNIVASC	Do Not Use Until Five Years After Release	123
valsartan	Do Not Use Until Five Years After Release	90
VASOTEC	Limited Use	123
WYTENSIN	⊘ Do Not Use	168
ZESTRIL	Limited Use	123

DRUGS FOR HEART FAILURE AND ANGINA

DEPONIT		108
digoxin		113
dipyridamole	⊘ Do Not Use Except After Valve Replacement	146
IMDUR		108
ISMO		108
ISORDIL		108
isosorbide dinitrate		108
isosorbide-5-mononitrate		108
LANOXICAPS		113
LANOXIN		113
MINITRAN		108
NITRO-BID		108
NITRODISC		108
NITRO-DUR		108
nitroglycerin		108
NITROSTAT		108
PERSANTINE	⊘ Do Not Use Except After Valve Replacement	146
SORBITRATE		108
TRANSDERM-NITRO		108

DRUGS FOR ABNORMAL HEART RHYTHM

amiodarone	Last Choice Drug	83
CORDARONE	Last Choice Drug	83
disopyramide	Limited Use	139
DURAQUIN	Limited Use	94

mexiletine	Limited Use	133
MEXITIL	Limited Use	133
NORPACE	Limited Use	139
procainamide	Limited Use	148
PROCANBID	Limited Use	148
QUINAGLUTE DURA-TABS	Limited Use	94
QUINIDEX	Limited Use	94
quinidine	Limited Use	94
tocainide	Limited Use	164
TONOCARD	Limited Use	164

CHOLESTEROL-LOWERING DRUGS

atorvastatin	Do Not Use Until Five Years After Release	130
BAYCOL	Do Not Use Until Five Years After Release	130
cerivastatin	Do Not Use Until Five Years After Release	130
cholestyramine	Limited Use	119
fluvastatin	Do Not Use Until Five Years After Release	130
gemfibrozil	⊘ Do Not Use	121
LESCOL	Do Not Use Until Five Years After Release	130
LIPITOR	Do Not Use Until Five Years After Release	130
LOCHOLEST	Limited Use	119
LOPID	⊘ Do Not Use	121
LORELCO	⊘ Do Not Use	122
lovastatin	Limited Use	130
MEVACOR	Limited Use	130
PRAVACHOL	Limited Use	130
pravastatin	Limited Use	130
probucol	⊘ Do Not Use	122
QUESTRAN	Limited Use	119
QUESTRAN LIGHT	Limited Use	119
simvastatin	Limited Use	130
ZOCOR	Limited Use	130

OTHER CARDIOVASCULAR DRUGS

CERESPAN	⊘ Do Not Use	81
COUMADIN		87
cyclandelate	⊘ Do Not Use	93
CYCLOSPASMOL	⊘ Do Not Use	93
isoxsuprine	⊘ Do Not Use	167
KAOCHLOR		111
KAON-CL		111
KATO		111
KAY CIEL		111

K-LOR		111
KLOTRIX	Limited Use	111
K-LYTE TABLETS		111
MICRO-K	Limited Use	111
papaverine	⊘ Do Not Use	81
PAVABID	⊘ Do Not Use	81
pentoxifylline	⊘ Do Not Use	166
potassium supplements		111
quinine	⊘ Do Not Use Except for Malaria	150
SLOW-K	Limited Use	111
TICLID	Last Choice Drug	162
ticlopidine	Last Choice Drug	162
TRENTAL	⊘ Do Not Use	166
VASODILAN	⊘ Do Not Use	167
warfarin		87

HIGH BLOOD PRESSURE

High blood pressure, or hypertension, is a major contributing factor to the development of strokes, heart attacks, kidney disease, and circulation disorders. Heart disease and stroke remain the first and third leading causes of death in the United States. More than 28 million Americans are estimated to have high blood pressure; this includes more than 22% of the population between the ages of 45 and 64.[1] The importance of high blood pressure, especially in older adults, has not always been appreciated. For a long time, an increase in blood pressure with age was considered helpful in maintaining blood flow as hardening of the arteries occurred. Studies have shown, however, that this increase in blood pressure can cause damage to organs and lead to a stroke or heart attack. Regardless of your age, reducing your blood pressure using diet and exercise, or diuretics or beta-blockers if drug treatment is necessary, reduces your risk of heart attack and stroke.

When your blood pressure is taken, you are given two numbers, which represent the systolic pressure and the diastolic pressure— 140/60 (mm Hg—millimeters of mercury, under pressure), for example. Systolic pressure, the upper number (140), reflects the pressure in the arteries as the heart contracts and pumps blood. As the arteries harden with age (arteriosclerosis), the systolic pressure increases. Diastolic pressure, the lower number (60), reflects the pressure in the arteries as the heart relaxes and fills with blood.

Either your systolic or your diastolic pressure can be elevated. Elevations of either one or both of these pressures can significantly increase your chance of having a stroke or heart attack.

Nondrug Treatment and Prevention of High Blood Pressure

Lowering high blood pressure should begin with methods that do not use drugs. Using one or more of these methods can often help reduce your blood pressure to the point where you do not need medication. Even if your high blood pressure does eventually require drugs, you should adhere to as many of the following recommendations as you can. A study of nutritional therapy showed that over one-third of people who previously needed drug treatment for high blood pressure were able to adequately control their blood pressure with nutritional therapy alone.[2] In addition, these methods are safer than using medication, since they have no adverse effects. Trying them will often make other beneficial contributions to your health.

1. Lose weight: One in five adults in the United States is at least 20% above "desirable" weight. Many people in this category who lose weight can reduce their blood pressure by 15%.

2. Reduce your salt intake: Changing your diet by not using your salt shaker and reducing your intake of processed and salty foods is a good first step.

3. Restrict alcohol: Cutting alcohol intake to, at most, one drink a day also can reduce blood pressure.

4. Exercise: Mild aerobic exercise such as walking 15 or 20 minutes a day at a comfortable pace will have a beneficial effect on heart and blood pressure.

5. Decrease your fat intake: Decreasing the amount of animal fat in your diet has a beneficial effect on blood pressure. Furthermore, a high-fat diet is a risk factor for heart disease independent of high blood pressure. Decreasing the amount of fat in your diet will therefore help reduce your overall risk of developing heart disease.

6. Increase the fiber in your diet: Diets with a high fiber content can lower blood pressure.[3] One study showed a drop of 10 mm Hg in systolic pressure and 5 mm Hg of diastolic pressure in people who took fiber supplements for two months, without any other dietary changes.[4] Fiber can be increased by eating more fruits, vegetables, and whole grains.

7. Biofeedback: Numerous studies have shown the value, in selected patients, of biofeedback as a way of reducing or eliminating the need for antihypertensive drugs.

8. Other methods: Increasing your potassium and calcium intake has been shown to have a beneficial effect on blood pressure, although this is somewhat controversial. If this is done through dietary means, however, it can have other health benefits and can be recommended as an overall healthy step.[5] (See p. 51 for foods that contain potassium and p. 601 for foods that contain calcium.)

A clinical trial was performed recently on people 60 to 80 years old with well-controlled blood pressures, who had been taking a high-blood-pressure-lowering drug for years. The results showed that keeping salt intake to 1,800 milligrams per day or less and losing a moderate amount of weight (on the order of 10 pounds) were responsible for further significant decreases in blood pressure while continuing drug treatment. At the end of the study more than 30% of the patients had lowered their blood pressure enough through salt reduction and weight loss to no longer require blood-pressure-lowering drugs. Salt reduction was equally effective in overweight and nonoverweight participants and was as effective as weight reduction in preventing recurrence of high blood pressure, need for a blood-pressure-lowering drug, or a cardiovascular event such as a stroke, heart attack, or chest pain (angina). Salt reduction combined with weight loss was more effective than either alone for control of high blood pressure, with or without the use of a blood-pressure-lowering drug.[6]

The results of this study and decades of extensive research now make it possible to speak in terms of preventing high blood pressure rather than treating it with drugs, which is defensive, mainly reactive, time-consuming, associated with adverse drug effects, costly, only partially successful, endless, and is not a cure. In the editorial that accompanied the study the author said: *"Hence, there is now evidence for a 'fare for all seasons,' to be consumed from postweaning through older age, to prevent adverse BP [blood pressure] levels, other major risk factors, and cardiovascular and other chronic diseases. This fare is delectable—high in fruits and vegetables; high in legumes and whole grains; high in fat-free and low-fat dairy products, poultry, fish, shellfish,* *and meats; high in all essential nutrients; reduced in salt; reduced in total fat, saturated fat, and cholesterol; with no more than 1 or 2 drinks per day for those who choose to ingest alcohol; and controlled in calories to prevent or correct obesity."[7]*

When Is Treatment Necessary?

Two things should be taken into account when considering whether your high blood pressure should be treated. One is the benefits of the treatment for your blood pressure, which vary depending on how high it is. The other consideration is the risks or the adverse effects of the treatment, which will vary depending on what is being considered.

Several studies have shown that the treatment of an elevated diastolic pressure does decrease your chance of having a stroke or heart attack. However, if only your systolic pressure is elevated, which often occurs in older adults, it is controversial as to what benefits are gained by treatment. Doctors generally agree that systolic blood pressure readings above a certain level are dangerous enough so that they require treatment. Treatment of systolic blood pressure below these levels is more controversial.

Blood Pressure *(Stages in Millimeters of mercury)*	Risk Group A *(No Risk Factors, No Organ Damage or Disease)*	Risk Group B *(At Least 1 Risk Factor, Not Including Diabetes, No Organ Damage or Disease)*	Risk Group C *(Organ Damage or Disease and/or Diabetes, with or Without Other Risk Factors)*
High-normal (130–139/85–89)	Lifestyle modification	Lifestyle modification	Drug therapy
Stage 1 (140–159/90–99)	Lifestyle modification (up to 12 months)	Lifestyle modification (up to 6 months)	Drug therapy
Stages 2 and 3 (greater than 160/ greater than 100)	Drug therapy	Drug therapy	Drug therapy

A person's blood pressure can be higher when measured at the doctor's office than when measured at home; feeling nervous probably contributes to the higher reading. Ask your doctor about the various methods available for home monitoring of blood pressure, so you can see if yours is lower at home. If so, it is possible that you actually do not have high blood pressure and do not have to be treated.

Classification and Treatment of Blood Pressure for Adults Age 18 and Older

In the chart at left, a risk factor refers to another disease, condition, or behavior that can by itself, in people without high blood pressure, increase the risk of heart attack or stroke. For example, smoking, high cholesterol, diabetes, being over 60 years of age, and a family history of cardiovascular disease are risk factors for heart attack and stroke. Organ damage refers to conditions caused by cardiovascular diseases such as an enlarged heart, a previous heart attack accompanied by chest pain (angina), heart vein bypass surgery or angioplasty, or heart failure. Also included as organ damage are stroke, kidney disease, artery disease, or eye damage caused by high blood pressure.

For example, a person with diabetes and a blood pressure of 142/94 plus an enlarged heart would be classified as having Stage 1 hypertension with organ disease and another risk factor (diabetes). This person would be categorized as Stage 1, Risk Group C, and recommended for immediate initiation of drug treatment.[8]

What Is "Normal" Blood Pressure for Older Adults?

There is no single level of pressure that separates "normal" from "abnormal." This surprises most people who ask what a good pressure is. The age of the person is a determining factor, as older people are able to tolerate higher blood pressure with fewer adverse effects than younger people.

It is a common misconception that a blood pressure over 140/90 is too high for older adults. (This misconception is often supported by the media, as in a *Washington Post* article on high blood pressure that stated that 64% of all people from age 65 to 74 had high blood pressure, defined as over 140/90.)[9] Although 140/90 may be a high blood pressure for younger adults, it is not too high for adults over 60 years of age. The current blood pressure guidelines for older people are listed on the following page.

Are Many Older Adults Being Given Antihypertensive Drugs Unnecessarily? One study found that 41% of patients 50 and older who were carefully taken off their high blood pressure medications did not need them, having normal blood pressure 11 months after the drug was stopped.[10]

Drug Treatment of High Blood Pressure

Regardless of your age, below or above 60, most of the time high blood pressure can be controlled with just one drug. The National Institutes of Health's National Heart, Lung and Blood Institute recommends beginning treatment with a mild water pill (diuretic) at a low dose. The safest and best studied of the diuretics is hydrochlorothiazide (see p. 100). The starting dose should be low—12.5 to 25 milligrams per day or even every other day. For older adults, in general, the rule for treating high blood pressure, like so many other drug treatments, is "start low and go slow." According to experts in prescribing for older adults, for mild hypertension (or heart failure) start with half the standard starting dose and increase gradually.

If a second drug is needed the National Heart, Lung, and Blood Institute recommends beta-blockers (see p. 52), although they are not as effective in older adults as they are in younger adults. Because of this, beta-blockers should never be used as the first drug in treating

GUIDELINES FOR TREATING HIGH BLOOD PRESSURE IN OLDER ADULTS

Diastolic Blood Pressure[11]	Treatment
Under 90 mm Hg	Does not have to be treated.
90–99 mm Hg	Mildly elevated blood pressure; it does not have to be treated with drugs, but nondrug measures can be started. Your blood pressure should be taken a few times during the next six months to make sure it has not increased.
100 mm Hg and over	Elevated blood pressure; it should be treated using nondrug measures first. If this is not effective, then drug treatment should be used. People over the age of 80 should discuss with their doctor whether their diastolic blood pressure is elevated enough to require treatment, as the cutoff level for treatment is debatable.
Systolic Blood Pressure[12]*	Treatment
140–160 mm Hg	Does not have to be treated. People over 60 have a higher systolic pressure than younger people. Although 140–160 mm Hg might be considered a high level in a younger person, it does not have to be treated in an older person.
160–180 mm Hg	Mildly elevated blood pressure; there is no one "best" type of treatment. Certainly, nondrug measures should be used; however, you may wish to discuss with your doctor whether a drug is necessary.
180 mm Hg and over	Most authorities agree that a systolic blood pressure of this level should be treated, beginning with nondrug measures and using drugs if necessary.

For older adults, the systolic pressure should not be reduced below 140 to 160 mm Hg with drugs. If you use a drug to control high blood pressure and this occurs, you should discuss with your doctor the need for decreasing the amount you take.

high blood pressure in older adults. *ACE inhibitors are also effective drugs to use as a second agent.* It is rarely necessary to take more than two drugs to treat high blood pressure. If you are taking more than two, a reassessment is indicated. Hydralazine (see p. 64), however, is a good agent to use if a third drug is required.

Common Adverse Effects of High Blood Pressure Drugs

The decision to use drugs to treat high blood pressure should be based on a consideration of both the benefits and the risks of the treatment. Therefore it is very important that you report any adverse effects of the drugs to your doctor, so that your situation can be reassessed.

These are some of the possible adverse effects of the various antihypertensive drugs:[13]

• Depression—especially with beta-blockers, reserpine, methyldopa, and clonidine (see *Drugs That Can Cause Depression, in Chapter 2,* p. 19).

• Sedation and fatigue—especially with beta-blockers, reserpine, methyldopa, and clonidine.

• Impotence and sexual dysfunction—especially with beta-blockers, methyldopa, and many other heart drugs (see *Drugs That Can Cause Sexual Dysfunction, in Chapter 2,* p. 28).

• Dizziness (from a drop in blood pressure after standing up, which can result in accidental falls and broken bones)—seen with all high blood pressure drugs to some degree, and especially with guanethidine, prazosin, and methyldopa. Older adults are more prone to this adverse effect because the internal blood pressure regulation system works more slowly as we age (see **Drugs That Can Cause Dizziness on Standing, in Chapter 2,** p. 26).

• Loss of appetite and nausea—especially with hydrochlorothiazide, digoxin, and potassium supplements (see **Drugs That Can Cause Loss of Appetite, Nausea, or Vomiting, in Chapter 2,** p. 30).

These and other adverse effects can occur with any medication for high blood pressure. Those listed occur most often. If you experience any effects, or just feel worse in general, tell your doctor. It is often better to tolerate a slightly higher blood pressure with no adverse effects from medication than to have a lower blood pressure along with serious effects from medication that will adversely affect your life.

For example, let's consider the steps in devising a treatment for a 75-year-old woman whose baseline blood pressure is 200/90 mm Hg:

1. She is first treated with 12.5 milligrams of hydrochlorothiazide. This results in a blood pressure of 170/90, and she feels quite well.

2. Her doctor attempts to lower her blood pressure further by adding another drug, propranolol, to her treatment. This results in a blood pressure of 160/90, but she "feels awful" and complains of fatigue and confusion.

3. Her doctor might consider discontinuing the propranolol and using another drug. A better idea might be to accept a blood pressure of 170/90 using hydrochlorothiazide alone or to lower it further with nondrug therapy.

Stopping Drug Treatment

Historically, patients have been taught that hypertension means treatment for life, although countless thousands of patients have abandoned their treatment without their doctors' knowledge or consent. For some patients, this may be

a dangerous idea, but for many others the treatment may no longer be needed. Two large studies in Australia and Britain have shown that one-third to one-half of patients with mild hypertension for whom treatment was stopped had normal blood pressures a year or more later.[14]

An editorial in the *British Medical Journal* stated, *"Treatment of hypertension is part of preventive medicine and like all preventive strategies, its progress should be regularly reviewed by whoever initiates it. Many problems could be avoided by not starting antihypertensive treatment until after prolonged observation.... Patients should no longer be told that treatment is necessarily for life: the possibility of reducing or stopping treatment should be mentioned at the outset."*[15]

This view is shared by American experts in hypertension who have stated that "once blood pressure has been normal for a year or more, a cautious decrease in antihypertensive dosage and renewed attention to nonpharmacologic treatment may be worth trying."[16]

RECOMMENDED DRUGS FOR TREATMENT OF HIGH BLOOD PRESSURE

First drug to use: a diuretic such as hydrochlorothiazide (Esidrix, HydroDiuril, or a generic)

Drug to add: a beta-blocker such as propranolol (Inderal, Inderal LA), an ACE inhibitor such as captopril (Capoten) or enalapril (Vasotec)

Another drug to add: hydralazine (Apresoline)

POTASSIUM SUPPLEMENTATION: DIET IS THE FIRST CHOICE

Who Needs Nondietary Potassium Supplementation?

Very few people actually need to take a potassium supplement or a potassium-sparing diuretic (amiloride, spironolactone, triamterene). If, however, you take digoxin, have severe liver disease, or take large doses of diuretics (water pills) for heart disease, eating a potassium-rich diet may not be sufficient to replace the potassium that you are losing. If you fall into one of these categories, it is very important for your doctor to precisely monitor and regulate the amount of potassium in your bloodstream. A potassium supplement or a potassium-sparing diuretic may be necessary. Read about the methods of increasing the potassium in your body discussed below and consult with your doctor about which will be best for you.

Who Does Not Need It?

Most people taking a thiazide diuretic (hydrochlorothiazide or metolazone, for example) for high blood pressure (hypertension) do not need potassium-sparing diuretics[17] or potassium supplements. This is especially true if treatment is started at a low dose (12.5 milligrams of hydrochlorothiazide for treatment of mild hypertension). Supplementing the diet with potassium-rich foods or beverages (see below) is sufficient to prevent low levels of potassium.[18]

Mild potassium deficiency (between 3.0 and 3.5 millimoles of potassium per liter of blood) can occur during diuretic therapy, but it usually has no symptoms and requires no treatment other than eating foods that are rich in potassium. Most people do not get severe potassium deficiency (less than 3.0 millimoles per liter) from treatment with diuretics. Comparisons of people eating a potassium-rich diet, people taking potassium supplements, and people taking potassium-sparing drugs have shown that (1) diet is the safest method of replacing potassium and (2) potassium supplements and potassium-sparing drugs return potassium levels to normal in only 50% of the users. Therefore, if you have mild potassium deficiency, eat a few bananas before risking the adverse effects of

potassium supplements or potassium-sparing drugs. Ask your doctor what your potassium levels were before and after you started diuretic treatment. You probably do not need a nondietary potassium supplement or potassium-sparing drug.

Three Ways to Increase Your Potassium Levels

The safest and least expensive way is to increase the amount of potassium-rich food in your *daily* diet. This will provide sufficient potassium replacement for the overwhelming majority of people taking diuretics (people who also take digoxin or who have liver disease may be exceptions).

Restricting sodium (salt) intake also helps to maintain potassium levels while lowering sodium levels. In fact, salt substitutes containing potassium chloride may be an additional source of potassium intake.[19] If you are already taking potassium supplements or potassium-sparing diuretics, consult your doctor before using salt substitutes. A dosage adjustment may be necessary to prevent too much potassium in the body, a potentially fatal condition.

Potassium supplements are a second method for replacing potassium, but these can cause serious adverse reactions. Potassium is an irritant to the mucous membranes that line the mouth, throat, stomach, and intestines. If not properly dissolved and dispersed in the digestive tract, potassium can come in contact with these membranes and cause bleeding, ulcers, and perforations. Use of potassium supplements, because of serious potential adverse effects, should be restricted to people who are eating plenty of potassium-rich foods, yet still have a low level of potassium in their blood (less than 3.0 millimoles per liter).[20]

There are several kinds of potassium supplements:

• **Liquids:** Liquid supplements are safer than tablets[21] because, when taken in a diluted form over a five- to ten-minute period, potassium is effectively dispersed in the digestive tract, and thus causes less stomach and intestinal irritation and ulceration. Packaged as a liquid, powder, or dissolvable tablet, all forms must be completely dissolved in at least one-half cup of cold water or juice before drinking, and then sipped slowly over five to ten minutes.

• **Extended-release tablets or capsules:** Although liquid supplements are safest, tablets and capsules are widely used to avoid the unpleasant taste of the liquids.[22] Rarely, but often unpredictably, these tablets and capsules can cause stomach and intestinal ulcers, bleeding, blockage, and perforation when the potassium in the tablets and capsules does not dissolve and comes in contact with the lining of the digestive tract.[23] Abdominal pain, diarrhea, nausea, vomiting, and heartburn have also been reported.[24] Because the amount of time required for food to be digested and travel through the digestive tract increases with age, older people are more likely to experience adverse effects with these tablets or capsules.[25,26] Increased transit time leaves more opportunity for an undissolved or partially dissolved tablet or capsule to damage mucous lining.

• **Enteric-coated tablets:** Avoid these. "Enteric-coated" potassium tablets are not reliably absorbed and have frequently been blamed for intestinal ulceration.[27]

The last method for increasing potassium levels is with a class of drugs called potassium-sparing diuretics. Examples of these drugs are spironolactone (ALDACTONE), triamterene (DYRENIUM), and amiloride (MIDAMOR). Potassium-sparing diuretics are also found in combination products such as Moduretic and Aldactazide. These should not be used for older adults. These drugs can cause potentially fatal adverse effects such as kidney failure and the retention of too much potassium, which causes irregular heartbeats and heart rhythm. Studies have shown that the potassium supple-

ments discussed above are equally effective and less dangerous than potassium-sparing diuretics, if nondietary potassium replacement is required.

If you are taking a potassium-sparing diuretic, you should never also use a potassium supplement or salt substitute containing potassium.[28] You should also not use an ACE inhibitor such as captopril (see p. 123) with potassium supplements because of the risk of high levels of potassium.[29] Too-high levels of potassium, a potentially fatal condition that may not produce warning symptoms, may develop rapidly.

POTASSIUM LEVELS IN MILLIEQUIVALENTS (MEQ) OF SELECTED FOODS AND POTASSIUM SUPPLEMENTS

Source	Amount	Potassium (mEq)
Peaches, dried, uncooked	1 cup	39
Raisins, dried, uncooked	1 cup	31
Dates, dried, cut	1 cup, pitted	29
Apricots, dried, uncooked	17 large halves	25
Figs, dried	7 medium	23
Prune juice, canned	1 cup	15
Watermelon	1 slice (1½ inches)	15
Banana	1 medium	14
Beef round	4 ounces	14
Cantaloupe	½ (5 inches in diameter)	13
Orange juice, fresh	1 cup	13
Turkey, roasted	3½ ounces	13
Klotrix Tabs	1 tablet	10
Kaon Cl-10	1 tablet	10
Milk, whole, 3.5% fat	1 cup	9
Slow-K	1 tablet	8
Kaon-Cl	1 tablet	6.7

FOODS HIGH IN POTASSIUM

All-bran cereals	Lentils
Almonds	Liver, beef
Apricots (dried)	Milk
Avocado	Molasses
Bananas	Peaches
Beans	Peanut butter
Beef	Peas
Broccoli	Pork
Brussels sprouts	Potatoes
Cantaloupe	Prunes (dried)
Carrots (raw)	Raisins
Chicken	Shellfish
Citrus fruits	Spinach
Coconut	Tomato juice
Crackers (rye)	Turkey
Dates and figs (dried)	Veal
Fish, fresh	Watermelon
Ham	Yams

BETA-BLOCKERS

Use

Beta-blockers are a class of drugs that are used to treat high blood pressure. A beta-blocker is often used as the drug of first choice for treating hypertension (high blood pressure) in young and middle-aged adults. A beta-blocker, however, is less effective in older adults. Therefore, hydrochlorothiazide (see p. 100), a diuretic (water pill), should be the drug of choice for treating hypertension in people 60 years old or older. If this drug is not sufficient to lower blood pressure, then a beta-blocker can be prescribed in addition to hydrochlorothiazide. (See p. 44 for a discussion of treatment strategies to lower blood pressure.) Some of the beta-blockers are also used to treat chest pain (angina), heart attacks, irregular heart rhythms, glaucoma, and migraine headaches.

Beta-blockers should not be taken if you have asthma, emphysema, chronic bronchitis, bronchospasm, allergies, congestive heart disease, or heart block. A baseline electrocardiogram (ECG, EKG) should be taken before a beta-blocker is first prescribed to be sure that you do not have heart block. Do not smoke while taking a beta-blocker (you shouldn't be smoking anyway). If you smoke, you might as well stop taking the beta-blocker. Not only will smoking aggravate some of the respiratory adverse effects, but it greatly reduces the level of drug in your body.

Beta-blockers may come as tablets or capsules in two forms. If you take the extended-release tablet or capsule, you should swallow them whole. Do not crush, break, or chew them before swallowing. If you do not take the extended-release form, the tablets may be crushed or the capsules opened and mixed with a teaspoon of applesauce or jelly to make them easier to swallow. It is important to schedule appointments regularly with your doctor so that he or she can check your progress and adjust your dosage. Make sure that you have enough medicine with you to last through weekends, holidays, or vacations. You may want to carry an extra prescription with you in case of emergency. Do not stop taking this medicine without checking with your doctor. Sudden withdrawal may cause a heart attack, chest pain (angina), or a rapid increase in your heart rate. If you are to reduce the amount of medicine you are taking, then your doctor should give you a schedule to help you gradually reduce the dosage.

Adverse Effects

Below are some general categories of adverse effects and a discussion of which beta-blockers are most or least likely to produce these effects. If you are having any of these adverse effects, ask your doctor about changing your prescription.

Effects on the Brain

Each of the beta-blockers has been reported to cause mental changes such as depression, nightmares, hallucinations, and insomnia in some people. These occur most frequently with people taking metoprolol, pindolol, or propranolol. Propranolol should be avoided by people who are depressed or have a past history of depression. Atenolol and nadolol may cause fewer of these reactions.

Breathing Difficulties

If you are experiencing breathing difficulty, call your doctor immediately. Beta-blockers can cause a spasm in the air passages of the lungs (bronchospasm) and bring on asthmatic wheezing. Therefore, beta-blockers should not be used if you have asthma, bronchospasm, chronic bronchitis, or emphysema. Atenolol and metoprolol are less likely to cause difficulty with breathing, but they are not always completely free of respiratory adverse effects.

Low Blood Sugar

Beta-blockers may mask signs of low blood sugar (such as blood pressure changes, increased heart rate). Diabetics on beta-blockers must learn to recognize sweating as a sign of low blood sugar. For these reasons, beta-blockers are not often used in diabetics. If you are diabetic and must take a beta-blocker, atenolol may be the best choice, since it does not delay recovery of normal blood glucose levels.

Liver Function Impairment

Atenolol and nadolol are the best choices because their primary method of elimination from the body does not involve the liver. In older adults, the liver does not work as well to break down drugs and other compounds so that they can be eliminated safely from the body.

Kidney Function Impairment

Metoprolol, timolol, propranolol, and labetalol are the best choices because their primary method of elimination from the body does not depend on the kidneys.

Raynaud's Syndrome or Problems with Blood Supply to the Extremities (Hands and Feet)

In addition to its beta-blocking properties, labetalol also dilates blood vessels and increases blood supply to the extremities. Raynaud's syndrome is the only reason to prefer labetalol over the other beta-blockers.[30]

Dizziness, Lightheadedness, Low Blood Pressure

Labetalol causes these adverse effects most often. The high incidence of adverse effects makes labetalol a beta-blocker drug of second choice in treating uncomplicated high blood pressure.

CALCIUM CHANNEL BLOCKERS

Despite the 1993 recommendations of the National Institutes of Health's National Heart, Lung, and Blood Institute that diuretics and beta-blockers should be used first in the treatment of mild to moderate high blood pressure, the calcium channel blockers remain the largest selling family of high-blood-pressure-lowering drugs in the U.S.[31]

There are four new members of the calcium channel blocking family on the market. These are amlodipine (NORVASC), felodipine (PLENDIL), nisoldipine (SULAR), and mibefradil (POSICOR). None of these drugs offer any therapeutic advantage over older calcium channel blockers. Amlodipine has been shown not to worsen heart failure and mibefradil is significantly more dangerous than other calcium channel blockers because of the additional risk of drug interactions. Mibefradil was eventually banned from the market on June 8, 1998 because of its dangers.

In 1995, Public Citizen's Health Research Group filed a petition with the Food and Drug Administration to add warnings to the labeling of all calcium channel blockers about the increased risk of heart attack and death. Our petition was based on three well conducted observational research studies.[32,33,34] Observational studies are frequently criticized by doctors who do not understand this type of research. Most of what we know about adverse drugs reactions and what we are likely to learn in the future comes from observational research. This type of research was used to show the link between cigarette smoking and lung cancer.

Our petition helped to bring about important labeling changes in February 1996 on one of the calcium channel blockers, the short-acting form of nifedipine. The labeling for this form of nifedipine now warns doctors that this product should not be used for the treatment of high blood pressure.

Since we filed our petition additional serious adverse effects have been associated with the use of calcium channel blockers. These include an increased risk of gastrointestinal bleeding in older adults.[35] Calcium channel blockers have been shown in some studies to increase the risk of cancer[36,37,38] including breast cancer in postmenopausal women.[39] However, another study has found no increase in the risk of cancer with the calcium channel blockers.[40]

CHOLESTEROL-LOWERING DRUGS

For People 70 or Older

It is clear that the relationship between moderately elevated cholesterol levels and increased risk of heart disease is not as clear as people get older. As geriatricians Fran Kaiser and John Morely have written: *"Given the uncertainty of the effects of cholesterol manipulation in older individuals, what should be the approach of the prudent geriatrician to hypercholesterolemia [elevated blood cholesterol*

levels]? In persons over 70 years of age, life-long dietary habits are often difficult to change and overzealous dietary manipulation may lead to failure to eat and subsequent malnutrition. Thus in this group minor dietary manipulations such as the addition of some oatmeal [or other sources of oat bran or soluble fiber] and beans and modest increases in the amount of fish eaten, may represent a rational approach. Recommending a modest increase in exercise would also seem appropriate. Beyond this, it would seem best to remember that the geriatrician's dictum is to use no drug for which there is not a clear indication."[41]

The use of cholesterol-lowering drugs in people 70 or older should be limited to patients with very high cholesterol levels (greater than 300 milligrams) and those who manifest cardiovascular disease (previous history of heart attack or angina).[42]

Older Adults Younger than 70

Some of the cholesterol-lowering drugs in the statin family have been shown to lower cardiac deaths and overall mortality. Lovastatin (MEVACOR), pravastatin (PRAVACHOL) and simvastatin (ZOCOR) have been shown to cause regression of heart lesions, and pravastatin and simvastatin have been shown to reduce, though by a small amount, coronary deaths and total mortality. However, even in those people who are under 70, drugs should not be the first choice for lowering cholesterol unless the levels are extremely high or other circumstances as discussed above exist.[43,44]

To lower cholesterol the first, safer, and less costly measure is to eat a low-fat diet, using mostly polyunsaturated fats (such as canola, corn, safflower, and sunflower oils) or monounsaturated fats (such as olive oil). A change from animal to vegetable proteins often corrects high cholesterol. However, it is inadvisable to go on a very low-fat diet. The main focus on cholesterol-lowering diets has been on saturated fat and cholesterol content, not soluble fiber. (When added to the diet, psyllium or oat bran is a safe, effective way of lowering cholesterol.) Exercise and weight reduction are also recommended. Conditions that aggravate high cholesterol, such as dependence on alcohol or tobacco, diabetes, high blood pressure, low magnesium or potassium, and thyroid disease, should be corrected before adding a cholesterol-reducing drug. If cholesterol remains high despite diet, add 10 grams of psyllium a day (see p. 380). Numerous studies have shown that psyllium, for example five grams twice a day, can significantly lower total cholesterol and LDL cholesterol.[45] Psyllium, a naturally occurring vegetable fiber, is clearly safer than any of the cholesterol-lowering drugs.

Cholesterol-Lowering Drugs and Cancer

Researchers from the University of California[46] have raised questions about the correlation between an increased risk of cancer and lifelong use of cholesterol-lowering drugs by millions of people who have no signs of illness other than an elevated blood cholesterol level. This research is based on animal studies and is sure to be controversial.

Animal studies consistently show a cancer-causing effect for the two most popular classes of cholesterol-lowering drugs, the fibrates or fibric acid derivatives, which include clofibrate (ATROMID-S) and gemfibrozil (LOPID), and the widely used statin drugs, fluvastatin (LESCOL), lovastatin (MEVACOR), pravastatin (PRAVACHOL), and simvastatin (ZOCOR). Evidence of a cancer-causing effect from these drugs based on clinical trials in humans is inconclusive because of inconsistent results and a follow-up period that, to date, is too short to detect some cancers which can take years to develop. The ultimate effect of cholesterol-lowering drugs in humans may not be known for decades.

As part of the Food and Drug Administration's requirements for getting a new drug approved, companies are required to report the result of cancer experiments on rodents (rats and mice). The most common technique is to give three groups of rodents different doses of a new drug for two years and then compare the incidence of cancer among these groups as well as with a fourth group that received a dummy drug called a placebo. Rats and mice are used because almost all known agents that cause cancer in humans have been found to cause it in these animals. The results of rodent studies are generally published in scientific journals, but are summarized in a product information sheet, or "package insert," distributed to the pharmacist with each prescription drug. You can get a package insert for any drug you are taking by asking your pharmacist for one.

Researchers have taken the rodent cancer data from the 1992 and 1994 editions of the *Physicians' Desk Reference*® (*PDR,* a compilation of package inserts available in many public libraries). The package inserts for cholesterol-lowering drugs show that all the fibrates and statins cause cancer in rats and mice. In most instances, cancer-causing dose levels corresponded to maximums recommended for humans.

How should consumers weigh the worrisome, but uncertain, risk of cancer based on animal studies against the demonstrated benefits of lowering cholesterol? With some caution.

On the one hand, the study's authors clearly state that they do not know whether or not treatment with these cholesterol-lowering drugs will lead to an increased rate of cancer in coming decades. They believe that, for patients with known heart disease, the recent studies suggest that benefits of cholesterol-lowering drugs exceed their risks, at least in men and in the short term (five years). Given the strength of this evidence, it is reasonable to treat high blood cholesterol with drugs in patients with heart or other atherosclerotic disease. On the other hand, for patients not at high short-term risk of heart disease (especially patients with life expectancies of more than 10 to 20 years), drug treatment should probably be avoided. For this group, the benefits of treatment are smaller and the potential risk of increased cancer in the decades after treatment is of greater concern. The authors suggest that cholesterol-lowering drug treatment should be avoided except in patients at high short-term risk of coronary heart disease.

The safest course is to control cholesterol through changes in diet and lifestyle rather than with drugs, because this way there is no potential risk of drug-induced cancer. People who have heart disease and high blood-cholesterol levels should not hesitate to use these drugs because their benefits outweigh the risks. At the same time, however, they should also try to control their cholesterol through diet and exercise.

We list the fibrate drug, gemfibrozil (p. 121) as **"Do Not Use."** This was done because there is no proof that gemfibrozil has any health benefit, such as lowering the chance of having a heart attack, for most people with high blood cholesterol or fat levels. The other fibrate, clofibrate is not listed in the book, but is required by the FDA to carry the following warning:

BECAUSE OF THE TUMORIGENICITY [CANCER-CAUSING POTENTIAL] OF CLOFIBRATE IN RODENTS AND THE POSSIBLE INCREASED RISK OF MALIGNANCY ASSOCIATED WITH CLOFIBRATE IN THE HUMAN, AS WELL AS THE INCREASED RISK OF CHOLELITHIASIS [GALLSTONES], AND BECAUSE THERE IS NOT, TO DATE, SUBSTANTIAL EVIDENCE OF A BENEFICIAL EFFECT ON CARDIOVASCULAR MORTALITY FROM CLOFIBRATE, THIS DRUG SHOULD BE USED ONLY [IN SPECIAL SITUATIONS].

If you must use a cholesterol-lowering drug, the fibrate family should generally be avoided.

DRUG PROFILES

 Do Not Use

ALTERNATIVE TREATMENT:
See Hydrochlorothizade, p. 100.

Nifedipine, Short-Acting Forms
ADALAT (Bayer)
PROCARDIA (Pfizer)

FAMILY: Calcium Channel Blockers (see p. 53)

Most of the evidence associating the calcium channel blockers with serious adverse reactions was with the short-acting form of nifedipine. This led the National Heart, Lung and Blood Institute to declare in August 1995 that "short-acting nifedipine should be used with great caution (if at all), especially at higher doses, in the treatment of hypertension, angina, and MI."[47] The countless injuries and deaths that occurred when short-acting nifedipine was used to treat chronic high blood pressure or high blood pressure emergencies were preventable tragedies. This form of nifedipine is approved by the FDA only for the treatment of chest pain (angina). It has never been approved to treat any type of high blood pressure, including high blood pressure emergencies. In fact, in 1985 an FDA advisory committee voted unanimously not to recommend that short-acting nifedipine be approved to treat high blood pressure emergencies.[48] An article in the *Journal of the American Medical Association* called for a moratorium on the use of short-acting nifedipine to treat high blood pressure emergencies.[49]

If you have high blood pressure, the best way to reduce or eliminate your need for medication is by improving your diet, losing weight, exercising, and decreasing your salt and alcohol intake. Mild hypertension can be controlled by proper nutrition and exercise. If these measures do not lower your blood pressure enough and you need medication, **hydrochlorothiazide, a water pill (see thiazide diuretics, p. 100), is the drug of choice, starting with a low dose of 12.5 milligrams daily.** It also costs less than other blood pressure drugs.

There is now good evidence that thiazide diuretics, such as hydrochlorothiazide, significantly decrease the rate of bone mineral loss in both men and women because they reduce the amount of calcium lost in the urine. An increasing number of researchers think that this will also decrease the number of fractures.[50]

If this drug does not lower your blood pressure enough, your doctor can prescribe a second type of drug called a beta-blocker (see p. 52) to accompany the hydrochlorothiazide. If you cannot take a beta-blocker, a drug from another family (calcium channel blockers) can be used instead.

Whatever drugs you take for high blood pressure, once your blood pressure has been normal for a year or more, a cautious decrease in dose and renewed attention to nondrug treatment may be worth trying, according to *The Medical Letter.*[51]

And an editorial in the *British Medical Journal* stated: *"Treatment of hypertension is part of preventive medicine and like all preventive strategies, its progress should be regularly reviewed by whoever initiates it. Many problems could be avoided by not starting antihypertensive treatment until after prolonged observation. . . . Patients should no longer be told that treatment is necessarily for life: the possibility of reducing or stopping treatment should be mentioned at the outset."*[52]

 Do Not Use

ALTERNATIVE TREATMENT:
See Hydrochlorothiazide, p. 100.

Spironolactone and Hydrochlorothiazide
ALDACTAZIDE (Searle)

FAMILY: Diuretics
Antihypertensives
(See High Blood Pressure, p. 44)

This product, a combination of spironolactone (see p. 58) and hydrochlorothiazide (see p. 100), is used to treat high blood pressure (hypertension). **Older adults should not use drugs that contain a fixed combination of spironolactone and hydrochlorothiazide.**

Spironolactone can cause severe adverse effects. It is especially dangerous for people with kidney disease.[53,54] **It can cause kidney failure, retention of too much potassium,**[55,56,57,58] **muscle paralysis,**[59] **and mental confusion**[60] **in older adults.** These effects may be fatal. Spironolactone has also been found to cause leukemia and liver, thyroid, testicular, and breast cancer in rats.[61]

In addition to spironolactone's dangers, there are good reasons not to use any fixed-combination drug for high blood pressure. A single drug is often enough to control high blood pressure. If a combination drug like this one is controlling your high blood pressure, it is quite possible that one drug alone would do the same job. There is no reason to put yourself at extra risk by taking drugs you do not need.

If you have high blood pressure, the best way to reduce or eliminate your need for medication is by improving your diet, losing weight, exercising, and decreasing your intake of salt and alcohol. Mild hypertension can be controlled by proper nutrition and exercise. If these measures do not lower your blood pressure enough and you need medication, **hydrochlorothiazide, a water pill (see thiazide diuretics, p. 100),**

is the drug of choice, starting with a low dose of 12.5 milligrams daily. It also costs less than other blood pressure drugs.

There is now good evidence that thiazide diuretics, such as hydrochlorothiazide, significantly decrease the rate of bone mineral loss in both men and women because they reduce the amount of calcium lost in the urine. An increasing number of researchers think that this will also decrease the number of fractures.[62]

If your high blood pressure is severe and hydrochlorothiazide alone does not control it, there are still better drug treatments than the combination of hydrochlorothiazide and spironolactone. The best treatment in this case is a combination of hydrochlorothiazide and a second type of drug called a beta-blocker, such as propranolol (see p. 154). If you can't take a drug in the beta-blocker family, another drug called a calcium channel blocker may be used instead. In either case, your doctor would prescribe the hydrochlorothiazide and the second drug separately, with the dose of each drug adjusted to meet your needs, rather than using a product that combines the drugs in advance in a fixed combination.

If you are taking this fixed-combination drug, ask your doctor about changing your prescription.

Whatever drugs you take for high blood pressure, once your blood pressure has been normal for a year or more, a cautious decrease in dose and renewed attention to nondrug treatment may be worth trying, according to *The Medical Letter.*[63]

And an editorial in the *British Medical Journal* stated: *"Treatment of hypertension is part of preventive medicine and like all preventive strategies, its progress should be regularly reviewed by whoever initiates it. Many problems could be avoided by not starting antihypertensive treatment until after prolonged observation. . . . Patients should no longer be told that treatment is necessarily for life: the possibility of reducing or stopping treatment should be mentioned at the outset."*[64]

━━━━━━━━

Limited Use

Spironolactone
ALDACTONE (Searle)

GENERIC: available
FAMILY: Diuretics
Antihypertensives
(See High Blood Pressure, p. 44)

Spironolactone (speer on oh *lak* tone) is a water pill (diuretic) that removes less of the mineral potassium from your body than other types of diuretics do. Doctors sometimes prescribe it for high blood pressure, instead of another diuretic, in the hope that it will prevent a potassium imbalance, but there is no guarantee that this will work.

Spironolactone can cause severe adverse effects. It is especially dangerous for people with kidney disease.[65,66] **It can cause kidney failure, retention of too much potassium,[67,68,69,70] muscle paralysis,[71] and mental confusion[72,73,74] in older adults.** These effects may be fatal. Spironolactone has also been found to cause leukemia as well as liver, thyroid, testicular, and breast cancer in rats.[75]

Because of its dangers, spironolactone is not the best drug for treating high blood pressure or water retention. Older adults should not use spironolactone just for its ability to keep potassium in the body. If you need extra potassium, you can adjust your diet or take potassium supplements. Both methods are equally effective[76] (see p. 49) and are safer than using spironolactone. The only reason for an older adult to use this drug is to control a rare condition in which the body releases too much aldosterone (a hormone that regulates potassium and sodium levels).

If you have high blood pressure, the best way to reduce or eliminate your need for medication is by improving your diet, losing weight, exercising, and decreasing your salt and alcohol intake. Mild hypertension can be controlled by proper nutrition and exercise. If these measures do not lower your blood pressure enough and you need medication, **hydrochlorothiazide, a water pill (see thiazide diuretics, p. 100), is the drug of choice, starting with a low dose of 12.5 milligrams daily.** It also costs less than other blood pressure drugs.

There is now good evidence that thiazide diuretics, such as hydrochlorothiazide, significantly decrease the rate of bone mineral loss in both men and women because they reduce the amount of calcium lost in the urine. An increasing number of researchers think that this will also decrease the number of fractures.[77]

If this drug does not lower your blood pressure enough, your doctor can prescribe a second type of drug called a beta-blocker (see p. 52) to accompany the hydrochlorothiazide. If you cannot take a beta-blocker, a drug from another family (calcium channel blockers) can be used instead.

Whatever drugs you take for high blood pressure, once your blood pressure has been normal for a year or more, a cautious decrease in dose and renewed attention to nondrug treatment may be worth trying, according to *The Medical Letter.*[78]

And an editorial in the *British Medical Journal* stated: *"Treatment of hypertension is part of preventive medicine and like all preventive strategies, its progress should be regularly reviewed by whoever initiates it. Many problems could be avoided by not starting antihypertensive treatment until after prolonged observation. . . . Patients should no longer be told that treatment is necessarily for life: the possibility of reducing or stopping treatment should be mentioned at the outset."*[79]

Before You Use This Drug

Tell your doctor if you have or have had:

- allergies to drugs
- diabetes
- heart, kidney, or liver problems
- menstrual problems
- breast enlargement

Tell your doctor about any other drugs you take, including aspirin, herbs, vitamins, and other nonprescription products.

When You Use This Drug

- Do not use potassium supplements, salt substitutes (potassium chloride), or potassium-rich foods.
- If you plan to have any surgery, including dental, tell your doctor that you take this drug.
- **Do not take any other drugs without first talking to your doctor—especially nonprescription drugs for appetite control, asthma, colds, coughs, hay fever, or sinus problems.**

HEAT STRESS ALERT

This drug can affect your body's ability to adjust to heat, putting you at risk of "heat stress." If you live alone, ask a friend to check on you several times during the day. Early signs of heat stress are dizziness, lightheadedness, faintness, and slightly high temperature. Call your doctor if you have any of these signs.

Drink more fluids (water, fruit and vegetable juices) than usual—even if you're not thirsty—unless your doctor has told you otherwise. Do not drink alcohol.

How to Use This Drug

- Take with food or milk to avoid stomach irritation.

• If you miss a dose, take it as soon as you remember, but skip it if it is almost time for the next dose. **Do not take double doses.**

• Do not store in the bathroom. Do not expose to heat, moisture, or strong light.

Interactions with Other Drugs

The following drugs are listed in the *Evaluations of Drug Interactions* 1997 as causing "highly clinically significant" or "clinically significant" interactions when used together with this drug. We have also included potentially serious interactions listed in the drug's FDA-approved professional product labeling or package insert. New scientific techniques have allowed researchers to predict some drug interactions before they have been documented in people. There may be other drugs, especially those in the families of drugs listed below, that also will react with this drug to cause severe adverse effects. The number of new drugs approved for marketing increases the chance of drug interactions, and new drug interactions are being identified with old drugs. Be vigilant. Make sure to tell your doctor and pharmacist the drugs you are taking and tell your doctor if you are taking any of these interacting drugs:

cholestyramine, digoxin, guanethidine, ISMELIN, K-LOR, KATO, LANOXICAPS, LANOXIN, LOCHOLEST, potassium chloride, QUESTRAN, SLOW-K.

Adverse Effects

Call your doctor immediately if you experience:

• **signs of potassium imbalance:** confusion, anxiety, irregular heartbeat, numbness or tingling in hands, feet, lips, difficulty breathing, unusual tiredness or weakness, heavy legs
• sore throat and fever

• skin rash or itching
• cough or hoarseness
• fever or chills
• lower back or side pain
• painful or difficult urination
• severe or continuing nausea, vomiting, or diarrhea
• postmenopausal bleeding
• breast enlargement or tenderness

Call your doctor if these symptoms continue:

• drowsiness
• diarrhea, stomach cramps
• inability to get or keep an erection
• unusual sweating
• voice deepening and breast tenderness, increased hair growth in women
• enlarged breasts in men
• irregular menstrual periods
• dry mouth, increased thirst
• nausea, vomiting
• mental confusion
• stumbling, clumsiness
• dizziness
• headache
• decreased sexual ability

Periodic Tests

Ask your doctor which of these tests should be done periodically while you are taking this drug:

• blood pressure
• complete blood count
• kidney function tests
• blood levels of potassium and sodium (weekly when first starting to use the drug)

Do Not Use

ALTERNATIVE TREATMENT:
See Hydrochlorothiazide, p. 100.

Methyldopa
ALDOMET (Merck)

FAMILY: Antihypertensives
(See High Blood Pressure, p. 44)

Methyldopa (meth ill *doe* pa) **is an outdated medicine for treating high blood pressure (hypertension) in older adults.** It can cause severe depression and is particularly dangerous for anyone with a history of depression. Methyldopa can also cause other severe adverse effects, including drug-induced parkinsonism (see p. 25), decreased mental sharpness, and autoimmune problems such as the destruction of blood cells and liver disease (hepatitis).

Many newer drugs are available that do not have methyldopa's severe adverse effects (see p. 44).

If you have high blood pressure, the best way to reduce or eliminate your need for medication is by improving your diet, losing weight, exercising, and decreasing your salt and alcohol intake. Mild hypertension can be controlled by proper nutrition and exercise. If these measures do not lower your blood pressure enough and you need medication, **hydrochlorothiazide, a water pill (see thiazide diuretics, p. 100), is the drug of choice starting with a low dose of 12.5 milligrams daily.** It also costs less than other blood pressure drugs.

There is now good evidence that thiazide diuretics, such as hydrochlorothiazide, significantly decrease the rate of bone mineral loss in both men and women because they reduce the amount of calcium lost in the urine. An increasing number of researchers think that this will also decrease the number of fractures.[80]

If this drug does not lower your blood pressure enough, your doctor can prescribe a second type of drug called a beta-blocker (see p. 52) to accompany the hydrochlorothiazide. If you cannot take a beta-blocker, a drug from another family (calcium channel blockers) can be used instead.

Whatever drugs you take for high blood pressure, once your blood pressure has been normal for a year or more, a cautious decrease in dose and renewed attention to nondrug treatment may be worth trying, according to *The Medical Letter.*[81]

And an editorial in the *British Medical Journal* stated: *"Treatment of hypertension is part of preventive medicine and like all preventive strategies, its progress should be regularly reviewed by whoever initiates it. Many problems could be avoided by not starting antihypertensive treatment until after prolonged observation. . . . Patients should no longer be told that treatment is necessarily for life: the possibility of reducing or stopping treatment should be mentioned at the outset."*[82]

Do Not Use

ALTERNATIVE TREATMENT:
See Hydrochlorothiazide, p. 100.

Methyldopa and Hydrochlorothiazide
ALDORIL (Merck)

FAMILY: Diuretics
Antihypertensives
(See High Blood Pressure, p. 44)

This product, a combination of methyldopa (see this page) and hydrochlorothiazide (see p. 100), is used to treat high blood pressure (hypertension). **Older adults should not use drugs that contain a fixed combination of methyldopa and hydrochlorothiazide.**

Methyldopa is an outdated medicine for treating high blood pressure (hypertension) in older adults. It can cause severe depression and is particularly dangerous to anyone with a history of depression. Methyldopa can also cause other severe adverse effects, including drug-induced parkinsonism (see p. 25), decreased mental sharpness, and autoimmune problems such as the destruction of blood cells and liver disease (hepatitis).

In addition to methyldopa's dangers, there are good reasons not to use any fixed-combination drug for high blood pressure. A single drug is often enough to control high blood pressure. If a combination drug like this one is controlling your high blood pressure, it is quite possible that one drug alone would do the same job. There is no reason to put yourself at extra risk by taking drugs you do not need.

If you have high blood pressure, the best way to reduce or eliminate your need for medication is by improving your diet, losing weight, exercising, and decreasing your salt and alcohol intake. Mild hypertension can be controlled by proper nutrition and exercise. If these measures do not lower your blood pressure enough and you need medication, **hydrochlorothiazide, a water pill (see thiazide diuretics, p. 100), is the drug of choice starting with a low dose of 12.5 milligrams daily.** It also costs less than other blood pressure drugs.

There is now good evidence that thiazide diuretics, such as hydrochlorothiazide, significantly decrease the rate of bone mineral loss in both men and women because they reduce the amount of calcium lost in the urine. An increasing number of researchers think that this will also decrease the number of fractures.[83]

Hydrochlorothiazide is one of the ingredients in this combination. The other ingredient, methyldopa, can cause severe adverse effects, as described above. If hydrochlorothiazide alone would control your high blood pressure, there is no reason to take the extra risk of using methyldopa as well.

If your high blood pressure is more severe and hydrochlorothiazide alone does not control it, there are still better drug treatments than this combination product. The best treatment in this case is a combination of hydrochlorothiazide and a second type of drug called a beta-blocker, such as propranolol (see p. 154). If you can't take a drug in the beta-blocker family, another drug called a calcium channel blocker may be used instead. In either case, your doctor would prescribe the hydrochlorothiazide and the second drug separately, with the dose of each drug adjusted to meet your needs, rather than using a product that combines the drugs in advance in a fixed combination.

If you are taking this fixed-combination drug, ask your doctor about changing your prescription.

Whatever drugs you take for high blood pressure, once your blood pressure has been normal for a year or more, a cautious decrease in dose and renewed attention to nondrug treatment may be worth trying, according to *The Medical Letter.*[84]

And an editorial in the *British Medical Journal* stated: *"Treatment of hypertension is part of preventive medicine and like all preventive strategies, its progress should be regularly reviewed by whoever initiates it. Many problems could be avoided by not starting antihypertensive treatment until after prolonged observation. . . . Patients should no longer be told that treatment is necessarily for life: the possibility of reducing or stopping treatment should be mentioned at the outset."*[85]

Limited Use

Hydralazine and Hydrochlorothiazide
APRESAZIDE (CIBA)

GENERIC: available

FAMILY: Diuretics
Antihypertensives
(See High Blood Pressure, p. 44)

This product, a combination of hydralazine (see p. 64) and hydrochlorothiazide (see p. 100), is used to treat high blood pressure (hypertension). Drugs containing a fixed combination of hydralazine and hydrochlorothiazide offer limited benefit.

Hydralazine is not the first-choice drug for treating high blood pressure because of its adverse effects. People with heart failure should not take it.[86] Common adverse effects of this drug include rapid heartbeat and abnormally low blood pressure, which may cause lightheadedness, fainting, and falling.[87] Hydralazine may worsen chest pain (angina).[88]

In addition to hydralazine's dangers, there are good reasons not to use any fixed-combination drug for high blood pressure. A single drug is often enough to control high blood pressure. If a combination drug like this one is controlling your high blood pressure, it is quite possible that one drug alone would do the same

job. There is no reason to put yourself at extra risk by taking drugs you do not need.

If you have high blood pressure, the best way to reduce or eliminate your need for medication is by improving your diet, losing weight, exercising, and decreasing your salt and alcohol intake. Mild hypertension can be controlled by proper nutrition and exercise. If these measures do not lower your blood pressure enough and you need medication, **hydrochlorothiazide, a water pill (see thiazide diuretics, p. 100), is the drug of choice starting with a low dose of 12.5 milligrams daily.** It also costs less than other blood pressure drugs.

There is now good evidence that thiazide diuretics, such as hydrochlorothiazide, significantly decrease the rate of bone mineral loss in both men and women because they reduce the amount of calcium lost in the urine. An increasing number of researchers think that this will also decrease the number of fractures.[89]

Hydrochlorothiazide is one of the ingredients in this combination. Hydralazine can cause severe adverse effects, as described above. If hydrochlorothiazide alone would control your blood pressure, there is no reason to take the extra risk of taking the second drug as well.

If your high blood pressure is more severe and hydrochlorothiazide alone does not control it, the best treatment is a combination of

---

WARNING

This fixed-combination drug should not be the first drug used to treat your high blood pressure. You may not need more than one drug. If you do need two drugs, the fixed-combination product may not contain the dose of each drug that is right for you. Your doctor has to regularly check your condition and reevaluate the effect of the drug(s) you take. This may mean adjusting doses, and even changing drugs, to ensure proper treatment. A fixed-combination drug may be the best drug for you, but it should be used only after you have tried each of its ingredients separately, in varying doses. If the doses that you need to control your high blood pressure match those in a fixed-combination product, use it. See Hydralazine, p. 64 and hydrochlorothiazide, p. 100, for more information on the use of these and other drugs and potentially harmful interactions.

hydrochlorothiazide and a second type of drug called a beta-blocker, such as propranolol (see p. 154). If you can't take a drug in the beta-blocker family, another drug called a calcium channel blocker may be used instead. In either case, your doctor would prescribe the hydrochlorothiazide and the second drug separately, with the dose of each drug adjusted to meet your needs, rather than using a product that combines the drugs in advance in a fixed combination.

If you are taking this fixed-combination drug, ask your doctor about changing your prescription.

Whatever drugs you take for high blood pressure, once your blood pressure has been normal for a year or more, a cautious decrease in dose and renewed attention to nondrug treatment may be worth trying, according to *The Medical Letter.*[90]

And an editorial in the *British Medical Journal* stated: *"Treatment of hypertension is part of preventive medicine and like all preventive strategies, its progress should be regularly reviewed by whoever initiates it. Many problems could be avoided by not starting antihypertensive treatment until after prolonged observation. . . . Patients should no longer be told that treatment is necessarily for life: the possibility of reducing or stopping treatment should be mentioned at the outset."*[91]

HEAT STRESS ALERT

This drug can affect your body's ability to adjust to heat, putting you at risk of "heat stress." If you live alone, ask a friend to check on you several times during the day. Early signs of heat stress are dizziness, lightheadedness, faintness, and slightly high temperature. Call your doctor if you have any of these signs.

Drink more fluids (water, fruit and vegetable juices) than usual—even if you're not thirsty—unless your doctor has told you otherwise. Do not drink alcohol.

PREGNANCY WARNING

This drug caused harm to developing fetuses in animal studies, or such studies were not done. Use during pregnancy only for clear medical reasons. Tell your doctor if you are pregnant or thinking of becoming pregnant before you take this drug.

Hydralazine
APRESOLINE (CIBA)

GENERIC: available

FAMILY: Antihypertensives
(See High Blood Pressure, p. 44)

Hydralazine (hye *dral* a zeen) is used to treat high blood pressure (hypertension), but it is not the first-choice drug for this purpose. People with coronary artery disease should not use hydralazine at all.[92]

If you have high blood pressure, the best way to reduce or eliminate your need for medication is by improving your diet, losing weight, exercising, and decreasing your salt and alcohol intake. Mild hypertension can be controlled by proper nutrition and exercise. If these measures do not lower your blood pressure enough and you need medication, **hydrochlorothiazide, a water pill (see thiazide diuretics, p. 100), is the drug of choice starting with a low dose of 12.5 milligrams daily.** It also costs less than other blood pressure drugs.

There is now good evidence that thiazide diuretics, such as hydrochlorothiazide, significantly decrease the rate of bone mineral loss in both men and women because they reduce the amount of calcium lost in the urine. An increasing number of researchers think that this will also decrease the number of fractures.[93]

If this drug does not lower your blood pressure enough, your doctor can prescribe a second type of drug called a beta-blocker (see p. 52) to accompany the hydrochlorothiazide. If you cannot take a beta-blocker, a drug from another family (calcium channel blockers) can be used instead.

Whatever drugs you take for high blood pressure, once your blood pressure has been normal for a year or more, a cautious decrease in dose and renewed attention to nondrug treatment may be worth trying, according to *The Medical Letter.*[94]

And an editorial in the *British Medical Journal* stated: *"Treatment of hypertension is part of preventive medicine and like all preventive strategies, its progress should be regularly reviewed by whoever initiates it. Many problems could be avoided by not starting antihypertensive treatment until after prolonged observation. . . . Patients should no longer be told that treatment is necessarily for life: the possibility of reducing or stopping treatment should be mentioned at the outset."*[95]

A major problem with hydralazine is that after you take it for 4 to 24 months, you are likely to develop a "tolerance" for it.[96] This means that as time goes on, the same amount of the drug will have less and less effect. Because of this problem, your doctor should try other drugs—a combination of a water pill (diuretic) and a beta-blocker such as propranolol (see p. 154)—before prescribing hydralazine. If this combination fails to bring your diastolic blood pressure below 100 millimeters of mercury, your doctor should then consider hydralazine.[97]

Hydralazine commonly causes a rapid heartbeat and below normal blood pressure, which may lead to lightheadedness, fainting, and a risk of falling. It may also make chest pain (angina) worse.[98]

The starting dose of hydralazine should be between 10 and 12.5 milligrams (mg), four times a day. The total daily dose should not go over 150 to 200 milligrams.[99] **If you have impaired kidney function, you should be taking a smaller dose.**

Before You Use This Drug

Do not use if you have or have had:

- aortic aneurysm
- disease of the arteries that nourish the heart
- disease of the blood vessels that nourish the brain
- rheumatic heart disease
- severe heart disease
- severe kidney disease

Tell your doctor if you have or have had:

- allergies to drugs
- congestive heart failure
- kidney disease

Tell your doctor about any other drugs you take, including aspirin, herbs, vitamins, and other nonprescription products.

When You Use This Drug

- Until you know how you react to this drug, do not drive or perform other activities requiring alertness.
- **Do not stop taking this drug suddenly. Your doctor must give you a schedule to decrease your dose gradually.**
- You may feel dizzy when rising from a lying or sitting position. When getting out of bed, hang your legs over the side of the bed for a few minutes, then get up slowly. When getting up from a chair, get up slowly and stay beside the chair until you are sure that you are not dizzy. (See p. 16.)
- If you plan to have any surgery, including dental, tell your doctor that you take this drug.
- **Do not take other drugs without talking to your doctor first—especially nonprescription drugs for appetite control, asthma, colds, coughs, hay fever, or sinus problems.**
- You may need more vitamin B_6 (pyridoxine) than usual. Ask your doctor about getting

more vitamin B$_6$ in your diet or about taking a supplement.

- Do not drink alcohol.

How to Use This Drug

- Take with food. Crush tablet and mix with food or drink, or swallow whole with water.
- Keep the liquid form in the refrigerator. Do not use it after 14 days or if its color changes. Replace it.
- If you miss a dose, take it as soon as you remember, but skip it if it is almost time for the next dose. **Do not take double doses.**
- Call your doctor if you miss two doses in a row.
- Do not store in the bathroom. Do not expose to heat, moisture, or strong light.

Interactions with Other Drugs

Some other drugs that you may be taking (either over-the-counter or prescription drugs) can interact with this one, causing adverse effects. Ask your doctor what these drugs are and let him or her know if you are taking any of them.

Adverse Effects

Call your doctor immediately if you experience:

- blisters on skin
- chest pain
- general discomfort or weakness
- muscle or joint pain
- numbness and tingling of hands and feet
- skin rash or itching
- sore throat and fever
- swelling of feet or lower legs
- swelling of lymph glands
- fever

Call your doctor if these symptoms continue:

- diarrhea or constipation

- loss of appetite
- nausea, vomiting
- rapid or irregular heartbeat
- redness or flushing of face
- shortness of breath on exertion
- dizziness, lightheadedness
- watering or irritated eyes
- headache
- stuffy nose (do not take any medication for this)

Periodic Tests

Ask your doctor which of these tests should be done periodically while you are taking this drug:

- blood pressure
- antinuclear antibody titer
- complete blood count
- direct Coombs' test
- lupus erythematosus (LE) cell preparation

PREGNANCY WARNING

This drug caused harm to developing fetuses in animal studies, or such studies were not done. Use during pregnancy only for clear medical reasons. Tell your doctor if you are pregnant or thinking of becoming pregnant before you take this drug.

Timolol
BLOCADREN (Merck)

GENERIC: available

FAMILY: Beta-blockers (See p. 52)
         Antihypertensives
         (See High Blood Pressure, p. 44)

Timolol (*tim* oh lole) has two forms for different uses: tablets for the heart (BLOCADREN) and drops for the eyes (TIMOPTIC, see p. 643). The tablet is used for high blood pressure (hypertension), chest pain (angina), and irregular heartbeats (arrhythmias), and to decrease the frequency of migraine headaches. **If you are over 60, you will generally need to take less than the usual adult dose of the tablet, especially if your liver function is impaired.** The eye drop is used for glaucoma.

Although this page discusses timolol primarily as a drug for heart and blood vessel disease, eye drop users may have some of the general adverse effects listed below, especially if the drops are used improperly. See p. 622 for instructions on using eye drugs properly.

For young adults with high blood pressure, doctors usually prescribe a drug in this family (a beta-blocker) before any other drug. But for African-Americans and older adults, these drugs are less effective as the sole treatment. For these groups of people, doctors usually prescribe another type of drug called a diuretic (water pill) to lower blood pressure, and add a beta-blocker, such as propranolol, as a second drug if the diuretic alone is not enough.

If you have high blood pressure, the best way to reduce or eliminate your need for medication is by improving your diet, losing weight, exercising, and decreasing your salt and alcohol intake. Mild hypertension can be controlled by proper nutrition and exercise. If these measures do not lower your blood pressure enough and you need medication, **hydrochlorothiazide, a water pill (see thiazide diuretics, p. 100), is the drug of choice starting with a low dose of 12.5 milligrams daily.** It also costs less than other blood pressure drugs.

There is now good evidence that thiazide diuretics, such as hydrochlorothiazide, significantly decrease the rate of bone mineral loss in both men and women because they reduce the amount of calcium lost in the urine. An increasing number of researchers think that this will also decrease the number of fractures.[100]

If this drug does not lower your blood pressure enough, your doctor can prescribe a second type of drug called a beta-blocker (see p. 52) to accompany the hydrochlorothiazide. If you cannot take a beta-blocker, a drug from another family (calcium channel blockers) can be used instead.

Whatever drugs you take for high blood pressure, once your blood pressure has been normal for a year or more, a cautious decrease in dose and renewed attention to nondrug treatment may be worth trying, according to *The Medical Letter.*[101]

And an editorial in the *British Medical Journal* stated: *"Treatment of hypertension is part of preventive medicine and like all preventive strategies, its progress should be regularly reviewed by whoever initiates it. Many problems could be avoided by not starting antihypertensive treatment until after prolonged observation. . . . Patients should no longer be told that treatment is necessarily for life: the possibility of reducing or stopping treatment should be mentioned at the outset."*[102]

All beta-blockers are similarly effective, although not necessarily interchangeable. If you are bothered by adverse effects when taking timolol, talk to your doctor about switching to another beta-blocker, such as propranolol, which is available generically. The adverse effects of these drugs vary widely, and each individual responds differently to each one. See p. 52 for a discussion of alternatives to timolol.

Timolol has been shown to cause an increased number of adrenal, lung, uterine, and breast cancers in rats.

Before You Use This Drug

Do not use if you have:

- congestive heart failure
- asthma
- emphysema or chronic bronchitis

Tell your doctor if you have or have had:

- allergies to drugs
- poor blood circulation

- diabetes
- difficulty breathing
- gout
- unusually slow heartbeat
- heart or blood vessel disease
- myasthenia gravis
- psoriasis
- kidney, liver, lung, or pancreas problems
- lupus erythematosus
- mental depression
- alcohol dependence
- Raynaud's syndrome
- thyroid problems

Tell your doctor about any other drugs you take, including aspirin, herbs, vitamins, and other nonprescription products.

When You Use This Drug

- **Learn to take your pulse, and get immediate medical help if your pulse slows to 50 beats per minute or slower, even if you are feeling well. Some people have suffered from slowed heart rate and heart failure while taking timolol.**
- Until you know how you react to this drug, do not drive or perform other activities requiring alertness.
- Be careful not to overexert yourself, even though your chest pain may feel better.
- **Do not stop taking this drug suddenly. Your doctor must give you a schedule to decrease your dose gradually, to prevent chest pain and possible heart attack.**
- You may feel dizzy when rising from a lying or sitting position. When getting out of bed, hang your legs over the side of the bed for a few minutes, then get up slowly. When getting up from a chair, get up slowly and stay beside the chair until you are sure that you are not dizzy. (See p. 16.)
- **Caution diabetics:** see p. 550.
- If you plan to have any surgery, including dental, tell your doctor that you take this drug.

- **Do not take other drugs without talking to your doctor first—especially non-prescription drugs for appetite control, asthma, colds, coughs, hay fever, or sinus problems.**

HEAT STRESS ALERT

This drug can affect your body's ability to adjust to heat, putting you at risk of "heat stress." If you live alone, ask a friend to check on you several times during the day. Early signs of heat stress are dizziness, lightheadedness, faintness, and slightly high temperature. Call your doctor if you have any of these signs.

Drink more fluids (water, fruit and vegetable juices) than usual—even if you're not thirsty—unless your doctor has told you otherwise. Do not drink alcohol.

How to Use This Drug

- Crush tablets and mix with water, or swallow whole with water.
- If you miss a dose, take it as soon as you remember, unless it is less than four hours until your next scheduled dose. **Do not take double doses.**
- Do not store in the bathroom. Do not expose to heat, moisture, or strong light.

Interactions with Other Drugs

The following drugs are listed in the *Evaluations of Drug Interactions* 1997 as causing "highly clinically significant" or "clinically significant" interactions when used together with this drug. We have also included potentially serious interactions listed in the drug's FDA-approved professional product labeling or package insert. New scientific techniques have allowed researchers to predict some drug inter-actions before they have been documented in people. There may be other drugs, especially those in the families of drugs listed below, that also will react with this drug to cause severe adverse effects. The number of new drugs approved for marketing increases the chance of drug interactions, and new drug interactions are being identified with old drugs. Be vigilant. Make sure to tell your doctor and pharmacist the drugs you are taking and tell your doctor if you are taking any of these interacting drugs:

ADRENALIN (also in bee sting kits), ALDOMET, amiodarone, CALAN SR, CATAPRES, chlorpromazine, cimetidine, clonidine, cocaine, CORDARONE, COUMADIN, COVERA-HS, ELIXOPHYLLIN, epinephrine, FLUOTHANE, furosemide, halothane, HUMALOG, HUMULIN, INDERAL, INDERAL LA, insulin, ISOPTIN SR, LASIX, LEVOTHROID, levothyroxine, lidocaine, lithium, LITHOBID, LITHONATE, methyldopa, mibefradil, MINIPRESS, NEMBUTAL, pentobarbital, POSICOR, prazosin, PRIMATENE MIST, propranolol, pseudoephedrine, RIFADIN, rifampin, RIMACTANE, SLO-BID, SUDAFED, SYNTHROID, TAGAMET, THEO-24, theophylline, THORAZINE, thyroid, tobacco, TUBARINE, tubocurarine, verapamil, VERELAN, warfarin, XYLOCAINE.

Adverse Effects

Call your doctor immediately if you experience:

- difficulty breathing and/or wheezing
- cold hands and feet
- depression
- slow heartbeat
- swelling of ankles, feet and/or lower legs

- back or joint pain
- chest pain
- confusion
- fever and sore throat
- hallucinations
- irregular heartbeat
- red, scaling or crusted skin
- skin rash
- unusual bleeding and bruising
- **signs of overdose**: slow heartbeat, severe dizziness, fast or irregular heartbeat, difficulty breathing, bluish-colored fingernails or palms of hands, convulsions
- headache

Call your doctor if these symptoms continue:

- decreased sexual ability
- dizziness or lightheadedness
- drowsiness
- trouble sleeping, nightmares, or vivid dreams
- unusual tiredness or weakness
- anxiety and/or nervousness
- itchiness
- nausea or vomiting
- numbness and/or tingling of fingers and/or toes
- stomach discomfort
- stuffy nose
- slow pulse

Call your doctor if these symptoms continue after you stop using the medication:

- chest pain
- irregular heartbeat
- general feeling of discomfort, illness, or weakness
- headache
- sudden shortness of breath
- sweating
- trembling

More adverse effects information appears on p. 52.

Periodic Tests

Ask your doctor which of these tests should be done periodically while you are taking this drug:

- complete blood count
- blood pressure and pulse rate
- heart function tests, such as electrocardiogram (ECG, EKG)
- kidney function tests
- liver function tests
- blood glucose levels
- eye pressure exams

PREGNANCY WARNING

This drug caused harm to developing fetuses in animal studies, or such studies were not done. Use during pregnancy only for clear medical reasons. Tell your doctor if you are pregnant or thinking of becoming pregnant before you take this drug.

Limited Use

Bumetanide
BUMEX (Roche)

GENERIC: not available

FAMILY: Diuretics
Antihypertensives
(See High Blood Pressure, p. 44)

Bumetanide (byoo *met* a nide) is a very strong "water pill" (diuretic) with many adverse effects. It is used to treat fluid retention and high blood pressure. If you are over 60, you should use bumetanide only for reducing fluid retention, and then only if you have decreased kidney function[103] and have already tried a milder drug such as hydrochlorothiazide (see p. 100) or the more proven and less expensive furosemide (see p. 116) without success.[104] People over 60 years old who have normal kidney function should rarely, if ever, use bumetanide.[105]

If you have high blood pressure, the best way to reduce or eliminate your need for medication is by improving your diet, losing weight, exercising, and decreasing your salt and alcohol intake. Mild hypertension can be controlled by proper nutrition and exercise. If these measures do not lower your blood pressure enough and you need medication, **hydrochlorothiazide, a water pill (see thiazide diuretics, p. 100), is the drug of choice starting with a low dose of 12.5 milligrams daily.** It also costs less than other blood pressure drugs.

There is now good evidence that thiazide diuretics, such as hydrochlorothiazide, significantly decrease the rate of bone mineral loss in both men and women because they reduce the amount of calcium lost in the urine. An increasing number of researchers think that this will also decrease the number of fractures.[106]

If hydrochlorothiazide alone does not work, your doctor should add a second drug, such as a beta-blocker, propranolol for example, (see p. 154) rather than switching you to a strong diuretic like bumetanide.[107]

Older adults are more likely than others to develop blood clots, shock,[108] dizziness, confusion, and insomnia, and have an increased chance of falling, while taking bumetanide.[109]

Whatever drugs you take for high blood pressure, once your blood pressure has been normal for a year or more, a cautious decrease in dose and renewed attention to nondrug treatment may be worth trying, according to *The Medical Letter*.[110]

And an editorial in the *British Medical Journal* stated: *"Treatment of hypertension is part of preventive medicine and like all preventive strategies, its progress should be regularly reviewed by whoever initiates it. Many prob-*

*lems could be avoided by not starting antihy-
pertensive treatment until after prolonged
observation. . . . Patients should no longer be
told that treatment is necessarily for life: the
possibility of reducing or stopping treatment
should be mentioned at the outset.*"[111]

Before You Use This Drug

Do not use if you have or have had:

- a sensitivity to sulfa drugs (sulfonamides)
  or yellow dye #5

Tell your doctor if you have or have had:

- allergies to drugs
- diabetes
- kidney, liver, or pancreas problems
- gout
- hearing loss
- recent heart attack
- lupus erythematosus
- salt- or sugar-restricted diet

*Tell your doctor about any other drugs you
take,* including aspirin, herbs, vitamins, and
other nonprescription products.

When You Use This Drug

- **Check with your doctor to make certain your fluid intake is adequate and
appropriate. Because bumetanide is a
very strong water pill, you are in danger
of becoming dehydrated.**
- You may feel dizzy when rising from a
lying or sitting position. When getting up from
bed, hang your legs over the side of the bed for
a few minutes, then get up slowly. When getting up from a chair, stay beside the chair
until you are sure that you are not dizzy. (See
p. 16.)
- **Bumetanide will cause your body to
lose potassium, an important mineral.** See
p. 49 for information on how to make sure you
get enough potassium.

- Bumetanide can cause a loss of hearing,
which is usually temporary but may be permanent. The risk of hearing loss is greater if you
are also using amphotericin B or an antibiotic
from the aminoglycoside family (see p. 635 for
two examples).
- If you plan to have any surgery, including
dental, tell your doctor that you take this drug.
- **Do not take other drugs without first
talking to your doctor—especially nonprescription drugs for appetite control,
asthma, colds, coughs, hay fever, or sinus
problems.**

HEAT STRESS ALERT

This drug can affect your body's ability to
adjust to heat, putting you at risk of "heat stress."
If you live alone, ask a friend to check on you several times during the day. Early signs of heat
stress are dizziness, lightheadedness, faintness,
and slightly high temperature. Call your doctor if
you have any of these signs.

Drink more fluids (water, fruit and vegetable
juices) than usual—even if you're not thirsty—
unless your doctor has told you otherwise. Do not
drink alcohol.

How to Use This Drug

- Take with food or milk to avoid stomach
irritation. Tablet may be crushed and mixed
with food or drink.
- If you are taking bumetanide more than
once a day, try to take the last dose before 6 P.M.
This will help you avoid interrupting your
sleep to go to the bathroom.
- If you miss a dose, take it as soon as you
remember, but skip it if it is almost time for the
next dose. **Do not take double doses.**
- Keep oral form from freezing.

• Do not store in the bathroom. Do not expose to heat, moisture, or strong light.

Interactions with Other Drugs

The following drugs are listed in the *Evaluations of Drug Interactions* 1997 as causing "highly clinically significant" or "clinically significant" interactions when used together with this drug. We have also included potentially serious interactions listed in the drug's FDA-approved professional product labeling or package insert. New scientific techniques have allowed researchers to predict some drug interactions before they have been documented in people. There may be other drugs, especially those in the families of drugs listed below, that also will react with this drug to cause severe adverse effects. The number of new drugs approved for marketing increases the chance of drug interactions, and new drug interactions are being identified with old drugs. Be vigilant. Make sure to tell your doctor and pharmacist the drugs you are taking and tell your doctor if you are taking any of these interacting drugs:

CAPOTEN, captopril, cephalexin, charcoal, chlorpropamide, cholestyramine, cisplatin, DIABINESE, digoxin, ELIXOPHYLLIN, INDERAL, INDERAL LA, KEFLEX, LANOXICAPS, LANOXIN, lithium, LITHOBID, LITHONATE, LOCHOLEST, PLATINOL, propranolol, QUESTRAN, SLO-BID, THEO-24, theophylline.

Adverse Effects

Call your doctor immediately if you experience:

• **signs of potassium loss**: dry mouth, increased thirst, irregular heartbeat, mood or mental changes, muscle cramps or pain, nausea, vomiting, unusual tiredness or weakness, weak pulse
  • skin rash or hives
  • chest pain
  • nipple tenderness
  • black, tarry stools
  • blood in urine or stools
  • cough or hoarseness
  • fever or chills
  • joint, lower back, or side pain
  • painful or difficult urination
  • pinpoint red spots on skin
  • ringing or buzzing in ears or hearing loss
  • severe stomach pain with nausea or vomiting
  • unusual bleeding or bruising
  • yellow eyes or skin

Call your doctor if these symptoms continue:

  • dizziness, lightheadedness
  • diarrhea
  • loss of appetite, upset stomach
  • headache
  • blurred vision
  • premature ejaculation or difficulty with erection
  • chest pain
  • redness or pain at place of injection

Periodic Tests

Ask your doctor which of these tests should be done periodically while you are taking this drug:

  • blood pressure
  • complete blood count
  • blood levels of sodium, potassium, chloride, calcium, sugar, and uric acid
  • liver function tests
  • kidney function tests

<table>
<tr><td>

PREGNANCY WARNING

This drug caused harm to developing fetuses in animal studies, or such studies were not done. Use during pregnancy only for clear medical reasons. Tell your doctor if you are pregnant or thinking of becoming pregnant before you take this drug.

</td></tr>
</table>

Limited Use

Verapamil
CALAN, CALAN SR, COVERA-HS (Searle)
ISOPTIN, ISOPTIN SR (Knoll)
VERELAN (Lederle)

GENERIC: available
FAMILY: Calcium Channel Blockers (See p. 53)

Verapamil (ver *ap* a mill) belongs to a family of drugs called calcium channel blockers. They are used primarily to treat chest pain (angina) and coronary artery disease, and also to lower blood pressure (hypertension) and improve irregular heartbeats (arrhythmias). Calcium channel blockers control, but do not cure, high blood pressure. These drugs may improve capacity for exercise and delay the need for heart surgery.

In 1995, Public Citizen's Health Research Group filed a petition with the Food and Drug Administration to add warnings to the labeling of all calcium channel blockers about the increased risk of heart attack and death. Our petition was based on three well conducted observational research studies.[112,113,114] Observational studies are frequently criticized by doctors who do not understand this type of research. Most of what we know about adverse drug reactions and what we are likely to learn in the future comes from observational research. This type of research was used to show the link between cigarette smoking and lung cancer.

Our petition helped to bring about important labeling changes in February 1996 on one of the calcium channel blockers, the short-acting form of nifedipine. The labeling for this form of nifedipine now warns doctors that this product should not be used for the treatment of high blood pressure.

Since we filed our petition additional serious adverse reactions have been associated with the use of calcium channel blockers. These include an increased risk of gastrointestinal bleeding in older adults.[115] Calcium channel blockers have been shown in some studies to increase the risk of cancer[116,117,118] including breast cancer in postmenopausal women.[119] However, another study has found no increase in the risk of cancer with the calcium channel blockers.[120]

Despite the 1993 recommendations of the National Institutes of Health's National Heart, Lung, and Blood Institute that diuretics and beta-blockers should be used first in the treatment of mild to moderate high blood pressure the calcium channel blockers remain the largest selling family of high-blood-pressure-lowering drugs in the U.S.[121]

Each calcium channel blocker differs in the likelihood of harmful adverse effects. Verapamil, more than other calcium channel blockers, commonly causes constipation. It is more apt to slow heart rate, depress heart contraction, and slow conduction than other calcium channel blockers, but is less likely to cause dizziness, flushing, headache, and swelling of legs and feet.[122]

Compared to other calcium channel blockers, certain individuals are more apt to get congestive heart failure from verapamil.[123] Older adults may be more sensitive to harmful effects. A dose of 40 milligrams of verapamil three times a day is recommended when older people, those with liver disease, or certain heart conditions start to take it. People with decreased kidney function should avoid the long-acting forms of verapamil[124] and may require a low dose. It is sometimes taken with other heart medications.

If you have high blood pressure, the best way to reduce or eliminate your need for medication is by improving your diet, losing weight, exercising, and decreasing your salt and alcohol intake. Mild hypertension can be controlled by proper nutrition and exercise. If these measures do not lower your blood pressure enough and you need medication, **hydrochlorothiazide, a water pill (see thiazide diuretics, p. 100), is the drug of choice starting with a low dose of 12.5 milligrams daily.** It also costs less than other blood pressure drugs.

There is now good evidence that thiazide diuretics, such as hydrochlorothiazide, significantly decrease the rate of bone mineral loss in both men and women because they reduce the amount of calcium lost in the urine. An increasing number of researchers think that this will also decrease the number of fractures.[125]

If this drug does not lower your blood pressure enough, your doctor can prescribe a second type of drug called a beta-blocker (see p. 52) to accompany the hydrochlorothiazide. If you cannot take a beta-blocker, a drug from this family (calcium channel blockers) can be used instead.

Whatever drugs you take for high blood pressure, once your blood pressure has been normal for a year or more, a cautious decrease in dose and renewed attention to nondrug treatment may be worth trying, according to *The Medical Letter.*[126]

And an editorial in the *British Medical Journal* stated: *"Treatment of hypertension is part of preventive medicine and like all preventive strategies, its progress should be regularly reviewed by whoever initiates it. Many prob-lems could be avoided by not starting antihypertensive treatment until after prolonged observation. . . . Patients should no longer be told that treatment is necessarily for life: the possibility of reducing or stopping treatment should be mentioned at the outset."*[127]

CALCIUM CHANNEL BLOCKERS ARE OVERUSED IN OLDER ADULT HEART ATTACK SURVIVORS

Research found that the calcium channel blockers are being overutilized by doctors treating older persons after a heart attack, while the beta-blocking drugs were being underutilized. None of the calcium channel blockers has been shown to improve survival in persons with heart disease. Some beta-blockers are approved by the Food and Drug Administration (FDA) to reduce the risk of death after a heart attack.

This research study looked at the use of calcium channel blockers and beta-blockers in 500 consecutive people being admitted to a nursing home. Heart diagnostic tests were done on all 500 at the time of admission. Of these people, 202 (40%) had experienced heart attacks. Only 17 (8%) were receiving a beta-blocker while 74 (37%) were receiving a calcium channel blocker.[128]

The beta-blockers approved by the FDA to reduce the risk of death after a heart attack are: atenolol (Tenormin), metoprolol (Lopressor, Toprol XL), propranalol (Inderal, Inderal LA), and timolol (Blocadren).

Before You Use This Drug

In certain conditions use of verapamil is not only risky, but it is also less apt to work well.[129]

Do not use if you have or have had:

- severe hypotension
- cardiogenic shock
- heart attack
- heartbeats which are too slow (bradycardia)

- heart block without a pacemaker
- heartbeats that are too rapid in association with Wolff-Parkinson-White syndrome
- heart failure[130]
- sick sinus syndrome

Tell your doctor if you have or have had:

- allergies to drugs
- aortic stenosis
- diabetes[131]
- heart, kidney or liver problems
- low blood pressure
- muscular dystrophy
- myasthenia gravis[132]

Tell your doctor about any other drugs you take, including aspirin, herbs, vitamins, and other nonprescription products.

If you now take a beta-blocker, your doctor may gradually take you off of it before starting a calcium channel blocker.[133]

When You Use This Drug

- **Learn to take your pulse, and get immediate help if your pulse slows to 50 beats per minute or slower, even if you are feeling well.**
- Until you know how you react to this drug, do not drive or perform other activities requiring alertness.
- Follow a diet recommended by your doctor.
- Have your doctor suggest exercises which avoid overexertion.
- **Do not stop taking calcium channel blockers suddenly. Contact your doctor for a schedule to decrease your drug gradually.**
- You may feel dizzy when rising from a lying or sitting position. If you are lying down, hang your legs over the side of the bed for a few minutes, then get up slowly. When getting up from a chair, stay by the chair until you are sure that you are not dizzy. (See p. 16.)

- If you plan to have any surgery, including dental, tell your doctor that you take this drug.
- **Do not take other drugs without talking to your doctor first—especially drugs for asthma, colds, cough, diet, hay fever, or sinus problems.**

How to Use This Drug

- Swallow tablets whole or break in half. Do not break, chew, or crush the long-acting capsule or tablet forms.
- Take long-acting forms with food or milk.
- If you miss a dose, take it as soon as you remember, but skip it if it is almost time for the next dose. **Do not take double doses.**
- Do not store in the bathroom. Do not expose to heat, moisture, or strong light.
- If you use a generic verapamil, request your pharmacist to dispense verapamil made by the same manufacturer each time.

Interactions with Other Drugs

The following drugs are listed in the *Evaluations of Drug Interactions* 1997 as causing "highly clinically significant" or "clinically significant" interactions when used together with this drug. We have also included potentially serious interactions listed in the drug's FDA-approved professional product labeling or package insert. New scientific techniques have allowed researchers to predict some drug interactions before they have been documented in people. There may be other drugs, especially those in the families of drugs listed below, that also will react with this drug to cause severe adverse effects. The number of new drugs approved for marketing increases the chance of drug interactions, and new drug interactions are being identified with old drugs. Be vigilant. Make sure to tell your doctor and pharmacist the drugs you are taking and tell your doctor if you are taking any of these interacting drugs:

alcohol, CALCIFEROL, calcium gluconate, carbamazepine, cimetidine, cyclosporine, DANTRIUM, dantrolene, digoxin, DILANTIN, DURAQUIN, ELIXOPHYLLIN, ergocalciferol, INDERAL, INDERAL LA, LANOXICAPS, LANOXIN, lithium, LITHOBID, LITHONATE, NEORAL, NORCURON, phenytoin, propranolol, QUINAGLUTE DURA-TABS, QUINIDEX, quinidine, RIFADIN, rifampin, RIMACTANE, SANDIMMUNE, SLO-BID, TAGAMET, TEGRETOL, THEO-24, theophylline, vecuronium.

If you stop taking verapamil, doses of interacting drugs may need to be adjusted.

Adverse Effects

Call your doctor immediately if you experience:

- bleeding, tender or swollen gums
- difficulty breathing
- chest pain
- convulsions, jerking movements of limbs
- fever
- severe headache
- heartbeat changes
- low blood pressure
- skin rash
- swelling of legs or feet
- unusual secretion of milk

Call your doctor if these symptoms continue:

- abdominal pain
- constipation
- flushing, feeling of warmth
- headache
- nausea
- unusual tiredness or weakness
- vivid or disturbing dreams
- fatigue
- heartburn

- impotence
- muscle pain or tenderness
- nausea
- frequent urination
- blurred vision

Periodic Tests

Ask your doctor which of these tests should be done periodically while you are taking this drug:

- blood pressure
- electrocardiogram (ECG, EKG)
- kidney function tests
- liver function tests
- pulse

PREGNANCY WARNING

This drug caused harm to developing fetuses in animal studies, or such studies were not done. Use during pregnancy only for clear medical reasons. Tell your doctor if you are pregnant or thinking of becoming pregnant before you take this drug.

Limited Use

Diltiazem
CARDIZEM, CARDIZEM CD
(Hoechst Marion Roussel)
DILACOR XR (Watson)
TIAZAC (Forest)

GENERIC: not available
FAMILY: Calcium Channel Blockers (See p. 53)

Diltiazem (dill *tie* a zem) belongs to a family of drugs called calcium channel blockers.

They are used primarily to treat chest pain (angina) and coronary artery disease, and also to lower high blood pressure (hypertension) and improve irregular heartbeats (arrhythmias). Calcium channel blockers control, but do not cure high blood pressure. These drugs may improve capacity for exercise and delay the need for heart surgery.

In 1995, Public Citizen's Health Research Group filed a petition with the Food and Drug Administration to add warnings to the labeling of all calcium channel blockers about the increased risk of heart attack and death. Our petition was based on three well conducted observational research studies.[134,135,136] Observational studies are frequently criticized by doctors who do not understand this type of research. Most of what we know about adverse drug reactions and what we are likely to learn in the future comes from observational research. This type of research was used to show the link between cigarette smoking and lung cancer.

Our petition helped to bring about important labeling changes in February 1996 on one of the calcium channel blockers, the short-acting form of nifedipine. The labeling for this form of nifedipine now warns doctors that this product should not be used for the treatment of high blood pressure.

Since we filed our petition additional serious adverse effects have been associated with the use of calcium channel blockers. These include an increased risk of gastrointestinal bleeding in older adults.[137] Calcium channel blockers have been shown in some studies to increase the risk of cancer[138,139,140] including breast cancer in postmenopausal women.[141] However, another study has found no increase in the risk of cancer with the calcium channel blockers.[142]

Despite the 1993 recommendations of the National Institutes of Health's National Heart, Lung, and Blood Institute that diuretics and beta-blockers should be used first in the treatment of mild to moderate high blood pressure the calcium channel blockers remain the largest selling family of high-blood-pressure-lowering drugs in the U.S.[143]

Each calcium channel blocker differs in the likelihood of harmful adverse effects. Compared to the other calcium channel blockers, diltiazem is less likely than verapamil to cause constipation. It is also less likely than the nifedipine group of channel blockers to cause severe headaches, rapid heartbeat, and swelling of the legs and feet.[144]

If you have high blood pressure, the best way to reduce or eliminate your need for medication is by improving your diet, losing weight, exercising, and reducing your salt and alcohol intake. Mild hypertension can be controlled by proper nutrition and exercise. If these measures do not lower your blood pressure enough and you need medication, **hydrochlorothiazide, a water pill (see thiazide diuretics, p. 100), is the drug of choice starting with a low dose of 12.5 milligrams daily.** It also costs less than other blood pressure drugs.

There is now good evidence that thiazide diuretics, such as hydrochlorothiazide, significantly decrease the rate of bone mineral loss in both men and women because they reduce the amount of calcium lost in the urine. An increasing number of researchers think that this will also decrease the number of fractures.[145]

If this drug does not lower your blood pressure enough, your doctor can prescribe a second type of drug called a beta-blocker (see p. 52) to accompany the hydrochlorothiazide. If you cannot take a beta-blocker, a drug from this family (calcium channel blockers) can be used instead.

Whatever drugs you take for high blood pressure, once your blood pressure has been normal for a year or more, a cautious decrease in dose and renewed attention to nondrug treatment may be worth trying, according to *The Medical Letter*.[146]

And an editorial in the *British Medical Journal* stated: *"Treatment of hypertension is part of preventive medicine and like all preventive strategies, its progress should be regularly reviewed by whoever initiates it. Many problems could be avoided by not starting antihypertensive treatment until after prolonged observation. . . . Patients should no longer be told that treatment is necessarily for life: the possibility of reducing or stopping treatment should be mentioned at the outset."*[147]

CALCIUM CHANNEL BLOCKERS ARE OVERUSED IN OLDER ADULT HEART ATTACK SURVIVORS

Research found that the calcium channel blockers are being overutilized by doctors treating older persons after a heart attack, while the beta-blocking drugs were being underutilized. None of the calcium channel blockers has been shown to improve survival in persons with heart disease. Some beta-blockers are approved by the Food and Drug Administration (FDA) to reduce the risk of death after a heart attack.

This research study looked at the use of calcium channel blockers and beta-blockers in 500 consecutive people being admitted to a nursing home. Heart diagnostic tests were done on all 500 at the time of admission. Of these people, 202 (40%) had experienced heart attacks. Only 17 (8%) were receiving a beta-blocker while 74 (37%) were receiving a calcium channel blocker.[148]

The beta-blockers approved by the FDA to reduce the risk of death after a heart attack are: atenolol (Tenormin), metoprolol (Lopressor, Toprol XL), propranalol (Inderal, Inderal LA), and timolol (Blocadren).

Before You Use This Drug

Do not take if you have or have had:

- aortic stenosis
- severe hypotension
- heart block without a pacemaker

- extremely low heart rate
- myocardial infarction (acute) and pulmonary congestion
- sick sinus syndrome

Tell your doctor if you have or have had:

- allergies to drugs
- heart, kidney or liver problems
- low blood pressure
- lung condition or breathing problems

Tell your doctor about any other drugs you take, including aspirin, herbs, vitamins, and other nonprescription products.

If you now take a beta-blocker, your doctor may gradually take you off of it before starting a calcium channel blocker.[149]

When You Use This Drug

- **Learn to take your pulse, and get immediate help if your pulse slows to 50 beats per minute or slower, even if you are feeling well.**
- Until you know how you react to this drug, do not drive or perform other activities requiring alertness.
- Follow a diet recommended by your doctor.
- Have your doctor suggest exercises which avoid overexertion.
- **Do not stop taking calcium channel blockers suddenly. Contact your doctor for a schedule to decrease your drug gradually.**
- If you plan to have any surgery, including dental, tell your doctor that you take this drug.
- **Do not take other drugs without talking to your doctor first—especially drugs for asthma, colds, cough, diet, hay fever, or sinus problems.**

How to Use This Drug

- Swallow capsule or tablet whole or break in half. Do not break, chew or crush the long-acting forms of the drug.

• Take on an empty stomach, at least one hour before or two hours after meals.

• If you miss a dose, take it as soon as you remember, but skip it if it is almost time for the next dose. **Do not take double doses.**

• Store this drug at room temperature with the lid on tightly.

• Do not store in the bathroom. Do not expose to heat, moisture, or strong light.

Interactions with Other Drugs

The following drugs are listed in the *Evaluations of Drug Interactions* 1997 as causing "highly clinically significant" or "clinically significant" interactions when used together with this drug. We have also included potentially serious interactions listed in the drug's FDA-approved professional product labeling or package insert. New scientific techniques have allowed researchers to predict some drug interactions before they have been documented in people. There may be other drugs, especially those in the families of drugs listed below, that also will react with this drug to cause severe adverse effects. The number of new drugs approved for marketing increases the chance of drug interactions, and new drug interactions are being identified with old drugs. Be vigilant. Make sure to tell your doctor and pharmacist the drugs you are taking and tell your doctor if you are taking any of these interacting drugs:

amiodarone, beta-blockers, optic, CALCIFEROL, calcium supplements, carbamazepine, CORDARONE, cyclosporine, DANTRIUM, dantrolene, digoxin, DILANTIN, disopyramide, DURAQUIN, ELIXOPHYLLIN, ergocalciferol, INDERAL, INDERAL LA, LANOXICAPS, LANOXIN, lithium, LITHOBID, LITHONATE, NEORAL, NORCURON, NORPACE, phenytoin, propranolol, QUINAGLUTE DURA-TABS, QUINIDEX, quinidine, RIFADIN, rifampin, RIMACTANE, SANDIMMUNE, SLO-BID, TEGRETOL, THEO-24, theophylline, vecuronium.

Adverse Effects

Call your doctor immediately if you experience:

• bleeding, tender, or swollen gums
• difficulty breathing
• chest pain
• convulsions, jerking movements of limbs
• fever
• severe headache
• heartbeat changes
• low blood pressure
• skin rash
• swelling of legs or feet

Call your doctor if these symptoms continue:

• abdominal pain
• constipation
• flushing, feeling of warmth
• headache
• nausea
• unusual tiredness or weakness
• vivid or disturbing dreams
• fatigue
• heartburn
• impotence
• muscle pain or tenderness
• nausea
• frequent urination
• blurred vision

Periodic Tests

Ask your doctor which of these tests should be done periodically while you are taking this drug:

• blood pressure
• heart function tests, such as electrocardiogram (ECG, EKG)

- kidney function tests
- liver function tests
- pulse

PREGNANCY WARNING

This drug caused harm to developing fetuses in animal studies, or such studies were not done. Use during pregnancy only for clear medical reasons. Tell your doctor if you are pregnant or thinking of becoming pregnant before you take this drug.

 Do Not Use

ALTERNATIVE TREATMENT:
See Hydrochlorothiazide, p. 100.

Clonidine
CATAPRES (Boehringer Ingelheim)

FAMILY: Antihypertensives
(See High Blood Pressure, p. 44)

Clonidine (*kloe* ni deen) is used to treat high blood pressure (hypertension). **It has severe adverse effects and should not be used.**

The main problem with clonidine is that missing only one or two doses of the drug can have serious effects, including sweating, tremors, flushing, and severe high blood pressure. Clonidine can also cause severe depression and is particularly dangerous for anyone with a history of depression. Nearly one-fourth of the people who use the patch form have a skin reaction.

If you have high blood pressure, the best way to reduce or eliminate your need for medica-tion is by improving your diet, losing weight, exercising, and decreasing your salt and alcohol intake. Mild hypertension can be controlled by proper nutrition and exercise. If these measures do not lower your blood pressure enough and you need medication, **hydrochlorothiazide, a water pill (see thiazide diuretics, p. 100), is the drug of choice starting with a low dose of 12.5 milligrams daily.** It also costs less than other blood pressure drugs.

There is now good evidence that thiazide diuretics, such as hydrochlorothiazide, significantly decrease the rate of bone mineral loss in both men and women because they reduce the amount of calcium lost in the urine. An increasing number of researchers think that this will also decrease the number of fractures.[150]

If this does not lower your blood pressure enough, your doctor can prescribe a second type of drug called a beta-blocker, such as propranolol (see p. 154), to accompany the hydrochlorothiazide. If you cannot take a beta-blocker, a drug from another family (calcium channel blockers) can be used instead.

Whatever drugs you take for high blood pressure, once your blood pressure has been normal for a year or more, a cautious decrease in dose and renewed attention to nondrug treatment may be worth trying, according to *The Medical Letter*.[151]

And an editorial in the *British Medical Journal* stated: *"Treatment of hypertension is part of preventive medicine and like all preventive strategies, its progress should be regularly reviewed by whoever initiates it. Many problems could be avoided by not starting antihypertensive treatment until after prolonged observation. . . . Patients should no longer be told that treatment is necessarily for life: the possibility of reducing or stopping treatment should be mentioned at the outset."*[152]

> **Do not suddenly stop using this drug.** Sudden withdrawal from clonidine can cause sweating, tremors, flushing, and even severe high blood pressure. This dangerous reaction may occur after missing only one or two doses. Ask your doctor for a schedule that reduces your dose of clonidine gradually over at least ten days, and even more slowly if symptoms occur. At the same time as you are reducing your dose of clonidine, your doctor should start you on another drug for high blood pressure.

Do Not Use

ALTERNATIVE TREATMENT:
Mild exercise, no smoking, extreme cleanliness of legs and feet.

Papaverine
CERESPAN (Rorer)
PAVABID (Hoechst Marion Roussel)

FAMILY: Vasodilators
(Blood Vessel Dilators)

Doctors prescribe papaverine (pa *pav* er een) to improve the blood circulation of people with certain types of blood vessel disease. The expectation is that better circulation will relieve pain (leg pain, for example) and improve mental function (by increasing blood flow to the brain). However, there is no evidence that papaverine prevents or relieves any disease of blood vessels to the brain, nor has it been shown to improve the mental or physical state of older or senile adults.[153] In fact, although this drug has been available for use and evaluation for many years, **it has not been proven effective for treating any condition.**[154,155] The American Medical Association's guide to drug therapy does not even suggest a dose for papaverine because "the

role of this agent in the treatment of peripheral vascular disease [disease of the blood vessels in the arms or legs] has not been established."[156]

In addition to being ineffective, papaverine has serious dangers. There is strong evidence that it can cause liver damage. In one study, one out of five people taking the drug developed liver damage.[157] **We recommend that you do not use papaverine because it can cause harmful adverse effects and has not been proven to have any benefit.**

> Studies have failed to show that this drug is effective.

Do Not Use

ALTERNATIVE TREATMENT:
See Hydrochlorothiazide, p. 100.

Clonidine and Chlorthalidone
COMBIPRES (Boehringer Ingelheim)

FAMILY: Diuretics
Antihypertensives
(See High Blood Pressure, p. 44)

This product, a combination of clonidine (see p. 80) and chlorthalidone (see p. 105), is used to treat high blood pressure. **Older adults should not use drugs containing a fixed combination of clonidine and chlorthalidone.**

Clonidine can cause severe depression, and can also cause a dangerous reaction if you miss only one or two doses (see box below). We do not recommend that any older adult use clonidine, and it is particularly dangerous for anyone with a history of depression.

Chlorthalidone puts the older adult user at such a high risk of adverse effects that the

World Health Organization has said it should not be used by people over 60.[158]

In addition to the risks of clonidine and chlorthalidone, there are good reasons not to use a fixed-combination drug for high blood pressure. A single drug is often enough to control high blood pressure. If a combination drug like this one is controlling your high blood pressure, it is quite possible that one drug alone would do the same job. There is no reason to put yourself at extra risk by taking drugs you do not need.

If you have high blood pressure, the best way to reduce or eliminate your need for medication is by improving your diet, losing weight, exercising, and decreasing your salt and alcohol intake. Mild hypertension can be controlled by proper nutrition and exercise. If these measures do not lower your blood pressure enough and you need medication, **hydrochlorothiazide, a water pill (see thiazide diuretics, p. 100), is the drug of choice starting with a low dose of 12.5 milligrams daily.** It also costs less than other blood pressure drugs.

There is now good evidence that thiazide diuretics, such as hydrochlorothiazide, significantly decrease the rate of bone mineral loss in both men and women because they reduce the amount of calcium lost in the urine. An increasing number of researchers think that this will also decrease the number of fractures.[159]

If your high blood pressure is more severe, and hydrochlorothiazide alone does not control it, the best treatment is a combination of hydrochlorothiazide and a second type of drug called a beta-blocker, such as propranolol (see p. 154). If you can't take a drug in the beta-blocker family, another drug called a calcium channel blocker may be used instead. In either case, your doctor would prescribe the hydrochlorothiazide and the second drug separately, with the dose of each drug adjusted to meet your needs, rather than using a product that combines the drugs in advance in a fixed combination.

If you are taking this fixed-combination drug, ask your doctor about changing your prescription.

Whatever drugs you take for high blood pressure, once your blood pressure has been normal for a year or more, a cautious decrease in dose and renewed attention to nondrug treatment may be worth trying, according to *The Medical Letter.*[160]

And an editorial in the *British Medical Journal* stated: *"Treatment of hypertension is part of preventive medicine and like all preventive strategies, its progress should be regularly reviewed by whoever initiates it. Many problems could be avoided by not starting antihypertensive treatment until after prolonged observation. . . . Patients should no longer be told that treatment is necessarily for life: the possibility of reducing or stopping treatment should be mentioned at the outset."*[161]

Do not suddenly stop using this drug. Sudden withdrawal from clonidine can cause sweating, tremors, flushing, and even severe high blood pressure. This dangerous reaction may occur after missing only one or two doses. Ask your doctor for a schedule that reduces your dose of clonidine gradually over at least ten days, and even more slowly if symptoms occur. At the same time as you are reducing your dose of clonidine, your doctor should start you on another drug for high blood pressure.

Last Choice Drug

Amiodarone
CORDARONE (Wyeth-Ayerst)

GENERIC: not available
FAMILY: Antiarrhythmics

Amiodarone (am ee *oh* da rone) is used to treat and prevent life-threatening irregular heartbeats, especially ventricular arrhythmias. It should be used only when other drugs or devices are ineffective or cannot be tolerated. It is best to start amiodarone in a hospital. Along with 200 mg of amiodarone, each tablet contains 75 mg of iodine. As with any medicine, the lowest effective dose should be used. Since the oral form may take up to three months to show effects, a loading dose is sometimes prescribed.

Amiodarone accumulates in the body, leading to a substantial number of potential adverse effects. More than 80% of people who take amiodarone experience adverse, sometimes fatal, effects. Amiodarone can cause toxic reactions in the liver, lung, thyroid, and ironically, the heart. People with advanced heart failure who take amiodarone are at extremely high risk for early sudden death.[162] Changes in vision are common.[163] Women are more prone to adverse effects.[164] So are those who develop low potassium. Injectable amiodarone can lower the blood pressure too much. Older people may be more sensitive to adverse effects on the thyroid,[165] while people under age 60 are more apt to develop skin reactions, including sunburn.[166] Fair-skinned individuals' skin may turn blue-gray in color.[167] Adverse effects are not dose related and most are not predictable. Many studies of amiodarone are small. One study shows a trend toward a lower mortality with amiodarone.[168] Long-term safety and effectiveness information is still forthcoming. Use of amiodarone should be weighed against the risk of alternative drugs or devices available. Cost is also a consideration.

Before You Use This Drug

Tell your doctor if you have or have had:

- allergies including iodine and lactose
- asthma
- autoimmune disorder
- blood pressure that is too high or too low
- bronchitis
- other heart problems, such as bradycardia, congestive heart failure, heart block, or sinus node impairment
- liver problems
- thyroid problems

Tell your doctor about any other drugs you take, including aspirin, herbs, vitamins, and other nonprescription products.
Before you start this drug request a thyroid test.

When You Use This Drug

- Wear identification that you take amiodarone.
- Protect yourself from sunburn, using a sun block like zinc oxide. Sunscreens don't protect against ultra-violet-B light. Wear protective brimmed hats, long sleeves and pants.
- If you plan to have any surgery, including dental, tell your doctor that you take this drug.

How to Use This Drug

- Swallow according to instructions. Injection should be given by a health professional.
- If you miss a dose, skip it. Notify your doctor if you miss two or more doses in a row. **Do not take double doses.**
- If you stop taking this medication, remember that adverse effects can still last for several weeks or months.
- Store tablets at room temperature.
- Do not store in the bathroom. Do not expose to heat, moisture, or strong light.

Interactions with Other Drugs

The following drugs are listed in the *Evaluations of Drug Interactions* 1997 as causing "highly clinically significant" or "clinically significant" interactions when used together with this drug. We have also included potentially serious interactions listed in the drug's FDA-approved professional product labeling or package insert. New scientific techniques have allowed researchers to predict some drug interactions before they have been documented in people. There may be other drugs, especially those in the families of drugs listed below, that also will react with this drug to cause severe adverse effects. The number of new drugs approved for marketing increases the chance of drug interactions and new drug interactions are being identified with old drugs. Be vigilant. Make sure to tell your doctor and pharmacist the drugs you are taking and tell your doctor if you are taking any of these interacting drugs:

antihistamines, antipsychotics, beta-blockers, calcium channel blockers, COUMADIN, digoxin, DILANTIN, diuretics, DURAQUIN, flecainide, grepafloxacin, LANOXICAPS, LANOXIN, mexiletine, MEXITIL, phenytoin, procainamide, PROCANBID, propafenone, QUINAGLUTE DURA-TABS, QUINIDEX, quinidine, RAXAR, RYTHMOL, sparfloxacin, TAMBOCOR, warfarin, ZAGAM.

Interactions with amiodarone can occur months after you stop taking amiodarone since it stays in the body.

Adverse Effects

Call your doctor immediately if you experience:

- difficulty breathing
- fever
- cough
- unusual and uncontrolled movements of the body

- coldness
- dry eyes
- heartbeat becoming faster, slower or irregular
- nervousness
- numbness in fingers or toes
- swelling or painful scrotum
- sensitivity to heat or sunlight
- skin rash, blue-gray color, cold, puffiness or irritation at site of injection
- difficulty sleeping
- sweating
- swelling of legs or feet
- tiredness
- vision changes, blurred or blue-green halos
- difficulty walking (weak arms and legs)
- undesired weight loss or gain
- yellowing of skin or eyes

Call your doctor if these symptoms continue:

- appetite loss
- constipation
- dizziness
- flushing of face
- hair loss
- headache
- nausea or vomiting
- decreased sexual ability and interest
- blue-gray skin tone
- sunburn
- bitter or metallic taste

Periodic Testing

Ask your doctor which of these tests should be done periodically while you are taking this drug:

- liver function tests
- chest examination
- broncoscopy
- chest x-ray
- heart function tests, such as electrocardiogram (ECG, EKG)
- gallium radionuclide scan
- eye examination

- plasma amiodarone determinations
- lung function determinations
- thyroid function determinations

PREGNANCY WARNING

This drug caused harm to developing fetuses in animal studies, or such studies were not done. Use during pregnancy only for clear medical reasons. Tell your doctor if you are pregnant or thinking of becoming pregnant before you take this drug.

Do Not Use Until Five Years After Release

Carvedilol (Do Not Use Until 2003)
COREG (SmithKline Beecham)

GENERIC: not available
FAMILY: Beta-blockers (see p. 52)

You should wait at least five years from the date of release to take any new drug unless it is one of those rare "breakthrough" drugs that offers you a documented therapeutic advantage over older proven drugs. New drugs are tested in a relatively small number of people before being approved, and serious adverse effects or life-threatening drug interactions may not be detected until the new drug has been taken by hundreds of thousands of people. A number of new drugs have been withdrawn within their first five years after release. Also, serious new adverse reaction warnings have been added to the labeling of a number of drugs, or new drug interactions have been detected, usually within five years after a drug's release.

Carvedilol (car *ved* i lole) is used to control blood pressure and delay the progression of mild or moderate heart failure. It belongs to the family of beta-blockers, specifically the alpha/beta-adrenergic blockers, in the same family as labetalol.

Carvedilol is approved for use in the treatment of certain types of mild or moderate congestive heart failure, in conjunction with other drugs, to reduce the progression of disease. Whether this drug improves survival is controversial.[169,170]

Starting with a low dose helps reduce adverse effects. The starting dose is 3.125 mg twice daily.[171] The dose can be increased at one- or two-week intervals if needed. Most older people need no more than 12.5 mg.[172] The total dose in a day should not exceed 50 mg, unless you weigh over 170 lb.[173] People with liver impairment should take a lower dose. The first dose commonly causes blood pressure to drop significantly. Older people are more likely to experience dizziness. Carvedilol may mask symptoms of low blood sugar. People with bronchial asthma and atrioventricular heart blocks (between the top and bottom parts of the heart), and Class IV heart failure should not take this drug. Whether carvedilol prolongs life is yet to be determined. Information on use in pregnancy, nursing, or children under age 18 is lacking.

If you have high blood pressure, the best way to reduce or eliminate your need for medication is by improving your diet, losing weight, exercising, and decreasing your salt and alcohol intake. Mild hypertension can be controlled by proper nutrition and exercise. If these measures do not lower your blood pressure enough and you need medication, **hydrochlorothiazide, a water pill (see thiazide diuretics, p. 100), is the drug of choice starting with a low dose of 12.5 milligrams daily.** It also costs less than other blood pressure drugs.

There is now good evidence that thiazide diuretics, such as hydrochlorothiazide, significantly decrease the rate of bone mineral loss in both men and women because they reduce the amount of calcium lost in the urine. An increasing number of researchers think that this will also decrease the number of fractures.[174]

If this drug does not lower your blood pressure enough, your doctor can prescribe a second type of drug called a beta-blocker (see p. 52) to accompany the hydrochlorothiazide. If you cannot take a beta-blocker, a drug from another family (calcium channel blockers) can be used instead.

Whatever drugs you take for high blood pressure, once your blood pressure has been normal for a year or more, a cautious decrease in dose and renewed attention to nondrug treatment may be worth trying, according to *The Medical Letter.*[175]

And an editorial in the *British Medical Journal* stated: *"Treatment of hypertension is part of preventive medicine and like all preventive strategies, its progress should be regularly reviewed by whoever initiates it. Many problems could be avoided by not starting antihypertensive treatment until after prolonged observation. . . . Patients should no longer be told that treatment is necessarily for life: the possibility of reducing or stopping treatment should be mentioned at the outset."*[176]

Carvedilol may be used along with diuretics and other heart medications. Doses of these medications may need to be adjusted when carvedilol is added.

Before You Use This Drug

Tell your doctor if you have or have had:

- allergies, including lactose intolerance
- asthma
- chronic bronchitis or emphysema
- diabetes
- heart or liver problems
- low blood pressure
- pregnant or nursing
- thyroid problems
- wear contact lenses[177]

Tell your doctor about any other drugs you take, including aspirin, herbs, vitamins, and other nonprescription products.

When You Use This Drug

- Have someone with you or to check on you after you take your first dose.
- Do not drink alcohol.
- Until you know how you react to this drug, do not drive or perform other activities requiring alertness.
- You may feel dizzy when rising from a lying or sitting position. When getting up from bed, hang your legs over the side of the bed for a few minutes, then get up slowly. When getting up from a chair, stay beside the chair until you are sure that you are not dizzy. (See p. 16.)
- Eat a low-fat, low-salt diet.
- Exercise regularly.
- If you plan to have any surgery, including dental, tell your doctor that you take this drug.

How to Use This Drug

- Swallow whole or half tablets, according to your dose. Take with food.
- If you miss a dose, take as soon as you remember but skip it if it is almost time for the next dose. **Do not take double doses.**
- Do not stop taking this medication without checking with your doctor. This medication should be stopped gradually, especially for people with ischemic heart disease.
- Store at room temperature.

Interactions with Other Drugs

The following drugs are listed in the *Evaluations of Drug Interactions* 1997 as causing "highly clinically significant" or "clinically significant" interactions when used together with this drug. We have also included potentially serious interactions listed in the drug's FDA-approved professional product labeling or package insert. New scientific techniques have allowed researchers to predict some drug interactions before they have been documented in people. There may be other drugs, especially those in the families of drugs listed below, that also will react with this drug to cause severe adverse effects. The number of new drugs approved for marketing increases the chance of drug interactions, and new drug interactions are being identified with old drugs. Be vigilant. Make sure to tell your doctor and pharmacist the drugs you are taking and tell your doctor if you are taking any of these interacting drugs:

> cimetidine, digoxin, LANOXICAPS, LANOXIN, RIFADIN, rifampin, RIMACTANE, TAGAMET.

Any other drug that affects your blood pressure, including alcohol, may add to the effects of carvedilol.

Adverse Effects

Call your doctor immediately if you experience:

- chest pain
- chills
- dizziness or fainting
- flu-like symptoms, such as sore throat, fever
- cold hands and feet
- heart pain, slower or more rapid heartbeat
- itching
- pain or tenderness in the right upper quadrant of the abdomen
- rash, blisters
- shortness of breath
- difficulty swallowing, swelling of tongue
- swelling of legs or feet
- dark urine
- yellowing of skin

Call your doctor if these symptoms continue:

- back pain
- increase in blood sugar
- coughing, wheezing
- diarrhea
- headache

- impotence
- tiredness
- weight gain

Ask your doctor which of these tests should be done periodically while you are taking this drug:

- liver function tests

_____

Warfarin
COUMADIN (Du Pont)

GENERIC: available

FAMILY: Anticoagulants

DRUG INTERACTION WARNING: INCREASED RISK OF BLEEDING WHEN ACETAMINOPHEN AND WARFARIN (COUMADIN) ARE TAKEN TOGETHER.

Acetaminophen may interact with warfarin to increase the risk of bleeding. This risk increases with increasing doses of acetaminophen. The risk of bleeding has been found to increase tenfold in people who were taking 28 or more regular strength acetaminophen tablets per week, or the equivalent of 18 or more extra-strength tablets per week, compared to those taking warfarin and no acetaminophen.[178] A regular strength tablet contains 325 milligrams of acetaminophen and extra-strength tablets contain 500 milligrams each of the drug.

Warfarin is a drug of considerable benefit after heart valve replacement and in preventing blood clots from a type of heart rhythm disturbance known as atrial fibrillation. It also reduces the risk of death, recurrent heart attacks, and stroke after a heart attack.

Based on this new evidence, if you are taking warfarin you should notify your doctor before taking any product containing acetaminophen.

Warfarin (*war* far in) reduces the blood's ability to clot (coagulate) and prevents blood clots from forming in the arteries and veins. It is prescribed for people with a history of abnormal blood clots or who are at high risk of having abnormal clots. **If you are over 60, you should generally be taking less than the usual adult dose,** to lower the risk of heavy bleeding (hemorrhage). Once you have taken warfarin for three months, your doctor should reevaluate your need to continue taking it.

If you do not take this drug properly, it can cause severe adverse effects (see Adverse Effects). **You must take warfarin exactly on schedule.** While taking warfarin, **your doctor should monitor your progress with regular blood tests to ensure that you are taking the most effective dose of the drug.**

Warfarin can interact with nearly all drugs. Its anti-clotting action is very difficult to control when other drugs are added or subtracted, or when another drug's dose is changed. Another medication may either increase or decrease warfarin's action. **While taking warfarin, do not take any other drugs, including nonprescription drugs (such as aspirin, cold remedies, antacids, laxatives), or change the dose of any drug that you currently take, without consulting your doctor first.**

Before You Use This Drug

Do not use if you have or have had:

- recent surgery
- aneurysm or dissecting aorta
- blood disorders
- active bleeding
- severe, uncontrolled high blood pressure

Tell your doctor if you have or have had:

- allergies to drugs
- heart problems, including atrial fibrillation, myocardial infarction, or stroke
- thromboembolism
- severe allergies
- ulcers
- kidney or liver problems
- polyarthritis
- recent radiation therapy
- vitamin C or K deficiency
- alcohol dependence
- severe inflammation of blood vessels
- subacute bacterial endocarditis (infection of the heart)
- diabetes
- recent injury
- childbirth
- spinal anesthesia
- a fall or blow to the body or head
- fever lasting more than a couple of days
- an IUD
- heavy or unusual menstrual bleeding
- medical or dental surgery
- severe or continuing diarrhea

Tell your doctor about any other drugs you take, including aspirin, herbs, vitamins, and other nonprescription products.

When You Use This Drug

- Wear a medical identification bracelet or carry a card stating that you take warfarin.
- Be very careful doing activities that may cause cuts or bleeding, such as shaving or cooking.
- Do not drink alcohol.
- Eat a normal, balanced diet. **Do not change your diet or take nutritional supplements or vitamins without first checking with your doctor.**
- If you plan to have any surgery, including dental, tell your doctor that you take this drug.
- **Do not take any other drugs, including nonprescription products (aspirin, cold remedies, antacids, laxatives), or change the dose of drugs you are taking, without consulting your doctor.**
- **Be sure to schedule regular doctor visits for blood tests.**

How to Use This Drug

• If you miss a dose, take it as soon as you remember, but skip it if you don't remember until the next day. **Do not take double doses.** Keep a record of missed doses and give the list to your doctor at each visit.

• Do not store in the bathroom. Do not expose to heat, moisture, or strong light.

Interactions with Other Drugs

The following drugs are listed in the *Evaluations of Drug Interactions* 1997 as causing "highly clinically significant" or "clinically significant" interactions when used together with this drug. We have also included potentially serious interactions listed in the drug's FDA-approved professional product labeling or package insert. New scientific techniques have allowed researchers to predict some drug interactions before they have been documented in people. There may be other drugs, especially those in the families of drugs listed below, that also will react with this drug to cause severe adverse effects. The number of new drugs approved for marketing increases the chance of drug interactions, and new drug interactions are being identified with old drugs. Be vigilant. Make sure to tell your doctor and pharmacist the drugs you are taking and tell your doctor if you are taking any of these interacting drugs:

acetaminophen, ADVIL, amiodarone, ANTABUSE, ANTURANE, AQUAMEPHYTON, aspirin, ATROMID-S, azathioprine, BACTRIM, GENUINE BAYER ASPIRIN, BUTAZOLIDIN, cefamandole, chloral hydrate, cholestyramine, cimetidine, CLINORIL, clofibrate, CORDARONE, COTRIM, cyclosporine, DARVON, DARVON-N, DIFLUCAN, disulfiram, DORIDEN, DURAQUIN, ECOTRIN, EDECRIN, EES, ERYTHROCIN, erythromycin, erythromycin estolate, ethacrynic acid, ethchlorvynol,

ETHMOZINE, etretinate, felbamate, FELBATOL, FLAGYL, fluconazole, flu shot (influenza virus vaccine), FULVICIN, GANTANOL, glucagon, glutethimide, GRIFULVIN, GRISACTIN, GRIS-PEG, griseofulvin, ibuprofen, IFEX, ifosfamide, ILOSONE, IMURAN, INDERAL, INDERAL LA, INDOCIN, indomethacin, ketoconazole, KONAKION, LOCHOLEST, lovastatin, LUMINAL, LYSODREN, MANDOL, methyltestosterone, metronidazole, MEVACOR, miconazole, mitotane, MONISTAT-DERM, MONISTAT 7, moricizine, MOTRIN, nafcillin, nalidixic acid, NEgGRAM, NEORAL, NIZORAL, NOCTEC, NOLVADEX, ORETON METHYL, phenobarbital, phenylbutazone, phytonadione, PLACIDYL, propoxyphene, propranolol, QUESTRAN, QUINAGLUTE DURA-TABS, QUINIDEX, quinidine, RIFADIN, rifampin, RIMACTANE, SANDIMMUNE, SEPTRA, SOLFOTON, sulfamethoxazole, sulfinpyrazone, sulindac, TAGAMET, tamoxifen, TEGISON, thyroid, trimethoprim/TYLENOL, UNIPEN, vitamin E.

Adverse Effects

Call your doctor immediately if you experience:

• **signs of overdose or bleeding including:** bleeding gums when brushing teeth, nosebleeds, unexplained bruising, unusually heavy bleeding from cuts or wounds, unusually heavy or unexpected menstrual bleeding, abdominal pain or swelling, sudden lightheadedness, weakness, loss of consciousness, backaches, blood in urine, bloody or tarry stools, constipation, headache, joint pain, stiffness or swelling, coughing up blood, vomiting blood or material that looks like coffee grounds
• abnormal bleeding
• bloody or cloudy urine

- difficult or painful urination or sudden decrease in amount of urine
- swelling of ankles, feet, or legs
- unusual weight gain
- blue/purple color of toes
- chills, fever, sore throat, or unusual tiredness
- dark urine, yellow eyes or skin
- diarrhea, nausea, or vomiting
- skin rash, hives, or itching
- sores or white spots in mouth or throat
- stomach cramps or pain

Call your doctor if this symptom continues:

- unusual hair loss

Periodic Tests

Ask your doctor which of these tests should be done periodically while you are taking this drug:

- prothrombin time (measure of how long it takes your blood to clot): daily for the first week on warfarin, weekly for the next three months, and monthly thereafter
- complete blood count
- stool tests for possible blood loss
- urine tests for possible blood loss

PREGNANCY WARNING

This drug should not be used if you are pregnant or are thinking of becoming pregnant. The risk of use of this drug in pregnant women clearly outweighs any possible benefit.

Do Not Use Until Five Years After Release

Losartan (Do Not Use Until 2001)
COZAAR (Merck)

Valsartan (Do Not Use Until 2003)
DIOVAN (Novartis)

Irbesartan (Do Not Use Until 2004)
AVAPRO (Sanofi)

Losartan and Hydrochlorothiazide
(Do Not Use Until 2001)
HYZAAR (Merck)

Irbesartan and Hydrochlorothiazide
(Do Not Use Until 2004)
AVAPRO HCT (Sanofi)

GENERIC: not available
FAMILY: Angiotensin II Antagonists
Antihypertensives
(See High Blood Pressure, p. 44)

You should wait at least five years from the date of release to take any new drug unless it is one of those rare "breakthrough" drugs that offers you a documented therapeutic advantage over older proven drugs. New drugs are tested in a relatively small number of people before being approved, and serious adverse effects or life-threatening drug interactions may not be detected until the new drug has been taken by hundreds of thousands of people. A number of new drugs have been withdrawn within their first five years after release. Also, serious new adverse reaction warnings have been added to the labeling of a number of drugs, or new drug interactions have been detected, usually within five years after a drug's release.

Losartan (loe *sar* tan), valsartan (val *sar* tan), and irbesartan (ir be *sar* tan) are used to reduce high blood pressure. These drugs are in a new family know as angiotensin II antagonists. Both the angiotensin II antagonists and the ACE inhibitors have an effect on a natural substance called angiotensin that can raise blood pressure. Losartan's effectiveness in lowering blood pressure is similar to the ACE inhibitor enalapril and to the beta-blocker atenolol.

Losartan was the first member of this family and its effectiveness is similar to enalapril and atenolol. The full effect of losartan may take a few weeks to develop.

To date the main adverse effect is dizziness. Like ACE inhibitors, losartan is less effective in most African-Americans. It also has the adverse effect of causing too high a potassium level. Losartan and other angiotensin II antagonists do not cause the dry, hacking cough that is sometimes an adverse effect seen with the ACE inhibitors. Long-term studies are needed to show whether losartan prolongs life by preventing stroke, heart attack, or premature death.

If you have high blood pressure, the best way to reduce or eliminate your need for medication is by improving your diet, losing weight, exercising, and decreasing your salt and alcohol intake. Mild hypertension can be controlled by proper nutrition and exercise. If these measures do not lower your blood pressure enough and you need medication, **hydrochlorothiazide, a water pill (see thiazide diuretics, p. 100, is the drug of choice, starting with a low dose of 12.5 milligrams daily.** It also costs less than other blood pressure drugs.

If you also take hydrochlorothiazide, buy it and losartan separately, until your doses of both medicines are stabilized. If your eventual dose is identical to the combination product of losartan with hydrochlorothiazide, compare the price of the combination with buying the hydrochlorothiaizde and losartan separately.

There is now good evidence that thiazide diuretics, such as hydrochlorothiazide, significantly decrease the rate of bone mineral loss in both men and women because they reduce the amount of calcium lost in the urine. An increasing number of researchers think that this will also decrease the number of fractures.[179]

If this drug does not lower your blood pressure enough, your doctor can prescribe a second type of drug called a beta-blocker (see p. 52) to accompany the hydrochlorothiazide. If you cannot take a beta-blocker, a drug from another family (calcium channel blockers) can be used instead.

Whatever drugs you take for high blood pressure, once your blood pressure has been normal for a year or more, a cautious decrease in dose and renewed attention to nondrug treatment may be worth trying, according to *The Medical Letter.*[180]

And an editorial in the *British Medical Journal* stated: *"Treatment of hypertension is part of preventive medicine and like all preventive strategies, its progress should be regularly reviewed by whoever initiates it. Many problems could be avoided by not starting antihypertensive treatment until after prolonged observation. . . . Patients should no longer be told that treatment is necessarily for life: the possibility of reducing or stopping treatment should be mentioned at the outset."*[181]

Before You Use This Drug

Tell your doctor if you have or have had:

- allergies
- cirrhosis or other liver problems
- diabetes
- heart or kidney problems
- sodium deficiency

Tell your doctor about any other drugs you take, including aspirin, herbs, vitamins, and other nonprescription products.

When You Use This Drug

- Continue to follow your diet, exercise regularly, and avoid undue stress. Do not use salt substitutes or salt-free milk.
- Drink fluids to prevent dehydration, especially when exercising during hot weather, or if you develop nausea, vomiting, or diarrhea.
- Do not drink alcohol, which can cause dehydration.

• The first time you take this drug have a friend stay with you until you know how you react.

• You may feel dizzy when rising from a lying or sitting position. When getting out of bed, hang your legs over the side of the bed for a few minutes, then get up slowly. When getting up from a chair, stay beside the chair until you are sure that you are not dizzy. (See p. 16.)

• Until you know how you react to this drug, do not drive or perform other activities that require alertness.

• Monitor your blood pressure periodically.

• **Do not take any other drugs without first talking to your doctor—especially nonprescription drugs for appetite control, asthma, colds, coughs, hay fever, or sinus problems.**

How to Use This Drug

• Swallow whole tablets. Take without regard for food.

• Do not suddenly stop taking without checking with your doctor to find out if you need to taper off these drugs.

• Do not store in the bathroom. Do not expose to heat, moisture, or strong light.

• If you miss a dose, take it as soon as you remember, but skip it if it is almost time for the next dose. **Do not take double doses.**

Interactions with Other Drugs

Some other drugs that you may be taking (either over-the-counter or prescription drugs) can interact with this one, causing adverse effects. Ask your doctor what these drugs are and let him or her know if you are taking any of them.

Adverse Effects

Call you doctor immediately if you experience:

• cough

• dizziness
• fever, cold, or sore throat
• hoarseness
• skin rash
• swelling of lips, eyes, face, hands or feet
• sudden trouble swallowing or breathing

Call your doctor if these symptoms continue:

• back pain
• diarrhea
• headache
• indigestion
• muscle cramps or pain
• nasal or sinus congestion
• sleep disturbance
• fatigue, weakness
• leg pain

Periodic Testing

Ask your doctor which of these tests should be done periodically while you are taking this drug:

• blood pressure
• renal function determinations

PREGNANCY WARNING

When used in pregnancy during the second and third trimesters, drugs that affect the renin-angiotensin system such as angiotensin II and ACE inhibitors can cause injury and even death to the developing fetus. You should always tell your doctor if you are pregnant or thinking of becoming pregnant before you take this drug.

Do Not Use

ALTERNATIVE TREATMENT:
Mild exercise, no smoking, extreme cleanliness of legs and feet.

Cyclandelate
CYCLOSPASMOL (Wyeth)

FAMILY: Vasodilators
(Blood Vessel Dilators)

It has taken more than 25 years for the Food and Drug Administration to have this ineffective drug removed from the market. The marketing approval for this drug in the United States was revoked effective January 2, 1997. However, the drug was not recalled, so supplies may still exist.

Doctors prescribed cyclandelate (sye *klan* de late) to improve the blood circulation of people with certain types of blood vessel disease. The expectation is that better circulation will relieve pain (leg pain, for example) and improve mental function (by increasing blood flow to the brain). However, there is no evidence that cyclandelate prevents or relieves any disease of blood vessels to the brain, nor has it been shown to improve the mental or physical state of older or senile adults.[182] In fact, although this drug had been available for use and evaluation for many years, it has not been proven effective for treating any condition.[183] The American Medical Association's guide to drug therapy did not even suggest a dose for cyclandelate because "the role of this agent in the treatment of peripheral vascular disease [disease of the blood vessels in the arms or legs] has not been established."[184]

Do Not Use

ALTERNATIVE TREATMENT:
See Hydrochlorothiazide, p. 100.

Reserpine and Chlorothiazide
DIUPRES (Merck Sharp & Dohme)
CHLOROSERPINE (Schein)

FAMILY: Diuretics
Antihypertensives
(See High Blood Pressure, p. 44)

This product, a combination of reserpine (see p. 152) and chlorothiazide (see p. 100), is used to treat high blood pressure (hypertension). **Older adults should not use drugs that contain a fixed combination of reserpine and chlorothiazide.**

Reserpine causes severe adverse effects that may occur during treatment and even months after you stop taking it. It has caused severe depression, in some cases leading to suicide. We do not recommend that any older adult use reserpine, and it is particularly dangerous for anyone with a history of depression. It also decreases mental sharpness in older adults.

In addition to the risks of reserpine, there are good reasons not to use any fixed-combination drug for high blood pressure. A single drug is often enough to control high blood pressure. If a combination drug like this one is controlling your high blood pressure, it is quite possible that one drug alone would do the same job. There is no reason to put yourself at extra risk by taking drugs you do not need.

If you have high blood pressure, the best way to reduce or eliminate your need for medication is by improving your diet, losing weight, exercising, and decreasing your salt and alcohol intake. Mild hypertension can be controlled by proper nutrition and exercise. If these measures do not lower your blood pressure enough and you need medication, **hydrochlorothiazide, a water pill (see thiazide diuretics, p. 100), is the drug of choice starting with a low dose of 12.5 milligrams daily.** It also costs less than other blood pressure drugs.

There is now good evidence that thiazide diuretics, such as hydrochlorothiazide, significantly decrease the rate of bone mineral loss in both men and women because they reduce the amount of calcium lost in the urine. An increasing number of researchers think that this will also decrease the number of fractures.[185]

If your high blood pressure is more severe, and hydrochlorothiazide alone does not control it, there are still better drug treatments than this combination product. The best treatment in this case is a combination of hydrochlorothiazide and a second type of drug called a beta-blocker such as propranolol (see p. 154). If you can't take a drug in the beta-blocker family, another drug called a calcium channel blocker may be used instead. In either case, your doctor would prescribe the hydrochlorothiazide and the second drug separately, with the dose of each drug adjusted to meet your needs, rather than using a product that combines the drugs in advance in a fixed combination.

If you are taking this fixed-combination drug, ask your doctor about changing your prescription.

Whatever drugs you take for high blood pressure, once your blood pressure has been normal for a year or more, a cautious decrease in dose and renewed attention to nondrug treatment may be worth trying, according to *The Medical Letter.*[186]

And an editorial in the *British Medical Journal* stated: *"Treatment of hypertension is part of preventive medicine and like all preventive strategies, its progress should be regularly reviewed by whoever initiates it. Many problems could be avoided by not starting antihypertensive treatment until after prolonged observation. . . . Patients should no longer be told that treatment is necessarily for life: the possibility of reducing or stopping treatment should be mentioned at the outset."*[187]

Limited Use

Quinidine
DURAQUIN (Parke-Davis)
QUINAGLUTE DURA-TABS (Berlex)
QUINIDEX (A.H. Robins)

GENERIC: available
FAMILY: Antiarrhythmics

Quinidine (*kwin* i deen) slows the heart rate and decreases irregular heartbeats (arrhythmias). It is often the first drug used to treat an irregular heartbeat. **If your kidney function is impaired, you will need to take less than the usual dose.**

WARNING! INCREASED RISK OF DEATH

In the National Heart, Lung, and Blood Institute's Cardiac Arrhythmia Suppression Trial (CAST) (a long-term, multi-centered, randomized, double-blind study), in patients with asymptomatic non-life-threatening ventricular (the large chambers of the heart) arrhythmias (rhythm disturbances) who had a heart attack more than six days, but less than two years previously, deaths or non-fatal cardiac arrest were seen in 7.7% of those patients treated with encainide or flecainide, members of the Class 1 group of antiarrhythmic drugs, compared to 3.0% in patients receiving an inactive sugar pill or placebo.

Because of the known ability of the Class 1 drugs, such as quinidine, to cause rhythm disturbances, and the lack of evidence of improved survival for any antiarrhythmic drug in patients without life-threatening heart rhythm disturbances, the use of the Class 1 drugs should be reserved for patients with life-threatening rhythm disturbances of the ventricles. These warnings now appear in the FDA-approved product labeling, or package insert, for all Class 1 drugs including: disopyramide (Norpace and generics), flecainide (Tambocor), mexiletine (Mexitil and generics), moricizine (Ethmozine), procainamide (Procanbid and generics), propafenone (Rythmol), quinidine (Duraquin, Quinaglute Dura-Tabs, Quinidex and generics), and tocainide (Tonocard).

Many people who are taking quinidine or another drug in its family have relatively mild disturbances in their heart rhythm and no symptoms of underlying heart disease. The vast majority of these people do not need these drugs, and there is no evidence that using them improves health. In fact, most of the drugs in this family have severe adverse effects that are sometimes worse, and even more life-threatening, than the irregular heartbeats they treat. All of these drugs can also cause new irregularities in your heartbeat.

If you have an irregular heartbeat, without any symptoms of underlying heart disease, you should not be exposed to the dangers of a drug that has no health benefit for your condition.[188] If you are taking quinidine or another drug in its family for an irregular heartbeat (arrhythmia), talk to your doctor and find out whether you also have symptoms of underlying heart disease. If not, discuss the possibility of stopping the drug.

Some people are very sensitive to quinidine and may have difficulty breathing, changes in vision, dizziness, fever, headache, ringing in ears, or skin rash when taking this drug. Since there is a narrow range between a helpful and a harmful amount of this drug, call your doctor immediately if you experience these adverse effects (as well as any of those listed under Adverse Effects).

Before You Use This Drug

Do not use if you have or have had:

- complete heart block
- digitalis toxicity with heart block

Tell your doctor if you have or have had:

- allergies to drugs
- asthma or emphysema
- incomplete heart block
- digitalis toxicity
- kidney or liver problems
- increased secretion of thyroid hormones
- low blood potassium
- myasthenia gravis
- psoriasis
- difficulty stopping bleeding

Tell your doctor about any other drugs you take, including aspirin, herbs, vitamins, and other nonprescription products.

When You Use This Drug

• **Do not stop taking this drug suddenly. Your doctor must give you a schedule to lower your dose gradually, to prevent serious changes in heart function.**

• Wear a medical identification bracelet or carry a card stating that you take quinidine.

• If you plan to have any surgery, including dental, tell your doctor that you take this drug.

How to Use This Drug

• Swallow extended-release tablets whole. Do not crush or break them. Take with **a full glass (eight ounces) of water.** Take your last dose of the day **with a full glass of water** at least an hour before bedtime. If your stomach gets irritated when you take this drug, you can take it with food or milk to help prevent that.

• If you miss a dose, take it as soon as you remember, but skip it if it is within two hours of your next scheduled dose. **Do not take double doses.**

Interactions with Other Drugs

The following drugs are listed in the *Evaluations of Drug Interactions* 1997 as causing "highly clinically significant" or "clinically significant" interactions when used together with this drug. We have also included potentially serious interactions listed in the drug's FDA-approved professional product labeling or package insert. New scientific techniques have allowed researchers to predict some drug interactions before they have been documented in people. There may be other drugs, especially those in the families of drugs listed below, that also will react with this drug to cause severe adverse effects. The number of new drugs approved for marketing increases the chance of drug interactions, and new drug interactions are being identified with old drugs. Be vigilant. Make sure to tell your doctor and pharmacist the drugs you are taking and tell your doctor if you are taking any of these interacting drugs:

amiodarone, CALAN SR, cimetidine, CORDARONE, COUMADIN, COVERA-HS, cyclosporine, digoxin, DILANTIN, grepafloxacin, ISOPTIN SR, ketoconazole, LANOXICAPS, LANOXIN, LUMINAL, NEORAL, NIZORAL, NORVIR, phenobarbital, phenytoin, propafenone, RAXAR, RIFADIN, rifampin, RIMACTANE, ritonavir, RYTHMOL, SANDIMMUNE, SERLECT, sertindole, SOLFOTON, sparfloxacin, TAGAMET, TUBARINE, tubocurarine, verapamil, VERELAN, warfarin, ZAGAM.

Adverse Effects

Call your doctor immediately if you experience:

• blurred—or any change—in vision
• dizziness or fainting
• fever
• severe headache
• ringing in ears or loss of hearing
• skin rash, hives, or itching
• painful joints
• wheezing, shortness of breath
• unusual bleeding or bruising
• unusually fast heartbeat
• unusual tiredness or weakness

Call your doctor if these symptoms continue:

• bitter taste in mouth
• confusion
• diarrhea
• flushing or itching skin
• loss of appetite
• nausea, vomiting, stomach pain

Periodic Tests

Ask your doctor which of these tests should be done periodically while you are taking this drug:

- blood pressure
- complete blood count
- heart function tests, such as electrocardiogram (ECG, EKG)
- kidney function tests
- liver function tests
- blood levels of potassium and quinidine

PREGNANCY WARNING

This drug caused harm to developing fetuses in animal studies, or such studies were not done. Use during pregnancy only for clear medical reasons. Tell your doctor if you are pregnant or thinking of becoming pregnant before you take this drug.

Limited Use

Triamterene and Hydrochlorothiazide
DYAZIDE (SmithKline Beecham)
MAXZIDE (Bertek)

GENERIC: available

FAMILY: Diuretics
Antihypertensives
(See High Blood Pressure, p. 44)

This product, a combination of triamterene (see p. 99) and hydrochlorothiazide (see p. 100), is used to treat high blood pressure (hypertension). **Older adults should never use drugs that contain a fixed combination of triamterene and hydrochlorothiazide as a first choice drug.** Triamterene can cause kidney stones, kidney failure, and retention of too much potassium (especially if potassium supplements are also given), adverse effects which may be fatal.[189,190] Because of these effects, we do not recommend that any older adult use triamterene, alone.

In addition to triamterene's dangers, there are good reasons not to use any fixed-combination drug for high blood pressure. A single drug is often enough to control high blood pressure. If a combination drug like this one is controlling your high blood pressure, it is quite possible that one drug alone would do the same job. There is no reason to put yourself at extra risk by taking drugs you do not need.

If you have high blood pressure, the best way to reduce or eliminate your need for medication is by improving your diet, losing weight, exercising, and decreasing your salt and alcohol intake. Mild hypertension can be controlled by proper nutrition and exercise. If these measures do not lower your blood pressure enough and you need medication, **hydrochlorothiazide, a water pill (see thiazide diuretics, p. 100), is the drug of choice starting with a low dose of 12.5 milligrams daily.** It also costs less than other blood pressure drugs.

There is now good evidence that thiazide diuretics, such as hydrochlorothiazide, significantly decrease the rate of bone mineral loss in both men and women because they reduce the amount of calcium lost in the urine. An increasing number of researchers think that this will also decrease the number of fractures.[191]

Since Dyazide and Maxzide contain 25 milligrams and 50 milligrams of hydrochlorothiazide respectively, it is not possible for older adults to start with a lower starting dose of 12.5 milligrams if either of these products are used. People responding to 12.5 milligrams of hydrochlorothiazide alone will have a lower risk of adverse effects and less need to use potassium supplements or a potassium-saving drug such as triamterene.

If hydrochlorothiazide alone would control your high blood pressure, there is no reason to take the extra risk of using triamterene as well.

If your high blood pressure is more severe, and hydrochlorothiazide alone does not control it, there are still better drug treatments than this combination product. The best treatment in this case is a combination of hydrochlorothiazide and a second type of drug called a beta-blocker such as propranolol (see p. 154). If you can't take a drug in the beta-blocker family, another drug called a calcium channel blocker may be used instead. In either case, your doctor would prescribe the hydrochlorothiazide and the second drug separately, with the dose of each drug adjusted to meet your needs, rather than using a product that combines the drugs in advance in a fixed combination.

If you are taking this fixed-combination drug, ask your doctor about changing your prescription.

Whatever drugs you take for high blood pressure, once your blood pressure has been normal for a year or more, a cautious decrease in dose and renewed attention to nondrug treatment may be worth trying, according to *The Medical Letter*.[192]

And an editorial in the *British Medical Journal* stated: *"Treatment of hypertension is part of preventive medicine and like all preventive strategies, its progress should be regularly reviewed by whoever initiates it. Many problems could be avoided by not starting antihypertensive treatment until after prolonged observation. . . . Patients should no longer be told that treatment is necessarily for life: the possibility of reducing or stopping treatment should be mentioned at the outset."*[193]

Do Not Use

ALTERNATIVE TREATMENT:
See Hydrochlorothiazide, p. 100.

Triamterene
DYRENIUM (SmithKline Beecham)

FAMILY: Diuretics
Antihypertensives
(See High Blood Pressure, p. 44)

Triamterene (trye *am* ter een) is a water pill (diuretic) that removes less potassium from your body than other types of diuretics do. Doctors sometimes prescribe it for high blood pressure, instead of another diuretic, in the hope that it will prevent a potassium imbalance. **It should not be used by older adults.** It can cause serious and sometimes fatal adverse effects such as kidney stones, kidney failure, retention of too much potassium in your body, and a drop in your body's production of blood cells (bone marrow depression).[194,195]

If you have high blood pressure, the best way to reduce or eliminate your need for medication is by improving your diet, losing weight, exercising, and decreasing your salt and alcohol intake. Mild hypertension can be controlled by proper nutrition and exercise. If these measures do not lower your blood pressure enough and you need medication, **hydrochlorothiazide, a water pill (see thiazide diuretics, p. 100), is the drug of choice starting with a low dose of 12.5 milligrams daily.** It also costs less than other blood pressure drugs.

There is now good evidence that thiazide diuretics, such as hydrochlorothiazide, significantly decrease the rate of bone mineral loss in both men and women because they reduce the amount of calcium lost in the urine. An increasing number of researchers think that this will also decrease the number of fractures.[196]

If you are taking triamterene, ask your doctor about switching to hydrochlorothiazide (see p. 100). If you need to replace potassium in your body because of potassium losses from other drugs, certain potassium supplements are less dangerous than a drug such as triamterene and are equally effective[197] (see p. 49).

If this drug does not lower your blood pressure enough, your doctor can prescribe a second type of drug called a beta-blocker (see p. 52) to accompany the hydrochlorothiazide. If you cannot take a beta-blocker, a drug from another family (calcium channel blockers) can be used instead.

Whatever drugs you take for high blood pressure, once your blood pressure has been normal for a year or more, a cautious decrease in dose and renewed attention to nondrug treatment may be worth trying, according to *The Medical Letter.*[198]

And an editorial in the *British Medical Journal* stated: *"Treatment of hypertension is part of preventive medicine and like all preventive strategies, its progress should be regularly reviewed by whoever initiates it. Many problems could be avoided by not starting antihypertensive treatment until after prolonged observation. . . . Patients should no longer be told that treatment is necessarily for life: the possibility of reducing or stopping treatment should be mentioned at the outset."*[199]

Do Not Use

ALTERNATIVE TREATMENT:
See Hydrochlorothiazide, p. 100.

Deserpidine and Methyclothiazide
ENDURONYL (Abbott)

FAMILY: Diuretics
Antihypertensives
(See High Blood Pressure, p. 44)

This product, a combination of deserpidine (de *ser* pi deen) and methyclothiazide (see p. 101), is used to treat high blood pressure. **Older adults should not use drugs containing a fixed combination of deserpidine and methyclothiazide.**

Deserpidine is in the same family of drugs as reserpine (see p. 152) and should not be used by older adults. Drugs in this family cause severe adverse effects during treatment and sometimes months after treatment has ended. Some people taking these drugs have suffered severe depression, in some cases leading to suicide. Deserpidine is particularly dangerous for anyone with a history of depression.[200] This drug can also cause decreased mental sharpness in older adults.

In addition to the risks of deserpidine, there are good reasons not to use any fixed-combination drug for high blood pressure. A single drug is often enough to control high blood pressure. If a combination drug like this one is controlling your high blood pressure, it is quite possible that one drug alone would do the same job. There is no reason to put yourself at extra risk by taking drugs you do not need.

If you have high blood pressure, the best way to reduce or eliminate your need for medication is by improving your diet, losing weight, exercising, and decreasing your salt and alcohol intake. Mild hypertension can be controlled by proper nutrition and exercise. If these measures do not lower your blood pressure enough and you need medication, **hydrochlorothiazide, a water pill (see thiazide diuretics, p. 100), is the drug of choice starting with a low dose of 12.5 milligrams daily.** It also costs less than other blood pressure drugs.

There is now good evidence that thiazide diuretics, such as hydrochlorothiazide, significantly decrease the rate of bone mineral loss in both men and women because they reduce the amount of calcium lost in the urine. An increasing number of researchers think that this will also decrease the number of fractures.[201]

If your high blood pressure is more severe, and hydrochlorothiazide alone does not control it, there are still better drug treatments than this combination product. The best treatment in this case is a combination of hydrochlorothiazide and a second type of drug called a beta-blocker such as propranolol (see p. 154). If you can't take a drug in the beta-blocker family, another drug called a calcium channel blocker may be used instead. In either case, your doctor would prescribe the hydrochlorothiazide and the second drug separately, with the dose of each drug adjusted to meet your needs, rather than using a product that combines the drugs in advance in a fixed combination.

If you are taking this fixed-combination drug, ask your doctor about changing your prescription.

Whatever drugs you take for high blood pressure, once your blood pressure has been normal for a year or more, a cautious decrease in dose and renewed attention to nondrug treatment may be worth trying, according to *The Medical Letter*.[202]

And an editorial in the *British Medical Journal* stated: *"Treatment of hypertension is part of preventive medicine and like all preventive strategies, its progress should be regularly reviewed by whoever initiates it. Many problems could be avoided by not starting antihypertensive treatment until after prolonged observation. . . . Patients should no longer be told that treatment is necessarily for life: the possibility of reducing or stopping treatment should be mentioned at the outset."*[203]

Hydrochlorothiazide (hye droe klor oh *thye* a zide)
ESIDRIX (Novartis)
HYDRODIURIL (Merck)

Limited Use (following drugs)

Chlorothiazide (klor oh *thye* a zide)
DIURIL (Merck)

Indapamide (in *dap* a mide)
LOZOL (Rhone-Poulenc Rorer)

Methyclothiazide (meth ee kloe *thye* a zide)
ENDURON (Abbott)

Metolazone (me *tole* a zone)
DIULO (Searle)
ZAROXOLYN (Pennwalt)

Trichlormethiazide (trye klor meth *eye* a zide)
METAHYDRIN (Merrell Marion Dow)
NAQUA (Schering)

GENERIC: available
FAMILY: Thiazide Diuretics
Antihypertensives
(See High Blood Pressure, p. 44)

Diuretics, commonly called "water pills," are used to treat high blood pressure (hypertension), congestive heart failure, and other conditions in which the body holds too much fluid.[204] All diuretics have potential adverse effects, commonly including loss of potassium and sodium from the body, harmful interactions with other drugs, and allergic reactions. Older adults also may suffer blood clots and shock, but this is rare.[205] Diuretics in this family (thiazide diuretics) are mild, which reduces the risk of dizziness, falling, and other adverse effects that you may suffer if your body loses too much fluid. It has recently been stated by an expert on hypertension in older adults that "thiazide diuretics [as the ones discussed on this page] are almost certainly safer than any of the other drugs available to treat hypertension."[206]

If you have high blood pressure, the best way to reduce or eliminate your need for medication is by improving your diet, losing weight, exercising, and decreasing your salt and alcohol intake. Mild hypertension can be controlled by proper nutrition and exercise. If these measures do not lower your blood pressure enough and you need medication, **hydrochloro-thiazide is the drug of choice starting with a low dose of 12.5 milligrams daily.** It also costs less than other blood pressure drugs.

There is now good evidence that thiazide diuretics, such as hydrochlorothiazide, significantly decrease the rate of bone mineral loss in both men and women because they reduce the amount of calcium lost in the urine. An increasing number of researchers think that this will also decrease the number of fractures.[207]

Hydrochlorothiazide has been studied more than the other diuretics in this family, is available in a generic form, usually costs less, and is just as effective as the other thiazide diuretics. If you are taking a thiazide diuretic other than hydrochlorothiazide, compare cost and then ask your doctor about switching.

If you are taking hydrochlorothiazide, you should not—in most cases—be taking more than 50 milligrams per day. Daily doses higher than 50 milligrams do not significantly improve blood pressure control and can make adverse effects worse.[208]

If your hypertension is severe, rather than mild, and has not responded to a drug in this family, you may need a stronger drug. See p. 44 for a discussion of the alternatives.

Whatever drugs you take for high blood pressure, once your blood pressure has been normal for a year or more, a cautious decrease in dose and renewed attention to nondrug treatment may be worth trying, according to *The Medical Letter.*[209]

And an editorial in the *British Medical Journal* stated: *"Treatment of hypertension is part of preventive medicine and like all preventive strategies, its progress should be regularly reviewed by whoever initiates it. Many problems could be avoided by not starting antihypertensive treatment until after prolonged observation. . . . Patients should no longer be told that treatment is necessarily for life: the possibility of reducing or stopping treatment should be mentioned at the outset."*[210]

Before You Use This Drug

Do not use if you have or have had:

- a sensitivity to sulfa drugs (sulfonamides) or thiazide drugs

Tell your doctor if you have or have had:

- allergies to drugs
- diabetes
- gout
- kidney, liver, or pancreas problems
- lupus erythematosus
- a salt- or sugar-restricted diet

Tell your doctor about any other drugs you take, including aspirin, herbs, vitamins, and other nonprescription products.

When You Use This Drug

- **Because these drugs help you lose water, you may become dehydrated. Check with your doctor to make certain your fluid intake is adequate and appropriate.**
- Stay out of the sun as much as possible, and call your doctor if you get a rash, hives, or skin reaction. These drugs can make you more sensitive to the sun.
- **These drugs may cause your body to lose potassium, an important mineral.** Potassium loss is worse when there is too much salt in your diet. See p. 49 for information on how to make sure you get enough potassium.
- You may feel dizzy when rising from a lying or sitting position. When getting out of bed, hang your legs over the side of the bed for a few minutes, then get up slowly. When getting up from a chair, stay beside the chair until you are sure that you are not dizzy. (See p. 16.)
- If you plan to have any surgery, including dental, tell your doctor that you take a thiazide diuretic.
- **Do not take any other drugs without first talking to your doctor—especially nonprescription drugs for appetite control, asthma, colds, coughs, hay fever, or sinus problems.**

HEAT STRESS ALERT

These drugs can affect your body's ability to adjust to heat, putting you at risk of "heat stress." If you live alone, ask a friend to check on you several times during the day. Early signs of heat stress are dizziness, lightheadedness, faintness, and slightly high temperature. Call your doctor if you have any of these signs.

Drink more fluids (water, fruit and vegetable juices) than usual—even if you're not thirsty—unless your doctor has told you otherwise. Do not drink alcohol.

How to Use This Drug

- Take with food or milk to avoid stomach irritation. Tablet may be crushed and mixed with food or drink.
- If you are taking a thiazide diuretic more than once a day, try to take the last dose before 6 P.M. This will help you avoid interrupting your sleep to go to the bathroom.
- If you miss a dose, take it as soon as you remember, but skip it if it is almost time for the next dose. **Do not take double doses.**
- Do not store in the bathroom. Do not expose to heat, moisture, or strong light.

Interactions with Other Drugs

The following drugs are listed in the *Evaluations of Drug Interactions* 1997 as causing "highly clinically significant" or "clinically significant" interactions when used together with this drug. We have also included potentially serious interactions listed in the drug's FDA-approved professional product labeling or package insert. New scientific techniques have allowed researchers to predict some drug interactions before they have been documented in people. There may be other drugs, especially those in the families of drugs listed below, that also will react with this drug to cause severe adverse effects. The number of

new drugs approved for marketing increases the chance of drug interactions, and new drug interactions are being identified with old drugs. Be vigilant. Make sure to tell your doctor and pharmacist the drugs you are taking and tell your doctor if you are taking any of these interacting drugs:

> calcium carbonate, CALTRATE, CAPOTEN, captopril, chlorpropamide, DIABINESE, digoxin, guanethidine, INDOCIN, indomethacin, ISMELIN, LANOXICAPS, LANOXIN, lithium, LITHOBID, LITHONATE, OS-CAL 500.

> The drugs listed above have reported interactions with hydrochlorothiazide. Not all of these interactions may have been reported for the other thiazide diuretics listed in this section. Always ask your doctor and pharmacist about specific interactions for the thiazide diuretic you are taking.

Adverse Effects

Call your doctor immediately if you experience:

- coughing, wheezing or hoarseness
- difficulty breathing
- dry mouth or increased thirst that does not go away quickly after you take a drink
- fever, chills
- irregular heartbeat, chest pain
- weak pulse
- mood or mental changes
- muscle cramps, pain
- nausea, vomiting
- unusual tiredness or weakness
- black, tarry stools
- blood in urine or stools
- joint, lower back or side pain
- painful or difficult urination

Call your doctor if these symptoms continue:

- dizziness, lightheadedness

- diarrhea
- loss of appetite, upset stomach
- headache
- blurred vision or "halo" effect
- premature ejaculation or difficulty with erection

Periodic Tests

Ask your doctor which of these tests should be done periodically while you are taking this drug:

- blood pressure
- complete blood count
- blood levels of sodium, potassium, chloride, calcium, sugar, and uric acid
- liver function tests
- kidney function tests

PREGNANCY WARNING

Metahydrin and Naqua caused harm to developing fetuses in animal studies, or such studies were not done. Use during pregnancy only for clear medical reasons. Tell your doctor if you are pregnant or thinking of becoming pregnant before you take any of these drugs.

 Do Not Use

ALTERNATIVE TREATMENT: *See Hydrochlorothiazide, p. 100.*

Reserpine and Hydrochlorothiazide
HYDROPRES (Merck)
HYDROSERPINE (Schein)

FAMILY: Diuretics
Antihypertensives
(See High Blood Pressure, p. 44)

This product, a combination of reserpine (see p. 152) and hydrochlorothiazide (see p. 100), is used to treat high blood pressure (hypertension). **Older adults should not use drugs that contain a fixed combination of reserpine and hydrochlorothiazide.**

Reserpine causes severe adverse effects that may occur during treatment and even months after you stop taking it. It has caused severe depression, in some cases leading to suicide. We do not recommend that any older adult use reserpine, and it is particularly dangerous for anyone with a history of depression.[211] It also decreases mental sharpness in older adults.

In addition to the risks of reserpine, there are good reasons not to use any fixed-combination drug for high blood pressure. A single drug is often enough to control high blood pressure. If a combination drug like this one is controlling your high blood pressure, it is quite possible that one drug alone would do the same job. There is no reason to put yourself at extra risk by taking drugs you do not need.

If you have high blood pressure, the best way to reduce or eliminate your need for medication is by improving your diet, losing weight, exercising, and decreasing your salt and alcohol intake. Mild hypertension can be controlled by proper nutrition and exercise. If these measures do not lower your blood pressure enough and you need medication, **hydrochlorothiazide, a water pill (see thiazide diuretics, p. 100), is the drug of choice starting with a low dose of 12.5 milligrams daily.** It also costs less than other blood pressure drugs.

There is now good evidence that thiazide diuretics, such as hydrochlorothiazide, significantly decrease the rate of bone mineral loss in both men and women because they reduce the amount of calcium lost in the urine. An increasing number of researchers think that this will also decrease the number of fractures.[212]

Hydrochlorothiazide is one of the ingredients in this combination. Reserpine can cause severe adverse effects, as described above. If hydrochlorothiazide alone would control your blood pressure, there is no reason to take the extra risk of taking the second drug as well.

If your high blood pressure is more severe, and hydrochlorothiazide alone does not control it, there are still better drug treatments than this combination product. The best treatment in this case is a combination of hydrochlorothiazide and a second type of drug called a beta-blocker, such as propranolol (see p. 154). If you can't take a drug in the beta-blocker family, another drug called a calcium channel blocker may be used instead. In either case, your doctor would prescribe the hydrochlorothiazide and the second drug separately, with the dose of each drug adjusted to meet your needs, rather than using a product that combines the drugs in advance in a fixed combination.

If you are taking this fixed-combination drug, ask your doctor about changing your prescription.

Whatever drugs you take for high blood pressure, once your blood pressure has been normal for a year or more, a cautious decrease in dose and renewed attention to nondrug treatment may be worth trying, according to *The Medical Letter.*[213]

And an editorial in the *British Medical Journal* stated: *"Treatment of hypertension is part of preventive medicine and like all preventive strategies, its progress should be regularly reviewed by whoever initiates it. Many problems could be avoided by not starting antihypertensive treatment until after prolonged observation. . . . Patients should no longer be told that treatment is necessarily for life: the possibility of reducing or stopping treatment should be mentioned at the outset."*[214]

Do Not Use

ALTERNATIVE TREATMENT:
See Hydrochlorothiazide, p. 100.

Chlorthalidone
HYGROTON (Rhone-Poulenc Rorer)

FAMILY: Diuretics
Antihypertensives
(See High Blood Pressure, p. 44)

Chlorthalidone (klor *thal* i doan) is used to remove water and salt from the body in order to lower blood pressure. **It should not be used by people over 60.** It can make you urinate more often, so that you may lose too much water, potassium, and magnesium which can be dangerous; it can also cause you to lose bladder control, which is both inconvenient and embarrassing. The risk of serious adverse effects is so high that the World Health Organization has said chlorthalidone should not be used by older adults.[215]

If you have high blood pressure, the best way to reduce or eliminate your need for medication is by improving your diet, losing weight, exercising, and decreasing your salt and alcohol intake. Mild hypertension can be controlled by proper nutrition and exercise. If these measures do not lower your blood pressure enough and you need medication, **hydrochlorothiazide, a water pill (see thiazide diuretics, p. 100), is the drug of choice starting with a low dose of 12.5 milligrams daily.** It also costs less than other blood pressure drugs.

There is now good evidence that thiazide diuretics, such as hydrochlorothiazide, significantly decrease the rate of bone mineral loss in both men and women because they reduce the amount of calcium lost in the urine. An increasing number of researchers think that this will also decrease the number of fractures.[216]

If this drug does not lower your blood pressure enough, your doctor can prescribe a second type

of drug called a beta-blocker (see p. 52) to accompany the hydrochlorothiazide. If you cannot take a beta-blocker, a drug from another family (calcium channel blockers) can be used instead.

If you use chlorthalidone, ask your doctor about changing your prescription to hydrochlorothiazide.

Whatever drugs you take for high blood pressure, once your blood pressure has been normal for a year or more, a cautious decrease in dose and renewed attention to nondrug treatment may be worth trying, according to *The Medical Letter.*[217]

And an editorial in the *British Medical Journal* stated: *"Treatment of hypertension is part of preventive medicine and like all preventive strategies, its progress should be regularly reviewed by whoever initiates it. Many problems could be avoided by not starting antihypertensive treatment until after prolonged observation. . . . Patients should no longer be told that treatment is necessarily for life: the possibility of reducing or stopping treatment should be mentioned at the outset."*[218]

Limited Use for High Blood Pressure

Terazosin
HYTRIN (Abbott)

GENERIC: not available
FAMILY: Antihypertensives
(See High Blood Pressure, p. 44)

Terazosin (tair *az* o sin) is used to control high blood pressure (hypertension) and treat the symptoms of benign prostatic hyperplasia (BPH) and is in a group of drugs called alpha adrenergic blocking agents. It does not cure hypertension.[219] According to *The Medical Letter*, this group of drugs is not a good first choice for hypertension.[220]

Terazosin relieves the symptoms of BPH by relaxing the muscles around the neck of the bladder and appears to work both for men with small and with large prostate glands.

When taken for high blood pressure, terazosin is sometimes combined with a water pill (thiazide diuretic, see p. 100) or a beta-blocker (see p. 52). The water pill works with terazosin to lower your blood pressure and helps decrease your body's retention of salt and water, but it also increases your risk of becoming dizzy or lightheaded.

Occasionally, a person will collapse and lose consciousness for a few minutes up to an hour after taking his or her first dose. This is more likely to happen to older adults, but several measures decrease the risk of fainting.[221,222] Your doctor should prescribe a first dose of no more than one milligram. Before you take the first dose, remove any object that would be dangerous if you fell onto it. It is wise to have a companion stay with you for a couple of hours after taking the first dose. Do not drive or attempt any hazardous task for 24 hours after the first dose.

Eat some food. If your diet allows, include a moderate amount of salt. Do not stand for a prolonged time. It is best to take your dose at bedtime.[223] Repeat these precautions any time your dose is increased, or if you restart the drug after an interruption in therapy, or if an additional blood pressure drug is prescribed for you. It may take eight weeks to reach the desired control of blood pressure using terazosin. Some individuals develop heart palpitations and rapid heartbeat with this medication. Be sure to report this to your doctor if it occurs.

If you have high blood pressure, the best way to reduce or eliminate your need for medication is by improving your diet, losing weight, exercising, and decreasing your salt and alcohol intake. Mild hypertension can be controlled by proper nutrition and exercise. If these measures do not lower your blood pressure enough and you need medication, **hydrochloro-thiazide, a water pill (see thiazide diuretics, p. 100), is the drug of choice starting with a low dose of 12.5 milligrams daily.** It also costs less than other blood pressure drugs.

There is now good evidence that thiazide diuretics, such as hydrochlorothiazide, significantly decrease the rate of bone mineral loss in both men and women because they reduce the amount of calcium lost in the urine. An increasing number of researchers think that this will also decrease the number of fractures.[224]

If this drug does not lower your blood pressure enough, your doctor can prescribe a second type of drug called a beta-blocker (see p. 52) to accompany the hydrochlorothiazide. If you cannot take a beta-blocker, a drug from another family (calcium channel blockers) can be used instead.

Whatever drugs you take for high blood pressure, once your blood pressure has been normal for a year or more, a cautious decrease in dose and renewed attention to nondrug treatment may be worth trying, according to *The Medical Letter.*[225]

And an editorial in the *British Medical Journal* stated: "*Treatment of hypertension is part of preventive medicine and like all preventive strategies, its progress should be regularly reviewed by whoever initiates it. Many problems could be avoided by not starting antihypertensive treatment until after prolonged observation. . . . Patients should no longer be told that treatment is necessarily for life: the possibility of reducing or stopping treatment should be mentioned at the outset.*"[226]

Before You Use This Drug

Tell your doctor if you have or have had:

- allergies to drugs
- angina (chest pain)
- heart disease
- kidney function impairment

- liver function impairment (dose should be decreased)
- a low-salt diet

Tell your doctor about any other drugs you take, including aspirin, herbs, vitamins, and other nonprescription products.

When You Use This Drug

- You may feel dizzy when rising from a lying or sitting position. If you are lying down, hang your legs over the side of the bed for a few minutes, then get up slowly. When getting up from a chair, stay by the chair until you are sure that you are not dizzy. (See p. 16.)
- If you plan to have any surgery, including dental, tell your doctor that you take this drug.
- Until you know how you react to this drug, do not drive or perform other activities that require alertness.
- **Do not take other drugs without talking to your doctor first—especially nonprescription drugs for appetite control, asthma, colds, coughs, hay fever, sinus problems, pain, or sleep.**

HEAT STRESS ALERT

This drug can affect your body's ability to adjust to heat, putting you at risk of "heat stress." If you live alone, ask a friend to check on you several times during the day. Early signs of heat stress are dizziness, lightheadedness, faintness, and slightly high temperature. Call your doctor if you have any of these signs.

Drink more fluids (water, fruit and vegetable juices) than usual—even if you're not thirsty—unless your doctor has told you otherwise. Do not drink alcohol.

How to Use This Drug

- Swallow tablets whole. Do not fast while taking this drug.

- Take at the same time every day, preferably at bedtime.
- Take even when you feel well.
- If your doctor directs taking terazosin twice a day, space your doses 10 to 12 hours apart.
- If you miss a dose, take it as soon as you remember, but skip it if it is almost time for the next dose. **Do not take double doses.**
- Store at room temperature with cap on tightly. Do not store in the bathroom. Do not expose to heat.
- Monitor your blood pressure periodically, both standing and lying down.[227]

Interactions with Other Drugs

The following drugs are listed in the *Evaluations of Drug Interactions* 1997 as causing "highly clinically significant" or "clinically significant" interactions when used together with this drug. We have also included potentially serious interactions listed in the drug's FDA-approved professional product labeling or package insert. New scientific techniques have allowed researchers to predict some drug interactions before they have been documented in people. There may be other drugs, especially those in the families of drugs listed below, that also will react with this drug to cause severe adverse effects. The number of new drugs approved for marketing increases the chance of drug interactions, and new drug interactions are being identified with old drugs. Be vigilant. Make sure to tell your doctor and pharmacist the drugs you are taking and tell your doctor if you are taking any of these interacting drugs:

digoxin, INDOCIN, indomethacin, LANOXICAPS, LANOXIN.

Adverse Effects

Call your doctor immediately if you experience:

- dizziness, lightheadedness

- fainting
- chest pain (angina)
- irregular heartbeat
- shortness of breath
- swelling of feet and lower legs
- inability to control urination
- numbness and tingling of hands and feet
- skin rash

Call your doctor if these symptoms continue:

- drowsiness
- headache
- lack of energy
- nausea, vomiting
- decreased sexual ability
- diarrhea or constipation
- dry cough
- nasal congestion
- pain in joints, arms, back, or legs
- unusual tiredness
- undesired weight gain
- blurred vision

Periodic Tests

Ask your doctor which of these tests should be done periodically while you are taking this drug:

- blood pressure

PREGNANCY WARNING

This drug caused harm to developing fetuses in animal studies, or such studies were not done. Use during pregnancy only for clear medical reasons. Tell your doctor if you are pregnant or thinking of becoming pregnant before you take this drug.

Isosorbide Dinitrate
ISORDIL (Wyeth-Ayerst)
SORBITRATE (Zeneca)

Isosorbide-5-mononitrate
ISMO (Wyeth-Ayerst)
IMDUR (Schering/Key)

Nitroglycerin
DEPONIT (Schwarz Pharma K-U)
MINITRAN (3-M)
NITRO-BID (Hoechst Marion Roussel)
NITRODISC (Searle)
NITRO-DUR (Key)
NITROSTAT (Parke-Davis)
TRANSDERM-NITRO (Novartis)

GENERIC: available
FAMILY: Nitrates

WARNING

If you are taking any member of the nitrate family of drugs you should not take sildenafil (Viagra), a drug used for sexual dysfunction. The use of sildenafil in men who were treated with a nitrate has resulted in deaths.

Isosorbide dinitrate (eye soe *sor* bide dye *nye* trate), isosorbide-5-mononitrate, the major breakdown product of isosorbide dinitrate, and nitroglycerin (nye troe *gli* ser in) are used to treat sudden severe attacks of chest pain (acute angina). They come in several different forms: tablets that dissolve under the tongue (sublingual), chewable tablets, tablets and capsules to be swallowed, and ointments and patches to be applied to the skin. For treating sudden attacks of chest pain, only the sublingual tablets, and certain chewable tablets are effective. The other dosage forms are used on a regular basis to prevent angina attacks from occurring, although the high doses of oral tablets and capsules needed to be effective make them less useful.

Wearing nitroglycerin patches continuously can lead to tolerance to nitroglycerin, which can be prevented or slowed by wearing patches for only 10 to 12 hours, instead of continuously. However, the nitrate-free interval may be associated with decreased tolerance to exercise, and the possibility of increased angina.[228]

Before You Use This Drug

Tell your doctor if you have or have had:

- allergies to any adhesives, drugs, or other materials
- glaucoma
- hemorrhage of a blood vessel supplying the head
- food absorption problem
- recent heart attack or stroke
- severe anemia
- trauma to the head
- kidney or liver problems
- overactive thyroid

Tell your doctor about any other drugs you take, including aspirin, herbs, vitamins, and other nonprescription products.

When You Use This Drug

- You may feel dizzy for a time, or faint, after taking these drugs, especially if you are upright and standing still. If you feel dizzy, put your head between your knees, breathe deeply, and move your arms and legs.
- Be careful not to overexert yourself, even though your chest pain may feel better.
- Do not drink alcohol.
- **If you are taking this drug regularly, do not stop taking it suddenly.** Your doctor must give you a schedule to lower your dose gradually, to prevent chest pain and possible heart attack.

- Until you know how you react to this drug, do not drive or perform other activities requiring alertness.
- *For patch:* Carry identification that you use nitroglycerin patches.
- If you seek emergency care, or have surgery, including dental, tell your doctor that you take nitroglycerin and the form you use.

HEAT STRESS ALERT

These drugs can affect your body's ability to adjust to heat, putting you at risk of "heat stress." If you live alone, ask a friend to check on you several times during the day. Early signs of heat stress are dizziness, lightheadedness, faintness, and slightly high temperature. Call your doctor if you have any of these signs.

Drink more fluids (water, fruit and vegetable juices) than usual—even if you're not thirsty—unless your doctor has told you otherwise. Do not drink alcohol.

How to Use This Drug

For sublingual form:

- Place tablet under tongue and allow it to dissolve. Do not chew, crush, or swallow. While tablet is dissolving, do not eat, drink, or smoke.
- Store tablets only in the original container with the lid on tightly. Nitroglycerin is very sensitive and can lose strength rapidly if not stored properly. Do not add any other drug, material, or object to the container that was not there originally. Protect from air, heat, moisture, and sunlight. This includes times you carry nitroglycerin with you, or otherwise store it away from home. Special stainless-steel containers are available to wear for emergency supplies of nitroglycerin. Once any container of nitroglycerin is opened, the supply should be replaced within six months.

• *For isosorbide dinitrate and mononitrate:* You should feel the drug's effect in five minutes. If the pain does not go away in 5 to 10 minutes, take a second tablet. If you still have chest pain after three tablets in 15 minutes, call your doctor or go to an emergency room immediately.

• *For nitroglycerin:* You should feel the drug's effect in five minutes. If the pain does not go away in five minutes, take a second tablet. If you still have chest pain after three tablets in 10 to 15 minutes, call your doctor or go to an emergency room immediately.

• **Do not take other drugs without talking to your doctor first—especially non-prescription drugs for appetite control, asthma, colds, coughs, hay fever, or sinus problems.**

For patch form:

• Open and prepare patch according to package instructions. Do not cut or trim the patch to adjust the dose.

• Select a site that is dry, on the chest, upper arm, or shoulders. Avoid areas that are broken, calloused, hairy, irritated or shaved. Do not use sites below the knee or elbow, or areas where movement or clothing is apt to dislodge the patch. The need to rotate sites has recently been questioned.

• Press adhesive side of patch to skin firmly.

• Replace patch if it loosens, or falls off.

• Leave on the amount of time specified by your doctor, then remove.

• Apply new patch at the same time each day.

• Discard used patch.

• Store unopened patches at room temperature. Do not expose to high temperatures or moisture. Do not store in a bathroom or refrigerator.

Interactions with Other Drugs

The following drugs are listed in the *Evaluations of Drug Interactions* 1997 as causing "highly clinically significant" or "clinically significant" interactions when used together with this drug. We have also included potentially serious interactions listed in the drug's FDA-approved professional product labeling or package insert. New scientific techniques have allowed researchers to predict some drug interactions before they have been documented in people. There may be other drugs, especially those in the families of drugs listed below, that also will react with this drug to cause severe adverse effects. The number of new drugs approved for marketing increases the chance of drug interactions, and new drug interactions are being identified with old drugs. Be vigilant. Make sure to tell your doctor and pharmacist the drugs you are taking and tell your doctor if you are taking any of these interacting drugs:

D.H.E-45, dihydroergotamine (with nitroglycerin), disopyramide, heparin, imipramine, NORPACE, sildenafil, TOFRANIL, VIAGRA.

Adverse Effects

Call your doctor immediately if you experience:

• **signs of overdose:** bluish lips, fingernails, or palms, dizziness or fainting, feeling of pressure in head, shortness of breath, unusual tiredness or weakness, weak and unusually fast heartbeat, fever, seizures
  • blurred vision
  • dry mouth
  • severe or prolonged headache
  • skin rash

Call your doctor if these symptoms continue:

  • dizziness, lightheadedness
  • nausea or vomiting
  • flushed face and neck
  • rapid pulse
  • burning, itching, or reddened skin

Periodic Tests

Ask your doctor which of these tests should be done periodically while you are taking this drug:

- blood pressure and pulse
- heart function tests, such as electrocardiogram (ECG, EKG)

PREGNANCY WARNING

This drug caused harm to developing fetuses in animal studies, or such studies were not done. Use during pregnancy only for clear medical reasons. Tell your doctor if you are pregnant or thinking of becoming pregnant before you take this drug.

Potassium Supplements (Nondietary)
Oral solution
KAY CIEL (Forest)
KAOCHLOR, KAON-CL (Savage)

Powder for oral solution
K-LOR (Abbott)
KATO (ICN)
K-LYTE TABLETS (Mead Johnson)

Limited Use (following drugs)

Extended-release capsules
MICRO-K (Robins)

Extended-release tablets
KLOTRIX (Apothecon) **SLOW-K** (Novartis)

GENERIC: available
FAMILY: Potassium Supplements (See p. 49)

If you need to get more of the mineral potassium (poe *tass* ee um), the safest and least expensive way is to eat more potassium-rich foods *daily* (see p. 49 for a discussion of dietary potassium). When researchers compared people eating a potassium-rich diet, people taking potassium supplements, and people taking drugs designed to keep potassium in the body, they found the following: (1) diet is the safest way to replace potassium and (2) potassium supplements and potassium-sparing drugs return potassium levels to normal in only half the people who use them.

Potassium supplements can cause stomach and intestinal ulcers, bleeding, blockage, and perforation. Because of these serious potential adverse effects, you should only take supplements if you have been eating plenty of potassium-rich foods yet still have a low level of potassium in your blood (less than 3.0 millimoles per liter of blood).[229] Also, you should only take potassium supplements if you have adequate kidney function. The safest form of potassium supplement is an oral solution (liquid) of potassium chloride, and you should only use other forms if you cannot tolerate the liquid. However, enteric-coated potassium products should never be taken.

Before You Use This Drug

Do not use if you have or have had:

- Addison's disease
- prolonged and severe diarrhea
- heart disease
- intestinal blockage
- kidney disease or decreased urine production
- stomach ulcer

Tell your doctor about any other drugs you take, including aspirin, herbs, vitamins, and other nonprescription products.

When You Use This Drug

• **If you have black, tarry stools or bloody vomit, call your doctor immediately.** These are signs of stomach or intestinal bleeding.

• Schedule regular appointments with your doctor to check your progress.

• Check with your doctor before using salt substitutes, low-salt milk, or other low-salt foods. Because these foods often contain potassium, your potassium supplement dose may have to be adjusted to avoid getting dangerously high levels of potassium in your blood.

• Ask your doctor whether you should supplement your diet with vitamin B_{12}. Your body may not be able to absorb this vitamin as well while you are taking potassium supplements.

How to Use This Drug

• Take with, or immediately after, meals. If you are taking extended-release tablets or capsules, swallow them whole, without chewing or crushing them. Take tablets with **a full glass (eight ounces) of water.** Take your last dose of the day with a full glass of water at least an hour before bedtime. Taking this drug with food may help prevent stomach irritation. If you are taking a solution, dissolvable tablet, or powder, dissolve it completely in at least one half glass (four ounces) of juice or cold water, then sip slowly over a five-to-ten minute period. Do not use tomato juice, which has a high salt content.

• Do not store in the bathroom. Do not expose to heat, moisture, or strong light. Do not allow the liquid form to freeze.

• If you miss a dose, take it within two hours of the time you were supposed to take it. Skip it if it is almost time for the next dose. **Do not take double doses.**

Interactions with Other Drugs

The following drugs are listed in the *Evaluations of Drug Interactions* 1997 as causing "highly clinically significant" or "clinically significant" interactions when used together with this drug. We have also included potentially serious interactions listed in the drug's FDA-approved professional product labeling or package insert. New scientific techniques have allowed researchers to predict some drug interactions before they have been documented in people. There may be other drugs, especially those in the families of drugs listed below, that also will react with this drug to cause severe adverse effects. The number of new drugs approved for marketing increases the chance of drug interactions, and new drug interactions are being identified with old drugs. Be vigilant. Make sure to tell your doctor and pharmacist the drugs you are taking and tell your doctor if you are taking any of these interacting drugs:

angiotensin converting enzyme (ACE) inhibitors, potassium sparing diuretics, salt substitutes.

Adverse Effects

Call your doctor immediately if you experience:

• confusion
• irregular heartbeat
• numbness or tingling in hands, feet, or lips
• unusual tiredness or weakness
• weakness or heaviness of legs
• difficulty breathing
• unexplained anxiety
• abdominal or stomach pain, cramping or soreness
• chest or throat pain
• bloody or black tarry stools

Call your doctor if these symptoms continue:

- diarrhea*
- nausea or vomiting*
- stomach pain*

These adverse effects can be reduced by taking potassium with food or by using more liquid (water or juice) to dilute it.

Periodic Tests

Ask your doctor which of these tests should be done periodically while you are taking this drug:

- heart function tests, such as electrocardiogram (ECG, EKG)
- kidney function tests
- blood potassium levels
- blood pH and bicarbonate levels

PREGNANCY WARNING

This drug caused harm to developing fetuses in animal studies, or such studies were not done. Use during pregnancy only for clear medical reasons. Tell your doctor if you are pregnant or thinking of becoming pregnant before you take this drug.

Digoxin
LANOXIN, LANOXICAPS (Glaxo Wellcome)

GENERIC: available
FAMILY: Digitalis Glycosides
Antiarrhythmics

Digoxin (di *jox* in) is usually used to treat heart failure, a condition in which the heart cannot pump enough blood through the body. The symptoms of heart failure are fatigue, difficulty breathing, swelling (especially in the legs and ankles), and rapid or "galloping" heart-beats. Digoxin is also used to slow certain kinds of abnormally fast heartbeats and to stabilize certain kinds of irregular heartbeats (arrhythmias).

Before prescribing digoxin for heart failure, your doctor should first try giving you another type of drug called a thiazide diuretic (water pill), see p. 100. You should only switch to digoxin if the diuretic does not control your symptoms well enough. **In general, if you are over 60, you should be taking a smaller daily dose than the usual 0.25 milligram,[230] especially if you have impaired kidney function.**

Anyone taking digoxin is at risk of toxic effects (digitalis toxicity). While you are taking digoxin, your doctor should regularly check the levels of the drug in your blood. You and your doctor should also watch for the subtle symptoms of toxicity: fatigue, loss of appetite, nausea and vomiting, problems with vision, bad dreams, nervousness, drowsiness, and hallucinations.[231] Other signs of toxicity are changes in heart rhythm, slow pulse, and lethargy. Since there is a narrow range between a helpful and a harmful amount of digoxin in your body, you should take the drug daily in the exact amount prescribed. If you get too much digoxin in your body, you may develop the effects listed above; if you get too little, you may develop symptoms of heart failure or a rapid heart rate.

Digoxin is often overprescribed for older adults.[232] One study of people using digoxin outside the hospital found that four out of ten people were getting no benefit from the drug.[233] Because of digoxin's toxic effects, taking the drug when it has no benefit is not only wasteful but also dangerous. As many as one in five digoxin users develops signs of toxic effects,[234] and much of this could be prevented if the people who did not need digoxin were taken off the drug. Evidence shows that **up to eight out of ten long-term digoxin users can stop**

using the drug successfully, under close
supervision by a doctor, with no harmful
results.[235] This is partly due to digoxin being
wrongly prescribed in the first place.

If you have used digoxin regularly for some
time, ask your doctor if you might be able to try
withdrawing from the drug. You are more likely to be able to stop taking digoxin if you meet
the following conditions:

1. You have used digoxin for a long time
   without your initial symptoms of heart
   failure coming back.
2. You have a normal heart rhythm.
3. You are not using digoxin to control an
   irregular heart rhythm.

There is no good way of knowing in advance
who can stop taking digoxin. People taking
digoxin to correct an irregular heart rhythm
should not attempt to stop taking the drug, but
most other people will benefit from a trial of
withdrawal under close supervision by a doctor.

Before You Use This Drug

Do not use if you have or have had:

- toxic effects from other digitalis preparations
- ventricular fibrillation

Tell your doctor if you have or have had:

- allergies to drugs
- high blood calcium level
- decreased thyroid hormones
- rheumatic fever
- heart block
- carotid sinus hypersensitivity
- high or low blood potassium level
- insufficient oxygen supply to the heart
- irregular or rapid heartbeat
- kidney or liver problems
- low blood magnesium level
- heart attack

- severe lung disease
- heart disease in which enlargement of the
  heart muscle decreases the heart's ability to
  pump blood (IHSS)

Tell your doctor about any other drugs you take, including aspirin, herbs, vitamins, and other nonprescription products.

When You Use This Drug

- **Learn to take your pulse, and get
  immediate medical help if your pulse
  slows to 60 beats per minute or less. Some
  people have suffered a slow heart rate
  and heart failure while using digoxin.**
- **Do not stop taking this drug suddenly.** Your doctor must give you a schedule to
  lower your dose gradually, to prevent serious
  changes in your heart function.
- Wear a medical identification bracelet or
  carry a card saying that you take digoxin.
- Eat a diet that is rich in potassium, adequate in magnesium, and low in salt and
  dietary fiber (see p. 49).
- **Do not take other drugs without talking to your doctor first—especially nonprescription drugs for appetite control,
  asthma, colds, coughs, hay fever, or sinus
  problems.**
- If you plan to have any surgery, including
  dental, tell your doctor that you take this drug.

How to Use This Drug

- Crush tablets and mix with water, or
  swallow whole with water. Take on an empty
  stomach, at least one hour before or two hours
  after meals.
- Measure the liquid form only with the specially marked dropper.
- If you miss a dose, do not take it. Wait
  until your next scheduled dose. **Do not take
  double doses.** If you miss two or more doses in
  a row, call your doctor.

Interactions with Other Drugs

The following drugs are listed in the *Evaluations of Drug Interactions* 1997 as causing "highly clinically significant" or "clinically significant" interactions when used together with this drug. We have also included potentially serious interactions listed in the drug's FDA-approved professional product labeling or package insert. New scientific techniques have allowed researchers to predict some drug interactions before they have been documented in people. There may be other drugs, especially those in the families of drugs listed below, that also will react with this drug to cause severe adverse effects. The number of new drugs approved for marketing increases the chance of drug interactions, and new drug interactions are being identified with old drugs. Be vigilant. Make sure to tell your doctor and pharmacist the drugs you are taking and tell your doctor if you are taking any of these interacting drugs:

ACHROMYCIN, ADVIL, ALDACTONE, aluminum hydroxide, amiodarone, AMPHOJEL, ANECTINE, AZULFIDINE, CALAN SR, CALCIJECT, calcium chloride injection, CAPOTEN, captopril, cholestyramine, CORDARONE, COVERA-HS, CUPRIMINE, cyclophosphamide, cyclosporine, CYTOXAN, DELTASONE, DEPEN, diazepam, DILANTIN, DURAQUIN, EES, ERYTHROCIN, erythromycin, furosemide, GAVISCON, hydroxychloroquine, ibuprofen, ISOPTIN SR, kaolin and pectin, KAO-SPEN, KAPECTOLIN, LASIX, LOCHOLEST, magnesium hydroxide, MATULANE, METICORTEN, metoclopramide, MINIPRESS, MOTRIN, neomycin, NEORAL, ONCOVIN, PANMYCIN, penicillamine, phenytoin, PHILLIPS' MILK OF MAGNESIA, PLAQUENIL, prazosin, prednisone, PRO-BANTHINE, procarbazine, propafenone, propantheline, QUESTRAN, QUINAGLUTE DURA-TABS, QUINIDEX, quinidine, REGLAN, RYTHMOL, SANDIMMUNE, spironolactone, succinylcholine, sulfasalazine, tetracycline, thyroid, VALIUM, VERELAN, verapamil, vincristine.

Adverse Effects

Call your doctor immediately if you experience:

- **signs of overdose**: loss of appetite, nausea, vomiting, lower stomach pain, diarrhea, irregular heartbeats, slow pulse, unusual tiredness or weakness, blurred vision or colored "halos," depression or confusion, drowsiness, headache, bad dreams, hallucinations, nervousness, skin rash or hives, fainting

Periodic Tests

Ask your doctor which of these tests should be done periodically while you are taking this drug:

- blood pressure and pulse rate
- heart function tests, such as electrocardiogram (ECG, EKG)
- kidney function tests
- liver function tests
- blood levels of potassium, magnesium and calcium
- blood levels of digoxin

PREGNANCY WARNING

This drug caused harm to developing fetuses in animal studies, or such studies were not done. Use during pregnancy only for clear medical reasons. Tell your doctor if you are pregnant or thinking of becoming pregnant before you take this drug.

Furosemide
LASIX (Hoechst Marion Roussel)

GENERIC: available

FAMILY: Diuretics
         Antihypertensives
         (See High Blood Pressure, p. 44)

Furosemide (fur *oh* se mide) is a very strong "water pill" (loop diuretic) with many adverse effects. It is used to treat fluid retention and high blood pressure. If you are over 60, you should be taking this drug only to reduce fluid retention, and then only if you have decreased kidney function and have tried milder drugs such as hydrochlorothiazide (see p. 100) without success. People over 60 years old who have normal kidney function should not use furosemide for any reason.[236]

The World Health Organization recommends that furosemide should not be used for the treatment of high blood pressure in older adults because it has been associated with the occurence of stroke.[237] Older adults are more likely than others to develop blood clots, shock,[238] dizziness, confusion, and insomnia, and to have an increased risk of falling, while taking furosemide.[239]

If you have high blood pressure, the best way to reduce or eliminate your need for medication is by improving your diet, losing weight, exercising, and decreasing your salt and alcohol intake. Mild hypertension can be controlled by proper nutrition and exercise. If these measures do not lower your blood pressure enough and you need medication, **hydrochlorothiazide, a water pill (see thiazide diuretics, p. 100), is the drug of choice starting with a low dose of 12.5 milligrams daily.** It also costs less than other blood pressure drugs.

There is now good evidence that thiazide diuretics, such as hydrochlorothiazide, significantly decrease the rate of bone mineral loss in both men and women because they reduce the amount of calcium lost in the urine. An increasing number of researchers think that this will also decrease the number of fractures.[240]

If hydrochlorothiazide alone does not work, your doctor should add a second drug such as a beta-blocker, for example propranolol (see p. 154) rather than switching you to a strong diuretic like furosemide.

Whatever drugs you take for high blood pressure, once your blood pressure has been normal for a year or more, a cautious decrease in dose and renewed attention to nondrug treatment may be worth trying, according to *The Medical Letter*.[243]

And an editorial in the *British Medical Journal* stated: "*Treatment of hypertension is part of preventive medicine and like all preventive strategies, its progress should be regularly reviewed by whoever initiates it. Many problems could be avoided by not starting antihypertensive treatment until after prolonged observation. . . . Patients should no longer be told that treatment is necessarily for life: the possibility of reducing or stopping treatment should be mentioned at the outset.*"[244]

Before You Use This Drug

Do not use if you have or have had:

- a sensitivity to sulfa drugs (sulfonamides) or yellow dye #5

Tell your doctor if you have or have had:

- allergies to drugs
- diabetes
- a recent heart attack
- gout
- kidney, liver, or pancreas problems
- hearing loss
- lupus erythematosus
- salt- or sugar-restricted diet

Tell your doctor about any other drugs you take, including aspirin, herbs, vitamins, and other nonprescription products.

WARNING: THIAMINE DEFICIENCY WITH FUROSEMIDE

Studies have shown that significant amounts of thiamine (vitamin B_1) are lost in the urine of people using furosemide (Lasix) and that patients therefore become thiamine deficient. The researchers found that replenishing thiamine, by taking one 100 milligram pill of thiamine hydrochloride daily for seven weeks, significantly improved heart function in patients who were using furosemide.[241,242] It is likely that after replacing the significant thiamine losses with these larger doses, the daily maintenence dose will be less. For now, however, **we recommend the use of 100 milligrams of thiamine hydrochloride a day for at least seven weeks in people who have used furosemide chronically.**

If there seems to be an improvement in your heart status, and your physician agrees, you should continue with a daily dose of about 50 milligrams of thiamine as long as you are taking furosemide.

When You Use This Drug

• **Check with your doctor to make certain your fluid intake is adequate and appropriate. Because furosemide is a very strong water pill, you are in danger of becoming dehydrated.**

• Stay out of the sun as much as possible, and call your doctor if you get a rash, hives, or any other skin reaction. Furosemide makes you more sensitive to the sun.

• **Furosemide will cause your body to lose potassium, an important mineral.** See p. 49 for a discussion of how to make sure you get enough.

• You may feel dizzy when rising from a lying or sitting position. When getting up from bed, hang your legs over the side of the bed for a few minutes, then get up slowly. When getting up from a chair, stay beside the chair until you are sure that you are not dizzy. (See p. 16.)

• Furosemide can cause a loss of hearing, which is usually temporary but may be permanent. The risk of hearing loss is greater if you are also using amphotericin B or an antibiotic from the aminoglycoside family (see p. 635 for two examples).

• If you plan to have any surgery, including dental, tell your doctor that you take this drug.

• **Do not take other drugs without first talking to your doctor—especially non-**prescription drugs for appetite control, asthma, colds, coughs, hay fever, or sinus problems.

HEAT STRESS ALERT

This drug can affect your body's ability to adjust to heat, putting you at risk of "heat stress." If you live alone, ask a friend to check on you several times during the day. Early signs of heat stress are dizziness, lightheadedness, faintness, and slightly high temperature. Call your doctor if you have any of these signs.

Drink more fluids (water, fruit and vegetable juices) than usual—even if you're not thirsty—unless your doctor has told you otherwise. Do not drink alcohol.

How to Use This Drug

• Take with food or milk to avoid stomach irritation. Tablets may be crushed and mixed with food or drink.

• If you are taking furosemide more than once a day, try to take the last dose before 6 P.M. This will help you avoid interrupting your sleep to go to the bathroom.

• If you miss a dose, take it as soon as you

remember, but skip it if it is almost time for the next dose. **Do not take double doses.**

• Do not store in the bathroom. Do not expose to heat, moisture, or strong light.

Interactions with Other Drugs

The following drugs are listed in the *Evaluations of Drug Interactions* 1997 as causing "highly clinically significant" or "clinically significant" interactions when used together with this drug. We have also included potentially serious interactions listed in the drug's FDA-approved professional product labeling or package insert. New scientific techniques have allowed researchers to predict some drug interactions before they have been documented in people. There may be other drugs, especially those in the families of drugs listed below, that also will react with this drug to cause severe adverse effects. The number of new drugs approved for marketing increases the chance of drug interactions, and new drug interactions are being identified with old drugs. Be vigilant. Make sure to tell your doctor and pharmacist the drugs you are taking and tell your doctor if you are taking any of these interacting drugs:

CAPOTEN, captopril, cephalothin, charcoal, cholestyramine, cisplatin, digoxin, ELIXOPHYLLIN, INDERAL, INDERAL LA, KEFLIN, LANOXICAPS, LANOXIN, lithium, LITHOBID, LITHONATE, LOCHOLEST, PLATINOL, propranolol, QUESTRAN, SLO-BID, THEO-24, theophylline.

Adverse Effects

Call your doctor immediately if you experience:

• dry mouth, increased thirst
• irregular heartbeat
• mood or mental changes

• muscle cramps, pain
• severe stomach pain with nausea, vomiting
• unusual tiredness or weakness
• weak pulse
• yellow vision
• cough or hoarseness
• fever or chills
• joint, back or side pain
• painful or difficult urination
• pinpoint red spots on skin
• any loss of hearing or ringing in ears
• skin rash or hives
• unusual bleeding or bruising
• yellow eyes or skin

Call your doctor if these symptoms continue:

• dizziness, lightheadedness
• diarrhea
• loss of appetite, upset stomach
• headache
• blurred vision
• premature ejaculation or difficulty with erection

Periodic Tests

Ask your doctor which of these tests should be done periodically while you are taking this drug:

• blood pressure
• complete blood count
• blood levels of sodium, potassium, chloride, calcium, sugar, and uric acid
• liver function tests
• kidney function tests
• hearing exam
• weight measurement

PREGNANCY WARNING

This drug caused harm to developing fetuses in animal studies, or such studies were not done. Use during pregnancy only for clear medical reasons. Tell your doctor if you are pregnant or thinking of becoming pregnant before you take this drug.

Limited Use

Cholestyramine
LOCHOLEST (Warner Chilcott)
QUESTRAN, QUESTRAN LIGHT (Bristol-Myers Squibb)

GENERIC: not available
FAMILY: Cholesterol-lowering Drugs (see p. 54)

Cholestyramine (coal es *tire* am ene) is used primarily to lower cholesterol, specifically low density lipoprotein (LDL). It works by binding bile acid in the intestines and therefore increasing the breakdown of cholesterol in the body. In middle-aged people it is clear that lowering cholesterol lessens the risk of coronary artery disease, but no cholesterol-lowering drug has been shown to lower overall death rates in this age group. In older adults the extent to which higher cholesterol levels contribute to heart disease and should be treated with drugs is much less clear. Cholestyramine helps control high cholesterol, but does not cure the condition. Besides removing cholesterol, cholestyramine may remove needed nutrients and medicines from your body, and actually increase triglycerides.[245] People over age 60 and those who take high doses are more likely to experience harmful effects from cholestyramine.[246]

The use of cholesterol-lowering drugs in people 70 or older should be limited to patients with very high cholesterol levels (greater than 300 milligrams) and those who manifest cardiovascular disease (previous history of heart attack or angina).[247]

The first, safer and less costly measure to lower cholesterol for people under 70 is to eat a low-fat diet, using mostly polyunsaturated fats (such as canola, corn, safflower, and sunflower oils), or monounsaturated fats (such as olive oil). A change from animal to vegetable proteins often corrects high cholesterol. However, it is inadvisable to go on a very low-fat diet. The main focus on cholesterol-lowering diets has been on saturated fat and cholesterol content, not soluble fiber. (When added to the diet, psyllium or oat bran is a safe, effective way of lowering cholesterol.) Exercise and weight reduction are also recommended. Conditions that aggravate high cholesterol, such as dependence on alcohol or tobacco, diabetes, high blood pressure, low magnesium or potassium, and thyroid disease should be corrected before adding a cholesterol-reducing drug. If cholesterol remains high despite diet, add 10 grams of psyllium a day (see p. 380).

Before You Use This Drug

Do not use if you have or have had:
- complete biliary obstruction

Tell your doctor if you have or have had:
- allergies to drugs
- bleeding disorders
- chronic constipation
- diabetes
- gallbladder problems
- heart, kidney or liver problems
- hemorrhoids
- osteoporosis
- phenylketonuria (PKU)
- thyroid disorder
- ulcers

Tell your doctor about any other drugs you take, including aspirin, herbs, vitamins, and other nonprescription products.

When taking cholestyramine it is important that your doctor knows all the drugs you take.

When You Use This Drug

- Tell any other doctor, dentist, nurse practitioner, or surgeon you see that you take cholestyramine.
- Tell your doctor whenever you start any new medication.
- If you take other medications, check with your doctor before you stop taking cholestyramine.
- Continue to follow a low-fat diet.
- Avoid constipation. Increase your fiber with more bran, fluids, fruits, or psyllium.[248] If constipation persists try a stool softener.

How to Use This Drug

- Take cholestyramine within half an hour of meals,[249] preferably before meals.[250]
- *If you take the bar form of cholestyramine,* chew thoroughly before swallowing. Drink plenty of fluids.
- *If you take the powder form of cholestyramine,* measure the dose, unless you use pre-measured packets. Color of the powder varies from batch to batch. Never swallow the dry form, but mix the powder in two or more ounces of water, milk, apple or orange juice. Stir vigorously, then shake. However, the mixture will not dissolve. To further improve flavor try stirring in a heavy fruit juice or pulpy fruits (applesauce, fruit cocktail, crushed pineapple), thin soups, or with milk in cold or hot cereal.[251] Chilling the mixture may aid the flavor. If you use a carbonated beverage stir slowly to reduce foaming.[252] Avoid taking with highly acidic drinks, such as Kool-Aid.[253] Swallow immediately. Do not hold or swish the mixture in your mouth.[254] To be sure all the medication is taken, rinse the container thoroughly and drink the remaining contents.[255]

- If you take any other medications, separate the times as far apart from cholestyramine as possible, but at least one hour before you take the cholestyramine, or four to eight hours after you take the cholestyramine.
- If you miss a dose, take as soon as you remember but skip it if it is almost time for the next dose. **Do not take double doses.**
- Store at room temperature. Close lid of bulk powder tightly.
- Do not store in the bathroom. Do not expose to heat, moisture, or strong light.

Interactions with Other Drugs

The following drugs are listed in the *Evaluations of Drug Interactions* 1997 as causing "highly clinically significant" or "clinically significant" interactions when used together with this drug. We have also included potentially serious interactions listed in the drug's FDA-approved professional product labeling or package insert. New scientific techniques have allowed researchers to predict some drug interactions before they have been documented in people. There may be other drugs, especially those in the families of drugs listed below, that also will react with this drug to cause severe adverse effects. The number of new drugs approved for marketing increases the chance of drug interactions, and new drug interactions are being identified with old drugs. Be vigilant. Make sure to tell your doctor and pharmacist the drugs you are taking and tell your doctor if you are taking any of these interacting drugs:

ALDACTONE, COUMADIN, CRYSTODIGIN, digitoxin, glipizide, GLUCOTROL, LEVOTHROID, levothyroxine, spironolactone, SYNTHROID, warfarin.

If you stop taking cholestyramine, your doctor will again review doses of your other drugs. Serious harm may occur if you stop taking cholestyramine while taking other medicines.

Adverse Effects

Call your doctor immediately if you experience:

- unusual bleeding or bruising
- black, tarry stools
- constipation
- inability to see as well at night
- severe stomach pain
- sudden weight loss

Call your doctor if these symptoms continue:

- belching or hiccups
- bloating
- diarrhea
- dizziness
- headache
- heartburn, indigestion, stomach pain
- irritation of skin, tongue, or anal area
- nausea or vomiting

Periodic Testing

Ask your doctor which of these tests should be done periodically while you are taking this drug:

- blood calcium, cholesterol, and triglyceride levels
- prothrombin time
- blood pressure

Do Not Use

ALTERNATIVE TREATMENT:
See Cholesterol-lowering Drugs, p. 54.

Gemfibrozil
LOPID (Parke-Davis)

FAMILY: Cholesterol-lowering Drugs (See p. 54)
See Psyllium, p. 380

Gemfibrozil (gem *fi* broe zil) is given to people who have high levels of cholesterol or fats in their blood, to lower those levels in the hope of preventing heart disease. Although gemfibrozil does lower the level of fats in your blood, it has little effect on cholesterol levels. More importantly, there is no evidence that it decreases your risk of sickness or death from heart disease. **In fact, there is no proof that gemfibrozil has any health benefit, such as lowering the chance of having a heart attack, for most people with high blood cholesterol or fat levels.**

Referring to a study in which some patients who had had a previous heart attack were given gemfibrozil, and some were given a placebo, a Food and Drug Administration physician summarized the results: *"showed adverse trends with higher total mortality, higher coronary deaths and higher coronary heart disease events in the gemfibrozil (Lopid) group compared to the placebo group. . . . Studies have repeatedly shown increased gallbladder toxicity and statistically increased appendectomies with gemfibrozil. . . . We are concerned about the potential for human carcinogenesis induced by long-term treatment with fibrates [such as gemfibrozil] based on animal findings at doses equal to those used with humans."*[256]

Other serious problems with this drug are seen if it is used in combination with the "statin" drugs such lovastatin (MEVACOR), pravastatin (PRAVACHOL), or simvastatin (ZOCOR), see p. 130. There are numerous reports of severe muscle damage, sometimes accompanied by life-threatening destruction of muscle and subsequent kidney damage.[257] Therefore, gemfibrozil and the "statin" drugs should not be used together.

The use of cholesterol-lowering drugs in people 70 or older should be limited to patients with very high cholesterol levels (greater than 300 milligrams) and those who manifest cardiovascular disease (previous history of heart attack or angina).[258]

The first, safer, and less costly measure to lower cholesterol for people under 70 is to eat a low-fat diet, using mostly polyunsaturated fats (such as canola, corn, safflower, and sunflower oils) or monounsaturated fats (such as olive oil). A change from animal to vegetable proteins often corrects high cholesterol. However, it is inadvisable to go on a very low-fat diet. The main focus on cholesterol-lowering diets has been on saturated fat and cholesterol content, not soluble fiber. (When added to the diet, psyllium or oat bran is a safe, effective way of lowering cholesterol.) Exercise and weight reduction are also recommended. Conditions that aggravate high cholesterol, such as dependence on alcohol or tobacco, diabetes, high blood pressure, low magnesium or potassium, and thyroid disease, should be corrected before adding a cholesterol-reducing drug. If cholesterol remains high despite diet, add 10 grams of psyllium a day (see p. 380).

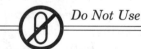

Do Not Use

ALTERNATIVE TREATMENT:
See Cholesterol-lowering Drugs, p. 54.

Probucol
LORELCO (Hoechst Marion Roussel)

FAMILY: Cholesterol-lowering Drugs (See p. 54)
    See Psyllium, p. 380

Probucol (pro *biew* call) was withdrawn from the market by its manufacturer in 1995. Commercial reasons were given by Hoechst Marion Roussel for the decision: sales, the company explained, have been declining in recent years because of competition from many new cholesterol-lowering drugs.

Factors other than competition may have been responsible for the decision, however. The FDA began considering withdrawal of probucol in 1994 but decided to await results of a long-term clinical trial that ultimately showed no

benefit from the drug in reversing the buildup of plaque in blood vessels. When this verdict came in, the agency asked the company to withdraw the drug. Hoechst Marion Roussel did not initially agree to the request, and the FDA scheduled a meeting to discuss issues of safety and efficacy—two criteria for drug marketing under the Food, Drug and Cosmetic Act. The company's decision followed the FDA's announcement of this meeting.

Probucol was not as effective at lowering undesirable low-density lipoprotein (LDL) cholesterol as other drugs. Also, probucol lowered desirable high-density lipoprotein (HDL) cholesterol. While taking probucol, heart rhythm disturbances and abnormal changes in heart conduction were seen causing serious adverse reactions.

The use of cholesterol-lowering drugs in people 70 or older should be limited to patients with very high cholesterol levels (greater than 300 milligrams) and those who manifest cardiovascular disease (previous history of heart attack or angina).[259]

The first, safer, and less costly measure to lower cholesterol for people under 70 is to eat a low-fat diet, using mostly polyunsaturated fats (such as canola, corn, safflower, and sunflower oils) or monounsaturated fats (such as olive oil). A change from animal to vegetable proteins often corrects high cholesterol. However, it is inadvisable to go on a very low-fat diet. The main focus on cholesterol-lowering diets has been on saturated fat and cholesterol content, not soluble fiber. (When added to the diet, psyllium or oat bran is a safe, effective way of lowering cholesterol.) Exercise and weight reduction are also recommended. Conditions that aggravate high cholesterol, such as dependence on alcohol or tobacco, diabetes, high blood pressure, low magnesium or potassium, and thyroid disease, should be corrected before adding a cholesterol-reducing drug. If cholesterol remains high despite diet, add 10 grams of psyllium a day (see p. 380).

Limited Use

Benazepril (ben *ay* ze pril)
LOTENSIN (Novartis)

Captopril (*kap* toe pril)
CAPOTEN (Bristol-Myers Squibb)

Enalapril (n *al* ap ril)
VASOTEC (Merck)

Fosinopril (foe *sin* oh pril)
MONOPRIL (Bristol-Myers Squibb)

Lisinopril (liss *sin* o prill)
PRINIVIL (Merck)
ZESTRIL (Stuart)

Quinapril (*kwin* a pril)
ACCUPRIL (Parke-Davis)

Ramipril (ra *mi* pril)
ALTACE (Hoechst Marion Rousel)

Do Not Use Until Five Years After Release

Moexipril (moe *ex* i pril)
(Do Not Use Until 2001)
UNIVASC (Schwarz)

Trandolapril (tran *dol* ap ril)
(Do Not Use Until 2002)
MAVIK (Knoll)

GENERIC: not available
FAMILY: Antihypertensives
(See High Blood Pressure, p. 44)

These drugs belong to a group of drugs for high blood pressure called angiotensin converting enzyme (ACE) inhibitors. Captopril, lisinopril and enalapril are the preferred ACE inhibitors because they have been on the market the longest.

You should wait at least five years from the date of release to take any new drug unless it is one of those rare "breakthrough" drugs that offers you a documented therapeutic advantage over older proven drugs. New drugs are tested in a relatively small number of people before being approved, and serious adverse effects or life-threatening drug interactions may not be detected until the new drug has been taken by hundreds of thousands of people. A number of new drugs have been withdrawn within their first five years after approval. Also, serious new adverse reaction warnings have been added to the labeling of a number of drugs, or new drug interactions have been detected, usually within the first five years after a drug's release.

ACE inhibitors are effective drugs for the treatment of high blood pressure (hypertension) and congestive heart failure in older adults. After a heart attack, treatment with an ACE inhibitor prevents subsequent heart failure and reduces morbidity and mortality.[260] In people with high blood pressure and kidney disease, ACE inhibitors, along with water pills, slow progressive kidney failure.[261,262,263] ACE inhibitors may also be the preferred class of drugs to control blood pressure in those people with kidney damage from diabetes.[264,265,266] They can cause dangerous adverse effects such as bone marrow depression and kidney disease and, therefore, should be taken in lower doses by older adults. This may amount to less than one-third the doses used in the past.

You are more likely to suffer harmful effects from ACE inhibitors if you have decreased kidney function, especially if you are dehydrated. Since older adults generally have some decrease in kidney function, these drugs may be especially dangerous for them. For this reason, they should not be the first choice for patients with kidney disease. In addition, patients taking a diuretic (water pill) should be watched carefully or, at their physician's discretion, be taken off that medication when an ACE inhibitor is started. Patients using potassium-sparing drugs (see below) should not use ACE inhibitors.

At times when using ACE inhibitors, the blood pressure goes too low, especially with the first dose. Older people are more likely to be sensitive to low blood pressure. A rare but potentially life-threatening reaction is angioedema, a sudden swelling of the face, lips, and particularly the tongue, which may last three days.[267,268] While this reaction usually occurs with the first dose, it can occur years later. Once angioedema occurs, all ACE inhibitors should be stopped.[269] In general, if you are over 60, you should be taking less than the usual adult dose. Since enalapril stays in the body longer than captopril, its adverse effects may last longer.

If you have high blood pressure, the best way to reduce or eliminate your need for medication is by improving your diet, losing weight, exercising, and decreasing your salt and alcohol intake. Mild hypertension can be controlled by proper nutrition and exercise. If these measures do not lower your blood pressure enough and you need medication, **hydrochlorothiazide, a water pill (see thiazide diuretics, p. 100), is the drug of choice starting with a low dose of 12.5 milligrams daily.** It also costs less than other blood pressure drugs.

There is now good evidence that another benefit of thiazide diuretics, such as hydrochlorothiazide, is that they significantly decrease the rate of bone mineral loss in both men and women because they reduce the amount of calcium lost in the urine. An increasing number of researchers think that this will also decrease the number of fractures.[270]

If this drug does not lower your blood pressure enough, your doctor can prescribe a second type of drug called a beta-blocker (see p. 52) to accompany the hydrochlorothiazide. If you cannot take a beta-blocker, a drug from another family (calcium channel blockers) can be used instead.

Whatever drugs you take for high blood pressure, once your blood pressure has been normal for a year or more, a cautious decrease in dose and renewed attention to nondrug treatment may be worth trying, according to *The Medical Letter.*[271]

And an editorial in the *British Medical Journal* stated: *"Treatment of hypertension is part of preventive medicine and like all preventive strategies, its progress should be regularly reviewed by whoever initiates it. Many problems could be avoided by not starting antihypertensive treatment until after prolonged observation. . . . Patients should no longer be told that treatment is necessarily for life: the possibility of reducing or stopping treatment should be mentioned at the outset."*[272]

Before You Use This Drug

Do not use if you have or have had:

- angioedema[273,274]
- severe kidney disease
- are taking a potassium-sparing drug such as spironolactone (ALDACTONE), triamterene (DYRENIUM—a Do Not Use drug) or triamterene and hydrochlorothiazide (DYAZIDE/MAXZIDE)

Tell your doctor if you have or have had:

- allergies to drugs
- an autoimmune disease such as lupus or scleroderma
- renal artery stenosis or generalized arteriosclerosis[275]
- asthma or other lung problems
- bone marrow depression
- cerebrovascular accident
- diabetes
- salt-restricted diet
- heart, kidney or liver problems
- high potassium levels

Tell your doctor about any other drugs you take, including aspirin, herbs, vitamins, and other nonprescription products.

When You Use This Drug

• If you take a diuretic, your doctor may taper you off of it, or lower your dose, a few days prior to starting one of these drugs. Take the first dose of any of these drugs under medical supervision. For hypertension, treatment supervision should last at least two hours and then an additional hour after your blood pressure has stabilized. Usually, this will be at a doctor's office. Have a companion stay with you until at least six hours has elapsed from your first dose.

• When taken for congestive heart failure, supervision should continue at least six hours. Many doctors prefer to start these drugs in a hospital.[276] You should be watched closely for two weeks.

• You should also be closely supervised whenever your dose of any of these drugs or diuretics is changed.

• You may feel dizzy when rising from a lying or sitting position. If you are lying down, hang your legs over the side of the bed for a few minutes, then get up slowly. When getting up from a chair, stay by the chair until you are sure that you are not dizzy. (See p. 16.)

• Drink plenty of fluids to avoid dehydration, especially when exercising, during spells of hot weather, or if you have nausea, vomiting or diarrhea. Call your doctor if it continues or becomes severe.

• **Do not take other drugs without talking to your doctor first—especially nonprescription drugs for appetite control, asthma, colds, coughs, hay fever, or sinus problems.**

• Be careful not to overexert yourself, even though your chest pain may feel better. Talk to your doctor about a safe exercise program.

• Until you know how you react to these drugs, do not drive or perform other activities requiring alertness. Do not drive after taking the first dose, or any time your dose changes.

• Maintain some sodium (salt) in your diet, but avoid excess salt. Do not use low-salt milk, or salt substitutes containing potassium. Check with your doctor before going on any kind of diet.[277] Do not drink alcohol.

• Take your blood pressure periodically. Having your blood pressure checked away from the doctor's office is good practice. If possible have your own automatic blood pressure measuring device but be sure to have both your blood pressure and the device checked by your doctor.

HEAT STRESS ALERT

This drug can affect your body's ability to adjust to heat, putting you at risk of "heat stress." If you live alone, ask a friend to check on you several times during the day. Early signs of heat stress are dizziness, lightheadedness, faintness, and slightly high temperature. Call your doctor if you have any of these signs.

Drink more fluids (water, fruit and vegetable juices) than usual—even if you're not thirsty—unless your doctor has told you otherwise. Do not drink alcohol.

COUGH ALERT

A common adverse effect, after taking ACE inhibitors for a few weeks, is a dry, hacking cough, especially in women. Check with your doctor about a four-day withdrawal from your ACE inhibitor to determine if this is the cause of your cough. This trial withdrawal can prevent unnecessary and sometimes costly tests and treatments.

• If you plan to have any surgery, including dental, tell your doctor that you take one of these drugs.

• Do not stop taking this drug suddenly. Your doctor must give you a schedule to lower your dose gradually.

How to Use This Drug

• Swallow tablets whole or break in half as prescribed. Take on an empty stomach at least one hour before meals.

• Take at the same time each day with the last dose at bedtime to control blood pressure overnight and decrease daytime drowsiness.

• Continue to take, even if you feel well.

• If you miss a dose, take it as soon as you remember but skip it if it is almost time for the next dose. **Do not take double doses**.

• Store at room temperature with lid on tightly.

• Do not store in the bathroom. Do not expose to heat, moisture, or strong light.

Interactions with Other Drugs

The following drugs are listed in the *Evaluations of Drug Interactions* 1997 as causing "highly clinically significant" or "clinically significant" interactions when used together with this drug. We have also included potentially serious interactions listed in the drug's FDA-approved professional product labeling or package insert. New scientific techniques have allowed researchers to predict some drug interactions before they have been documented in people. There may be other drugs, especially those in the families of drugs listed below, that also will react with this drug to cause severe adverse effects. The number of new drugs approved for marketing increases the chance of drug interactions, and new drug interactions are being identified with old drugs. Be vigilant. Make sure to tell your doctor and pharmacist the drugs you are taking and tell your doctor if you are taking any of these interacting drugs:

ADVIL, alcohol, ALDACTONE, amiloride, aspirin, GENUINE BAYER ASPIRIN, chlorpromazine, digoxin, potassium-sparing type diuretics, DYRENIUM, ECOTRIN, furosemide, ibuprofen, INDOCIN, indomethacin, KATO, K-LOR, LANOXICAPS, LANOXIN, LASIX, lithium, LITHOBID, LITHONATE, MIDAMOR, MOTRIN, potassium, SLOW-K, spironalactone, triamterene, THORAZINE.

Adverse Effects

Seek emergency help if you experience:

• difficulty breathing
• sudden swelling of eyes, face, lips, throat, tongue

Call your doctor immediately if you experience:

• chest pain or angina
• confusion
• dizziness, lightheadedness
• fainting
• fever or chills
• irregular heartbeat
• hoarseness
• joint pain
• a feeling of heaviness or weakness in your legs, awkwardness when walking
• nervousness
• numbness or tingling in hands, feet, lips
• skin rash
• difficulty swallowing
• swelling of hands, face, mouth, ankles, feet
• stomach pain
• itchiness
• yellow eyes or skin

Call your doctor if these symptoms continue:

- diarrhea
- cough or dry, tickling sensation in throat
- fatigue, unusual tiredness
- headache
- nausea, vomiting
- altered or lost sense of taste, loss of appetite
- urinary pain, or change in frequency or quantity of urine

Periodic Tests

Ask your doctor which of these tests should be done periodically while you are taking this drug:

- blood pressure
- kidney function tests
- urinary protein
- white blood cell count

PREGNANCY WARNING

When used in pregnancy during the second and third trimesters, ACE inhibitors can cause injury and even death to the developing fetus. You should always tell your doctor if you are pregnant or thinking of becoming pregnant before you take this drug.

Limited Use

Benazepril and Hydrochlorothiazide
LOTENSIN HCT (Novartis)

Captopril and Hydrochlorothiazide
CAPOZIDE (Bristol-Myers Squibb)

Lisinopril and Hydrochlorothiazide
PRINZIDE (Merck)
ZESTORETIC (Zeneca)

Enalapril and Hydrochlorothiazide
VASERETIC (Merck)

GENERIC: not available
FAMILY: Diuretics
Antihypertensives
(See High Blood Pressure, p. 44)

ACE inhibitors are effective drugs for the treatment of high blood pressure (hypertension) and congestive heart failure in older adults. They can also cause dangerous adverse effects such as bone marrow depression and kidney disease and, therefore, should be taken in lower doses by older adults. These lower doses may amount to less than one-third of the amount of medication used in the past.

You are more likely to suffer harmful effects from ACE inhibitors if you have decreased kidney function, especially if you are *dehydrated*. Since older adults generally have some decrease in kidney function, these drugs may be especially dangerous for them. For this reason, they should not be the first choice for patients with kidney disease. In addition, patients taking a diuretic (water pill) should be watched carefully or, at their physician's discretion, be taken off that medication, when an ACE inhibitor is started. Patients using potassium-sparing drugs (see below) should not use ACE inhibitors.

These products—a combination of either 25 or 50 milligrams of captopril (see p. 123) with either 15 or 25 milligrams of hydrochlorothiazide (see p. 100), 20 milligrams of lisinopril (see p. 123) with either 12.5 or 25 milligrams of hydrochlorothiazide, 10 milligrams of enalapril (see p. 123) with 25 milligrams of hydrochlorothiazide, or 5 milligrams, 10 milligrams or 20 milligrams of benazepril with 6.25 milligrams, 12.5 milligrams or 25 milligrams of hydrochlorothiazide—are used to treat high blood pressure (hypertension). Older adults should never use drugs that contain a fixed combination of one of these drugs and hydrochlorothiazide as a first choice. Captopril can cause kidney failure, bone marrow depression, and, like all ACE inhibitors, can cause cough in 5 to 20% of users.[278]

There are good reasons not to use any fixed-combination drug for high blood pressure. A single drug is often enough to control high blood pressure. If a combination drug like one of these is controlling your high blood pressure, it is quite possible that one drug alone would do the same job. There is no reason to put yourself at extra risk by taking drugs you do not need.

If you have high blood pressure, the best way to reduce or eliminate your need for medication is by improving your diet, losing weight, exercising, and decreasing your salt and alcohol intake. Mild hypertension can be controlled by proper nutrition and exercise. If these measures do not lower your blood pressure enough and you need medication, **hydrochlorothiazide, a water pill (see thiazide diuretics, p. 100), is the drug of choice starting with a low dose of 12.5 milligrams daily.** It also costs less than other blood pressure drugs.

There is now good evidence that thiazide diuretics, such as hydrochlorothiazide, significantly decrease the rate of bone mineral loss in both men and women because they reduce the amount of calcium lost in the urine. An increasing number of researchers think that this will also decrease the number of fractures.[279]

PREGNANCY WARNING

When used in pregnancy during the second and third trimesters, ACE inhibitors can cause injury and even death to the developing fetus. You should always tell your doctor if you are pregnant or thinking of becoming pregnant before you take this drug.

If your high blood pressure is more severe, and hydrochlorothiazide alone does not control it, the choice of a beta-blocker, (see p. 52), a calcium channel blocker (see p. 53), or an ACE inhibitor (see p. 123) depends on your condition. Depending on the drug that suits you, your doctor would prescribe the hydrochlorothiazide and the second drug separately, with the dose of each drug adjusted to meet your needs, rather than using a product that combines the drugs in advance in this fixed combination. If you are taking both drugs, compare the total price of each drug separately. The separate drugs may prove less expensive than this combination product. The separate drugs are also more flexible should your dose of either drug need to be changed.

Whatever drugs you take for high blood pressure, once your blood pressure has been normal

---

WARNING

A fixed-combination drug should not be the first drug used to treat your high blood pressure. You may not need more than one drug. If you do need two drugs, the fixed-combination product may not contain the dose of each drug that is right for you. Your doctor has to regularly check your condition and reevaluate the effect of the drug(s) you take. This may mean adjusting doses, and even changing drugs, to ensure proper treatment. This fixed-combination drug may be the best drug for you, but it should be used only after you have tried each of its ingredients separately, in varying doses. If the doses that you need to control your high blood pressure match those in this fixed-combination product, use it if the combination drug is more convenient.

for a year or more, a cautious decrease in dose and renewed attention to nondrug treatment may be worth trying, according to *The Medical Letter.*[280]

And an editorial in the *British Medical Journal* stated: *"Treatment of hypertension is part of preventive medicine and like all preventive strategies, its progress should be regularly reviewed by whoever initiates it. Many problems could be avoided by not starting antihypertensive treatment until after prolonged observation. . . . Patients should no longer be told that treatment is necessarily for life: the possibility of reducing or stopping treatment should be mentioned at the outset."*[281]

HEAT STRESS ALERT

This drug can affect your body's ability to adjust to heat, putting you at risk of "heat stress." If you live alone, ask a friend to check on you several times during the day. Early signs of heat stress are dizziness, lightheadedness, faintness, and slightly high temperature. Call your doctor if you have any of these signs.

Drink more fluids (water, fruit and vegetable juices) than usual—even if you're not thirsty—unless your doctor has told you otherwise. Do not drink alcohol.

COUGH ALERT

A common adverse effect, after taking ACE inhibitors for a few weeks, is a dry, hacking cough, especially in women. Check with your doctor about a four-day withdrawal from your ACE inhibitor to determine if this is the cause of your cough. This trial withdrawal can prevent unnecessary, and sometimes costly, tests and treatments.

 Do Not Use

ALTERNATIVE TREATMENT:
See Hydrochlorothiazide, p. 100.

Amlodipine and Benazepril
LOTREL (Novartis)

Diltiazem and Enalapril
TECZEM (Hoechst Marion Roussel)

Felodipine and Enalapril
LEXXEL (Astra Merck)

Verapamil and Trandolapril
TARKA (Knoll)

FAMILY: Calcium Channel Blockers (See p. 53)

These products are fixed combinations of a calcium channel blocker and an angiotensin converting enzyme (ACE) inhibitor drug. We have listed these drugs as **Do Not Use** because they are combinations that do not contain a first choice drug for the treatment of high blood pressure such as a diuretic or beta-blocker.

There are good reasons not to use any fixed-combination drug for high blood pressure. A single drug is often enough to control high blood pressure. If a combination drug like this one is controlling your high blood pressure, it is quite possible that one drug alone would do the same job. There is no reason to put yourself at extra risk by taking drugs you do not need.

If you have high blood pressure, the best way to reduce or eliminate your need for medication is by improving your diet, losing weight, exercising, and decreasing your salt and alcohol intake. Mild hypertension can be controlled by proper nutrition and exercise. If these measures do not lower your blood pressure enough and you need medication, **hydrochlorothiazide, a water pill (see thiazide diuretics, p. 100), is the drug of choice starting with a low dose of 12.5**

milligrams daily. It also costs less than other blood pressure drugs.

There is now good evidence that thiazide diuretics, such as hydrochlorothiazide, significantly decrease the rate of bone mineral loss in both men and women because they reduce the amount of calcium lost in the urine. An increasing number of researchers think that this will also decrease the number of fractures.[282]

If your high blood pressure is more severe, and hydrochlorothiazide alone does not control it, the best treatment is a combination of hydrochlorothiazide and a second type of drug called a beta-blocker, such as propranolol (see p. 154). If you can't take a drug in the beta-blocker family, another drug called a calcium channel blocker may be used instead. In either case, your doctor would prescribe the hydrochlorothiazide and the second drug separately, with the dose of each drug adjusted to meet your needs, rather than using a product that combines the drug in a fixed combination.

If you are taking this fixed-combination drug, ask your doctor about changing your prescription.

Whatever drugs you take for high blood pressure, once your blood pressure has been normal for a year or more, a cautious decrease in dose and renewed attention to nondrug treatment may be worth trying, according to *The Medical Letter.*[283]

And an editorial in the *British Medical Journal* stated: *"Treatment of hypertension is part of preventive medicine and like all preventive strategies, its progress should be regularly reviewed by whoever initiates it. Many problems could be avoided by not starting antihypertensive treatment until after prolonged observation. . . . Patients should no longer be told that treatment is necessarily for life: the possibility of reducing or stopping treatment should be mentioned at the outset."*[284]

Limited Use

Lovastatin (low vah *stat* in)
MEVACOR (Merck)

Pravastatin (prav ah *stat* in)
PRAVACHOL (Bristol-Myers Squibb)

Simvastatin (*sim* va stat in)
ZOCOR (Merck) *take pm*

Do Not Use Until Five Years After Release

Cerivastatin (cer iv ah *stat* in)
(Do Not Use Until 2004)
BAYCOL (Bayer)

Fluvastatin (*floo* va sta tin)
(Do Not Use Until 2000)
LESCOL (Novartis)

Atorvastatin (a *tor* va sta tin)
(Do Not Use Until 2003)
LIPITOR (Warner-Lambert)

GENERIC: not available
FAMILY: Cholesterol-lowering Drugs (See p. 54)

You should wait at least five years from the date of release to take any new drug unless it is one of those rare "breakthrough" drugs that offers you a documented therapeutic advantage over older proven drugs. New drugs are tested in a relatively small number of people before being approved, and serious adverse effects or life-threatening drug interactions may not be detected until the new drug has been taken by hundreds of thousands of people. A number of new drugs have been withdrawn within their first five years after release. Also, serious new adverse reaction warnings have been added to the labeling of a number of drugs, or new drug interactions have been detected, usually within the first five years after a drug's release.

The "statin" drugs lower cholesterol by preventing the body from making as much cholesterol, specifically low-density lipoprotein (LDL) cholesterol. In middle-aged people it is clear that lowering cholesterol lessens the risk of coronary artery disease. Lovastatin, pravastatin and simvastatin have been shown to cause regression of heart lesions, and pravastatin and simvastatin have been shown to reduce—though by a small amount—coronary and total mortality.[285] In older adults, the extent to which higher cholesterol levels contribute to heart disease and should be treated with drugs is much less clear. These drugs control high cholesterol, but do not cure any condition. They may prevent atherosclerosis.[286]

Drug-induced muscle injury, or rhabdomyolysis, is a known adverse effect of all statin cholesterol-lowering drugs. Rhabdomyolysis is usually accompanied by pain, tenderness, and weakness in the affected muscles. The most important consequences of rhabdomyolysis, however, are not those on the muscle themselves. As muscle cells break down, they release substances that can cause injury to the kidneys, sometimes permanent but even when reversible, sometimes requiring temporary hemodialysis (mechanical filtering of the blood). If muscle cells break down rapidly enough, released potassium can cause lethal heart rhythm disturbances. A number of drugs can interact with the statin drugs that can increase the likelihood of drug-induced muscle injury. See the section on drug interactions.

This family of drugs is generally better tolerated than other cholesterol-lowering drugs, according to *The Medical Letter.*[287] Still, these drugs commonly cause gastrointestinal problems. Of particular concern is the possibility of liver toxicity, including hepatitis. Therefore, liver function tests should be done every six weeks in patients on therapy. In animals these drugs have produced cancers. Long-term effects of interfering with the body's making of cholesterol are not known.[288,289,290] This family

of drugs is not effective for the homozygous familial type of high blood cholesterol.[291]

The use of cholesterol-lowering drugs in people 70 or older should be limited to patients with very high cholesterol levels (greater than 300 milligrams) and those who manifest cardiovascular disease (previous history of heart attack or angina).[292]

The first, safer, and less costly measure to lower cholesterol for people under 70 is to eat a low-fat diet, using mostly polyunsaturated fats (such as canola, corn, safflower, and sunflower oils) or monounsaturated fats (such as olive oil). A change from animal to vegetable proteins often corrects high cholesterol. However, it is inadvisable to go on a very low-fat diet. The main focus on cholesterol-lowering diets has been on saturated fat and cholesterol content, not soluble fiber. (When added to the diet, psyllium or oat bran is a safe, effective way of lowering cholesterol.) Exercise and weight reduction are also recommended. Conditions that aggravate high cholesterol, such as dependence on alcohol or tobacco, diabetes, high blood pressure, low magnesium or potassium, and thyroid disease, should be corrected before adding a cholesterol-reducing drug. If cholesterol remains high despite diet, add 10 grams of psyllium a day (see p. 380). These drugs are usually reserved for people who do not respond to other drugs. However, choice of a drug in older adults must be individualized.

Before You Use This Drug

Do not use if you have:

- active liver disease

Tell your doctor if you have or have had:

- allergies to drugs
- alcohol dependence
- cataracts
- low blood pressure

- metabolic, hormone or mineral imbalance
- severe infections
- serious injuries
- kidney or liver problems
- organ transplant or other major surgery
- seizures

Tell your doctor about any other drugs you take, including aspirin, herbs, vitamins, and other nonprescription products.

When You Use This Drug

- Continue to eat a low-fat diet.
- If you plan to have any surgery, including dental, tell your doctor that you take this drug.

How to Use This Drug

- Swallow tablet whole. If you take one of these drugs once daily, take it with the evening meal. If you are taking more than one dose a day take it with meals or snacks.
- If you miss a dose, take it as soon as you remember but skip it if it is almost time for the next dose. **Do not take double doses.**
- Do not store in the bathroom. Do not expose to heat, moisture, or strong light. Store tablets at room temperature.
- If you also take cholestyramine (LO-CHOLEST, QUESTRAN) or colestipol (COLESTID), take these drugs at least one hour before, or four hours after taking the other drugs.[293]

Interactions with Other Drugs

The following drugs are listed in the *Evaluations of Drug Interactions* 1997 as causing "highly clinically significant" or "clinically significant" interactions when used together with this drug. We have also included potentially serious interactions listed in the drug's FDA-approved professional product labeling or package insert. New scientific techniques have allowed researchers to predict some drug interactions before they have been documented in people. There may be other drugs, especially those in the families of drugs listed below, that also will react with this drug to cause severe adverse effects. The number of new drugs approved for marketing increases the chance of drug interactions, and new drug interactions are being identified with old drugs. Be vigilant. Make sure to tell your doctor and pharmacist the drugs you are taking and tell your doctor if you are taking any of these interacting drugs:

cholestyramine, cimetidine, COUMADIN, cyclosporine, EES, ERYTHROCIN, erythromycin, gemfibrozil, LOCHOLEST, LOPID, mibefradil, NEORAL, niacin (this refers to very large doses to lower cholesterol, not usual dietary amounts of niacin), NICOBID, NICOLAR, omeprazole, POSICOR, PRILOSEC, QUESTRAN, RIFADIN, rifampin, RIMACTANE, SANDIMMUNE, SLO-NIACIN, TAGAMET, warfarin.

Adverse Effects

Call your doctor immediately if you experience:

- fever
- muscle aches, cramps
- severe stomach pain
- unusual tiredness or weakness
- blurred vision

Call your doctor if these symptoms continue:

- constipation or diarrhea
- dizziness
- gas, heartburn
- headache

- nausea
- skin rash
- stomach pain
- decreased sexual ability
- trouble sleeping

Periodic Tests

Ask your doctor which of these tests should be done periodically while you are taking this drug:

- blood cholesterol and creatinine kinase tests
- eye exam
- liver function tests

PREGNANCY WARNING

This drug should not be used if you are pregnant or are thinking of becoming pregnant. The risk of use of this drug in pregnant women clearly outweighs any possible benefit.

Limited Use

Mexiletine
MEXITIL (Boehringer Ingelheim)

GENERIC: not available
FAMILY: Antiarrhythmics

Mexiletine (mex *ill* et een) slows rapid heartbeat and stabilizes irregular heartbeats (arrhythmias). Mexiletine prevents recurrence of ventricular arrhythmias, such as premature heartbeats. It can prevent sudden death. Mexiletine belongs to the same family of drugs as lidocaine (XYLOCAINE).

WARNING! INCREASED RISK OF DEATH

In the National Heart, Lung, and Blood Institute's Cardiac Arrhythmia Suppression Trial (CAST) (a long-term, multi-centered, randomized, double-blind study), in patients with asymptomatic non-life-threatening ventricular (the large chambers of the heart) arrhythmias (rhythm disturbances) who had a heart attack more than six days, but less than two years previously, deaths or non-fatal cardiac arrest were seen in 7.7% of those patients treated with encainide or flecainide, members of the Class 1 group of antiarrhythmic drugs, compared to 3.0% in patients receiving an inactive sugar pill or placebo.

Because of the known ability of the Class 1 drugs, such as mexiletine, to cause rhythm disturbances, and the lack of evidence of improved survival for any antiarrhythmic drug in patients without life-threatening heart rhythm disturbances, the use of the Class 1 drugs, such as Mexiletine, should be reserved for patients with life-threatening rhythm disturbances of the ventricles. These warnings now appear in the FDA-approved product labeling, or package insert, for all Class 1 drugs including: disopyramide (Norpace and generics), flecainide (Tambocor), mexiletine (Mexitil and generics), moricizine (Ethmozine), procainamide (Procanbid and generics), propafenone (Rythmol), quinidine (Duraquin, Quinaglute Dura-Tabs, Quinidex and generics), and tocainide (Tonocard).

It is as effective as quinidine for some, but not all, arrthymias[294] and sometimes is used beneficially with quinidine.[295] Mexiletine has little risk of organ toxicity but has a high risk of non-cardiac adverse effects.[296] However, these adverse effects often cause people to stop taking mexiletine.[297,298] Lower doses can reduce unwanted effects. People with decreased liver function should take a lower dose. At times mexiletine actually worsens some types of arrhythmias. It is not for use in minor arrhythmias. Use of mexiletine with procainamide (Procanbid) is of little or no value.[299]

Before You Use This Drug

Do not use if you have or have had:

- cardiogenic shock
- heart block of 2nd or 3rd degree without a pacemaker

Tell your doctor if you have or have had:

- allergies to drugs
- angina
- congestive heart failure[300]
- heart block or other heart problems
- kidney[301] or liver problems
- low blood pressure
- myocardial infarction
- pacemaker
- seizures

Tell your doctor about any other drugs you take, including aspirin, herbs, vitamins, and other nonprescription products.

When You Use This Drug

- Until you know how you react to this drug, do not drive or perform other activities requiring alertness. This drug may cause blurred vision and drowsiness.

- You may feel dizzy when rising from a lying or sitting position. If you are lying down, hang your legs over the side of the bed for a few minutes, then get up slowly. When getting up from a chair, stay by the chair until you are sure that you are not dizzy. (See p. 16.)
- Ask your doctor to recommend exercises suitable to your condition.
- Quit smoking, or at least try to cut down on smoking.
- Carry identification stating that you take mexiletine.
- If you plan to have any surgery, including dental, tell your doctor that you take this drug.

How to Use This Drug

- Swallow capsule whole. Take with food, milk, or antacids to lessen stomach upset. Space doses evenly apart. Antacids with calcium or magnesium may slow absorption of mexiletine. If you use these antacids, be consistent in usage, and avoid large doses.
- If you miss a dose, take it as soon as you remember but skip it if it is less than four hours until your next scheduled dose. **Do not take double doses.**
- Store at room temperature with lid on firmly.
- Do not store in the bathroom. Do not expose to heat, moisture, or strong light.

Interactions with Other Drugs

The following drugs are listed in the *Evaluations of Drug Interactions* 1997 as causing "highly clinically significant" or "clinically significant" interactions when used together with this drug. We have also included potentially serious interactions listed in the drug's FDA-approved professional product labeling or package insert. New scientific techniques have allowed researchers to predict some drug interactions before they have been documented in people. There may be other drugs, especially those in the families of drugs listed below, that also will react with this drug to cause severe adverse effects. The number of new drugs approved for marketing increases the chance of drug interactions, and new drug interactions are being identified with old drugs. Be vigilant. Make sure to tell your doctor and pharmacist the drugs you are taking and tell your doctor if you are taking any of these interacting drugs:

amiodarone, CORDARONE, cimetidine,[302] cyclosporine, ELIXOPHYLLIN, grepafloxacin, NEORAL, RAXAR, SANDIMMUNE, SLO-BID, sparfloxacin, TAGAMET, THEO-24, theophylline,[303,304,305] ZAGAM.

Mexiletine intensifies the effect of caffeine. Eliminate or reduce your intake of beverages containing caffeine.

Adverse Effects

Call your doctor immediately if you experience:

- unusual bleeding or bruising
- difficulty breathing
- chest pain
- fainting
- fever, chills
- unusually fast or slow heartbeat
- seizures
- sore throat

Call your doctor if these symptoms continue:

- abdominal pain
- confusion
- constipation, diarrhea
- depression
- dizziness, lightheadedness
- dry mouth

- headache
- heartburn
- impotence
- nausea, vomiting, loss of appetite
- nervousness
- numbness or tingling of fingers, toes
- pain in joints
- ringing in ears
- skin rash, yellowing of skin
- problems sleeping
- slurred speech
- swelling of hands or feet
- trembling of hands
- unsteadiness, trouble walking
- unusual tiredness or weakness
- decrease in urination
- blurred vision

Periodic Tests

Ask your doctor which of these tests should be done periodically while you are taking this drug:

- blood pressure
- blood mexiletine levels
- electrocardiogram (ECG, EKG)
- liver function tests

PREGNANCY WARNING

This drug has caused harm to developing fetuses in animal studies, or such studies were not done. Use during pregnancy only for clear medical reasons. Tell your doctor if you are pregnant or thinking of becoming pregnant before you take this drug.

Prazosin
MINIPRESS (Pfizer)

GENERIC: available
FAMILY: Antihypertensives
(See High Blood Pressure, p. 44)

Prazosin (*pra* zoe sin) is used to treat sudden congestive heart failure and to reduce high blood pressure (hypertension). It is effective for sudden congestive heart failure but is not the best drug for high blood pressure.[306] After a few days of taking prazosin, you are likely to develop a "tolerance" for it, which means that the same dose has less and less effect.[307] This problem limits prazosin's usefulness for long-term therapy. Some long-term studies have found that prazosin is no more effective than a sugar pill (placebo).[308]

When taken for high blood pressure, prazosin is most effective when combined with a water pill (thiazide diuretic, see p. 100) or a beta-blocker (see p. 52). The water pill or beta-blocker works with the prazosin to lower your blood pressure and helps to decrease your body's retention of salt and water, but it also increases your risk of becoming dizzy or light-headed.[309]

Occasionally, a person will collapse and lose consciousness for a few minutes to an hour after taking his or her first dose of prazosin.[310] This is more likely to happen to older adults, people on a low-salt diet, and people who are taking other high blood pressure drugs.[311] To decrease your risk of fainting, your doctor should prescribe a first dose of no more than one milligram, and you should take that dose at bedtime.[312,313] After taking the first dose, wait at least four hours before driving or doing anything else that requires alertness.

In general, your daily dose of prazosin should be no more than 6 to 10 milligrams. Some doctors prescribe daily doses as high as 20 to 40 milligrams, but doses higher than 6 to 10 milligrams increase the risk of harmful adverse effects without increasing the drug's benefit.[314]

If you have high blood pressure, the best way to reduce or eliminate your need for medication is by improving your diet, losing weight, exercising, and decreasing your salt and alcohol intake. Mild hypertension can be controlled by proper nutrition and exercise. If these measures do not lower your blood pressure enough and you need medication, **hydrochlorothiazide, a water pill (see thiazide diuretics, p. 100), is the drug of choice starting with a low dose of 12.5 milligrams daily.** It also costs less than other blood pressure drugs.

There is now good evidence that thiazide diuretics, such as hydrochlorothiazide, significantly decrease the rate of bone mineral loss in both men and women because they reduce the amount of calcium lost in the urine. An increasing number of researchers think that this will also decrease the number of fractures.[315]

If this drug does not lower your blood pressure enough, your doctor can prescribe a second type of drug called a beta-blocker (see p. 52) to accompany the hydrochlorothiazide. If you cannot take a beta-blocker, a drug from another family (calcium channel blockers) can be used instead.

Whatever drugs you take for high blood pressure, once your blood pressure has been normal for a year or more, a cautious decrease in dose and renewed attention to nondrug treatment may be worth trying, according to *The Medical Letter.*[316]

And an editorial in the *British Medical Journal* stated: *"Treatment of hypertension is part of preventive medicine and like all preventive strategies, its progress should be regularly reviewed by whoever initiates it. Many prob-*

lems could be avoided by not starting antihypertensive treatment until after prolonged observation. . . . Patients should no longer be told that treatment is necessarily for life: the possibility of reducing or stopping treatment should be mentioned at the outset.[317]

Before You Use This Drug

Tell your doctor if you have or have had:

- allergies to drugs
- angina (chest pain)
- heart disease
- kidney function impairment
- liver function impairment (dose should be decreased)
- a low-salt diet

Tell your doctor about any other drugs you take, including aspirin, herbs, vitamins, and other nonprescription products.

When You Use This Drug

- You may feel dizzy when rising from a lying or sitting position. When getting out of bed, hang your legs over the side of the bed for a few minutes, then get up slowly. When getting up from a chair, get up slowly and stay beside the chair until you are sure that you are not dizzy. (See p. 16.)
- If you plan to have any surgery, including dental, tell your doctor that you take this drug.
- Until you know how you react to this drug, do not drive or perform other activities requiring alertness.
- **Do not take other drugs without talking to your doctor first—especially nonprescription drugs for appetite control, asthma, colds, coughs, hay fever, or sinus problems.**

HEAT STRESS ALERT

This drug can affect your body's ability to adjust to heat, putting you at risk of "heat stress." If you live alone, ask a friend to check on you several times during the day. Early signs of heat stress are dizziness, lightheadedness, faintness, and slightly high temperature. Call your doctor if you have any of these signs.

Drink more fluids (water, fruit and vegetable juices) than usual—even if you're not thirsty—unless your doctor has told you otherwise. Do not drink alcohol.

How to Use This Drug

- Crush tablet and mix with water, or swallow whole with water.
- If you miss a dose, take it as soon as you remember, but skip it if it is almost time for the next dose. **Do not take double doses.**
- Do not store in the bathroom. Do not expose to heat, moisture, or strong light.

Interactions with Other Drugs

The following drugs are listed in the *Evaluations of Drug Interactions* 1997 as causing "highly clinically significant" or "clinically significant" interactions when used together with this drug. We have also included potentially serious interactions listed in the drug's FDA-approved professional product labeling or package insert. New scientific techniques have allowed researchers to predict some drug interactions before they have been documented in people. There may be other drugs, especially those in the families of drugs listed below, that also will react with this drug to cause severe adverse effects. The number of new drugs approved for marketing increases the chance of drug interactions, and new drug interactions are being identified with old drugs. Be vigilant. Make sure to tell your doctor and pharmacist the drugs you are taking and tell your doctor if you are taking any of these interacting drugs:

digoxin, INDERAL, INDERAL LA, INDOCIN, indomethacin, LANOXICAPS, LANOXIN, propranolol.

Adverse Effects

Call your doctor immediately if you experience:

- dizziness, lightheadedness
- fainting
- chest pain (angina)
- irregular heartbeat
- shortness of breath
- swelling of feet and lower legs
- weight gain from salt and water retention
- inability to control urination
- numbness and tingling of hands and feet
- skin rash
- painful, inappropriate erection

Call your doctor if these symptoms continue:

- drowsiness
- headache
- lack of energy
- nausea, vomiting
- decreased sexual ability
- diarrhea or constipation
- dry mouth
- nervousness
- unusual tiredness or weakness
- frequent urge to urinate

Periodic Tests

Ask your doctor which of these tests should be done periodically while you are taking this drug:

- blood pressure

PREGNANCY WARNING

This drug caused harm to developing fetuses in animal studies, or such studies were not done. Use during pregnancy only for clear medical reasons. Tell your doctor if you are pregnant or thinking of becoming pregnant before you take this drug.

 Do Not Use

ALTERNATIVE TREATMENT:
See Hydrochlorothiazide, p. 100.

Amiloride and Hydrochlorothiazide
MODURETIC (Merck)

FAMILY: Diuretics
Antihypertensives
(See High Blood Pressure, p. 44)

This product, a combination of amiloride (a *mill* oh ride) and hydrochlorothiazide (see p. 100), is used to treat high blood pressure (hypertension). **Older adults should not use drugs that contain a fixed combination of amiloride and hydrochlorothiazide.**

Thiazides with amiloride may produce high potassium in the blood and substantial sodium depletion.[318]

There are good reasons not to use any fixed-combination drug for high blood pressure. A single drug is often enough to control high blood pressure. If a combination drug like this one is controlling your high blood pressure, it is quite possible that one drug alone would do the same job. There is no reason to put yourself at extra risk by taking drugs you do not need.

If you have high blood pressure, the best way to reduce or eliminate your need for medication is by improving your diet, losing weight, exercising, and decreasing your salt and alcohol intake. Mild hypertension can be controlled by proper nutrition and exercise. If these measures do not lower your blood pressure enough and you need medication, **hydrochlorothiazide, a water pill (see thiazide diuretics, p. 100), is the drug of choice starting with a low dose of 12.5 milligrams daily.** It also costs less than other blood pressure drugs.

There is now good evidence that thiazide diuretics, such as hydrochlorothiazide, significantly decrease the rate of bone mineral loss in both men and women because they reduce the amount of calcium lost in the urine. An increasing number of researchers think that this will also decrease the number of fractures.[319]

Hydrochlorothiazide, is one of the ingredients in this combination. If your high blood pressure is more severe, and hydrochlorothiazide alone does not control it, there are still better drug treatments than this combination product. The best treatment in this case is a combination of hydrochlorothiazide and a second type of drug called a beta-blocker like propranolol (see p. 154). If you can't take a drug in the beta-blocker family, another drug called a calcium channel blocker may be used instead. In either case, your doctor would prescribe the hydrochlorothiazide and the second drug separately, with the dose of each drug adjusted to meet your needs, rather than using a product that combines the drugs in advance in a fixed combination.

If you are taking this fixed-combination drug, ask your doctor about changing your prescription.

Whatever drugs you take for high blood pressure, once your blood pressure has been normal for a year or more, a cautious decrease in dose and renewed attention to nondrug treatment may be worth trying, according to *The Medical Letter.*[320]

And an editorial in the *British Medical Journal* stated: *"Treatment of hypertension is part of preventive medicine and like all preventive strategies, its progress should be regularly reviewed by whoever initiates it. Many problems could be avoided by not starting antihypertensive treatment until after prolonged observation. . . . Patients should no longer be told that treatment is necessarily for life: the possibility of reducing or stopping treatment should be mentioned at the outset."*[321]

Limited Use

Disopyramide
NORPACE (Searle)

GENERIC: available
FAMILY: Antiarrhythmics

Disopyramide (dye soe *peer* a mide) slows the heart rate and stabilizes irregular heartbeats (arrhythmias). Because it has serious adverse effects, your doctor should not prescribe disopyramide unless you have already tried safer antiarrhythmic drugs such as quinidine (see p. 94) without success.

Disopyramide is linked to a high incidence of congestive heart failure and problems with urination, so people with these medical problems should not use the drug.[322] Since there is a narrow range between a helpful and a harmful amount of this drug in your body, call your doctor immediately if you experience these adverse effects or any of those listed under Adverse Effects. **If you have decreased kidney function, you should be taking less than the usual dose of disopyramide.**[323]

Many people who are taking disopyramide or another drug in its family have relatively mild disturbances in their heart rhythm and no symptoms of underlying heart disease. The vast majority of these people do not need these drugs, and there is no evidence that using them improves health. In fact, most of the drugs in this family have severe adverse effects that are sometimes worse and even more life-threatening than the irregular heartbeats they treat. All of these drugs can also cause new irregularities in your heartbeat.

If you have an irregular heartbeat without any symptoms of underlying heart disease, you should not be exposed to the dangers of a drug that has no health benefit for your condition.[324] If you are taking disopyramide or another drug in its family for an irregular heartbeat (arrhythmia), talk to your doctor and find out whether you also have symptoms of underlying heart disease. If not, discuss the possibility of stopping the drug.

WARNING: SPECIAL MENTAL AND PHYSICAL ADVERSE EFFECTS

Older adults are especially sensitive to the harmful anticholinergic (See Glossary p. 768) effects of disopyramide. Drugs in this family should not be used unless absolutely necessary.

Mental Effects: confusion, delirium, short-term memory problems, disorientation, and impaired attention.

Physical Effects: dry mouth, constipation, difficulty urinating (especially for a man with an enlarged prostate), blurred vision, decreased sweating with increased body temperature, sexual dysfunction, and worsening of glaucoma.

Before You Use This Drug

Do not use if you have or have had:

- complete heart block
- shock due to heart failure

Tell your doctor if you have or have had:

- allergies to drugs

- diabetes
- any heart problems
- enlarged prostate gland
- glaucoma
- kidney function impairment
- liver function impairment
- too much or too little blood potassium
- myasthenia gravis
- urinary obstruction

Tell your doctor about any other drugs you take, including aspirin, herbs, vitamins, and other nonprescription products.

When You Use This Drug

- Until you know how you react to this drug, do not drive or perform other activities requiring alertness. Disopyramide may cause dizziness.

- You may feel dizzy when rising from a lying or sitting position. When getting out of bed, hang your legs over the side of the bed for a few minutes, then get up slowly. When getting up from a chair, get up slowly and stay beside the chair until you are sure that you are not dizzy. (See p. 16.)

- **Do not stop taking this drug suddenly. Your doctor must give you a schedule to lower your dose gradually, to prevent serious changes in heart function.**

- Wear a medical identification bracelet or carry a card stating that you take disopyramide.

- If you plan to have any surgery, including dental, tell your doctor that you take this drug.

How to Use This Drug

- Swallow extended-release tablets whole. Do not crush or break.

- Take with food or milk to decrease stomach upset.

- If you miss a dose, take it as soon as you remember, but skip it if it is less than four hours (eight hours if you are taking extended-

---

WARNING! INCREASED RISK OF DEATH

In the National Heart, Lung, and Blood Institute's Cardiac Arrhythmia Suppression Trial (CAST) (a long-term, multi-centered, randomized, double-blind study) in patients with asymptomatic non-life-threatening ventricular (the large chambers of the heart) arrhythmias (rhythm disturbances) who had a heart attack more than six days, but less than two years previously, deaths or non-fatal cardiac arrest were seen in 7.7% of those patients treated with encainide or flecainide, members of the Class 1 group of antiarrhythmic drugs, compared to 3.0% in patients receiving an inactive sugar pill or placebo.

Because of the known ability of the Class 1 drugs, such as disopyramide, to cause rhythm disturbances, and the lack of evidence of improved survival for any antiarrhythmic drug in patients without life-threatening heart rhythm disturbances, the use of the Class 1 drugs should be reserved for patients with life-threatening rhythm disturbances of the ventricles. These warnings now appear in the FDA-approved product labeling, or package insert, for all Class 1 drugs including: disopyramide (Norpace and generics), flecainide (Tambocor), mexiletine (Mexitil and generics), moricizine (Ethmozine), procainamide (Procanbid and generics), propafenone (Rythmol), quinidine (Duraquin, Quinaglute Dura-tabs, Quinidex and generics), and tocainide (Tonocard).

---

release capsules) until your next scheduled dose. **Do not take double doses.**

• Do not store in the bathroom. Do not expose to heat, moisture, or strong light.

Interactions with Other Drugs

The following drugs are listed in the *Evaluations of Drug Interactions* 1997 as causing "highly clinically significant" or "clinically significant" interactions when used together with this drug. We have also included potentially serious interactions listed in the drug's FDA-approved professional product labeling or package insert. New scientific techniques have allowed researchers to predict some drug interactions before they have been documented in people. There may be other drugs, especially those in the families of drugs listed below, that also will react with this drug to cause severe adverse effects. The number of new drugs approved for marketing increases the chance of drug interactions, and new drug interactions are being identified with old drugs. Be vigilant. Make sure to tell your doctor and pharmacist the drugs you are taking and tell your doctor if you are taking any of these interacting drugs:

charcoal, DILANTIN, EES, ERYTHROCIN, erythromycin, grepafloxacin, ISORDIL, isosorbide (dinitrate), phenytoin, RAXAR, SORBITRATE, sparfloxacin, ZAGAM.

Adverse Effects

Call your doctor immediately if you experience:

• difficulty urinating
• chest pains
• confusion
• dizziness or fainting
• muscle weakness
• shortness of breath
• swelling of feet or lower legs
• unusually fast or slow heartbeat
• rapid weight gain
• eye pain
• depression
• sore throat and fever
• yellow eyes and skin
• **signs of low blood sugar:** anxious feeling, chills, cold sweats, confusion, cool pale skin, drowsiness, headache, hunger, nausea, nervousness, rapid heartbeat, shakiness, unsteady walk, unusual tiredness or weakness

Call your doctor if these symptoms continue:

- dry mouth, throat, eyes, or nose (relieve by sucking ice or chewing sugarless gum)
- bloating or stomach pain
- blurred vision
- decreased sexual ability
- loss of appetite
- frequent urge to urinate
- constipation

Periodic Tests

Ask your doctor which of these tests should be done periodically while you are taking this drug:

- blood pressure
- heart function tests, such as electrocardiogram (ECG, EKG)
- kidney function tests
- liver function tests
- blood levels of glucose and potassium
- eye pressure exams

PREGNANCY WARNING

This drug caused harm to developing fetuses in animal studies, or such studies were not done. Use during pregnancy only for clear medical reasons. Tell your doctor if you are pregnant or thinking of becoming pregnant before you take this drug.

Limited Use

Amlodipine (am *loe* di peen)
NORVASC (Pfizer)

Felodipine (fe *loe* di peen)
PLENDIL (Astra Merck)

Isradipine (is *rad* ip ene)
DYNACIRC, DYNACIRC CR (Novartis)

Nicardipine (nick *card* ip ene)
CARDENE, CARDENE SR
(Roche/Wyeth-Ayerst)

Nifedipine (nye *fed* i peen)
ADALAT CC (Bayer)
PROCARDIA XL (Pfizer)

Do Not Use Until Five Years After Release

Nisoldipine (nis *old* i peen)
(Do Not Use Until 2002)
SULAR (Zeneca)

GENERIC: in some strengths of nifedipine only
FAMILY: Calcium Channel Blockers (dihydropyridines)
(See p. 53)

You should wait at least five years from the date of release to take any new drug unless it is one of those rare "breakthrough" drugs that offers you a documented therapeutic advantage over older proven drugs. New drugs are tested in a relatively small number of people before being approved, and serious adverse effects or life-threatening drug interactions may not be detected until the new drug has been taken by hundreds of thousands of people. A number of new drugs have been withdrawn within their first five years after release. Also, serious new adverse reaction warnings have been added to the labeling of a number of drugs, or new drug interactions have been detected, usually within the first five years after a drug's release.

These drugs belong to a family of drugs called calcium channel blockers. They are used primarily to treat chest pain (angina) and coronary artery disease and also to lower blood pressure (hypertension). Calcium channel blockers control, but do not cure high blood pressure. These drugs may improve capacity for exercise and delay the need for heart surgery.

There are three new members of the dihydropyridine calcium channel blocking family on the market. These are amlodipine, felodipine, and nisoldipine. None of these drugs offer any therapeutic advantage over older calcium channel blockers.

In 1995, Public Citizen's Health Research Group filed a petition with the Food and Drug Administration to add warnings to the labeling of all calcium channel blockers about the increased risk of heart attack and death. Our petition was based on three well conducted observational research studies.[325,326,327] Observational studies are frequently criticized by doctors who do not understand this type of research. Most of what we know about adverse drugs reactions and what we are likely to learn in the future comes from observational research. This type of research was used to show the link between cigarette smoking and lung cancer.

Our petition helped to bring about important labeling changes in February 1996 on one of the calcium channel blockers, the short-acting form of nifedipine. The labeling for this form of nifedipine now warns doctors that this product should not be used for the treatment of high blood pressure.

Since we filed our petition additional serious adverse effects have been associated with the use of calcium channel blockers. These include an increased risk of gastrointestinal bleeding in older adults.[328] Calcium channel blockers have been shown in some studies to increase the risk of cancer[329,330,331] including breast cancer in postmenopausal women.[332] However, another study has found no increase in the risk of cancer with the calcium channel blockers.[333]

Despite the 1993 recommendations of the National Institutes of Health's National Heart, Lung, and Blood Institute that diuretics and beta-blockers should be used first in the treatment of mild to moderate high blood pressure the calcium channel blockers remain the largest selling family of high-blood-pressure-lowering drugs in the U.S.[334]

Each calcium channel blocker differs in the likelihood of harmful adverse effects. Although this group of calcium channel blockers is less likely than verapamil to cause constipation, it is more apt to cause dizziness, flushing, headaches, rapid heartbeat, and swelling of legs and feet compared to other calcium channel blockers.[335] These adverse effects can seriously limit use.

Older adults are more apt to have decreased kidney function, and may require a low dose of calcium channel blockers. Sometimes calcium channel blockers are used with a water pill or beta-blocker (see p. 52).

The American Medical Association reports nifedipine and nicardipine are more effective for angina than verapamil and diltiazem.[336]

If you have high blood pressure, the best way to reduce or eliminate your need for medication is by improving your diet, losing weight, exercising, and decreasing your salt and alcohol intake. Mild hypertension can be controlled by proper nutrition and exercise. If these measures do not lower your blood pressure enough and you need medication, **hydrochlorothiazide, a water pill (see thiazide diuretics, p. 100), is the drug of choice starting with a low dose of 12.5 milligrams daily.** It also costs less than other blood pressure drugs.

There is now good evidence that thiazide diuretics, such as hydrochlorothiazide, significantly decrease the rate of bone mineral loss in both men and women because they reduce the amount of calcium lost in the urine. An increasing number of researchers think that this will also decrease the number of fractures.[337]

If this drug does not lower your blood pressure enough, your doctor can prescribe a second type of drug called a beta-blocker (see p. 52) to accompany the hydrochlorothiazide. If you cannot take a beta-blocker, a drug from another family (calcium channel blockers) can be used instead.

Whatever drugs you take for high blood pressure, once your blood pressure has been normal for a year or more, a cautious decrease in dose and renewed attention to nondrug treatment may be worth trying, according to *The Medical Letter.*[338]

And an editorial in the *British Medical Journal* stated: *"Treatment of hypertension is part of preventive medicine and like all preventive strategies, its progress should be regularly reviewed by whoever initiates it. Many problems could be avoided by not starting antihypertensive treatment until after prolonged observation. . . . Patients should no longer be told that treatment is necessarily for life: the possibility of reducing or stopping treatment should be mentioned at the outset."*[339]

Before You Use This Drug

Do not use if you have or have had:

- severe hypotension

Tell your doctor if you have or have had:

- allergies to drugs
- aortic stenosis
- diabetes
- heart, kidney or liver problems
- hypokalemia
- mental depression
- narrowing of GI tract (*with nifedipine only*)
- low blood pressure

Tell your doctor about any other drugs you take, including aspirin, herbs, vitamins, and other nonprescription products. Be sure to include the name of any eyedrops which you use.

If you are taking a beta-blocker, your doctor may gradually take you off of it before starting a calcium channel blocker.[340]

When You Use This Drug

- **Learn to take your pulse, and get immediate help if your pulse slows to 50 beats per minute or slower, even if you are feeling well.**
- Periodically check your blood pressure one or two hours after you take a dose, and again eight hours after your last dose.
- Follow a diet recommended by your doctor.
- Have your doctor suggest exercises which avoid overexertion.
- **Do not stop taking calcium channel blockers suddenly. Contact your doctor for a schedule to decrease your drug gradually.**
- You may feel dizzy when rising from a lying or sitting position. If you are lying down, hang your legs over the side of the bed for a few minutes, then get up slowly. When getting up from a chair, stay by the chair until you are sure that you are not dizzy. (See p. 16.)
- If you plan to have any surgery, including dental, tell your doctor that you take this drug.
- **Do not take other drugs without talking to your doctor first—especially drugs for asthma, colds, cough, diet, hay fever, or sinus problems.**

How to Use This Drug

- Swallow capsule or tablet whole. Do not break, chew or crush long-acting forms of this drug.
- Be aware that the shell, empty of the drug, of some forms will pass in your stool.
- If you miss a dose, take it as soon as you remember, but skip it if it is almost time for the next dose. **Do not take double doses.**
- Do not store in the bathroom. Do not expose to heat, moisture, or strong light.

Interactions with Other Drugs

The following drugs are listed in the *Evaluations of Drug Interactions* 1997 as causing "highly clinically significant" or "clinically significant" interactions when used together with this drug. We have also included potentially serious interactions listed in the drug's FDA-approved professional product labeling or package insert because new scientific techniques have allowed researchers to predict some drug interactions before they have been documented in people. There may be other drugs, especially those in the families of drugs listed below, that also will react with this drug to cause severe adverse effects. The number of new drugs approved for marketing increases the chance of drug interactions, and new drug interactions are being identified with old drugs. Be vigilant. Make sure to tell your doctor and pharmacist the drugs you are taking and tell your doctor if you are taking any of these interacting drugs:

amiodarone, CALCIFEROL, calcium, carbamazepine, cimetidine, CORDARONE, cyclosporine, DANTRIUM, dantrolene, digoxin, DILANTIN, DURAQUIN, ELIXOPHYLLIN, ergocalciferol, INDERAL, INDERAL LA, LANOXICAPS, LANOXIN, lithium, LITHONATE, LITHOBID, NEORAL, NORCURON, phenytoin, propranolol, QUINAGLUTE DURA-TABS, QUINIDEX, quinidine, RIFADIN, rifampin, RIMACTANE, SANDIMMUNE, SLO-BID, TAGAMET, TEGRETOL, THEO-24, theophylline, vecuronium.

The drugs listed above have reported interactions with nifedipine. Not all of these interactions may have been reported for the other, newer calcium channel blockers listed in this section. Always ask your doctor and pharmacist about specific interactions for the calcium channel blocker you are taking.

Adverse Effects

Call your doctor immediately if you experience:

- chest pain
- dizziness
- irregular heartbeat
- pounding headache[341]
- fiery red discoloration of knees or ankles[342]
- swelling of legs and feet
- yellowing of skin or eyes
- problems urinating[343]
- breathing difficulty
- coughing or wheezing
- skin rash
- bleeding, tender or swollen gums
- fainting
- painful swollen joints (*with nifedipine only*)
- trouble seeing (*with nifedipine only*)

Call your doctor if these symptoms continue:

- drowsiness
- dry mouth
- flushing and feeling of warmth
- headache
- indigestion
- muscle cramps
- nausea
- numbness
- redness, heat, or pain in the fingers (This is more apt to happen during warm weather or while in bed at night.[344] If this occurs, dip your hands in cold water.)
- skin rash
- feeling of weakness
- constipation, diarrhea
- dizziness, lightheadedness

Periodic Tests

Ask your doctor which of these tests should be done periodically while you are taking this drug:

- blood pressure
- heart function tests, such as electrocardiogram (ECG, EKG)
- kidney function tests
- liver function tests

Do Not Use
(Except after valve replacement)

ALTERNATIVE TREATMENT FOR ANGINA:
See Propranolol, p. 154.

Dipyridamole
PERSANTINE (Boehringer Ingelheim)

FAMILY: Blood-clotting Inhibitor

Dipyridamole (dye peer *id* a mole) is used to reduce blood-clot formation and for other heart and blood conditions. **This drug has not been proven to have any health benefit** except in one study involving a certain type of heart surgery—heart valve replacement. It is also sometimes given in combination with aspirin to prevent a stroke, but there is no proof that this combination works any better than aspirin alone. There is no convincing evidence that dipyridamole will prevent or relieve any disease of the blood vessels supplying the brain, decrease the

The National Academy of Sciences has determined that this drug lacks evidence of effectiveness.

severity or frequency of chest pain (angina), or improve the mental or physical state of older or senile people.

Do Not Use

ALTERNATIVE TREATMENT:
See Hydrochlorothiazide, p. 100.

Mibefradil
POSICOR (Roche)

FAMILY: Antihypertensives
Calcium Channel Blockers (See p. 53)

Mibefradil was removed from the market on June 8, 1998 because of numerous serious injuries and deaths.

Mibefradil (mi *bef* ra dil), a new calcium channel blocker drug, is chemically distinct from other members of this family used for high blood pressure (hypertension) and chest pain (angina). It is the ninth calcium channel blocker to be marketed in the U.S. Like other members of the calcium channel blocker family it is not known whether the long-term use of mibefradil will reduce the risk of heart attack and stroke.

A controversy arose during the FDA advisory committee meeting to evaluate the scientific evidence to support the approval of mibefradil. Some members of the committee were concerned that the drug caused changes in the electrical conduction patterns of the heart (ECG, EKG changes) that could lead to potentially fatal heart rhythm disturbances. Committee members voting against the approval of mibefradil wanted to wait until mid-1998 for the results of a large clinical trial that would answer the question about potential heart rhythm disturbances. This would have been the wise decision, since there is no documented evidence to indicate that mibefradil offers any therapeutic advantage over other calcium channel blockers. However, the advisory committee voted 5 to 3 to recommend approval of the drug.

Within six months of mibefradil's introduction, doctors were informed of additional serious warnings and dangerous drug interactions with mibefradil. The drug may cause extremely low heart rates in some people, and, when taken with certain cholesterol-lowering drugs in the "statin" family (see p. 130) there is a risk of muscle injury that can be life-threatening.

If you have high blood pressure, the best way to reduce or eliminate your need for medication is by improving your diet, losing weight, exercising, and decreasing your salt and alcohol intake. Mild hypertension can be controlled by proper nutrition and exercise. If these measures do not lower your blood pressure enough and you need medication, **hydrochlorothiazide, a water pill (see thiazide diuretics, p. 100), is the drug of choice starting with a low dose of 12.5 milligrams daily.** It also costs less than other blood pressure drugs.

There is now good evidence that thiazide diuretics, such as hydrochlorothiazide, significantly decrease the rate of bone mineral loss in both men and women because they reduce the amount of calcium lost in the urine. An increasing number of researchers think that this will also decrease the number of fractures.[345]

If this drug does not lower your blood pressure enough, your doctor can prescribe a second type of drug called a beta-blocker (see p. 52) to accompany the hydrochlorothiazide. If you cannot take a beta-blocker, a drug from another family (calcium channel blockers) can be used instead.

Whatever drugs you take for high blood pressure, once your blood pressure has been normal for a year or more, a cautious decrease in dose and renewed attention to nondrug treatment may be worth trying, according to *The Medical Letter.*[346]

And an editorial in the *British Medical Journal* stated: *"Treatment of hypertension is part of preventive medicine and like all preventive strategies, its progress should be regularly reviewed by whoever initiates it. Many problems could be avoided by not starting antihypertensive treatment until after prolonged observation. . . . Patients should no longer be told that treatment is necessarily for life: the possibility of reducing or stopping treatment should be mentioned at the outset."*[347]

In 1995, Public Citizen's Health Research Group filed a petition with the Food and Drug Administration to add warnings to the labeling of all calcium channel blockers about the increased risk of heart attack and death. Our petition was based on three well conducted observational research studies.[348,349,350] Observational studies are frequently criticized by doctors who do not understand this type of research. Most of what we know about adverse drugs reactions and what we are likely to learn in the future comes from observational research. This type of research was used to show the link between cigarette smoking and lung cancer.

Our petition helped to bring about important labeling changes in February 1996 on one of the calcium channel blockers, the short-acting form of nifedipine. The labeling for this form of nifedipine now warns doctors that this product should not be used for the treatment of high blood pressure.

Since we filed our petition additional, serious adverse effects have been associated with the use of calcium channel blockers. These include an increased risk of gastrointestinal bleeding in older adults.[351] Calcium channel blockers have been shown in some studies to increase the risk of cancer[352,353,354] including breast cancer in postmenopausal women.[355] However, another study has found no increase in the risk of cancer with the calcium channel blockers.[356]

Despite the 1993 recommendations of the

National Institutes of Health's National Heart, Lung, and Blood Institute that diuretics and beta-blockers should be used first in the treatment of mild to moderate high blood pressure, the calcium channel blockers remain the largest selling family of high-blood-pressure-lowering drugs in the U.S.[357]

Limited Use

Procainamide
PROCANBID (Parke-Davis)

GENERIC: available
FAMILY: Antiarrhythmics

Procainamide (proe *kane* a mide) slows the heart rate and stabilizes irregular heartbeats (arrhythmias). Since this drug frequently causes a disease called lupus erythematosus, as well as other adverse effects, it is not the best choice for long-term treatment of irregular heartbeats.[358] For long-term use, your doctor should first try quinidine, a safer drug in this family (see p. 94). **If your kidney or liver function is impaired, you should be taking less than the usual dose.**[359]

Many people who are taking procainamide or another drug in its family have relatively mild disturbances in their heart rhythm and no symptoms of underlying heart disease. The vast majority of these people do not need these drugs, and there is no evidence that using them improves health. In fact, most of the drugs in this family have severe adverse effects that are sometimes worse and even more life-threatening than the irregular heartbeats they treat. All of these drugs can also cause new irregularities in your heartbeat.

If you have an irregular heartbeat without any symptoms of underlying heart disease, you should not be exposed to the dangers of a drug that has no health benefit for your condition.[360] If you are taking procainamide or another drug in its family for an irregular heartbeat (arrhythmia), talk to your doctor and find out whether you also have symptoms of underlying heart disease. If not, discuss the possibility of stopping the drug.

Since there is a narrow range between a helpful and a harmful amount of this drug in your body, call your doctor immediately if you experience adverse effects (see Adverse Effects).

Before You Use This Drug

Do not use if you have or have had:

- complete heart block
- digitalis toxicity with heart block

Tell your doctor if you have or have had:

- allergies to drugs
- asthma or emphysema
- digitalis toxicity
- incomplete heart block
- kidney or liver problems
- lupus erythematosus
- myasthenia gravis

Tell your doctor about any other drugs you take, including aspirin, herbs, vitamins, and other nonprescription products.

When You Use This Drug

- Until you know how you react to this drug, do not drive or perform other activities requiring alertness. Procainamide may cause dizziness.
- **Do not stop taking this drug suddenly. Your doctor must give you a schedule to lower your dose gradually, to prevent serious changes in heart function.**
- Wear a medical identification bracelet or carry a card stating that you take procainamide.

WARNING! INCREASED RISK OF DEATH

In the National Heart, Lung, and Blood Institute's Cardiac Arrhythmia Suppression Trial (CAST) (a long-term, multi-centered, randomized, double-blind study) in patients with asymptomatic non-life-threatening ventricular (the large chambers of the heart) arrhythmias (rhythm disturbances) who had a heart attack more than six days, but less than two years previously, deaths or non-fatal cardiac arrest were seen in 7.7% of those patients treated with encainide or flecainide, members of the Class 1 group of antiarrhythmic drugs, compared to 3.0% in patients receiving an inactive sugar pill or placebo.

Because of the known ability of the Class 1 drugs, such as procainamide, to cause rhythm disturbances, and the lack of evidence of improved survival for any antiarrhythmic drug in patients without life-threatening heart rhythm disturbances, the use of the Class 1 drugs should be reserved for patients with life-threatening rhythm disturbances of the ventricles. These warnings now appear in the FDA-approved product labeling, or package insert, for all Class 1 drugs including: disopyramide (Norpace and generics), flecainide (Tambocor), mexiletine (Mexitil and generics), moricizine (Ethmozine), procainamide (Procanbid and generics), propafenone (Rythmol), quinidine (Duraquin, Quinaglute Dura-Tabs, Quinidex and generics), and tocainide (Tonocard).

• If you plan to have any surgery, including dental, tell your doctor that you take this drug.

How to Use This Drug

• Swallow extended-release tablets whole. Do not crush or break them.

• Take with food or milk to decrease stomach upset.

• Store procainamide in a dry place. Do not store in the bathroom or refrigerator. Do not expose to heat, moisture, or strong light.

• If you miss a dose, take it as soon as you remember, but skip it if it is less than two hours until your next scheduled dose. **Do not take double doses.**

Interactions with Other Drugs

The following drugs are listed in the *Evaluations of Drug Interactions* 1997 as causing "highly clinically significant" or "clinically significant" interactions when used together with this drug. We have also included potentially serious interactions listed in the drug's FDA-approved professional product labeling or package insert. New scientific techniques have allowed researchers to predict some drug interactions before they have been documented in people. There may be other drugs, especially those in the families of drugs listed below, that also will react with this drug to cause severe adverse effects. The number of new drugs approved for marketing increases the chance of drug interactions, and new drug interactions are being identified with old drugs. Be vigilant. Make sure to tell your doctor and pharmacist the drugs you are taking and tell your doctor if you are taking any of these interacting drugs:

amiodarone, cimetidine, CORDARONE, cyclosporine, grepafloxacin, NEORAL, RAXAR, SANDIMMUNE, sparfloxacin, TAGAMET, ZAGAM.

Adverse Effects

Call your doctor immediately if you experience:

• **signs of overdose:** confusion, dizziness, fainting, drowsiness, nausea and vomiting, unusual decrease in urination, unusually fast or irregular heartbeat

• **signs of lupus-like syndrome:** fever,

chills, joint pain or swelling, pain with breathing, skin rash or itching

- hallucinations or depression
- sore mouth, gums, or throat
- unusual bleeding or bruising
- unusual tiredness or weakness

Call your doctor if these symptoms continue:

- diarrhea
- loss of appetite
- dizziness or lightheadedness

Periodic Tests

Ask your doctor which of these tests should be done periodically while you are taking this drug:

- complete blood count
- heart function tests, such as electrocardiogram (ECG, EKG)
- blood pressure
- liver function tests
- blood levels of procainamide and NAPA (a metabolite of procainamide)
- antinuclear antibody test (if this is positive ask your doctor about changing your drug, since a positive value is often linked with a lupus-like syndrome)

PREGNANCY WARNING

This drug caused harm to developing fetuses in animal studies, or such studies were not done. Use during pregnancy only for clear medical reasons. Tell your doctor if you are pregnant or thinking of becoming pregnant before you take this drug.

Do Not Use
(Except for treatment of malaria)

ALTERNATIVE TREATMENT:
Exercise and painkillers.

Quinine

FAMILY: Leg Cramp Treatment

Quinine (*kwye* nine) **is used to treat nighttime leg cramps, but there is no convincing evidence that it is safe and effective for this purpose.**[361] Repeated use of quinine can cause a group of adverse effects that is called cinchonism that includes ringing in the ears, headache, nausea, and abnormal vision. It can also affect the gastrointestinal tract, the nervous system, the cardiovascular system, and the skin. It can cause fatal bleeding disorders due to low levels of blood platelets. Because of its risks and its lack of proven effectiveness, quinine should not be used to treat leg cramps.

Quinine is useful for malaria, but it is not often prescribed in the United States for this purpose.

Do Not Use

ALTERNATIVE TREATMENT:
See Hydrochlorothiazide, p. 100.

Reserpine and Chlorthalidone
REGROTON (USV)
DEMI-REGROTON (USV)

FAMILY: Diuretics
Antihypertensives
(See High Blood Pressure, p. 44)

This product, a combination of reserpine (see p. 152) and chlorthalidone (see p. 105), is used to treat high blood pressure (hypertension). **Older adults should not use drugs that**

contain a fixed combination of reserpine and chlorthalidone.

Reserpine causes severe adverse effects (see p. 152) that may occur during treatment and even months after you stop taking it. It has caused severe depression, in some cases leading to suicide. We do not recommend that any older adult use reserpine, and it is particularly dangerous for anyone with a history of depression.[362] It also decreases mental sharpness in older adults.

Chlorthalidone puts the older adult user at such a high risk of adverse effects that the World Health Organization has said it should not be used by people over 60.[363] We do not recommend that any older adult use chlorthalidone.

In addition to the risks of reserpine and chlorthalidone, there are good reasons not to use any fixed-combination drug for high blood pressure. A single drug is often enough to control high blood pressure. If a combination drug like this one is controlling your high blood pressure, it is quite possible that one drug alone would do the same job. There is no reason to put yourself at extra risk by taking drugs you do not need.

If you have high blood pressure, the best way to reduce or eliminate your need for medication is by improving your diet, losing weight, exercising, and decreasing your salt and alcohol intake. Mild hypertension can be controlled by proper nutrition and exercise. If these measures do not lower your blood pressure enough and you need medication, **hydrochlorothiazide, a water pill (see thiazide diuretics, p. 100), is the drug of choice starting with a low dose of 12.5 milligrams daily.** It also costs less than other blood pressure drugs.

There is now good evidence that thiazide diuretics, such as hydrochlorothiazide, significantly decrease the rate of bone mineral loss in both men and women because they reduce the amount of calcium lost in the urine. An increasing number of researchers think that this will also decrease the number of fractures.[364]

If your high blood pressure is more severe, and hydrochlorothiazide alone does not control it, there are still safer drug treatments than this combination product. The best treatment in this case is a combination of hydrochlorothiazide and a second type of drug called a beta-blocker, such as propranolol (see p. 154). If you can't take a drug in the beta-blocker family, another drug called a calcium channel blocker may be used instead. In either case, your doctor would prescribe the hydrochlorothiazide and the second drug separately, with the dose of each drug adjusted to meet your needs, rather than using a product that combines the drugs in advance in a fixed combination.

If you are taking this fixed-combination drug, ask your doctor about changing your prescription.

Whatever drugs you take for high blood pressure, once your blood pressure has been normal for a year or more, a cautious decrease in dose and renewed attention to nondrug treatment may be worth trying, according to *The Medical Letter.*[365]

And an editorial in the *British Medical Journal* stated: *"Treatment of hypertension is part of preventive medicine and like all preventive strategies, its progress should be regularly reviewed by whoever initiates it. Many problems could be avoided by not starting antihypertensive treatment until after prolonged observation. . . . Patients should no longer be told that treatment is necessarily for life: the possibility of reducing or stopping treatment should be mentioned at the outset."*[366]

ALTERNATIVE TREATMENT:
See Hydrochlorothiazide, p. 100.

Reserpine

FAMILY: Antihypertensives
(See High Blood Pressure, p. 44)

Reserpine (re *ser* peen) is sometimes used to treat severe high blood pressure (hypertension) in older adults. **It should not be used because it has severe adverse effects, including depression, dizziness, drowsiness, flushed skin, and slow pulse. These may occur while taking reserpine and can last or even begin many months after treatment has ended.** Some people taking reserpine have become so severely depressed that they have committed suicide. People who have a history of depression should never take reserpine.[367] The drug can also cause decreased mental sharpness in older adults.

Mental depression caused by reserpine can be difficult to recognize because it occurs very gradually. Symptoms of depression include feelings of hopelessness, helplessness, and rejection, lack of self-worth, inability to sleep in the morning, vivid dreams, nightmares, and loss of appetite.

Stop taking reserpine and contact your doctor immediately if you have any of these symptoms.

If you have high blood pressure, the best way to reduce or eliminate your need for medication is by improving your diet, losing weight, exercising, and decreasing your salt and alcohol intake. Mild hypertension can be controlled by proper nutrition and exercise. If these measures do not lower your blood pressure enough and you need medication, **hydrochlorothiazide, a water pill (see thiazide diuretics, p. 100), is the drug of choice starting with a low dose of 12.5 milligrams daily.** It also costs less than other blood pressure drugs.

There is now good evidence that thiazide diuretics, such as hydrochlorothiazide, significantly decrease the rate of bone mineral loss in both men and women because they reduce the amount of calcium lost in the urine. An increasing number of researchers think that this will also decrease the number of fractures.[368]

If this drug does not lower your blood pressure enough, your doctor can prescribe a second type of drug called a beta-blocker (see p. 52) to accompany the hydrochlorothiazide. If you cannot take a beta-blocker, a drug from another family (calcium channel blockers) can be used instead.

Whatever drugs you take for high blood pressure, once your blood pressure has been normal for a year or more, a cautious decrease in dose and renewed attention to nondrug treatment may be worth trying, according to *The Medical Letter.*[369]

And an editorial in the *British Medical Journal* stated: *"Treatment of hypertension is part of preventive medicine and like all preventive strategies, its progress should be regularly reviewed by whoever initiates it. Many problems could be avoided by not starting antihypertensive treatment until after prolonged observation. . . . Patients should no longer be told that treatment is necessarily for life: the possibility of reducing or stopping treatment should be mentioned at the outset."*[370]

ALTERNATIVE TREATMENT:
See Hydrochlorothiazide, p. 100.

Reserpine and Hydroflumethiazide
SALUTENSIN (Roberts)

FAMILY: Diuretics
Antihypertensives
(See High Blood Pressure, p. 44)

This product, a combination of reserpine (see p. 152) and hydroflumethiazide (hye droe floo meth *eye* a zide), is used to treat high blood pressure. **Older adults should not use drugs containing a fixed combination of reserpine and hydroflumethiazide.**

Reserpine causes severe adverse effects (see p. 152) that may occur during treatment and even months after you stop taking it. It has caused severe depression, in some cases leading to suicide. We do not recommend that any older adult use reserpine, and it is particularly dangerous for anyone with a history of depression.[371] It also decreases mental sharpness in older adults.

In addition to the risks of reserpine, there are good reasons not to use any fixed-combination drug for high blood pressure. A single drug is often enough to control high blood pressure. If a combination drug like this one is controlling your high blood pressure, it is quite possible that one drug alone would do the same job. There is no reason to put yourself at extra risk by taking drugs you do not need.

If you have high blood pressure, the best way to reduce or eliminate your need for medication is by improving your diet, losing weight, exercising, and decreasing your salt and alcohol intake. Mild hypertension can be controlled by proper nutrition and exercise. If these measures do not lower your blood pressure enough and you need medication, **hydrochlorothiazide, a water pill (see thiazide diuretics, p. 100), is the drug of choice starting with a low dose of 12.5 milligrams daily.** It also costs less than other blood pressure drugs.

There is now good evidence that thiazide diuretics, such as hydrochlorothiazide, significantly decrease the rate of bone mineral loss in both men and women because they reduce the amount of calcium lost in the urine. An increasing number of researchers think that this will also decrease the number of fractures.[372]

Hydrochlorothiazide is a better choice than hydroflumethiazide because it is equally effective, less expensive, and milder. If your high blood pressure is more severe, and hydrochlorothiazide alone does not control it, there are still better drug treatments than this combination product. The best treatment in this case is a combination of hydrochlorothiazide and a second type of drug called a beta-blocker, such as propranolol (see p. 154). If you can't take a drug in the beta-blocker family, another drug called a calcium channel blocker may be used instead. In either case, your doctor would prescribe the hydrochlorothiazide and the second drug separately, with the dose of each drug adjusted to meet your needs, rather than using a product that combines the drugs in advance in a fixed combination.

If you are taking this fixed-combination drug, ask your doctor about changing your prescription.

Whatever drugs you take for high blood pressure, once your blood pressure has been normal for a year or more, a cautious decrease in dose and renewed attention to nondrug treatment may be worth trying, according to *The Medical Letter.*[373]

And an editorial in the *British Medical Journal* stated: *"Treatment of hypertension is part of preventive medicine and like all preventive strategies, its progress should be regularly reviewed by whoever initiates it. Many problems could be avoided by not starting antihypertensive treatment until after prolonged observation. . . . Patients should no longer be told that treatment is necessarily for life: the possibility of reducing or stopping treatment should be mentioned at the outset."*[374]

━━━━━━

Acebutolol (ace ah *butte* o lall)
SECTRAL (Wyeth-Ayerst)

Atenolol (a *ten* ah lole)
TENORMIN (Zeneca)

Betaxolol (bait *ax* o loll)
KERLONE (Searle)

Bisoprolol (bis *oh* proe lol)
ZEBETA (Lederle)

Carteolol (*kar* tee oh lole)
CARTROL (Abbott)

Metoprolol (me *toe* proe lale)
LOPRESSOR (Novartis)
TOPROL XL (Astra)

Nadolol (*nay* doe lole)
CORGARD (Mylan)

Penbutolol (pen *byoo* toe lole)
LEVATOL (Schwarz)

Pindolol (*pin* doe lole)
VISKEN (Novartis)

Propranolol (proe *pran* oh lole)
INDERAL, INDERAL LA (Wyeth-Ayerst)

Limited Use (following drug)

Labetalol (la *bet* a lole)
NORMODYNE (Schering)
TRANDATE (Glaxo Wellcome)

GENERIC: available
FAMILY: Beta-blockers (see p. 52)
Antihypertensives
(See High Blood Pressure, p. 44)

Beta-blocking drugs are used to treat high blood pressure (hypertension), chest pain (angina), heart attacks, irregular heartbeats (arrhythmias), to decrease the frequency of migraine headaches, and for tremors of unknown origin. If you are over 60, you will generally need to take less than the usual adult dose, especially if your kidney function is impaired.

Four new beta-blockers have come on the market. These are bisoprolol, carteolol, carvedilol (see p. 85), and penbutolol. None of these four new drugs offers any documented therapeutic advancement over the older beta-blockers.

For young adults with high blood pressure, doctors usually prescribe a drug in this family before any other drug. But for African-Americans and older adults, these drugs are less effective as the sole treatment. For these groups of people, doctors usually prescribe another type of drug called a diuretic (water pill) to lower blood pressure, and add a beta-blocker as a second drug if the diuretic alone is not enough.

If you have high blood pressure, the best way to reduce or eliminate your need for medication is by improving your diet, losing weight, exercising, and decreasing your salt and alcohol intake. Mild hypertension can be controlled by proper nutrition and exercise. If these measures do not lower your blood pressure enough and you need medication, **hydrochlorothiazide, a water pill (see thiazide diuretics, p. 100), is the drug of choice starting with a low dose of 12.5 milligrams daily.** It also costs less than other blood pressure drugs.

There is now good evidence that thiazide diuretics, such as hydrochlorothiazide, significantly decrease the rate of bone mineral loss in both men and women because they reduce the amount of calcium lost in the urine. An increasing number of researchers think that this will also decrease the number of fractures.[375]

If this drug does not lower your blood pressure enough, your doctor can prescribe a beta-blocker to accompany the hydrochlorothiazide. All beta-blockers are similarly effective, although not necessarily interchangeable. If you are bothered by adverse effects when taking one of these drugs, talk to your doctor about switching to another beta-blocker, such as propranolol, which is available generically. The adverse effects of these drugs vary widely, and each individual responds differently to each one. See p. 44 for a discussion of alternatives to these drugs. If you cannot take a beta-blocker, a drug from another family (calcium channel blockers) can be used instead.

Whatever drugs you take for high blood pressure, once your blood pressure has been normal for a year or more, a cautious decrease in dose and renewed attention to nondrug treatment may be worth trying, according to *The Medical Letter.*[376]

And an editorial in the *British Medical Journal* stated: *"Treatment of hypertension is part of preventive medicine and like all preventive strategies, its progress should be regularly reviewed by whoever initiates it. Many problems could be avoided by not starting antihypertensive treatment until after prolonged observation. . . . Patients should no longer be told that treatment is necessarily for life: the possibility of reducing or stopping treatment should be mentioned at the outset."*[377]

Before You Use This Drug

Do not use if you have:

- congestive heart failure
- asthma
- emphysema or chronic bronchitis

Tell your doctor if you have or have had:

- allergies to drugs
- gout
- alcohol dependence
- mental depression
- kidney, liver, lung, or pancreas disease
- diabetes
- lupus erythematosus
- difficulty breathing

- poor blood circulation
- Raynaud's syndrome
- thyroid problems
- myasthenia gravis
- psoriasis

Tell your doctor about any other drugs you take, including aspirin, herbs, vitamins, and other nonprescription products.

When You Use This Drug

- **Learn to take your pulse, and get immediate medical help if your pulse slows to 50 beats per minute or slower, even if you are feeling well. Some people have suffered from slowed heart rate and heart failure while taking these drugs.**
- Until you know how you react to this drug, do not drive or perform other activities requiring alertness.
- Be careful not to overexert yourself, even though your chest pain may feel better.
- **Do not stop taking this drug suddenly.** Your doctor must give you a schedule to decrease your dose gradually, to prevent chest pain and possible heart attack.
- You may feel dizzy when rising from a lying or sitting position. When getting out of bed, hang your legs over the side of the bed for a few minutes, then get up slowly. When getting up from a chair, get up slowly and stay beside the chair until you are sure that you are not dizzy. (See p. 16.)
- **Caution diabetics:** see p. 550.
- If you plan to have any surgery, including dental, tell your doctor that you take this drug.
- **Do not take other drugs without talking to your doctor first—especially nonprescription drugs for appetite control, asthma, colds, coughs, hay fever, or sinus problems.**

HEAT STRESS ALERT

This drug can affect your body's ability to adjust to heat, putting you at risk of "heat stress." If you live alone, ask a friend to check on you several times during the day. Early signs of heat stress are dizziness, lightheadedness, faintness, and slightly high temperature. Call your doctor if you have any of these signs.

Drink more fluids (water, fruit and vegetable juices) than usual—even if you're not thirsty—unless your doctor has told you otherwise. Do not drink alcohol.

How to Use This Drug

• Extended release dosage forms must not be crushed; others can be crushed and mixed with water, or swallowed whole with water.

• If you miss a dose, take it as soon as you remember, but skip it if it is less than eight hours until your next scheduled dose. **Do not take double doses.**

Interactions with Other Drugs

The following drugs are listed in the *Evaluations of Drug Interactions* 1997 as causing "highly clinically significant" or "clinically significant" interactions when used together with this drug. We have also included potentially serious interactions listed in the drug's FDA-approved professional product labeling or package insert. New scientific techniques have allowed researchers to predict some drug interactions before they have been documented in people. There may be other drugs, especially those in the families of drugs listed below, that also will react with this drug to cause severe adverse effects. The number of new drugs approved for marketing increases the chance of drug interactions, and new drug interactions are being identified with old drugs. Be vigilant.

Make sure to tell your doctor and pharmacist the drugs you are taking and tell your doctor if you are taking any of these interacting drugs:

ALDOMET, amiodarone, CALAN SR, CATAPRES, chlorpromazine, cimetidine, clonidine, cocaine, CORDARONE, COUMADIN, COVERA-HS, ephedrine, ELIXOPHYLLIN, FLUOTHANE, fluoxetine, furosemide, halothane, HUMALOG, HUMULIN, INDOCIN, indomethacin, insulin, ISOPTIN SR, LASIX, lidocaine, lithium, LITHOBID, LITHONATE, methyldopa, MINIPRESS, prazosin, PROZAC, SLO-BID, TAGAMET, theophylline, THEO-24, THORAZINE, TUBARINE, tubocurarine, verapamil, VERELAN, warfarin, XYLOCAINE.

The drugs listed above have reported interactions with propranolol. Not all of these interactions may have been reported for the other newer beta-blockers listed in this section. Always ask your doctor and pharmacist about specific interactions for the beta-blocker you are taking.

Adverse Effects

Call your doctor immediately if you experience:

• difficulty breathing
• cold hands or feet
• depression
• skin rash
• swelling of ankles, feet, or legs
• slow pulse
• back or joint pain
• chest pain
• confusion
• dark urine
• fever and sore throat

- hallucinations
- irregular heartbeat
- red, scaling or crusted skin
- unusual bleeding and bruising
- yellow eyes or skin
- convulsions
- bluish-colored fingernails or palms

Call your doctor if these symptoms continue:

- headache
- dizziness, lightheadedness
- nausea, vomiting, diarrhea — *some*
- unusual tiredness or weakness
- disturbed sleep, nightmares
- decreased sexual ability

More adverse effects information appears on p. 52.

Periodic Tests

Ask your doctor which of these tests should be done periodically while you are taking this drug:

- complete blood count
- blood pressure and pulse rate
- heart function tests, such as electrocardiogram (ECG, EKG)
- kidney function tests
- liver function tests
- blood glucose levels

PREGNANCY WARNING

Tenormin, Kerlone, Cartrol, Lopressor, Toprol XL, Corgard, Levatol, Inderal, Normodyne and Trandate caused harm to developing fetuses in animal studies, or such studies were not done. Use during pregnancy only for clear medical reasons. Tell your doctor if you are pregnant or thinking of becoming pregnant before you take any of these drugs.

 Do Not Use

ALTERNATIVE TREATMENT:
See Hydrochlorothiazide, p. 100.

Reserpine, Hydralazine, and Hydrochlorothiazide
SER-AP-ES (Novartis)

FAMILY: Diuretics
Antihypertensives
(See High Blood Pressure, p. 44)

This product, a combination of reserpine (see p. 152), hydralazine (see p. 64), and hydrochlorothiazide (see p. 100), is used to treat high blood pressure (hypertension). **Older adults should not use drugs that contain a fixed combination of reserpine, hydralazine, and hydrochlorothiazide.**

Reserpine causes severe adverse effects (see p. 152) that may occur during treatment and even months after you stop taking it. It has caused severe depression, in some cases leading to suicide. We do not recommend that any older adult use reserpine, and it is particularly dangerous for anyone with a history of depression.[378] It also decreases mental sharpness in older adults.

Hydralazine is not the first-choice drug for treating hypertension because of its adverse effects. Common adverse effects include rapid heartbeat and below normal blood pressure, which may cause lightheadedness, fainting, and falls. Hydralazine may worsen chest pain (angina).[379]

In addition to the risks of reserpine and hydralazine, there are good reasons not to use any fixed-combination drug for high blood pressure. A single drug is often enough to control high blood pressure. If a combination drug like this one is controlling your high blood pressure, it is quite possible that one drug alone would do the same job. There is no reason to put yourself at extra risk by taking drugs you do not need.

If you have high blood pressure, the best way to reduce or eliminate your need for medication is by improving your diet, losing weight, exercising, and decreasing your salt and alcohol intake. Mild hypertension can be controlled by proper nutrition and exercise. If these measures do not lower your blood pressure enough and you need medication, **hydrochlorothiazide, a water pill (see thiazide diuretics, p. 100), is the drug of choice starting with a low dose of 12.5 milligrams daily.** It also costs less than other blood pressure drugs.

There is now good evidence that thiazide diuretics, such as hydrochlorothiazide, significantly decrease the rate of bone mineral loss in both men and women because they reduce the amount of calcium lost in the urine. An increasing number of researchers think that this will also decrease the number of fractures.[380]

Hydrochlorothiazide is one of the ingredients in this combination. Reserpine and hydralazine can cause severe adverse effects, as described above. If hydrochlorothiazide alone would control your blood pressure, there is no reason to take the extra risk of taking the other two drugs as well.

If your high blood pressure is more severe and hydrochlorothiazide alone does not control it, there are still better drug treatments than this combination product. The best treatment in this case is a combination of hydrochlorothiazide and a second type of drug called a beta-blocker, such as propranolol (see p. 154). If you can't take a drug in the beta-blocker family, another drug called a calcium channel blocker may be used instead. In either case, your doctor would prescribe the hydrochlorothiazide and the second drug separately, with the dose of each drug adjusted to meet your needs, rather than using a product that combines the drugs in advance in a fixed combination.

If you are taking this fixed-combination drug, ask your doctor about changing your prescription.

Whatever drugs you take for high blood pressure, once your blood pressure has been normal for a year or more, a cautious decrease in dose and renewed attention to nondrug treatment may be worth trying, according to *The Medical Letter.*[381]

And an editorial in the *British Medical Journal* stated: *"Treatment of hypertension is part of preventive medicine and like all preventive strategies, its progress should be regularly reviewed by whoever initiates it. Many problems could be avoided by not starting antihypertensive treatment until after prolonged observation. . . . Patients should no longer be told that treatment is necessarily for life: the possibility of reducing or stopping treatment should be mentioned at the outset."*[382]

Limited Use

Guanfacine
TENEX (Robins)

GENERIC: not available
FAMILY: Antihypertensives
          (See High Blood Pressure, p. 44)

Guanfacine (gwawn *fas* seen) helps lower high blood pressure. It is not the first or second choice, but is reserved for use when other high blood pressure drugs do not work. In most studies with guanfacine, it is used along with diuretics (water pills), and no studies have yet established the appropriate dose of guanfacine when used alone.[383] Guanfacine controls, but does not cure high blood pressure. Nor does guanfacine improve your memory.[384,385]

A report in the *The American Journal of Medical Sciences* states that adrenergic blockers, such as guanfacine, should be used sparingly.[386] The same article finds any value of guanfacine over clonidine (a **Do Not Use** drug, see p. 80) to be marginal, and the cost of guanfacine compared to generic clonidine to be considerably higher. Tolerance to guanfacine can develop within a year, requiring an increased dose (and expense) for the same effect. Tolerance slows somewhat after the second year. Unfortunately, adverse effects increase with an increased dose. Guanfacine is not the drug of choice for people with congestive heart failure.[387]

In older people guanfacine tends to stay in the body longer. Older people also may be more sensitive to drowsiness and a low blood pressure when taking guanfacine.

If you have high blood pressure, the best way to reduce or eliminate your need for medication is by improving your diet, losing weight, exercising, and decreasing your salt and alcohol intake. Mild hypertension can be controlled by proper nutrition and exercise. If these measures do not lower your blood pressure enough and you need medication, **hydrochlorothiazide, a water pill (see thiazide diuretics, p. 100), is the drug of choice starting with a low dose of 12.5 milligrams daily.** It also costs less than other blood pressure drugs.

There is now good evidence that thiazide diuretics, such as hydrochlorothiazide, significantly decrease the rate of bone mineral loss in both men and women because they reduce the amount of calcium lost in the urine. An increasing number of researchers think that this will also decrease the number of fractures.[388]

If this drug does not lower your blood pressure enough, your doctor can prescribe a second type of drug called a beta-blocker, such as propranolol (see p. 154) to accompany the hydrochlorothiazide. If you cannot take a beta-blocker, a drug from another family (calcium channel blockers) can be used instead.

Whatever drugs you take for high blood pressure, once your blood pressure has been normal for a year or more, a cautious decrease in dose and renewed attention to nondrug treatment may be worth trying, according to *The Medical Letter.*[389]

And an editorial in the *British Medical Journal* stated: *"Treatment of hypertension is part of preventive medicine and like all preventive strategies, its progress should be regularly reviewed by whoever initiates it. Many problems could be avoided by not starting antihypertensive treatment until after prolonged observation. . . . Patients should no longer be told that treatment is necessarily for life: the possibility of reducing or stopping treatment should be mentioned at the outset."*[390]

Before You Use This Drug

Do not use if you have or have had:

- sick sinus node syndrome[391]

Tell your doctor if you have or have had:

- allergies to drugs
- cerebrovascular disease
- mental depression
- diabetes[392,393]
- heart, kidney, or liver problems
- myocardial infarction

Tell your doctor about any other drugs you take, including aspirin, herbs, vitamins, and other nonprescription products.

When You Use This Drug

- You may feel dizzy when rising from a lying or sitting position. If you are lying down, hang your legs over the side of the bed for a few minutes, then get up slowly. When getting up from a chair, stay by the chair until you are sure that you are not dizzy. (See p. 16.)
- Until you know how you react to this drug, do not drive or perform other tasks requiring mental alertness. Drowsiness is especially common when first starting guanfacine.
- Have your blood pressure taken periodically, including just before your daily dose.
- Eat a diet low in salt. Restrict calories if overweight.

• Check with your doctor before using non-prescription drugs to assure that the ingredients do not interact with guanfacine.

• If you have emergency medical care, or plan to have any surgery, including dental, tell your doctor that you take this drug.

How to Use This Drug

• Swallow tablet whole. Take at bedtime since it may cause drowsiness.

• Continue to take guanfacine, even if you feel well.

• If you miss a dose, take it as soon as you remember, but skip it if it is almost time for the next dose. If you miss two or more days in a row, check with your doctor. **Do not take double doses.**

• **Do not suddenly stop taking this drug. Ask your doctor for a schedule to lower your dose gradually.**

• Store at room temperature with the lid on tightly. Do not expose to heat and light.

Interactions with Other Drugs

Some other drugs that you may be taking (either over-the-counter or prescription drugs) can interact with this one, causing adverse effects. Ask your doctor what these drugs are and let him or her know if you are taking any of them.

Adverse Effects

Get emergency help if you have signs of overdose:

• difficulty breathing
• extreme dizziness, faintness
• slow heartbeat
• unusually severe tiredness, weakness

Call your doctor immediately if you experience:

• confusion
• depression
• numbness
• skin rash

Call your doctor if these symptoms continue:

• constipation, diarrhea
• dizziness
• drowsiness
• dry mouth
• burning, dry, or itching eyes
• headache
• leg cramps
• itching
• nausea, vomiting
• ringing in ears
• sexual problems, impotence
• insomnia
• sweating
• swelling of legs or eyes[394]
• thirst[395]
• unusual tiredness, weakness
• urinary incontinence
• vision changes
• weight change[396,397]

Call your doctor immediately if signs of withdrawal occur. This usually happens two to seven days after more than one dose is missed, or guanfacine is suddenly stopped. Withdrawal may be aggravated if your dose was large, or you also took a beta-blocker along with guanfacine.[398] Withdrawal symptoms include:

• anxiety, nervousness, restlessness, tenseness
• a rise in blood pressure
• chest pain
• irregular heartbeat
• nausea, vomiting
• increased saliva
• shaking or trembling of fingers and hands
• disturbed sleep
• stomach cramps
• sweating

Periodic Tests

Ask your doctor which tests should be done periodically while you are taking this drug:

* blood pressure

 Do Not Use

ALTERNATIVE TREATMENT:
See Hydrochlorothiazide, p. 100.

Atenolol and Chlorthalidone
TENORETIC (Zeneca)

FAMILY: Diuretics
Antihypertensives
(See High Blood Pressure, p. 44)

This product, a combination of atenolol (see p. 154 and chlorthalidone (see p. 105), is used to treat high blood pressure. **Older adults should not use drugs containing a fixed combination of atenolol and chlorthalidone.**

Chlorthalidone puts the older adult user at such a high risk of adverse effects that the World Health Organization has said it should not be used by people over 60.[399]

In addition to the risks of chlorthalidone, there are good reasons not to use a fixed-combination drug for high blood pressure. A single drug is often enough to control high blood pressure. If a combination drug like this one is controlling your high blood pressure, it is quite possible that one drug alone would do the same job. There is no reason to put yourself at extra risk by taking drugs you do not need.

If you have high blood pressure, the best way to reduce or eliminate your need for medication is by improving your diet, losing weight, exercising, and decreasing your salt and alcohol intake. Mild hypertension can be controlled by proper nutrition and exercise. If these measures do not lower your blood pressure enough and you need medication, **hydrochloro-thiazide, a water pill (see thiazide diuretics, p. 100), is the drug of choice starting with a low dose of 12.5 milligrams daily.** It also costs less than other blood pressure drugs.

There is now good evidence that thiazide diuretics, such as hydrochlorothiazide, significantly decrease the rate of bone mineral loss in both men and women because they reduce the amount of calcium lost in the urine. An increasing number of researchers think that this will also decrease the number of fractures.[400]

If your high blood pressure is more severe, and hydrochlorothiazide alone does not control it, the best treatment is a combination of hydrochlorothiazide and a second type of drug called a beta-blocker, such as propranolol (see p. 154. If you can't take a drug in the beta-blocker family, another drug called a calcium channel blocker may be used instead. In either case, your doctor would prescribe the hydrochlorothiazide and the second drug separately, with the dose of each drug adjusted to meet your needs, rather than using a product that combines the drugs in advance in a fixed combination.

If you are taking this fixed-combination drug, ask your doctor about changing your prescription.

Whatever drugs you take for high blood pressure, once your blood pressure has been normal for a year or more, a cautious decrease in dose and renewed attention to nondrug treatment may be worth trying, according to *The Medical Letter.*[401]

And an editorial in the *British Medical Journal* stated: *"Treatment of hypertension is part of preventive medicine and like all preventive strategies, its progress should be regularly reviewed by whoever initiates it. Many problems could be avoided by not starting antihypertensive treatment until after prolonged observation. . . . Patients should no longer be told that treatment is necessarily for life: the possibility of reducing or stopping treatment should be mentioned at the outset."*[402]

Last Choice Drug

Ticlopidine
TICLID (Roche)

GENERIC: not available
FAMILY: Drugs to Prevent Stroke

Ticlopidine (tye *kloe* pi deen) is approved by
the FDA to prevent stroke in people who
already had strokes or have signs of developing a stroke. It should not be used by people
who can take aspirin. It is also frequently
used for prevention of stroke and clot formation after a procedure in which a thin tube
called a *stent* is implanted to keep narrowed
heart vessels open. However, this is *not* an
FDA-approved use for this drug.

Ticlopidine prolongs bleeding time so blood
clots are less apt to form. The dose of ticlopidine is adjusted according to bleeding time.
Although somewhat more effective than
aspirin in preventing strokes, ticlopidine causes significantly more adverse effects than
aspirin, including life-threatening blood disorders. It lowers the white blood cell count,
increasing risk of infections, and can injure the
ability of bone marrow to make red blood cells.
Ticlopidine also increases cholesterol about
10%. It should only be used by people who are
allergic to aspirin. Ticlopidine should not be
used by people who have had bleeding ulcers or
liver disease. Anyone with kidney problems
may need lower doses of ticlopidine.

Over half the individuals who take ticlopidine have had gastrointestinal adverse
effects.[403] Older people are even more likely to
experience adverse effects, especially gastrointestinal effects, such as nausea and diarrhea.
Severe blood disorders have been reported,
most frequently in women over 75 years of
age.[404]

Worldwide, through 1994, a total of 645
cases of serious blood disorders had been
associated with the use of ticlopidine. Of
these 645 cases, 102 (16%) resulted in death.
Since ticlopidine was first marketed in late
1991 through March 1995, the FDA had
received 209 reports associating various
types of blood disorders with this drug. Of 188
people for whom complete information was
available, 36, (19%) had died. In reports to
the FDA, onset of the blood disorder occurred
about 30 to 45 days after starting ticlopidine.
In some of the reports people had been taking
other drugs that can cause blood disorders,
but most had no known causes other than
ticlopidine. After stopping the drug, the bone
marrow's ability to make blood cells returned
to normal in most people.[405]

Before You Use This Drug

Tell your doctor if you have or have had:

- allergies, including aspirin and iodine
- bleeding problems or blood disorders
- high cholesterol
- gingivitis
- hemophilia
- kidney or liver problems
- surgery
- ulcers

Tell your doctor about any other drugs you take, including aspirin, herbs, vitamins, and other nonprescription products.

When You Use This Drug

- Wear identification that you use ticlopidine.
- Check with your doctor before taking any nonprescription drugs.
- If you plan to have any surgery, including dental, tell your doctor that you take this drug. It is recommended that ticlopidine be discontinued for two weeks before any surgery, including dental surgery.

How to Use This Drug

- Swallow whole tablets. Take with food. Do not take at the same time as antacids.
- If you miss a dose, take it as soon as you remember but skip it if it is almost time for the next dose. **Do not take double doses.**
- Do not store in the bathroom. Do not expose to heat, moisture, or strong light.

Interactions with Other Drugs

The following drugs are listed in the *Evaluations of Drug Interactions* 1997 as causing "highly clinically significant" or "clinically significant" interactions when used together with this drug. We have also included potentially serious interactions listed in the drug's FDA-approved professional product labeling or package insert. New scientific techniques have allowed researchers to predict some drug interactions before they have been documented in people. There may be other drugs, especially those in the families of drugs listed below, that also will react with this drug to cause severe adverse effects. The number of new drugs approved for marketing increases the chance of drug interactions, and new drug interactions are being identified with old drugs. Be vigilant. Make sure to tell your doctor and pharmacist the drugs you are taking and tell your doctor if you are taking any of these interacting drugs:

ABBOKINASE, ADVIL, ALEVE, ANAPROX, ANSAID, aspirin, GENUINE BAYER ASPIRIN, cimetidine, CLINORIL, COUMADIN, DAYPRO, diclofenac, digoxin, DILANTIN, ECOTRIN, ELIXOPHYLLIN, etodolac, FELDENE, fenoprofen, flurbiprofen, heparin, ibuprofen, INDOCIN, indomethacin, KABIKINASE, ketoprofen, ketorolac, LANOXICAPS, LANOXIN, LODINE, LUMINAL, meclofenamate, MECLOMEN, MOTRIN, nabumetone, NALFON, NAPROSYN, naproxen, OCUFEN, ORUDIS, oxaprozin, phenobarbital, phenytoin, piroxicam, RELAFEN, SLO-BID, SOLFOTON, STREPTASE, streptokinase, sulindac, TAGAMET, THEO-24, theophylline, TOLECTIN, tolmetin, TORADOL, urokinase, VOLTAREN, warfarin.

Adverse Effects

Call your doctor immediately if you experience:

- abdominal or stomach pain or swelling
- back pain
- bleeding of any kind
- bruising, pinpoint red spots or purple areas on skin
- coordination difficulties
- coughing up blood
- diarrhea
- dizziness
- fever, chills
- headache
- hives or itching
- heavy menstrual flow
- joint pain or swelling
- paralysis
- ringing or buzzing in ears
- skin rash
- sore throat
- difficulty speaking, stammering
- black, tarry, bloody, or pale stools
- dark urine
- sores, ulcers or white spots in mouth
- vomiting blood or material that looks like coffee grounds
- yellowing of skin or eyes
- blood in eyes or urine
- blistering, peeling or loosening of the skin, lips or mucous membranes

- nosebleeds
- decreased alertness
- general feeling of discomfort or illness
- heavy bleeding from cuts or wounds

Call your doctor if these symptoms continue:

- abdominal pain
- diarrhea
- dizziness
- gas or indigestion
- nausea
- vomiting

Periodic Tests

Ask your doctor which of these tests should be done periodically while you are taking this drug:

- bleeding time and platelet count
- complete blood count
- white blood cell differentials

Limited Use

Tocainide
TONOCARD (Astra Merck)

GENERIC: not available

FAMILY: Antiarrhythmics

Tocainide (toe *kay* nide) slows the heart rate and stabilizes irregular heartbeats (arrhythmias). Because it has severe adverse effects, your doctor should not prescribe tocainide unless you have already tried safer drugs in its family, such as quinidine (see p. 94), without success. **If you have impaired liver or kidney function, you should be taking less than the usual dose.**

Tocainide most commonly causes harmful effects in the digestive tract and central nervous system. These effects include nausea, vomiting, dizziness, tremor, confusion, and a "pins-and-needles" sensation on the skin.[406] Three of the most serious possible adverse effects are bone marrow depression, hepatitis (liver disease), and inflammation of the lungs.[407]

Many people who are taking tocainide or another drug in its family have relatively mild disturbances in their heart rhythm and no symptoms of underlying heart disease. The vast majority of these people *do not need these drugs,* and there is no evidence that using them improves health. In fact, most of the drugs in this family have severe adverse effects that are sometimes worse and even more life-threatening than the irregular heartbeats they treat. All of these drugs can also cause *new* irregularities in your heartbeat.

If you have an irregular heartbeat without any symptoms of underlying heart disease, you should not be exposed to the dangers of a drug that has no health benefit for your condition.[408] If you are taking tocainide or another drug in its family for an irregular heartbeat (arrhythmia), talk to your doctor and find out whether you also have symptoms of underlying heart disease. If not, discuss the possibility of stopping the drug.

Before You Use This Drug

Do not use if you have or have had:

- allergic reaction to lidocaine (see p. 346)
- complete heart block

Tell your doctor if you have or have had:

- allergies to drugs
- congestive heart failure
- kidney or liver disease

Tell your doctor about any other drugs you take, including aspirin, herbs, vitamins, and other nonprescription products.

When You Use This Drug

• Until you know how you react to this drug, do not drive or perform other activities requiring alertness. Tocainide may cause dizziness.

• You may feel dizzy when rising from a lying or sitting position. When getting out of bed, hang your legs over the side of the bed for a few minutes, then get up slowly. When getting up from a chair, get up slowly and stay beside the chair until you are sure that you are not dizzy. (See p. 16.)

• **Do not stop taking this drug suddenly. Your doctor must give you a schedule to lower your dose gradually, to prevent serious changes in heart function.**

• Wear a medical identification bracelet or carry a card stating that you take tocainide.

• If you plan to have any surgery, including dental, tell your doctor that you take this drug.

How to Use This Drug

• Take with food or milk to reduce stomach upset.

• If you miss a dose, take it as soon as you remember if it is within four hours otherwise skip it until your next scheduled dose. **Do not take double doses.**

• Do not store in the bathroom. Do not expose to heat, moisture, or strong light.

Interactions with Other Drugs

The following drugs are listed in the *Evaluations of Drug Interactions* 1997 as causing "highly clinically significant" or "clinically significant" interactions when used together with this drug. We have also included potentially serious interactions listed in the drug's FDA-approved professional product labeling or package insert. New scientific techniques have allowed researchers to predict some drug interactions before they have been documented in people. There may be other drugs, especially those in the families of drugs listed below, that also will react with this drug to cause severe adverse effects. The number of new drugs approved for marketing increases the chance of drug interactions, and new drug interactions are being identified with old drugs. Be vigilant. Make sure to tell your doctor and pharmacist the drugs you are taking and tell your doctor if you are taking any of these interacting drugs:

amiodarone, cimetidine, CORDARONE, cyclosporine, ELIXOPHYLLIN, INDERAL, INDERAL LA, grepafloxacin, NEORAL, propranolol, RAXAR, SANDIMMUNE, SLO-BID, sparfloxacin, TAGAMET, THEO-24, theophylline, ZAGAM.

Adverse Effects

Call your doctor immediately if you experience:

• trembling or shaking
• cough or shortness of breath
• fever, chills, or sore throat
• unusual bleeding or bruising
• irregular heartbeats
• blisters on skin
• peeling or scaling of skin
• severe skin rash
• sores in mouth

Call your doctor if these symptoms continue:

• dizziness or lightheadedness
• loss of appetite

WARNING! INCREASED RISK OF DEATH

In the National Heart, Lung, and Blood Institute's Cardiac Arrhythmia Suppression Trial (CAST) (a long-term, multi-centered, randomized, double-blind study) in patients with asymptomatic non-life-threatening ventricular (the large chambers of the heart) arrhythmias (rhythm disturbances) who had a heart attack more than six days, but less than two years previously, deaths or non-fatal cardiac arrest were seen in 7.7% of those patients treated with encainide or flecainide, members of the Class 1 group of antiarrhythmic drugs, compared to 3.0% in patients receiving an inactive sugar pill or placebo.

Because of the known ability of the Class 1 drugs such as tocainide to cause rhythm disturbances, and the lack of evidence of improved survival for any antiarrhythmic drug in patients without life-threatening heart rhythm disturbances, the use of the Class 1 drugs should be reserved for patients with life-threatening rhythm disturbances of the ventricles. These warnings now appear in the FDA-approved product labeling, or package insert, for all Class 1 drugs including: disopyramide (Norpace and generics), flecainide (Tambocor), mexiletine (Mexitil and generics), moricizine (Ethmozine), procainamide (Procanbid and generics), propafenone (Rythmol), quinidine (Duraquin, Quinaglute Dura-Tabs, Quinidex and generics), and tocainide (Tonocard).

- nausea or vomiting
- blurred vision
- confusion
- headache
- nervousness
- numbness or tingling of fingers or toes
- skin rash
- sweating

Periodic Tests

Ask your doctor which of these tests should be done periodically while you are taking this drug:

- complete blood count
- heart function tests, such as electrocardiogram (ECG, EKG)
- chest X-ray

PREGNANCY WARNING

This drug caused harm to developing fetuses in animal studies, or such studies were not done. Use during pregnancy only for clear medical reasons. Tell your doctor if you are pregnant or thinking of becoming pregnant before you take this drug.

 Do Not Use

ALTERNATIVE TREATMENT:
Mild exercise, no smoking, extreme cleanliness of legs and feet.

Pentoxifylline
TRENTAL (Hoechst Marion Roussel)

FAMILY: Blood Flow Improvers

Pentoxifylline (pen tox *if* i lin) is advertised as a drug to relieve leg cramps caused by poor blood circulation (intermittent claudication). The manufacturer claims that the drug improves the flow of blood through the blood vessels by making red blood cells more flexible. Studies have shown, however, that exercise is more effective than pentoxifylline in reducing these cramps.[409] There is no convincing evidence that pentoxifylline is very effective in improving blood circulation.

Pentoxifylline may also have serious dangers. **One medical center recently reported two cases in which pentoxifylline caused fatal damage to patients' bone marrow.**[410] Animal studies have shown that rats develop benign breast tumors when taking this drug.

According to the Hospital Pharmacy Therapeutics Committee at the University of California, San Francisco Medical Center, studies are inconclusive as to the benefit of this drug.[411]

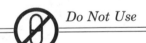

Do Not Use

ALTERNATIVE TREATMENT:
Mild exercise, no smoking, extreme cleanliness of legs and feet.

Isoxsuprine
VASODILAN (Geneva)

FAMILY: Vasodilators
(Blood Vessel Dilators)

Doctors prescribe isoxsuprine (eye *sox* syoo preen) to improve the blood circulation of people with certain types of blood vessel disease. The expectation is that better circulation will relieve pain (leg pain, for example) and improve mental function (by increasing blood flow to the brain). However, **isoxsuprine has not been proven effective for these problems.** It does not improve the flow of blood to

calf muscles in people with diseased blood vessels, nor does it help leg cramps caused by poor blood circulation (intermittent claudication).[412] In fact, although this drug has been available for use and evaluation for many years, **it has not been proven effective for treating any condition.**[413] The American Medical Association's guide to drug therapy does not even suggest a dose for isoxsuprine because "the role of this agent in the treatment of peripheral vascular disease [disease of the blood vessels in the arms or legs] has not been established."[414]

Isoxsuprine's adverse effects include headache, nausea, chills, flushing, tingling and burning sensations of the skin, heart flutter, and stomach and intestinal problems. **We recommend that you do not use isoxsuprine because it can cause harmful adverse effects and has not been proven to have any benefit.**

The National Academy of Sciences has found that isoxsuprine and a related drug called cyclandelate lack evidence of effectiveness.

WARNING

Isoxsuprine can cause or worsen high blood pressure. It is especially dangerous for people who have high blood pressure, heart disease, diabetes, or thyroid disease. People over 60 are more likely than younger people to experience effects on the heart and blood pressure, restlessness, nervousness, and confusion.

Do Not Use

ALTERNATIVE TREATMENT:
See Hydrochlorothiazide, p. 100.

Guanabenz
WYTENSIN (Wyeth-Ayerst)

FAMILY: Antihypertensives
(See High Blood Pressure, p. 44)

Guanabenz (*gwahn* a benz) is used to treat high blood pressure (hypertension). **It has severe adverse effects and should not be used.**

The main problem with guanabenz is that missing only *one* or *two* doses of the drug can have serious effects, including sweating, tremors, flushing, and severe high blood pressure. Guanabenz can also cause severe depression and is particularly dangerous for anyone with a history of depression.

If you have high blood pressure, the best way to reduce or eliminate your need for medication is by improving your diet, losing weight, exercising, and decreasing your salt and alcohol intake. Mild hypertension can be controlled by proper nutrition and exercise. If these measures do not lower your blood pressure enough and you need medication, **hydrochlorothiazide, a water pill (see thiazide diuretics, p. 100), is the drug of choice starting with a low dose of 12.5 milligrams daily.** It also costs less than other blood pressure drugs.

There is now good evidence that thiazide diuretics, such as hydrochlorothiazide, significantly decrease the rate of bone mineral loss in both men and women because they reduce the amount of calcium lost in the urine. An increasing number of researchers think that this will also decrease the number of fractures.[415]

If this does not lower your blood pressure enough, your doctor can prescribe a second type of drug called a beta-blocker (see p. 52) to accompany the hydrochlorothiazide. If you cannot take a beta-blocker, a drug from another family (calcium channel blockers) can be used instead.

Whatever drugs you take for high blood pressure, once your blood pressure has been normal for a year or more, a cautious decrease in dose and renewed attention to nondrug treatment may be worth trying, according to *The Medical Letter.*[416]

And an editorial in the *British Medical Journal* stated: *"Treatment of hypertension is part of preventive medicine and like all preventive strategies, its progress should be regularly reviewed by whoever initiates it. Many problems could be avoided by not starting antihypertensive treatment until after prolonged observation. . . . Patients should no longer be told that treatment is necessarily for life: the possibility of reducing or stopping treatment should be mentioned at the outset."*[417]

Do not suddenly stop using this drug. Ask your doctor for a schedule that lowers your dose gradually over at least ten days, and more slowly if you begin to have withdrawal symptoms. Another drug for high blood pressure should be started at the same time.[418]

Limited Use

Bisoprolol and Hydrochlorothiazide
ZIAC (Lederle)

Metoprolol and Hydrochlorothiazide
LOPRESSOR HCT (Novartis)

Nadolol and Bendroflumethiazide
CORZIDE (Mylan)

Propranolol (extended release) and Hydrochlorothiazide
INDERIDE LA (Wyeth-Ayerst)

Timolol and Hydrochlorothiazide
TIMOLIDE (Merck)

GENERIC: not available
FAMILY: Antihypertensives (combinations)
(See High Blood Pressure, p. 44)

WARNING

A fixed-combination drug should not be the first drug used to treat your high blood pressure. You may not need more than one drug. If you do need two drugs, the fixed-combination product may not contain the dose of each drug that is right for you. Your doctor has to regularly check your condition and reevaluate the effect of the drug(s) you take. This may mean adjusting doses, and even changing drugs, to ensure proper treatment. This fixed-combination drug may be the best drug for you, but it should be used only after you have tried each of its ingredients separately, in varying doses. If the doses that you need to control your high blood pressure match those in this fixed-combination product, use it if the combination drug is more convenient.

If you have high blood pressure, the best way to reduce or eliminate your need for medication is by improving your diet, losing weight, exercising, and decreasing your salt and alcohol intake. Mild hypertension can be controlled by proper nutrition and exercise. If these measures do not lower your blood pressure enough and you need medication, **hydrochlorothiazide, a water pill (see thiazide diuretics, p. 100), is the drug of choice starting with a low dose of 12.5 milligrams daily.** It also costs less than other blood pressure drugs.

There is now good evidence that thiazide diuretics, such as hydrochlorothiazide, significantly decrease the rate of bone mineral loss in both men and women because they reduce the amount of calcium lost in the urine. An increasing number of researchers think that this will also decrease the number of fractures.[419]

If your high blood pressure is more severe, and hydrochlorothiazide alone does not control it, the best treatment is a combination of hydrochlorothiazide and a second type of drug called a beta-blocker, such as propranolol (see p. 154). If you can't take a drug in the beta-blocker family, another drug called a calcium channel blocker may be used instead. In either case, your doctor would prescribe the hydrochlorothiazide and the second drug separately, with the dose of each drug adjusted to meet your needs, rather than using a product that combines the drug in a fixed combination.

If you are taking one of these fixed-combination drugs, ask your doctor about changing your prescription.

Whatever drugs you take for high blood pressure, once your blood pressure has been normal for a year or more, a cautious decrease in dose and renewed attention to nondrug treatment may be worth trying, according to *The Medical Letter.*[420]

And an editorial in the *British Medical Journal* stated: *"Treatment of hypertension is part of preventive medicine and like all preventive strategies, its progress should be regularly reviewed by whoever initiates it. Many problems could be avoided by not starting antihypertensive treatment until after prolonged observation. . . . Patients should no longer be told that treatment is necessarily for life: the possibility of reducing or stopping treatment should be mentioned at the outset.*[421]

PREGNANCY WARNING

Lopressor HCT, Corzide, Inderide LA, and Timolide caused harm to developing fetuses in animal studies, or such studies were not done. Use during pregnancy only for clear medical reasons. Tell your doctor if you are pregnant or thinking of becoming pregnant before you take any of these drugs.

NOTES FOR DRUGS FOR HEART CONDITIONS

1. *Statistical Abstract of the United States* 1997. U.S. Department of Commerce, Economics and Statistics Administration, Bureau of the Census, Table 218, p. 143.

2. Stamler R, Stamler J, Grimm R, Gosch FC, Elmer P, Dyer A, et al. Nutritional therapy for high blood pressure. *Journal of the American Medical Association* 1987; 257:1484–91.

3. 1984 Joint National Committee on Detection, Evaluation, and Treatment of High Blood Pressure. Nonpharmacological approaches to the control of high blood pressure: final report of the Subcommittee on Nonpharmacological Therapy. *Hypertension* 1986; 8:454–5.

4. Schlamowitz P, Halberg T, Warnoe O, Wilstrup F, Ryttig K. Treatment of mild to moderate hypertension with dietary fibre. *Lancet* 1987; 8559:622–3.

5. Eichner E. Nonpharmacological therapy of hypertension. *Internal Medicine* 1987; 8:155–61.

6. Whelton PK, Appel LJ, Espeland MA, Applegate WB, Ettinger WH, Kostis JB, et al. Sodium reduction and weight loss in the treatment of hypertension in older persons. *Journal of the American Medical Association* 1998; 279:839–46.

7. Stamler J. Setting the TONE for ending the hypertension epidemic. *Journal of the American Medical Association* 1998; 279:878–9.

8. National High Blood Pressure Education Program. The Sixth Report of the Joint National Committee on Prevention, Detection, Evaluation, and Treatment of High Blood Pressure. *Archives of Internal Medicine* 1997; 157:2413–46.

9. Squires S. Medical pressure cooker: doctors debate what to do about hypertension, *Washington Post* Health Section, February 10, 1987.

10. Hansen AG, Jensen H, Langesen LP, Peterson A. Withdrawal of antihypertensive drugs in the elderly. *Acta Medica Scandivica* 1982; 676:178–85.

11. Cohobanian A. Antihypertensive therapy in evolution. *New England Journal of Medicine* 1986; 314:1701–2.

12. Rowe J. Systolic hypertension in the elderly. *New England Journal of Medicine* 1983; 309:1246–7.

13. Vestal RE, ed. *Drug Treatment in the Elderly*. Sydney, Australia: ADIS Health Science Press, 1984:77–88.

14. Burton R. Withdrawing antihypertensive treatment: hypertension may settle with time. *British Medical Journal* 1991; 303:324–5.

15. Ibid.

16. *The Medical Letter on Drugs and Therapeutics.* New York: The Medical Letter Inc., 1991; 33:33–8.

17. *The Medical Letter on Drugs and Therapeutics.* New York: The Medical Letter Inc., 1981; 23:3.

18. *The Medical Letter on Drugs and Therapeutics.* New York: The Medical Letter Inc., 1978; 20:30.

19. Ibid.

20. Harrington JT, Isner JM, Kassirer JP. Our national obsession with potassium. *American Journal of Medicine* 1982; 73:155–9.

21. *The Medical Letter on Drugs and Therapeutics,* 1981, op. cit., p. 71.

22. Ibid, p. 3.

23. Ibid, p. 71.

24. Ibid, p. 3.

25. Ibid.

26. Kastrup EK, ed. *Facts and Comparisons.* St. Louis: J.B. Lippincott Co., July 1987:15a.

27. AMA Department of Drugs. *AMA Drug Evaluations.* 5th ed. Chicago: American Medical Association, 1983:1111.

28. *The Medical Letter on Drugs and Therapeutics,* 1981, op. cit., p. 3.

29. *Drug and Therapeutics Bulletin* 1992; 29:87–91.

30. Conversation with Dr. Andrew Herxheimer, Charing Cross Hospital, Editor, *Drug and Therapeutics Bulletin,* October 21, 1986.

31. Siegel D, Lopez J. Trends in antihypertensive drug use in the United States. *Journal of the American Medical Association* 1997; 278:1745–8.

32. Psaty BM, Heckbert SR, Koepsell TD, Siscovick DS, Raghunathan TE, Weiss NS, et al. The risk of myocardial infarction associated with antihypertensive drug therapies. *Journal of the American Medical Association* 1995; 274:620–5.

33. Pahor M, Guralnik JM, Corti M-C, Foley DJ, Carbonin P, Havlik RJ. Long-term survival and use of antihypertensive medications in older persons. *Journal of the American Geriatrics Society* 1995; 43:1191–7.

34. Furberg CD, Psaty BM, Meyer JV. Nifedipine dose-related increase in mortality in patients with coronary heart disease. *Circulation* 1995; 92:1326–31.

35. Pahor M, Guralnik JM, Furberg CD, Carbonin P, Havlik RJ. Risk of gastrointestinal haemorrhage with calcium antagonists in hypertensive persons over 67 years old. *Lancet* 1996; 347:1061–5.

36. Pahor M, Guralnik JM, Ferrucci L, Corti M-C, Salive ME, Cerhan JR, et al. Calcium-channel blockade and incidence of cancer in aged populations. *Lancet* 1996; 348: 493–7.

37. Hardell L, Fredrikson M, Axelson O. Case-control study on colon cancer regarding previous diseases and drug intake. *International Journal of Oncology* 1996; 8:439–44.

38. Pahor M, Guralnik JM, Salive ME, Corti M-C, Carbonin P, Havlik RJ. Do calcium channel blockers increase the risk of cancer? *American Journal of Hypertension* 1996; 9:695–9.

39. Fitzpatrick AL, Daling JR, Furberg CD, Kronmal RA, Weissfeld JL. Use of calcium channel blockers and breast carcinoma risk in postmenopausal women. *Cancer* 1997; 80:1438–47.

40. Rosenberg L, Rao RS, Palmer JR, Strom BL, Stolley PD, Zauber AG, et al. Calcium channel blockers and the risk of cancer. *Journal of the American Medical Association* 1998; 279:1000–4.

41. Kaiser FE, Morley JE. Cholesterol can be lowered in older persons: should we care? *Journal of the American Geriatric Society* 1990; 38:84–5.

42. American College of Physicians. Geriatrics: nutritional issues. Medical Knowledge Self-Assessment Program IX, 1991.

43. Hebert PR, Gaziano JM, Chan KS, Hennekens CH. Cholesterol lowering with statin drugs, risk of stroke, and total mortality. *Journal of the American Medical Association* 1997; 278:313–21.

44. Shepherd J, Cobbe SM, Ford I, Isles CG, Lorimer AR, Macfarlane PW, et al. Prevention of coronary heart disease with pravastatin in men with hypercholesterolemia. *New England Journal of Medicine* 1995; 333:1301–7.

45. Levin WEG, Miller VT, Muesing RA, Stoy DB, Balm TK, LaRosa JC. Comparison of psyllium hydrophilic mucilloid and cellulose as adjuncts to a prudent diet in the treatment of mild to moderate hypercholesterolemia. *Archives of Internal Medicine* 1990; 150:1822–7.

46. Newman TB, Hulley SB. Carcinogenicity of lipid-lowering drugs. *Journal of the American Medical Association* 1996; 275: 55–60.

47. National Heart, Lung, and Blood Institute, Public Health Service, U.S. Department of Health and Human Services. New analyses regarding the safety of calcium channel blockers: a statement for health professionals. August 31, 1995.

48. Messerli FH, Kowey P, Grodzicki T. Sublingual nifedipine for hypertensive emergencies. *Lancet* 1991; 338:881[letter].

49. Grossman E, Messerli FH, Grodzicki T, Kowey P. Should a moratorium be placed on sublingual nifedipine capsules given for hypertensive emergencies and pseudoemergencies? *Journal of the American Medical Association* 1996; 276:1328–31.

50. Wasnich R, Davis J, Ross P, Vogel J. Effect of thiazide on rates of bone mineral loss: a longitudinal study. *British Medical Journal* 1991; 301:1303–5.

51. *The Medical Letter on Drugs and Therapeutics,* 1991, op. cit.

52. Burton, op. cit.

53. Greenblatt DJ, Koch-Weser J. Adverse reactions to spironolactone. *Journal of the American Medical Association* 1973; 225:40–3.

54. Neal TJ, Lynn KL, Bailey RR. Spironolactone-associated aggravation of renal function impairment. *New Zealand Medical Journal* 1976; 83:147–9.

55. Greenblatt, op. cit.

56. Pongpaew C, Songkhla RN, Kozam RL. Hyperkalemic cardiac arrythmia secondary to spironolactone. *Chest* 1973; 63:1023–5.

57. Yap V, Patel A, Thomsen J. Hyperkalemia with cardiac arrythmia: induction by salt substitutes, spironolactone and azotemia. *Journal of the American Medical Association* 1976; 236:2775–6.

58. Davies DM, ed. *Textbook of Adverse Drug Reactions.* Oxford: Oxford University Press, 1977:237.

59. Udezue EO, Harrold BP. Hyperkalaemic paralysis due to spironolactone. *Postgraduate Medical Journal* 1980; 56:254–5.

60. *Physicians' Desk Reference.* 41st ed. Oradell, N.J.: Medical Economics Company, 1987:1540–1.

61. *Physicians' Desk Reference.* 40th ed. Oradell, N.J.: Medical Economics Company, 1986:1675.

62. Wasnich, op. cit.

63. *The Medical Letter on Drugs and Therapeutics,* 1991, op. cit..

64. Burton, op. cit.

65. Greenblatt, op. cit.

66. Neal, op. cit.

67. Greenblatt, op. cit.

68. Pongpaew, op. cit.

69. Yap, op. cit.

70. Davies, op. cit.

71. Udezue, op. cit.

72. Greenblatt, op. cit.

73. *Physicians' Desk Reference,* 1987, op. cit.

74. *Physicians' Desk Reference,* 1986, op. cit., p. 1677.

75. Ibid, p. 1675.

76. Papademetriou V, Burris J, Kukich S, Freis ED. Effectiveness of potassium chloride or triamterene in thiazide hypokalemia. *Archives of Internal Medicine* 1985; 145:1986–90.

77. Wasnich, op. cit.

78. *The Medical Letter on Drugs and Therapeutics,* 1991, op. cit.

79. Burton, op. cit.

80. Wasnich, op. cit.

81. *The Medical Letter on Drugs and Therapeutics,* 1991, op. cit.

82. Burton, op. cit.

83. Wasnich, op. cit.

84. *The Medical Letter on Drugs and Therapeutics,* 1991, op. cit.

85. Burton, op. cit.

86. Orland MJ, Saltman RJ eds. *Manual of Medical Therapeutics.* 25th ed. Boston: Little Brown and Company, 1986:57–69.

87. Ibid, p. 89–104.

88. Ibid.

89. Wasnich, op. cit.

90. *The Medical Letter on Drugs and Therapeutics,* 1991, op. cit.

91. Burton, op. cit.

92. Orland, op. cit.

93. Wasnich, op. cit.

94. *The Medical Letter on Drugs and Therapeutics,* 1991, op. cit.

95. Burton, op. cit.

96. *The Medical Letter on Drugs and Therapeutics.* New York: The Medical Letter Inc., 1984; 26:116.

97. Vestal, op. cit.

98. Orland, op. cit., p. 89–104.

99. Vestal, op. cit.

100. Wasnich, op. cit.

101. *The Medical Letter on Drugs and Therapeutics,* 1991, op. cit.

102. Burton, op. cit.

103. Lynn KL, Bailey RR, Swainson CP, Sainsbury R, Low WI. Renal failure with potassium-sparing diuretics. *New Zealand Medical Journal* 1985; 98:629–33.

104. *The Medical Letter on Drugs and Therapeutics.* New York: The Medical Letter, Inc., 1983; 25:62.

105. Vestal, op. cit.

106. Wasnich, op. cit.

107. Conversation with Dr. Andrew Herxheimer, op. cit.

108. *USP DI, Drug Information for the Health Care Provider.* 6th ed. Rockville MD: The United States Pharmacopeial Convention, Inc., 1986:704.

109. *Drug Intelligence and Clinical Pharmacy* July/August 1983; 17:539.

110. *The Medical Letter on Drugs and Therapeutics,* 1991, op. cit.

111. Burton, op. cit.

112. Psaty, op. cit.

113. Pahor, 1995, op. cit.

114. Furberg, op. cit.

115. Pahor, *Lancet,* 1996; 347, op. cit.

116. Pahor, *Lancet,* 1996; 348, op. cit.

117. Hardell, op. cit.

118. Pahor, *American Journal of Hypertension,* op. cit.

119. Fitzpatrick, op. cit.

120. Rosenberg, op. cit.

121. Siegel, op. cit.

122. Laverenne J. Effets indesirables des inhibiteurs calciques. *Therapie* 1989; 44:197.

123. AMA Department of Drugs. *AMA Drug Evaluations Annual 1992.* Chicago: American Medical Association, 1992:541.

124. Pritza DR, Bierman MH, Hammeke MD. Acute toxic effects of sustained-release verapamil in chronic renal failure. *Archives of Internal Medicine* 1991; 151:2081–4.

125. Wasnich, op. cit.

126. *The Medical Letter on Drugs and Therapeutics,* 1991, op. cit.

127. Burton, op. cit.

128. Aronow WS. Prevalence of use of beta-blockers and of calcium channel blockers in older patients with prior myocardial infarction at the time of admission to a nursing home. *Journal of the American Geriatrics Society* 1996; 44:1075–7.

129. Kuhn M, Schriger DL. Verapamil administration to patients with contraindications: is it associated with adverse outcomes? *Annals of Emergency Medicine* 1991; 20:1094–9.

130. Gheorghiade M. Calcium channel blockers in the management of myocardial infarction patients. *Henry Ford Hospital Medical Journal* 1991; 39:210–6.

131. Ferrier C, Ferrari P, Weidmann P, Keller U, Beretta-Piccoli C, Riesen WF. Antihypertensive therapy with Ca2+. *Diabetes Care* 1991; 14:911–4.

132. Swash M, Ingram DA. Adverse effect of verapamil in myasthenia gravis. *Muscle & Nerve* 1992; 15:396–8.

133. *USP DI, Drug Information for the Health Care Professional.* 12th ed. Rockville MD: The United States Pharmacopeial Convention, Inc., 1992:779–90.

134. Psaty, op. cit.

135. Pahor, 1995, op. cit.

136. Furberg, op. cit.

137. Pahor, *Lancet,* 1996; 347, op. cit.

138. Pahor, *Lancet,* 1996; 348, op. cit.

139. Hardell, op. cit.

140. Pahor, *American Journal of Hypertension,* op. cit.

141. Fitzpatrick, op. cit.

142. Rosenberg, op. cit.

143. Siegel, op. cit.

144. Laverenne, op. cit.

145. Wasnich, op. cit.

146. *The Medical Letter on Drugs and Therapeutics,* 1991, op. cit.

147. Burton, op. cit.

148. Aronow, op. cit.

149. *USP DI,* 1992, op. cit.

150. Wasnich, op. cit.

151. *The Medical Letter on Drugs and Therapeutics,* 1991, op. cit.

152. Burton, op. cit.

153. *The Medical Letter on Drugs and Therapeutics.* New York: The Medical Letter, Inc., 1976, 18:38–9.

154. AMA, 1983, op. cit., p. 678–9.

155. Gilman AG, Goodman LS, Rall TW, Murad F, eds. *The Pharmacological Basis of Therapeutics.* 7th ed. New York: Macmillan, 1985: 823.

156. AMA, 1983, op. cit., p. 678–9.

157. Ronnov-Jessen V, Tjernlund A. Hepatotoxicity due to treatment with papaverine. *New England Journal of Medicine* 1969; 281:1333–5. Zimmerman HJ. Papaverine revisited as a hepatotoxin. Same ref :1364–5.

158. Vestal, op. cit., p. 40.

159. Wasnich, op. cit.

160. *The Medical Letter on Drugs and Therapeutics,* 1991, op. cit.

161. Burton, op. cit.

162. Middlekauff HR, Stevenson WG, Saxon LA, Stevenson LW. Amiodarone and torsades de pointes in patients with advanced heart failure. *American Journal of Cardiology* 1995; 76:499–502.

163. Shukla R, Jowett NI, Thompson DR, Pohl JEF. Side effects with amiodarone therapy. *Postgraduate Medicine Journal* 1994; 70:492–8.

164. Makkar RR, Fromm BS, Steinman, RT, Meissner MD, Lehmann MH. Female gender as a risk factor for torsades de pointes associated with cardiovascular drugs. *Journal of the American Medical Association* 1993; 270:2590–7.

165. *USP DI, Drug Information for the Health Care Professional.* 16th ed. Rockville, MD: The United States Pharmacopeial Convention, Inc., 1996:83–7.

166. Tisdale JE, Follin SL, Ordelova A, Webb CR. Risk factors for the development of specific noncardiovascular adverse effects associated with amiodarone. *Journal of Clinical Pharmacology* 1995; 35:351–6.

167. *USP DI,* 1996, op. cit.

168. Singh SN, Fletcher RD, Fisher SG, Singh BN, Lewis HD, Deedwania PC, et al. Amiodarone in patients with congestive heart failure and asymptomatic ventricular arrhythmia. *New England Journal of Medicine* 1995; 333: 77–82.

169. Moyé LA, Abernethy D. Carvedilol in patients with chronic heart failure. *New England Journal of Medicine* 1996; 335:1318 [letter].

170. Pfeffer MA, Stevenson LW. b-adrenergic blockers and survival in heart failure. *New England Journal of Medicine* 1996; 334:1396–7[editorial].

171. Dunn CJ, Lea AP, Wagstaff AJ. Carvediolol: A reappraisal of its pharmacological properties and therapeutic use in cardiovascular disorders. *Drugs* 1997; 54:161–85.

172. McTavish D, Campoli-Richards D, Sorkin EM. Carvedilol: A review of its pharmacodynamic and pharmokinetic properties, and therapeutic efficacy. *Drugs* 1993; 45:232–58.

173. Dunn, op. cit.

174. Wasnich, op. cit.

175. *The Medical Letter on Drugs and Therapeutics,* 1991, op. cit.

176. Burton, op. cit.

177. Kastrup EK, ed. *Facts and Comparisons.* St. Louis: J.B. Lippincott Co., December 1995:159m.

178. Hylek EM, Heiman H, Skates SJ, Sheehan MA, Singer DE. Acetaminophen and other risk factors for excessive warfarin anticoagulation. *Journal of the American Medical Association* 1998; 279:657–62.

179. Wasnich, op. cit.

180. *The Medical Letter on Drugs and Therapeutics,* 1991, op. cit.

181. Burton, op. cit.

182. *The Medical Letter on Drugs and Therapeutics,* 1976, op. cit.

183. Gilman, op. cit.

184. AMA, 1983, op. cit., p. 678–9.

185. Wasnich, op. cit.

186. *The Medical Letter on Drugs and Therapeutics,* 1991, op. cit.

187. Burton, op. cit.

188. Nygaard TW, Sellers TD, Cook TS, Marco JP. Adverse reactions to antiarrythmic drugs during therapy for ventricular arrythmias. *Journal of the American Medical Association* 1986; 256:57.

189. Lynn, op. cit.

190. Davies, op. cit.

191. Wasnich, op. cit.

192. *The Medical Letter on Drugs and Therapeutics,* 1991, op. cit.

193. Burton, op. cit.

194. Lynn, op. cit.

195. Davies, op. cit.

196. Wasnich, op. cit.

197. Papademetriou, op. cit.

198. *The Medical Letter on Drugs and Therapeutics,* 1991, op. cit.

199. Burton, op. cit.

200. *Physicians' Desk Reference,* 1987, op. cit., p. 516.

201. Wasnich, op. cit.

202. *The Medical Letter on Drugs and Therapeutics,* 1991, op. cit.

203. Burton, op. cit.

204. *Physicians' Desk Reference,* 1986, op. cit., p. 1353.

205. *USP DI,* 1986, op. cit.

206. Morgan T, Adam W, Hodgson M. Adverse reactions to long-term diuretic therapy for hypertension. *Journal of Cardiovascular Pharmacology* 1984; 6:S269.

207. Wasnich, op. cit.

208. *The Medical Letter on Drugs and Therapeutics,* 1984, op. cit., p. 107.

209. *The Medical Letter on Drugs and Therapeutics,* 1991, op. cit.

210. Burton, op. cit.

211. Gilman, op. cit., p. 209.

212. Wasnich, op. cit.

213. *The Medical Letter on Drugs and Therapeutics,* 1991, op. cit.

214. Burton, op. cit.

215. Vestal, op. cit., p. 40

216. Wasnich, op. cit.

217. *The Medical Letter on Drugs and Therapeutics,* 1991, op. cit.

218. Burton, op. cit.

219. Cohen JD. Long-term efficacy and safety of terazosin alone and in combination with other antihypertensive agents. *American Heart Journal* 1991; 122:919–25.

220. *The Medical Letter on Drugs and Therapeutics,* 1991, op. cit., p. 15–6.

221. Gilman, AG, Rall TW, Nies AS, Taylor, P, eds. *The Pharmacological Basis of Therapeutics.* 8th ed. New York: Pergamon Press 1990: 226–7.

222. *USP DI,* 1992, op. cit., p. 2591–3

223. Titmarsh S, Monk JP. Terazosin: a review of its pharmacodynamic and pharmacokinetic properties, and therapeutic efficacy in essential hypertension. *Drugs* 1987; 33:461–77.

224. Wasnich, op. cit.

225. *The Medical Letter on Drugs and Therapeutics,* 1991, op. cit., p. 33–8.

226. Burton, op. cit.

227. Gilman, 1990, op. cit.

228. *The Medical Letter on Drugs and Therapeutics.* New York: The Medical Letter Inc, 1994; 36:111–4.

229. Harrington, op. cit.

230. Vestal, op. cit., p. 66.

231. *The Medical Letter on Drugs and Therapeutics.* New York: The Medical Letter Inc., 1979, 21:44.

232. Carlson KJ. An analysis of physicians' reasons for prescribing long-term digitalis therapy in outpatients. *Journal of Chronic Diseases* 1985; 389: 733–9.

233. Lee DC. Heart failure in outpatients: A randomized trial of digoxin versus placebo. *New England Journal of Medicine* 1982; 306:699–705.

234. AMA, 1983, op. cit., p. 606.

235. Fleg J, Lakatta E. How useful is digitalis in patients with congestive heart failure and sinus rhythm? *International Journal of Cardiology* 1984; 6:295–305.

236. Vestal, op. cit., p. 77–8.

237. *Drugs for the Elderly* 2nd edition. Copenhagen, Denmark: World Health Organization, 1997.

238. *USP DI,* 1986, op. cit.

239. *Drug Intelligence and Clinical Pharmacy,* op. cit.

240. Wasnich, op. cit.

241. Seligmann H, Halkin H, Rauchfleisch S, Kaufmann N, Motro M, Vered Z, et al. Thiamine deficiency in patients with congestive heart failure receiving long-term furosemide therapy: a pilot study. *American Journal of Medicine* 1991; 91:151–5.

242. Shimon I, Almog S, Vered Z, Seligmann H, Shefi M, Peleg E, et al. Improved left ventricular function after thiamine supplementation in patients with congestive heart failure receiving long-term furosemide therapy. *American Journal of Medicine* 1995; 98:485–90.

243. *The Medical Letter on Drugs and Therapeutics,* 1991, op. cit., p. 33–8.

244. Burton, op. cit.

245. Jay RH, Rampling MW, Betteridge DJ. Abnormalities of blood rheology in familial hypercholesterolaemia: effects of treatment. *Atherosclerosis* 1990; 85:249–56.

246. *USP DI,* 1992, op. cit., p. 921–3.

247. American College of Physicians, op. cit.

248. *The Medical Letter on Drugs and Therapeutics,* 1991, op. cit., p. 1–4.

249. Orland MJ, Saltmar RF, eds. *Manual of Medical Therapeutics.* 26th ed. St. Louis: Washington University 1989:421.

250. *The Medical Letter on Drugs and Therapeutics,* 1991, op. cit., p. 1–4.

251. *USP DI,* 1992, op. cit., p. 921–3.

252. American Society of Hospital Pharmacists, American Hospital Formulary Service Drug Information. Bethesda, MD, 1992:939–42.

253. Curtis DM, Driscoll DJ, Goldman DH, Weidman WH. Loss of dental enamel in a patient taking cholestyramine. *Mayo Clinic Proceedings* 1991; 66:1131.

254. Ibid.

255. *USP DI,* 1992, op. cit., p. 921–3.

256. Statement by Ross Pierce, M.D., FDA Supervisory Medical Officer to NIH Consensus Development Conference Panel on Triglycerides, High Density Lipoprotein and Coronary Heart Disease, February, 25, 1992.

257. Pierce LR, Wysowski DK, Gross TP. Myopathy and rhabdomyolysis associated with lovastatin-gemfibrozil combination therapy. *Journal of the American Medical Association* 1990; 264:71–5.

258. American College of Physicians, op. cit.

259. Ibid.

260. Pfeffer MA, Braunwald E, Moyé LA, Basta L, Brown EJ, Cuddy TE, et al., for the SAVE Investigators. Effect of captopril on mortality and morbidity in patients with left ventricular dysfunction after myocardial infarction: results of the Survival and Ventricular Enlargement Trial. *New England Journal of Medicine* 1992; 327:669–77.

261. Lewis EJ, Hunsicker LG, Bain RP, Rohde RD, for the Collaborative Study Group. The effect of angiotensin-converting-enzyme inhibition on diabetic nephropathy. *New England Journal of Medicine* 1993; 329:1456–62.

262. Maschio G, Alberti D, Janin G, Locatelli F, Mann JFE, Motolese M, et al., for the Angiotensin-Converting-Enzyme Inhibition in Progressive Renal Insufficiency Study Group. Effect of the angiotensin-converting-enzyme inhibitor benazepril on the progression of chronic renal insufficiency. *New England Journal of Medicine* 1996; 334:939–45.

263. Giatras I, Lau J, Levey AS, for the Angiotensin-Converting Enzyme Inhibition and Progressive Renal Disease Study Group. Effect of angiotensin-converting enzyme inhibitors on the progression of nondiabetic renal disease: a meta-analysis of randomized trials. *Annals of Internal Medicine* 1997; 127:337–45.

264. Lewis, op. cit.

265. Ravid M, Lang R, Rachmani R, Lishner M. Long-term renoprotective effect of angiotensin-converting enzyme inhibition in non-insulin-dependent diabetes mellitus: a 7-year follow-up study. *Archives of Internal Medicine* 1996; 156:286–9.

266. Kasiske BL, Kalil RSN, Ma JZ, Liao M, Keane WF. Effect of antihypertensive therapy on the kidney in patients with diabetes: a meta-regression analysis. *Annals of Internal Medicine* 1993; 118:129–38.

267. Gannon TH, Eby TL. Angioedema from angiotensin converting enzyme inhibitors: a cause of upper airway obstruction. *Laryngoscope* 1990; 100:1156–60.

268. Roberts JR, Wuerz RC. Clinical characteristics of angiotensin-converting enzyme inhibitor-induced angioedema. *Annals of Emergency Medicine* 1991; 20:555–8 [abstract].

269. Ibid.

270. Wasnich, op. cit.

271. *The Medical Letter on Drugs and Therapeutics* 1991, op. cit., p. 33–8.

272. Burton, op. cit.

273. American Society of Hospital Pharmacists, op. cit., 866–74.

274. Roberts, op. cit.

275. Sterner G. Renal artery stenosis and ACE inhibitor (letter). *Journal of Internal Medicine* 1990; 228:541.

276. American Society of Hospital Pharmacists, op. cit.

277. Stoltz ML, Andrews CE. Severe hyperkalemia during very low-calorie diets and angiotensin converting enzyme use. *Journal of the American Medical Association* 1990; 264:2737–8 [letter].

278. *The Medical Letter on Drugs and Therapeutics*, 1991, op. cit., p. 33–8.

279. Wasnich, op. cit.

280. *The Medical Letter on Drugs and Therapeutics*, 1991, op. cit., p. 33–8.

281. Burton, op. cit.

282. Wasnich, op. cit.

283. *The Medical Letter on Drugs and Therapeutics*, 1991, op. cit., p. 33–8.

284. Burton, op. cit.

285. *The Medical Letter on Drugs and Therapeutics.* New York: The Medical Letter Inc., 1998; 40:13–4.

286. Illingworth DR. Clinical implications of new drugs for lowering plasma cholesterol concentrations. *Drugs* 1991; 41:151–60.

287. *The Medical Letter on Drugs and Therapeutics.* New York, The Medical Letter, Inc. 1992; 34:57–8.

288. Illingworth, op. cit.

289. McTavish D, Sorkin EM. Pravastatin: a review of its pharmacological properties and therapeutic potential in hypercholesterolaemia. *Drugs* 1991; 42:65–89.

290. *The Medical Letter on Drugs and Therapeutics*, 1991, op. cit., p. 18–20.

291. McTavish, 1991, op. cit.

292. American College of Physicians, op. cit.

293. *The Medical Letter on Drugs and Therapeutics*, 1991, op. cit., p. 18–20.

294. Frank MJ, Watkins LO, Prisant LM, Smith MS, Russell SL, Abdulla AM, et al. Mexiletine versus quinidine as first-line antiarrhythmia therapy: results from consecutive trials. *Journal of Clinical Pharmacology* 1991; 31:222–8.

295. Dukes MNG, Beeley L. *Side Effects of Drugs Annual* 15, Amsterdam: Elsevier, 1991:178–80.

296. Podrid PJ, Kowey PR, Frishman WH, Arnold RJG, Kaniecki DJ, Beck JR, et al. Comparative cost-effectiveness analysis of quinidine, procainamide and mexiletine. *The American Journal of Cardiology* 1991; 68:1662–7.

297. Frank, op. cit.

298. Dukes, op. cit.

299. Widerhorn J, Sager PT, Rahimtoola SH, Bhandari AK. The role of combination therapy with mexiletine and procainamide in patients with inducible sustained ventricular tachycardia refractory to intravenous procainamide. *PACE* 1991; 14:420 [abstract].

300. Gottlieb SS, Weinberg M. Comparative hemodynamic effects of mexiletine and quinidine in patients with severe left ventricular dysfunction. *American Heart Journal* 1991; 122:1368 [abstract].

301. Dukes, op. cit.

302. Olin BR, ed. *Facts and Comparisons.* St. Louis: J.B. Lippincott Co., September 1992: 610–3.

303. Hurwitz A, Vacek JL, Botteron GW, Sztern MI, Hughes EM, Jayaraj A. Mexiletine effects on theophylline disposition. *Clinical Pharmacology and Therapeutics* 1991; 50:299–307.

304. Stoysich AM, Mohiuddin SM, Destache CJ, Nipper HC, Hilleman DE. Influence of mexiletine on the pharmacokinetics of theophylline in healthy volunteers. *Journal of Clinical Pharmacology* 1991; 31:354–7.

305. Ueno K, Miyai K, Kato M, Kawaguchi Y, Suzuki T. Mechanism of interaction between theophylline and mexiletine. *DICP, The Annals of Pharmacotherapy* 1991; 25:727–30.

306. *The Medical Letter on Drugs and Therapeutics*, 1984, op. cit., p. 116.

307. Orland, op. cit., p. 89–104.

308. *The Medical Letter on Drugs and Therapeutics*, 1984, op. cit., p. 116.

309. Kastrup, op. cit., p.160–70.

310. *The Medical Letter on Drugs and Therapeutics.* New York: The Medical Letter, Inc., 1977; 19:1.

311. Gilman, 1985, op. cit., p. 793.

312. Orland, op. cit., p. 57–69.

313. Kastrup, op. cit., p. 160–170.

314. *Drugs for the Elderly*, op. cit.

315. Wasnich, op. cit.

316. *The Medical Letter on Drugs and Therapeutics*, 1991, op. cit., p. 33–8.

317. Burton, op. cit.

318. *Drugs for the Elderly.* Copenhagen, Denmark: World Health Organization, 1985.

319. Wasnich, op. cit.

320. *The Medical Letter on Drugs and Therapeutics*, 1991, op. cit., p. 33–8.

321. Burton, op. cit.

322. Vestal, op. cit., p. 77–88.

323. Ibid.

324. Nygaard, op. cit.

325. Psaty, op. cit.

326. Pahor, 1995, op. cit.

327. Furberg, op. cit.

328. Pahor, *Lancet*, 1996; 347, op. cit.

329. Pahor, *Lancet*, 1996; 348, op. cit.

330. Hardell, op. cit.

331. Pahor, *American Journal of Hypertension*, op. cit.

332. Fitzpatrick, op. cit.

333. Rosenberg op. cit.

334. Siegel, op. cit.

335. Laverenne, op. cit.

336. AMA, 1992, op. cit., p. 511.

337. Wasnich, op. cit.

338. *The Medical Letter on Drugs and Therapeutics*, 1991, op. cit., p. 33–8.

339. Burton, op. cit.

340. *USP DI*, 1992, op. cit., p. 779–90.

341. Webster J, Petrie JC, Jeffers TA, Roy-Chaudhury P, Crichton W, Witte K, et al. Nicardipine sustained release in hypertension. *British Journal of Clinical Pharmacology* 1991; 32:433–9.

342. Ibid.

343. Dukes MNG, Beeley L. *Side Effects of Drugs Annual* 13, Amsterdam: Elsevier, 1989:158.

344. Dukes MNG, Beeley L. *Side Effects of Drugs Annual* 14, Amsterdam: Elsevier, 1990:165

345. Wasnich, op. cit.

346. *The Medical Letter on Drugs and Therapeutics*, 1991, op. cit., p. 33–8.

347. Burton, op. cit.

348. Psaty, op. cit.

349. Pahor, 1995, op. cit.

350. Furberg, op. cit.

351. Pahor, *Lancet,* 1996; 347, op. cit.

352. Pahor, *Lancet,* 1996; 348, op. cit.

353. Hardell, op cit.

354. Pahor, *American Journal of Hypertension,* op. cit.

355. Fitzpatrick, op cit.

356. Rosenberg, op. cit.

357. Siegel, op. cit.

358. AMA, 1983, op. cit., p. 637.

359. Vestal, op. cit., p. 66.

360. Nygaard, op. cit.

361. AMA, 1983, op. cit., p. 638.

362. Gilman, 1985, op. cit., p. 209.

363. Vestal, op. cit., p. 40.

364. Wasnich, op. cit.

365. *The Medical Letter on Drugs and Therapeutics,* 1991, op. cit., p. 33–8.

366. Burton, op. cit.

367. Gilman, 1985, op. cit., p. 209.

368. Wasnich, op. cit.

369. *The Medical Letter on Drugs and Therapeutics,* 1991, op. cit., p. 33–8.

370. Burton, op. cit.

371. Gilman, 1985, op. cit., p. 209.

372. Wasnich, op. cit.

373. *The Medical Letter on Drugs and Therapeutics,* 1991, op. cit., p. 33–8.

374. Burton, op. cit.

375. Wasnich, op. cit.

376. *The Medical Letter on Drugs and Therapeutics,* 1991, op. cit., p. 33–8.

377. Burton, op. cit.

378. Gilman, 1985, op. cit., p. 209.

379. Orland, op. cit., p. 89–104.

380. Wasnich, op. cit.

381. *The Medical Letter on Drugs and Therapeutics,* 1991, op. cit., p. 33–8.

382. Burton, op. cit.

383. Olin, op. cit., p. 738.

384. McEntee WJ, Crook T, Jenkyn LR, Petrie W, Larrabee GJ, Coffey DJ. Treatment of age-associated memory impairment with guanfacine. *Psychopharmacology Bulletin* 1991; 27:41–6.

385. Wilson MF, Blackshear J, Parsons OA, Lovallo WR, Mathur P. Antihypertensive efficacy of guanfacine and methyldopa in patients with mild to moderate essential hypertension. *Journal of Clinical Pharmacology* 1991; 31:318–26.

386. Mosqueda-Garcia R. Guanfacine: a second generation alpha 2-adrenergic blocker. *The American Journal of the Medical Sciences* 1990; 299:73–6.

387. Oster JR, Epstein M. Use of centrally acting sympatholytic agents in the management of hypertension. *Archives of Internal Medicine* 1991; 151:1638–44.

388. Wasnich, op. cit.

389. *The Medical Letter on Drugs and Therapeutics,* 1991, op. cit., p. 33–8.

390. Burton, op. cit.

391. Oster, op. cit.

392. O'Byrne S, Feely J. Effects of drugs on glucose tolerance in non-insulin-dependent diabetics (part I). *Drugs* 1990; 40:6–18.

393. Oster, op. cit.

394. Ibid.

395. San L, Cami J, Peri JM, Mata R, Porta M. Efficacy of clonidine, guanfacine and methadone in the rapid detoxification of heroin addicts: a controlled clinical trial. *British Journal of Addiction* 1990; 85:141–7.

396. Levin, op. cit.

397. Mosqueda-Garcia, op. cit.

398. Oster, op. cit.

399. Vestal, op. cit., p. 40.

400. Wasnich, op. cit.

401. *The Medical Letter on Drugs and Therapeutics,* 1991, op. cit., p. 33–8.

402. Burton, op. cit.

403. Desager J. Clinical pharmacokinetics of ticlopidine. *Clinical Pharmacokinetics* 1994; 26: 347–55.

404. Wysowski DK, Bacsanyi J. Blood dyscrasias and hematologic reactions in ticlopidine users. *Journal of the American Medical Association* 1996; 276:952.

405. Ibid.

406. Roden DM, Woosley RL. Drug therapy tocainide. *New England Journal of Medicine* 1986; 315:41.

407. *The Medical Letter on Drugs and Therapeutics.* New York: The Medical Letter Inc., 1985; 27:10.

408. Nygaard, op. cit.

409. *The Medical Letter on Drugs and Therapeutics,* 1984, op. cit., p. 103.

410. Mass RD, Venook AP, Linker CA. Pentoxifylline and aplastic anemia. *Annals of Internal Medicine* 1987; 107:428.

411. *Pharmacy and Therapeutics Forum* 1987:4.

412. AMA, 1983, op. cit., p. 678–9.

413. Gilman, 1985, op. cit., p. 823.

414. AMA, 1983, op. cit., p. 678–9.

415. Wasnich, op. cit.

416. *The Medical Letter on Drugs and Therapeutics,* 1991, op. cit., p. 33–8.

417. Burton, op. cit.

418. Gilman, 1985, op. cit., p. 792

419. Wasnich, op. cit.

420. *The Medical Letter on Drugs and Therapeutics,* 1991, op. cit., p. 33–8.

421. Burton, op. cit.

Mind Drugs

Tranquilizers and Sleeping Pills	**178**
Antipsychotic Drugs	**187**
Depression	**196**

DRUG LISTINGS

TRANQUILIZERS AND SLEEPING PILLS

Drug	Recommendation	Page
alprazolam	⊘ Do Not Use Except for Panic Disorder	222
AMBIEN	Limited Use	201
ATIVAN	⊘ Do Not Use	222
BUSPAR	Limited Use	206
buspirone	Limited Use	206
butabarbital	⊘ Do Not Use	208
BUTISOL	⊘ Do Not Use	208
CENTRAX	⊘ Do Not Use	222
chlordiazepoxide	⊘ Do Not Use	222
clorazepate	⊘ Do Not Use	222
DALMANE	⊘ Do Not Use	222
diazepam	⊘ Do Not Use	222
DORAL	⊘ Do Not Use	222
EQUANIL	⊘ Do Not Use	216
estazolam	⊘ Do Not Use	222
flurazepam	⊘ Do Not Use	222
halazepam	⊘ Do Not Use	222
HALCION	⊘ Do Not Use	222
LIBRIUM	⊘ Do Not Use	222
lorazepam	⊘ Do Not Use	222
meprobamate	⊘ Do Not Use	216
MILTOWN	⊘ Do Not Use	216
NEMBUTAL	⊘ Do Not Use	208
oxazepam	Limited Use	242
PAXIPAM	⊘ Do Not Use	222
pentobarbital	⊘ Do Not Use	208
prazepam	⊘ Do Not Use	222
PROSOM	⊘ Do Not Use	222
quazepam	⊘ Do Not Use	222
RESTORIL	⊘ Do Not Use	222
SERAX	Limited Use	242
temazepam	⊘ Do Not Use	222
TRANXENE	⊘ Do Not Use	222
triazolam	⊘ Do Not Use	222
VALIUM	⊘ Do Not Use	222
XANAX	⊘ Do Not Use Except for Panic Disorder	222
zolpidem	Limited Use	201

DRUGS FOR DEPRESSION

Drug	Recommendation	Page
amitriptyline	⊘ Do Not Use	216
amitriptyline and chlordiazepoxide	⊘ Do Not Use	224
amitriptyline and perphenazine	⊘ Do Not Use	250
amoxapine	Limited Use	203
ASENDIN	Limited Use	203
AVENTYL		230
bupropion	Limited Use	251
desipramine		230
DESYREL	Limited Use	211
doxepin	Limited Use	203
EFFEXOR	Limited Use	213
ELAVIL	⊘ Do Not Use	216
ESKALITH	Limited Use	217
fluoxetine		233
fluvoxamine	Do Not Use Until Five Years After Release	233

imipramine	Limited Use	203
LIMBITROL	⊘ Do Not Use	224
lithium	Limited Use	217
LITHOBID	Limited Use	217
LITHONATE	Limited Use	217
LUDIOMIL	Limited Use	225
LUVOX	Do Not Use Until Five Years After Release	233
maprotiline	Limited Use	225
mirtazapine	Do Not Use Until Five Years After Release	237
nefazodone	Limited Use	245
NORPRAMIN		230
nortriptyline		230
PAMELOR		230
paroxetine	Limited Use	233
PAXIL	Limited Use	233
PROZAC		233
REMERON	Do Not Use Until Five Years After Release	237
sertraline	Limited Use	233
SERZONE	Limited Use	245
SINEQUAN	Limited Use	203
TOFRANIL	Limited Use	203
trazodone	Limited Use	211
TRIAVIL	⊘ Do Not Use	250
venlafaxine	Limited Use	213
WELLBUTRIN	Limited Use	251
ZOLOFT	Limited Use	233

DRUGS FOR SCHIZOPHRENIA AND OTHER PSYCHOSES

chlorpromazine	Limited Use	247
clozapine	Last Choice Drug	209
CLOZARIL	Last Choice Drug	209
fluphenazine	Limited Use	247
HALDOL	Limited Use	219
haloperidol	Limited Use	219
MELLARIL	Limited Use	247
NAVANE	Limited Use	227
olanzapine	Limited Use	253
PROLIXIN	Limited Use	247
RISPERDAL	Limited Use	239
risperidone	Limited Use	239
STELAZINE	Limited Use	247
thioridazine	Limited Use	247
thiothixene	Limited Use	227
THORAZINE	Limited Use	247
trifluoperazine	Limited Use	247
ZYPREXA	Limited Use	253

TRANQUILIZERS AND SLEEPING PILLS

Tranquilizers (minor tranquilizers or antianxiety pills) and sleeping pills are discussed together because the most commonly used drugs in both classes belong to the same family of chemicals, called benzodiazepines. *Many of the benzodiazepines, along with another sleeping pill, zolpidem (AMBIEN), were among the 200 most dispensed drugs in community pharmacies in 1997. Zolpidem is not a benzodiazepine but has many of the same effects, including the potential to cause drug-induced dependence.*

Older adults have a much more difficult time eliminating benzodiazepines and similar drugs from their bloodstreams and these drugs can thus accumulate in their bodies. Also older adults are more sensitive to the effects of many of these drugs than are younger adults. For older adults the risk of serious adverse drug effects is significantly increased. Serious adverse effects may include: unsteady gait, dizziness, falling (causing an increased risk of hip fractures), increased risk of an auto accident, drug-induced or drug-affected impairment of thinking, memory loss, and addiction.

Despite these significantly increased risks, sleeping pills and minor tranquilizers are prescribed much more often for older adults than they are for younger adults, for much longer periods of time, and usually not at the reduced dose that could decrease the risks.

Commonly used sleeping pills or tranquilizers, in addition to the benzodiazepines, include the following:

- Buspirone (BUSPAR)
- Barbiturates: According to the World Health Organization, these drugs should not be used by older adults for anxiety or sleep disorders.[1] (Phenobarbital can be used for the treatment of convulsions or seizures.)
- Meprobamate (MILTOWN, EQUANIL)

- Hydroxyzine (ATARAX, VISTARIL) as a sleeping pill or tranquilizer
- Glutethimide (DORIDEN)
- Chloral hydrate (NOCTEC)
- Methyprylon (NOLUDAR)
- Diphenhydramine (BENADRYL, SOMINEX FORMULA)

How Often Are These Drugs Prescribed for Older Adults?

Minor Tranquilizers

Three surveys have determined what percentage of noninstitutionalized older adults use minor tranquilizers. Although one is regional (the west coast of Florida), one is statewide (Tennessee), and one is national, they came up with remarkably similar findings on overall minor tranquilizer use:

- In Florida, 15.6% of people 65 and older had used minor tranquilizers during the year the study was done. Of these, 39% had used them daily and 78% had used the pills for more than a year.[2]
- In Tennessee, 21% of noninstitutionalized Medicaid patients 65 and older had used minor tranquilizers during the year of the study.[3]
- A national study found that 16.9% of people 65 and older had used a minor tranquilizer during the previous year, and that 5.2% of all people 65 and older had used minor tranquilizers daily for at least a year.[4]

If we apply the national figure of 16.9% users (which falls between the other two) to the entire U.S. population 65 and over (33 million people in 1996),[5] there are 5.6 million people 65 and older using minor tranquilizers. *One and a half million people are using these drugs every day for at least a year.*

One of the most striking findings of the national study was that a much larger propor-

tion of older tranquilizer users (30%) were using the drugs on a long-term (longer than one year) daily basis than were users in the younger age groups (14% of people age 35–49 using tranquilizers used them daily for one year or more). The authors of the study attribute this finding to more physical health problems in older people. They said, however, that this does not "necessarily justify the long-term duration of use."[6]

This seriously understates a major public health problem. Even though 1.5 million older adults (65 and older) use minor tranquilizers daily for at least one year continuously, there is no evidence that any of these drugs are effective for more than four months. Furthermore, most, if not all, people using these drugs for more than several months become addicted. Therefore, drug-induced falls, impairment of memory and thinking, and other adverse effects, especially in older adults, also occur with these drugs that have no proven long-term benefits. (See later sections for more information on benefits and risks.)

In 1985, for example, patients 60 and older filled approximately 21.3 million prescriptions for benzodiazepine minor tranquilizers (Valium, Librium, Tranxene, Serax, Centrax, Paxipam, Ativan, and Xanax) in retail pharmacies. Since the number of people 60 and over using benzodiazepine minor tranquilizers is approximately 5.8 million,* this means that the average person 60 and older who used benzodiazepine tranquilizers filled more than three prescriptions a year. This totals approximately 160 pills a year, enough for one month's to five months' use.[7]

Based on 39.53 million people 60 and over, 16.9% using minor tranquilizers of which 86% are benzodiazepines, assuming that the rate of use in people 60 to 64 is the same as in the 65 and older group

Older adults are clearly being "tranquilized" far more frequently than younger adults. Whereas people 60 and older make up just 16.5% of the U.S. population, 35.7% of the prescriptions for minor tranquilizers are for people in this age group.[8]

Sleeping Pills

Two of the studies mentioned above reported on prescription sleeping pill use among the elderly and again came to the same conclusions about the extraordinary rate of use.

In Florida, 6.3% of people 65 years or older used sleeping pills during the year of the study. Of these users, 32% took them daily, almost 90% of these daily users had been using the drugs for a year or longer. Thus, 1.77% of all people 65 or older had been taking sleeping pills daily for at least a year.[9]

The study in Tennessee found that 5% of non-institutionalized people 65 to 84 years of age had used a sleeping pill in the past year, agreeing closely with the 6.3% rate of use in Florida.[10]

Again applying these findings on a national basis, if 6.3% of all those 65 or older are using sleeping pills, this amounts to 2.07 million prescription sleeping pill users, including 584,000 who have been using these pills daily for at least a year. An even larger number has been using sleeping pills daily for at least one month, based on the Florida findings. Thus, it is estimated that more than half a million people 65 or older are using prescription sleeping pills for one month or longer, although there is no evidence that these drugs are effective for more than two to four weeks at the longest.[11,12]

The use of these medications in institutions is even higher: 16% of patients 65 to 84 years old in Tennessee nursing homes received sleeping pills.[13] In another nursing home study,[14] 25.2% received them, and the percentage of older adults on sleeping pills in the hospital is even higher.

A study in the prestigious New York Hospital, of Cornell Medical School, found that 46% of patients on the medical wards had prescriptions written specifically for sleep, and that 31% actually were given a dose at least once during their hospitalization. On the surgical service an even larger percentage—96% of patients—not varying according to age, had prescriptions written, and 88% actually were given the drugs.[15]

In short, although people 60 and older make up one-sixth (16.6%) of the population, they are prescribed more than one-half (51%) of the sleeping medications. Most of these (75%) are the benzodiazepine sleeping pills such as Dalmane, Halcion, and Restoril.[16]

How Much Use Is Justified in View of the Significant Risks?

Minor Tranquilizers

Although minor tranquilizers are prescribed more often and for longer periods of time for older adults than for younger adults, studies have shown that, if anything, older adults have lower levels of "psychic distress" or serious "life crisis" than younger adults. Worse yet, since older adults usually take more prescription drugs for the direct treatment of physical diseases, the prescribing of tranquilizers is all the more dangerous because of possibly dangerous interactions.

In 1979, Roche, maker of Valium, Librium, and Dalmane, sent doctors brochures encouraging the use of Valium for older adults as "an important component of treatment programs for the relief of excessive geriatric anxiety and psychic tension."[17]

Faced with falling sales of Valium, the early 1980s saw Roche (and other drug makers) aggressively pursue the older adult market share. A series of handsomely illustrated brochures entitled "Roche Seminars on Aging," was mailed to doctors in 1982. Roche recommended Valium as appropriate for the elderly with "limited" coping skills, facing "not only the constraints brought about by their own reduced capabilities, but also those imposed by the social structure and environment."

The campaign worked because the rate of use of minor tranquilizers in people 60 and over increased significantly between 1980 and 1985, especially in older women.[18]

The fact that more than 1.7 million people 65 and older use minor tranquilizers daily for at least a year is the best evidence that they are being overprescribed.[19] Given that there is no evidence that any of these drugs are effective for more than four months, the number of older adults whose use of these drugs exceeds four months is even greater. As mentioned above, the average number of pills (160), that each of the 10 million minor tranquilizer users 60 and over gets per year, is enough for one to five months of use.

In a discussion about the use of tranquilizers and sleeping pills by older adults, World Health Organization (WHO) experts said the following: *"Anxiety is a normal response to stress and only when it is severe and disabling should it lead to drug treatment. Long-term treatment . . . is rarely effective and should be avoided. . . . Short-term use (less than two weeks) will minimize the risk of dependence."*

They concluded by saying that *"discussion of the problems of sleeplessness and anxiety and the drawbacks of drug therapy will often help the patient to come to terms with his or her problem without the need to resort to drugs."*[20]

Two studies on alternatives to the use of minor tranquilizers further highlight how much of the present use is unnecessary. Ninety patients, suffering mainly from anxiety, were randomly divided into two groups when they went to see their family doctors. The first group was given the usual dose of one of the benzodiazepine tranquilizers. The other group was given a small dose of a much safer treatment consisting solely of "listening, explanation, advice, and reassurance." The two treatments were equally effective in relieving the anxiety, but those receiving the informal counseling were more satisfied with their treatment than those given minor tranquilizers.[21]

In a second study, patients with anxiety were either given one of three different tranquilizers or a placebo (sugar pill). At the end of a month, with weekly evaluations of their anxiety levels being made by the patients themselves and by professional evaluators, the results showed "all four treatments to be efficacious in their therapeutic effects on relieving anxiety."[22] That is, placebos worked as well as tranquilizers.

Sleeping Pills

As seen with minor tranquilizers, the clearest evidence that there is dangerous overprescribing and misprescribing of sleeping medications to older adults comes from the estimated one-half million people who have been taking these drugs daily for at least a month. Since there is no evidence these drugs are effective for longer than this period of time, all of these people are getting the full risks of these drugs without the benefits.

In addition, as discussed above, the average number of benzodiazepine sleeping pills obtained per user is enough for five months, five to ten times longer than the drugs have been shown to be effective. Conservatively then, 80 to 90% of the use of these pills is a dangerous waste.

The increases in the use of these drugs by older adults, noted above, flies strongly in the face of the conclusions and recommendations of an exhaustive study by the National Academy of Sciences' Institute of Medicine in 1979.[23]

Speaking generally about the use of these drugs, the study concluded that: *"hypnotics (sleeping medications) should have only a limited place in contemporary medical practice: it is difficult to justify much of the current prescribing of sleeping medication. As a standard of prudent ambulatory medical care, the committee favors the prescription of only very limited numbers of sleeping pills for use for a few nights at a time. . . . Hypnotic drugs should be selected carefully and prescribed cautiously, if at all, for patients . . . who are old."*

Commenting specifically on sleeping pill use by older adults, the authors said: *"Of particular concern is the regular and prolonged use by this group of sleep-inducing medications that are of dubious value, and that add new hazards to their already complicated drug intake regimens."*

Although older people tend to complain more than younger people about sleeping problems, the study found that the time it takes to fall asleep does not increase with age, and that the total sleep time decreases very little, if at all. Older people who go to bed early and take cat naps during the daytime often do have sleeping problems. But, the study concluded, "it is this pattern of daytime sleep that must be changed instead of treating the night time insomnia that results from it."

According to Dr. Marshall Folstein, a Johns Hopkins psychiatrist and expert in Alzheimer's disease, *"it is extraordinarily rare to find an older person who actually requires them [sleeping pills]."*[24]

A further threat is posed by high doses. A study of sleeping pill dose and age found that a majority (almost 80%) of people 65 and over were using the "overdose" amount of 30 milligrams a night of Dalmane even though 15 milligrams is recommended for older adults. (In this book we list Dalmane as a **Do Not Use** drug.) In view of the limited use of these drugs recommended by the National Academy of Sciences, the current and increasing prescribing of sleeping medications for older adults—especially the extensive prolonged-use patterns discussed above—poses a serious threat to their health.

What Are the Main Risks of Sleeping Pills and Tranquilizers?

Drug-induced dependence, daytime sedation, confusion, memory loss, increased risk of an auto accident, poor coordination resulting in falls and hip fractures, impaired learning abil-

ity, slurred speech, and even death are adverse effects of these drugs. They are more likely to occur when these drugs are taken in combination with alcohol or other depressant drugs. They can happen to anyone at any age.

Older adults, however, cannot clear many of these drugs from their systems as rapidly as younger people can. They are also more sensitive to the drugs' adverse effects. Despite this evidence, older adults (1) are more likely to be given a prescription for tranquilizers or sleeping pills, (2) are not usually given the reduced dose that would at least diminish the odds of serious adverse effects, and (3) are prescribed these drugs for longer periods of time than are younger people. Therefore, it is not surprising that older adults are at much greater risk of suffering from adverse effects, and, when they occur, they are much more serious.

One of the biggest impediments to discovering and eliminating these drug-induced problems is their frequent attribution to the aging process instead of to the drugs. The onset of impaired intelligence with memory loss, confusion, or impaired learning, or the onset of loss of coordination in a younger person will more likely prompt an inquiry leading to the drug as culprit. But the same symptoms in an older person, especially if they develop more slowly, are often dismissed with a familiar remark, "Well, he (or she) is just growing old, what do you expect?" This lack of suspicion allows the drug to keep doing damage because the doctor keeps up the prescription.

Hip Fractures

A study of 1,021 older adults with hip fractures found that 14% of these life-threatening injuries are attributable to the use of mind-affecting drugs, including sleeping pills and minor tranquilizers, antipsychotics, and antidepressants.[25]

There are approximately 227,000 hip fractures each year in the United States, virtually all in older adults.[26] Since the above study found that 14% of hip fractures are drug-induced, this means that if the results of the study are projected nationally, approximately 32,000 hip fractures a year in older adults are caused by the use of mind-affecting drugs. Of these, about 30%, or almost 10,000 hip fractures a year, are caused by sleeping pills and minor tranquilizers, particularly the long-acting drugs such as Valium, Librium, and Dalmane.

Another study on fractures in older adults found that the increased occurrence of falls resulting in such fractures could often be reduced by removing the offending drug.[27]

Automobile Crashes which Caused Injuries

A study involving 495 automobile crashes by older drivers in which an injury occurred found that a significant number of such crashes by older adults aged 65–84 were attributable to the use of benzodiazepine tranquilizers and cyclic antidepressants. The study was particularly impressive because its findings were strengthened by observing that the rate of crashes which caused injuries increased in the same group of people when they were using these drugs as opposed to when they were not using the drugs. The majority of the excess number of auto crashes were attributable to the benzodiazepines. The authors, stating that the study findings may be generalizable to the population at large, found that if the association is causal, out of the 217,000 crashes that cause injuries that occur each year among elderly drivers, at least 16,000 are attributable to psychoactive drug use (specifically benzodiazepines and tricyclic antidepressants).[28]

Drug-induced or Drug-worsened Senility (Decreased Mental Functioning)

Drug-induced impairment of thinking is one of the most reversible, or treatable, forms of dementia. It is a by-product of the increased use of drugs during the past few decades. Among the 33 million people 65 and over in the United States,[29] approximately 5 out of every 100 have dementia, with an estimated one of these five due to "reversible" conditions such as treatable diseases (thyroid disease, for example) or adverse effects of drugs.[30]

A study of 308 older adults with significant intellectual impairment found that in 11.4% of these people the problem was caused or worsened by a drug.[31] This study, the first to ever systematically analyze this problem, revealed that after stopping the use of the dementia-causing drugs, all persons had long-term improvement of their mental function. The most common class of drugs to cause the impairment of mental function was the sleeping pill/tranquilizer group. It accounted for 46% of the drug-induced or drug-worsened dementia.

The University of Washington researchers who did the study had two further observations:

1. "Most patients had used these drugs for years, and the side effect of cognitive (mental) impairment developed insidiously as a 'late' complication of a drug begun at an earlier age.

2. The improvement experienced by patients in this study was usually surprising to family and caregivers. The patients noted an improved sense of well-being and were better able to care for themselves."

If these important findings are applied to all of the estimated 1.43 million Americans 65 and over who have dementia, there are 163,000 people whose mental impairment has either been entirely caused by or worsened by drugs. For approximately 75,000 older adults, their impaired mental functioning is caused by sleeping pills or minor tranquilizers.

Drug-induced Dependence

Drug-induced dependence is often called addiction by drug companies and doctors who seek to shift blame to the patients who were prescribed a drug, but were not told that the drug could cause physical dependence. The withdrawal from drug-induced dependence includes symptoms of sweating, nervousness or, when more severe, hallucinations or seizures which are often accompanied by psychological dependence.

The myth used to be that only people who were prone to addiction, as judged by a prior history of alcoholism or other drug problems, would possibly become addicted to benzodiazepine tranquilizers or sleeping pills. Even then they would have to use very large doses of these drugs for a long period of time before addiction could occur.

This attitude, intended to cover up a major national problem, was "pushed" by the president of Hoffman-la Roche, the world's biggest benzodiazepine maker (Valium, Librium, and Dalmane). Testifying in 1979 before U.S. Senate hearings on the abuse of these drugs, Robert Clark said that "true addiction is probably exceedingly unusual and, when it occurs, is probably confined to those individuals with abuse-prone personalities who ingest very large amounts."[32]

It was clear then and is now even clearer that a large fraction, probably the overwhelming majority, of people who use any of the benzodiazepines at the recommended dose for more than one or two months will become *dependent*.

Another study showed that a large proportion of people became *dependent* on these drugs and experienced an unpleasant withdrawal syndrome when they suddenly stopped taking the drug (as opposed to gradually tapering the dose to reduce, if not eliminate, the withdrawal symptoms). The only difference between addiction to the longer-acting drugs such as Valium and Dalmane, and the shorter-acting drugs such as Ativan and Serax was the time, after the drug was suddenly stopped, that it took before withdrawal symptoms occurred. With the longer-acting drugs the day of worst symptoms was the tenth; for the shorter-acting drugs it was

the first. Withdrawal symptoms included anxiety, headache, insomnia, tension, sweating, difficulty concentrating, tremor, fear, and fatigue.

The authors of the study concluded that *"when withdrawal was abrupt, symptoms were more frequent and more severe than when a gradual tapering technique was used. . . . there is little justification for abrupt withdrawal."*[33]

Serious Breathing Problems

Another serious adverse effect of the benzodiazepines is their effect on respiration. One effect of these drugs has to do with *sleep apnea,* a common condition in older adults in which, for varying periods of time while asleep, breathing stops. Dr. William Dement, an expert in sleep research, has found that older people with sleep apnea who use sleeping medications can stop breathing for much longer—dangerously longer—periods of time as a result of the respiration-suppressing effects of the drugs. He told a government task force on sleeping problems that people over 65 should not use Dalmane because of the risk of worsening sleep apnea.[34]

A second problem in this category affects people with *severe lung disease.* Anyone with severe lung disease should not use benzodiazepines because they decrease the urge to breathe, which can be life-threatening.[35] Asthmatics should also avoid benzodiazepine sleeping pills and tranquilizers.

Other Adverse Effects[36]

Frequent: drowsiness and lack of coordination that can affect walking or driving a car.

Occasional: confusion, forgetfulness, excitement instead of sedation, rebound insomnia (more difficulty sleeping when the drug wears off), or, especially with triazolam (HALCION), excitement instead of sedation.

Rare: low blood pressure, bone marrow toxicity, liver disease, allergies and rage reactions.

Reducing the Risks from Sleeping Pills and Tranquilizers

The best way to reduce the risks of these powerful drugs is avoid using them for most of the conditions for which they are now prescribed, especially in older adults.

Alternatives for Anxiety

According to noted British psychiatrist, Dr. Malcolm Lader: *"Until recently most anxious patients in the United Kingdom were treated with tranquilizers, usually a benzodiazepine. However, recognition that these drugs can cause dependence even at normal therapeutic dosages has led to a re-evaluation of drug therapy, and the value of non-pharmacologic treatments is increasingly being recognized."*[37]

Two British doctors use a nondrug alternative for the treatment of mild to moderate anxiety (and similar problems). They say that *". . . the best treatment is likely to be brief counselling provided by the general practitioner or by another professional working in the practice. Such counseling need not be intensive or specially skilled. It should always include careful assessment of the causes of the patient's distress. Once these have been identified, anxiety may often be reduced to tolerable levels by means of explanation, exploration of feelings, reassurance, and encouragement."*[38]

What else can be done? Talking to nonmedical people—a friend, a spouse, a relative, a member of the clergy, may help to identify causes of anxiety and potential solutions. Gathering the courage to talk about difficult concerns will generally be a better solution than taking pills. For some people, a specialized form of psychotherapy can treat anxiety. If indeed, medication is needed it is best to see a psychiatrist. Getting regular exercise can also help relieve anxiety.

In addition, the use of foods, beverages, and over-the-counter (nonprescription) or prescription drugs that have significant stimulant effects can also cause a chemically-induced anxiety that can be remedied. (See the list of such substances below, under alternatives for sleeping problems.)

Alternatives for Sleeping Problems

Experts in sleep and aging have recently stated that:

• Many old people have exaggerated expectations of what sleep should be like and they "spend too much time in bed chasing sleep."

• Many older people use sleep as an escape from boredom.

• "It's extraordinarily rare to find an old person who actually requires [sleeping pills]."[39]

If the cause of the sleeping problem is depression (see p. 196 for other problems that go along with depression), the depression should be addressed rather than simply treating the symptom by prescribing sleeping medication. If the cause is a medical condition, with pain as one of the components, the pain has to be treated rather than using a sleeping pill to induce sleep despite the pain. In the case of senile brain disease, such as Alzheimer's, the sleep disturbance will probably not respond to sleeping medications.[40]

Other causes of sleeping problems that can also be "treated" without using drugs include the following:

• Daytime napping or going to bed too early.

• Inaccurate idea of how much sleep you require each night. If you do not feel tired during the day, you had enough sleep the night before.

• Environmental factors such as light and noise. A quieter, darker room may promote a more restful sleep.

• Drinking stimulants—coffee, tea, or cola beverages—or eating chocolate within eight hours of when you want to sleep.

• Lack of a nighttime routine. A warm bath, a pleasant book, a light but bland snack, no working just before going to bed or while in bed are ways to encourage sleep.

Drugs can produce stimulating effects and a chemically-induced anxiety:

• *Over-the-counter (nonprescription) drugs:* Sleeplessness can be caused by caffeine, found in Anacin and other drugs, PPA (phenylpropanolamine), the stimulants found in Actifed, Contac, Sudafed and other decongestant products, and the ingredients in many asthma drugs.
• *Prescription drugs:* Sleeping problems may be caused by asthma drugs containing theophylline or aminophylline such as Slo-bid and Somophyllin, amphetamines such as Dexedrine and diet pills, steroids such as cortisone and prednisone, thyroid drugs, and the withdrawal from the use of sleeping pills, tranquilizers, and antidepressants. (See p. 24 in Chapter 2 for a list of drugs that can cause insomnia.)

If you have a sleeping problem and use one of these drugs, or if the problem began when you started using another drug, talk to your doctor. Tell him or her all the drugs (over-the-counter and prescription) you are taking. It might be possible to change the drug or lower the dosage to help you sleep. Returning to sleeping pills to get past withdrawal effects will only place you in a vicious cycle.

Which Tranquilizers or Sleeping Pills Should You Use, If Any?

Although we strongly discourage the use of these drugs in most situations, especially for older adults, there are some perfectly competent physicians who, in very well-defined circumstances and for very short periods of time, will prescribe them. But even the labeling approved by the Food and Drug Administration for all of the tranquilizers has to state, "Anxiety or tension associated with the stress of everyday life usually does not require treatment with an anxiolytic [tranquilizer]."[41] (See the seven rules for safer use, below.)

As mentioned at the beginning of this chapter, older adults should never use barbiturates as sleeping pills or tranquilizers. Other drugs such as meprobamate (MILTOWN, EQUANIL), hydroxyzine (VISTARIL, ATARAX) for sleep, glutethimide (DORIDEN), chloral hydrate (NOCTEC) and methyprylon (NOLUDAR) should also not be used.[42]

This leaves buspirone (BUSPAR, see p. 206) and the benzodiazepines, with the eight benzodiazepine drugs marketed primarily as tranquilizers and five as sleeping pills. All of these drugs are equally effective in tranquilizing or promoting sleep. "Calling some anti-anxiety drugs and others hypnotics (sleeping pills) has more to do with marketing than with pharmacology."[43]

These 13 benzodiazepine drugs are different from each other, and the difference has to do with the different ways in which they are dangerous for older adults. The World Health Organization specifically recommends that older adults should not use what is the most widely prescribed sleeping pill, DALMANE (flurazepam), "owing to a high incidence of adverse effects."[44]

Seven other benzodiazepines are also more slowly cleared out of the body, especially in older adults, and can therefore accumulate, leading to higher blood levels and increased risks. These drugs, which also should be avoided by older adults, are diazepam (VALIUM), chlordiazepoxide (LIBRIUM), clorazepate (TRANXENE), prazepam (CENTRAX), halazepam (PAXIPAM), quazepam (DORAL) and estazolam (PROSOM).

Another widely used sleeping pill, triazolam (HALCION), should also be avoided by older adults because it is so short-acting that it can cause rebound insomnia (increased sleeping problems when the drug effect has worn off), anxiety, serious amnesia (forgetfulness or memory loss) and violent, aggressive behavior. In 1992, Public Citizen's Health Research Group petitioned the Food and Drug Administration to ban Halcion. The sleeping pill estazolam (PROSOM) is in the same class as Halcion and, according to *The Medical Letter,* there is no reason to use it.[45] It also has the disadvantage of slow clearance from the body.

In a discussion of which of these drugs are best for older adults, it was stated that oxazepam (SERAX) and temazepam (RESTORIL) were the drugs of choice.[46] It has also been stated that "oxazepam (SERAX) may be the safest benzodiazepine for the older patient" because "oxazepam may offer the advantages of a short half-life and the absence of active metabolites" (that is, chemicals the body converts the drug into which can also have adverse effects).[47] In addition, studies have shown that oxazepam has much less of a "street" drug abuse potential than, for example, diazepam (VALIUM).[48,49]

In an article on how 11 of these benzodiazepines compare with one another as far as memory loss (a serious problem especially in older adults), geriatric drug expert Dr. Peter Lamy stated that oxazepam had less memory impairment than all other benzodiazepines except clorazepate,[50] a long-acting tranquilizer which should not be used by older adults for reasons mentioned above.

For other patients—not older adults—temazepam and clorazepate can also be used. In addition, the sleeping pill zolpidem (AMBIEN), discussed on p. 201, can also be used for those under 60. However, as mentioned in the profile on this drug, although it is technically not a benzodiazepine—the family containing Librium and Valium—it may still cause addiction and it should not be used for more than one to three weeks.

In summary, the only prescription tranquilizers or sleeping pills that we advise for **limited use,** in the older adult are buspirone (BUSPAR) and oxazepam, available generically, and under the brand name of Serax.

ANTIPSYCHOTIC DRUGS: ANOTHER GROUP OF DANGEROUSLY OVERUSED DRUGS

Antipsychotic drugs, also called neuroleptic drugs or major tranquilizers, are properly and successfully used to treat serious psychotic mental disorders, the most common of which is schizophrenia. Schizophrenia is a disease in which people have lost touch with reality, often see or hear things which are not there (hallucinations), believe things which are not true (delusions), often have severe mood problems such as depression, lose their expressiveness of feeling ("flat affect"), and in general, have disorders of thinking. Psychoses include other mental disorders which involve abnormal perceptions of reality such as hallucinations and delusions. Schizophrenia and the other psychoses are much less common in older adults than in younger adults, according to studies done by the National Institute of Mental Health.

We do not recommend the use of any benzodiazepines other than oxazepam. Here is how the large proportion of older adults who are using these drugs to their physical and mental detriment can stop using them, more safely.

If you have been taking any of these drugs for longer than several weeks continuously, there is a good chance that you have become addicted. Stopping the drugs suddenly (going "cold turkey") is a bad idea. With the help of your doctor, work out a schedule for slowly tapering down the amount of tranquilizer or sleeping pill by an average of 5 to 10% each day. Keep a written record of the dosage reduction schedule with you. This will greatly reduce the difficulty of stopping the use of these drugs.

Whereas about 1.12% of people aged 18 to 44 have been found to have active schizophrenia (symptoms in last six months) and 0.6% of 45- to 64-year-olds have this diagnosis, only 0.1% of people 65 and older are diagnosed as having active schizophrenia.[52] In other words, active schizophrenia is only one-tenth to one-fifth as common in older adults as in younger adults.

In younger adults, an alarming number of those with schizophrenia who could and often have previously benefited from antipsychotic drugs are not receiving them. They are seen, among other places, on the streets and in homeless shelters. In older adults, the problem is gross overuse by people who are not psychotic, not underuse.

Drugs That Can Cause Psychoses (Hallucinations) or Delirium

For anyone of any age who has recently become psychotic (has hallucinations, for example) or developed delirium, there should be careful questioning to see if this serious mental problem might have been drug-induced before the person is started on antipsychotic drugs. In someone who is 60

RULES FOR SAFER USE OF OXAZEPAM

(This is the only benzodiazepine we believe should be prescribed for older adults.)

1. The dose should be one-third to one-half the dose for younger people.[51] This means that the highest starting dose for older adults should be 7.5 milligrams, one to three times a day, if used as a tranquilizer, or 7.5 milligrams at bedtime, if used as a sleeping pill. (This is 1/2 of a 15 milligram tablet, generically available.)

2. Ask your doctor to limit the size of the prescription to seven days' worth of pills.

3. Ask your doctor to write *NO REFILL* on the prescription so that you will not be inclined (because of the "good chemical feelings" these pills may provide) to refill the prescription five times without seeing the doctor again. This dangerously lax refill policy is perfectly legal because oxazepam and other similar drugs are not very carefully controlled by the government. By urging your doctor to write *NO REFILL* you are making sure that he or she will reevaluate your condition after you use oxazepam for a short time. You want to discuss how you are doing with your anxiety or sleeping problem, rather than continuing to take the drug without a reevaluation. Continuing to take oxazepam without talking to your doctor could be the first step to addiction or other drug-induced problems.

4. At the end of the first day, and every day you use oxazepam, evaluate what you have done, on your own or by talking to others, to find out what is making you anxious. This includes evaluation of what you have done to alter the internal or external circumstances causing your anxiety. Keep a record of these evaluations. As soon as possible, try reducing the dose, in consultation with your doctor. Since you only have enough medication for one week, it is unlikely that you will have become addicted this quickly.

5. Do not drive a car or operate dangerous machinery while using oxazepam.

6. Do not drink alcohol. The combination of this drug with alcohol dangerously increases the effects of both. An overdose of oxazepam in combination with alcohol can be fatal.

7. Before using oxazepam, make sure that your doctor knows if you are taking other drugs with a sedative or "downer" effect, such as antidepressants, antipsychotics, antihistamines, narcotic painkillers, epilepsy medications, barbiturates, or other sleeping medications. Oxazepam taken with other drugs with sedative effects dangerously increases the risks of both.

years old or older, there is a strong likelihood that the recent onset of hallucinations, delirium, or other behavior which is like schizophrenia is due either to the effects of the drugs listed below or withdrawal from addiction to alcohol, barbiturates, or other sleeping pills or tranquilizers. Commonly used drugs which cause psychotic symptoms such as hallucinations or delirium include the following:[53]

• Analgesics/Narcotics such as indomethacin (INDOCIN), ketamine (KETALAR), morphine (ROXANOL), pentazocine (TALWIN), propoxyphene (DARVON), and salicylates (aspirin)

• Antibiotics and other anti-infective agents such as acyclovir (ZOVIRAX), amantadine (SYMMETREL), amphotericin B (FUNGIZONE), chloroquine (ARALEN), cycloserine (SEROMYCIN), dapsone, ethionamide (TRECATOR-SC), isoniazid (INH), nalidixic acid (NEGGRAM), penicillin G, podophyllum (PODOFIN), quinacrine (ATABRINE), and thiabendazole (MINTEZOL)

• Anticonvulsants such as ethosuximide (ZARONTIN), phenytoin (DILANTIN), and primidone (MYSOLINE)

• Allergy drugs such as antihistamines (CHLOR-TRIMETON, DIMETANE, etc.)

• Antiparkinsonians such as levodopa and carbidopa (SINEMET), bromocriptine (PARLODEL), and levodopa (LARODOPA)

• Asthma drugs such as albuterol (PROVENTIL, VENTOLIN)

• Drugs for depression such as trazodone (DESYREL) and tricyclic antidepressants such as amitriptyline (ELAVIL) and doxepin (SINEQUAN)

• Heart drugs such as digitalis preparations (LANOXIN, etc.), lidocaine (XYLOCAINE), procainamide (PROCANBID), and tocainide (TONOCARD)

• High blood pressure drugs such as clonidine (CATAPRES), methyldopa (ALDOMET),

prazosin (MINIPRESS), and propranolol (INDERAL)

• Nasal decongestants such as ephedrine, oxymetazoline (AFRIN), phenylephrine (NALDECON), and pseudoephedrine (SUDAFED)

• Drugs such as amphetamines, PCP, barbiturates, cocaine, and crack

• Sedatives/Tranquilizers such as alprazolam (XANAX), diazepam (VALIUM), ethchlorvynol (PLACIDYL), and triazolam (HALCION)

• Steroids such as dexamethasone (DECADRON) and prednisone (DELTASONE).

• Other drugs such as atropine, aminocaproic acid (AMICAR), baclofen (LIORESAL), cimetidine (TAGAMET), ranitidine (ZANTAC), disulfiram (ANTABUSE), methylphenidate (RITALIN), methysergide (SANSERT), metrizamide (AMIPAQUE), phenelzine (NARDIL), thyroid hormones, and vincristine (ONCOVIN)

How Often Are Antipsychotic Drugs Used in Older Adults?

Older adults, especially those in nursing homes, are prescribed a dangerously excessive amount of powerful antipsychotic drugs. This has resulted in hundreds of thousands of unnecessary cases of severe, disabling, and often irreversible adverse reactions. Although schizophrenia, the most common justifiable use for antipsychotic drugs is much less common in older adults than younger adults, people under 60 get about 4 prescriptions a year per 100 people of the antipsychotic drugs. But people over 60, with much less schizophrenia and other psychoses, get more than 10 prescriptions per 100 people a year.[54]

A study of older adults (ages 65 to 84) on Medicaid found that about 5% of those in the community and 39% of those in nursing homes had received a prescription for antipsychotic drugs during the previous year.[55] An earlier study by the same researchers[56] found that 30.1% of

Medicaid nursing home patients had received at least three months' worth of antipsychotic drugs during the year of the study.

Even if a more recent, and lower, estimate of the percentage of nursing home residents who are chronically prescribed antipsychotic drugs is used—22.9%—this means that approximately 300,000 of the 1.3 million U.S. nursing home residents 65 and over (*Health: United States 1987*) take these drugs for at least three or four months continuously.[57] In addition, one third of noninstitutionalized people getting these drugs are estimated to be using them for at least three or four months continuously,[58] adding another 450,000 older adults to the number of potential victims.[59] Thus, an estimated 750,000 people 65 or older, not even including those older people in mental hospitals, are regularly using antipsychotic drugs, even though the total number of people 65 and over with schizophrenia (not in mental hospitals) is only approximately 92,000.[60] Thus, 92,000 of the 750,000 older adults regularly using antipsychotic drugs—less than one eighth (12.3%)—actually have schizophrenia. Put another way, more than 80% of the use of antipsychotic drugs in older adults is unnecessary.

In addition to these 750,000 people over 65 chronically using antipsychotic drugs (although fewer than 100,000 are schizophrenic), there are more than one million additional people 65 and over in nursing homes and in the community getting prescriptions for antipsychotic drugs for less than three or four months continuously.[61] Thus, a total of approximately 1.7 million people 65 and over get a prescription for an antipsychotic drug each year, according to these estimates.

What Are These Antipsychotic Drugs Being Prescribed for, If Not for Schizophrenia and Other Psychoses?

A group of physicians and other health professionals who specialize in geriatric pharma-cology have stated that: *"The usefulness of antipsychotic medications in nonpsychotic, elderly patients has been questioned. . . . The high frequency of toxic reactions to these drugs is well documented, with many older patients who take them experiencing orthostatic hypotension [low blood pressure on sitting or standing], Parkinson's syndrome, tardive dyskinesia [see p. 192], akathisia [see p. 193], worsened confusion, dry mouth, constipation, oversedation, and urinary incontinence."*[62]

One of the more common purposes for which antipsychotic drugs are blatantly misused is as a sedative in nursing home patients.[63] Other unjustifiable uses include controlling the overall level of disturbance in older demented (nonpsychotic) patients,[64] and for treating chronic anxiety.[65] Two different studies concluded that often the most mentally alert and least physically disabled people are given these drugs.[66,67] This is consistent with the charge that these drugs are being used more for the convenience of the nursing home staff or other caretaker than for the needs of the patients.

Another study found that "80% of elderly demented persons are receiving tranquilizers (antipsychotic drugs) unnecessarily."[68] Other researchers concluded that antipsychotics are "frequently prescribed inappropriately as sedatives to elderly patients" and that "using these drugs incorrectly or for unnecessarily prolonged periods enhances the probability of developing this virtually untreatable, disfiguring syndrome" (referring to tardive dyskinesia).[69]

After finding that overall there were no significant benefits for antipsychotic drugs in elderly demented patients, one group of researchers concluded that "because of the apparently limited therapeutic efficacy of antipsychotic medication, it is especially important to search for possible social and environmental solutions for behavioral disturbances in this population."[70]

In other words, medical professionals should attempt to find out what it is in the environment that may be causing or contributing to the problems older people are having and, if possible, change it, rather than endanger their health with these powerful drugs. A perfect example is the use of antipsychotic drugs at the end of the day to treat the so-called "sundowner syndrome." As the end of the day approaches, some nursing home or hospital patients become agitated, restless or confused, and may wander about. A careful study of the characteristics of people with this problem found that they were much more likely to have been in their present room for less than one month, to have come to the nursing home or hospital more recently, and were awakened much more on the evening shift. The implication was that changes in the management of these patients by nurses and other staff could reduce the problem without resorting to the use of antipsychotic drugs.[71]

A review of the use of antipsychotic drugs in older adults confirmed that their most common use was to control agitation, wandering, belligerence, and sleeplessness. But this "disturbed" behavior is sometimes an appropriate response to changes in the environment or physical changes in the older adult. Treating the physical problem or changing the environment may lessen the need to resort to the antipsychotic drugs.[72]

Another important category of misprescribing of antipsychotic drugs in older adults is for depression, instead of, or in addition to antidepressants. A study of older adults found that in those for whom antipsychotic drugs were prescribed as treatment for depression there was an alarmingly high incidence of tardive dyskinesia (see p. 192) and the authors recommended that doctors "should be cautious in prescribing neuroleptic [antipsychotic] drugs for these patients."[73]

Two other drugs—prochlorperazine (COMPAZINE) and promethazine (PHENERGAN), which are from the same family as the antipsychotics (phenothiazines)—are mainly used for treating nonpsychotic (especially gastrointestinal) disorders and both are significantly overused. Discussions of their use appear on p. 366 and p. 385.

Has Federal Regulation Improved the Use of Antipsychotic Drugs in Nursing Homes?

The Omnibus Budget Reconciliation Act of 1987 (OBRA-87) included provisions for regulating the use of psychotropic medications, particularly antipsychotics, in long-term care facilities. Several surveys conducted since the enactment of OBRA-87 suggest that the use of these powerful drugs in elderly nursing home residents is being curtailed.

A review of prescription and medical records in eight nursing homes conducted between August 1994 and March 1996 found that of a total of 1,573 residents, 279 were taking antipsychotic drugs (17.7%). Of these 279, 70.9% were receiving the drug for an appropriate reason, 90.1% were prescribed the drug within the recommend dosage limits, and appropriate target symptoms were documented in 90.4% of these residents.[74]

A 1996 survey conducted in a 514-bed nursing home affiliated with a large medical school found that after implementation of OBRA-87 the prescribing of antidepressants increased significantly, coinciding with a reduction in the use of antianxiety agents and sedative-hypnotic drugs, and a substantial decrease in the prescribing of antipsychotic drugs. The total number of residents who received any type of psychotropic medication decreased, and over time a trend toward the use of drugs recommended for older adults emerged.[75]

It appears that at least some nursing homes are complying with regulations intended to ensure that psychotropic drugs are used properly in nursing home residents and that the total number of residents receiving these drugs may be declining.

Benefits and Risks of
Antipsychotic Drugs

For the small fraction of older adults taking antipsychotic drugs appropriately, that is for the treatment of psychotic illnesses such as schizophrenia, the significant risks are more than balanced out by the proven benefits for those people who respond. But at least 80% of the use of these drugs in older adults is inappropriate. Either the drugs are ineffective, as in the treatment of senile dementia, or unnecessary, as in their frequent uses to sedate or control nonpsychotic behavior that is often responsive to nondrug approaches.

Thus, well over one million older adults are being prescribed antipsychotic drugs, often for months or years continuously, for unjustified purposes, and they are suffering the consequences of risks without benefits.

What Are the Main Adverse Effects of Antipsychotic Drugs?

Falls and hip fractures

Approximately 16,000 older adults a year suffer from drug-induced hip fractures, attributable to the use of antipsychotic drugs. In one study, the main category of drugs responsible for falls leading to hip fractures was antipsychotic drugs.[76] Fifty-two percent of those hip fractures attributable to the use of mind-affecting drugs were due to antipsychotic drug use. (Also, see section on minor tranquilizers and sleeping pills, p. 178.)

Nerve problems

Tardive dyskinesia: This is the most common, serious, and often irreversible adverse effect of antipsychotic drugs. It is characterized by involuntary movements of the lips, tongue, and sometimes the fingers, toes, and trunk.[77] Older adults are at increased risk for this adverse effect, and it may occur in as many as 40% of people over the age of 60 taking antipsychotic drugs.[78]

Tardive dyskinesia is more common and more severe in older adults. The majority of cases are irreversible and often result in immobility, difficulty chewing and swallowing, and eventually weight loss and dehydration. None of the antipsychotic drugs has a lower chance of causing this problem than others.[79]

In most studies of elderly patients, the incidence of tardive dyskinesia in people taking antipsychotic medications is between 30 and 35%. However, a recent study found that in those elderly patients who had never before been given an antipsychotic drug, the incidence of tardive dyskinesia was 60% in those patients given the drugs for depression, significantly higher than in older adults getting these drugs for other purposes.[80]

Another study estimated that there were 192,718 people in the United States who had developed tardive dyskinesia attributable to antipsychotic drugs.[81] Of these, 54,284 cases occurred in nursing homes. If 80% of these exposures to antipsychotic drugs were unnecessary, more than 43,000 people in nursing homes developed tardive dyskinesia unnecessarily because they should not have been given these drugs. An additional 112,854 people not in an institution also suffered from tardive dyskinesia induced by antipsychotic drugs. According to national drug prescribing data, approximately 33% of the prescriptions for the drugs were in people over the age of 60.[82] Thus, an additional 37,000 noninstitutionalized older adults appear to have developed tardive dyskinesia from these drugs. If the prescriptions for 80% of these people are unnecessary, another 30,000 cases of tardive dyskinesia which should have been avoided, have occurred. Thus, there are approximately 73,000 cases of tardive dyskinesia, in older adults which are the result of poor prescribing practices by physicians.

To date, no drug has been found to be effective in treating tardive dyskinesia, thus making its prevention extremely important.

Drug-induced parkinsonism: Drug-induced parkinsonism involves the following symptoms: difficulty speaking or swallowing; loss of balance; mask-like face; muscle spasms; stiffness of arms or legs; trembling and shaking; unusual twisting movements of body.

Although many people believe that parkinsonism is one of the inevitable consequences of growing old, a large proportion of the cases seen in older adults are caused by drugs. A study found that 51% of 93 patients referred for evaluation of newly developed parkinsonism had drug-induced diseases.[83] One-fourth of patients with drug-induced parkinsonism could not walk when first seen by their doctors, and 45% required hospital admission. The parkinsonism cleared in 66% of the patients, but 11% continued to have the disease a year after the drug was stopped. An additional 25% who had cleared initially went on to develop classic Parkinson's disease, leading the authors to speculate that, for this latter 25%, these drugs were "unmasking" a disease which might have showed up later.

Even more disturbing is the finding in another study in which 36% of patients with drug-induced parkinsonism had been started on antiparkinson drugs to treat the disease! Because the doctors had not considered the possibility that a drug was responsible for the disease, they assumed that the patients had classic Parkinson's disease and treated the parkinsonism with another drug instead of stopping the one responsible for the disease in the first place.[84]

Another way of looking at this serious problem is to ask what proportion of patients who take antipsychotic drugs or other drugs which can also cause these problems (Phenergan, Compazine, and Reglan) get drug-induced parkinsonism. In various groups of patients in whom this has been studied, the range is from 15 to 52%.[85] In one study, 26% of older adults (60 and over) taking haloperidol (HALDOL) devel-

oped drug-induced parkinsonism.[86] Other studies have shown an overall incidence of 15.4% but, among patients over 60, the incidence was approximately 40%.[87] In the same study, 90% of the cases of drug-induced parkinsonism began within 72 days after starting the drug.

In older persons the symptoms of an adverse drug reaction may be mistaken for a new disease or attributed to the normal process of aging. The chance of such misinterpretation is more likely when symptoms of an adverse reaction are indistinguishable from an illness common in the elderly, such as Parkinson's disease.

A study published in the *Journal of the American Medical Association* reported that the likelihood of being treated for Parkinson's disease increases threefold in elderly patients taking the antinausea drug metoclopramide. The most troubling finding of this study, according to the authors, was the extent to which adverse metoclopramide reactions were treated with levodopa-containing drugs carrying increased risk of toxicity at greater cost, but offering little likelihood of benefit.[88]

Restless leg (akathisia): Another very common adverse effect of these drugs is the restless leg syndrome, in which the person restlessly paces around and describes having the "jitters." When seated, the patient often taps his or her feet. Not infrequently, this might be interpreted as needing *more* antipsychotic medicine. Instead of reducing the dose of the drug or stopping it entirely, more of the drug causing the problem may be used.

Weakness and muscle fatigue (akinesia): The most common of this group of drug-induced nerve problems (extrapyramidal reactions) is when the patient appears listless, disinterested, and depressed. This drug-induced problem is often misdiagnosed as primary depression, and the patient is put on antidepressant drugs. Giving these drugs along with the antipsychotic drugs even further increases the risk of serious adverse effects. Once again, instead of recognizing a drug-induced problem and either stopping or lowering the dose of the drug, another drug is added making things even worse.

Although seen as a component of parkinsonism, akinesia can also occur on its own. Additional problems can include infrequent blinking, slower swallowing of saliva with subsequent drooling, and a lack of facial expression.

As a general rule, if any elderly person on psychoactive medication—sleeping pills, antianxiety tranquilizers, antidepressants, or antipsychotic drugs—appears to be doing poorly, first think about reducing the dose or stopping the drug rather than adding another drug.

Anticholinergic adverse effects

The two types of anticholinergic effects (see Glossary, p. 768.) are those affecting the brain, such as confusion, delirium, short-term memory problems, disorientation, and impaired attention and those affecting the rest of the body. The latter type includes dry mouth, constipation, retention of urine (especially in men with an enlarged prostate), blurred vision, decreased sweating with increased body temperature, sexual dysfunction, and worsening of glaucoma. These adverse effects are much more common in the so-called high-dose antipsychotic drugs (see chart below).

Sedation

Sedation is one of the most common adverse effects of the antipsychotic drugs, especially with the high-dose drugs. Since these drugs are often improperly prescribed as sleeping pills, older adults will often have a decreased level of functioning during the day. In nonpsychotic older adults, the largest group being given these drugs, the quality of sleep is extremely unpleasant. The frightening aspects of this drug-induced disturbed sleep can last up to 24 hours after a single dose.

Hypotensive effects: lowering of blood pressure to levels that are too low

Orthostatic (postural) hypotension, or the fall in blood pressure which occurs when someone stands up suddenly, is a common adverse effect of antipsychotic drugs, especially in older adults. It can be even more troublesome if the person is already at increased risk for this problem because he or she is taking other drugs to treat high blood pressure. As a result

ADVERSE EFFECTS OF ANTIPSYCHOTIC DRUGS

Generic/Brand Name	Sedative	Anticholinergic (dry mouth, urine retention, confusion)	Extrapyramidal (parkinsonism)	Hypotensive
chlorpromazine/THORAZINE	strong	strong	moderate	strong
thioridazine/MELLARIL	strong	strong	mild	moderate
trifluoperazine/STELAZINE	mild	mild	strong	moderate
fluphenazine/PROLIXIN	mild	mild	strong	mild
haloperidol/HALDOL	mild	mild	strong	mild
loxapine/LOXITANE	mild	mild	strong	mild
thiothixene/NAVANE	mild	mild	strong	moderate
clozapine/CLOZARIL	strong	strong	mild	strong
olanzapine/ZYPREXA	mild	moderate	mild	strong
risperidone/RISPERDAL	strong	mild	strong	moderate

mild = mild adverse effects
moderate = moderate adverse effects
strong = strong adverse effects[89]

of such a drug-induced drop in blood pressure, falls which result in injury, heart attacks, and strokes can occur. For this reason, before starting one of these drugs, the person's blood pressure should be taken both in the lying position and after standing for two minutes. This should be repeated after the person has used the drug for several weeks. People taking these drugs should rise *slowly* from a lying position and wear supportive stockings to help prevent hypotension. This adverse effect is also seen more often with the use of the higher dose drugs, such as chlorpromazine (THORAZINE), but occurs with all of the antipsychotic drugs.

Other adverse effects

Other adverse effects include weight gain, poor ability to withstand high or low temperatures (because these drugs affect the body's temperature regulation center), increased sensitivity to sunlight and other skin problems, bone marrow toxicity, and abnormal heart rhythms.

How To Reduce the Risks of These Antipsychotic Drugs

• *Give antipsychotic drugs only to people who need them*. The majority, at least 80%, of older adults being prescribed these drugs should not be getting them, and the serious adverse effects are just as harmful in them as in the small fraction of people for whom the drugs are appropriate (people with schizophrenia). Thus, the most effective way of reducing the risk of these drugs for most older adults is to stop using them. Unless the patient has schizophrenia or another psychotic condition, beginning to use them or continuing to use them provides significant risks without compensating benefits. These drugs are also not effective for psychoses seen with senile dementia.[90] As discussed on p. 192, the use of these powerful drugs for older people who have depression is fraught with a high incidence— 60%—of tardive dyskinesia.

Antipsychotic drugs should never be used as sleeping pills or to treat anxiety.

• *Start with the lowest possible dose*. For older adults this is usually one-tenth to two-fifths the dose for younger adults. Use the drug for as short a period of time as possible.[91] If, however, the use of antipsychotic drugs is indicated, the first thing to realize is that as is the case for many drugs for older adults, the starting dose and, very likely, the eventually used dose should be lower than the dose for younger adults. There are three reasons why this is so for the antipsychotic drugs:

First, kidney function in older adults decreases, which means that the drugs last longer in the body. They get more "mileage" out of a given dose. Second, because of a decrease in an important brain chemical, dopamine, as people age, there is an increased risk in older adults of the adverse effects, such as drug-induced parkinsonism or akinesia. Third, because of another change in brain metabolism with aging, there is an increased sensitivity to the anticholinergic (see Glossary, p. 768) effects of these drugs, such as confusion, delirium, dry mouth, difficulty urinating, constipation and worsening of glaucoma.[92]

• *Pay attention to the adverse effect profile of the drugs* (see comparison chart on p. 194). As mentioned previously, the antipsychotic drugs are all quite similar in their effectiveness for treating psychoses, but differ mainly in the spectrum of their adverse effects. The chart shows a great difference in the severity of the adverse reactions, depending on whether the drug is a less potent or more potent one.

At the top of the list is the less potent, higher dose chlorpromazine (THORAZINE). It causes more sedative, anticholinergic, and hypotensive effects, but has a relatively lower risk of the extrapyramidal effects, such as restless leg and drug-induced parkinsonism. In the middle of the list are more potent, lower dose drugs, such as haloperidol (HALDOL) and thiothixene (NAVANE). They cause fewer sedative, anticholinergic, and hypotensive adverse effects, but have a higher risk of the extrapyramidal adverse effects, such as drug-induced parkinsonism. At the bottom of the list are drugs which have more recently come on the market.

Since all of these drugs are equally effective, the choice depends on which adverse effects would likely be or are most intolerable. For a person with a tendency to become faint or dizzy upon standing (orthostatic, postural hypotension), the addition of Thorazine with its high risk of lowering blood pressure would not be a good idea. Instead, if drug treatment is really necessary, one of the more potent drugs with fewer hypotensive and sedative effects might be a better choice. Similarly, people who already have trouble walking or who have trouble with their posture would be at much greater risk if they developed one of the extrapyramidal adverse effects of Haldol, Navane, or the other more potent antipsychotic drugs. Therefore, these people would probably do better on one of the less potent drugs with fewer extrapyramidal adverse effects. The most important consideration is to adjust the dose or change or discontinue drugs when and if adverse effects occur. This is especially true when the adverse effects are as bad or worse than the original reason for starting the drug.

DEPRESSION: WHEN ARE DRUGS CALLED FOR AND WHICH ONES SHOULD YOU USE?

Should Everyone Who Is Sad or Depressed Take Antidepressants?

Although depression is the most common mental illness in older adults, everyone who is sad or depressed is not a candidate for these powerful drugs.

Kinds of Depression

Drug-induced depression

Ironically, one of the kinds of depression that should not be treated with drugs is depression *caused* by other kinds of drugs. If someone is depressed and the depression started after beginning a new drug, it may well be drug-caused. Commonly used drugs known to cause depression include the following:

• Barbiturates such as phenobarbital
• Tranquilizers such as diazepam (VALIUM) and triazolam (HALCION)
• Heart drugs containing reserpine (SER-AP-ES and others)
• Beta-blockers such as propranolol (INDERAL)
• High blood pressure drugs such as clonidine (CATAPRES), methyldopa (ALDOMET), and prazosin (MINIPRESS)
• Drugs for treating abnormal heart rhythms such as disopyramide (NORPACE)
• Ulcer drugs such as cimetidine (TAGAMET) and ranitidine (ZANTAC)
• Antiparkinsonians such as levodopa (LARODOPA) and bromocriptine (PARLODEL)
• Corticosteroids such as cortisone (CORTONE) and prednisone (DELTASONE)
• Anticonvulsants such as phenytoin (DILANTIN), ethosuximide (ZARONTIN), and primidone (MYSOLINE)
• Antibiotics such as cycloserine (SEROMYCIN), ethionamide (TRECATOR-SC), ciprofloxacin (CIPRO) and metronidazole (FLAGYL)
• Diet drugs such as amphetamines (during withdrawal from the drug)
• Painkillers or arthritis drugs such as pentazocine (TALWIN), indomethacin (INDOCIN), and ibuprofen (MOTRIN, ADVIL)
• The acne drug isotretinoin (ACCUTANE)
• Other drugs including metrizamide (AMIPAQUE), a drug used for diagnosing slipped discs, and disulfiram (ANTABUSE), the alcoholism treatment drug.[93]

The remedy for this kind of depression is to reduce the dose of the drug or stop it altogether if possible. If necessary, switch to another drug that does not cause depression.

Another major cause of drug-induced depression is alcoholism, the treatment of which is difficult.

Situational or reactive depression

Other causes of depression which should not be treated with antidepressant drugs are the "normal" reactions to life problems, such as the loss of a spouse, friend, relative, or job, or other situations that normally make almost anyone sad. If the depression is clearly a response to overwhelming life crises, antidepressants have little value. Other options such as support from family and friends, psychotherapy with a mental health professional, or a change in your environment, are worth exploring.[94] Doing something nice for yourself, talking with a friend, and exercising every day can help you get through these difficult situations.

Medical conditions that can cause depression

Older adults (or anyone) who appear depressed may have a thyroid disorder, a type of cancer, such as pancreatic, bowel, brain, or lymph node (lymphoma), viral pneumonia, or hepatitis.[95,96] In addition, there is evidence that people who have had a stroke or who have Parkinson's disease or Alzheimer's disease may become depressed and, in some cases, may respond to antidepressant drugs.[97]

A major depressive episode: the kind that will usually respond to drugs

If a depressed mood accompanied by several of the following problems has been present for at least several weeks, and a careful history, physical exam, and lab tests have ruled out specific causes of depression, true primary depression is probably the diagnosis. The problems are sadness that impairs normal functioning, difficulty concentrating, low self-esteem, guilt, suicidal thoughts, extreme fatigue, low energy level or agitation, sleep disturbances (increased or decreased), or appetite disturbance (increased or decreased) with associated weight change.[98] Since suicidal thoughts and attempts often characterize depression, the possibility of suicide using antidepressant drugs has to be kept in mind and only a small number of pills (see p. 200) prescribed at one time. Another way of describing the pervasive nature of this kind of severe depression is that the person displays—and relates if asked—a sense of "helplessness, hopelessness, worthlessness and uselessness . . . as well as intense feelings of guilt over real or imagined shortcomings or indiscretions."[99]

Although depression in older adults is usually unipolar (depression alone), occasionally there is a bipolar pattern with alternation of depression and mania. The latter shows up as an elated mood, rapid flow of ideas, and increased "energy." The patient, often seeming hyperactive during this manic phase, can be intrusive, have an infectious sense of humor, and may show poor judgment in business or personal affairs, not infrequently going on spending sprees.[100] Lithium is often successfully used to treat people with bipolar disease (see p. 217).

Serious depressive illness is far less frequent in the elderly. According to data from the National Institute of Mental Health, while nearly 4% of people age 25 to 44 have had a major depression recently, fewer than 1% of people 65 and over have had this misfortune. In spite of this, about one-third of antidepressants are prescribed for people 60 and over even though they make up just one-sixth of the population.

Some of this apparent "overtreatment" may be due to failing to diagnose drug-induced depression and, instead, the use of a second drug to treat the depression caused by the first.

Other Uses—Usually Inappropriate—for Antidepressants

In addition to drug-induced depression, medical conditions which can cause depression and situational or reactive depression—none of which merit treatment with antidepressants—there are other circumstances in which antidepressants are inappropriately dished out. In one community-based study, more than 50% of older people who had been taking antidepressants for a year or more had been started without a clear history of depression. Of these, one-half (or one out of four of all people using antidepressants) were using antidepressants as a sleeping pill and others were given the drugs as alternatives to tranquilizers.[101] In view of the significant adverse effects of these drugs, their use for such purposes will cause risks which will outweigh the benefits.

What Is the Best and Worst Treatment for Severe Depression?

Everyone with the kind of severe depression described above should be evaluated by a mental health professional to determine what kind of psychotherapy would best supplement the antidepressant drugs that are going to be used.

The decision as to which drug is best will depend largely on choosing one with the fewest adverse effects, since all antidepressants are equally effective.[102] If depression has occurred previously and responded to one of the drugs without too many adverse effects, that would be the best one to try first. Otherwise, the table on p. 200 compares the 11 tricyclic antidepressants that are listed in this book as well as fluoxetine (PROZAC) and bupropion (WELLBUTRIN).

The Main Risks of Antidepressant Drugs

The four most common groups of adverse effects are anticholinergic, sedative, hypotensive (blood-pressure-lowering), and those effects on heart rate or rhythm. Two serious risks arising from the adverse effects are hip fractures and automobile crashes.

Hip fractures

A study of 1,021 older adults with hip fractures found that 14% of these life-threatening injuries are attributable to the use of mind-affecting drugs, including sleeping pills and minor tranquilizers, antipsychotics, and antidepressants.[103]

There are approximately 227,000 hip fractures each year in the United States, virtually all in older adults.[104] Since the above study found that 14% of hip fractures are drug-induced, this means that if the results of the study are projected nationally, approximately 32,000 hip fractures a year in older adults are caused by the use of mind-affecting drugs. Approximately 60% of these hip fractures are caused by antidepressant drugs.

The selective serotonin reuptake inhibitor (SSRI) antidepressants such as Prozac, Zoloft, and Paxil (see p. 233) are promoted as having fewer adverse effects than the older tricyclic antidepressants such as Elavil (see p. 216) and Tofranil (see p. 203). Canadian researchers recently reported that the SSRIs do not offer any advantage over the older antidepressants with regards to the risk of hip fracture.[105]

Automobile crashes that cause injury

A study involving 495 automobile crashes in older drivers in which an injury occurred found that a significant number of such crashes in older adults aged 65–84 were attributable to the use of benzodiazepine tranquilizers and tricyclic antidepressants. The study was particularly impressive because its findings were strengthened by observing that the rate of crashes that caused injury increased in the same group of people when they were using these drugs as opposed to when they were not using the drugs. The majority of the excess number of auto crashes that caused injury were attributable to the benzodiazepines. The authors, stating that the study findings may be generalizable to the population at large, found that if the association is causal, at least 16,000 auto crashes that caused injury each year in older drivers are attributable to psychoactive drug use (specifically benzodiazepines and tricyclic antidepressants) out of the 217,000 crashes that caused injury that occur each year among elderly drivers.[106]

ANTICHOLINERGIC EFFECTS

WARNING: SPECIAL MENTAL AND PHYSICAL ADVERSE EFFECTS

Older adults are especially sensitive to the harmful anticholinergic (see Glossary, p. 768) effects of tricyclic antidepressants. Drugs in this family should not be used unless absolutely necessary.

Mental Effects: confusion, delirium, short-term memory problems, disorientation, and impaired attention.

Physical Effects: dry mouth, constipation, difficulty urinating (especially for a man with an enlarged prostate), blurred vision, decreased sweating with increased body temperature, sexual dysfunction, and worsening of glaucoma.

Sedative effects

Most older adults who think they have a sleeping problem do not have the kind of severe depression that justifies the use of these drugs. (See p. 185 for a discussion of nondrug treatments for sleeplessness.) Nevertheless, if the sleep disorder is a consequence of severe depression, the "adverse effect" of sedation may be useful as long as it does not produce too much sedation, with the risk of falling. This is an important consideration especially in people who already have some impairment of thinking, increased confusion, disorientation, and agitation.[107]

Hypotensive effects: lowering of blood pressure to levels that are too low

Orthostatic (postural) hypotension, or the fall in blood pressure that occurs when someone stands up suddenly, is a common adverse effect of antidepressants, especially in older adults. It can be even more troublesome if the person is already at increased risk for this problem because he or she is taking other drugs to treat high blood pressure. As a result of such a drug-induced drop in blood pressure, falls that result in injury, heart attacks, and strokes can occur. For this reason, before starting treatment with one of these antidepressants, blood pressure should be taken both in the lying position and after standing for two minutes. This should be repeated after using the drug for several weeks.

Drug-induced parkinsonism

Like the antipsychotic drugs, many antidepressants can also cause drug-induced parkinsonism (see p. 193). Drug-induced parkinsonism involves the following symptoms: difficulty speaking or swallowing; loss of balance; mask-like face; muscle spasms; stiffness of arms or legs; trembling and shaking; unusual twisting movements of body.

Effects on heart rate and rhythm

These drugs can cause the heart to speed up. They can also cause a slowing down in the conduction of electricity through the heart, which is especially dangerous if someone already has heart block.[108] For this reason, a baseline electrocardiogram should be taken before starting any antidepressant therapy.

Mania induced by serotonin reuptake inhibitors

All currently available antidepressant drugs appear able to induce hypomanic and manic reactions.[109,110] This is a serious concern for people taking the serotonin reuptake inhibitor group of antidepressants which includes the selective serotonin reuptake inhibitors (SSRIs) such as fluoxetine[111] but also the antidepressants such as nefazodone that have a combined effect on serotonin and norepinephrine reuptake.[112] This reaction can be severe having psychotic features or requiring patients to be secluded for extreme agitation.[113]

ADVERSE EFFECTS OF ANTIDEPRESSANTS

Generic/Brand Names	Anticholinergics*	Sedative	Hypotensive Effect	Heart Rate/ Rhythm
fluoxetine/PROZAC**	none	none	none	none
paroxetine/PAXIL**	none	none	none	none
sertraline/ZOLOFT**	none	none	none	none
fluvoxamine/LUVOX**	none	none	none	none
bupropion/WELLBUTRIN**	mild	none	none	none
desipramine/NORPRAMIN	mild	mild	mild	mild
nortriptyline/AVENTYL, PAMELOR	moderate	mild	mild	mild
amoxapine/ASENDIN	moderate	mild	moderate	moderate
maprotiline/LUDIOMIL	moderate	moderate	moderate	mild
trazodone/DESYREL	mild	moderate	moderate	moderate
imipramine/TOFRANIL	moderate	moderate	moderate	moderate
doxepin/SINEQUAN	moderate	strong	moderate	moderate
amitriptyline/ELAVIL	strong	strong	moderate	strong

mild = mild adverse effects
moderate = moderate adverse effects
strong = strong adverse effects

* see p. 199
** There is inadequate information for these drugs in older people to ensure that the risk of the adverse effects is as low as it appears; there is more information about nortriptyline and desipramine as far as their reduced amount of adverse effects on older adults in comparison with the drugs listed above them.

These listings are a composite of comparative ratings of 11 of these drugs by four other researchers[114] and information from the references listed for fluoxetine and bupropion on the drug profiles.

As can be seen from the chart below, the drugs with the fewest overall adverse effects in older adults are desipramine (NORPRAMIN), which has a "mild" for all four kinds of adverse effects, and nortriptyline (AVENTYL, PAMELOR), which is "mild" for three of the four. Fluoxetine (PROZAC) and bupropion (WELLBUTRIN) may have as few or fewer adverse effects as desipramine and nortriptyline but adequate comparative studies on older adults have not yet been published. The drug with the worst adverse effects profile in older adults is amitriptyline (ELAVIL), with "strong" adverse effects for three of the four categories. We list this drug as **Do Not Use.**

If the adverse effects of whichever drug is selected are too severe, or if the drug does not seem to be working, talk to your doctor about switching to a drug less likely to cause the troublesome effects.

How To Reduce the Adverse Effects of Any of these Antidepressants

• Have a baseline electrocardiogram and blood pressure taken before starting.[115]
• Start with a dose of one-third to one-half the usual adult dose, meaning 15–25 milligrams a day, at bedtime. Increase the dose very slowly.[116] It may take three weeks to see an effect. A trial with one of these drugs should continue until it either works or causes persistent adverse effects.[117]
• Get a prescription for only one week's worth of pills since more pills increase the chance of a successful suicide attempt by people who are severely depressed.[118]
• Lower the dose gradually, as symptoms dictate, after successful treatment for several months.[119]

It is important to realize that long-term treatment with antidepressants is not always necessary even when the drug is being used to treat the kind of serious depression for which its use is proper. In one study, after patients had been successfully treated for four months with antidepressants, half were continued on their drugs and the other half were switched to a placebo. After an additional two months, most of the patients—either on the actual drug or the placebo—were still doing well, only about one-fourth, the same in both groups, had relapsed.[120]

Other recommendations for more effective and safer use of these drugs include:[121]

1. When starting a drug for a specific depressive illness, the doctor should monitor your response carefully to see if a different dose [or drug] should be used.

2. It should be made clear to you that depression can be an episodic illness, that recovery is expected and that the treatment will probably eventually be stopped.

3. If treatment with drugs is started as a trial in possible depression, you should be informed that it is a trial and that treatment will continue for a specified time, depending on the response of key symptoms.

4. The possibility of adverse effects should be evaluated carefully before these drugs are used primarily as sleeping pills or as an alternative to tranquilizers in the elderly.

DRUG PROFILES

Limited Use

Zolpidem
AMBIEN (Searle)

GENERIC: not available
FAMILY: Hypnotic/sedative

Zolpidem (*zole* pi dem) is used for short-term relief of insomnia. Although not classified as a benzodiazepine (related to Valium), zolpidem shares many similarities with that family of drugs.[122] Like the benzodiazepine family of drugs, zolpidem can cause drowsiness. Since it can be habit-forming, zolpidem is a controlled substance. Unlike the benzodiazepine family of drugs, zolpidem lacks most muscle relaxant and anticonvulsant action. Zolpidem is recommended to be used for one to three weeks. It acts quickly and stays in the body a short time, but in older people remains somewhat longer than in younger people. The recommended dose for older people is 5 mg. No additional benefit is gained by higher doses, which are more apt to cause adverse effects. People with kidney problems may require a lower dose. Older individuals are more apt to experience confusion or fall while taking zolpidem.

The best way to reduce the risks from sleeping pills and tranquilizers is to avoid them if at all possible. Before taking one of these powerful medications, see p. 185 for nondrug alternatives to try before using either sleeping pills or tranquilizers.

Before You Use This Drug

Tell your doctor if you have or have had:

- alcohol or drug abuse problems
- allergies to any drugs or lactose intolerance
- kidney or liver problems
- mental depression or suicidal feelings
- smoked
- sleep apnea

Tell your doctor about any other drugs you take, including asprin, herbs, vitamins, and other nonprescription products.

When You Use This Drug

• Until you know how you react to this drug do not drive or perform other activities requiring alertness.

• Do not drink alcohol or use other drugs that can cause drowsiness.

How to Use This Drug

• Do not take until ready to go to bed. Do not take at all if you will not get a full night's sleep, for example needing to wake up after a plane ride of less than eight hours.

• Take on an empty stomach. Food slows absorption.

• Do not increase the dose.

• Do not store in the bathroom. Do not expose to heat, moisture, or strong light.

• If you miss a dose, take it as soon as you remember, but skip it if it is almost time for the next dose. **Do not take double doses.**

• If you decide to stop taking this drug after several weeks or months, check with your doctor about a plan to taper off zolpidem.

Interactions with Other Drugs

The following drugs are listed in the *Evaluations of Drug Interactions* 1997 as causing "highly clinically significant" or "clinically significant" interactions when used together with this drug. We have also included potentially serious interactions listed in the drug's FDA-approved professional product labeling or package insert. New scientific techniques have allowed researchers to predict some drug interactions before they have been documented in people. There may be other drugs, especially those in the families of drugs listed below, that also will react with this drug to cause severe adverse effects. The number of new drugs approved for marketing increases the chance of drug interactions, and new drug interactions are being identified with old drugs. Be vigilant. Make sure to tell your doctor and pharmacist the drugs you are taking and tell your doctor if you are taking any of these interacting drugs:

Central nervous system (CNS) depressant drugs including alcohol, antidepressants, antihistamines, antipsychotics, some blood pressure medications (reserpine, methyldopa, beta-blockers), motion sickness medications, muscle relaxants, narcotics, sedatives, sleeping pills and tranquilizers.

Adverse Effects

Call your doctor immediately if you experience:

• difficulty breathing
• irregular heartbeat
• clumsiness or unsteadiness
• swelling of face
• confusion
• dizziness or falls
• depression
• unusual excitement or nervousness
• hallucinations
• insomnia
• memory loss
• vision changes

Call your doctor if these symptoms continue:

• back pain or muscle aches
• diarrhea
• drowsiness during the day
• drugged feeling
• dry mouth
• flu-like symptoms
• headache
• nausea or vomiting
• sleepwalking[123]
• rash

Call your doctor if these symptoms continue after you stop taking the drug:

• abdominal or stomach cramps
• agitation, nervousness or feelings of panic
• flushing

- lightheadedness
- muscle cramps
- nausea or vomiting
- worsening of mental or emotional problems
- seizures
- sweating, tremors
- unusual tiredness or weakness

One hazard of taking zolpidem continuously for longer than several weeks is drug-induced dependence. **Do not stop taking your drug suddenly.** With the help of your doctor, work out a schedule for slowly decreasing the amount of the drug you take by about 5 to 10% each day. Keep a written record of the dosage reduction schedule with you. These steps will make it much easier to become drug free without developing distressing symptoms of drug withdrawal.

Limited Use

Amoxapine (a *mox* a peen)
ASENDIN (Lederle)

Doxepin (*dox* e pin)
SINEQUAN (Pfizer)

Imipramine (im *ip* ra meen)
TOFRANIL (Novartis)

GENERIC: available
FAMILY: Antidepressants (See p. 196 for discussion of depression.)

These medications are used to treat severe depression that is not caused by other drugs, by alcohol, or by emotional losses (such as a death in the family). You should *not* be taking them for anxiety or mild depression, or as a sleeping pill. Because these drugs have more harmful adverse effects (see chart, p. 200) than the two antidepressants desipramine and nortriptyline

(see p. 230), we consider them to be of limited use to older adults.

If you are over 60, you will generally need to take one-third to one-half the dose used by younger adults. If the initial dose is not enough and needs to be increased, this should be done very slowly.

Amoxapine can cause tardive dyskinesia—uncontrolled movements of the jaws, tongue, and lips—an effect also seen with antipsychotic drugs (see p. 192). Doxepin has especially strong sedative effects.

The length of time it takes an antidepressant to work can overlap with the time of spontaneous recovery, especially if the depression is situational—caused by a death or other external circumstances. The majority of people lift themselves out of depression with friends, or activities such as exercise, work, reading, play, art, travel, and spiritual resources. If depression is not overcome by these measures, seek help from mental health professionals, such as therapists or psychiatrists. Antidepressant drugs should be reserved for depression that is major and does not respond to psychotherapy alone.

WARNING: SPECIAL MENTAL AND PHYSICAL ADVERSE EFFECTS

Older adults are especially sensitive to the harmful anticholinergic (see Glossary, p. 768) effects of antidepressants such as these. Drugs in this family should not be used unless absolutely necessary.

Mental Effects: confusion, delirium, short-term memory problems, disorientation, and impaired attention.

Physical Effects: dry mouth, constipation, difficulty urinating (especially for a man with an enlarged prostate), blurred vision, decreased sweating with increased body temperature, sexual dysfunction, and worsening of glaucoma.

Before You Use This Drug

Tell your doctor if you have or have had:

- allergies to drugs
- alcohol dependence
- asthma
- bipolar disorder (manic-depressive illness) or schizophrenia
- blood disorders
- convulsions (seizures)
- difficulty urinating or enlarged prostate
- glaucoma
- heart or blood vessel disease
- high blood pressure
- schizophrenia
- kidney or liver problems
- overactive thyroid
- stomach or intestinal disease

Tell your doctor about any other drugs you take, including aspirin, herbs, vitamins, and other nonprescription products.

Ask your doctor to check your blood pressure, once while you are lying down and once after you have been standing up for at least two minutes, and to do an electrocardiogram.

When You Use This Drug

- **Do not stop taking this drug suddenly. Your doctor must give you a schedule to lower your dose gradually, to prevent withdrawal symptoms** such as headache, mood change, nausea, vomiting, diarrhea, or trouble sleeping and vivid dreams.
- Until you know how you react to this drug, do not drive or perform other activities requiring alertness. These drugs may cause blurred vision and drowsiness.
- It may take several weeks before you can tell that these drugs are working. If the drug works, talk with your doctor about gradually lowering the dose.
- Do not smoke. Smoking may increase the drug's effects on your heart.

- Do not drink alcohol or use other drugs that can cause drowsiness.
- You may feel dizzy when rising from a lying or sitting position. When getting out of bed, hang your legs over the side of the bed for a few minutes, then get up slowly. When getting up from a chair, stay beside the chair until you are sure that you are not dizzy. (See p. 16.)
- Check with your doctor before taking any other drugs, prescription or nonprescription. These drugs frequently interact with other drugs.
- The effects of these drugs may last for up to a week after you stop taking them. Avoid alcohol and heed all other warnings for this time period.
- If you plan to have any surgery, including dental, tell your doctor that you take one of these drugs.

How to Use This Drug

- Take with food to reduce stomach upset.
- If you are taking any other drugs, take them one to two hours before you take your antidepressant.
- Capsules may be opened and mixed with food or drink.
- Do not store in the bathroom. Do not expose to heat, moisture, or strong light.
- *If you miss a dose, use the following guidelines:* If you are taking more than one dose a day of one of these drugs, take the missed dose as soon as you remember, but skip it if it is almost time for the next dose.

If you are taking your drug only once a day at bedtime, and you go to sleep without taking that dose, do not take it in the morning. Instead, call your doctor.

Do not take double doses.

Interactions with Other Drugs

The following drugs are listed in the *Evaluations of Drug Interactions* 1997 as causing "highly clinically significant" or "clinically significant" interactions when used together with this drug. We have also included potentially serious interactions listed in the drug's FDA-approved professional product labeling or package insert. New scientific techniques have allowed researchers to predict some drug interactions before they have been documented in people. There may be other drugs, especially those in the families of drugs listed below, that also will react with this drug to cause severe adverse effects. The number of new drugs approved for marketing increases the chance of drug interactions, and new drug interactions are being identified with old drugs. Be vigilant. Make sure to tell your doctor and pharmacist the drugs you are taking and tell your doctor if you are taking any of these interacting drugs:

ADRENALIN (also in bee sting kits), alcohol, cimetidine, CYTOMEL, epinephrine, guanethidine, IMDUR, ISMELIN, ISMO, ISORDIL, isosorbide, liothyronine, MELLARIL, nitroglycerin (sublingual), NITROBID, NITROSTAT, PARNATE, PRIMATENE MIST, SORBITRATE, TAGAMET, tramadol, thioridazine, tolazamide, TOLINASE, TRANSDERM-NITRO, TRIOSTAT, tranylcypromine, ULTRAM.

Adverse Effects

Call your doctor immediately if you experience:

- **signs of overdose:** confusion, severe drowsiness, fever, hallucinations, restlessness and agitation, seizures, breathing difficulty, irregular heartbeat, unusual tiredness, weakness, vomiting, enlarged pupils
  - irregular blood pressure
  - loss of bladder control
  - severe muscle stiffness
  - pale skin
  - blurred vision

- constipation
- confusion, delirium, or hallucinations
- decreased sexual ability
- difficulty in speaking or swallowing
- eye pain
- fainting
- loss of balance control
- mask-like face
- difficulty urinating
- shakiness or trembling
- shuffling walk
- slowed movements
- stiffness of arms and legs
- anxiety
- breast enlargement in both males and females
- hair loss
- inappropriate secretion of milk
- increased sensitivity to sunlight
- irritability
- twitching muscle
- red or brownish spots on skin
- ringing or buzzing in the ears
- skin rash and itching
- sore throat and fever
- swelling of face and tongue
- swelling of testicles
- trouble with teeth or gums
- yellow skin or eyes

For amoxapine only:

- **signs of tardive dyskinesia:** lip smacking, chewing movements, puffing of cheeks, rapid, darting tongue movements, uncontrolled movements of arms or legs

Call your doctor if these symptoms continue:

- diarrhea
- dizziness
- dry mouth
- headache
- heartburn
- insomnia
- nausea or vomiting
- increased appetite for sweets

- unpleasant taste in mouth
- weight gain
- trouble sleeping

Call your doctor if these symptoms continue after you stop taking the drugs:

- headache
- irritability
- nausea and vomiting
- diarrhea
- restlessness or unusual excitement
- insomnia

Periodic Tests

Ask your doctor which of these tests should be done periodically while you are taking this drug:

- complete blood count
- blood pressure
- pulse
- glaucoma tests
- liver function tests
- kidney function tests
- heart function tests such as electrocardiogram (ECG, EKG)
- dental exams (at least twice yearly)
- plasma tricyclic determinations

PREGNANCY WARNING

Asendin caused harm to developing fetuses in animal studies, or such studies were not done. Use during pregnancy only for clear medical reasons. Tell your doctor if you are pregnant or thinking of becoming pregnant before you take this drug.

Limited Use

Buspirone
BUSPAR (Bristol-Myers Squibb)

GENERIC: not available
FAMILY: Tranquilizers (see p. 178)

Buspirone (*bu* spire own) is an antianxiety agent, which differs chemically from the benzodiazepine drugs (see p. 178) and appears to lack the potential for addiction common to this family of drugs, such as Xanax and Valium. While buspirone is less apt than the benzodiazepines to cause drowsiness, drowsiness remains a common side effect. Although buspirone is preferred for older adults, compared to other drugs available,[124] information about buspirone is limited, and much is still unknown including its long-term safety and effectiveness.[125,126] Adverse effects are often paradoxical (drowsiness or insomnia, anorexia or weight gain). While buspirone is used for short-term anxiety, it takes a few weeks to work. In some people buspirone may increase anxiety, rather than alleviate it.[127] A decision to use buspirone should be reviewed periodically.

Anxiety is a universal emotion closely allied with appropriate fears.[128] No drug is useful for the stress of everyday living. Try nondrug therapies for anxiety first. Explore preventable causes of anxiety, such as overuse of caffeine, as well as medical/physical causes. Drugs may control but do not cure anxiety.

If you already take a benzodiazepine (see p. 178) or antidepressant (see p. 196), your doctor should taper you off those drugs before trying buspirone. However, if you have already taken a benzodiazepine, the buspirone is less likely to be effective.[129]

The best way to reduce the risks from sleeping pills and tranquilizers is to avoid them if at all possible. Before taking one of these powerful medications, see p. 185 for nondrug alternatives to try before using either sleeping pills or tranquilizers.

Before You Use This Drug

Tell your doctor if you have or have had:

- allergies to drugs
- alcohol or drug dependence
- high blood pressure
- kidney or liver problems
- thyroid disease

Tell your doctor about any other drugs you take, including aspirin, herbs, vitamins, and other nonprescription products.

When You Use This Drug

- Do not drink alcohol or use other drugs that can cause drowsiness.
- Until you know how you react to this drug, do not drive or perform other activities that require alertness. Buspirone may cause blurred vision and drowsiness.
- If you plan to have any surgery, including dental, tell your doctor that you take this drug.
- Do not take other drugs without checking with your doctor first—especially nonprescription drugs for appetite control, colds, coughs, hay fever, sinus problems, or sleep.

How to Use This Drug

- Swallow drug whole, or break in half to ease swallowing.
- If you miss a dose, take it as soon as you remember, but skip it if it is almost time for the next dose. **Do not take double doses.**
- Do not store in the bathroom. Do not expose to heat, moisture, or strong light.

Interactions with Other Drugs

The following drugs are listed in the *Evaluations of Drug Interactions* 1997 as causing "highly clinically significant" or "clinically significant" interactions when used together with this drug. We have also included potentially serious interactions listed in the drug's FDA-approved professional product labeling or package insert. New scientific techniques have allowed researchers to predict some drug interactions before they have been documented in people. There may be other drugs, especially those in the families of drugs listed below, that also will react with this drug to cause severe adverse effects. The number of new drugs approved for marketing increases the chance of drug interactions, and new drug interactions are being identified with old drugs. Be vigilant. Make sure to tell your doctor and pharmacist the drugs you are taking and tell your doctor if you are taking any of these interacting drugs:

Taking buspirone with any MAO (monoamine oxidase) inhibitors may increase your blood pressure. Do not take buspirone for at least 10 days after stopping any of these monoamine oxidase (MAO) inhibitors: deprenyl, ELDEPRYL, furazolidone, FUROXONE, isocarboxazid, MARPLAN, MATULANE, NARDIL, PARNATE, phenelzine, procarbazine, selegiline, tranylcypromine.

Adverse Effects

Call your doctor immediately if you experience:

- **signs of overdose**: severe dizziness, severe drowsiness, dry mouth, severe nausea and vomiting, unusually small pupils
- chest pain

- confusion or depression
- fast or pounding heartbeat
- sore throat or fever
- muscle weakness
- numbness, tingling, pain or weakness in hands or feet
- uncontrolled movements of the body

Call your doctor if these symptoms continue:

- anger, hostility
- blurred vision
- dizziness, lightheadedness
- constipation or diarrhea
- sleep or dream disturbance[130]
- drowsiness
- headache
- dry mouth
- involuntary movements
- muscle pain, spasms, cramps, stiffness
- nasal congestion
- numbness
- restlessness, nervousness, insomnia, nightmares
- ringing in ears
- sweating
- unusual weakness, tiredness
- upset stomach
- urinary problems

Periodic Tests

Ask your doctor which of these tests should be done periodically while you are taking this drug:

- kidney function tests
- liver function tests

 Do Not Use

ALTERNATIVE TREATMENT:
See nondrug approaches, p. 185, Oxazepam, p. 242, and Buspirone, p. 206. See also Tranquilizers and Sleeping Pills, p. 178.

Butabarbital
BUTISOL (Wallace)

Pentobarbital
NEMBUTAL (Abbott)

FAMILY: Barbiturates
         Sleeping Pills

Butabarbital (byoo ta *bar* bi tal) and pentobarbital (pen toe *bar* bi tal) are used to promote sleep and to relieve tension and anxiety. **You should not use these drugs because they are addictive and cause serious adverse effects.** The World Health Organization has designated them as drugs that older adults should not use.[131]

One hazard of taking butabarbital or pentobarbital continuously for longer than several weeks is drug-induced dependence. **Do not stop taking your drug suddenly.** With the help of your doctor, work out a schedule for slowly decreasing the amount of the drug you take by about 5 to 10% each day. Keep a written record of the dosage reduction schedule with you. These steps will make it much easier to become drug free without developing distressing symptoms of drug withdrawal.

The best way to reduce the risks from sleeping pills and tranquilizers is to avoid them if at all possible. Before taking one of these powerful medications, see p. 185 for nondrug alternatives to try before using either sleeping pills or tranquilizers.

Last Choice Drug

Clozapine
CLOZARIL (Novartis)

GENERIC: not available

FAMILY: Antipsychotics (See p. 187)

Clozapine (*kloe* za peen) is a drug used to treat schizophrenia. Clozapine is the first atypical antipsychotic, in the same family with olanzapine. While all antipsychotics usually improve symptoms such as agitation, delusions, hallucinations, and suspiciousness, atypical antipsychotics tend to improve "negative" symptoms such as apathy, disorientation, emotional withdrawal, and lack of pleasure, more than older antipsychotics. Although the risk of movement disorders is not eliminated with atypical antipsychotics, these drugs have a lower risk of these types of disorders, especially at higher doses.

The most serious risk of this drug is a lowering of the number of white blood cells called agranulocytosis. Clozapine is dispensed only in one week supplies to assure that monitoring of white blood cells is done, and the dose adjusted if necessary. Dry mouth or excess saliva can cause dental problems. Older people are more apt to develop dizziness. Rare, sometimes fatal effects include neuroleptic malignant syndrome (NMS). Symptoms are fever, profuse sweating, and rigid muscles. Clozapine is not recommended for women who are pregnant or breast-feeding, or in children under age 16.

Before You Use This Drug

Tell your doctor if you have or have had:

- allergies, including lactose and iodine
- blood disorders
- bone marrow problems
- depression of the central nervous system
- glaucoma (narrow-angle)
- gastrointestinal problems
- enlarged prostate or difficulty urinating

- heart, kidney or liver problems
- malnourishment
- pregnancy or nursing
- seizures

Tell your doctor about any other drugs you take, including aspirin, herbs, vitamins, and other nonprescription products.

When You Use This Drug

- Do not drink alcohol or use other drugs that can cause drowsiness.
- Do not smoke.
- Until you know how you react to this drug, do not drive or perform other activities that require alertness.
- You may feel dizzy when rising from a lying or sitting position. When getting out of bed, hang your legs over the side of the bed for a few minutes, then get up slowly. When getting up from a chair, stay beside the chair until you are sure that you are not dizzy. (See p. 16.)
- Use sugarless gum, ice, or saliva substitutes to relieve dry mouth.
- Check with your doctor before stopping clozapine. Ask for a schedule to taper off this drug.
- If you plan to have any surgery, including dental, tell your doctor that you take this drug.

How to Use This Drug

- Swallow tablet according to dose.
- If you miss a dose take it as soon as you remember but skip it if it is almost time for the next dose. **Do not take double doses**.
- Store at room temperature below 86°F. Do not store in the bathroom. Do not expose to heat, moisture, or strong light.

Interactions with Other Drugs

The following drugs are listed in the *Evaluations of Drug Interactions* 1997 as causing "highly clinically significant" or "clinically significant" interactions when used together with

this drug. We have also included potentially serious interactions listed in the drug's FDA-approved professional product labeling or package insert. New scientific techniques have allowed researchers to predict some drug interactions before they have been documented in people. There may be other drugs, especially those in the families of drugs listed below, that also will react with this drug to cause severe adverse effects. The number of new drugs approved for marketing increases the chance of drug interactions, and new drug interactions are being identified with old drugs. Be vigilant. Make sure to tell your doctor and pharmacist the drugs you are taking and tell your doctor if you are taking any of these interacting drugs:

Central nervous system (CNS) depressant drugs including alcohol, antidepressants, antihistamines, some blood pressure medications (reserpine, methyldopa, beta-blockers), motion sickness medications, muscle relaxants, narcotics, sedatives, sleeping pills, and tranquilizers.

Other drugs that can interact with clozapine are: bone marrow depressants, diazepam, EES, ERYTHROCIN, erythromycin, fluvoxamine, lithium, LITHOBID, LITHONATE, LUVOX, VALIUM.

Adverse Effects

Call your doctor immediately if you experience:

- unusual anxiety, nervousness
- bleeding, bruising
- blood pressure decreases or increases
- difficulty breathing
- chills
- confusion
- dizziness, fainting
- fever, sweating

- hallucinations
- irregular heartbeat
- severe or continuing headaches
- lip-smacking
- muscle stiffness
- restlessness
- seizures
- skin becomes pale
- sore throat
- tremor
- uncontrollable movements of arms, legs, or tongue
- unusual tiredness, weakness
- difficulty urinating
- vision changes
- sores, ulcers or white spots on lips or mouth
- yellowing of skin or eyes[132]
- puffiness of cheeks
- watering of the mouth
- decreased sexual ability
- depression
- severe drowsiness

Call your doctor if these symptoms continue:

- abdominal discomfort
- heartburn
- constipation
- nausea or vomiting
- sleeping disturbance
- stuttering
- weight gain

Periodic Tests

Ask your doctor which of these tests should be done periodically while you are taking this drug:

- white blood cell and differential counts

RISK OF SEIZURE

It has been estimated that a seizure will occur in 5% of people using clozapine for one year.

Limited Use

Trazodone
DESYREL (Apothecon)

GENERIC: available
FAMILY: Antidepressants (See p. 196 for discussion of depression.)

Trazodone (*traz* oh done) is used to treat severe depression that is not caused by other drugs, by alcohol, or by emotional losses (such as a death in the family). You should *not* be taking this drug for anxiety or mild depression, or as a sleeping pill. Because trazodone has more harmful adverse effects (see chart, p. 200) than the two antidepressants desipramine and nortriptyline (see p. 230), we consider it to be of limited use to older adults.

If you are over 60, you will generally need to take one-third to one-half the dose used by younger adults. If the initial dose is not enough and needs to be increased, this should be done very slowly.

Trazodone can cause painful, prolonged penile erections (priapism) in men. If you suffer this reaction, stop taking the drug and notify your doctor.

The length of time it takes an antidepressant to work can overlap with the time of spontaneous recovery, especially if the depression is situational—caused by a death or other external circumstances. The majority of people lift themselves out of depression with friends, or activities such as exercise, work, reading, play, art, travel, and spiritual resources. If depression is not overcome by these measures, seek help from mental health professionals, such as therapists or psychiatrists. Antidepressant drugs should be reserved for depression that is major and does not respond to psychotherapy alone.

WARNING: SPECIAL MENTAL AND PHYSICAL ADVERSE EFFECTS

Older adults are especially sensitive to the harmful anticholinergic (see Glossary, p. 768) effects of antidepressants. Drugs in this family should not be used unless absolutely necessary.

Mental Effects: confusion, delirium, short-term memory problems, disorientation, and impaired attention.

Physical Effects: dry mouth, constipation, difficulty urinating (especially for a man with an enlarged prostate), blurred vision, decreased sweating with increased body temperature, sexual dysfunction, and worsening of glaucoma.

Before You Use This Drug

Tell your doctor if you have or have had:

- allergies to drugs
- alcohol dependence
- kidney or liver problems
- retention of urine or enlarged prostate
- heart rhythm disturbance
- fever or sore throat

Tell your doctor about any other drugs you take, including aspirin, herbs, vitamins, and other nonprescription products.

Ask your doctor to check your blood pressure, once while you are lying down and once after you have been standing up for at least two minutes, and to do an electrocardiogram.

When You Use This Drug

• **Do not stop taking this drug suddenly. Your doctor must give you a schedule to lower your dose gradually, to prevent withdrawal symptoms** such as headache, mood change, nausea, vomiting, diarrhea, or trouble sleeping and vivid dreams.

• Until you know how you react to this drug, do not drive or perform other activities requiring alertness. This drug may cause blurred vision and drowsiness.

• It may take several weeks before you can tell that this drug is working. If the drug works, talk with your doctor about gradually lowering the dose.

• Do not smoke. Smoking may increase the drug's effects on your heart.

• Do not drink alcohol or use other drugs that can cause drowsiness.

• You may feel dizzy when rising from a lying or sitting position. When getting out of bed, hang your legs over the side of the bed for a few minutes, then get up slowly. When getting up from a chair, stay beside the chair until you are sure that you are not dizzy. (See p. 16.)

• Check with your doctor before taking any other drugs, prescription or nonprescription. This drug frequently interacts with other drugs.

• The effects of this drug may last for up to a week after you stop taking it. Avoid alcohol and heed all other warnings for this time period.

• If you plan to have any surgery, including dental, tell your doctor that you take this drug.

How to Use This Drug

• Take with food to reduce stomach upset. Taking trazodone with food will also reduce dizziness and lightheadedness.

• If you are taking any other drugs, take them one to two hours before you take your antidepressant.

• Do not store in the bathroom. Do not expose to heat, moisture, or strong light.

• If you miss a dose take it as soon as you remember, but skip it if it is less than four hours until your next scheduled dose. **Do not take double doses.**

Interactions with Other Drugs

The following drugs are listed in the *Evaluations of Drug Interactions* 1997 as causing "highly clinically significant" or "clinically significant" interactions when used together with this drug. We have also included potentially serious interactions listed in the drug's FDA-approved professional product labeling or package insert. New scientific techniques have allowed researchers to predict some drug interactions before they have been documented in people. There may be other drugs, especially those in the families of drugs listed below, that also will react with this drug to cause severe adverse effects. The number of new drugs approved for marketing increases the chance of drug interactions, and new drug interactions are being identified with old drugs. Be vigilant. Make sure to tell your doctor and pharmacist the drugs you are taking and tell your doctor if you are taking any of these interacting drugs:

Central nervous system (CNS) depressant drugs including alcohol, antidepressants, antihistamines, antipsychotics, some blood pressure medications (reserpine, methyldopa, beta-blockers), motion sickness medications, muscle relaxants, narcotics, sedatives, sleeping pills, and tranquilizers.

Adverse Effects

Call your doctor immediately if you experience:

- **signs of overdose:** confusion, severe drowsiness, fever, hallucinations, restlessness and agitation, seizures, shortness of breath, trouble breathing, irregular heartbeat, unusual tiredness, weakness, nausea and vomiting
  - painful, inappropriate erection of the penis
  - muscle tremors
  - fainting
  - skin rash
  - unusual excitement

Call your doctor if these symptoms continue:

- dizziness
- dry mouth
- headache
- unpleasant taste in mouth
- blurred vision
- constipation
- diarrhea
- muscle aches or pains

Periodic Tests

Ask your doctor which of these tests should be done periodically while you are taking this drug:

- complete blood count
- blood pressure
- heart function tests, an electrocardiogram (ECG, EKG)
- leukocyte and neutrophil counts

PREGNANCY WARNING

This drug caused harm to developing fetuses in animal studies, or such studies were not done. Use during pregnancy only for clear medical reasons. Tell your doctor if you are pregnant or thinking of becoming pregnant before you take this drug.

Limited Use

Venlafaxine
EFFEXOR (Wyeth-Ayerst)

GENERIC: not available

FAMILY: Antidepressants (See p. 196 for discussion of depression.)

Venlafaxine (ven la *fax* een) is used to treat major depression. Antidepressants improve symptoms of depression, but do not cure depression. Venlafaxine blocks the neurotransmitters serotonin and norepinephrine. Adverse effects can be minimized by starting with low doses of 25 mg. a day.[133] It takes about two weeks for improvement, several weeks for the full effect. If improvement is inadequate, the dose can be increased at intervals of no less than four days up to 150 mg. a day. The maximum total daily dose is 375 mg. People with kidney or liver problems or older adults should take a lower dose.

Some adverse effects are more likely to occur with higher doses. With prolonged use, a decrease in saliva can cause cavities and other dental problems. A serious, sometimes fatal, effect is called serotonin syndrome. Symptoms include restlessness, shivering, lack of coordination, and profuse sweating. Venlafaxine is not recommended for women who are pregnant or breast-feeding, or children under age 18.

The length of time it takes an antidepressant to work can overlap with the time of spontaneous recovery, especially if the depression is situational—caused by a death or other external circumstances. The majority of people lift themselves out of depression with friends, or activities such as exercise, work, reading, play, art, travel, and spiritual resources. If depression is not overcome by these measures, seek help from mental health professionals, such as therapists or psychiatrists. Antidepressant drugs should be reserved for depression that is major and does not respond to psychotherapy alone.

Before You Use This Drug

Tell your doctor if you have or have had:

- allergies, including lactose intolerance
- drug abuse
- blood pressure problems
- heart, kidney or liver problems
- nursing
- seizures

Tell your doctor about any other drugs you take, including aspirin, herbs, vitamins, and other nonprescription products.

When You Use This Drug

- Do not drink alcohol or use other drugs that can cause drowsiness.
- Until you know how you react to this drug, do not drive or perform other activities that require alertness.
- You may feel dizzy when rising from a lying or sitting position. When getting out of bed, hang your legs over the side of the bed for a few minutes, then get up slowly. When getting up from a chair, stay beside the chair until you are sure that you are not dizzy. (See p. 16.)
- Use sugarless gum, ice, or saliva substitute if you develop a dry mouth.
- Have your doctor assess your need to continue taking this drug periodically.
- If you plan to have any surgery, including dental, tell your doctor that you take this drug.

How to Use This Drug

- Swallow whole or half tablets, according to dose. Take at regular intervals with food.
- If you miss a dose, take it as soon as you remember, unless it is within two hours of the next dose. **Do not take double doses.**
- Do not suddenly stop taking this drug since you could develop signs of withdrawal,

such as dizziness, headache and nausea. Check with your doctor about tapering your dose.
- Store tablets at room temperature below 104°F. Do not store in the bathroom. Do not expose to heat, moisture, or strong light.

Interactions with Other Drugs

The following drugs are listed in the *Evaluations of Drug Interactions* 1997 as causing "highly clinically significant" or "clinically significant" interactions when used together with this drug. We have also included potentially serious interactions listed in the drug's FDA-approved professional product labeling or package insert. New scientific techniques have allowed researchers to predict some drug interactions before they have been documented in people. There may be other drugs, especially those in the families of drugs listed below, that also will react with this drug to cause severe adverse effects. The number of new drugs approved for marketing increases the chance of drug interactions, and new drug interactions are being identified with old drugs. Be vigilant. Make sure to tell your doctor and pharmacist the drugs you are taking and tell your doctor if you are taking any of these interacting drugs:

Do not take venlafaxine within 14 days of stopping or starting these monoamine oxidase (MAO) inhibitors: deprenyl, ELDEPRYL, furazolidone, FUROXONE, isocarboxazid, MARPLAN, MATULANE, NARDIL, PARNATE, phenelzine, procarbazine, selegiline, tranylcypromine.

Central nervous system (CNS) depressant drugs including alcohol, antidepressants, antihistamines, antipsychotics, some blood pressure medications (reserpine, methyldopa, beta-blockers), motion sickness medications, muscle relaxants, narcotics, sedatives, sleeping pills and tranquilizers.

Adverse Effects

Call your doctor immediately if you experience:

- agitation
- blood pressure increases
- breathing difficulty
- chest pain
- confusion
- seizures
- decreased sexual desire or ability
- depression
- diarrhea
- dizziness
- extreme drowsiness, tiredness or weakness
- uncontrolled excitement and activity
- fainting or lightheadedness
- fever
- headache
- more rapid or pounding heartbeat
- uncoordination
- itching or skin rash
- lockjaw
- menstrual changes
- mood or mental changes
- rash
- restlessness
- ringing or buzzing in ears
- swelling of legs or feet
- twitching
- difficulty urinating
- vision changes

Call your doctor if these symptoms continue:

- abnormal dreams
- anxiety, nervousness
- constipation
- dry mouth
- insomnia
- loss of appetite
- nausea or vomiting
- runny nose
- stomach pain
- taste changes
- tingling sensation
- tiredness, weakness
- weight loss

Call your doctor if these symptoms continue after you stop taking the drug:

- blood pressure increases or decreases
- difficulty breathing
- dizziness
- excitement
- fever
- headache
- impotence
- itching
- lockjaw
- menstrual changes
- rash
- ringing in ears
- seizures
- difficulty urinating
- vision changes
- nausea
- nervousness
- tiredness or weakness

Periodic Tests

Ask your doctor which of these tests should be done periodically while you are taking this drug:

- blood pressure

PREGNANCY WARNING

This drug caused harm to developing fetuses in animal studies, or such studies were not done. Use during pregnancy only for clear medical reasons. Tell your doctor if you are pregnant or thinking of becoming pregnant before you take this drug.

Do Not Use

ALTERNATIVE TREATMENT:
For depression, see Nortriptyline and
Desipramine, p. 230.

Amitriptyline
ELAVIL (Zeneca)

FAMILY: Antidepressants (See p. 196 for discussion of
depression.)

Amitriptyline (a mee *trip* ti leen) is used to
treat depression, but we do not recommend its
use because it has more harmful adverse
effects than any other drug in its family (see
chart, p. 200). If you need an antidepressant
drug, either nortriptyline or desipramine is a
better choice (see p. 230).

The length of time it takes an antidepressant
to work can overlap with the time of spontaneous recovery, especially if the depression is situational—caused by a death or other external
circumstances. The majority of people lift themselves out of depression with friends, or activities such as exercise, work, reading, play, art,
travel, and spiritual resources. If depression is
not overcome by these measures, seek help from

WARNING: SPECIAL MENTAL AND PHYSICAL ADVERSE EFFECTS

Older adults are especially sensitive to the harmful anticholinergic effects (see Glossary, p. 768) of
antidepressants such as amitriptyline. Drugs in
this family should not be used unless absolutely
necessary.

Mental Effects: confusion, delirium, short-term
memory problems, disorientation, and impaired
attention.

Physical Effects: dry mouth, constipation, difficulty urinating (especially for a man with an
enlarged prostate), blurred vision, decreased
sweating with increased body temperature, sexual
dysfunction, and worsening of glaucoma.

---

mental health professionals, such as therapists
or psychiatrists. Antidepressant drugs should be
reserved for depression that is major and does
not respond to psychotherapy alone.

If you use amitripyline, ask your doctor about
switching to another antidepressant. **Do not stop
taking this drug suddenly.** Your doctor must give
you a schedule to lower your dose *gradually,* to
prevent withdrawal symptoms such as headache,
mood change, nausea, vomiting, diarrhea, or trouble sleeping and vivid dreams.

Do Not Use

ALTERNATIVE TREATMENT:
See nondrug approaches, p. 185, Oxazepam, p. 242,
and Buspirone, p. 206. See also Tranquilizers
and Sleeping Pills, p. 178.

Meprobamate
EQUANIL (Wyeth-Ayerst)
MILTOWN (Wallace)

FAMILY: Antianxiety Drugs

Meprobamate (me proe *ba* mate) is a tranquilizer. It is commonly misused to relieve occasional,
short-term anxiety. **If you are suffering anxiety and tension from the stress of everyday
life, you usually do not need an antianxiety
drug.** There are safer ways to relieve such anxiety. If you do need a drug for anxiety, oxazepam
(see p. 242) or buspirone (see p. 206) is a better
choice than meprobamate.

Long-term treatment (longer than four
months) of anxiety with meprobamate is rarely
effective. It also puts you at risk of developing
harmful adverse effects such as: drowsiness,
dizziness, unsteady gait, with an increased risk
of falls and hip fractures, impairment of thinking, memory loss, and addiction.

One hazard of taking meprobamate continuously for longer than several weeks is drug-induced dependence. **Do not stop taking your drug suddenly.** With the help of your doctor, work out a schedule for slowly decreasing the amount of the drug you take by about 5 to 10% each day. Keep a written record of the dosage reduction schedule with you. These steps will make it much easier to become drug free without developing distressing symptoms of drug withdrawal.

Limited Use

Lithium
ESKALITH (SmithKline Beecham)
LITHOBID (Solvay)
LITHONATE (Solvay)

GENERIC: available
FAMILY: Antimanic Drugs (See p. 196 for discussion of depression.)

Lithium (*lith* ee um) is used to treat manic episodes of manic depression, a condition in which a person's mood swings severely from normal to elated to depressed. It is also used to prevent or decrease the intensity of future manic episodes.

If you are over 60, you generally need to take less than the usual adult dose. Your doctor should frequently measure the levels of lithium in your blood.

Even when the amount of lithium in an older person's body is no more than is needed for it to work, the drug may cause harm to the central nervous system. Ideally, you should only use lithium if you have a normal salt (sodium) intake and normal heart and kidney function.[134]

Before You Use This Drug

Tell your doctor if you have or have had:

- allergies to drugs
- heart or blood vessel disease
- Parkinson's disease
- epilepsy, seizures
- enlarged prostate or difficulty urinating
- kidney disease
- diabetes
- goiter, thyroid disease
- overactive parathyroid glands
- recent severe infection
- organic brain disease
- schizophrenia
- psoriasis
- a current low-salt diet
- leukemia

Tell your doctor about any other drugs you take, including aspirin, herbs, vitamins, and other nonprescription products.

When You Use This Drug

- It may take one to three weeks before you can tell that this drug is working.
- **Do not stop taking this drug suddenly. Your doctor must give you a schedule to lower your dose gradually, to prevent withdrawal symptoms.**
- See your doctor regularly to make sure that the drug is working and that you are not developing adverse effects. Your doctor should regularly measure the amount of drug in your body.
- Follow diet recommended by your doctor to avoid weight gain.
- Until you know how you react to this drug, do not drive or perform other activities requiring alertness. Lithium may cause blurred vision, drowsiness, fainting, or slow your reaction time.
- If you plan to have any surgery, including dental, tell your doctor that you take this drug.

HEAT STRESS ALERT

This drug can affect your body's ability to adjust to heat, putting you at risk of "heat stress." If you live alone, ask a friend to check you several times during the day. Early signs of heat stress are dizziness, lightheadedness, faintness, and slightly high temperature. Call your doctor if you have these signs.

Drink more fluids (water, fruit and vegetable juices) than usual—even if you're not thirsty—unless your doctor has told you otherwise. Do not drink alcohol.

How to Use This Drug

- Swallow extended-release tablets whole.
- Do not store in the bathroom. Do not expose to heat, moisture, or strong light. Do not let the liquid form freeze.
- If you miss a dose, take it as soon as you remember, but skip it if it is less than four hours until your next scheduled dose. If you are taking extended-release tablets, skip the missed dose if it is less than six hours until your next scheduled dose. **Do not take double doses**.

Interactions with Other Drugs

The following drugs are listed in the *Evaluations of Drug Interactions* 1997 as causing "highly clinically significant" or "clinically significant" interactions when used together with this drug. We have also included potentially serious interactions listed in the drug's FDA-approved professional product labeling or package insert. New scientific techniques have allowed researchers to predict some drug interactions before they have been documented in people. There may be other drugs, especially those in the families of drugs listed below, that also will react with this drug to cause severe adverse effects. The number of new drugs approved for marketing increases the chance of drug interactions, and new drug interactions are being identified with old drugs. Be vigilant. Make sure to tell your doctor and pharmacist the drugs you are taking and tell your doctor if you are taking any of these interacting drugs:

acetazolamide, ACHROMYCIN, ADVIL, ALDOMET, ALEVE, ANAPROX, caffeine, CALAN SR, carbamazepine, chlorothiazide, chlorpromazine, COVERA-HS, DIAMOX, DIURIL, ELIXOPHYLLIN, enalapril, FLAGYL, fluoxetine, HALDOL, haloperidol, ibuprofen, imipramine, IMITREX, INDOCIN, indomethacin, ISOPTIN SR, LOPRESSOR, MAZANOR, mazindol, MELLARIL, metaprolol, methyldopa, metronidazole, MOTRIN, NAPROSYN, naproxen, PANMYCIN, PIMA, potassium iodide, PROZAC, SANOREX, SLO-BID, sumatriptan, SUMYCIN, TEGRETOL, tetracycline, THEO-24, theophylline, thioridazine, THORAZINE, TOFRANIL, VASOTEC, verapamil, VERELAN.

Adverse Effects

Call your doctor immediately if you experience:

- **signs of overdose:** *early signs* are diarrhea, drowsiness, loss of appetite, muscle weakness, nausea or vomiting, slurred speech, trembling; *late signs* are blurred vision, clumsiness, confusion, dizziness, seizures, trembling, increased amount of urine
- **signs of parkinsonism:** difficulty speaking or swallowing, loss of balance, mask-like

face, muscle spasms, stiffness of arms or legs, trembling and shaking, unusual twisting movements of body
- **signs of low thyroid hormone levels:** dry, rough skin, hair loss, hoarseness, swelling of feet or lower legs, swelling of neck (goiter), increased sensitivity to cold, fatigue, depression, unusual excitement
  - fainting
  - difficulty breathing
  - fast heartbeat, irregular pulse
  - unusual weight gain
  - blue color and pain in fingers or toes
  - cold limbs
  - headache
  - eye pain, visual problems
  - nausea, vomiting
  - unusual tiredness or weakness
  - noises in ear

Call your doctor if these symptoms continue:

- increased amount of urine or loss of bladder control
- increased thirst
- mild nausea
- trembling of hands
- skin rash, acne
- bloated feeling
- fatigue

Periodic Tests

Ask your doctor which of these tests should be done periodically while you are taking this drug:

- white blood cell counts
- blood levels of lithium (more often if taking other drugs)
- blood levels of calcium
- electrocardiogram
- kidney function tests
- thyroid function tests
- weight evaluation

- Parathyroid hormone and calcium levels may rise above normal after long-term lithium therapy.

Limited Use

Haloperidol
HALDOL (Ortho-McNeil)

GENERIC: available
FAMILY: Antipsychotics (see p. 187)

Haloperidol (ha loe *per* i dole) is effective for treating mental illnesses called psychoses, including schizophrenia. It should not be used to treat anxiety, to treat the loss of mental abilities (for example due to Alzheimer's disease) in nonpsychotic people, to sedate, or to control restless behavior or other problems in nonpsychotic people. Haloperidol should also be used sparingly, if at all, for treating depression in older people since the incidence of tardive dyskinesia (involuntary movements of parts of the body), an often disabling adverse effect of this drug, is 60% in older adults with depression who are given antipsychotic drugs.[135]

The antipsychotics can cause serious adverse effects, including tardive dyskinesia, drug-induced parkinsonism (see p. 193), the "jitters," and weakness and muscle fatigue (see Adverse Effects).

The chart on p. 194 shows the major differences among the various antipsychotic drugs. If your doctor has prescribed one of these drugs and it is causing an unwanted side effect, use this chart to find alternative drugs that cause less of that particular effect.

Whichever of these drugs you use, you should be taking between one-tenth and one-fifth of the dose used for younger adults.

WARNING: SPECIAL MENTAL AND PHYSICAL ADVERSE EFFECTS

Older adults are especially sensitive to the harmful anticholinergic (see Glossary, p. 768) effects of antipsychotic drugs such as haloperidol. Drugs in this family should not be used unless absolutely necessary.

Mental Effects: confusion, delirium, short-term memory problems, disorientation, and impaired attention.

Physical Effects: dry mouth, constipation, difficulty urinating (especially for a man with an enlarged prostate), blurred vision, decreased sweating with increased body temperature, sexual dysfunction, and worsening of glaucoma.

Before You Use This Drug

Tell your doctor if you have or have had:

- allergies to drugs
- alcohol dependence
- glaucoma
- heart or blood vessel disease
- Parkinson's disease
- epilepsy, seizures
- kidney or liver problems
- overactive thyroid
- difficulty urinating
- lung disease

Tell your doctor about any other drugs you take, including aspirin, herbs, vitamins, and other nonprescription products.

When You Use This Drug

- It may take two to three weeks before you can tell that your drug is working.
- **Do not stop taking your drug suddenly. Your doctor must give you a schedule to lower your dose gradually, to prevent withdrawal symptoms such as nausea, vomiting, and stomach upset.**

- Until you know how you react to this drug, do not drive or perform other activities requiring alertness. These drugs may cause blurred vision, drowsiness, and fainting.
- Do not drink alcohol or use other drugs that can cause drowsiness.
- You may feel dizzy when rising from a lying or sitting position. When getting out of bed, hang your feet over the side of the bed for a few minutes, then get up slowly. When getting out of a chair, stay by the chair until you are sure that you are not dizzy. (See p. 16.)
- If you plan to have any surgery, including dental, tell your doctor that you take this drug.

How to Use This Drug

- Take with food or **a full glass (eight ounces) of milk or water** to prevent stomach upset.
- Do not store in the bathroom. Do not expose to heat, moisture, or strong light. Do not let the liquid form freeze.
- If you take antacids or diarrhea drugs, take them at least two hours apart from taking your antipsychotic drug.
- If you miss a dose, take it as soon as you remember, but skip it if it is almost time for the next dose. **Do not take double doses.**

Interactions with Other Drugs

The following drugs are listed in the *Evaluations of Drug Interactions* 1997 as causing "highly clinically significant" or "clinically significant" interactions when used together with this drug. We have also included potentially serious interactions listed in the drug's FDA-approved professional product labeling or package insert. New scientific techniques have allowed researchers to predict some drug interactions before they have been documented in people. There may be other drugs, especially those in the families of drugs listed below, that also will react with this drug to cause severe adverse effects. The number of new drugs approved for marketing increases the chance of drug interactions, and new drug interactions are being identified with old drugs. Be vigilant. Make sure to tell your doctor and pharmacist the drugs you are taking and tell your doctor if you are taking any of these interacting drugs:

> alcohol, carbamazepine, COGNEX, LARODOPA, levodopa, lithium, LITHOBID, LITHONATE, pergolide, PERMAX, tacrine, TEGRETOL.

Central nervous system (CNS) depressant drugs including alcohol, antidepressants, antihistamines, antipsychotics, some blood pressure medications (reserpine, methyldopa, beta-blockers), motion sickness medications, muscle relaxants, narcotics, sedatives, sleeping pills and tranquilizers.

Adverse Effects

Call your doctor immediately if you experience:

- **signs of tardive dyskinesia:** lip smacking, chewing movements, puffing of cheeks, rapid, darting tongue movements, uncontrolled movements of arms or legs
- **signs of parkinsonism:** difficulty speaking or swallowing, loss of balance, mask-like face, muscle spasms, stiffness of arms or legs, trembling and shaking, unusual twisting movements of body
- **signs of restless leg (akathisia):** restless pacing, a feeling of the "jitters"
- **signs of akinesia:** weakness, muscular fatigue, listlessness, depression. Although often confused with true depression, akinesia is actually the most common of a group of adverse effects called extrapyramidal effects (see p. 193).
- change or blurred vision
- difficulty urinating

- **signs of neuroleptic malignant syndrome:** troubled or fast breathing, high or low blood pressure, increased sweating, loss of bladder control, muscle stiffness, seizures, unusual tiredness, weakness, fast heartbeat, irregular pulse, pale skin
- fever and sore throat
- yellow eyes or skin
- skin rash
- fainting
- hives or itching
- hallucinations
- restlessness and the need to keep moving
- decreased thirst
- unusual bleeding or bruising
- hot dry skin or lack of sweating
- blinking or spasms of eyelids
- **signs of overdose of *haloperidol:*** severe breathing problems, dizziness, severe drowsiness, muscle stiffness or jerking, unusual tiredness or weakness

Call your doctor if these symptoms continue:

- changes in menstrual period
- constipation
- dry mouth
- swelling or pain in breasts
- unusual secretion of milk
- decreased sexual ability
- decreased sweating
- weight gain
- increased skin sensitivity to sun
- nausea or vomiting

Periodic Tests

Ask your doctor which of these tests should be done periodically while you are taking this drug:

- liver function tests
- observation for early signs of tardive dyskinesia
- reevaluation of need for the drug
- observation for the early signs of dehydration
- complete blood count

PREGNANCY WARNING

This drug caused harm to developing fetuses in animal studies, or such studies were not done. Use during pregnancy only for clear medical reasons. Tell your doctor if you are pregnant or thinking of becoming pregnant before you take this drug.

DECREASED SWEATING

Haloperidol may make you sweat less, causing your body temperature to increase. Use extra care not to become overheated during exercise or hot weather while you are taking one of these medications, since overheating may result in heat stroke. Also, hot baths or saunas may make you feel dizzy or faint while you are taking this medicine.

 Do Not Use

ALTERNATIVE TREATMENT:
See nondrug approaches, p. 185, Buspirone, p. 206, and Oxazepam, p. 242.

Chlordiazepoxide (klor dye az e *pox* ide)
LIBRIUM (Roche)

Clorazepate (klor *az* e pate)
TRANXENE (Abbott)

Diazepam (dye *az* e pam)
VALIUM (Roche)

Estazolam (est *as* oh lamb)
PROSOM (Abbott)

Flurazepam (flure *az* e pam)
DALMANE (Roche)

Halazepam (hal *az* e pam)
PAXIPAM (Schering)

Lorazepam (lor *az* e pam)
ATIVAN (Wyeth-Ayerst)

Prazepam (*praz* e pam)
CENTRAX (Parke-Davis)

Quazepam (*kwayz* e pam)
DORAL (Wallace)

Temazepam (tem *az* e pam)
RESTORIL (Novartis)

Triazolam (trye *ay* zoe lam)
HALCION (Pharmacia & Upjohn)

Do Not Use Except for Panic Disorder

Alprazolam (al *praz* oh lam)
XANAX (Pharmacia & Upjohn)

FAMILY: Benzodiazepine Sleeping Pills and Tranquilizers (see p. 178)

These 12 sleeping pills and tranquilizers all belong to the benzodiazepine (ben zoe dye *az* e

---

WARNING:

DO NOT USE ALPRAZOLAM (XANAX) EXCEPT FOR PANIC DISORDER

Panic Disorder and related conditions must be evaluated by the appropriate mental health professional. Specialized psychotherapy decreases the need for drugs for this condition. A psychiatrist may be able to prescribe less hazardous medications for this condition.

peen) family. Although they are widely used for older adults, they present significantly higher risks to people over 60 and lack proven long-term benefits. These drugs can cause unsteady gait, dizziness, falling—with an increased risk of hip fractures—automobile accidents that cause injury, impairment of thinking and memory loss, and addiction. While some of these sleeping pills stay in the body so long you can still be sedated during the daytime, other drugs in this family stay in the body such a short time you can get rebound insomnia and become confused the following day. **Many older people who use these drugs should not be taking them. They have significant risks and are often prescribed unnecessarily.**

Based on our review of the benzodiazepine drugs, which are all effective but differ in their degree of safety, we recommend **(for limited use only)** *oxazepam* (see p. 242) as the safest drug in this family for older adults who truly need a tranquilizer or sleeping pill. The nonbenzodiazepine, buspirone (BUSPAR), see p. 206, is also suggested for limited use.

These 13 benzodiazepine drugs (oxazepam and the 12 listed above) are different from each other, and the difference has to do with the different ways in which they are dangerous for older adults.

The World Health Organization specifically recommends that older adults should not use the most widely prescribed sleeping pill, flurazepam (DALMANE), "owing to a high incidence of adverse effects."[136] Seven other benzodiazepines are also cleared out of the body more slowly, especially in older adults, and can therefore accumulate, leading to increased risks. These drugs, which also should be avoided by older adults, include diazepam (VALIUM), chlordiazepoxide (LIBRIUM), clorazepate (TRAXENE), prazepam (CENTRAX), halazepam (PAXIPAM), quazepam (DORAL), and estazolam (PROSOM).

Another widely used sleeping pill, triazolam (HALCION), should also be avoided by older adults because it is so short-acting that it can cause rebound insomnia (increased sleeping problems when the drug effect has worn off), anxiety, serious amnesia (forgetfulness or memory loss) and violent, aggressive behavior. In 1992, Public Citizen's Health Research Group petitioned the Food and Drug Administration to ban Halcion. The sleeping pill estazolam (PROSOM) is in the same chemical sub-class as Halcion and, according to *The Medical Letter,* there is no reason to use it.[137] It also has the disadvantage of slow clearance from the body.

In a discussion of which of these drugs are best for older adults, it was stated that oxazepam (SERAX) and temazepam (RESTORIL) were the drugs of choice.[138] But it has also been stated that "oxazepam (SERAX) may be the safest benzodiazepine for the older patient" because **"oxazepam may offer the advantages of a short half-life and the absence of active metabolites"** (that is, chemicals into which the body converts the drug which can also have adverse effects).[139] In addition, studies have shown that oxazepam has much less of a "street" drug abuse potential than, for example, diazepam (VALIUM).[140,141]

If you are taking a tranquilizer or sleeping pill other than buspirone or oxazepam, ask your doctor to reevaluate your need for this drug. If you do need such a drug, you should be taking one of these two.

The best way to reduce the risks from sleeping pills and tranquilizers is to avoid them if at all possible. Before taking one of these powerful medications, see p. 185 for nondrug alternatives to try before using either sleeping pills or tranquilizers.

One hazard of taking benzodiazepines continuously for longer than several weeks is drug-induced dependence. **Do not stop taking your drug suddenly.** With the help of your doctor, work out a schedule for slowly decreasing the amount of the drug you take by about 5 to 10% each day. Keep a written record of the dosage reduction schedule with you. These steps will make it much easier to become drug free without developing distressing symptoms of drug withdrawal.

Do Not Use

ALTERNATIVE TREATMENT:
For depression, see Nortriptyline and Desipramine, p. 230.

Amitriptyline and Chlordiazepoxide
LIMBITROL (Roche)

FAMILY: Antidepressants (See p. 196 for discussion of depression.)
Antianxiety Drugs

The brand-name drug Limbitrol contains a fixed combination of an antidepressant, amitriptyline (see p. 216), and a benzodiazepine (tranquilizer or antianxiety drug), chlordiazepoxide (see p. 222). It is used to treat moderate to severe depression associated with moderate to severe anxiety. We do not recommend that you use it, for several reasons.

First, combining an antidepressant with a benzodiazepine has not been shown to produce a more effective drug.[142] Second, taking these two drugs together raises the risk of harmful adverse effects. Chlordiazepoxide might increase the harmful anticholinergic effects of amitriptyline (see box below), and amitriptyline could increase the drowsiness caused by chlordiazepoxide.[143] Third, the anti-depressant in this combination, amitriptyline, has more adverse effects than any other drug in its family (see chart, p. 200) and should not be used by older adults, either alone or in a combination such as this one.

If you use Limbitrol, ask your doctor if your treatment can be changed. Do not stop taking this drug suddenly. Your doctor may want to reduce your dose gradually over one or two months before you completely stop taking Limbitrol.

The length of time it takes an antidepressant to work can overlap with the time of spontaneous recovery, especially if the depression is situational—caused by a death or other external circumstances. The majority of people lift themselves out of depression with friends, or activities such as exercise, work, reading, play, art, travel, and spiritual resources. If depression is not overcome by these measures, seek help from mental health professionals, such as therapists or psychiatrists. Antidepressant drugs should be reserved for depression that is major and does not respond to psychotherapy alone.

WARNING: SPECIAL MENTAL AND PHYSICAL ADVERSE EFFECTS

Older adults are especially sensitive to the harmful anticholinergic (see Glossary, p. 768) effects of tricyclic antidepressants such as amitriptyline. Drugs in this family should not be used unless absolutely necessary.

Mental Effects: confusion, delirium, short-term memory problems, disorientation, and impaired attention.

Physical Effects: dry mouth, constipation, difficulty urinating (especially for a man with an enlarged prostate), blurred vision, decreased sweating with increased body temperature, sexual dysfunction, and worsening of glaucoma.

Limited Use

Maprotiline
LUDIOMIL (Novartis)

GENERIC: available

FAMILY: Antidepressants (See p. 196 for discussion of depression.)

Maprotiline (ma *proe* ti leen) is used to treat severe depression that is not caused by other drugs, by alcohol, or by emotional losses (such as a death in the family). You should *not* be taking it for anxiety or mild depression, or as a sleeping pill. Because maprotiline has more harmful adverse effects (see chart, p. 200) than the two antidepressants desipramine and nortriptyline (see p. 230), we consider it to be of limited use to older adults.

If you are over 60, you will generally need to take one-third to one-half the dose used by younger adults. If the initial dose is not enough and needs to be increased, this should be done very slowly.

The length of time it takes an antidepressant to work can overlap with the time of spontaneous recovery, especially if the depression is situational—caused by a death or other external circumstances. The majority of people lift themselves out of depression with friends, or activities such as exercise, work, reading, play, art, travel, and spiritual resources. If depression is not overcome by these measures, seek help from mental health professionals, such as therapists or psychiatrists. Antidepressant drugs should be reserved for depression that is major and does not respond to psychotherapy alone.

Before You Use This Drug

Tell your doctor if you have or have had:

- allergies to drugs
- alcohol dependence
- asthma

> ### WARNING: SPECIAL MENTAL AND PHYSICAL ADVERSE EFFECTS
>
> Older adults are especially sensitive to the harmful anticholinergic (see Glossary, p. 768) effects of antidepressants such as maprotiline. Drugs in this family should not be used unless absolutely necessary.
>
> *Mental Effects:* confusion, delirium, short-term memory problems, disorientation, and impaired attention.
>
> *Physical Effects:* dry mouth, constipation, difficulty urinating (especially for a man with an enlarged prostate), blurred vision, decreased sweating with increased body temperature, sexual dysfunction, and worsening of glaucoma.

- difficulty urinating or enlarged prostate
- glaucoma
- severe mental illness
- stomach or intestinal problems
- heart attack
- heart or blood vessel disease
- thyroid disease
- epilepsy or seizures
- liver problems

Tell your doctor about any other drugs you take, including aspirin, herbs, vitamins, and other nonprescription products.
Ask your doctor to check your blood pressure, once while you are lying down and once after you have been standing up for at least two minutes, and to do an electrocardiogram.

When You Use This Drug

- **Do not stop taking this drug suddenly. Your doctor must give you a schedule to lower your dose gradually, to prevent withdrawal symptoms** such as headache, mood change, nausea, vomiting, diarrhea, or trouble sleeping and vivid dreams.

• Until you know how you react to this drug, do not drive or perform other activities requiring alertness. This drug may cause blurred vision and drowsiness.

• It may take several weeks before you can tell that this drug is working. If the drug works, talk with your doctor about lowering the dose gradually.

• Do not smoke. Smoking may increase the drug's effects on your heart.

• Do not drink alcohol or use other drugs that can cause drowsiness.

• You may feel dizzy when rising from a lying or sitting position. When getting out of bed, hang your legs over the side of the bed for a few minutes, then get up slowly. When getting up from a chair, stay beside the chair until you are sure that you are not dizzy. (See p. 16.)

• Check with your doctor before taking any other drugs, prescription or nonprescription. This drug frequently interacts with other drugs.

• The effects of these drugs may last for up to a week after you stop taking them. Avoid alcohol and heed all other warnings for this time period.

• If you plan to have any surgery, including dental, tell your doctor that you take this drug.

How to Use This Drug

• Take with food to reduce stomach upset.

• If you are taking any other drugs, take them one to two hours before you take your antidepressant.

• Do not store in the bathroom. Do not expose to heat, moisture, or strong light.

• *If you miss a dose, use the following guidelines:* If you are taking more than one dose a day take the missed dose as soon as you remember, but skip it if it is almost time for the next dose.

If you are taking your drug only once a day at bedtime, and you go to sleep without taking that dose, do not take it in the morning. Instead, call your doctor.

Do not take double doses.

Interactions with Other Drugs

The following drugs are listed in the *Evaluations of Drug Interactions* 1997 as causing "highly clinically significant" or "clinically significant" interactions when used together with this drug. We have also included potentially serious interactions listed in the drug's FDA-approved professional product labeling or package insert. New scientific techniques have allowed researchers to predict some drug interactions before they have been documented in people. There may be other drugs, especially those in the families of drugs listed below, that also will react with this drug to cause severe adverse effects. The number of new drugs approved for marketing increases the chance of drug interactions, and new drug interactions are being identified with old drugs. Be vigilant. Make sure to tell your doctor and pharmacist the drugs you are taking and tell your doctor if you are taking any of these interacting drugs:

ADRENALIN (also in bee sting kits), alcohol, cimetidine, CYTOMEL, epinephrine, guanethidine, IMDUR, ISMELIN, ISMO, ISORDIL, isosorbide, liothyronine, MELLARIL, NITRO-BID, nitroglycerin (sublingual), NITROSTAT, PARNATE, PRIMATENE MIST, SORBITRATE, TAGAMET, thioridazine, tolazamide, TOLINASE, tramadol, TRANSDERM-NITRO, tranylcypromine, TRIOSTAT, ULTRAM.

Adverse Effects

Call your doctor immediately if you experience:

• **signs of overdose:** confusion, severe drowsiness, fever, hallucinations, muscle stiffness or weakness, restlessness and agitation, seizures, trouble breathing, irregular heartbeat, unusual tiredness, weakness, vomiting
- skin rash, redness, swelling, or itching
- nausea or vomiting
- weight loss
- breast enlargement in both males and females
- delirium
- unusual secretion of milk
- constipation (severe)
- fainting
- shakiness or trembling
- difficulty urinating
- sore throat and fever
- unusual excitement
- yellow eyes or skin
- swelling of testicles

Call your doctor if these symptoms continue:

- blurred vision
- decreased sexual ability or interest
- dizziness or lightheadedness
- dry mouth
- headache
- constipation (mild)
- diarrhea
- heartburn
- increased appetite and weight gain
- increased sensitivity to sunlight
- increased sweating
- trouble sleeping

Periodic Tests

Ask your doctor which of these tests should be done periodically while you are taking this drug:

- complete blood count
- blood pressure
- heart function tests
- liver function tests
- dental exams (at least twice yearly)

Limited Use

Thiothixene
NAVANE (Pfizer)

GENERIC: available
FAMILY: Antipsychotics (see p. 187)

Thiothixene (thye oh *thix* een) is effective for treating mental illnesses called psychoses, including schizophrenia. It should not be used to treat anxiety, to treat the loss of mental abilities (for example, due to Alzheimer's disease) in nonpsychotic people, to sedate, or to control restless behavior or other problems in nonpsychotic people. Thiothixene should also be used sparingly, if at all, for treating depression in older people since the incidence of tardive dyskinesia (involuntary movements of parts of the body), an often disabling adverse effect of this drug, is 60% in older adults with depression who are given antipsychotic drugs.[144]

The antipsychotics can cause serious adverse effects, including tardive dyskinesia, drug-induced parkinsonism (see p. 193), the "jitters," and weakness and muscle fatigue (see Adverse Effects).

The chart on p. 194 shows the major differences among the various antipsychotic drugs. If your doctor has prescribed one of these drugs and it is causing an unwanted side effect, use this chart to find alternative drugs that cause less of that particular effect.

Whichever of these drugs you use, you should be taking between one-tenth and one-fifth of the dose used for younger adults.

Before You Use This Drug

Tell your doctor if you have or have had:

- allergies to drugs
- alcohol dependence
- blood disease
- enlarged prostate or difficulty urinating
- glaucoma
- heart or blood vessel disease
- lung disease or breathing problems
- Parkinson's disease
- epilepsy, seizures
- stomach ulcer
- liver disease
- Reye's syndrome
- seizure

Tell your doctor about any other drugs you take, including aspirin, herbs, vitamins, and other nonprescription products.

When You Use This Drug

- It may take two to three weeks before you can tell that your drug is working.

- **Do not stop taking your drug sudden- ly. Your doctor must give you a schedule to lower your dose gradually, to prevent withdrawal symptoms such as nausea, vomiting, and stomach upset.**
- Until you know how you react to this drug, do not drive or perform other activities requir- ing alertness. This drug may cause blurred vision, drowsiness, and fainting.
- Do not drink alcohol or use other drugs that can cause drowsiness.
- You may feel dizzy when rising from a lying or sitting position. When getting out of bed, hang your feet over the side of the bed for a few minutes, then get up slowly. When get- ting out of a chair, stay by the chair until you are sure that you are not dizzy. (See p. 16.)
- If you plan to have any surgery, including dental, tell your doctor that you take this drug.

How to Use This Drug

- Take with food or **a full glass (eight ounces) of milk or water** to prevent stomach upset.
- Do not store in the bathroom. Do not expose to heat, moisture, or strong light. Do not let the liquid form freeze.
- If you take antacids or diarrhea drugs, take them at least one hour apart from taking your antipsychotic drug.
- If you miss a dose, take it as soon as you remember, but skip it if it is almost time for the next dose. **Do not take double doses.**

Interactions with Other Drugs

The following drugs are listed in the *Evalua- tions of Drug Interactions* 1997 as causing "highly clinically significant" or "clinically significant" interactions when used together with this drug. We have also included poten- tially serious interactions listed in the drug's FDA-approved professional product labeling or package insert. New scientific techniques have allowed researchers to predict some drug interactions before they have been documented in people. There may be other drugs, especially those in the families of drugs listed below, that also will react with this drug to cause severe adverse effects. The number of new drugs approved for marketing increases the chance of drug interactions, and new drug interactions are being identified with old drugs. Be vigilant. Make sure to tell your doctor and pharmacist the drugs you are taking and tell your doctor if you are taking any of these interacting drugs:

ADRENALIN (also in bee sting kits), alcohol, DURAQUIN, epinephrine, LARODOPA, levodopa, PRIMATENE MIST, QUINAGLUTE DURA-TABS, QUINIDEX, quinidine, SINEMET.

Central nervous system (CNS) depressant drugs including alcohol, antidepressants, antihistamines, antipsychotics, some blood pressure medications (reserpine, methyldopa, beta-blockers), motion sickness medications, muscle relaxants, narcotics, sedatives, sleeping pills and tranquilizers.

Adverse Effects

Call your doctor immediately if you experience:

- **signs of tardive dyskinesia:** lip smacking, chewing movements, puffing of cheeks, rapid, darting tongue movements, uncontrolled movements of arms or legs
- **signs of parkinsonism:** difficulty speaking or swallowing, loss of balance, mask-like face, muscle spasms, stiffness of arms or legs, trembling and shaking, unusual twisting movements of body
- **signs of restless leg (akathisia):** restless pacing, a feeling of the "jitters"
- **signs of akinesia:** weakness, muscular fatigue, listlessness, depression. Although often confused with true depression, akinesia is actually the most common of a group of adverse effects called extrapyramidal effects (see p. 193).
- changed or blurred vision
- difficulty urinating
- **signs of neuroleptic malignant syndrome:** troubled or fast breathing, high or low blood pressure, increased sweating, loss of bladder control, muscle stiffness, seizures, unusual tiredness, weakness, fast heartbeat, irregular pulse, pale skin
- fever and sore throat
- yellow eyes or skin
- skin rash
- fainting
- **signs of overdose:** severe breathing problems, severe dizziness, severe drowsiness, fever, muscle stiffness or jerking, seizures, unusual excitement, unusually fast heartbeat, tiny pupils

Call your doctor if these symptoms continue:

- constipation
- decreased sweating
- dry mouth
- increased appetite and weight
- increased skin sensitivity to sun
- stuffy nose
- changes in menstrual period
- decreased sexual ability
- swelling or pain in breasts in males and females
- unusual secretion of milk

Periodic Tests

Ask your doctor which of these tests should be done periodically while you are taking this drug:

- complete blood count
- eye examinations
- liver function tests
- observation for early signs of tardive dyskinesia
- reevaluation of need for the drug
- urine tests for bile and bilirubin

DECREASED SWEATING

Thiothixene may make you sweat less, causing your body temperature to increase. Use extra care not to become overheated during exercise or hot weather while you are taking one of these medications, since overheating may result in heat stroke. Also, hot baths or saunas may make you feel dizzy or faint while you are taking this medicine.

Desipramine
NORPRAMIN (Hoechst Marion Roussel)

Nortriptyline
AVENTYL (Lilly)
PAMELOR (Novartis)

GENERIC: available
FAMILY: Antidepressants (See p. 196 for discussion of depression.)

Desipramine (dess *ip* ra meen) and nortriptyline (nor *trip* ti leen) are used to treat severe depression that is not caused by other drugs, by alcohol, or by emotional losses (such as a death in the family). These two drugs produce fewer sedative effects and fewer harmful anticholinergic adverse effects (see box below) than some other antidepressants, and some clinicians suggest trying one of these two drugs before other drugs in their family (see p. 200 for comparison with other antidepressants). You should *not* be taking these drugs for mild depression or anxiety, or as a sleeping pill.

If you are over 60, you will generally need to take one-third to one-half the dose used for younger adults. If the initial dose is not enough and must be increased, this should be done very slowly under the guidance of your doctor. Your doctor should monitor the level of the drug in your bloodstream, because there is a point at which a higher drug level produces

less benefit.

The length of time it takes an antidepressant to work can overlap with the time of spontaneous recovery, especially if the depression is situational—caused by a death or other external circumstances. The majority of people lift themselves out of depression with friends, or activities such as exercise, work, reading, play, art, travel, and spiritual resources. If depression is not overcome by these measures, seek help from mental health professionals, such as therapists or psychiatrists. Antidepressant drugs should be reserved for depression that is major and does not respond to psychotherapy alone.

WARNING: SPECIAL MENTAL AND PHYSICAL ADVERSE EFFECTS

Older adults are especially sensitive to the harmful anticholinergic (see Glossary, p. 768) effects of tricyclic antidepressants such as desipramine and nortriptyline. Drugs in this family should not be used unless absolutely necessary.

Mental Effects: confusion, delirium, short-term memory problems, disorientation, and impaired attention.

Physical Effects: dry mouth, constipation, difficulty urinating (especially for a man with an enlarged prostate), blurred vision, decreased sweating with increased body temperature, sexual dysfunction, and worsening of glaucoma.

Before You Use This Drug

Tell your doctor if you have or have had:

- allergies to drugs
- alcohol dependence
- asthma
- blood disorders
- heart or blood vessel disease
- epilepsy, seizures
- stomach or intestinal disease

- glaucoma
- kidney, liver, or thyroid problems
- manic-depressive illness, schizophrenia, or paranoia
- retention of urine or enlarged prostate

Tell your doctor about any other drugs you take, including aspirin, herbs, vitamins, and other nonprescription products.

Ask your doctor to check your blood pressure, once while you are lying down and once after you have been standing up for at least two minutes, and to do an electrocardiogram.

When You Use This Drug

- **Do not stop taking your drug suddenly. Your doctor must give you a schedule to lower your dose gradually, to prevent withdrawal symptoms** such as headache, mood change, nausea, vomiting, diarrhea, or trouble sleeping and vivid dreams.
- Do not smoke. Smoking may increase the drug's effects on your heart.
- Until you know how you react to this drug, do not drive or perform other activities requiring alertness. These drugs may cause blurred vision and drowsiness.
- It may take several weeks before you can tell that these drugs are working. If the drug works, talk with your doctor about lowering the dose gradually.
- Do not drink alcohol or use other drugs that can cause drowsiness.
- You may feel dizzy when rising from a lying or sitting position. When getting out of bed, hang your legs over the side of the bed for a few minutes, then get up slowly. When getting up from a chair, stay by the chair until you are sure that you are not dizzy. (See p. 16.)
- Check with your doctor before taking any other drugs, prescription or nonprescription. These drugs frequently interact with other drugs.
- The effects of these drugs may last for up to a week after you stop taking them. Avoid

alcohol and heed all other warnings for this time period.
- If you plan to have any surgery, including dental, tell your doctor that you take this drug.

How to Use This Drug

- Take with food to reduce stomach upset.
- If you are taking other drugs, take them one to two hours before taking your antidepressant.
- Capsules may be opened and mixed with food or drink.
- Do not store in the bathroom. Do not expose to heat, moisture, or strong light.
- *If you miss a dose, use the following guidelines:* If you are taking your drug more than once a day, take the missed dose as soon as you remember, but skip it if it is almost time for your next scheduled dose.

If you are taking your drug only once a day at bedtime and you go to sleep without taking that dose, do not take it in the morning. Instead, call your doctor.

Do not take double doses.

Interactions with Other Drugs

The following drugs are listed in the *Evaluations of Drug Interactions* 1997 as causing "highly clinically significant" or "clinically significant" interactions when used together with this drug. We have also included potentially serious interactions listed in the drug's FDA-approved professional product labeling or package insert. New scientific techniques have allowed researchers to predict some drug interactions before they have been documented in people. There may be other drugs, especially those in the families of drugs listed below, that also will react with this drug to cause severe adverse effects. The number of new drugs approved for marketing increases the chance of drug interactions, and new drug interactions are being identified with old drugs. Be vigilant.

Make sure to tell your doctor and pharmacist the drugs you are taking and tell your doctor if you are taking any of these interacting drugs:

ADRENALIN (also in bee sting kits), cimetidine, CYTOMEL, epinephrine, guanethidine, IMDUR, INDERAL, INDERAL LA, ISMELIN, ISMO, ISORDIL, isosorbide, liothyronine, MELLARIL, nitroglycerin (sublingual), NITRO-BID, NITROSTAT, PARNATE, PRIMATENE MIST, propranolol, SORBITRATE, TAGAMET, thioridazine, tolazamide, TOLINASE, TRANSDERM-NITRO, tranylcypromine, TRIOSTAT.

Adverse Effects

Call your doctor immediately if you experience:

- **signs of overdose:** confusion, severe drowsiness, fever, hallucinations, restlessness and agitation, seizures, shortness of breath, trouble breathing, unusually fast, slow, or irregular heartbeat, unusual tiredness, weakness, vomiting, enlarged pupils
- **signs of parkinsonism:** difficulty speaking or swallowing, loss of balance, mask-like face, muscle spasms, stiffness of arms or legs, trembling and shaking, unusual twisting movements of body
  - irregular blood pressure
  - loss of bladder control
  - severe muscle stiffness
  - pale skin
  - blurred vision
  - constipation
  - confusion, delirium, or hallucinations
  - decreased sexual ability
  - difficulty in speaking or swallowing
  - eye pain
  - fainting
  - loss of balance control

- mask-like face
- difficulty urinating
- shakiness or trembling
- shuffling walk
- slowed movements
- stiffness of arms and legs
- anxiety
- breast enlargement in both males and females
- hair loss
- unusual secretion of milk
- increased sensitivity to sunlight
- irritability
- muscle twitching
- red or brownish spots on skin
- ringing or buzzing in the ears
- skin rash and itching
- sore throat and fever
- swelling of face and tongue
- swelling of testicles
- trouble with teeth or gums
- yellow skin or eyes

Call your doctor if these symptoms continue:

- diarrhea
- dizziness
- dry mouth
- headache
- heartburn
- insomnia
- nausea or vomiting
- increased appetite for sweets
- unpleasant taste in mouth
- weight gain
- trouble sleeping

Call your doctor if these symptoms continue after you have stopped taking the drugs:

- headache
- irritability
- nausea and vomiting
- diarrhea
- restlessness or unusual excitement
- insomnia

Periodic Tests

Ask your doctor which of these tests should be done periodically while you are taking this drug:

- complete blood count
- pulse
- blood pressure
- glaucoma tests
- desipramine blood levels
- liver function tests
- kidney function tests
- heart function tests such as electrocardiogram (ECG, EKG)
- dental exams, at least twice yearly

You should wait at least five years from the date of release to take any new drug unless it is one of those rare "breakthrough" drugs that offers you a documented therapeutic advantage over older proven drugs. New drugs are tested in a relatively small number of people before being released, and serious adverse effects, or life-threatening drug interactions may not be detected until the new drug has been taken by hundreds of thousands of people. A number of new drugs have been withdrawn within their first five years after approval. Also, warnings about serious new adverse reactions have been added to the labeling of a number of drugs, or new drug interactions have been detected, usually within the first five years after a drug's release.

Fluoxetine
PROZAC (Dista)

Limited Use (following drugs)

Paroxetine
PAXIL (SmithKline Beecham)

Sertraline
ZOLOFT (Pfizer)

Do Not Use Until Five Years After Release

Fluvoxamine (Do Not Use Until 2000)
LUVOX (Solvay)

GENERIC: not available

FAMILY: Selective Serotonin Reuptake Inhibitor (SSRI) Antidepressants (See p. 196 for discussion of depression.)

Fluoxetine (floo *ox* uh teen), paroxetine (pa *rox* uh teen), sertraline (*ser* tral leen), and fluvoxamine (floo *vox* uh meen) all belong to the family of antidepressants known as selective serotonin reuptake inhibitors (SSRIs). Fluoxetine, paroxetine, and sertraline are approved to treat severe depression and obsessive compulsive disorder. Fluoxetine is also approved for the eating disorder bulimia, and paroxetine and sertraline for the treatment of panic disorder. Fluvoxamine is only approved for obsessive compulsive disorder at this time.

Fluoxetine, paroxetine, and sertraline are used to treat severe depression that is not caused by other drugs, by alcohol, or by emotional losses (such as a death in the family). These are effective medications in many patients including some whose depression has not improved on other drugs. Fluoxetine appears to be most appropriate for patients who are at special risk from the fatigue, low blood pressure, dry mouth, and constipation caused by other antidepressants. It is safer in overdoses than some other antidepressants, but there is no evidence that the death rate from suicides with antidepressants has decreased with the widespread use of fluoxetine and the other SSRI antidepressants.[145] Only limited data on fluoxetine's safety and efficacy in older adults are available.

Fluoxetine and the other SSRIs may reduce the risk of suicide in depressed patients. However, there have been a few reports that fluoxetine may actually induce suicidal thoughts in selected patients, although this has not been confirmed.[146] Public Citizen's Health Research Group petitioned the Food and Drug Administration in 1991 to require a box warning in the professional product labeling for fluoxetine warning doctors that a small minority of persons taking the drug have experienced intense, violent, suicidal thoughts, agitation, and impulsivity after starting treatment with the drug. You should *not* take this drug for mild depression or anxiety, or as a sleeping pill.

A review of 64 randomized controlled trials comparing SSRIs to the older tricyclic antidepressants such as imipramine (TOFRANIL) found similar benefit from the new and older drugs. When the results of many clinical trials were pooled, called a meta-analysis, no clear benefit was found for the new drugs over the older antidepressants. The adverse effects of the new and old antidepressants have little in common except for withdrawal symptoms. For example, SSRIs are less likely than the tricyclic drugs to cause sedation, anticholinergic effects (see p. 194), and heart rhythm disturbances. On the other hand, SSRIs' adverse effects commonly affect the gastrointestinal tract, especially causing nausea and diarrhea, and may also cause insomnia, agitation, extrapyramidal symptoms (drug-induced parkinsonism), and withdrawal effects.

One group of adverse effects is traded for another between the SSRIs and tricyclic antidepressants and there does not appear to be any difference in the proportion of people who can tolerate these two groups of antidepressants. When the number of people who stopped taking an antidepressant in 58 clinical trials were studied there was no clinically important difference between the SSRIs and the tricyclic and related antidepressants.[147]

When you take these medicines you may experience some adverse effects. The most frequently reported include nausea, anxiety, headache, and insomnia. These adverse effects tend to be worst at the start of treatment, and improve over a few weeks. Akathisia, or symptoms of restlessness, constant pacing, and purposeless movements of the feet and legs, may also occur. Dry mouth, sweating, diarrhea, tremor, loss of appetite, and dizziness are also common adverse effects.

Elderly patients, and those who experience troublesome agitation, anxiety, or insomnia at the recommended daily dose of 20 mg should start at lower doses (e.g,. 5 mg). Many consultants to *The Medical Letter* think that the manufacturer's dosage recommendations are too high.[148] A liquid form of the medicine is now available for lower doses.

The length of time it takes an antidepressant to work can overlap with the time of spontaneous recovery, especially if the depression is situational—caused by a death or other external circumstances. The majority of people lift themselves out of depression with friends, or activities such as exercise, work, reading, play, art, travel, and spiritual resources. If depression is not overcome by these measures, seek help from mental health professionals, such as therapists or psychiatrists. Antidepressant drugs should be reserved for depression that is major and does not respond to psychotherapy alone.

WARNING

A small number of people taking fluoxetine have experienced intense, violent, suicidal thoughts, agitation, and impulsivity. Whether their symptoms were induced by fluoxetine or were related to their underlying psychological problems is unclear. As with any other antidepressant, fluoxetine should only be used under close medical supervision. Patients are advised to consider telling relatives and friends about their use of this drug and the risk of suicidal obsession and self-injurious behavior.

Do not take fluoxetine, paroxetine, sertraline, or fluvoxamine with monoamine oxidase (MAO) inhibitors (see Interactions with Other Drugs) because the combinations may produce a syndrome of rising temperature, tremor, and seizures.

Before You Use This Drug

Tell your doctor if you have or have had:

- allergies to drugs
- suicidal thoughts or actions
- kidney or liver problems
- diabetes
- epilepsy or seizures
- brain disease or damage

Tell your doctor about any other drugs you take, including aspirin, herbs, vitamins, and other nonprescription products.

When You Use This Drug

- Until you know how you react to these drugs, do not drive or perform other activities requiring alertness. These drug may cause drowsiness.
- Do not drink alcohol or take other drugs that can cause drowsiness.
- You may feel dizzy when rising from a lying or sitting position. When getting out of bed, hang your legs over the side of the bed for a few minutes, then get up slowly. When getting up from a chair, stay by the chair until you are sure that you are not dizzy. (See p. 16.)
- Stop taking these drugs and check with your doctor as soon as possible if you develop skin rash or hives.
- If you develop dryness of the mouth, take sips of water. If dry mouth persists for more than two weeks, check with your doctor.
- Check with your doctor before you take any other drugs, prescription or nonprescription. These drugs frequently interact with other drugs.

- The effects of these drugs may last for several weeks after you stop taking them. Do not drink alcohol and heed all other warnings for this time period.

How to Use This Drug

- Measure liquid with a calibrated teaspoon.
- Capsules may be opened and mixed with food or drink. Food does not affect the extent of absorption, although rate may be slightly decreased.
- If you are taking other drugs, take them one to two hours before taking one of these drugs.
- If you miss a dose, skip the missed dose, and continue with your next scheduled dose. **Do not take double doses**.
- Store both forms at room temperature with cap on tightly.
- Do not store in the bathroom. Do not expose to heat, moisture, or strong light.

Interactions with Other Drugs

The following drugs are listed in the *Evaluations of Drug Interactions* 1997 as causing "highly clinically significant" or "clinically significant" interactions when used together with this drug. We have also included potentially serious interactions listed in the drug's FDA-approved professional product labeling or package insert. New scientific techniques have allowed researchers to predict some drug interactions before they have been documented in people. There may be other drugs, especially those in the families of drugs listed below, that also will react with this drug to cause severe adverse effects. The number of new drugs approved for marketing increases the chance of drug interactions, and new drug interactions are being identified with old drugs. Be vigilant. Make sure to tell your doctor and pharmacist the drugs you are taking and tell your doctor if you are taking any of these interacting drugs:

At least two weeks should elapse between stopping a monoamine oxidase (MAO) inhibitor and starting one of these drugs. You should wait at least five weeks after stopping one of these drugs and starting one of these MAO inhibitors: deprenyl, ELDEPRYL, furazolidone, FUROXONE, isocarboxazid, MARPLAN, MATULANE, NARDIL, PARNATE, phenelzine, procarbazine, selegiline, tranylcypromine.

Other interacting drugs are: alprazolam, astemizole, DESYREL, DILANTIN, HISMANAL, lithium, LITHOBID, LITHONATE, marijuana, phenytoin, trazodone, XANAX.

Central nervous system (CNS) depressant drugs including: alcohol, antidepressants, antihistamines, antipsychotics, some blood pressure medications (reserpine, methyldopa, beta-blockers), motion sickness medications, muscle relaxants, narcotics, sedatives, sleeping pills and tranquilizers. These drugs can increase the blood levels of other antidepressants, potentially increasing adverse effects from those medications.

Adverse Effects

Call your doctor immediately if you experience:

- **signs of overdose:** agitation and restlessness, convulsions, seizures, unusual excitement, severe nausea and vomiting, severe drowsiness, dry mouth, irritability, large pupils, fast heartbeat
- **signs of allergic reaction or serum sickness-like syndrome:** skin rash or hives associated with burning or tingling in fingers, hands, or arms, chills or fever, swollen glands, joint or muscle pain, swelling of feet or lower legs, or trouble breathing

- **signs of hypoglycemia:** anxiety, chills, cold sweats, confusion, cool, pale skin, difficulty in concentration, drowsiness, excessive hunger, fast heartbeat, headache, nervousness, shakiness, unsteady walk, unusual tiredness or weakness
- suicidal thoughts or behavior
- chills or fever
- joint or muscle pain
- skin rash, hives, or itching
- difficulty breathing
- cold sweats
- confusion
- excessive hunger
- unusual excitement
- swollen glands
- swelling of feet or lower legs
- difficulty speaking
- dry mouth
- decreased sexual drive
- stomach or abdominal cramps
- gas
- tiredness or weakness
- trouble sleeping
- mania

Call your doctor if these symptoms continue:

- anxiety and nervousness
- nausea, vomiting, or diarrhea
- increased or decreased appetite or weight loss
- constipation
- frequent urination
- change in taste
- drowsiness
- dizziness
- headache
- increased sweating
- disturbing dreams
- changes in vision
- chest pain
- irregular or fast heartbeat
- stuffy nose
- cough
- impaired concentration
- trembling or quivering

- feeling of warmth or heat
- flushing or redness of skin, especially on face and neck

Periodic Tests

Ask your doctor which of these tests should be done periodically while you are taking this drug:

- supervision of depression with suicidal tendencies

WARNING

WITHDRAWAL REACTIONS WITH SELECTIVE SEROTONIN REUPTAKE INHIBITOR ANTIDEPRESSANTS (SSRIS)

A withdrawal reaction has been reported with all SSRI antidepressants. The symptoms generally start within one to three days after stopping the drug, and generally resolve within one to two weeks after the drug has been discontinued. Withdrawal symptoms may occur even when the dosage of the drug is gradually decreased. The main symptoms of this reaction are: dizziness, vertigo, uncoordination, nausea and vomiting, and flu-like symptoms that include fatigue, lethargy, muscle pain and chills.

This reaction appears to be most common with paroxetine, and to a lesser extent with sertraline and fluoxetine.[149] Withdrawal has also been reported with fluvoxamine. Because this is the newest SSRI how often the withdrawal reaction occurs is unknown.

PREGNANCY WARNING

Luvox caused harm to developing fetuses in animal studies, or such studies were not done. Use during pregnancy only for clear medical reasons. Tell your doctor if you are pregnant or thinking of becoming pregnant before you take this drug.

Do Not Use Until Five Years After Release

Mirtazapine (Do Not Use Until 2002)
REMERON (Organon)

GENERIC: not available

FAMILY: Antidepressants
(See p. 196 for discussion of depression.)

Mirtazapine (mir *taz* a peen) is used to treat major depression. Mirtazapine resembles a hybrid of other types of antidepressants, namely both tricyclic (TCA) and selective serotonin reuptake inhibitors (SSRIs). Mirtazapine blocks receptors of the neurotransmitters serotonin and norepinephrine. In drug studies about 20% more people improved taking mirtazapine than improved taking a placebo (sugar pills).[150]

Older people and those with liver or kidney problems may need a lower dose of mirtazapine. Over half the people who take mirtazapine experience prolonged drowsiness. Mirtazapine can cause a blood disorder which lowers the number of white blood cells. Called agranulocytosis, it is a serious, sometimes fatal, adverse effect. Another potential life-threatening effect is serotonin syndrome. Symptoms include sweating, shivering, and uncoordination. Mirtazapine is not recommended for women who are pregnant or children under 18.

Published information about this drug is sparse. With so many other antidepressants available, it is wiser to use an antidepressant with better known safety and effectiveness.

The length of time it takes an antidepressant to work can overlap with the time of spontaneous recovery, especially if the depression is situational—caused by a death or other external circumstances. The majority of people lift themselves out of depression with friends, or activities such as exercise, work, reading, play, art, travel, and spiritual resources. If depression is not overcome by these measures, seek help from mental health professionals, such as therapists or psychiatrists. Antidepressant drugs should be reserved for depression that is major and does not respond to psychotherapy alone.

Before You Use This Drug

Tell your doctor if you have or have had:

- allergies
- heart, kidney or liver problems
- nursing
- seizures

Tell your doctor about any other drugs you take, including aspirin, herbs, vitamins, and other nonprescription products.

When You Use This Drug

- Do not drink alcohol or use other drugs that can cause drowsiness.
- Until you know how you react to this drug, do not drive or perform other activities that require alertness.
- You may feel dizzy when rising from a lying or sitting position. When getting out of bed, hang your legs over the side of the bed for a few minutes, then get up slowly. When getting up from a chair, stay beside the chair until you are sure that you are not dizzy. (See p. 16.)
- Have your doctor reassess your need to continue taking mirtazapine periodically.
- If you plan to have any surgery, including dental, tell your doctor that you take this drug.

How to Use This Drug

- Swallow half or whole tablets, according to dose. Take at bedtime. Take with or without food.
- If you miss a dose, take it as soon as you remember but skip it if it is almost time for the next dose. **Do not take double doses.**
- Do not suddenly stop taking this drug. Check with your doctor.
- Store at room temperature, below 77°F. Do not store in the bathroom. Do not expose to heat, moisture, or strong light.

Interactions with Other Drugs

The following drugs are listed in the *Evaluations of Drug Interactions* 1997 as causing "highly clinically significant" or "clinically significant" interactions when used together with this drug. We have also included potentially serious interactions listed in the drug's FDA-approved professional product labeling or package insert. New scientific techniques have allowed researchers to predict some drug interactions before they have been documented in people. There may be other drugs, especially those in the families of drugs listed below, that also will react with this drug to cause severe adverse effects. The number of new drugs approved for marketing increases the chance of drug interactions, and new drug interactions are being identified with old drugs. Be vigilant. Make sure to tell your doctor and pharmacist the drugs you are taking and tell your doctor if you are taking any of these interacting drugs:

Do not take mirtazapine within 14 days after stopping or starting any of these monoamine oxidase (MAO) inhibitors: deprenyl, ELDEPRYL, furazolidone, FUROXONE, isocarboxazid, MARPLAN, MATULANE, NARDIL, PARNATE, phenelzine, procarbazine, selegiline, tranylcypromine.

Central nervous system (CNS) depressant drugs including alcohol, antidepressants, antihistamines, antipsychotics, some blood pressure medications (reserpine, methyldopa, beta-blockers), motion sickness medications, muscle relaxants, narcotics, sedatives, sleeping pills and tranquilizers.

Adverse Effects

Call your doctor immediately if you experience:

- agitation
- chills, shivering
- excitement
- confusion
- dizziness
- fever
- more rapid heartbeat
- uncoordination
- mouth is inflamed or has sores
- seizures
- sore throat
- suicidal thoughts
- sweating
- twitching
- menstrual pain or missed periods
- mood or mental changes
- shortness of breath
- swelling of feet or ankles

Call your doctor if these symptoms continue:

- constipation
- drowsiness
- dry mouth
- weakness
- weight gain
- abdominal pain
- abnormal dreams
- back pain
- frequent urge to urinate
- sensitivity to touch and pain
- increased thirst
- low blood pressure
- muscle pain
- nausea, vomiting
- trembling, shaking

Ask your doctor which of these tests should be done periodically while you are taking this drug:

- blood tests

You should wait at least five years from the date of release to take any new drug unless it is one of those rare "breakthrough" drugs that offers you a documented therapeutic advantage over older proven drugs. New drugs are tested in a relatively small number of people before being approved, and serious adverse effects, or life-threatening drug interactions may not be detected until the new drug has been taken by hundreds of thousands of people. A number of new drugs have been withdrawn within their first five years after release. Also, warnings about serious new adverse reactions have been added to the labeling of a number of drugs, or new drug interactions have been detected, usually within the first five years after a drug's release.

PREGNANCY WARNING

This drug caused harm to developing fetuses in animal studies, or such studies were not done. Use during pregnancy only for clear medical reasons. Tell your doctor if you are pregnant or thinking of becoming pregnant before you take this drug.

Limited Use

Risperidone
RISPERDAL (Janssen)

GENERIC: not available
FAMILY: Antipsychotics (see p. 187)

Risperidone (ris *per* i done) is used to treat, but not cure, mental illnesses such as psychosis, especially schizophrenia. Risperidone has about the same effectiveness as haloperidol and clozapine. Older people should start with

0.5 mg doses. If needed, the dose of risperidone is gradually increased over several days or weeks. The maximum dose for older people is 3 mg a day. Lower doses should also be taken by people with kidney or liver problems or low blood pressure.

Doses of 3.5 mg a day and higher can cause serious adverse effects similar to ones experienced with haloperidol.[151,152] Doses greater than 6 mg have not proved to be more effective. Older people are at increased risk for adverse effects. These include NMS (neuroleptic malignant syndrome) characterized by fever, profuse sweating, rigid muscles, fast or irregular heartbeat, and kidney failure. Risperidone can also cause you to sunburn more readily, gain weight, and change the amount of saliva in your mouth causing cavities. Some adverse effects can be averted by lowering doses. Information about long-term effects of risperidone is still sparse. Continued use should be reassessed periodically. The cost of risperidone is high compared to generic haloperidol. If you switch from other drugs to risperidone, the time the drugs overlap should be minimal.

Before You Use This Drug

Tell your doctor if you have or have had:

- allergies
- blood pressure that is low
- breast cancer
- dehydration
- heart, kidney or liver problems
- hypovolemia
- Parkinson's disease
- seizures
- brain tumor
- drug overdose or abuse
- intestinal obstruction
- Reye's syndrome

Tell your doctor about any other drugs you take, including aspirin, herbs, vitamins, and other nonprescription products.

When You Use This Drug

- Until you know how you react to this drug, do not drive or perform other activities that require alertness. Risperidone can cause drowsiness, dizziness, and blurred vision.
- When you first take risperidone try to have someone stay with you in case you become very weak from lowering of your blood pressure.
- Do not drink alcohol or use other central nervous system (CNS) depressants including antidepressants, antihistamines, antipsychotics, some blood pressure medications, (reserpine, methyldopa, beta-blockers), motion sickness medications, muscle relaxants, narcotics, sedatives, sleeping pills, and tranquilizers.
- You may feel dizzy when rising from a lying or sitting position. When getting out of bed, hang your legs over the side of the bed for a few minutes, then get up slowly. When getting up from a chair, stay beside the chair until you are sure that you are not dizzy. (See p. 16.)
- Protect yourself from sun. Use sun block that protects against both ultraviolet A and B and/or wear wide brim hats, sunglasses, long sleeves, and long slacks. Avoid sunlamps, tanning beds and tanning booths.
- Avoid heatstroke from exercise, hot baths, or hot weather. Drink adequate fluids during hot weather.
- Chew sugarless gum, candy, or ice or use a saliva substitute if you develop dryness in your mouth. If dryness continues more than two weeks, check with your doctor or dentist.
- Keep regular appointments with your doctor.
- If you plan to have any surgery, including dental, tell your doctor that you take this drug.

How to Use This Drug

- Swallow tablets or solution. Take without regard to food.
- If you miss a dose, take it as soon as you remember but skip it if it is almost time for the next dose. **Do not take double doses.**

- Check with your doctor before decreasing your dose or stopping risperidone.
- Store at room temperature below 104°F. Do not store in the bathroom. Do not expose to heat, moisture, or strong light.

Interactions with Other Drugs

The following drugs are listed in the *Evaluations of Drug Interactions* 1997 as causing "highly clinically significant" or "clinically significant" interactions when used together with this drug. We have also included potentially serious interactions listed in the drug's FDA-approved professional product labeling or package insert. New scientific techniques have allowed researchers to predict some drug interactions before they have been documented in people. There may be other drugs, especially those in the families of drugs listed below, that also will react with this drug to cause severe adverse effects. The number of new drugs approved for marketing increases the chance of drug interactions, and new drug interactions are being identified with old drugs. Be vigilant. Make sure to tell your doctor and pharmacist the drugs you are taking and tell your doctor if you are taking any of these interacting drugs:

> bromocriptine, carbamazepine, clozapine, CLOZARIL, LARODOPA, levodopa, PARLODEL, TEGRETOL. Because risperidone may cause low blood pressure (hypotension), it may enhance the blood-pressure-lowering effects of drugs used to treat high blood pressure.

Adverse Effects

Call your doctor immediately if you experience:

- anxiety, nervousness
- decrease in appetite
- arms or legs feel weak or stiff
- back pain
- bleeding
- blood pressure becomes irregular
- unusual secretion of milk
- difficulty breathing
- puffy cheeks
- chest pain
- dandruff
- difficulty concentrating or remembering
- dizziness
- drowsiness
- unusual facial expression
- fever
- trembling or shaking of hands or fingers
- irregular heartbeat
- lips smack or pucker
- menstrual changes
- mood changes, including aggressive behavior or uncontrolled excitement
- muscles become stiff
- penis erection is painful or prolonged
- restlessness, need to keep moving
- seizures
- sexual desire declines
- shuffling walk or loss of balance
- skin itches, becomes oily or pale, bruises or rash appears
- difficulty sleeping
- uncontrolled movements of arms, back, face, legs, neck, or trunk
- difficulty swallowing or speaking
- extreme thirst
- tic-like, twisting, or twitching movements of body
- rapid or darting movement of tongue
- difficulty urinating
- vision blurs or changes, eyes blink uncontrollably, inability to move eyes
- uncontrolled tiredness or weakness

Call your doctor if these symptoms continue:

- abdominal pain
- constipation

- cough
- diarrhea
- dry mouth
- headache
- heartburn
- joint pain
- nausea
- runny nose
- increase in saliva (watering of mouth)
- skin becomes dry or darkens
- sleep and dreams increase
- sore throat
- sunburn
- undesired weight gain or loss
- vomiting

Periodic Tests

Ask your doctor which of these tests should be done periodically while you are taking this drug:

- abnormal movement determinations

DECREASED SWEATING

Risperidone may make you sweat less, causing your body temperature to increase. Use extra care not to become overheated during exercise or hot weather while you are taking one of these medications, since overheating may result in heat stroke. Also, hot baths or saunas may make you feel dizzy or faint while you are taking this medicine.

Limited Use

Oxazepam
SERAX (Wyeth-Ayerst)

GENERIC: available

FAMILY: Benzodiazepine Sleeping Pills and Tranquilizers (see p. 178)

Oxazepam (ox *az* e pam) is used to treat anxiety and is the only sleeping pill or tranquilizer in its family that we recommend for older adults. Because oxazepam, like all the drugs in its family, is addictive, you should not be taking it to relieve the stress of daily life (see information in the box below). There are safer ways to deal with occasional and short-term tension, nervousness, and sleeplessness (see p. 185). Only in a very limited number of circumstances is a sleeping pill or tranquilizer really necessary.

Oxazepam, like Valium, Dalmane and Librium (see p. 222), belongs to a family of drugs called benzodiazepines (ben zoe dye *az* e peens). It is safer than these other drugs, and may be the safest benzodiazepine for older adults, because it is short-acting rather than long-acting, meaning that it is eliminated more quickly from your body. This reduces the risk that it will accumulate in your bloodstream and reach dangerously high levels, causing harmful adverse effects. Another reason that oxazepam is safer than other drugs in its family is that your body does not convert it into chemicals called active metabolites that can produce adverse effects.[153]

Studies show that there is much less potential for abusing oxazepam than for abusing diazepam (VALIUM).[154,155] Oxazepam also may have a lower risk of addiction than benzodiazepines that act over a shorter period of time, such as lorazepam (ATIVAN), alprazolam (XANAX), and triazolam (HALCION).[156]

Oxazepam can cause adverse effects common to all benzodiazepines, and older adults are more likely to experience certain ones: confusion, drowsiness, and uncoordination that can result in falls and hip fractures. Oxazepam causes no less memory impairment than any benzodiazepine, other than clorazepate, a long-acting drug.[157]

One hazard of taking oxazepam continuously for longer than several weeks is drug-induced dependence. **Do not stop taking your drug suddenly.** With the help of your doctor, work out a schedule for slowly decreasing the amount of the drug you take by about 5 to 10% each day. Keep a written record of the dosage reduction schedule with you. These steps will make it much easier to become drug free without developing distressing symptoms of drug withdrawal.

RULES FOR SAFER USE OF OXAZEPAM

1. Use a low dose. The dose should be one-third to one-half the dose used for younger people. This means that the highest starting dose for older adults should be 7.5 milligrams one to three times a day, if used as a tranquilizer, or 7.5 milligrams at bedtime, if used as a sleeping pill. The generic tablet form of oxazepam is only available in a 15 milligram tablet, which should be broken in half to get a 7.5 milligram dose. This is one-half of a 15 milligram tablet, available generically.

2. Ask your doctor to limit the amount of your prescription to seven days' worth of pills.

3. Ask your doctor to write *NO REFILL* on your prescription, so that you will not be inclined (because of the "good chemical feelings" these pills may provide) to refill the prescription five times without seeing the doctor again. This dangerously lax refill policy is perfectly legal because oxazepam and other similar drugs are not very carefully controlled by the government.

By urging your doctor to write *NO REFILL* you are making sure that he or she will reevaluate your condition after you use oxazepam for a short time. You will want to discuss how you are doing with your anxiety or sleeping problem, rather than continuing to take the drug without a reevaluation. Continuing to take oxazepam without talking to your doctor could be the first step to addiction or other drug-induced problems.

4. At the end of the first day and every day that you use oxazepam, evaluate what you have done, on your own or by talking to others, to learn what makes you anxious. Evaluate what you have done to change the internal or external circumstances causing your anxiety. Keep a record of these evaluations. Talk to your doctor about reducing the dose of oxazepam as soon as a reduction seems appropriate. Since you only have enough medication for one week, it is unlikely that you will have become addicted this quickly.

5. Do not drive a car or operate dangerous machinery while using oxazepam.

6. Do not drink alcohol. Combining oxazepam and alcohol dangerously increases the effects of both. An overdose of oxazepam in combination with alcohol can be fatal.

7. Before using oxazepam, tell your doctor if you are taking other drugs with a sedative or "downer" effect, such as antidepressants, antipsychotics, antihistamines, narcotic painkillers, epilepsy medications, barbiturates, or other sleeping medications. Combining oxazepam with other drugs that have sedative effects dangerously increases the risks of both drugs.

The best way to reduce the risks from sleeping pills and tranquilizers is to avoid them if at all possible. Before taking one of these powerful medications, see p. 185 for nondrug alternatives to try before using either sleeping pills or tranquilizers.

Before You Use This Drug

Tell your doctor if you have or have had:

- allergies to drugs
- kidney or liver problems
- brief periods of not breathing during sleep (sleep apnea)
- lung disease or breathing problems
- alcohol or drug dependence
- mental depression or illness
- myasthenia gravis
- glaucoma
- epilepsy, seizures
- porphyria
- brain disease
- difficulty swallowing
- hyperactivity

Tell your doctor about any other drugs you take, including aspirin, herbs, vitamins, and other nonprescription products.

When You Use This Drug

- Do not take more than prescribed. Oxazepam is addictive.
- Do not drink alcohol or use other drugs that can cause drowsiness.
- Until you know how you react to this drug, do not drive or perform other activities requiring alertness. Oxazepam may cause drowsiness. **People who take drugs in this family may be more likely to have traffic accidents.**
- If you plan to have any surgery, including dental, tell your doctor that you take this drug.

How to Use This Drug

- Crush tablet and mix with food or water, or swallow whole. Take with food.
- If you miss a dose, take it if you remember within one hour of the time you were supposed to take it. Skip it if more than an hour has passed. **Do not take double doses.**
- Do not store in the bathroom. Do not expose to heat, moisture, or strong light.

Interactions with Other Drugs

The following drugs are listed in the *Evaluations of Drug Interactions* 1997 as causing "highly clinically significant" or "clinically significant" interactions when used together with this drug. We have also included potentially serious interactions listed in the drug's FDA-approved professional product labeling or package insert. New scientific techniques have allowed researchers to predict some drug interactions before they have been documented in people. There may be other drugs, especially those in the families of drugs listed below, that also will react with this drug to cause severe adverse effects. The number of new drugs approved for marketing increases the chance of drug interactions, and new drug interactions are being identified with old drugs. Be vigilant. Make sure to tell your doctor and pharmacist the drugs you are taking and tell your doctor if you are taking any of these interacting drugs:

alcohol, BENADRYL, digoxin, diphenhydramine, KETALAR, ketamine, LANOXICAPS, LANOXIN, SOMINEX FORMULA.

Adverse Effects

Call your doctor immediately if you experience:

- **signs of overdose:** prolonged confusion, severe drowsiness, slurred speech, shakiness, staggering, slow heartbeat, shortness of breath, trouble breathing, extreme weakness

- confusion, hallucinations
- trouble sleeping
- unusual excitement, irritability
- mental depression
- skin rash, itching
- sore throat and fever
- yellow eyes or skin
- ulcers or sores in mouth or throat that last
- unusual bleeding or bruising
- clumsiness, unsteadiness, or falling
- seizures
- low blood pressure
- unusual tiredness or weakness
- impaired memory
- muscle weakness
- uncontrolled movements

Call your doctor if these symptoms continue:

- blurred or changed vision
- dizziness, lightheadedness
- constipation or diarrhea
- drowsiness
- difficulty urinating
- headache
- dry mouth, increased thirst, or unusual mouth watering
- nausea or vomiting
- slurred speech
- joint or chest pain
- fast heartbeat
- nasal congestion
- abdominal or stomach cramps
- muscle spasms
- change in sex drive or performance

Call your doctor if these symptoms continue after you stop taking this drug:

- irritability, nervousness
- trouble sleeping
- abdominal or stomach cramps
- confusion
- irregular heartbeat
- increased sense of hearing
- increased sensitivity to touch and pain
- sweating

- loss of reality, feelings of distrust or depression
- muscle cramps
- nausea or vomiting
- sensitivity to light
- tingling, burning or prickly sensation
- trembling
- confusion
- seizures
- hallucinations

Limited Use

Nefazodone
SERZONE (Bristol-Myers Squibb)

GENERIC: not available

FAMILY: Antidepressants (See p. 196 for discussion of depression.)

Nefazodone (ne *faz* ah done) is used to treat depression. It improves, but does not cure depression. Nefazodone inhibits the neurotransmitters serotonin and norepinephrine. Nefazodone belongs to the same family as trazodone.

The adverse effects of nefazodone may increase with higher doses. Dangerous, life-threatening, drug interactions can occur with certain antihistamines and stomach medications. Nefazodone is not recommended for women who are pregnant or breast-feeding, or children under age 18.

The length of time it takes an antidepressant to work can overlap with the time of spontaneous recovery, especially if the depression is situational—caused by a death or other external circumstances. The majority of people lift themselves out of depression with friends, or activities such as exercise, work, reading, play, art, travel, and spiritual resources. If depression is not overcome by these measures, seek help from mental health professionals, such as therapists or psychiatrists. Antidepressant drugs should be reserved for depression that is major and does not respond to psychotherapy alone.

Before You Use This Drug

Tell your doctor if you have or have had:

- allergies
- drug abuse
- heart or liver problems
- manic depression or bipolar disorder
- nursing

Tell your doctor about any other drugs you take, including aspirin, herbs, vitamins, and other nonprescription products.

When You Use This Drug

- Do not drink alcohol or use other drugs that can cause drowsiness.
- Until you know how you react to this drug, do not drive or perform other activities that require alertness.
- You may feel dizzy when rising from a lying or sitting position. When getting out of bed, hang your legs over the side of the bed for a few minutes, then get up slowly. When getting up from a chair, stay beside the chair until you are sure that you are not dizzy. (See p. 16.)
- Have your doctor periodically reassess your need to continue taking this drug.
- If you plan to have any surgery, including dental, tell your doctor that you take this drug.
- If you miss a dose, take it as soon as you remember, but skip it if it is almost time for the next dose. **Do not take double doses.**

How to Use This Drug

- Do not store in the bathroom. Do not expose to heat, moisture, or strong light.

Interactions with Other Drugs

The following drugs are listed in the *Evaluations of Drug Interactions* 1997 as causing "highly clinically significant" or "clinically sig-

nificant" interactions when used together with this drug. We have also included potentially serious interactions listed in the drug's FDA-approved professional product labeling or package insert. New scientific techniques have allowed researchers to predict some drug interactions before they have been documented in people. There may be other drugs, especially those in the families of drugs listed below, that also will react with this drug to cause severe adverse effects. The number of new drugs approved for marketing increases the chance of drug interactions, and new drug interactions are being identified with old drugs. Be vigilant. Make sure to tell your doctor and pharmacist the drugs you are taking and tell your doctor if you are taking any of these interacting drugs:

Do not take nefazodone within 14 days of using any of these monoamine oxidase (MAO) inhibitors: ELDEPRYL, furazolidone, FUROXONE, isocarboxazid, MARPLAN, MATULANE, NARDIL, PARNATE, phenelzine, procarbazine, selegiline, tranylcypromine.

Other drugs that can interact with nefazodone include: alcohol, alprazolam, astemizole, cisapride, digoxin, HALCION, HALDOL, haloperidol, HISMANAL, INDERAL, INDERAL LA, LANOXICAPS, LANOXIN, midazolam, propranolol, PROPULSID, SELDANE, terfenadine, triazolam, VERSED, XANAX.

Avoid taking lovastatin (MEVACOR) and simvastatin (ZOCOR) with nefazodone.[158]

Adverse Effects

Call your doctor immediately if you experience:

- agitation
- decreased blood pressure

- clumsiness or unsteadiness
- confusion
- dizziness
- more rapid heartbeat
- hives, rash
- persistent erection of the penis
- sore throat
- suicidal thoughts
- tremors
- vision changes
- difficulty urinating
- memory problems

Call your doctor if these symptoms continue:

- constipation or diarrhea
- drowsiness
- dry mouth
- headache
- impotence
- insomnia
- nausea
- ringing in ears
- tiredness, weakness
- increased appetite or weight gain
- tingling sensation
- taste changes
- flushing or feeling of warmth

PREGNANCY WARNING

This drug caused harm to developing fetuses in animal studies, or such studies were not done. Use during pregnancy only for clear medical reasions. Tell your doctor if you are pregnant or thinking of becoming pregnant before you take this drug.

Limited Use

Chlorpromazine (klor *proe* ma zeen)
THORAZINE (SmithKline Beecham)

Fluphenazine (floo *fen* a zeen)
PROLIXIN (Apothecon)

Thioridazine (thye oh *rid* a zeen)
MELLARIL (Novartis)

Trifluoperazine (trye floo oh *pair* a zeen)
STELAZINE (SmithKline Beecham)

GENERIC: available
FAMILY: Antipsychotics (see p. 187)

These drugs are in a group called phenothiazines (fee noe *thye* a zeens) that are effective for treating mental illnesses called psychoses, including schizophrenia. They should not be used to treat anxiety, to treat the loss of mental abilities (for example due to Alzheimer's disease) in nonpsychotic people, to sedate, or to control restless behavior or other problems in nonpsychotic people. They should also be used sparingly, if at all, for treating depression in older people since the incidence of tardive dyskinesia (involuntary movements of parts of the body), an often disabling adverse effect of these drugs, is 60% in older adults with depression who are given antipsychotic drugs.[159]

These antipsychotics can cause serious adverse effects, including tardive dyskinesia, drug-induced parkinsonism (see p. 193), the "jitters," and weakness and muscle fatigue (see Adverse Effects).

The chart on p. 194 shows the major differences among these drugs. If your doctor has prescribed one of these drugs and it is causing an unwanted side effect, use this chart to find alternative drugs that cause less of that particular effect.

Whichever of these drugs you use, you should be taking between one-tenth and one-fifth of the dose used for younger adults.

WARNING: SPECIAL MENTAL AND PHYSICAL ADVERSE EFFECTS

Older adults are especially sensitive to the harmful anticholinergic (see Glossary, p. 768) effects of antipsychotic drugs such as these. Drugs in this family should not be used unless absolutely necessary.

Mental Effects: confusion, delirium, short-term memory problems, disorientation, and impaired attention.

Physical Effects: dry mouth, constipation, difficulty urinating (especially for a man with an enlarged prostate), blurred vision, decreased sweating with increased body temperature, sexual dysfunction, and worsening of glaucoma.

Before You Use These Drugs

Tell your doctor if you have or have had:

- allergies to drugs
- alcohol dependence
- blood disease
- breast cancer
- enlarged prostate or difficulty urinating
- heart or blood vessel disease
- Parkinson's disease
- lung disease
- epilepsy, seizures
- glaucoma
- liver disease
- stomach ulcer
- Reye's syndrome

Tell your doctor about any other drugs you take, including aspirin, herbs, vitamins, and other nonprescription products.

When You Use This Drug

- It may take two to three weeks before you can tell that your drug is working.

- **Do not stop taking your drug suddenly. Your doctor must give you a schedule to lower your dose gradually, to prevent withdrawal symptoms such as nausea, vomiting, and stomach upset.**
- Until you know how you react to this drug, do not drive or perform other activities requiring alertness. These drugs may cause blurred vision, drowsiness, and fainting.
- Do not drink alcohol or use other drugs that can cause drowsiness.
- You may feel dizzy when rising from a lying or sitting position. When getting out of bed, hang your feet over the side of the bed for a few minutes, then get up slowly. When getting out of a chair, stay by the chair until you are sure that you are not dizzy. (See p. 16.)
- If you plan to have any surgery, including dental, tell your doctor that you take this drug.

How to Use This Drug

- Take with food or **a full glass (eight ounces) of milk or water** to prevent stomach upset.
- Do not store in the bathroom. Do not expose to heat, moisture, or strong light. Do not let the liquid form freeze.
- If you take antacids or diarrhea drugs, take them at least two hours apart from taking your antipsychotic drug.
- Swallow extended-release chlorpromazine capsules whole.
- If you miss a dose, take it as soon as you remember, but skip it if it is almost time for the next dose. **Do not take double doses.**

Interactions with Other Drugs

The following drugs are listed in the *Evaluations of Drug Interactions* 1997 as causing "highly clinically significant" or "clinically significant" interactions when used together with

this drug. We have also included potentially serious interactions listed in the drug's FDA-approved professional product labeling or package insert. New scientific techniques have allowed researchers to predict some drug interactions before they have been documented in people. There may be other drugs, especially those in the families of drugs listed below, that also will react with this drug to cause severe adverse effects. The number of new drugs approved for marketing increases the chance of drug interactions, and new drug interactions are being identified with old drugs. Be vigilant. Make sure to tell your doctor and pharmacist the drugs you are taking and tell your doctor if you are taking any of these interacting drugs:

> AEROSPORIN, alcohol, amphetamines, ANECTINE, benztropine, bromocriptine, CAPOTEN, captopril, carbamazepine, cimetidine, COGENTIN, DEMEROL, desipramine, DEXEDRINE, diazoxide, guanethidine, INDERAL, INDERAL LA, ISMELIN, lithium, LITHOBID, LITHONATE, meperidine, NORPRAMIN, PARLODEL, polymyxin B, PROGLYCEM, propranolol, RIFADIN, rifampin, RIMACTANE, succinylcholine, TAGAMET, TEGRETOL.

Adverse Effects

Call your doctor immediately if you experience:

* **signs of tardive dyskinesia:** lip smacking, chewing movements, puffing of cheeks, rapid, darting tongue movements, uncontrolled movements of arms or legs
* **signs of parkinsonism:** difficulty speaking or swallowing, loss of balance, mask-like face, muscle spasms, stiffness of arms or legs, trembling and shaking, unusual twisting movements of body

* **signs of restless leg (akathisia):** restless pacing, a feeling of the "jitters"
* **signs of akinesia:** weakness, muscular fatigue, listlessness, depression. Although often confused with true depression, akinesia is actually the most common of a group of adverse effects called extrapyramidal effects (see p. 193).
* changed or blurred vision
* difficulty urinating
* **signs of neuroleptic malignant syndrome:** troubled or fast breathing, high or low blood pressure, increased sweating, loss of bladder control, muscle stiffness, seizures, unusual tiredness, weakness, fast heartbeat, irregular pulse, pale skin
* fever and sore throat
* yellow eyes or skin
* skin rash
* fainting
* abnormal bleeding or bruising
* sore mouth or gums
* nightmares

Call your doctor if these symptoms continue:

* blurred vision
* change in color vision or difficulty seeing at night
* difficulty in speaking or swallowing
* fainting
* inability to move eyes
* loss of balance control
* abdominal or stomach pains
* aching muscles and joints
* confusion
* fever and chills
* muscle weakness
* nausea, vomiting, or diarrhea
* painful, inappropriate penile erection
* skin discoloration
* severe itching
* sore throat and fever
* yellow eyes or skin
* dry mouth
* sensitivity of skin to sunlight

Periodic Tests

Ask your doctor which of these tests should be done periodically while you are taking this drug:

- complete blood count
- blood pressure
- eye tests
- liver function tests
- observation for early signs of tardive dyskinesia
- reevaluation of need for the drug
- urine tests for bile and bilirubin

DECREASED SWEATING

Drugs such as chlorpromazine (Thorazine), fluphenazine (Prolixin), prochlorperazine (Compazine), thioridazine (Mellaril), and trifluoperazine (Stelazine) may make you sweat less, causing your body temperature to increase. Use extra care not to become overheated during exercise or hot weather while you are taking one of these medications, since overheating may result in heat stroke. Also, hot baths or saunas may make you feel dizzy or faint while you are taking this medicine.

SENSITIVITY TO COLD

Drugs such as chlorpromazine (Thorazine), fluphenazine (Prolixin), prochlorperazine (Compazine), thioridazine (Mellaril), and trifluoperazine (Stelazine) may make you more sensitive to cold temperatures. Dress warmly during cold weather. Be careful during prolonged exposure to cold, such as in winter sports or swimming in cold water.

 Do Not Use

ALTERNATIVE TREATMENT:
For depression, see Nortriptyline and Desipramine, p. 230.

Amitriptyline and Perphenazine
TRIAVIL (Merck)

FAMILY: Antidepressants (See p. 196 for discussion of depression.)
Antipsychotics (see p. 187)

The brand name product Triavil contains a fixed combination of an antidepressant, amitriptyline (see p. 216), and an antipsychotic, perphenazine. It is used to treat moderate to severe anxiety, agitation, and depression. We do not recommend that you use it, for several reasons.

First, although Triavil is available in different strengths, the dose of each of its two ingredients is fixed and may not exactly fit your needs. **Second, combining an antipsychotic with an antidepressant has not been shown to produce a more effective drug.**[160] Third, using this combination raises the risk of harmful adverse effects, since it may cause any of the adverse effects of either of its ingredients, including severe drowsiness and other anticholinergic effects (see box below).[161] And fourth, the antidepressant ingredient in this combination, amitriptyline, has more adverse effects than any other drug in its family (see chart, p. 200) and should not be used by older adults either alone or in combinations such as this one.

The length of time it takes an antidepressant to work can overlap with the time of sponta-

---

If you use Triavil, talk to your doctor about changing your treatment. **Do not stop taking this drug suddenly.** Your doctor may want to give you a schedule to lower your dose *gradually* to prevent withdrawal symptoms, such as headache, mood change, nausea, vomiting, diarrhea, or trouble sleeping and vivid dreams.

neous recovery, especially if the depression is situational—caused by a death or other external circumstances. The majority of people lift themselves out of depression with friends, or activities such as exercise, work, reading, play, art, travel, and spiritual resources. If depression is not overcome by these measures, seek help from mental health professionals, such as therapists or psychiatrists. Antidepressant drugs should be reserved for depression that is major and does not respond to psychotherapy alone.

WARNING: SPECIAL MENTAL AND PHYSICAL ADVERSE EFFECTS

Older adults are especially sensitive to the harmful anticholinergic (see Glossary, p. 768) effects of tricyclic antidepressants such as amitriptyline. Drugs in this family should not be used unless absolutely necessary.

Mental Effects: confusion, delirium, short-term memory problems, disorientation, and impaired attention.

Physical Effects: dry mouth, constipation, difficulty urinating (especially for a man with an enlarged prostate), blurred vision, decreased sweating with increased body temperature, sexual dysfunction, and worsening of glaucoma.

Limited Use

Bupropion
WELLBUTRIN (Glaxo Wellcome)

GENERIC: not available

FAMILY: Antidepressants (See p. 196 for a discussion of depression.)

Bupropion (byu *pro* pee on) is used to treat severe depression that is not caused by other drugs, alcohol, or emotional losses (such as

---

EXTREME CAUTION

Bupropion has been approved by the Food and Drug Administration (FDA) for smoking cessation for people 18 years of age and older under the brand name Zyban (see p. 739). Zyban and Wellbutrin are exactly the same drug. Taking Zyban and Wellbutrin together will increase the risk of seizure. See the warning about bupropion-induced seizure below.

---

death in the family). It can take four weeks to be effective. Bupropion controls, but does not cure depression. Although it has been used for several years in some people,[162] the manufacturer does not recommend use beyond six weeks. Bupropion is related to amphetamines and diethylpropion (TENUATE, TEPANIL), but purportedly is not habit-forming. Although bupropion is preferred for the elderly by some doctors,[163] it has not been studied much in older people.

Weight loss is a common side effect. A number of people become restless when taking bupropion.

Higher doses increase likelihood of harmful effects. With doses more than 450 milligrams per day the risk of seizures increases tenfold and no one should take more than 450 mg per day.[164] Bupropion was temporarily banned in the United States for that reason. People age 60 and over are more likely to experience adverse effects, such as heart complications. Due to age-related decrease in kidney and liver function, the lowest effective dose should be used.

The length of time it takes an antidepressant to work can overlap with the time of spontaneous recovery, especially if the depression is situational—caused by a death or other external circumstances. The majority of people lift themselves out of depression with friends, or activities such as exercise, work, reading, play, art, travel, and spiritual resources. If depression is not overcome by these measures, seek help from mental health professionals, such as therapists or psychiatrists. Antidepressant drugs should be reserved for depression that is major and does not respond to psychotherapy alone.

WARNING: SPECIAL MENTAL AND PHYSICAL ADVERSE EFFECTS

Older adults are especially sensitive to the harmful anticholinergic (see Glossary, p. 768.) effects of antidepressants such as bupropion. Drugs in this family should not be used unless absolutely necessary.

Mental Effects: confusion, delirium, short-term memory problems, disorientation, and impaired attention.

Physical Effects: dry mouth, constipation, difficulty urinating (especially for a man with an enlarged prostate), blurred vision, decreased sweating with increased body temperature, sexual dysfunction, and worsening of glaucoma.

Before You Use This Drug

Do not use if you have or have had:

- eating disorders, such as anorexia or bulimia
- seizures

Tell your doctor if you have or have had:

- allergies to drugs
- bipolar disorder (manic depression)
- drug abuse
- electroshock therapy[165]
- head injury
- heart, kidney or liver problems

- myocardial infarction
- psychosis
- tumor of the central nervous system
- brain tumor
- seizures

Tell your doctor about any other drugs you take, including aspirin, herbs, vitamins, and other nonprescription products.

When You Use This Drug

- Until you know how you react to this drug, do not drive or perform other activities requiring alertness.
- Do not drink alcohol.

How to Use This Drug

- Swallow tablet whole. Take with food to lessen stomach upset.
- Space doses evenly apart during the day, but avoid taking at bedtime.
- If you miss a dose, take it as soon as you remember, but skip it if it is within four hours of the next dose. **Do not take double doses.**
- Store tablets at room temperature with lid on firmly.
- Do not store in the bathroom. Do not expose to heat, moisture, or strong light. Do not expose to high heat.

Interactions with Other Drugs

The following drugs are listed in the *Evaluations of Drug Interactions* 1997 as causing "highly clinically significant" or "clinically significant" interactions when used together with this drug. We have also included potentially serious interactions listed in the drug's FDA-approved professional product labeling or package insert. New scientific techniques have allowed researchers to predict some drug interactions before they have been documented in people. There may be other drugs, especially those in the families of drugs listed below, that also will react with this drug to cause severe adverse effects. The number of new drugs approved for marketing increases the chance of drug interactions, and new drug interactions are being identified with old drugs. Be vigilant. Make sure to tell your doctor and pharmacist the drugs you are taking and tell your doctor if you are taking any of these interacting drugs:

Do not take bupropion within 14 days of starting or stopping these monoamine oxidase (MAO) inhibitors: deprenyl, ELDEPRYL, furazolidone, FUROXONE, isocarboxazid, MARPLAN, MATULANE, NARDIL, PARNATE, phenelzine, procarbazine, selegiline, tranylcypromine.

These drugs also can interact with bupropion: alcohol, amitriptyline, chlorpromazine, clozapine, CLOZARIL, DESYREL, ELAVIL, fluoxetine, HALDOL, haloperidol, lithium, LITHOBID, LITHONATE, loxapine, LOXITANE, LUDIOMIL, maprotiline, MOBAN, molindone, NAVANE, NORVIR, PROZAC, ritonavir, thiothixene, THORAZINE, trazodone.

Adverse Effects

Call your doctor immediately if you experience:

- agitation, anxiety
- seizures
- convulsions
- fainting
- hallucinations
- severe headache
- irregular or fast heartbeat
- insomnia, restlessness
- skin rash, itching

Call your doctor if these symptoms continue:

- anger, hostility
- low or high blood pressure
- constipation, diarrhea
- dizziness
- drowsiness
- dry mouth or increased saliva
- fever, chills
- impotence
- uncoordination
- inflammation of the mouth
- loss of appetite, weight loss
- muscle spasms, tremor, twitching
- nausea or vomiting
- tinnitus, ringing in ears[166]
- increased sweating
- weight change
- unusual tiredness, sleep disturbance
- tremor
- difficulty concentrating
- increase in frequency of urination, especially at night, or difficult urination
- blurred vision

Periodic Tests

Ask your doctor which of these tests should be done periodically while you are taking this drug:

- kidney function tests
- liver function tests
- supervision for suicidal tendencies

Limited Use

Olanzapine
ZYPREXA (Lilly)

GENERIC: not available
FAMILY: Antipsychotics (see p. 187)

Olanzapine (oh *lan* za peen) is an antipsychotic used to treat schizophrenia, and related psychoses. This drug is chemically similar to clozapine and may work in a similar way to clozapine.[167]

All antipsychotics tend to improve symptoms, such as hallucinations, agitation, delusions, suspiciousness, and disorganized thinking. Atypical antipsychotics better improve the "negative" symptoms of schizophrenia, such as apathy, emotional withdrawal, lack of pleasure, and disorientation than older antipsychotics. Newer antipsychotics are less likely to cause adverse effects on equilibrium and muscle tone, often called movement disorders, at moderate doses. However, in higher doses these medications can cause serious adverse effects.

Drowsiness and weight gain are the most common adverse effects with olanzapine. Women, the elderly, and Asians are more prone to adverse effects. A rare, but potentially fatal effect is neuroleptic malignant syndrome (NMS). Symptoms of NMS are fever, profuse sweating, rigid muscles, fast or irregular heartbeat, and kidney failure.

Olanzapine has not been studied in children under age 18. Women who are breastfeeding should not take olanzapine. Long-term effects are not yet known. Many studies are as yet unpublished.[168]

Before You Use This Drug

Tell your doctor if you have or have had:

- allergies, including lactose intolerance
- low blood pressure
- diabetes
- heart or liver problems
- pregnant or nursing
- seizures

Tell your doctor about any other drugs you take, including aspirin, herbs, vitamins, and other nonprescription products.

When You Use This Drug

- Have someone stay with you or contact you after you take the first dose, in case you become dizzy or faint.
- Do not drink alcohol or use other drugs that can cause drowsiness.
- Do not smoke.
- Until you know how you react to this drug, do not drive or perform other activities that require alertness.
- You may feel dizzy when rising from a lying or sitting position. When getting out of bed, hang your legs over the side of the bed for a few minutes, then get up slowly. When getting up from a chair, stay beside the chair until you are sure that you are not dizzy. (See p. 16.)
- Avoid dehydration. Drink plenty of fluids, especially during hot weather, or if you have nausea, vomiting, or diarrhea.
- Chew sugarless gum, ice, or use saliva substitutes if you develop a dry mouth.
- Have your doctor reassess your need to continue taking this drug periodically.
- If you plan to have any surgery, including dental, tell your doctor that you take this drug.

How to Use This Drug

- Swallow tablet whole. Take with or without food.
- If you miss a dose, take it as soon as you remember but skip it if it is almost time for the next dose. **Do not take double doses.**
- Store at room temperature below 80°F. Do not store in the bathroom. Do not expose to heat, moisture, or strong light.

Interactions with Other Drugs

The following drugs are listed in the *Evaluations of Drug Interactions* 1997 as causing "highly clinically significant" or "clinically significant" interactions when used together with this drug. We have also included potentially

serious interactions listed in the drug's FDA-approved professional product labeling or package insert. New scientific techniques have allowed researchers to predict some drug interactions before they have been documented in people. There may be other drugs, especially those in the families of drugs listed below, that also will react with this drug to cause severe adverse effects. The number of new drugs approved for marketing increases the chance of drug interactions, and new drug interactions are being identified with old drugs. Be vigilant. Make sure to tell your doctor and pharmacist the drugs you are taking and tell your doctor if you are taking any of these interacting drugs:

Central nervous system depressant (CNS) drugs including: alcohol, antidepressants, antihistamines, antipsychotics, some blood pressure medications (reserpine, methyldopa, beta-blockers), motion sickness medications, muscle relaxants, narcotics, sedatives, sleeping pills, and tranquilizers.

Other drugs that can interact with olanzapine include: carbamazepine, charcoal, LARODOPA, levodopa, omeprazole, PRILOSEC, RIFADIN, rifampin, RIMACTANE, TEGRETOL.

Adverse Effects

Call your doctor immediately if you experience:

- difficulty swallowing
- chest pain
- agitation, hostility
- stiff arms or legs
- dizziness
- excess saliva
- fever
- fast or irregular heartbeat
- involuntary movements of hands

- pain in abdomen, back, chest, joints, or throat
- restlessness
- swelling of legs or feet
- tremor

Call your doctor if these symptoms continue:

- constipation
- drowsiness
- dry mouth
- nasal congestion
- nausea or vomiting
- sleep disturbances
- sweating, increased perspiration
- vision changes
- weight gain

Ask your doctor which of these tests should be done periodically while you are taking this drug:

- liver function tests

DECREASED SWEATING

Olanzapine may make you sweat less, causing your body temperature to increase. Use extra care not to become overheated during exercise or hot weather while you are taking this medication, since overheating may result in heat stroke. Also, hot baths or saunas may make you feel dizzy or faint while you are taking this medicine.

PREGNANCY WARNING

This drug caused harm to developing fetuses in animal studies, or such studies were not done. Use during pregnancy only for clear medical reasons. Tell your doctor if you are pregnant or thinking of becoming pregnant before you take this drug.

NOTES FOR MIND DRUGS

1. *Drugs for the Elderly*. 2nd ed. Copenhagen, Denmark: World Health Organization, 1997:119.

2. Stewart RB, May FE, Hale WE, Marks RG. Psychotropic drug use in an ambulatory elderly population. *Gerontology* 1982; 28:328–35.

3. Ray WA. Prescribing patterns of drugs for the elderly. In *Pharmaceuticals for the Elderly*. Pharmaceutical Manufacturers Association, 1986.

4. Mellinger GD, Balter MB, Uhlenhuth EH. Prevalence and correlates of the long-term regular use of anxiolytics. *Journal of the American Medical Association* 1984; 251:375–79. Of those people 65 and older who were using minor tranquilizers, 30.5% had been using them every day for at least 12 months.

5. *Statistical Abstracts of the United States*. U.S. Department of Commerce, 1997.

6. Mellinger, op. cit.

7. *National Prescription Audit*, I.M.S., Inc. Ambler, Pennsylvania, 1986.

8. *National Disease and Therapeutic Index*, I.M.S., Inc. Ambler, Pennsylvania, 1985.

9. Stewart, op. cit.

10. Ray, op. cit.

11. *Sleeping Pills, Insomnia, and Medical Practice*. Institute of Medicine, National Academy of Sciences, 1979.

12. Solomon F, White C, Arron D, Mendelson W. Sleeping pills, insomnia and medical practice. *New England Journal of Medicine* 1979; 300:803–8.

13. Ray, op. cit.

14. Ingman SR, Lawson IR, Pierpaoli PG, Blake P. A survey of the prescribing and administration of drugs in a long-term care institution for the elderly. *Journal of the American Geriatric Society* 1975; 23:309–16.

15. Perry SW, Wu A. Rationale for the use of hypnotic agents in a general hospital. *Annals of Internal Medicine* 1984; 100:441–6.

16. *Drug Utilization in the U.S.* Department of Health and Human Services, Food and Drug Administration, December 1986.

17. Hoffman-LaRoche mailing to physicians: "The later years . . . an optimistic outlook," 1979.

18. *Drug Utilization in the U.S.*, op. cit.

19. The fact that there are more than 1.7 million daily users 60 and over who use these drugs for a year or more is calculated as follows: 5.2% of people use minor tranquilizers daily for one year or more (Mellinger, op. cit.) and the 1996 U.S. population of people 60 and over was 33 million people (*Statistical Abstracts*, op. cit.). 5.2% of 33 is 1.7 million.

20. *Drugs for the Elderly*, op. cit.

21. Catalan J, Gath D, Edmonds G, Ennis J. The effects of non-prescribing of anxiolytics in general practice—I: controlled evaluation of psychiatric and social outcome. *British Journal of Psychiatry* 1984; 144:593–602.

22. Zung WK, Daniel JT, King RE, Moore DT. A comparison of prazepam, diazepam, lorazepam and placebo in anxious outpatients in non-psychiatric private practices. *Journal of Clinical Psychiatry* 1981; 42:280–1.

23. *Sleeping Pills, Insomnia, and Medical Practice*, op. cit.

24. Kolata G. Elderly become addicts to drug-induced sleep. *The New York Times*, February 1, 1992, p. 5.

25. Ray WA, Griffin MR, Schaffner W, Baugh DK, Melton J. Psychotropic drug use and the risk of hip fracture. *New England Journal of Medicine* 1987; 316:363–9.

26. Riggs BL, Melton LJ III. Involutional osteoporosis. *New England Journal of Medicine* 1986; 314:1676–86.

27. Buchner DM, Larson DB. Falls and fractures in patients with Alzheimer-type dementia. *Journal of the American Medical Association* 1987; 257:1492–5.

28. Ray WA, Fought RL, Decker MD. Psychoactive drugs and the risk of injurious motor vehicle crashes in elderly drivers. *American Journal of Epidemiology* 1992; 136:873–83.

29. *Statistical Abstracts of the United States*, op. cit.

30. Beck JC, Benson DF, Scheibel AB, Spar JE, Rubenstein LZ. Dementia in the elderly: The silent epidemic. *Annals of Internal Medicine* 1982; 97:231–41.

31. Larson EB, Kukull WA, Buchner D, Reifler BV. Adverse drug reactions associated with global cognitive impairment in elderly persons. *Annals of Internal Medicine* 1987; 107:169–73.

32. *Use and Misuse of Benzodiazepines*. Hearing before the Subcommittee on Health and Scientific Research of the Committee on Labor and Human Resources, United States Senate, September 10, 1979.

33. Busto U, Sellers EM, Naranjo CA, Cappell H, Sanchez-Craig M, Sykora K. Withdrawal reaction after long-term therapeutic use of benzodiazepines. *New England Journal of Medicine* 1986; 315:854–9.

34. Dement W. Presentation before the Health, Education and Welfare Joint Coordinating Council for Project Sleep. July 28, 1980.

35. Lakshminarayan S, Saohn SA, Hudson LD, Weil JV. Effect of diazepam on ventilatory response. *Clinical Pharmacology and Therapeutics* 1976; 20:178–83.

36. *The Medical Letter on Drugs and Therapeutics*. New York: The Medical Letter Inc., 1986; 28:99–106.

37. Lader M. Anxiety and its treatment. *Scrip Magazine* October 1992:46–8.

38. Catalan, op. cit.

39. Kolata, op. cit.

40. *Sleeping Pills, Insomnia, and Medical Practice*, op. cit.

41. *Physicians' Desk Reference*. 41st ed. Oradell, N.J.: Medical Economics Company, 1987. The FDA-approved labeling for all benzodiazepine tranquilizers states that there is no evidence of effectiveness for more than four months.

42. Vestal RE, ed. *Drug Treatment in the Elderly*. Sydney, Australia: ADIS Health Science Press, 1984:317–37.

43. *The Medical Letter on Drugs and Therapeutics*. New York: The Medical Letter Inc., 1981; 23:41–3.

44. *Drugs for the Elderly*, op. cit.

45. *The Medical Letter on Drugs and Therapeutics*. New York: The Medical Letter Inc., 1991; 33:91.

46. Avorn JL, Lamy PP, Vestal RE. Prescribing for the elderly—safely. *Patient Care* June 1982:14–62.

47. Vestal, op. cit.

48. Bergman U, Griffiths RR. Relative abuse of diazepam and oxazepam: Prescription forgeries and theft loss reports in Sweden. *Drug & Alcohol Dependence* 1986; 16:293–301.

49. Griffiths RR, McLeod DR, Bigelow GE, Liebson IA, Nowowieski P. Comparison of diazepam and oxazepam: preference, liking and extent of abuse. *Journal of Pharmaceutical and Experimental Therapeutics* 1984; 229:501–8.

50. Lamy PP. Pharmacological considerations in the treatment of Alzheimer's disease. *Geriatric Medicine Today* 1987; 6:29–53.

51. Vestal, op. cit.

52. National Institute of Mental Health. Epidemiological Catchment Area Data from 1981–1982.

53. *The Medical Letter on Drugs and Therapeutics* 1986, op. cit., p. 81–6.

54. *National Disease and Therapeutic Index,* I.M.S., Inc. Ambler, Pennsylvania. Data is from 1984–1985.

55. Ray, 1986, op. cit.

56. Ray WA, Federspiel CF, Schaffner W. A study of antipsychotic drug use in nursing homes: Epidemiological evidence suggesting misuse. *American Journal of Public Health* 1980; 70:485–91.

57. Morgenstern H, Glazer WM, Niedzwiecki D, Nourjah P. The impact of neuroleptic medication on tardive dyskinesia. *American Journal of Public Health* 1987; 77:717–24. 22.9% of the estimated 1.3 million nursing home residents 65 and over 300,000 people *(Statistical Abstracts of the United States,* 1986), are being given the antipsychotic drugs chronically.

58. Ibid.

59. The 450,000 estimate is based on the total U.S. non-institutionalized population 65 and over (27 million, *Statistical Abstracts of the United States*) multiplied by the estimates in Ray, 1986, op. cit., of community antipsychotic drug use—about 5% for all adults 65 and over multiplied by one-third because one-third of non-institutionalized people using these drugs use them for three or four months or more (Morgenstern, op. cit.).

60. Estimate of total number of schizophrenics 65 years and over in the U.S. comes from multiplying the number of people 65 and over living in the community, 27 million, times 0.1%, the percentage of those 65 and over with active schizophrenia, to get 27,000 older non-institutionalized adults with schizophrenia. Then add the estimated number of nursing home residents 65 and over with schizophrenia (5% x 1.3 million = 65,000) for an estimated total of 92,000. All other psychotic disorders, such as the manic phase of manic depressive psychosis, which had a measured rate of 0.0 in people over 65 in the national survey of mental illness referred to at National Institute of Mental Health, op. cit, are not likely to add up to more than several thousand people 65 and over.

61. Again, using the estimates in Ray, 1986, op. cit., that for all people 65 and over in nursing homes, 39% get an antipsychotic drug and that 22.9% of all 65 and over nursing home residents, as in Morgenstern, op. cit., are chronic users, then 39% minus 22.9%, or 16.1%, are using these drugs for fewer than three or four months. Since there are 1.3 million residents 65 and over in nursing homes, multiplied by 16.1% gives a total of 209,000 non-chronic antipsychotic drug users in nursing homes. Similarly, using Ray, 1986, op. cit., finding that approximately 5% of all people 65 and over in the community are getting antipsychotic drugs and, from Morgenstern, op. cit., that 2/3 are non-chronic users, 900,000 non-institutionalized people 65 and over are also getting these drugs. 209,000 plus 900,000 equals 1,109,000 people.

62. Beers M, Avorn J, Soumerai SB, Everitt DE, Sherman DS, Salem S. Psychoactive medication use in intermediate-care facility residents. *Journal of the American Medical Association* 1988; 260:3016–20.

63. Ray, 1980, op. cit.

64. Barnes R, Veith R, Okinoto J, Raskind M, Gumbrecht G. Efficacy of antipsychotic medicines in behaviorally disturbed dementia patients. *American Journal of Psychiatry* 1982; 139:1170–4.

65. Grimes JD. Drug-induced parkinsonism and tardive dyskinesia in non-psychiatric patients. *Canadian Medical Association Journal* 1982; 126:468.

66. Cooper JW, Francisco GE. Psychotropic drug usage in long term care facility geriatric patients, *Hospital Formulary* 1981; 16:407–13.

67. Ingman, op. cit.

68. Barton R, Hurst L. Unnecessary use of tranquilizers in elderly patients. *British Journal of Psychiatry* 1966; 112:989–90.

69. Shamoian CA. Psychogeriatrics. *Medical Clinics of North America* 1983; 67:361–78.

70. Reference 61, op. cit.

71. Evans LK. Sundown syndrome in institutionalized elderly. *Journal of the American Geriatrics Society* 1987; 35:101–8.

72. Peabody CE, Warner MD, Whiteford HA, Hollister LE. Neuroleptics and the elderly. *Journal of the American Geriatrics Society* 1987; 35:233–8.

73. Yassa R, Nastase C, Dupont D, Thibeau M. Tardive dyskinesia in elderly psychiatric patients: a five-year study. *American Journal of Psychiatry* 1992; 149:1206–11.

74. Llorente MD, Olsen EJ, Leyva O, Silverman MA, Lewis JE, Rivero J. Use of antipsychotic drugs in nursing homes: current compliance with OBRA regulations. *Journal of the American Geriatrics Society* 1998; 46:198–201.

75. Lantz MS, Giambanco V, Buchalter EN. A ten-year review of the effect of OBRA-87 on psychotropic prescribing practices in an academic nursing home. *Psychiatric Services* 1996; 47:951–5.

76. Ray, 1987, op. cit.

77. *The Medical Letter on Drugs and Therapeutics,* 1986, op. cit., p. 104.

78. Evans, op. cit.

79. Barton, op. cit.

80. Yassa, op. cit.

81. Ray, 1980, op. cit.

82. *The Medical Letter on Drugs and Therapeutics,* 1986, op. cit., p. 81–6.

83. Stephen PJ, Williamson J. Drug-induced parkinsonism in the elderly. *The Lancet* 1984; ii:1082–3.

84. Grimes, op. cit.

85. Donlon PT, Stenson RL. Neuroleptic induced extrapyramidal symptoms. *Diseases of the Nervous System* 1976; 37:629–35.

86. Ibid.

87. Ayd FJ. A survey of drug-induced extrapyramidal reactions. *Journal of the American Medical Association* 1961; 175:102–8.

88. Avorn J, Gurwitz JH, Bohn RL, Mogun H, Monane M, Walker A. Increased incidence of levodopa therapy following metoclopramide use. *Journal of the American Medical Association* 1995; 274:1780–2.

89. Mild, strong, and medium rankings of adverse effects are the rankings from these souces: Gilman AG, Goodman LS, Rall TW, Murad F, eds. *The Pharmacological Basis of Therapeutics.* 7th ed. New York: Macmillan, 1985.; Vestal, op. cit.; Everitt DE, Avorn J. Drug prescribing for the elderly. *Archives of Internal Medicine* 1986; 146:2393–6. Young LY, Koda-Kimble MA, eds. *Applied Therapeutics: The Clinical Use of Drugs.* 6th ed. Vancouver, WA: Applied Therapeutics, Inc., 1995. Carter CS, Mulsant BH, Sweet RA, Maxwell RA, Coley K, Ganguli R, et al. Pharmacoeconomics made simple. *Psychopharmacology Bulletin* 1995; 31:719–25. Knable MB, Heinz A, Raedler T, Weinberger DR. Extrapyramidal side effects with risperidone and haloperidol at comparable D2 receptor occupancy levels. *Psychiatry Research: Neuroimaging Section* 1997; 75:91–101.

90. Ingman, op. cit.

91. Vestal, op. cit.

92. Salzman C. A primer on geriatric psychopharmacology. *American Journal of Psychiatry* 1982; 139:67–74.

93. *The Medical Letter on Drugs and Therapeutics,* 1986, op. cit., p. 81–5.

94. Avorn, 1982, op. cit.

95. Thompson TL, Moran MG, Nies AS. Psychotropic drug use in the elderly. *New England Journal of Medicine* 1983; 308:194–8.

96. Thomas P. Primary care; Depressed elderly's best hope. *Medical World News* July 13, 1987:38–52.

97. Ibid.

98. American Psychiatric Association. *Diagnostic and Statistical Manual of Mental Disorders, Fourth Edition.* Washington, DC: American Psychiatric Association, 1994.

99. Salzman C. Clinical guidelines for the use of antidepressant drugs in geriatric patients. *Journal of Clinical Psychiatry* 1985; 46:38–44.

100. Shamoian, op. cit.

101. Duncan AJ, Campbell AJ. Antidepressant drugs in the elderly: are the indications as long term as the treatment? *British Medical Journal* 1988; 296:1230–2.

102. Shamoian, op. cit.

103. Ray, 1987, op. cit.

104. Riggs, op. cit.

105. Lui B, Anderson G, Mittmann N, To T, Axcell T, Shear N. Use of selective serotonin-reuptake inhibitors of tricyclic antidepressants and risk of hip fractures in elderly people. *Lancet* 1998; 351:1303-7.

106. Ray, 1992, op. cit.

107. Vestal, op. cit.

108. Ibid.

109. Dubin H, Spier S, Giannandrea P. Nefazodone-induced mania. *American Journal of Psychiatry* 1997; 154:578–9[letter].

110. Wehr TA, Goodwin FK. Can antidepressants cause mania and worsen the course of affective illness? *American Journal of Psychiatry* 1987; 144:1403–11.

111. Howland RH. Induction of mania with serotonin reuptake inhibitors. *Journal of Clinical Psychopharmacology* 1996; 16:425–7.

112. Dubin, op. cit.

113. Howland, op. cit.

114. Rankings of adverse effects are the averages of rankings from Vestal, op. cit; Thompson, op. cit; Salzman, op. cit.; Everitt, op. cit.

115. Avorn, 1982, op. cit.

116. Ibid.

117. Thompson, op. cit.

118. Shamoian, op. cit.

119. Vestal, op. cit.

120. Georgotas A, McCue RE. Relapse of depressed patients after effective continuation therapy. *Journal of Affective Disorders* 1989; 17:159.

121. Duncan, op. cit.

122. American Society of Health System Pharmacists. *American Hospital Formulary Service Drug Information,* Bethesda, MD, 1996:1744–7.

123. *The Medical Letter on Drugs and Therapeutics.* New York: The Medical Letter Inc., 1996: 38:59–61.

124. *Drugs of Choice.* New Rochelle, NY: The Medical Letter, Inc., 1991:29–39.

125. *The Medical Letter on Drugs and Therapeutics,* 1986, op. cit., p. 117–8.

126. Buspirone—a radical advance in the treatment of anxiety? *Lancet* 1988; 1:804–6.

127. American Society of Hospital Pharmacists. *American Hospital Formulary Service Drug Information,* Bethesda, MD, 1992:1355–61.

128. Gilman AG, Rall TW, Nies AS, Taylor P, eds. *The Pharmacological Basis of Therapeutics.* 8th ed. New York: Pergamon Press, 1990:428.

129. Dukes MNG, Beeley L. *Side Effects of Drugs Annual* 12, Amsterdam: Elsevier, 1988:45–6.

130. Manfredi RL, Kales A, Vgontzas AN, Bixler EO, Isaac MA, Falcone CM. Buspirone: sedative or stimulant effect? *American Journal of Psychiatry* 1991; 148:1213–7.

131. *Drugs for the Elderly,* op. cit.

132. MacFarlane B, Davies S, Mannan K, Sarsam R, Pariente D, Dooley J. Fatal acute fulminant liver failure due to clozapine: A case report and review of clozapine-induced hepatotoxicity. *Gastroenterology* 1997; 112:1707–9.

133. Cohen LJ. Rational drug use in the treatment of depression. *Pharmacotherapy* 1997; 17:45–61.

134. Gilman, 1985, op. cit.

135. Yassa, op. cit.

136. *Drugs for the Elderly,* op. cit.

137. *The Medical Letter on Drugs and Therapeutics,* 1991, op. cit.

138. Avorn, 1982, op. cit.

139. Vestal, op. cit.

140. Bergman, op. cit.

141. Griffiths, op. cit.

142. *Drug and Therapeutics Bulletin,* August 13, 1984, p. 62.

143. Shinn AF, Shrewsbury RP. *Evaluations of Drug Interactions.* 3rd ed. St. Louis, Toronto, Princeton: The C.V. Mosby Company, 1985:282.

144. Yassa, op. cit.

145. Owens D. Benefits of new drugs are exaggerated. *British Medical Journal* 1994; 309:1281–2.

146. Teicher MH, Glod C, Cole JO. Emergence of intense suicidal preoccupation during fluoxetine treatment. *American Journal of Psychiatry* 1990; 147:207–10.

147. Owens, op. cit.

148. *The Medical Letter on Drugs and Therapeutics.* New York: The Medical Letter Inc., 1990; 32:83–5.

149. SSRIs and withdrawal syndrome. *Australian Adverse Drug Reactions Bulletin* 1996; 15:3.

150. *The Medical Letter on Drugs and Therapeutics,* 1996, op. cit., p. 113–4.

151. Carter, op. cit.

152. Knable, op. cit.

153. Vestal, op. cit.

154. Bergman, op. cit.

155. Griffiths, op. cit.

156. Tyrer P, Murphy S. The place of benzodiazepines in psychiatric practice. *British Journal of Psychiatry* 1987; 151:719–23.

157. Lamy, op. cit.

158. Hansten PD, Horn JR. Drug interactions analysis and management. *Applied Therapeutics,* Vancouver, WA, 1997; 1:I.64.

159. Yassa, op. cit.

160. *Drug and Therapeutics Bulletin,* op. cit.

161. *USP DI, Drug Information for the Health Care Provider.* 6th ed. Rockville MD: The United States Pharmacopeial Convention, Inc., 1986:240.

162. Harsch HH. Bupropion. *American Family Physician* 1991; 43:1789–90.

163. Gelenberg AJ. Imperfect drugs in an imperfect world. *Journal of Clinical Psychiatry* 1992; 53:39–40.

164. Davidson J. Seizures and bupropion: a review. *Journal of Clinical Psychiatry* 1989; 50:256–61.

165. Rudorfer MV, Manji HK, Potter WZ. Bupropion, ECT, and dopaminergic overdrive. *American Journal of Psychiatry* 1991; 148:1101–2 [letter].

166. Settle EC. Tinnitus related to bupropion treatment. *Journal of Clinical Psychiatry* 1991; 52:352.

167. *The Medical Letter on Drugs and Therapeutics.* New York: The Medical Letter Inc., 1997: 39:5–6.

168. Fulton B, Goa KL. Olanzapine, a review of its pharmacological properties and therapeutic efficacy in the management of schizophrenia and related psychoses. *Drugs* 1997; 53:281–98.

Painkillers and Arthritis Drugs

Salicylates **261**
Narcotics **264**
Arthritis and Inflammation **265**

DRUG LISTINGS

NONSTEROIDAL ANTI-INFLAMMATORY DRUGS (NSAIDS)

ADVIL		311
ANAPROX		317
ANSAID (oral tablets)		270
ARTHROPAN	Limited Use	336
ASCRIPTIN	⊘ Do Not Use	280
ASCRIPTIN A/D	⊘ Do Not Use	280
aspirin		275
BAYER ASPIRIN (GENUINE BAYER)		275
bromfenac	⊘ Do Not Use	292
buffered aspirin	⊘ Do Not Use	280
BUFFERIN	⊘ Do Not Use	280
BUTAZOLIDIN	⊘ Do Not Use	281
choline salicylate	Limited Use	336
choline and magnesium salicylates	Limited Use	336
CLINORIL	Limited Use	281
DAYPRO	Limited Use	314
diclofenac	Limited Use	343
diflunisal	⊘ Do Not Use	291
DISALCID	⊘ Do Not Use	291
DOAN'S PILLS	Limited Use	336
DOLOBID	⊘ Do Not Use	291
DURACT	⊘ Do Not Use	292
EASPRIN		275
ECOTRIN		275
etodolac	Limited Use	303
FELDENE	⊘ Do Not Use	298
fenoprofen	Limited Use	314
flurbiprofen		270
ibuprofen		311
INDOCIN	⊘ Do Not Use	302
indomethacin	⊘ Do Not Use	302
ketoprofen		320
ketorolac	⊘ Do Not Use	335
LODINE	Limited Use	303
magnesium salicylate	Limited Use	336
meclofenamate	Limited Use	306
MECLOMEN	Limited Use	306
MEDIPREN		311
MOTRIN		311
nabumetone	Limited Use	303
NALFON	Limited Use	314
NAPROSYN		317
naproxen		317
NORGESIC FORTE	⊘ Do Not Use	319
NUPRIN		311
OCUFEN (eye solution)		270
orphenadrine, aspirin and caffeine	⊘ Do Not Use	319
ORUDIS		320
oxaprozin	Limited Use	314
phenylbutazone	⊘ Do Not Use	281
piroxicam	⊘ Do Not Use	298

RELAFEN	Limited Use	303
salsalate	⊘ Do Not Use	291
sulindac	Limited Use	281
TOLECTIN	Limited Use	332
tolmetin	Limited Use	332
TORADOL	⊘ Do Not Use	335
TRILISATE	Limited Use	336
VOLTAREN	Limited Use	343

NON-NARCOTIC PAINKILLERS

acetaminophen	338
lidocaine	346
TYLENOL	338
XYLOCAINE	346

NARCOTIC-CONTAINING PAINKILLERS

acetaminophen and codeine		340
acetaminophen and hydrocodone		274
acetaminophen and oxycodone		323
aspirin and oxycodone		324
aspirin with codeine		273
BANCAP-HC		274
butalbital, acetaminophen and caffeine	⊘ Do Not Use	297
butalbital, caffeine and aspirin	⊘ Do Not Use	299
butalbital, caffeine, aspirin and codeine	⊘ Do Not Use	299
butorphanol	⊘ Do Not Use	331
codeine		284
DARVOCET-N	⊘ Do Not Use	288
DARVON	⊘ Do Not Use	288
DARVON COMPOUND	⊘ Do Not Use	288
DARVON COMPOUND-65	⊘ Do Not Use	288
DARVON-N	⊘ Do Not Use	288
DEMEROL		289
dihydrocodeine, aspirin and caffeine	⊘ Do Not Use	331
DILAUDID		289
DURAGESIC	Limited Use	293
ESGIC	⊘ Do Not Use	297
fentanyl patches	Limited Use	293
FIORICET	⊘ Do Not Use	297
FIORINAL	⊘ Do Not Use	299
FIORINAL WITH CODEINE	⊘ Do Not Use	299
hydromorphone		289
meperidine		289
pentazocine	⊘ Do Not Use	332
pentazocine and naloxone	⊘ Do Not Use	332
PERCOCET		323
PERCODAN		324
PERCODAN-DEMI		324
propoxyphene	⊘ Do Not Use	288
propoxyphene and acetaminophen	⊘ Do Not Use	288
propoxyphene, aspirin and caffeine	⊘ Do Not Use	288
STADOL	⊘ Do Not Use	331
STADOL NS	⊘ Do Not Use	331
SYNALGOS-DC	⊘ Do Not Use	331
TALWIN	⊘ Do Not Use	332
TALWIN-NX	⊘ Do Not Use	332
tramadol	⊘ Do Not Use	342
TYLENOL NO. 3		340
TYLOX		323
ULTRAM	⊘ Do Not Use	342
VICODIN		274
WYGESIC	⊘ Do Not Use	288

DRUGS FOR ARTHRITIS AND GOUT

allopurinol	Limited Use	347
aurothioglucose	Limited Use	329
BENEMID	Limited Use	278
colchicine	Limited Use	286
gold sodium thiomalate	Limited Use	329
hydroxychloroquine	Limited Use	325
methotrexate	Limited Use	327
MINOCIN	Last Choice Drug	309
minocycline	Last Choice Drug	309
MYOCHRYSINE	Limited Use	329
PLAQUENIL	Limited Use	325
probenecid	Limited Use	278
RHEUMATREX DOSE PACK	Limited Use	327
SOLGANAL	Limited Use	329
ZYLOPRIM	Limited Use	347

IMMUNOSUPPRESSANTS

azathioprine	Limited Use	299
IMURAN	Limited Use	299

SALICYLATES

The salicylates are used to relieve pain and to reduce fever and inflammation. Aspirin, a nonsteroidal anti-inflammatory drug (NSAID), is the most well-known and frequently used salicylate. Other salicylates discussed in this book are salsalate and choline and magnesium salicylates.

Aspirin

Aspirin is the common name for a chemical called acetylsalicylic acid, or A.S.A. (as it is still known in Canada and some other countries).

Aspirin, used as directed, is perhaps the most effective non-narcotic remedy, prescription or nonprescription, for pain, fever, and inflammation. Unfortunately, certain people should not use aspirin.

Aspirin Allergies

Some people are allergic to aspirin and may experience a wide variety of reactions, including hives, rash, swollen lymph nodes, generalized swelling, severe breathing difficulties, or a drop in blood pressure. Simple stomach discomfort following the use of aspirin or any other medication, however, does not indicate that you have an allergy.

Asthmatics seem to be particularly prone to aspirin allergies, as well as allergies to calcium carbaspirin, another member of the salicylate family.

If you have ever had an allergic reaction to aspirin or any other drug, be sure to tell your doctor. This kind of reaction can also occur in response to other related medications, which include prescription drugs containing salicylates or similar ingredients.

Aspirin and the Digestive Tract

Aspirin is a locally irritating, corrosive substance, which when used for a long time or in high doses can increase the likelihood of developing peptic ulcers[1] (in the lower part of the esophagus, the stomach, or the beginning of the small intestine). If you have ulcers, inflammation of the stomach (gastritis), or any form of stomach discomfort, you should not be taking even small quantities of aspirin, in any form.

Aspirin and Bleeding

Aspirin causes bleeding in the stomach; over time, it can weaken the body's ability to slow and contain bleeding. Taking aspirin for a few days can increase the amount of bleeding during childbirth, after tooth extraction, and during surgery. Aspirin should not be taken for at least five days before surgery, even in small doses. Persons with serious liver disease, vitamin K deficiency or blood clotting disorders, or persons already taking blood thinners (anticoagulants, such as warfarin and heparin) or other drugs should not take aspirin without strict supervision of a doctor or other health professional.

Aspirin should not be taken in very large doses (more than 12 regular-strength 325-milligram or 5-grain tablets per day) or for more than a few days without the supervision of a doctor. Even small doses used over a long period of time may leave certain predisposed individuals at an increased risk of serious bleeding after wounds or cuts.

Aspirin Preparations and Use

Aspirin is highly advertised, and there are many different brands from which to choose. We recommend plain generic aspirin for intermittent use, such as for an occasional headache.

Enteric-coated aspirin (coated so it does not dissolve in the stomach) causes much less blood loss than regular or buffered aspirin.[2] For this reason, we recommend generic enteric-coated aspirin for everyone on long-term aspirin therapy, such as for arthritis. Although a generic form of enteric-coated aspirin is available, it is more expensive than plain aspirin, but still less expensive than most other drugs for long-term treatment of arthritis. High-dose enteric-coated aspirin is now available (EASPRIN from Parke-Davis), but you pay for convenience.

National Institutes of Health arthritis expert Dr. Paul Plotz has said, referring to the treatment of arthritis when long-term use of aspirin is needed: *Enteric-coated aspirin is the best form of the drug. Indeed since the gastrointestinal side effects, the principal drawback of plain aspirin, are so much reduced and the drug is so well absorbed, enteric-coated aspirin is a close to perfect nonsteroidal inflammatory drug. It is available in several sizes and can be given twice a day with adequate serum [blood] levels.*[3]

Enteric-coated aspirin should not be used for occasional problems, such as headaches, because it is absorbed more slowly than regular aspirin and takes more time to relieve pain.

Alka-Seltzer® contains aspirin and buffering agents and is much less irritating to the stomach than regular or buffered aspirin, but it is quite expensive and contains a great deal of salt (sodium).[4] If you have to restrict your intake of salt or take a salicylate for a long time, do not use Alka-Seltzer®. Since this drug contains aspirin, do not use it as an antacid.

Taking aspirin with food or after meals can decrease stomach upset. If you are on a high-dose salicylate treatment together with antacids, do not suddenly change (start or stop) the way that you take antacids without talking to your doctor first.

If you take aspirin or another salicylate regularly, the level of drug in your blood may have to be checked to make sure that you are taking the best dose. You should also have regular checkups and ask your doctor about the necessity of certain tests including hematocrit (a blood test), kidney and liver function tests, and hearing tests. Also ask if you should take vitamin C or vitamin K.

Salicylates should *not* be used by anyone with acute liver or kidney failure. They should be discontinued by anyone who has chronic liver or kidney disease if there is any sign of a worsening condition.[5] If you develop ringing in your ears or persistent stomach pain after using aspirin for a long time, call your doctor.

When you buy aspirin, make sure it is pure white and does not contain broken tablets. If it smells like vinegar, do not use it. Do not store your drug in the bathroom medicine cabinet because the heat or moisture might cause it to deteriorate and lose its effectiveness. Keep it away from heat and direct light.

ASPIRIN/REYE'S SYNDROME ALERT

Do not use this product for treating chicken pox, flu, or flu-like illness. It will increase the risk of contracting Reye's syndrome, a rare but often fatal disease.

This warning appears in this book on the profiles of drugs that contain aspirin and other salicylates. Although most cases of Reye's syndrome are in children, some occur up to age 40. People under 40 who have chicken pox, flu, or flu-like illness and need a drug simply to relieve pain or reduce fever should use acetaminophen (TYLENOL, for example) rather than aspirin.

What You Don't Know About Nonsteroidal Anti-Inflammatory Drugs (NSAIDs) Can Hurt You

Gastrointestinal (GI) bleeding and perforation are common and serious adverse effects of NSAIDs. These adverse reactions can lead to hospitalization and potentially death. About one-third of all bleeding ulcers in older adults are linked with this family of drugs. The most important factors predisposing people to GI toxicity from NSAIDs are the type and dose of drug (and use of two NSAIDs together), which can increase the risk up to twentyfold. Other risk factors include a history of ulcer, anticoagulants (blood thinners), steroid drugs, smoking, alcohol use, and older age.[6]

An ingenious study published in 1996 involving patients who had bled while taking an NSAID supports a principle long held by Public Citizen's Health Research Group: patients who are informed about the risks of their drugs and instructed what to do if an adverse reaction should occur can avoid serious drug-induced injury.[7]

In the study, patients who had experienced GI bleeding and were subsequently hospitalized knew less about the adverse effects of NSAIDs or what to do when they occurred than those using these drugs that did not have GI bleeding. Fewer patients who bled (16%) than those that did not (41%) remembered having been told of the potential adverse effects of NSAIDs or about what steps to take if they developed an adverse effect (4% versus 21%). Faithful obedience (compliance) in taking an NSAID was more common in patients who bled (96%) than in those who did not (70%). In addition, 18 (36%) of those who bled had experienced stomach pain before bleeding and all but two had continued to take the drug, while only 15 (15%) of those who did not bleed had stomach pain, of whom 10 had subsequently reduced their intake of the NSAID.

> **WARNING**
>
> **NONSTEROIDAL ANTI-INFLAMMATORY DRUG (NSAID) INDUCED GASTROIN-TESTINAL TOXICITY**
>
> All members of the NSAID family of drugs can cause gastrointestinal toxicity that can lead to gastrointestinal bleeding and hospitalization or death. The risk of gastrointestinal toxicity from these drugs increases with increasing doses and the length of treatment.
>
> If the following symptoms develop while you are taking an NSAID, stop the drug immediately and contact your doctor: severe abdominal or stomach pain, cramping, or burning, severe and continuing nausea, heartburn, or indigestion, bloody or black, tarry stools, vomiting blood or material that looks like coffee grounds, or spitting up blood.

NARCOTICS

Narcotic drugs are prescribed to relieve pain and cough, to treat diarrhea not caused by poisoning, and to cause drowsiness before an operation. These drugs are addictive and have many adverse effects, and their use should be limited to the lowest dose for the shortest period of time except in the case of terminally ill people with extraordinary pain.

Use

Pain relief is the primary legitimate use of narcotics, which are effective for moderate to severe pain that has not responded to non-narcotic painkillers such as aspirin and other salicylates, acetaminophen, or nonsteroidal anti-inflammatory drugs (NSAIDs). Narcotics can be used alone or in combination with these drugs.

Most of the time when someone is able to swallow, they should first try a non-narcotic drug such as aspirin taken by mouth. If aspirin alone is not effective, it can be combined with a narcotic, such as codeine. These two drugs work in different ways and, when they are used together, they generally relieve pain that would otherwise require a higher dose of narcotic, while causing fewer adverse effects.[8] A sedative or antianxiety drug is just as effective as a narcotic, without causing vomiting like narcotics can.

Because narcotics are addictive and have many adverse effects, many doctors do not prescribe them freely. This reserve is not always appropriate. In the case of severe pain from late-stage cancer that has spread throughout the body, the pain is often under-treated as far as the use of narcotics is concerned. In an editorial in the *New England Journal of Medicine*, Dr. Marcia Angell wrote: *"Pain is soul destroying. No patient should have to endure intense pain unnecessarily. The quality of mercy is essential to the practice of medicine; here, of all places, it should not be strained."*[9]

Wanted and Unwanted Effects of Narcotics

Narcotics affect the central nervous system, producing pain relief and drowsiness as well as less desirable effects. Older adults may require less than the usual adult dose to produce desired effects because of their bodies' greater sensitivity to the drugs. Some of the adverse effects frequently seen in older adults are slow or troubled breathing (narcotics should never be given to anyone with depressed breathing), stimulation or confusion,[10] and hallucinations and unpleasant dreams (seen more in people using pentazocine).[11]

Other adverse effects are: dizziness, drowsiness, feeling faint or lightheaded, nausea or vomiting (which might go away if you lie down for a while), blurry vision or change in vision (double vision), constipation (more often seen with long-term use and with codeine), difficult or painful urination, or need to urinate often, general feeling of discomfort or illness, headache, dry mouth, loss of appetite, bad or unusual dreams, red or flushed face (more often with meperidine or methadone), redness, swelling, pain, or burning at place of injection, stomach pain or cramps, trouble sleeping, abnormal decrease in amount of urine, abnormal increase in sweating (more often with meperidine and methadone), abnormal nervousness, restlessness, tiredness, or weakness, and sexual problems.

Narcotics will add to the effects of alcohol and other drugs that slow down the nervous system: antidepressants, antihistamines, antipsychotics, some blood pressure medications (reserpine, methyldopa, beta-blockers), motion sickness medications, muscle relaxants, narcotics, sedatives, sleeping pills and tranquilizers. Do not take any of these drugs or drink alcohol when you are taking a narcotic, unless your doctor has told you otherwise.

One hazard of taking narcotics continuously for longer than several weeks is drug-induced dependence. Do not stop taking your drug suddenly. With the help of your doctor, work out a schedule for slowly decreasing the amount of the drug you take by about 5 to 10% each day. Keep a written record of the dosage reduction schedule with you. These steps will make it much easier to become drug free without developing distressing symptoms of drug withdrawal. Common withdrawal symptoms include body aches, diarrhea, goosebumps, loss of appetite, nausea or vomiting, nervousness or restlessness, runny nose, shivering or trembling, sneezing, cramps, trouble sleeping, unexplained fever, abnormal increase in sweating or yawning, abnormal irritability, abnormally fast heartbeat or weakness.

Taking Narcotics

Taking narcotics by mouth is preferred and is usually effective unless the pain is very severe.[12] The drugs can also be given in injections into the muscle or under the skin, intravenously into the bloodstream, alone or mixed with a solution, or into the spinal cord.

Morphine sulfate is available as extended-release tablets which must be swallowed whole, but tablets of the other narcotics can be crushed. Meperidine sulfate oral solution should be mixed with a half glass of water before you drink it to decrease possible numbness of your mouth and throat.

If you are on a regular dosing schedule and you miss a dose, take it as soon as possible. But if it is almost time for the next dose, skip the missed dose and go back to the regular schedule. Do not take double doses. Drink plenty of liquids, as this may help decrease constipation. Call your doctor if you do not have a bowel movement for several days and feel uncomfortable. If you have diarrhea, do not take a drug to stop it. Instead, ask your doctor what to do.

ARTHRITIS AND INFLAMMATION

Arthritis literally means an inflammation of a joint and is a blanket term for a number of ailments with differing significance, various causes, and diverse symptoms. Such conditions are usually characterized by pain when moving or putting weight on the joint. Inflammation (pain, heat, redness, and swelling) may or may not be present.

Pain, stiffness, swelling, or tenderness in any joint, or in the neck or lower back, which lasts longer than six weeks, warrants a trip to the doctor to determine the cause of the problem. A long delay in seeking help may result in irreversible damage to joints.

You should seek medical attention for pain in a joint immediately if:

- Joint pain or swelling is very sudden and intense;
- Joint pain follows an injury (you may have a fracture near the joint); or
- Joint problems are accompanied by a fever above 100°F (38°C).

At least 31.6 million Americans suffer from some form of arthritis. The three most common types are rheumatoid arthritis, osteoarthritis, and gout. Each has a different cause, treatment, and probable outcome.

Rheumatoid Arthritis

Rheumatoid arthritis is an inflammation of the joints caused by disturbances in the body's immune system (which defends it against disease) and can occur at any age. Its victims are more likely to be female and include infants, teenagers, and middle-aged and older adults. It is often characterized by morning stiffness, along with pain and swelling in the joints of fingers, ankles, knees, wrists, and elbows, which improves as the day goes on. The distribution of affected joints is usually symmetrical; that is, if your right wrist is afflicted, your left wrist will probably be afflicted as well.

Treatment

There is no cure for rheumatoid arthritis, but the inflammation may be controlled under medical supervision. Drug therapy draws from two broad categories: the anti-inflammatory drugs and the antirheumatic drugs.

Anti-inflammatory drugs: Anti-inflammatory drugs can be further divided into *nonsteroidal* and *steroidal* drugs. Nonsteroidal anti-inflammatory drugs (NSAIDs) work by inhibiting formation of chemicals in the body that cause pain, fever, and inflammation. NSAIDs can be either salicylate, such as aspirin, or nonsalicylate, such as ibuprofen (MOTRIN, ADVIL, NUPRIN, MEDIPRIN).

For rheumatoid arthritis, enteric-coated aspirin is the first choice medication of many doctors. The amount of aspirin required to reduce the inflammation of arthritis, however, approaches levels at which a small proportion

ANTI-INFLAMMATORY DRUGS

1. **Nonsteroids**
   salicylates
   - aspirin
   - salsalate
   nonsalicylates
   - bromfenac (withdrawn from the market June 1998)
   - choline and magnesium salicylates
   - diclofenac
   - diflunisal
   - etodolac
   - fenoprofen
   - flurbiprofen
   - ibuprofen
   - indomethacin
   - ketoprofen
   - ketorolac
   - meclofenamate
   - nabumetone
   - naproxen
   - oxaprozin
   - phenylbutazone
   - piroxicam
   - salsalate
   - sulindac
   - tolmetin
2. **Steroids**
   - cortisone
   - prednisone

ANTIRHEUMATIC DRUGS

1. **Gold salts**
   - auranofin
   - aurothioglucose
   - gold sodium thiomalate
2. **Antimalarial drugs**
   - chloroquine
   - hydroxychloroquine
3. **Sulfasalazine**
4. **Penicillamine**
5. **Cytotoxic drugs**
   - azathioprine
   - cyclophosphamide
   - methotrexate
6. **Minocycline**

of people may experience undesirable adverse effects. (High-dose aspirin therapy should never be started without medical supervision to determine the correct dose and to achieve the most therapeutic effect with the fewest adverse effects.)

Aspirin works when it is present in the bloodstream at a certain level, which varies among users. Effective blood levels of aspirin range between 15 and 30 milligrams per deciliter (tenth of a liter of blood). To achieve this level, between 9 and 23 regular (325 milligrams) aspirin tablets must be taken daily (3.0 to 7.5 grams of aspirin).[13] If you are taking aspirin, the level of the drug in your blood should be monitored periodically to prevent toxicity (poisoning). Signs of aspirin toxicity include ringing in the ears, rapid breathing (hyperventilation), mental confusion, shortness of breath, swelling of feet or lower legs (edema), dizziness, headache, nausea or vomiting, sweating, and thirst. These symptoms should be reported to your doctor immediately.

For chronic use, such as in treatment of rheumatoid arthritis, we strongly recommend generic enteric-coated aspirin (the brand name version, ECOTRIN, is almost twice as expensive). Studies have shown that enteric-coated aspirin provides the same amount of aspirin in the body but sharply decreases the amount of bleeding in comparison with plain aspirin.[14]

In addition to being as effective as any other arthritis drug in its family (nonsteroidal anti-inflammatory drugs), generic enteric-coated aspirin is less than one-fifth as expensive as piroxicam (Pfizer's FELDENE), another NSAID. We recommend that piroxicam should not be used because of its increased risk of often fatal ulcers, intestinal perforation, and bleeding.

An early 1998 sampling of retail prices for various aspirin and nonaspirin arthritis drugs in drugstores in Washington, D.C. showed extraordinary differences between aspirin and others, except for ibuprofen. The most expensive drug was piroxicam ($100 a month, or

$1,200 a year for one 20-mg pill per day). The least expensive was generic enteric-coated aspirin ($11.97 a month, or $143.64 a year for a dose of 3 grams a day). Generic ibuprofen, at a dose of one 400-milligram pill three times a day, costs $18.98 a month or $227 a year. Naproxen (Syntex's NAPROSYN) costs $99.59 a month or $1,188 a year for a dose of two 375-mg pills a day.

Drug	Doses	Cost per Month
piroxicam (Feldene)	20 mg	$100.00
piroxicam (generic)	20 mg	$33.79
naproxen (Naprosyn)	1000 mg	$99.59
generic ibuprofen	3200 mg	$18.98
generic enteric-coated aspirin	4000 mg	$11.97

All prescription NSAIDs for rheumatoid arthritis are much more expensive than aspirin, have significant adverse effects, and are no more effective than aspirin. Like aspirin, other NSAIDs may also cause gastrointestinal bleeding or impair kidney function. Unless you have an allergy to aspirin or have experienced gastrointestinal problems while taking aspirin, enteric-coated aspirin is the drug of choice for rheumatoid arthritis. If you have had an allergic reaction or stomach problems after taking aspirin, however, another NSAID may be better tolerated. Read the information on individual NSAIDs for recommendations and adverse effects. Then discuss these choices with your doctor.

Steroids: The other type of anti-inflammatory drugs, steroids, are very important hormones that have two functions: controlling inflammation and regulating vital body functions. They are not generally recommended first for treatment of rheumatoid arthritis. Steroids may be useful, however, for older adults who cannot take or do not respond to an NSAID. They can be locally injected into a joint if a specific joint is causing considerable pain.

Whenever possible, steroids are to be avoided because they are associated with numerous adverse effects (see p. 651), including an increased risk of developing the bone-weakening disease, osteoporosis (which is more likely to affect thin, small-boned white women).

Antirheumatic drugs: In contrast with the anti-inflammatory drugs just described, the antirheumatic drugs not only relieve symptoms, but may also slow the rheumatic disease process itself. Antirheumatic drugs, such as gold salts, should be reserved for people who have active rheumatoid arthritis that does not respond to salicylates or other NSAIDs because some form of toxicity is seen in more than 50% of people taking antirheumatic drugs.

Regardless of the drug therapy chosen by you and your doctor, an exercise program and physical therapy should be designed within the limits of pain. This will help to strengthen muscular action and maintain or improve range of motion in the joints.

Inflammation also occurs in other rheumatologic diseases such as ankylosing spondylitis, scleroderma, temporal arteritis, and polymyalgia rheumatica. Therapy follows the same general anti-inflammatory guidelines that are used to treat rheumatoid arthritis.

Osteoarthritis

Osteoarthritis is the most common type of arthritis, and is usually related to the aging of the joint *or prior injury.* Often a mild condition, it may cause no symptoms or only occasional joint pain and stiffness. Most of the time osteoarthritis is not crippling, although a few people experience considerable pain and disability. It occasionally progresses to a point at which walking is difficult. Osteoarthritis frequently occurs in the finger joints, where it causes knobby bumps, and the spine, where it induces bone-like growths. These, however, do not commonly cause serious problems.

Osteoarthritis can often be treated without medical supervision.

Unlike rheumatoid arthritis, osteoarthritis is a degenerative joint disease that does not always have inflammation as a symptom. Obesity (being excessively overweight) aggravates the wear and tear on the inside surface of the joint. Not surprisingly, the most severe form of osteoarthritis is the type that affects the joints that bear the body's weight, such as the hips and the knees. A marked improvement is often seen after weight loss and an exercise program that helps to preserve full range of movement in the affected joints.

Treatment

Enteric-coated aspirin is the best and least expensive way to relieve the pain of osteoarthritis. Unlike rheumatoid arthritis, which requires high doses of aspirin to reduce inflammation, two 325-mg tablets four times a day is often sufficient to control osteoarthritic pain in adults. Other pain relievers, including acetaminophen, are recommended for the person who cannot take aspirin. Be aware that in contrast to aspirin, acetaminophen relieves pain, but it is not effective in reducing inflammation. Therefore, we do not recommend the use of acetaminophen for the treatment of arthritis unless it is clear that you have osteoarthritis which does not have a significant amount of inflammation.

Topical (skin) preparations marketed for treating arthritis (external salicylate-containing painkillers, such as Aspercreme and Myoflex) have no place in arthritis treatment. Salicylates (including aspirin) exert their effect on joints by absorption into the bloodstream. This is best done by swallowing tablets, not by applying cream.

Exercise should put an affected joint through its full range of motion. Swimming and walking are particularly good for this. You can start immediately and gradually improve your strength and flexibility. Under medical supervision, severe osteoarthritis is sometimes treated with physical therapy, orthopedic devices and, in extreme cases, surgery.

Gout

Gout is related to the formation of uric acid crystals in the joints. White blood cells respond to the crystals by releasing certain enzymes into the joint space. The release of these enzymes causes the intense pain and inflammation of an acute attack of gout. The big toe is a common location of gouty pain. Medical treatment by a professional is required, and is usually sought, as the pain typically comes on suddenly and is often severe.

Treatment

Gout therapy can be divided into treatment of acute (sudden) attacks and prevention of uric acid crystal formation. Colchicine relieves an acute attack by inhibiting the white blood cell response. NSAIDs are also effective for treating an acute attack, but require 12 to 24 hours before their onset of action. If you suffer from frequent attacks, or if your uric acid blood levels remain high between attacks, your doctor may prescribe either allopurinol or probenecid to reduce the uric acid in your body. Allopurinol decreases the amount of uric acid produced by the body. Probenecid increases the amount of uric acid that is eliminated by the body.

People who have gout should not use aspirin and other salicylates. Be aware that over-the-counter (nonprescription) products that contain aspirin cause retention of uric acid, and may result in a worsening of gouty arthritis. Aspirin also reduces the effectiveness of several anti-gout medications, for example probenecid.

Infectious Arthritis

Infectious arthritis occurs when a joint is invaded by bacteria, causing it to become red, hot, and swollen. It may be difficult to distinguish this type of arthritis from other types, as it frequently occurs in patients with other kinds of arthritis.

Treatment

This type of infection is almost always accompanied by fever and requires antibiotics, as directed by a physician, as soon as possible; otherwise the joint may be destroyed by the infectious process. No nonprescription preparations are appropriate as the sole treatment for infectious arthritis.

ALCOHOL WARNINGS ON ALL NONPRESCRIPTION PAIN RELIEVERS

The FDA has proposed regulations requiring alcohol warnings for all over-the-counter (OTC) pain relievers which include aspirin, other salicylates, acetaminophen, ibuprofen, ketoprofen, and naproxen sodium. The proposal includes the following warning statements:

For Acetaminophen-Containing Products
"Alcohol warning: If you drink three or more alcoholic beverages daily, you should ask your doctor whether you should take [the product name] or other pain relievers. [Product name] may increase your risk of liver damage."

For Aspirin, Carbaspirin calcium, Choline salicylate, Ibuprofen, Ketoprofen, Magnesium salicylate, Naproxen sodium and Sodium salicylate-Containing Products
"Alcohol Warning: If you drink three or more alcoholic beverages daily, ask your doctor whether you should take [the product name] or other pain relievers. [Product name] may increase your risk of stomach bleeding."

Some OTC pain relievers already carry an alcohol warning. This regulation is long overdue.

DRUG PROFILES

Flurbiprofen
ANSAID oral tablets (UpJohn)
OCUFEN eye solution (Allergan)

GENERIC: available
FAMILY: Nonsteroidal Anti-inflammatory Drugs "NSAIDs"
Arthritis Drugs (see p. 265)

Flurbiprofen (fler bih *pro* fen) belongs to the family of drugs called nonsteroidal anti-inflammatory drugs, shortened to NSAIDs (*n* sayds), often used to treat arthritis in older adults. NSAIDs can cause serious harm, even fatalities, from bleeding in the stomach or intestines. Bleeding can occur at any time and without warning and older people are more likely to experience adverse effects from bleeding. Older adults are also more likely to have reduced liver and kidney function. Some doctors believe people over age 70 should be started with half the usual dose of drugs in this group.[15]

Flurbiprofen is used to treat mild to moderate symptoms of rheumatoid arthritis, osteoarthritis, and bursitis. Your doctor may prescribe other arthritis drugs as well. The drug is used in drop form to dilate the eyes during cataract surgery. **In general, if you are over 60, you should take less than the usual adult dose, especially if you have decreased kidney function.**

Although flurbiprofen relieves symptoms, it does not cure any condition, nor delay progress of disease and can mask symptoms of infection. Flurbiprofen belongs to the same family as ibuprofen (see p. 311) and aspirin (see p. 275).

Aspirin is just as effective and less costly than other NSAIDs and is the drug of choice for treating pain, fever, and inflammation in people who do not have ulcers, gastritis (inflammation of the stomach), or an allergy to aspirin. Some rheumatologists (arthritis specialists) prefer aspirin to other NSAIDs for treating rheumatoid arthritis.[16]

If you are taking flurbiprofen ask your doctor if you can switch to taking enteric-coated asprin (asprin coated so it won't dissolve in the stomach) twice a day. If you cannot take asprin, ask about switching to another drug in this family such as ibuprofen (see p. 311). Each person responds differently to different NSAIDS.

WARNING

NONSTEROIDAL ANTI-INFLAMMATORY DRUG (NSAID) INDUCED GASTROINTESTINAL TOXICITY

All members of the NSAID family of drugs can cause gastrointestinal toxicity that can lead to gastrointestinal bleeding and hospitalization or death. The risk of gastrointestinal toxicity from these drugs increases with increasing doses and the length of treatment.

If the following symptoms develop while you are taking an NSAID, stop the drug immediately and contact your doctor: severe abdominal or stomach pain, cramping, or burning, severe and continuing nausea, heartburn, or indigestion, bloody or black, tarry stools, vomiting blood or material that looks like coffee grounds, or spitting up blood.

Before You Use This Drug

Do not use if you have or have had:

- an allergic reaction to aspirin, any other NSAID or iodides[17]
- herpes simplex (for eye drops)[18]
- alcohol dependence
- peptic ulcer
- nasal polyps

Tell your doctor if you have or have had:

- allergies to drugs
- heart, kidney or liver problems
- hemophilia or other bleeding problems
- high blood pressure

- anemia
- asthma
- diabetes
- stomach or intestinal problems
- tobacco use
- tuberculosis[19]

Tell your doctor about any other drugs you take, including aspirin, herbs, vitamins, and other nonprescription products.

When You Use This Drug

- Do not drink alcohol. It irritates the stomach lining and increases the risk of stomach bleeding.
- Call your doctor immediately if you have flu-like symptoms (chills, fever, muscle aches or pains) shortly before or with a skin rash. This may indicate a serious reaction to flurbiprofen.
- You may feel dizzy when rising from a lying or sitting position. If you are lying down, hang your legs over the side of the bed for a few minutes, then get up slowly. When getting up from a chair, stay by the chair until you are sure that you are not dizzy. (See p. 16.)
- Until you know how you react to this drug, do not drive or perform other activities requiring alertness.
- If you plan to have any surgery, including dental, tell your doctor that you take this drug.

How to Use This Drug

- Take with food to reduce stomach irritation.
- Take with **a full glass (eight ounces) of water.** Do not lie down for 30 minutes afterwards.
- If you miss a dose, take it as soon as possible, but skip it if it is almost time for the next dose. **Do not take double doses.**
- Instill eye drops according to instructions of your surgeon. Your eyes may sting temporarily.
- Store both tablets and eye drops at room temperature with cap on firmly. Do not expose to heat or light.

Interactions with Other Drugs

The following drugs are listed in the *Evaluations of Drug Interactions* 1997 as causing "highly clinically significant" or "clinically significant" interactions when used together with this drug. We have also included potentially serious interactions listed in the drug's FDA-approved professional product labeling or package insert. New scientific techniques have allowed researchers to predict some drug interactions before they have been documented in people. There may be other drugs, especially those in the families of drugs listed below, that also will react with this drug to cause severe adverse effects. The number of new drugs approved for marketing increases the chance of drug interactions, and new drug interactions are being identified with old drugs. Be vigilant. Make sure to tell your doctor and pharmacist the drugs you are taking and tell your doctor if you are taking any of these interacting drugs:

bendroflumethiazide, BENEMID, CAPOTEN, captopril, COUMADIN, cyclosporine, DEXATRIM, digoxin, DILANTIN, DYAZIDE, DYRENIUM, GARAMYCIN, gentamicin, gold sodium thiomalate, INDERAL, INDERAL LA, ketorolac, LANOXICAPS, LANOXIN, lithium, LITHOBID, LITHONATE, MAXZIDE, methotrexate, MINIPRESS, MYOCHRYSINE, NATURETIN, NEORAL, phenylpropanolamine, phenytoin, prazosin, probenecid, propranolol, RHEUMATREX DOSE PACK, SANDIMMUNE, TORADOL, triamterene, triamterene and hydrochlorothiazide, warfarin.

Adverse Effects

Call your doctor immediately if you experience:

- back pain[20]
- abdominal pain or swelling
- appetite loss
- bloody, black, tarry or light stools

- blood pressure increase or decrease
- difficulty breathing
- unusual bruising
- chest pain
- chills
- confusion
- cough or hoarseness
- depression
- drowsiness
- pain, dryness, redness, irritation or swelling of the eyes
- facial skin color changes
- fever
- forgetfulness
- gastrointestinal pain, cramping or burning
- swollen glands
- headache
- hearing change or ringing or buzzing
- heartburn
- hives on face, eyelids or tongue
- indigestion
- lower back, neck or side pain
- unusually heavy menstrual bleeding
- muscle cramps or pain
- nausea, vomiting
- nosebleeds, running nose or sneezing
- pinpoint red spots on skin
- skin rash, hives, itching, scaling
- sore throat
- sores, ulcers, or white spots on lips or in mouth
- difficulty speaking
- difficulty swallowing
- swelling of face, lips, tongue, fingers, lower legs or feet
- continuing thirst
- burning throat or chest
- unusual tiredness or weakness
- difficulty urinating
- dark, bloody or cloudy urine
- vision change
- vomiting blood or material that looks like coffee grounds
- rapid weight gain
- yellow eyes or skin

Call your doctor if these symptoms continue:

- anxiety
- constipation, diarrhea, gas
- dizziness
- drowsiness
- flushing or hot flashes
- irregular heartbeat
- insomnia
- irritated or dry mouth
- muscle weakness
- nervousness, irritability
- sunburn
- sweating
- bitter taste
- trembling
- weakness

Periodic Tests

Ask your doctor which of these tests should be done periodically while you are taking this drug:

- kidney function tests
- liver function tests
- stool tests for possible blood loss
- hematocrit and/or hemoglobin test
- blood concentrations of creatinine, potassium, and urea nitrogen
- white blood cell count
- upper GI diagnostic tests
- ophthalmologic exams

PREGNANCY WARNING

This drug caused harm to developing fetuses in animal studies, or such studies were not done. Use during pregnancy only for clear medical reasons. Tell your doctor if you are pregnant or thinking of becoming pregnant before you take this drug.

Aspirin with Codeine

GENERIC: available

FAMILY: Painkillers
Fever Reducers
Nonsteroidal Anti-inflammatory Drugs "NSAIDs"
Narcotics (see p. 264)

Aspirin (see p. 275) and codeine (see p. 284) are both effective painkillers. Together, they produce a rational combination drug that relieves pain better than aspirin alone, but has less risk of adverse effects than the larger amount of codeine that would be needed if codeine were used alone. This combination is available in capsules and tablets.

Although this combination is the best drug for some situations, it is overused. Many people who are prescribed this combination would get pain relief from aspirin alone, and would avoid the harmful adverse effects codeine can have—drug-induced dependence and constipation. So before taking this drug, ask your doctor about trying plain aspirin first.

ASPIRIN/REYE'S SYNDROME ALERT

Do not use this product for treating chicken pox, flu, or flu-like illness. It will increase the risk of contracting Reye's syndrome, a rare but often fatal disease.

This drug can increase the risk of hip fracture.[21]

One hazard of taking codeine continuously for longer than several weeks is drug-induced dependence. **Do not stop taking your drug suddenly.** With the help of your doctor, work out a schedule for slowly decreasing the amount of the drug you take by about 5 to 10% each day. Keep a written record of the dosage reduction schedule with you. These steps will make it much easier to become drug free without developing distressing symptoms of drug withdrawal.

WARNING

NONSTEROIDAL ANTI-INFLAMMATORY DRUG (NSAID) INDUCED GASTROINTESTINAL TOXICITY

All members of the NSAID family of drugs can cause gastrointestinal toxicity that can lead to gastrointestinal bleeding and hospitalization or death. The risk of gastrointestinal toxicity from these drugs increases with increasing doses and the length of treatment.

If the following symptoms develop while you are taking an NSAID, stop the drug immediately and contact your doctor: severe abdominal or stomach pain, cramping, or burning, severe and continuing nausea, heartburn, or indigestion, bloody or black, tarry stools, vomiting blood or material that looks like coffee grounds, or spitting up blood.

PREGNANCY WARNING

This drug caused harm to developing fetuses in animal studies, or such studies were not done. Use during pregnancy only for clear medical reasons. Tell your doctor if you are pregnant or thinking of becoming pregnant before you take this drug.

Acetaminophen and Hydrocodone
BANCAP-HC (Forest)
VICODIN (Knoll)

GENERIC: available

FAMILY: Painkillers
         Fever Reducers
         Narcotics (see p. 264)

Acetaminophen (see p. 338) and hydrocodone (hye droe *koe* done) are painkillers. Acetaminophen also reduces fever, but it does not relieve the redness, stiffness, or swelling of rheumatoid arthritis or other conditions that cause inflammation. Hydrocodone acts similarly to the narcotic drug codeine.

Together, these two drugs produce a rational combination that relieves pain better than acetaminophen alone, but has less risk of adverse effects than the larger dose of hydrocodone that would be needed if hydrocodone were used alone. This combination is available in tablets and in capsules.

Although this drug is the best choice in some situations, it is overused. Many people who are prescribed this combination would get pain relief from acetaminophen alone, and would avoid the danger of becoming addicted to hydrocodone. So before taking this drug, ask your doctor about trying plain acetaminophen first.

One hazard of taking hydrocodone continuously for longer than several weeks is drug-induced dependence. **Do not stop taking your drug suddenly.** With the help of your doctor, work out a schedule for slowly decreasing the amount of the drug you take by about 5 to 10% each day. Keep a written record of the dosage reduction schedule with you. These steps will make it much easier to become drug free without developing distressing symptoms of drug withdrawal.

DRUG INTERACTION WARNING

INCREASED RISK OF BLEEDING WHEN ACETAMINOPHEN AND WARFARIN (COUMADIN) ARE TAKEN TOGETHER

Acetaminophen may interact with warfarin to increase the risk of bleeding. This risk increases with increasing doses of acetaminophen. The risk of bleeding has been found to increase tenfold in people who were taking 28 or more regular strength acetaminophen tablets per week, or the equivalent of 18 or more extra-strength tablets per week compared to those taking warfarin and no acetaminophen.[22] A regular strength tablet contains 325 milligrams of acetaminophen and extra-strength tablets contain 500 milligrams each of the drug.

Warfarin is a drug of considerable benefit after heart valve replacement and in preventing blood clots from a type of heart rhythm disturbance known as atrial fibrillation. It also reduces the risk of death, recurrent heart attacks, and stroke after a heart attack.

Based on this new evidence, if you are taking warfarin, you should notify your doctor before taking any product containing acetaminophen.

WARNING

There have been a number of case reports of liver damage involving a possible drug interaction between isoniazid, a medication used to prevent and treat tuberculosis, and acetaminophen, an over-the-counter painkiller and the active ingredient in Tylenol. Isoniazid alone, especially as people get older, has been documented to cause liver damage. Acetaminophen, alone in large doses or probably in combination with alcohol, also increases the risk of liver damage. The combination of acetaminophen with isoniazid, according to the authors of these case reports, may also be dangerous.[23]

If you are taking isoniazid for tuberculosis or have a positive TB skin test and are using the drug, consult your physician before using acetaminophen or any combination product containing acetaminophen. Discuss alternatives to acetaminophen with your physician.[24]

PREGNANCY WARNING

This drug caused harm to developing fetuses in animal studies, or such studies were not done. Use during pregnancy only for clear medical reasons. Tell your doctor if you are pregnant or thinking of becoming pregnant before you take this drug.

Aspirin/Acetylsalicylic Acid
GENUINE BAYER ASPIRIN Plain 325 mg
(Glenbrook)
**ECOTRIN Enteric-coated 325 mg
and 500 mg** (SmithKline Consumer Products)
EASPRIN 975 mg (Parke-Davis)

GENERIC: available (except 975 mg product)
FAMILY: Painkillers
Nonsteroidal Anti-inflammatory Drugs "NSAIDs"
Salicylates (see p. 261)
Fever Reducers

Aspirin (*as* pir in) belongs to the family of drugs called nonsteroidal anti-inflammatory drugs, shortened to NSAIDs (*n* sayds), often used to treat arthritis in older adults. NSAIDs can cause serious harm, even fatalities, from bleeding in the stomach or intestines. Bleeding can occur at any time and without warning and older people are more likely to experience adverse effects from bleeding. Older adults are also more likely to have reduced liver and kidney function. Some doctors believe people over age 70 should be started with half the usual dose of drugs in this group.[25]

Aspirin relieves mild to moderate pain and reduces fever and inflammation. When you take aspirin for pain or fever, you are only treating *symptoms* of an underlying problem such as an infection. You are *not* treating the underlying problem itself. **You should not take aspirin if you have ulcers, a severely irritated stomach, gout, severe anemia, hemophilia or other bleeding problems, if you take an anticoagulant drug such as heparin or warfarin, or if you are allergic to aspirin or similar painkillers.**

There are several forms of aspirin for different situations. If you take aspirin only occasionally, plain, generic aspirin is best. For long-term use, we strongly recommend aspirin that is "enteric-coated" (coated so it does not dissolve in the stomach), since it helps prevent the stomach bleeding that aspirin can cause and it can be taken twice a day. We do not recommend buffered aspirin (see p. 280), since it is no better than plain aspirin and is more costly.

In general, you should not take aspirin to reduce a fever until the cause of the fever is known. It is rarely *necessary* to reduce a fever, but if a fever is having harmful effects or is making you extremely uncomfortable, it can be treated with aspirin.[26] When you are taking aspirin for a fever, you should take it regularly (every three to four hours), and stop taking it when the underlying problem goes away or is controlled through other treatment.

If you have arthritis, either plain or enteric-coated aspirin may be the first drug your doctor prescribes. As long as you can tolerate high doses of aspirin for a long time, it is the best treatment. It might take two to three weeks or longer before aspirin is maximally effective. If the dose you are taking at first is not high enough, it should be increased slowly—more slowly for older adults than it would be for younger people. **In general, people over 60 should take less than the usual adult dose because of the risk of harmful adverse effects, such as stomach and intestinal problems.**

If you have joint pain and think that you might have arthritis, **do not try to treat yourself.** See your doctor. There are several kinds of arthritis, and different types require different treatments (see p. 265). **High-dose aspirin therapy can be dangerous if it is not monitored by a doctor.**

Doctors sometimes prescribe aspirin as a preventive measure for illnesses such as heart disease. If you have had a heart attack or are at risk of having sudden chest pain (unstable angina pectoris), your doctor may prescribe low, daily doses of aspirin to help prevent heart attacks. Aspirin also reduces the risk of stroke and death for some men who have had decreased blood flow to the brain (this has not been proven for women). Do not take aspirin for this purpose unless your doctor has prescribed it for you.

ASPIRIN/REYE'S SYNDROME ALERT

Do not use this product for treating chicken pox, flu, or flu-like illness. It will increase the risk of contracting Reye's syndrome, a rare but often fatal disease.

WARNING

NONSTEROIDAL ANTI-INFLAMMATORY DRUG (NSAID) INDUCED GASTROINTESTINAL TOXICITY

All members of the NSAID family of drugs can cause gastrointestinal toxicity that can lead to gastrointestinal bleeding and hospitalization or death. The risk of gastrointestinal toxicity from these drugs increases with increasing doses and the length of treatment.

If the following symptoms develop while you are taking an NSAID, stop the drug immediately and contact your doctor: severe abdominal or stomach pain, cramping, or burning, severe and continuing nausea, heartburn, or indigestion, bloody or black, tarry stools, vomiting blood or material that looks like coffee grounds, or spitting up blood.

Before You Use This Drug

Tell your doctor if you have or have had:

- allergies to drugs
- a reaction to aspirin, other salicylates, or nonsteroidal anti-inflammatory drugs such as ibuprofen or naproxen
- bleeding problems
- ulcer or other stomach problems
- kidney, liver, or heart problems
- asthma, allergies, or nasal polyps
- anemia
- glucose-6-phosphate dehydrogenase deficiency

- gout
- overactive thyroid
- high blood pressure

Tell your doctor about any other drugs you take, including aspirin, herbs, vitamins, and other nonprescription products.

When You Use This Drug

- Do not drink alcohol. This combination increases the risk of stomach or intestinal bleeding.
- Never take more than the amount prescribed by your doctor or recommended on the package label.
- **Caution diabetics:** see p. 550.
- If you are treating yourself, call your doctor if your symptoms do not improve or if you have a fever that lasts more than three days or returns.
- Do not take aspirin for five days before any surgery, unless your doctor tells you otherwise. Aspirin interferes with your body's ability to stop bleeding.
- If you are on long-term or high-dose treatment, you should have regular checkups.
- Never place aspirin directly on teeth or gums because it irritates these tissues.
- Do not chew aspirin within one week after you have had any type of surgery in your mouth.

How to Use This Drug

- Take tablets and capsules with **a full glass (eight ounces) of water.** Do not lie down for 30 minutes.
- Take with food to decrease stomach upset.
- If you miss a dose, take it as soon as you remember, but skip it if it is almost time for the next dose. **Do not take double doses.**

Interactions with Other Drugs

The following drugs are listed in the *Evaluations of Drug Interactions* 1997 as causing "highly clinically significant" or "clinically significant" interactions when used together with this drug. We have also included potentially serious interactions listed in the drug's FDA-approved professional product labeling or package insert. New scientific techniques have allowed researchers to predict some drug interactions before they have been documented in people. There may be other drugs, especially those in the families of drugs listed below, that also will react with this drug to cause severe adverse effects. The number of new drugs approved for marketing increases the chance of drug interactions, and new drug interactions are being identified with old drugs. Be vigilant. Make sure to tell your doctor and pharmacist the drugs you are taking and tell your doctor if you are taking any of these interacting drugs:

acetazolamide, alcohol, aluminum hydroxide/magnesium hydroxide, ANTURANE, CAPOTEN, captopril, chlorpropamide, COUMADIN, DEPAKENE/DEPAKOTE, DIABINESE, DIAMOX, GARAMYCIN, gentamicin, heparin, ketorolac, MAALOX, MAALOX TC, magaldrate, MEDROL, methotrexate, methylprednisolone, RHEUMATREX DOSE PACK, RIOPAN, sulfinpyrazone, TORADOL, valproic acid, warfarin.

Adverse Effects

Call your doctor immediately if you experience:

- **signs of overdose:** bluish discoloration or flushing or redness of skin, coughing, difficulty swallowing, severe or continuing headache, ringing or buzzing in ears, loss of hearing, severe or continuing diarrhea, dizziness or lightheadedness, confusion, extreme drowsiness, nausea or vomiting, stomach pain, abnormal increase in sweating, abnormally fast or deep breathing, abnormal thirst, abnormal or uncontrolled flapping of hands, vision problems, bloody urine, seizures, hallucinations, nervousness or excitement, trouble breathing, unexplained fever, skin rash, hives or itching

- vomiting material that looks bloody or like coffee grounds
- bloody or black, tarry stools
- wheezing, tightness in chest, or trouble breathing
- fainting or dizzy spells

Call your doctor if these symptoms continue:

- heartburn, indigestion, nausea, or stomach pain
- abnormal weakness or fatigue
- decreased urination

Periodic Tests

Ask your doctor which of these tests should be done periodically while you are taking this drug:

- liver function tests
- hematocrit determinations
- salicylate concentrations

PREGNANCY WARNING

This drug caused harm to developing fetuses in animal studies, or such studies were not done. Use during pregnancy only for clear medical reasons. Tell your doctor if you are pregnant or thinking of becoming pregnant before you take this drug.

Limited Use

Probenecid
BENEMID (Merck)

GENERIC: available

FAMILY: Antigout Drugs (see p. 265)
Antibiotic Therapy Aid

Probenecid (proe *ben* e sid) helps to prevent gout attacks. Gout occurs in people who have high levels of uric acid in their body, and an attack occurs when crystals of uric acid form in your joints and your body releases chemicals in response to the crystals. This causes pain and inflammation. Probenecid works by causing more uric acid to leave your body through the kidneys, thereby lowering the level of uric acid in your blood.

Probenecid will not relieve a gout attack that has already started. If you are taking probenecid, keep taking it during an attack, even if another drug is prescribed to treat the attack.

After you start using probenecid, you may still have gout attacks for a while. Keep taking the drug. If you take it regularly, the attacks gradually will become less frequent and less painful, and they may stop completely after several months.

Probenecid can increase your risk of getting kidney stones. To help prevent kidney stones while using probenecid, drink at least 10 to 12 full glasses (eight ounces each) of fluid each day, unless your doctor tells you otherwise. Too much vitamin C (see p. 614) also increases your risk of kidney stones, so do not take vitamin C supplements while taking probenecid unless you have checked with your doctor.

Before You Use This Drug

Tell your doctor if you have or have had:

- allergies to drugs
- kidney problems
- kidney stones
- blood disease
- stomach ulcer

- cancer being treated by antineoplastics or radiation

Tell your doctor about any other drugs you take, including aspirin, herbs, vitamins, and other nonprescription products.

When You Use This Drug

- Do not take aspirin and other drugs in its family (salicylates, see p. 261) because they may make probenecid less effective.
- Do not drink alcohol. Alcohol increases the amount of uric acid in your blood and it may make your gout attacks more frequent and more difficult to control. It also increases the likelihood of stomach problems.
- **Caution diabetics:** Probenecid may cause false results in copper sulfate urine sugar tests (Clinitest). It will not interfere with glucose enzymatic urine sugar tests (Clinistix).

How to Use This Drug

- Take with food to decrease stomach upset. If this does not work and your stomach continues to be upset, check with your doctor.
- Do not store in the bathroom. Do not expose to heat, moisture, or strong light.
- If you miss a dose, take it as soon as you remember, but skip it if you don't remember until the next day. **Do not take double doses.**

Interactions with Other Drugs

The following drugs are listed in the *Evaluations of Drug Interactions* 1997 as causing "highly clinically significant" or "clinically significant" interactions when used together with this drug. We have also included potentially serious interactions listed in the drug's FDA-approved professional product labeling or package insert. New scientific techniques have allowed researchers to predict some drug interactions before they have been documented in people. There may be other drugs, especially those in the families of drugs listed below, that also will react with this drug to cause severe adverse effects. The number of new drugs approved for marketing increases the chance of drug interactions, and new drug interactions are being identified with old drugs. Be vigilant. Make sure to tell your doctor and pharmacist the drugs you are taking and tell your doctor if you are taking any of these interacting drugs:

aspirin, GENUINE BAYER ASPIRIN, cephalothin, DILOR, dyphylline, ECOTRIN, INDOCIN, indomethacin, KEFLIN, LUFYLLIN, methotrexate, RETROVIR, RHEUMATREX DOSE PACK, zidovudine (AZT).

Adverse Effects

Call your doctor immediately if you experience:

- **signs of overdose:** convulsions, severe vomiting, trouble breathing, puffiness or swelling of eyelids, changes in skin color of face, skin rash, hives or itching
  - bloody or cloudy urine
  - difficult or painful urination
  - back or rib pain
  - difficulty breathing
  - unusual weight gain
  - swelling of feet, legs, fingers or face
  - sore throat and fever
  - unusual bleeding or bruising
  - unusual tiredness or weakness
  - decrease in amount of urine
  - yellow eyes or skin
  - cough or hoarseness
  - sores, ulcers or white spots on lips or mouth
  - swollen and/or painful glands

Call your doctor if these symptoms continue:

- headache
- joint pain, redness or swelling
- loss of appetite
- nausea or vomiting

- dizziness
- flushing or redness of face
- frequent urge to urinate
- sore gums

Periodic Tests

Ask your doctor which of these tests should be done periodically while you are taking this drug:

- blood and urine levels of uric acid

 Do Not Use

ALTERNATIVE TREATMENT:
See Plain or Enteric-coated Aspirin, p. 275.

Buffered Aspirin
BUFFERIN (Bristol-Myers)
ASCRIPTIN, ASCRIPTIN A/D (Rorer)

FAMILY: Painkillers
Nonsteroidal Anti-inflammatory Drugs "NSAIDs"
Fever Reducers
Salicylates (see p. 261)

Buffered aspirin is aspirin with a "buffer" or "acid neutralizer" added. Advertisements for buffered aspirin claim that it relieves pain faster than plain aspirin because it is absorbed better, and also that it is less irritating to the stomach and intestines than plain aspirin. These claims cannot be justified.

The amount of buffer in buffered aspirin is very small, only a fraction of the amount found in even one teaspoon of many antacids. A Food and Drug Administration advisory committee found that although buffered aspirin may be absorbed more quickly than plain aspirin, it does *not* provide much faster pain relief. The committee also found *no* evidence that buffered aspirin is any gentler to the stomach than plain aspirin.[27] Alka-Seltzer®, a brand of buffered aspirin, should not be taken by anyone whose salt (sodium) intake has been limited.

If you take aspirin only occasionally, plain generic aspirin (see p. 275) is better than buffered, because it is much less expensive (about one-quarter of the price of Bufferin or Ascriptin) and relieves pain just as quickly. If you are taking aspirin for a long period of time, such as for arthritis, you should use generic enteric-coated aspirin, which actually does decrease the amount of irritation and bleeding in the stomach and which is also much less expensive than Bufferin or Ascriptin.

ASPIRIN/REYE'S SYNDROME ALERT

Do not use this product for treating chicken pox, flu, or flu-like illness. It will increase the risk of contracting Reye's syndrome, a rare but often fatal disease.

WARNING

NONSTEROIDAL ANTI-INFLAMMATORY DRUG (NSAID) INDUCED GASTROINTESTINAL TOXICITY

All members of the NSAID family of drugs can cause gastrointestinal toxicity that can lead to gastrointestinal bleeding and hospitalization or death. The risk of gastrointestinal toxicity from these drugs increases with increasing doses and the length of treatment.

If the following symptoms develop while you are taking an NSAID, stop the drug immediately and contact your doctor: severe abdominal or stomach pain, cramping, or burning, severe and continuing nausea, heartburn, or indigestion, bloody or black, tarry stools, vomiting blood or material that looks like coffee grounds, or spitting up blood.

Do Not Use

ALTERNATIVE TREATMENT:
See Enteric-coated Aspirin, p. 275.

Phenylbutazone
BUTAZOLIDIN (Geigy)

FAMILY: Nonsteroidal Anti-inflammatory Drugs "NSAIDs"
Arthritis Drugs (see p. 265)

Phenylbutazone (fen ill *byoo* ta zone) belongs to the family of drugs called nonsteroidal anti-inflammatory drugs, shortened to NSAIDs (*n* sayds), often used to treat arthritis in older adults. NSAIDs can cause serious harm, even fatalities, from bleeding in the stomach or intestines. Bleeding can occur at any time and without warning and older people are more likely to experience adverse effects from bleeding. Older adults are also more likely to have reduced liver and kidney function. Some doctors believe people over age 70 should be started with half the usual dose of drugs in this group.[28]

Phenylbutazone relieves the pain and inflammation of rheumatoid arthritis and acute gout. **Do not use this drug.** Phenylbutazone is still being prescribed and sold but the World Health Organization has said that the drug should not be used by older people.[29] **The drug has caused numerous deaths and produces severe adverse effects.** It is toxic (poisonous) to bone marrow and can kill white blood cells.

Aspirin (see p. 275) is just as effective and less costly than other NSAIDs and is the drug of choice for treating pain, fever, and inflammation in people who do not have ulcers, gastritis (inflammation of the stomach), or an allergy to aspirin. Some rheumatologists (arthritis specialists) prefer aspirin to other NSAIDs for treating rheumatoid arthritis.[30]

If you are taking phenylbutazone ask your doctor if you can switch to taking enteric-coated aspirin (aspirin coated so it won't dissolve in the stomach) twice a day. If you cannot take aspirin, ask about switching to another drug in this family such as ibuprofen (see p. 311). Each person responds differently to different NSAIDs.

WARNING

NONSTEROIDAL ANTI-INFLAMMATORY DRUG (NSAID) INDUCED GASTROINTESTINAL TOXICITY

All members of the NSAID family of drugs can cause gastrointestinal toxicity that can lead to gastrointestinal bleeding and hospitalization or death. The risk of gastrointestinal toxicity from these drugs increases with increasing doses and the length of treatment.

If the following symptoms develop while you are taking an NSAID, stop the drug immediately and contact your doctor: severe abdominal or stomach pain, cramping, or burning, severe and continuing nausea, heartburn, or indigestion, bloody or black, tarry stools, vomiting blood or material that looks like coffee grounds, or spitting up blood.

Limited Use

Sulindac
CLINORIL (Merck)

GENERIC: available
FAMILY: Nonsteroidal Anti-inflammatory Drugs "NSAIDs"
Arthritis Drugs (see p. 265)

Sulindac (sul *in* dak) belongs to the family of drugs called nonsteroidal anti-inflammatory drugs, shortened to NSAIDs (*n* sayds), often used to treat arthritis in older adults. NSAIDs can cause serious harm, even fatalities, from bleeding in the stomach or intestines. Bleeding can occur at any time and without warning and older people are more likely to experience adverse effects from bleeding. Older adults are also more likely to have reduced liver and kidney function. Some doctors believe people over age 70 should be started with half the usual dose of drugs in this group.[31]

Sulindac is used mainly to relieve the pain and inflammation of rheumatoid arthritis, osteoarthritis, and acute gout. **In general, if you are over 60, you should take less than the usual adult dose, especially if you have decreased kidney function.** Like indomethacin (see p. 302), to which it is chemically related, sulindac can cause headaches, drowsiness, and dizziness.

For most people, sulindac has no proven advantage over other drugs in this family. However, it may do less harm to the kidneys than other NSAIDs. Because of this, people with kidney disease may be able to take sulindac even if they can't take other drugs in its family, as long as they don't also have liver disease.[32]

Aspirin (see p. 275) is just as effective and less costly than other NSAIDs and is the drug of choice for treating pain, fever, and inflammation in people who do not have ulcers, gastritis (inflammation of the stomach), or an allergy to aspirin. Some rheumatologists (arthritis experts) prefer aspirin to other NSAIDs for treating rheumatoid arthritis.[33]

If you are taking sulindac, ask your doctor if you can switch to taking enteric-coated aspirin (aspirin coated so it won't dissolve in the stomach) twice a day. If you can't take aspirin, ask about switching to another drug in this family such as ibuprofen (see p. 311). Each person responds differently to different NSAIDs.

WARNING

NONSTEROIDAL ANTI-INFLAMMATORY DRUG (NSAID) INDUCED GASTROINTESTINAL TOXICITY

All members of the NSAID family of drugs can cause gastrointestinal toxicity that can lead to gastrointestinal bleeding and hospitalization or death. The risk of gastrointestinal toxicity from these drugs increases with increasing doses and the length of treatment.

If the following symptoms develop while you are taking an NSAID, stop the drug immediately and contact your doctor: severe abdominal or stomach pain, cramping, or burning, severe and continuing nausea, heartburn, or indigestion, bloody or black, tarry stools, vomiting blood or material that looks like coffee grounds, or spitting up blood.

Before You Use This Drug

Do not use if you have or have had:

- an allergic reaction to aspirin, any other NSAID or iodides[34]
- peptic ulcers
- alcohol dependence
- nasal polyps

Tell your doctor if you have or have had:

- allergies to drugs
- heart, kidney, or liver problems
- hemophilia or other bleeding problems
- high blood pressure
- anemia
- asthma
- diabetes
- stomach or intestinal problems
- tobacco use

Tell your doctor about any other drugs you take, including aspirin, herbs, vitamins, and other nonprescription products.

When You Use This Drug

• Do not drink alcohol. It irritates the stomach lining and increases the risk of stomach bleeding.

• Call your doctor immediately if you have flu-like symptoms (chills, fever, muscle aches or pains) shortly before or with a skin rash. This may indicate a serious reaction to sulindac.

• You may feel dizzy when rising from a lying or sitting position. If you are lying down, hang your legs over the side of the bed for a few minutes, then get up slowly. When getting up from a chair, stay by the chair until you are sure that you are not dizzy. (See p. 16.)

• If you plan to have any surgery, including dental, tell your doctor that you take this drug.

How to Use This Drug

• Take with food to reduce stomach irritation.

• Take with **a full glass (eight ounces) of water.** Do not lie down for 30 minutes afterwards.

• If you miss a dose, take it as soon as possible, but skip it if it is almost time for the next dose. **Do not take double doses.**

• Store at room temperature, with lid on tightly. Do not store in the bathroom. Do not expose to moisture or heat.

Interactions with Other Drugs

The following drugs are listed in the *Evaluations of Drug Interactions* 1997 as causing "highly clinically significant" or "clinically significant" interactions when used together with this drug. We have also included potentially serious interactions listed in the drug's FDA-approved professional product labeling or package insert. New scientific techniques have allowed researchers to predict some drug interactions before they have been documented in people. There may be other drugs, especially those in the families of drugs listed below, that also will react with this drug to cause severe adverse effects. The number of new drugs approved for marketing increases the chance of drug interactions, and new drug interactions are being identified with old drugs. Be vigilant. Make sure to tell your doctor and pharmacist the drugs you are taking and tell your doctor if you are taking any of these interacting drugs:

COUMADIN, cyclosporine, DILANTIN, ketorolac, labetalol, methotrexate, MINIPRESS, NEORAL, NORMODYNE, phenytoin, prazosin, RHEUMATREX DOSE PACK, SANDIMMUNE, TORADOL, TRANDATE, warfarin.

Adverse Effects

Call your doctor immediately if you experience:

• abdominal pain or swelling
• appetite loss
• bloody, black, tarry or light-colored stools
• blood pressure increase or decrease
• difficulty breathing
• unusual bruising
• chest pains
• chills
• confusion
• convulsions
• cough or hoarseness
• depression
• diarrhea
• drowsiness
• facial skin color changes
• fainting
• fever
• flushing
• gastrointestinal pain, cramping or burning
• swollen glands
• headache
• hearing change or ringing or buzzing
• heartburn
• hives on face, eyelids or tongue
• indigestion

- lower back, neck or side pain or stiffness
- unusually heavy menstrual bleeding
- muscle cramps or pain
- nausea, vomiting
- nosebleeds
- numbness, tingling, pain or weakness in hands or feet
- pinpoint red spots on skin
- psychotic reaction
- skin rash, hives, itching, scaling
- sore throat
- sores, ulcers, or white spots on lips or in mouth
- spitting blood
- sweating
- swelling of face, lips, tongue, fingers, lower legs or feet
- continuous thirst
- irritated tongue
- unusual tiredness or weakness
- difficulty urinating
- bloody, dark or cloudy urine
- vision change
- vomiting blood or material that looks like coffee grounds
- rapid weight gain
- yellow eyes or skin

Call your doctor if these symptoms continue:

- constipation, gas
- dizziness
- irregular heartbeat
- insomnia
- irritated or dry mouth
- muscle weakness
- nervousness, irritability
- sunburn
- bitter taste
- weakness
- lightheadedness

Periodic Tests

Ask your doctor which of these tests should be done periodically while you are taking this drug:

- kidney function tests
- liver function tests
- stool tests for possible blood loss
- hematocrit and/or hemoglobin test
- blood concentrations of creatinine, potassium, and urea nitrogen
- white blood cell count
- upper GI diagnostic tests
- ophthalmologic exams

Codeine

GENERIC: available

FAMILY: Narcotics (see p. 264)

Codeine (*koe* deen) relieves mild to moderate pain and also suppresses coughing. **Do not use codeine if you have a history of serious constipation.**

> One hazard of taking codeine continuously for longer than several weeks is drug-induced dependence. **Do not stop taking your drug suddenly.** With the help of your doctor, work out a schedule for slowly decreasing the amount of the drug you take by about 5 to 10% each day. Keep a written record of the dosage reduction schedule with you. These steps will make it much easier to become drug free without developing distressing symptoms of drug withdrawal.

Before You Use This Drug

Tell your doctor if you have or have had:

- allergies to drugs
- an unusual reaction to any narcotics
- brain disease or head injury
- colitis (inflammation of the colon)
- emphysema, asthma, or other lung disease
- enlarged prostate or trouble urinating
- gallbladder disease or gallstones
- heart, kidney, or liver problems
- seizures

- underactive thyroid or adrenal gland
- alcohol or drug abuse
- emotional problems

Tell your doctor about any other drugs you take, including aspirin, herbs, vitamins, and other nonprescription products.

When You Use This Drug

- Do not drink alcohol or take any drugs that make you drowsy unless you have checked with your doctor first. When codeine is combined with these substances, it will make you even more drowsy, which puts you at risk of having accidents.
- Do not drive or perform other activities that require alertness because this drug may make you drowsy, dizzy, or lightheaded.
- If this drug seems less effective after a few weeks of use, **do not increase the dose.** Call your doctor instead.
- If you use this drug for a long time, have regular checkups.
- You may feel dizzy when rising from a lying or sitting position. If you are lying down, hang your legs over the side of the bed for a few minutes, then get up slowly. When getting up from a chair, stay by the chair until you are sure that you are not dizzy. (See p. 16.)
- If you plan to have any surgery, including dental, tell your doctor that you take this drug.

This drug can increase the risk of hip fracture.[35]

How to Use This Drug

- Protect liquid form from freezing.
- If you miss a dose, take it as soon as you remember, but skip it if it is almost time for the next dose. **Do not take double doses.**
- Do not store in the bathroom. Do not expose to heat, moisture, or strong light.

Interactions with Other Drugs

The following drugs are listed in the *Evaluations of Drug Interactions* 1997 as causing "highly clinically significant" or "clinically significant" interactions when used together with this drug. We have also included potentially serious interactions listed in the drug's FDA-approved professional product labeling or package insert. New scientific techniques have allowed researchers to predict some drug interactions before they have been documented in people. There may be other drugs, especially those in the families of drugs listed below, that also will react with this drug to cause severe adverse effects. The number of new drugs approved for marketing increases the chance of drug interactions, and new drug interactions are being identified with old drugs. Be vigilant. Make sure to tell your doctor and pharmacist the drugs you are taking and tell your doctor if you are taking any of these interacting drugs:

carbamazepine, chlorpromazine, cimetidine, COUMADIN, NARDIL, PENTOTHAL, phenelzine, TAGAMET, TEGRETOL, thiopental, THORAZINE, TUBARINE, tubocurarine, warfarin.

Adverse Effects

Call your doctor immediately if you experience:

- **signs of overdose:** cold, clammy skin, seizures, severe dizziness or drowsiness, nervousness or restlessness, confusion, small pupils, unconsciousness, abnormally low blood pressure, slow heartbeat, slow or troubled breathing, severe weakness
- feelings of unreality
- hallucinations
- skin rash, hives, or itching

- depression or other mood or mental change
- ringing sound in ears
- slow, irregular, or troubled breathing
- swollen, red or flushed face
- trembling or uncontrolled or rigid muscle movements
- abnormal (slow, fast, or pounding) heartbeat
- increased sweating
- headache
- loss of appetite
- unusual excitement, nervousness or restlessness

Call your doctor if these symptoms continue:

- dizziness
- drowsiness
- confusion
- feeling faint or lightheaded
- nausea or vomiting
- constipation
- nightmares or insomnia
- difficulty urinating
- vision changes

Call your doctor if these symptoms continue after you stop taking this drug:

- body aches
- diarrhea
- irregular heartbeat
- fever, runny nose or sneezing
- insomnia
- loss of appetite
- nausea or vomiting
- nervousness, restlessness or irritability
- enlarged pupils
- sweating
- trembling or shivering
- weakness

Periodic Tests

Ask your doctor which of these tests should be done periodically while you are taking this drug:

- respiratory function tests

Limited Use

Colchicine

GENERIC: available
FAMILY: Antigout Drugs (see p. 265)

Colchicine (*kol* chi seen) prevents and treats gout attacks, and reduces inflammation and relieves pain from acute gouty arthritis.

Gout occurs in people who have high levels of uric acid in their body, and an attack occurs when crystals of uric acid form in the joints and the body responds by releasing harmful chemicals. This causes pain and inflammation.

Colchicine prevents and treats attacks by decreasing the amount of chemicals that your body releases into the joints. It does not lower the level of uric acid in your body, which is the root cause of the problem. Colchicine has several harmful adverse effects (see Adverse Effects) and you may be better off taking large doses of an anti-inflammatory drug such as naproxen (a nonsteroidal anti-inflammatory drug, see p. 317), which has fewer harmful effects. Stop taking colchicine and call your doctor immediately if you have diarrhea, nausea, vomiting, or stomach pain. **Older adults are more susceptible to colchicine's adverse effects. If you have decreased kidney function, you should be on a low dose of colchicine in order to reduce adverse effects such as muscle and nerve damage.**[36]

Before You Use This Drug

Tell your doctor if you have or have had:

- allergies to drugs
- alcohol abuse
- bone marrow depression or blood cell diseases
- heart, kidney, or liver problems
- severe intestinal disease
- ulcer or other stomach problem

Tell your doctor about any other drugs you take, including aspirin, herbs, vitamins, and other nonprescription products.

When You Use This Drug

- **Do not take more than prescribed, even if the pain is not relieved or if you do not experience adverse effects.**
- Do not drink alcohol. Alcohol increases the amount of uric acid in your blood and may make your gout attacks more frequent or more difficult to control. It also increases the likelihood of stomach problems.

How to Use This Drug

- If you take other drugs to prevent gout attacks and your doctor prescribes colchicine when you have an attack, keep taking the other drugs as directed by your doctor.
- *If you take colchicine only when you have an attack:* Take it at the first sign of attack. Stop taking it as soon as pain is relieved or if you experience nausea, vomiting, stomach pain, or diarrhea. Do not take it more often than every three days, unless your doctor tells you otherwise.
- *If you take colchicine regularly to prevent attacks:* Increase your dose, as directed by your doctor, at the first sign of an attack. Stop taking the larger dose as soon as pain is relieved or if you experience nausea, vomiting, stomach

pain, or diarrhea. After the attack is over, return to your regular dose.
- Do not store in the bathroom. Do not expose to heat, moisture, or strong light.
- If you miss a dose, take it as soon as you remember, but skip it if it is almost time for the next dose. **Do not take double doses.**

Interactions with Other Drugs

Some other drugs that you may be taking (either over-the-counter or prescription drugs) can interact with this one, causing adverse effects. Ask your doctor what these drugs are and let him or her know if you are taking any of them.

Adverse Effects

Call your doctor immediately if you experience:

- **signs of overdose:** bloody urine, burning feeling in stomach, throat, or skin, seizures, diarrhea, fever, mood or mental changes, severe muscle weakness, sudden decrease in amount of urine, difficulty breathing, severe vomiting
- numbness or tingling in fingers or toes
- skin rash or hives
- sore throat and fever
- unusual bleeding or bruising
- unusual tiredness or weakness

Call your doctor if these symptoms continue:

- loss of appetite
- unusual hair loss

Periodic Tests

Ask your doctor which of these tests should be done periodically while you are taking this drug:

- complete blood count

PREGNANCY WARNING

This drug caused harm to developing fetuses in animal studies, or such studies were not done. Use during pregnancy only for clear medical reasons. Tell your doctor if you are pregnant or thinking of becoming pregnant before you take this drug.

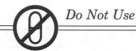

Do Not Use

ALTERNATIVE TREATMENT:
See Aspirin, p. 275, and Codeine, p. 284.

Propoxyphene
DARVON, DARVON-N (Lilly)

Propoxyphene and Acetaminophen
DARVOCET-N (Lilly)
WYGESIC (Wyeth-Ayerst)

Propoxyphene, Aspirin, and Caffeine
DARVON COMPOUND
DARVON COMPOUND-65 (Lilly)

FAMILY: Narcotics (see p. 264)

Propoxyphene (proe *pox* i feen) is a narcotic that relieves mild to moderate pain. **We recommend that you do not use it because it is no more effective than aspirin (see p. 275) or codeine (see p. 284) and it is much more dangerous than aspirin.** If you have taken aspirin for your pain and it has not worked, propoxyphene will probably not do any better.[37] In fact, some studies say that propoxyphene by itself is no more effective than a sugar pill (placebo).[38] Most studies show that propoxyphene is less effective than aspirin **and that it has a potential for addiction and overdose.**[39]

Many people who have taken propoxyphene have become dependent on the drug without knowing it. Thousands of these people have died, some through accidental overdoses. Sev-

eral experts on drug prescribing for older adults have recommended that propoxyphene not be taken by this group.[40]

These drugs can increase the risk of hip fracture.[41]

WARNING

There have been a number of case reports of liver damage involving a possible drug interaction between isoniazid, a medication used to prevent and treat tuberculosis, and acetaminophen, an over-the-counter painkiller and the active ingredient in Tylenol. Isoniazid alone, especially as people get older, has been documented to cause liver damage. Acetaminophen, alone in large doses, or probably in combination with alcohol, also increases the risk of liver damage. The combination of acetaminophen with isoniazid, according to the authors of these case reports, may also be dangerous.[42]

If you are taking isoniazid for tuberculosis or have a positive TB skin test and are using the drug, consult your physician before using acetaminophen or any combination product containing acetaminophen. Discuss alternatives to acetaminophen with your physician.[43]

One hazard of taking propoxyphene continuously for longer than several weeks is drug-induced dependence. **Do not stop taking your drug suddenly.** With the help of your doctor, work out a schedule for slowly decreasing the amount of the drug you take by about 5 to 10% each day. Keep a written record of the dosage reduction schedule with you. These steps will make it much easier to become drug free without developing distressing symptoms of drug withdrawal.

Meperidine
DEMEROL (Sanofi)

Hydromorphone
DILAUDID (Knoll)

GENERIC: available

FAMILY: Narcotics (see p. 264)

Meperidine (me *per* i deen) is a narcotic drug that relieves moderate to severe pain. Do not take this drug if you have taken antidepressant monoamine oxidase inhibitors within the past two weeks (see Interactions with Other Drugs). **In general, if you are over 60, you should take less than the usual adult dose of meperidine, especially if you have kidney disease.**

Hydromorphone (hye droe *mor* fone), another narcotic, is related to morphine. Like morphine, it relieves severe pain (such as pain from many kinds of cancer) that is not helped by non-narcotic drugs.

One hazard of taking meperidine or hydromorphone continuously for longer than several weeks is drug-induced dependence. **Do not stop taking your drug suddenly.** With the help of your doctor, work out a schedule for slowly decreasing the amount of the drug you take by about 5 to 10% each day. Keep a written record of the dosage reduction schedule with you. These steps will make it much easier to become drug free without developing distressing symptoms of drug withdrawal.

Before You Use This Drug

Tell your doctor if you have or have had:

- allergies to drugs
- an unusual reaction to any narcotics
- brain disease or head injury
- colitis (inflammation of the colon)
- emphysema, asthma, or other lung disease
- enlarged prostate or trouble urinating
- gallbladder disease or gallstones
- heart, kidney, or liver problems
- seizures
- underactive thyroid or adrenal gland
- alcohol or drug abuse
- emotional problems

Tell your doctor about any other drugs you take, including aspirin, herbs, vitamins, and other nonprescription products.

When You Use This Drug

- Do not drink alcohol or take any drugs that make you drowsy without talking to your doctor. The narcotics will add to their effects, putting you at risk.
- Avoid driving or other activities that require alertness because these drugs may make you drowsy, dizzy, or lightheaded.
- If your drug seems less effective after a few weeks of use, **do not increase the dose.** Call your doctor instead.
- If you use a narcotic for a long time, have regular checkups.
- You may feel dizzy when rising from a lying or sitting position. If you are lying down, hang your legs over the side of the bed for a few minutes, then get up slowly. When rising from a chair, stay by the chair until you are sure that you are not dizzy. (See p. 16.)
- If you plan to have any surgery, including dental, tell your doctor that you take this drug.

How to Use This Drug

- *Liquid form of meperidine:* Mix with a half glass (four ounces) of water and drink the mixture. The water will lessen the numbness that this drug can cause in your mouth and throat.
- *Suppository form of hydromorphone:* Remove wrapper, moisten suppository with water, lie on side, and insert into rectum.
- Do not store tablets in the bathroom. Heat and moisture can damage the drug.
- Store suppositories in the refrigerator.

• Prevent liquid form and suppositories from freezing.

• If you miss a dose, take it as soon as you remember, but skip it if it is almost time for the next dose. **Do not take double doses.**

Interactions with Other Drugs

The following drugs are listed in the *Evaluations of Drug Interactions* 1997 as causing "highly clinically significant" or "clinically significant" interactions when used together with this drug. We have also included potentially serious interactions listed in the drug's FDA-approved professional product labeling or package insert. New scientific techniques have allowed researchers to predict some drug interactions before they have been documented in people. There may be other drugs, especially those in the families of drugs listed below, that also will react with this drug to cause severe adverse effects. The number of new drugs approved for marketing increases the chance of drug interactions, and new drug interactions are being identified with old drugs. Be vigilant. Make sure to tell your doctor and pharmacist the drugs you are taking and tell your doctor if you are taking any of these interacting drugs:

carbamazepine, chlorpromazine, cimetidine, COUMADIN, NARDIL, PENTOTHAL, phenelzine, RIFADIN, rifampin, RIMACTANE, TAGAMET, TEGRETOL, thiopental, THORAZINE, TUBARINE, tubocurarine, warfarin.

At least two weeks should elapse after you stop taking a monoamine oxidase (MAO) inhibitor and start taking demerol. The same is true if you stop taking demerol and then start one of these MAO inhibitors: deprenyl, ELDEPRYL, furazolidone, FUROXONE, isocarboxazid, MARPLAN, MATULANE, NARDIL, PARNATE, phenelzine, procarbazine, selegiline, tranylcypromine.

Adverse Effects

Call your doctor immediately if you experience:

• **signs of overdose:** cold, clammy skin, seizures, severe dizziness or drowsiness, nervousness or restlessness, confusion, small pupils, unconsciousness, abnormally low blood pressure, slow heartbeat, slow or troubled breathing, severe weakness
• feelings of unreality
• hallucinations
• skin rash, hives, or itching
• depression or other mood or mental change
• ringing sound in ears
• slow, irregular, or troubled breathing
• swollen, red or flushed face
• trembling or uncontrolled or rigid muscle movements
• abnormal (slow, fast, or pounding) heartbeat
• increased sweating
• headache
• loss of appetite
• unusual excitement, nervousness or restlessness

Call your doctor if these symptoms continue:

• dizziness
• drowsiness
• confusion
• feeling faint or lightheaded
• nausea or vomiting
• constipation
• nightmares or insomnia
• difficulty urinating
• vision changes

Call your doctor if these symptoms continue after you stop taking this drug:

• body aches
• diarrhea
• irregular heartbeat
• fever, runny nose or sneezing

- insomnia
- loss of appetite
- nausea or vomiting
- nervousness, restlessness or irritability
- enlarged pupils
- sweating
- trembling or shivering
- weakness

Periodic Tests

Ask your doctor which of these tests should be done periodically while you are taking this drug:

- respiratory function test

PREGNANCY WARNING

Dilaudid caused harm to developing fetuses in animal studies, or such studies were not done. Use during pregnancy only for clear medical reasons. Tell your doctor if you are pregnant or thinking of becoming pregnant before you take this drug.

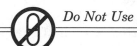 *Do Not Use*

ALTERNATIVE TREATMENT:
See Enteric-coated Aspirin, p. 275.

Salsalate
DISALCID (3M)

FAMILY: Salicylates (see p. 261)

Salsalate (*sal* sa late) belongs to the same family as aspirin and, like aspirin, relieves pain and reduces fever. Salsalate may cause fewer stomach problems than aspirin, but it may not be as effective and has the same potential adverse effects (see p. 261).[44] **It has no advantage over enteric-coated aspirin (see p. 275)**

and is more expensive.[45] For the vast majority of people, aspirin is the drug of choice and salsalate should not be used.

ASPIRIN/REYE'S SYNDROME ALERT

Do not use this product for treating chicken pox, flu, or flu-like illness. It will increase the risk of contracting Reye's syndrome, a rare but often fatal disease.

  Do Not Use

ALTERNATIVE TREATMENT:
See Enteric-coated Aspirin, p. 275.

Diflunisal
DOLOBID (Merck)

FAMILY: Nonsteroidal Anti-inflammatory Drugs "NSAIDs" Arthritis Drugs (see p. 265)

Diflunisal (dye *floo* ni sal) belongs to the family of drugs called nonsteroidal anti-inflammatory drugs, shortened to NSAIDs (*n* sayds), often used to treat arthritis in older adults. NSAIDs can cause serious harm, even fatalities, from bleeding in the stomach or intestines. Bleeding can occur at any time and without warning and older people are more likely to experience adverse effects from bleeding. Older adults are also more likely to have reduced liver and kidney function. Some doctors believe people over age 70 should be started with half the usual dose of drugs in this group.[46]

Diflunisal, like aspirin, relieves pain and inflammation. **It should not be used because it has no advantage over enteric-coated aspirin (see p. 275) and is much more expensive.**[47] Enteric-coated aspirin (aspirin coated so that it does not dissolve in the stomach) is the best drug for long-term treatment, such as for arthritis.

Aspirin (see p. 275) is just as effective and less costly than other NSAIDs and is the drug of choice for treating pain, fever, and inflammation in people who do not have ulcers, gastritis (inflammation of the stomach), or an allergy to aspirin. Some rheumatologists (arthritis specialists) prefer aspirin to other NSAIDs for treating rheumatoid arthritis.[48]

If you are taking diflunisal, ask your doctor if you can switch to taking enteric-coated aspirin (aspirin coated so it won't dissolve in the stomach) twice a day. If you cannot take aspirin, ask about switching to another drug in this family such as ibuprofen (see p. 311). Each person responds differently to different NSAIDs.

 Do Not Use

ALTERNATIVE TREATMENT:
Ibuprofen or combination painkillers containing a narcotic with acetaminophen.

Bromfenac
DURACT (Wyeth)

FAMILY: Nonsteroidal Anti-inflammatory drugs "NSAIDs"
Arthritis Drugs (see p. 265)

Bromfenac was withdrawn from the market in June 1998 because of liver toxicity that resulted in liver transplants and deaths.

Bromfenac (*brom* fen ac) belongs to the family of drugs called nonsteroidal anti-inflammatory drugs, shortened to NSAIDs (*n* sayds), often used to treat arthritis in older adults. NSAIDs can cause serious harm, even fatalities, from bleeding in the stomach or intestines. Bleeding can occur at any time and without warning and older people are more likely to experience adverse effects from bleeding. Older adults are also more likely to have reduced liver and kidney function. Some doctors believe people over age 70 should be started with half the usual dose of drugs in this group.[49]

Bromfenac was approved only for the short-term (10 days) treatment of acute pain because of the risk of liver toxicity. This drug should never have been approved by the Food and Drug Administration (FDA). After only seven months on the market the FDA issued a warning telling doctors of severe liver toxicity with bromfenac in people who had taken the drug for longer than the recommended 10 days of treatment. The FDA had received reports of jaundice (yellowing of the skin or whites of the eyes), potentially fatal hepatitis (inflammation

WARNING

NONSTEROIDAL ANTI-INFLAMMATORY DRUG (NSAID) INDUCED GASTROINTESTINAL TOXICITY

All members of the NSAID family of drugs can cause gastrointestinal toxicity that can lead to gastrointestinal bleeding and hospitalization or death. The risk of gastrointestinal toxicity from these drugs increases with increasing doses and the length of treatment.

If the following symptoms develop while you are taking an NSAID, stop the drug immediately and contact your doctor: severe abdominal or stomach pain, cramping, or burning, severe and continuing nausea, heartburn, or indigestion, bloody or black, tarry stools, vomiting blood or material that looks like coffee grounds, or spitting up blood.

of the liver) and liver failure. Some of those people experiencing liver failure required liver transplants.[50]

Bromfenac has been shown in clinical trials to be about as effective as acetaminophen with oxycodone or ibuprofen in relieving pain. Promotion to doctors emphasizes bromfenac mainly as a "nonnarcotic," downplaying that it is an NSAID which can produce all of the gastrointestinal, including liver toxicity, and other adverse effects associated with this family of drugs. In clinical trials, conducted before the drug was approved, 3% of those taking bromfenac in longer-term trials developed elevated liver enzymes, a signal of possible liver toxicity.

The Medical Letter on Drugs and Therapeutics, a highly respected independent source of drug information, said about bromfenac: "Whether the new drug offers any advantage over much less expensive NSAID alternatives remains to be established."[51] We agree, and would add that there is no medical reason why you should be taking bromfenac for the short-term treatment of pain when ibuprofen and combination pain relievers like acetaminophen with oxycodone are just as effective, safer, and less expensive.

Aspirin (see p. 275) is just as effective and less costly than other NSAIDs and is the drug of choice for treating pain, fever, and inflammation in people who do not have ulcers, gastritis (inflammation of the stomach), or an allergy to aspirin. Some rheumatologists (arthritis specialists) prefer aspirin to other NSAIDs for treating rheumatoid arthritis.[52]

If you are taking bromfenac ask your doctor if you can switch to taking enteric-coated aspirin (aspirin coated so it won't dissolve in the stomach) twice a day. If you cannot take aspirin, ask about switching to another drug in this family such as ibuprofen (see p. 311). Each person responds differently to different NSAIDs.

WARNING

NONSTEROIDAL ANTI-INFLAMMATORY DRUG (NSAID) INDUCED GASTROINTESTINAL TOXICITY

All members of the NSAID family of drugs can cause gastrointestinal toxicity that can lead to gastrointestinal bleeding and hospitalization or death. The risk of gastrointestinal toxicity from these drugs increases with increasing doses and the length of treatment.

If the following symptoms develop while you are taking an NSAID, stop the drug immediately and contact your doctor: severe abdominal or stomach pain, cramping, or burning, severe and continuing nausea, heartburn, or indigestion, bloody or black, tarry stools, vomiting blood or material that looks like coffee grounds, or spitting up blood.

Limited Use

Fentanyl Patches
DURAGESIC Transdermal Therapeutic System (Janssen)

GENERIC: not available
FAMILY: Narcotics (see p. 264)

Fentanyl (*fen* ta nil) is a synthetic narcotic that relieves pain. Most studies about fentanyl focus on the injectable form used during surgery. Fewer studies have been done on the transdermal (patch) form, and even fewer studies have been done on older people using fentanyl patches.

Fentanyl patches, which slowly release medication over three days, are used for chronic pain, such as cancer pain. Pain relief usually improves sleep. People with swallowing difficulties or poor veins benefit from the topical application. Others find the patch convenient. However, fentanyl is not a band-aid for mild or intermittent pain, and is not usually used until doses of oral morphine have become high and frequent. The first dose of fentanyl is usually 25 mcg. (this refers to the number of micrograms released each hour). Doses must be estimated according to prior use of other analgesics. Older people usually need less fentanyl than younger people. It may take a few days until adequate pain relief is achieved. During the transition, other shorter acting analgesics relieve breakthrough pain. One drawback of the patches is less flexibility in doses, which are currently limited to four sizes and their combinations. People who lose weight may need to have their dose lowered, since fentanyl is stored in fat tissue.

Fentanyl is not recommended for those weighing less than 110 lbs. Common adverse effects of fentanyl are nausea, vomiting, constipation, and skin irritation from the adhesive on the patch. Fentanyl patches are not recommended after surgery due to risk of severe respiratory problems. Like morphine, fentanyl is a controlled substance and could be habit forming. The fentanyl patches costs are more than short-acting oral morphine, similar to long-acting oral morphine, and usually less than injectable morphine which involves costs for supplies and equipment.

One hazard of taking fentanyl continuously for longer than several weeks is drug-induced dependence. **Do not stop taking your drug suddenly.** With the help of your doctor, work out a schedule for slowly decreasing the amount of drug you take by about 5 to 10% each day. Keep a written record of the dosage reduction schedule with you. These steps will make it much easier to become drug free without developing distressing symptoms of drug withdrawal.

Before You Use This Drug

Tell your doctor if you have or have had:

- allergies to medications or adhesives
- emphysema, asthma or other lung problems
- colitis or inflammatory bowel disease
- diarrhea
- alcohol or drug abuse
- gallbladder problems
- head injuries or brain tumor
- kidney or liver problems
- skin problems
- gastrointestinal problems
- thyroid problems
- slow heartbeat
- emotional problems
- enlarged prostate or difficulty urinating

Tell your doctor about any other drugs you take, including aspirin, herbs, vitamins, and other nonprescription products.

When You Use This Drug

- Avoid constipation. Drink plenty of water or fluids. Eat fiber. Take a stool softener. If constipation develops you may need a laxative or enema.
- Until you know how you react to fentanyl avoid driving or performing other activities requiring alertness as fentanyl can cause drowsiness.
- Avoid drinking alcohol which adds to central nervous system (CNS) effects of fentanyl.
- Until your dose of fentanyl stabilizes you may need another short-acting pain reliever for breakthrough pain.
- If you plan to have any surgery, including dental, tell your doctor that you take this drug.
- Do not use heating pads, electric blankets, heated water beds, hot tubs, saunas or heat lamps. These could cause fentanyl to be too rapidly absorbed, especially if devices slip onto the patch while you sleep.
- You may feel dizzy when rising from a lying or sitting position. When getting out of

bed, hang your legs over the side of the bed for a few minutes, then get up slowly. When getting up from a chair, stay beside the chair until you are sure that you are not dizzy. (See p. 16.)

• If nausea develops, try lying down until it subsides.

• You may wear fentanyl patches while bathing, showering, or swimming, but do not rub the patch vigorously or stay for a prolonged time in hot water. If the patch loosens or dislodges, discard it, and apply new patch on a dry area.

• If you sleep or nap near someone else, cover the area of the patch with clothing. Otherwise, the patch could transfer to the other person. This has caused children to receive overdoses.

How to Use This Drug

• Prepare the site with water. Clip hair if necessary. Do not shave the site or use soap, alcohol or lotions. Do not apply to areas that are burned, cut, or irritated.

• Remove liner just before using. Take care not to touch the adhesive surface. Wash any area where the medication unintentionally touches with clean water.

• Do not use if seal is broken, or patch is otherwise damaged or cut.

• Apply entire patch to dry skin above the waist. Press firmly with palm of hand for 30 seconds, especially around the edges.

• If applying more than one patch do not let edges overlap or touch.[53] Rotate site of application, preferably on the opposite side of the body.

• Change patch every three days, unless your doctor tells you to change at a different frequency.

• Do not apply more than the prescribed dose.

• Fold used patches in half with adhesive layer inside the fold. Flush down toilet, or otherwise dispose of in secure manner.

• Wash hands.

• Do not stop using abruptly. A gradual reduction prevents withdrawal symptoms. Even if you stop using fentanyl patches, some of the drug can remain in older people for a few days.[54]

• Do not store in the bathroom. Do not expose to heat, moisture, or strong light.

Interactions with Other Drugs

The following drugs are listed in the *Evaluations of Drug Interactions* 1997 as causing "highly clinically significant" or "clinically significant" interactions when used together with this drug. We have also included potentially serious interactions listed in the drug's FDA-approved professional product labeling or package insert. New scientific techniques have allowed researchers to predict some drug interactions before they have been documented in people. There may be other drugs, especially those in the families of drugs listed below, that also will react with this drug to cause severe adverse effects. The number of new drugs approved for marketing increases the chance of drug interactions, and new drug interactions are being identified with old drugs. Be vigilant. Make sure to tell your doctor and pharmacist the drugs you are taking and tell your doctor if you are taking any of these interacting drugs:

People who take monoamine oxidase inhibitors should be off these drugs for 14 days before starting fentanyl.[55] These include: deprenyl, ELDEPRYL, furazolidone, FUROXONE, isocarboxazid, MARPLAN, MATULANE, NARDIL, PARNATE, phenelzine, procarbazine, selegiline, tranylcypromine.

Central nervous system (CNS) depressant drugs including alcohol, antidepressants, antihistamines, antipsychotics, some blood pressure medications (reserpine, methyldopa, beta-blockers), motion sickness medications, muscle relaxants, narcotics, sedatives, sleeping pills, and tranquilizers. Doses of fentanyl and any of these drugs may need to be lowered by 50%. If any of these drugs are discontinued while you use fentanyl, adjustments in doses may be required.

Naltrexone (REVIA) blocks the effects of fentanyl.

Adverse Effects

Call you doctor immediately if you experience:

- abdominal pain
- breathing or speaking problems (If you care for a person who uses fentanyl patches, and their breathing slows while sleeping, try to waken them. If breathing does not improve once awake, call their doctor)[56]
  - chest pain or change in heartbeat
  - confusion
  - dizziness, uncoordination, or fainting
  - fever of 102°F or more (your dose may be lowered temporarily)[57]
  - hallucinations
  - restlessness or nervousness
  - skin becomes cold, red, swollen, blistered or itches severely
  - spitting blood
  - thoughts become combative or suspicious
  - difficulty urinating
  - mental or mood changes
  - unusual bruising
  - swollen glands

Call your doctor if these symptoms continue:

- decreased appetite
- confusion
- constipation
- diarrhea
- dizziness
- unusual dreams
- drowsiness

- dry mouth
- headache
- nausea or vomiting
- red or itchy skin, sweating, tingling or burning sensation
- weakness
- abdominal or stomach pain
- indigestion, gas

Call your doctor if these symptoms continue after you stop taking the drug:

- diarrhea
- increased heartbeat
- nervousness, restlessness, irritability
- nausea, vomiting
- enlarged pupils
- shivering or sweating
- fever, runny nose, or sneezing
- stomach cramps
- insomnia
- weakness

Periodic Tests

Ask your doctor which of these tests should be done periodically while you are taking this drug:

- blood pressure
- heart rate
- respiratory rate
- serum concentration levels
- degree of sedation

PREGNANCY WARNING

This drug caused harm to developing fetuses in animal studies, or such studies were not done. Use during pregnancy only for clear medical reasons. Tell your doctor if you are pregnant or thinking of becoming pregnant before you take this drug.

Do Not Use

ALTERNATIVE TREATMENT:
See Acetaminophen, p. 338.

Butalbital, Acetaminophen, and Caffeine
ESGIC (Forest)
FIORICET (Novartis)

FAMILY: Painkillers
Narcotics (see p. 264)

This combination of butalbital (byoo *tal* bi tal), acetaminophen (see p. 338), and caffeine (ka *feen*) is marketed for tension headaches. When taking this product you are, in fact, taking three drugs, each with its own cautions, adverse effects, and drug interactions. Like other fixed-combination products, this combination curtails the ability to vary doses of each drug—irrationally combining in this case one ineffective drug (caffeine), one effective painkiller (acetaminophen), and one excessively dangerous drug (butalbital).

Caffeine has not proven effective in relieving pain. It can aggravate incontinence, produce insomnia, and lead to dependence-causing withdrawal headaches.

Butalbital is a barbiturate, and because of the serious adverse effects and addictive nature of all barbiturates, older adults should not use it and therefore should not take Esgic or Fioricet.

Acetaminophen is an effective painkiller, available separately without a prescription (see p. 338), as is aspirin (see p. 275).

One hazard of taking butalbital continuously for longer than several weeks is drug-induced dependence. **Do not stop taking your drug suddenly.** With the help of your doctor, work out a schedule for slowly decreasing the amount of the drug you take by about 5 to 10% each day. Keep a written record of the dosage reduction schedule with you. These steps will make it much easier to become drug free without developing distressing symptoms of drug withdrawal.

WARNING

There have been a number of case reports of liver damage involving a possible drug interaction between isoniazid, a medication used to prevent and treat tuberculosis, and acetaminophen, an over-the-counter painkiller and the active ingredient in Tylenol. Isoniazid alone, especially as people get older, has been documented to cause liver damage. Acetaminophen, alone in large doses or probably in combination with alcohol, also increases the risk of liver damage. The combination of acetaminophen with isoniazid, according to the authors of these case reports, may also be dangerous.[58]

If you are taking isoniazid for tuberculosis or have a positive TB skin test and are using the drug, consult your physician before using acetaminophen or any combination product containing acetaminophen. Discuss alternatives to acetaminophen with your physician.[59]

Do Not Use

ALTERNATIVE TREATMENT:
See Enteric-coated Aspirin, p. 275.

Piroxicam
FELDENE (Pfizer)

FAMILY: Nonsteroidal Anti-inflammatory Drugs "NSAIDs"
Arthritis Drugs (see p. 265)

Piroxicam (peer *ox* i cam) belongs to the family of drugs called nonsteroidal anti-inflammatory drugs, shortened to NSAIDs (*n* sayds), often used to treat arthritis in older adults. NSAIDs can cause serious harm, even fatalities, from bleeding in the stomach or intestines. Bleeding can occur at any time and without warning and older people are more likely to experience adverse effects from bleeding. Older adults are also more likely to have reduced liver and kidney function. Some doctors believe people over age 70 should be started with half the usual dose of drugs in this group.[60]

Piroxicam relieves pain and inflammation caused by two kinds of arthritis, rheumatoid arthritis and osteoarthritis. **It has caused serious adverse effects and numerous deaths**, especially in older adults.[61,62] **People over 60 are more likely than other users of this drug to suffer stomach and intestinal bleeding, ulcers, and perforations.** These adverse effects have occurred *even* when patients were taking only the recommended dose. People in all age groups have had **serious skin reactions, some of which have been fatal**, while taking piroxicam.

Although piroxicam is appealing because you only have to take it once a day, this "convenience" is *not* an advantage for older adults. Older adults eliminate drugs from their bodies more slowly than younger people, so a large once-a-day dose may not be eliminated as easily as smaller doses taken throughout the day. As a result, dangerous levels of the drug can accumulate in the bloodstream.

After receiving many reports of adverse reactions in older people taking piroxicam, the Canadian drug regulatory agency recommended that people over 65 start with a dose of 10 milligrams per day. This is half the U.S. recommended dose for adults.

Instead of piroxicam, we recommend equally effective and less dangerous drugs such as aspirin (see p. 275). Aspirin is just as effective and less costly than other NSAIDs and is the drug of choice for treating pain, fever, and inflammation in people who do not have ulcers, gastritis (inflammation of the stomach), or an allergy to aspirin. Some rheumatologists (arthritis specialists) still prefer aspirin to other NSAIDs for treating rheumatoid arthritis.[63]

If you are taking piroxicam, ask your doctor whether you can switch to taking enteric-coated aspirin (aspirin coated so it does not dissolve in the stomach) twice a day. If you cannot take aspirin, ask about switching to another, safer drug in this family such as ibuprofen (see p. 311). Each person may respond differently to different NSAIDs.

WARNING

NONSTEROIDAL ANTI-INFLAMMATORY DRUG (NSAID) INDUCED GASTROINTESTINAL TOXICITY

All members of the NSAID family of drugs can cause gastrointestinal toxicity that can lead to gastrointestinal bleeding and hospitalization or death. The risk of gastrointestinal toxicity from these drugs increases with increasing doses and the length of treatment.

If the following symptoms develop while you are taking an NSAID, stop the drug immediately and contact your doctor: severe abdominal or stomach pain, cramping, or burning, severe and continuing nausea, heartburn, or indigestion, bloody or black, tarry stools, vomiting blood or material that looks like coffee grounds, or spitting up blood.

Do Not Use

ALTERNATIVE TREATMENT:
See Aspirin, p. 275, and Acetaminophen, p. 338.

Butalbital, Caffeine, and Aspirin
FIORINAL (Novartis)
Butalbital, Caffeine, Aspirin, and Codeine
FIORINAL WITH CODEINE (Novartis)

FAMILY: Painkillers
Narcotics (see p. 264)

These are combination drugs composed of butalbital (*byoo* tal bi tal), caffeine (ka *feen*), aspirin (see p. 275), and (in the case of Fiorinal with Codeine) codeine (see p. 284). Both of these combination drugs are used to relieve pain. They do contain two effective painkillers, aspirin and codeine, but they are *irrational* combinations because they also contain one ineffective drug (caffeine) and one excessively dangerous one (butalbital). We recommend that you do not use either of these drugs.

Caffeine has *not* been proven effective in relieving pain. Butalbital is a barbiturate, and because of the serious adverse effects and addictive nature of all barbiturates, older adults should not use Fiorinal or Fiorinal with Codeine.[64]

Aspirin and codeine, both effective painkillers, are available separately as well as combined with each other (see p. 273). There is no reason to take a product that combines these two useful painkillers with excessively dangerous butalbital and ineffective caffeine. It is much better to take plain aspirin (see p. 275) or acetaminophen (see p. 338), or, if necessary, aspirin or acetaminophen combined with codeine (see pp. 273, 340). Codeine can cause constipation and is addictive, so it should only be used if aspirin or acetaminophen alone does not work.

One hazard of taking butalbital or codeine continuously for longer than several weeks is drug-induced dependence. **Do not stop taking your drug suddenly.** With the help of your doctor, work out a schedule for slowly lowering the amount of the drug you take by about 5 to 10% each day. Keep a written record of the dosage reduction schedule with you. These steps will make it much easier to become drug free without developing distressing symptoms of drug withdrawal.

ASPIRIN/REYE'S SYNDROME ALERT

Do not use these products for treating chicken pox, flu, or flu-like illness. They will increase the risk of contracting Reye's syndrome, a rare but often fatal disease.

Fiorinal with Codeine can increase the risk of hip fracture.[65]

Limited Use

Azathioprine
IMURAN (Glaxo Wellcome)

GENERIC: unavailable in tablets
FAMILY: Immunosuppressants

Azathioprine (aze *thy* o prin) is a potent drug reserved for severe conditions. It prevents rejection of transplanted organs, particularly kidneys, by suppressing the immune system. While azathioprine is also used in multiple sclerosis, severe skin diseases, and a number of other conditions, it is not yet approved for those conditions in the U.S. When all other treatments (rest, anti-inflammatory drugs, gold compounds) fail to relieve rheumatoid arthritis, azathioprine may slow damage to the joints and control symptoms but does not cure any condition. It is an alternative when surgery for some disabling arthritis cannot be done, and to lower the dose of steroids, often given along with azathioprine. It may take several weeks or even a few months for improvement to show.

Older people with age-related decrease in kidney function are more likely to need a low dose. In all ages, the lowest effective dose should be used.

During the first couple of weeks of therapy with azathioprine, nausea is common. Since azathioprine affects your immune system, you may get infections, which can be fatal, more easily. Azathioprine increases the risk of skin cancer, cervical cancer, Karposi's sarcoma, and leukemia.[66] These risks increase when the drug is used for transplants, and rises after the drug has been used for five years.[67] Azathioprine can also irritate your pancreas, damage your bone marrow, and harm your liver enough to be life-threatening. This liver damage is more apt to happen to men.[68] Lowering the dose may reverse some of these problems.

Before You Use This Drug

Because your risk of developing cancer would rise, discuss the benefit/risk balance of using azathioprine with your doctor if you are taking or have previously taken:

ALKERAN, chlorambucil, cyclophosphamide, CYTOXAN, LEUKERAN, melphalan.

Tell your doctor if you have or have had:
- allergies to drugs
- chicken pox presently or a recent exposure
- gout
- hepatitis zoster
- herpes
- infection

- kidney or liver problems
- pancreatitis
- radiation therapy
- xanthine oxidase deficiency

Tell your doctor about any other drugs you take, including aspirin, herbs, vitamins, and other nonprescription products.

When You Use This Drug

- Keep your appointments for lab work. For the first two months blood tests should be done at least weekly, and at least monthly thereafter.
- Avoid places and people that expose you to bacterial or viral infections. During flu seasons avoid crowds. Report the first sign of any infection to your doctor: cough, hoarseness, fever, chills, lower back or side pain, or painful or difficult urination.
- Practice good hygiene. Wash your hands before touching your eyes or the inside of your nose.
- Check with your dentist about teeth cleaning methods suited to your condition. Check with your physician before having dental work done.
- Be cautious using knives, razors, nail clippers, and other sharp objects.
- Avoid engaging in contact sports, moving heavy objects, and activities where you might get bruised.
- Continue to rest, get physical therapy, and use anti-inflammatory drugs if you have rheumatoid arthritis.
- If you undergo emergency care, or surgery, including dental, tell your doctor that you take azathioprine.
- If you must take allopurinol, your dose of azathioprine should be reduced to one-fourth the usual dose.

How to Use This Drug

- Swallow tablet whole or break in half. If you take azathioprine once a day, take it at bedtime to reduce stomach upset. Otherwise, take it with food or after a meal.

• If your doctor prescribes a suspension, shake it well before measuring.

• *If you miss a dose, use the following guidelines:* If you take the drug once a day, do not take the missed dose, nor double the next dose.

If you take the drug several times a day, then take it as soon as you remember or double the next dose only. Check with your doctor if you miss more than one dose.

• Store tablets at room temperature with lid on firmly. Do not expose to light and heat. Store other forms according to the prescription label.

Interactions with Other Drugs

The following drugs are listed in the *Evaluations of Drug Interactions* 1997 as causing "highly clinically significant" or "clinically significant" interactions when used together with this drug. We have also included potentially serious interactions listed in the drug's FDA-approved professional product labeling or package insert. New scientific techniques have allowed researchers to predict some drug interactions before they have been documented in people. There may be other drugs, especially those in the families of drugs listed below, that also will react with this drug to cause severe adverse effects. The number of new drugs approved for marketing increases the chance of drug interactions, and new drug interactions are being identified with old drugs. Be vigilant. Make sure to tell your doctor and pharmacist the drugs you are taking and tell your doctor if you are taking any of these interacting drugs:

COUMADIN, warfarin. (Do not suddenly stop taking azathioprine or warfarin. Check with your doctor.)

Avoid live virus vaccines, such as polio vaccines, for at least three months after stopping azathioprine. Not only might the vaccine be ineffective, but you may be more apt to have adverse reactions to the vaccine. It is very important that you not come in close contact with anyone else, such as your grandchildren, getting live virus vaccines. If you must come in contact, wear a mask over your mouth and nose. Let someone else change and dispose of their diapers.

Adverse Effects

Call your doctor immediately if you experience:

• bloody or black, tarry or pale stools
• bleeding or bruising
• difficulty breathing
• chills
• cough, hoarseness
• severe diarrhea
• dizziness
• fever
• rapid heartbeat
• severe nausea or vomiting
• pain in lower back, muscles, joints, side, or stomach
• pinpoint red spots, redness, blisters on skin
• sores in mouth or lips
• swelling of feet or legs
• unusual tiredness or weakness
• painful or difficult urination
• dark or bloody urine
• yellowing of eyes or skin

Call your doctor if these symptoms continue:

• abdominal pain
• constipation
• depression[69]
• hair loss
• headache
• heartburn
• loss of appetite
• low blood pressure
• nausea and vomiting

- skin rash, itching
- unusually deep suntan[70]
- blurred vision[71]

Adverse effects may persist after azathioprine is stopped.

Periodic Tests

Ask your doctor which of these tests should be done periodically while you are taking this drug:

- complete blood count

    Do Not Use

ALTERNATIVE TREATMENT:
See Enteric-coated Aspirin, p. 275.

Indomethacin
INDOCIN (Merck)

FAMILY: Nonsteroidal Anti-inflammatory Drugs "NSAIDs"
Arthritis Drugs (see p. 265)

Indomethacin (in doe *meth* a sin) belongs to the family of drugs called nonsteroidal anti-inflammatory drugs, shortened to NSAIDs (*n* sayds), often used to treat arthritis in older adults. NSAIDs can cause serious harm, even fatalities, from bleeding in the stomach or intestines. Bleeding can occur at any time and without warning and older people are more likely to experience adverse effects from bleeding. Older adults are also more likely to have reduced liver and kidney function. Some doctors believe people over age 70 should be started with half the usual dose of drugs in this group.[72]

Indomethacin relieves the pain and inflammation of rheumatoid arthritis and acute gout and reduces fever. **This drug is not recommended for older adults.**[73] It can cause depression, mood changes, and confusion. Indomethacin may also make epilepsy or Parkinson's disease worse, cause more stomach and intestinal bleeding than aspirin, and hide the signs of any infection you might have.[74,75,76]

Aspirin (see p. 275) is just as effective and less costly than other NSAIDs and is the drug of choice for treating pain, fever, and inflammation in people who do not have ulcers, gastritis (inflammation of the stomach), or an allergy to aspirin. Some rheumatologists (arthritis specialists) prefer aspirin to other NSAIDs for treating rheumatoid arthritis.[77]

If you are taking indomethacin, ask your doctor whether you can switch to taking enteric-coated aspirin (aspirin coated so it does not dissolve in the stomach) twice a day. If you can't take aspirin, ask about switching to another, safer drug in this family such as ibuprofen (see p. 311). Each person responds differently to different NSAIDs.

WARNING

NONSTEROIDAL ANTI-INFLAMMATORY DRUG (NSAID) INDUCED GASTROINTESTINAL TOXICITY

All members of the NSAID family of drugs can cause gastrointestinal toxicity that can lead to gastrointestinal bleeding and hospitalization or death. The risk of gastrointestinal toxicity from these drugs increases with increasing doses and the length of treatment.

If the following symptoms develop while you are taking an NSAID, stop the drug immediately and contact your doctor: severe abdominal or stomach pain, cramping, or burning, severe and continuing nausea, heartburn, or indigestion, bloody or black, tarry stools, vomiting blood or material that looks like coffee grounds, or spitting up blood.

Limited Use

Etodolac
LODINE (Wyeth-Ayerst)

Nabumetone
RELAFEN (SmithKline Beecham)

GENERIC: not available

FAMILY: Nonsteroidal Anti-inflammatory Drugs "NSAIDs"
Arthritis Drugs (see p. 265)

Etodolac (et *o* dole ac) and Nabumetone (na *byoo* me tone) belong to the family of drugs called nonsteroidal anti-inflammatory drugs, shortened to NSAIDs (*n* sayds) often used to treat arthritis in older adults. NSAIDs can cause serious harm, even fatalities, from bleeding in the stomach or intestines. Bleeding can occur at any time, without warning and older people are more likely to experience adverse effects from bleeding. Older adults are also more likely to have reduced liver and kidney function. Some doctors believe people over age 70 should be started with half the usual dose of drugs in this group.[78]

Etodolac is used to treat mild to moderate pain and symptoms of osteoarthritis and of rheumatoid arthritis. Nabumetone belongs to the same chemical group of NSAIDs as etodolac and is also approved for osteroarthritis and rheumatoid arthritis.

SmithKline Beecham Pharmaceutical, the manufacturer of nabumetone, was cited by the Food and Drug Administration's (FDA) Division of Drug Marketing, Advertising, and Communications for distributing false and misleading advertising about the safety of this drug. The company was distributing copies of medical journal articles claiming that nabumetone causes a relatively low incidence of ulcers, one of the most common and serious adverse effects of NSAIDs. These articles were based on nonclinical studies (those done in the laboratory), when in fact, there is no evidence from human studies to support such a claim.[79]

In general, if you are over 60, you should take less than the usual adult dose of these drugs, especially if you have decreased kidney function. It takes about half an hour for the drug to begin working.

Etodolac and nabumetone are comparable in effectiveness to other NSAIDs, such as aspirin and several prescription drugs. Like other NSAIDs, these drugs relieve symptoms, but do not cure any condition. Because NSAIDs relieve pain and inflammation and reduce fever, these drugs can mask signs of infection. When taking etodolac, older people also tend to get more indigestion.[80]

Compared to other new drugs, etodolac received a higher rate of adverse drug reports in Britain, including deaths.[81] Etodolac can impair liver function, may prolong bleeding time, and damage bone marrow. Etodolac can cause severe damage to the kidneys, even kidney failure. This is more likely in older adults.[82]

Enteric-coated aspirin is the best and least expensive way to relieve the pain of osteoarthritis. Unlike the treatment of rheumatoid arthritis, which requires high doses of aspirin to reduce inflammation, two 325-mg aspirin tablets four times a day is often sufficient to control osteoarthritic pain in adults. Other pain relievers, including acetaminophen, are recommended for the person who cannot take aspirin.

For the treatment of osteoarthritis, *The Medical Letter* states that etodolac may offer no advantage over the painkiller acetaminophen (TYLENOL), which does not cause gastrointestinal ulcers or bleeding and costs less.[83]

Be aware that in contrast to aspirin, acetaminophen relieves pain, but is not effective in reducing inflammation. Therefore, we do not recommend the use of acetaminophen for the treatment of arthritis unless it is clear that you have osteoarthritis which does not have a significant amount of inflammation.

WARNING

NONSTEROIDAL ANTI-INFLAMMATORY DRUG (NSAID) INDUCED GASTROIN-TESTINAL TOXICITY

All members of the NSAID family of drugs can cause gastrointestinal toxicity that can lead to gastrointestinal bleeding and hospitalization or death. The risk of gastrointestinal toxicity from these drugs increases with increasing doses and the length of treatment.

If the following symptoms develop while you are taking an NSAID, stop the drug immediately and contact your doctor: severe abdominal or stomach pain, cramping, or burning, severe and continuing nausea, heartburn, or indigestion, bloody or black, tarry stools, vomiting blood or material that looks like coffee grounds, or spitting up blood.

Before You Use This Drug

Do not use if you have or have had:

- an allergic reaction to aspirin, any other NSAID or iodides[84]
- alcohol dependence
- peptic ulcer
- nasal polyps

Tell your doctor if you have or have had:

- allergies to drugs
- heart, kidney or liver problems
- hemophilia or other bleeding problems
- high blood pressure
- tobacco use
- diabetes
- asthma
- anemia
- stomach or intestinal problems

Tell your doctor about any other drugs you take, including aspirin, herbs, vitamins, and other nonprescription products.

When You Use This Drug

- If you smoke, try to quit, since adverse effects of etodolac occur more often in smokers.[85]
- Do not drink alcohol. It irritates the stomach lining and increases the risk of stomach bleeding.
- Call your doctor immediately if you have flu-like symptoms (chills, fever, muscle aches or pains) shortly before or with a skin rash. This may indicate a serious reaction to etodolac.
- You may feel dizzy when rising from a lying or sitting position. If you are lying down, hang your legs over the side of the bed for a few minutes, then get up slowly. When getting up from a chair, stay by the chair until you are sure that you are not dizzy. (See p. 16.)
- Do not drive or perform other activities that require alertness because this drug may make you drowsy, dizzy, or lightheaded.
- If you plan to have any surgery, including dental, tell your doctor that you take this drug.

How to Use This Drug

- Take with food to reduce stomach irritation.
- Take with **a full glass (eight ounces) of water**. Do not lie down for 30 minutes afterwards.
- If you miss a dose, take it as soon as possible, but skip it if it is almost time for the next dose. **Do not take double doses.**
- Store at room temperature with lid on firmly. Do not store in the bathroom. Do not expose to moisture.

Interactions with Other Drugs

The following drugs are listed in the *Evaluations of Drug Interactions* 1997 as causing "highly clinically significant" or "clinically significant" interactions when used together with this drug. We have also included potentially serious interactions listed in the drug's FDA-approved professional product labeling or package insert. New scientific techniques have allowed researchers to predict some drug interactions before they have been documented in people. There may be other drugs, especially those in the families of drugs listed below, that also will react with this drug to cause severe adverse effects. The number of new drugs approved for marketing increases the chance of drug interactions, and new drug interactions are being identified with old drugs. Be vigilant. Make sure to tell your doctor and pharmacist the drugs you are taking and tell your doctor if you are taking any of these interacting drugs:

aspirin, atenolol, GENUINE BAYER ASPIRIN, BENEMID, CEFOBID, cefoperazone, COUMADIN, DYAZIDE, DYRENIUM, ECOTRIN, enalapril, INDOCIN, indomethacin, ketorolac, lithium, LITHOBID, LITHONATE, MAXZIDE, methotrexate, probenecid, RHEUMATREX DOSE PACK, TENORMIN, TORADOL, triamterene, triamterene and hydrochlorothiazide, VASOTEC, warfarin.

Adverse Effects

Call your doctor immediately if you experience:

- abdominal pain or swelling
- appetite loss
- bloody, black or light-colored tarry stools
- increase or decrease in blood pressure
- difficulty breathing
- unusual bruising
- chest pain
- chills
- confusion
- cough or hoarseness
- depression
- diarrhea
- pain, redness, irritation or swelling of the eyes
- facial skin color changes
- fainting
- fever
- gastrointestinal pain, cramping or burning

- swollen glands
- hearing change or ringing or buzzing
- heartburn
- hives on face, eyelids or tongue
- indigestion
- lower back or side pain
- unusually heavy menstrual bleeding
- muscle cramps or pain
- nausea, vomiting
- pinpoint red spots on skin
- skin rash, blisters, hives, itching, scaling
- sore throat
- sores, ulcers, or white spots on lips or in mouth
- spitting blood
- stomach tenderness
- difficulty swallowing
- swelling of face, lips, tongue, fingers, lower legs or feet
- continuing thirst
- burning in throat or chest
- irritated tongue
- unusual tiredness or weakness
- difficulty urinating
- bloody, dark or cloudy urine
- vision change
- vomiting blood or material that looks like coffee grounds
- rapid weight gain
- yellow eyes or skin

Call your doctor if these symptoms continue:

- anxiety
- constipation, gas
- dizziness
- drowsiness
- eyes sensitive to light
- flushing or hot flashes
- headache
- irregular heartbeat
- insomnia
- lightheadedness
- irritated or dry mouth
- nervousness, irritability

- sunburn
- sweating
- bitter taste
- trembling
- weakness

Periodic Tests

Ask your doctor which of these tests should be done periodically while you are taking this drug:

- kidney function tests
- liver function tests
- stool tests for possible blood loss
- hematocrit and/or hemoglobin test
- blood concentrations of creatinine, potassium, urea nitrogen levels
- white blood cell counts
- upper GI diagnostic tests
- ophthalmologic exams

PREGNANCY WARNING

This drug caused harm to developing fetuses in animal studies, or such studies were not done. Use during pregnancy only for clear medical reasons. Tell your doctor if you are pregnant or thinking of becoming pregnant before you take this drug.

Limited Use

Meclofenamate
MECLOMEN (Parke-Davis)

GENERIC: available

FAMILY: Nonsteroidal Anti-inflammatory Drugs "NSAIDs"
Arthritis Drugs (see p. 265)

Meclofenamate (me kloe *fen* am ate) belongs to the family of drugs called nonsteroidal anti-inflammatory drugs, shortened to NSAIDs

(*n* sayds), often used to treat arthritis in older adults. NSAIDs can cause serious harm, even fatalities, from bleeding in the stomach or intestines. Bleeding can occur at any time and without warning and older people are more likely to experience adverse effects from bleeding. Older adults are also more likely to have reduced liver and kidney function. Some doctors believe people over age 70 should be started with half the usual dose of drugs in this group.[86]

Meclofenamate is used mainly to relieve the pain and inflammation of two kinds of arthritis, rheumatoid arthritis and osteoarthritis. **In general, if you are over 60, you should take less than the usual adult dose, especially if you have decreased kidney function.**

Meclofenamate can cause stomach and intestinal problems, such as severe diarrhea.[87] It has also been linked with a few cases of serious blood cell abnormalities.[88] These blood cell abnormalities can occasionally be cured if they are caught early, so if you are taking meclofenamate, watch for the warning signs: fever and sore throat, ulcers (sores) in the mouth, easy bruising, and skin rashes. If you have any of these symptoms while taking this drug, call your doctor immediately. Stop taking meclofenamate immediately if you have a rash.

Aspirin (see p. 275) is just as effective and less costly than other NSAIDs and is the drug of choice for treating pain, fever, and inflammation in people who do not have ulcers, gastritis (inflammation of the stomach), or an allergy to aspirin. Some rheumatologists (arthritis specialists) prefer aspirin to other drugs in its family for treating rheumatoid arthritis.[89] Meclofenamate should be used only if enteric-coated aspirin (see p. 275) and safer drugs in the NSAID family, such as ibuprofen and naproxen (see pp. 311, 317), do not provide relief.[90]

If you are taking meclofenamate, ask your doctor if you can switch to taking enteric-coated aspirin (aspirin coated so it will not dissolve in the stomach) twice a day. If you cannot take aspirin and are having trouble with adverse effects on meclofenamate, ask if you can switch to another NSAID such as ibuprofen (see p. 311). Each person responds differently to different NSAIDs.

WARNING

NONSTEROIDAL ANTI-INFLAMMATORY DRUG (NSAID) INDUCED GASTROINTESTINAL TOXICITY

All members of the NSAID family of drugs can cause gastrointestinal toxicity that can lead to gastrointestinal bleeding and hospitalization or death. The risk of gastrointestinal toxicity from these drugs increases with increasing doses and the length of treatment.

If the following symptoms develop while you are taking an NSAID, stop the drug immediately and contact your doctor: severe abdominal or stomach pain, cramping, or burning, severe and continuing nausea, heartburn, or indigestion, bloody or black, tarry stools, vomiting blood or material that looks like coffee grounds, or spitting up blood.

Before You Use This Drug

Do not use if you have or have had:

- an allergic reaction to aspirin, any other NSAID or iodides[91]
- peptic ulcers
- alcohol dependence
- nasal polyps

Tell your doctor if you have or have had:

- allergies to drugs
- heart, kidney, or liver problems
- hemophilia or other bleeding problems
- high blood pressure
- asthma

- anemia
- diabetes
- stomach or intestinal problems
- tobacco use
- epilepsy (seizures)
- mental depression or other psychiatric conditions
- Parkinson's disease
- lupus erythematosus

Tell your doctor about any other drugs you take, including aspirin, herbs, vitamins, and other nonprescription products.

When You Use This Drug

- Do not drink alcohol. It irritates the stomach lining and increases the risk of stomach bleeding.
- Call your doctor immediately if you have flu-like symptoms (chills, fever, muscle aches or pains) shortly before or with a skin rash. This may be a sign of a serious reaction to meclofenamate.
- You may feel dizzy when rising from a lying or sitting position. If you are lying down, hang your legs over the side of the bed for a few minutes, then get up slowly. When getting up from a chair, stay by the chair until you are sure that you are not dizzy. (See p. 16)
- If you plan to have any surgery, including dental, tell your doctor that you take this drug.

How to Use This Drug

- Take with food to reduce stomach irritation.
- Take with **a full glass (eight ounces) of water**. Do not lie down for 30 minutes afterwards.
- If you miss a dose, take it as soon as possible, but skip it if it is almost time for the next dose. **Do not take double doses.**
- Store at room temperature, with lid on tightly. Do not expose to moisture or heat. Do not store in the bathroom.

Interactions with Other Drugs

The following drugs are listed in the *Evaluations of Drug Interactions* 1997 as causing "highly clinically significant" or "clinically significant" interactions when used together with this drug. We have also included potentially serious interactions listed in the drug's FDA-approved professional product labeling or package insert. New scientific techniques have allowed researchers to predict some drug interactions before they have been documented in people. There may be other drugs, especially those in the families of drugs listed below, that also will react with this drug to cause severe adverse effects. The number of new drugs approved for marketing increases the chance of drug interactions, and new drug interactions are being identified with old drugs. Be vigilant. Make sure to tell your doctor and pharmacist the drugs you are taking and tell your doctor if you are taking any of these interacting drugs:

bendroflumethiazide, CAPOTEN, captopril, COUMADIN, cyclosporine, digoxin, DILANTIN, GARAMYCIN, gentamicin, gold sodium thiomalate, INDERAL, INDERAL LA, ketorolac, LANOXICAPS, LANOXIN, lithium, LITHOBID, LITHONATE, methotrexate, MINIPRESS, MYOCHRYSINE, NATURETIN, NEORAL, ORINASE, phenytoin, prazosin, propranolol, RHEUMATREX DOSE PACK, SANDIMMUNE, tolbutamide, TORADOL, warfarin.

Adverse Effects

Call your doctor immediately if you experience:

- abdominal pain or swelling
- bloody, black, tarry or light-colored stools
- increase or decrease in blood pressure
- difficulty breathing
- unusual bruising
- chest pains
- chills
- cough or hoarseness
- depression
- pain, dryness, redness, irritation or swelling of the eyes
- fever
- gastrointestinal pain, cramping or burning
- swollen glands
- heartburn
- indigestion
- lower back, neck or side pain
- muscle cramps or pain
- nausea, vomiting
- numbness, tingling, pain or weakness in hands or feet
- pinpoint red spots on skin
- ringing or buzzing in ears
- skin rash, hives, itching, scaling
- sore throat
- sores, ulcers, or white spots on lips or in mouth
- swelling of face, lips, tongue, fingers, lower legs or feet
- continuous thirst
- unusual tiredness or weakness
- difficulty urinating
- dark, bloody or cloudy urine
- vision change
- vomiting blood or material that looks like coffee grounds
- rapid weight gain

Call your doctor if these symptoms continue:

- decreased appetite
- constipation, diarrhea, gas
- dizziness
- headache
- irregular heartbeat
- irritated or dry mouth
- bitter taste
- weakness

Periodic Tests

***Ask your doctor which of these tests should
be done periodically while you are taking
this drug:***

- kidney function tests
- liver function tests
- stool tests for possible blood loss
- hematocrit and/or hemoglobin test
- blood concentrations of creatinine,
  potassium, and urea nitrogen
- white blood cell count
- upper GI diagnostic tests
- ophthalmologic exams

━━━━━━━

Last Choice Drug (in Rheumatoid Arthritis)

Minocycline
MINOCIN (Lederle)

GENERIC: not available

FAMILY: Tetracyclines (see p. 474)
Antibiotics (see p. 468)

Minocycline (mi noe *sye* kleen) is a member of the
family of antibiotics known as tetracyclines. A
large, well-done, controlled clinical trial lasting
48 weeks has shown a beneficial effect with
minocycline compared to a placebo (inactive
sugar pill) in the treatment of rheumatoid arthritis.[92] The trial was sponsored by the National
Institutes of Health and involved 219 people
who, on average, had rheumatoid arthritis for
eight years. People in the trial could have taken
other disease modifying antiarthritic drugs such
as oral or injectable gold, D-penicillamine, azathioprine, methotrexate, or sulfasalazine but
were not allowed to use these drugs for four
weeks before or during the study. More than 30%
of the people in the trial required oral steroid
drugs to control their arthritis symptoms.

At the end of the 48 week study, more people
in the minocycline group than in the placebo
group showed improvement in joint swelling
(54% vs 39%) and joint tenderness (56% vs
41%). Those taking minocycline also showed
greater improvement in the laboratory tests
used to monitor rheumatoid arthritis.

No one knows what causes rheumatoid
arthritis, but one theory is that some cases may
be caused by a persistent hard-to-treat infection. However, minocycline and other tetracyclines have several non-antibiotic effects that
may explain the drugs' effect in rheumatoid
arthritis. These include anti-inflammatory and
antioxidant effects.

Using minocycline for the treatment of
rheumatoid arthritis is not an FDA-approved
use for this drug and would be called an "off-
label" or unapproved use for the drug. This
means that the FDA has not reviewed the drug
for this use and deemed it safe and effective for
the treatment of rheumatoid arthritis. This
does not mean that your doctor is prohibited
from prescribing minocycline for rheumatoid
arthritis, but you should be informed that you
are receiving a drug for an "off-label" use and
insist that your doctor inform you of the potential risks and benefits of this drug.

WARNING

The use of tetracyclines during tooth development (last half of pregnancy, infancy, and childhood to the age of eight years) may cause
permanent discoloration of the teeth.

Before You Use This Drug

Tell your doctor if you have or have had:

- allergies to drugs
- an unusual reaction to tetracycline or another drug in its family, such as doxycycline

- kidney or liver problems
- diabetes insipidous

Tell your doctor about any other drugs you take, including aspirin, herbs, vitamins, and other nonprescription products.

When You Use This Drug

- Until you know how you react to this drug, do not drive or perform other activities requiring alertness.
- Stay out of the sun as much as possible, and call your doctor if you get a rash, hives, or any other skin reaction. Minocycline and other tetracyclines make you more sensitive to the sun.
- Do not eat or drink milk or other dairy products, and do not take antacids or iron, vitamin, or mineral supplements for a few hours before and after you take each dose of tetracycline. These substances can keep your body from absorbing the drug, which makes it less effective.
- If you plan to have any surgery, including dental, tell your doctor that you take this drug.

How to Use This Drug

- Take on an empty stomach (at least one hour before or two hours after a meal) for best absorption of the drug into your body. Take with **a full glass (eight ounces) of water.** Take your last dose of the day at least an hour before bedtime.
- Keep the container closed tightly and in a dry place. Do not store in the bathroom. Do not expose to heat, moisture, or strong light. Do not use if the appearance or taste has changed.
- Take at least two hours apart from any other drug you are taking.
- If you miss a dose, take it as soon as you remember, but skip it if it is almost time for the next dose. **Do not take double doses.**

Interactions with Other Drugs

The following drugs are listed in the *Evaluations of Drug Interactions* 1997 as causing "highly clinically significant" or "clinically significant" interactions when used together with this drug. We have also included potentially serious interactions listed in the drug's FDA-approved professional product labeling or package insert. New scientific techniques have allowed researchers to predict some drug interactions before they have been documented in people. There may be other drugs, especially those in the families of drugs listed below, that also will react with this drug to cause severe adverse effects. The number of new drugs approved for marketing increases the chance of drug interactions, and new drug interactions are being identified with old drugs. Be vigilant. Make sure to tell your doctor and pharmacist the drugs you are taking and tell your doctor if you are taking any of these interacting drugs:

aluminum hydroxide, AMPHOJEL, calcium carbonate, CALTRATE, digoxin, FEOSOL, ferrous sulfate, LANOXICAPS, LANOXIN, lithium, LITHOBID, LITHONATE, magnesium hydroxide, methoxyflurane, oral contraceptives, OS–CAL 500, PENTHRANE, PHILLIPS' MILK OF MAGNESIA, SLOW FE.

Adverse Effects

Call your doctor immediately if you experience:

- abdominal pain
- skin rash, increased sensitivity of skin to sun (increased sunburn)
- nausea or vomiting
- discoloration of skin or mucous membranes
- headache
- loss of appetite
- vision changes
- yellowing skin

Call your doctor if these symptoms continue:

- stomach cramps or burning sensation in the stomach
- diarrhea
- sore or discolored mouth or tongue
- itching in the genital or rectal area
- dizziness, clumsiness, lightheadedness or unsteadiness

PREGNANCY WARNING

This drug caused harm to developing fetuses in animal studies, or such studies were not done. Use during pregnancy only for clear medical reasons. Tell your doctor if you are pregnant or thinking of becoming pregnant before you take this drug.

Ibuprofen
Prescription:
MOTRIN (Pharmacia & Upjohn)
Nonprescription:
ADVIL (Whitehall-Robins)
NUPRIN (Bristol-Myers Products)
MEDIPREN (McNeil Consumer Products)

GENERIC: available
FAMILY: Nonsteroidal Anti-inflammatory Drugs "NSAIDs"
Arthritis Drugs (see p. 265)

Ibuprofen (eye byoo *proe* fen) belongs to the family of drugs called nonsteroidal anti-inflammatory drugs, shortened to NSAIDs (*n* sayds), often used to treat arthritis in older adults. NSAIDs can cause serious harm, even fatalities, from bleeding in the stomach or intestines. Bleeding can occur at any time and without warning and older people are more likely to experience adverse effects from bleeding. Older adults are also more likely to have reduced liver and kidney function. Some doc-

tors believe people over age 70 should be started with half the usual dose of drugs in this group.[93]

Ibuprofen is used to treat fever and pain, including pain caused by two kinds of arthritis, osteoarthritis and rheumatoid arthritis. **In general, if you are over 60, you should take less than the usual adult dose, especially if you have decreased kidney function.**

WARNING

NONSTEROIDAL ANTI-INFLAMMATORY DRUG (NSAID) INDUCED GASTROINTESTINAL TOXICITY

All members of the NSAID family of drugs can cause gastrointestinal toxicity that can lead to gastrointestinal bleeding and hospitalization or death. The risk of gastrointestinal toxicity from these drugs increases with increasing doses and the length of treatment.

If the following symptoms develop while you are taking an NSAID, stop the drug immediately and contact your doctor: severe abdominal or stomach pain, cramping, or burning, severe and continuing nausea, heartburn, or indigestion, bloody or black, tarry stools, vomiting blood or material that looks like coffee grounds, or spitting up blood.

Aspirin (see p. 275) is just as effective and less costly than other NSAIDs and is the drug of choice for treating pain, fever, and inflammation in people who do not have ulcers, gastritis (inflammation of the stomach), or an allergy to aspirin. Some rheumatologists (arthritis specialists) prefer aspirin to other NSAIDs for treating rheumatoid arthritis.[94]

If you cannot use enteric-coated aspirin (aspirin coated so that it does not dissolve

in the stomach), ibuprofen is generally the best second-choice drug because it has been studied longer than other drugs in this family and appears to have a good safety record. If you cannot take enteric-coated aspirin and are also bothered by adverse effects when taking ibuprofen, talk to your doctor about switching to another drug in this family. Each person responds differently to different NSAIDs.

Before You Use This Drug

Do not use if you have or have had:

- an allergic reaction to aspirin, any other NSAID or iodides[95]
- peptic ulcers
- alcohol dependence
- nasal polyps

Tell your doctor if you have or have had:

- allergies to drugs
- heart, kidney, or liver problems
- hemophilia or other bleeding problems
- high blood pressure
- anemia
- asthma
- diabetes
- stomach or intestinal problems
- tobacco use

Tell your doctor about any other drugs you take, including aspirin, herbs, vitamins, and other nonprescription products.

When You Use This Drug

- Do not drink alcohol. It irritates the stomach lining and increases the risk of stomach bleeding.
- Call your doctor immediately if you have flu-like symptoms (chills, fever, muscle aches or pains) shortly before or at the same time as a skin rash. This may be a sign of a serious reaction to ibuprofen.
- You may feel dizzy when rising from a lying or sitting position. If you are lying down, hang your legs over the side of the bed for a few minutes, then get up slowly. When getting up from a chair, stay by the chair until you are sure that you are not dizzy. (See p. 16.)
- If you plan to have any surgery, including dental, tell your doctor that you take this drug.

How to Use This Drug

- Take with food to reduce stomach irritation.
- Take with a full glass (eight ounces) of water. Do not lie down for 30 minutes afterwards.
- If you miss a dose, take it as soon as possible, but skip it if it is almost time for the next dose. Do not take double doses.
- Store at room temperature, with lid on tightly. Do not store in the bathroom. Do not expose to moisture or heat.

Interactions with Other Drugs

The following drugs are listed in the *Evaluations of Drug Interactions* 1997 as causing "highly clinically significant" or "clinically significant" interactions when used together with this drug. We have also included potentially serious interactions listed in the drug's FDA-approved professional product labeling or package insert. New scientific techniques have allowed researchers to predict some drug interactions before they have been documented in people. There may be other drugs, especially those in the families of drugs listed below, that also will react with this drug to cause severe adverse effects. The number of new drugs approved for marketing increases the chance of drug interactions, and new drug interactions are being identified with old drugs. Be vigilant.

Make sure to tell your doctor and pharmacist the drugs you are taking and tell your doctor if you are taking any of these interacting drugs:

bendroflumethiazide, BENEMID, CAPOTEN, captopril, COUMADIN, cyclosporine, digoxin, DILANTIN, GARAMYCIN, gentamicin, INDERAL, INDERAL LA, ketorolac, labetalol, LANOXICAPS, LANOXIN, lithium, LITHOBID, LITHONATE, methotrexate, MINIPRESS, NATURETIN, NEORAL, NORMODYNE, phenytoin, prazosin, probenecid, propranolol, RHEUMATREX DOSE PACK, SANDIMMUNE, TORADOL, TRANDATE, warfarin.

Adverse Effects

Call your doctor immediately if you experience:

- abdominal pain or swelling
- appetite loss
- bloody or black, tarry stools
- increase or decrease in blood pressure
- difficulty breathing
- unusual bruising
- chest pain
- chills
- confusion
- cough or hoarseness
- depression
- drowsiness
- pain, dryness, redness, irritation or swelling of the eyes
- facial skin color changes
- fever
- gastrointestinal pain, cramping or burning
- swollen glands
- hallucinations
- headache
- hearing change or ringing or buzzing
- heartburn
- hives on face, eyelids or tongue
- indigestion
- lower back, neck or side pain
- unusually heavy menstrual bleeding
- muscle cramps or pain
- nausea, vomiting
- nosebleeds, runny nose or sneezing
- numbness, tingling, pain, or weakness in hands or feet
- pinpoint red spots on skin
- skin rash, blisters, hives, itching, scaling
- sore throat
- sores, ulcers, or white spots on lips or in mouth
- swelling of face, lips, tongue, fingers, lower legs or feet
- unusual tiredness or weakness
- difficulty urinating
- bloody or cloudy urine
- vision change
- vomiting blood or material that looks like coffee grounds
- rapid weight gain
- yellow eyes or skin

Call your doctor if these symptoms continue:

- constipation, diarrhea, gas
- dizziness
- flushing or hot flashes
- irregular heartbeat
- insomnia
- nervousness, irritability
- sunburn
- sweating

Periodic Tests

Ask your doctor which of these tests should be done periodically while you are taking this drug:

- kidney function tests
- liver function tests
- stool tests for possible blood loss

- hematocrit and/or hemoglobin test
- blood concentrations of creatinine, potassium, and urea nitrogen
- white blood cell count
- upper GI diagnostic tests
- ophthalmologic exams

Limited Use

Fenoprofen
NALFON (Dista)

Oxaprozin
DAYPRO (Searle)

GENERIC: available for fenoprofen

FAMILY: Nonsteroidal Anti-inflammatory Drugs "NSAIDs"
Arthritis Drugs (see p. 265)

Fenoprofen (fen oh *proe* fen) and oxaprozin (ox a *proe* zin) belong to the family of drugs called nonsteroidal anti-inflammatory drugs, shortened to NSAIDs (*n* sayds), and share a chemical similarity. Both drugs are used to treat arthritis in older adults. NSAIDs can cause serious harm, even fatalities, from bleeding in the stomach or intestines. Bleeding can occur at any time and without warning and older people are more likely to experience adverse effects from bleeding. Older adults are also more likely to have reduced liver and kidney function. Some doctors believe people over age 70 should be started with half the usual dose of drugs in this group.[96]

Fenoprofen and oxaprozin are used mainly to relieve the pain and inflammation of two kinds of arthritis, rheumatoid arthritis and osteoarthritis, but these are not the best drugs for this purpose. **In general, if you are over 60, you should take less than the usual adult dose of these drugs.**

Fenoprofen causes kidney disease in a large percentage of people who take it, compared with other NSAIDs,[97] so you should not take it if you have impaired kidney function.[98] If you have impaired hearing and take this drug for a long time, you should have periodic hearing tests.[99] Oxaprozin can also cause kidney damage.

Aspirin (see p. 275) is just as effective and less costly than other NSAIDs and is the drug of choice for treating pain, fever, and inflammation in people who do not have ulcers, gastritis (inflammation of the stomach), or an allergy to aspirin. Some rheumatologists (arthritis specialists) prefer aspirin to other drugs in this family for treating rheumatoid arthritis.[100] Fenoprofen or oxaprozin should be used only if enteric-coated aspirin (see p. 275) and other safe drugs in this family, such as ibuprofen and naproxen (see pp. 311, 317), do not work.

If you are taking fenoprofen or oxaprozin, ask your doctor whether you can switch to taking enteric-coated aspirin (aspirin coated so it won't dissolve in the stomach) twice a day. If you can't take aspirin and are having trouble with adverse effects of fenoprofen, ask if you can switch to another drug in this family such as ibuprofen. Each person responds differently to different NSAIDs.

WARNING

NONSTEROIDAL ANTI-INFLAMMATORY DRUG (NSAID) INDUCED GASTROINTESTINAL TOXICITY

All members of the NSAID family of drugs can cause gastrointestinal toxicity that can lead to gastrointestinal bleeding and hospitalization or death. The risk of gastrointestinal toxicity from these drugs increases with increasing doses and the length of treatment.

If the following symptoms develop while you are taking an NSAID, stop the drug immediately and contact your doctor: severe abdominal or stomach pain, cramping, or burning, severe and continuing nausea, heartburn, or indigestion, bloody or black, tarry stools, vomiting blood or material that looks like coffee grounds, or spitting up blood.

Before You Use This Drug

Do not use if you have or have had:

- an allergic reaction to aspirin, any other NSAID or iodides[101]
- peptic ulcers
- alcohol dependence
- nasal polyps or asthma

Tell your doctor if you have or have had:

- allergies to drugs
- heart, kidney, or liver problems
- hemophilia or other bleeding problems
- high blood pressure
- anemia
- asthma
- diabetes
- stomach or intestinal problems
- tobacco use

Tell your doctor about any other drugs you take, including aspirin, herbs, vitamins, and other nonprescription products.

When You Use This Drug

- Do not drink alcohol. It irritates the stomach lining and increases the risk of stomach bleeding.
- Call your doctor immediately if you have flu-like symptoms (chills, fever, muscle aches or pains) shortly before or with a skin rash. This may be a sign of a serious reaction to fenoprofen.
- You may feel dizzy when rising from a lying or sitting position. If you are lying down, hang your legs over the side of the bed for a few minutes, then get up slowly. When getting up from a chair, stay by the chair until you are sure that you are not dizzy. (See p. 16.)
- If you plan to have any surgery, including dental, tell your doctor that you take this drug.

How to Use This Drug

- Taking with food may reduce stomach irritation, but it will also decrease the drug's effectiveness.
- Take with **a full glass (eight ounces) of water.** Do not lie down for 30 minutes afterward.
- If you miss a dose, take it as soon as possible, but skip it if it is almost time for the next dose. **Do not take double doses.**
- Store at room temperature, with lid on tightly. Do not store in the bathroom. Do not expose to moisture or heat.

Interactions with Other Drugs

The following drugs are listed in the *Evaluations of Drug Interactions* 1997 as causing "highly clinically significant" or "clinically significant" interactions when used together with this drug. We have also included potentially serious interactions listed in the drug's FDA-approved professional product labeling or package insert. New scientific techniques have allowed researchers to predict some drug interactions before they have been documented in people. There may be other drugs, especially those in the families of drugs listed below, that also will react with this drug to cause severe adverse effects. The number of new drugs approved for marketing increases the chance of drug interactions, and new drug interactions are being identified with old drugs. Be vigilant. Make sure to tell your doctor and pharmacist the drugs you are taking and tell your doctor if you are taking any of these interacting drugs:

bendroflumethiazide, BENEMID, CAPOTEN, captopril, COUMADIN, cyclosporine, digoxin, DILANTIN, GARAMYCIN, gentamicin, gold sodium thiomalate INDERAL, INDERAL LA, ketorolac, LANOXICAPS, LANOXIN, lithium, LITHOBID, LITHONATE, methotrexate, MINIPRESS, MYOCHRYSINE, NATURETIN, NEORAL, phenytoin, prazosin, probenecid, propranolol, RHEUMATREX DOSE PACK, SANDIMMUNE, TORADOL, warfarin.

Adverse Effects

Call your doctor immediately if you experience:

- abdominal pain or swelling
- appetite loss
- bloody, black tarry or light stools
- blood pressure increase or decrease
- difficulty breathing
- unusual bruising
- chest pain
- chills
- confusion
- convulsions
- cough or hoarseness
- depression, disorientation
- pain, redness, irritation or swelling of the eyes
- facial skin color changes
- fever
- gastrointestinal pain, cramping or burning
- swollen glands
- hearing change or ringing or buzzing
- heartburn
- hives on face, eyelids or tongue
- indigestion
- lower back, neck or side pain
- muscle cramps or pain
- nausea, vomiting
- pinpoint red spots on skin
- rectal bleeding
- skin rash, hives, itching, scaling
- sore throat
- sores, ulcers, or white spots on lips or in mouth
- swelling of face, lips, tongue, fingers, lower legs or feet
- continuous thirst
- unusual tiredness or weakness
- difficulty urinating
- bloody, dark, or cloudy urine
- vision change

- vomiting blood or material that looks like coffee grounds
- rapid weight gain
- yellow eyes or skin

Call your doctor if these symptoms continue:

- constipation, diarrhea, gas
- dizziness
- drowsiness
- headache
- irregular heartbeat
- insomnia
- irritated or dry mouth
- nervousness, irritability
- sweating

Periodic Tests

Ask your doctor which of these tests should be done periodically while you are taking this drug:

- kidney function tests
- liver function tests
- stool tests for possible blood loss
- hematocrit and/or hemoglobin test
- blood concentrations of creatinine, potassium, and urea nitrogen
- white blood cell count
- hearing tests, for prolonged use
- upper GI diagnostic tests
- ophthalmologic exams

Naproxen
NAPROSYN, ANAPROX (Roche)

GENERIC: available

FAMILY: Nonsteroidal Anti-inflammatory Drugs "NSAIDs"
Arthritis Drugs (see p. 265)

Naproxen (na *prox* en) belongs to the family of drugs called nonsteroidal anti-inflammatory drugs, shortened to NSAIDs (*n* sayds), often used to treat arthritis in older adults. NSAIDs can cause serious harm, even fatalities, from bleeding in the stomach or intestines. Bleeding can occur at any time and without warning and older people are more likely to experience adverse effects from bleeding. Older adults are also more likely to have reduced liver and kidney function. Some doctors believe people over age 70 should be started with half the usual dose of drugs in this group.[102]

Naproxen relieves mild to moderate pain and symptoms of osteoarthritis, rheumatoid arthritis, ankylosing spondylitis, tendonitis, bursitis, and sudden gout attacks. **In general, if you are over 60, you should take less than the usual adult dose, especially if you have decreased kidney function.**

Aspirin (see p. 275) is just as effective and less costly than other NSAIDs and is the drug of choice for treating pain, fever, and inflammation in people who do not have ulcers, gastritis (inflammation of the stomach), or an allergy to aspirin. Some rheumatologists (arthritis specialists) prefer aspirin to other NSAIDs for treating rheumatoid arthritis.[103]

If you cannot take twice-a-day enteric-coated aspirin (aspirin coated so it will not dissolve in the stomach), naproxen may be a good alternative. If you cannot take enteric-coated aspirin and are also bothered by adverse effects when taking naproxen, talk to your doctor about switching to another drug in this family such as ibuprofen (see p. 311). Each person responds differently to different NSAIDs.

WARNING

NONSTEROIDAL ANTI-INFLAMMATORY DRUG (NSAID) INDUCED GASTROINTESTINAL TOXICITY

All members of the NSAID family of drugs can cause gastrointestinal toxicity that can lead to gastrointestinal bleeding and hospitalization or death. The risk of gastrointestinal toxicity from these drugs increases with increasing doses and the length of treatment.

If the following symptoms develop while you are taking an NSAID, stop the drug immediately and contact your doctor: severe abdominal or stomach pain, cramping, or burning, severe and continuing nausea, heartburn, or indigestion, bloody or black, tarry stools, vomiting blood or material that looks like coffee grounds, or spitting up blood.

Before You Use This Drug

Do not use if you have or have had:

- an allergic reaction to aspirin, any other NSAID or iodides[104]
- peptic ulcers
- alcohol dependence
- nasal polyps or asthma

Tell your doctor if you have or have had:

- allergies to drugs
- heart, kidney, or liver problems
- hemophilia or other bleeding problems
- high blood pressure
- anemia
- asthma
- diabetes
- stomach or intestinal problems
- tobacco use

Tell your doctor about any other drugs you take, including aspirin, herbs, vitamins, and other nonprescription products.

When You Use This Drug

• Do not drink alcohol. It irritates the stomach lining and increases the risk of stomach bleeding.

• Call your doctor immediately if you have flu-like symptoms (chills, fever, muscle aches or pains) shortly before or with a skin rash. This may indicate a serious reaction to naproxen.

• You may feel dizzy when rising from a lying or sitting position. If you are lying down, hang your legs over the side of the bed for a few minutes, then get up slowly. When getting up from a chair, stay by the chair until you are sure that you are not dizzy. (See p. 16.)

• If you plan to have any surgery, including dental, tell your doctor that you take this drug.

How to Use This Drug

• Take with food to reduce stomach irritation.

• Take with **a full glass (eight ounces) of water**. Do not lie down for 30 minutes afterwards.

• If you miss a dose, take it as soon as possible, but skip it if it is almost time for the next dose. **Do not take double doses.**

• Store at room temperature, with lid on tightly. Do not store in the bathroom. Do not expose to moisture or heat.

Interactions with Other Drugs

The following drugs are listed in the *Evaluations of Drug Interactions* 1997 as causing "highly clinically significant" or "clinically significant" interactions when used together with this drug. We have also included potentially serious interactions listed in the drug's FDA-approved professional product labeling or package insert. New scientific techniques have allowed researchers to predict some drug interactions before they have been documented in people. There may be other drugs, especially those in the families of drugs listed below, that also will react with this drug to cause severe adverse effects. The number of new drugs approved for marketing increases the chance of drug interactions, and new drug interactions are being identified with old drugs. Be vigilant. Make sure to tell your doctor and pharmacist the drugs you are taking and tell your doctor if you are taking any of these interacting drugs:

bendroflumethiazide, BENEMID, CAPOTEN, captopril, COUMADIN, cyclosporine, digoxin, DILANTIN, GARAMYCIN, gentamicin, gold sodium thiomalate, INDERAL, INDERAL LA, INDOCIN, indomethacin, ketorolac, LANOXICAPS, LANOXIN, lithium, LITHOBID, LITHONATE, methotrexate, MINIPRESS, MYOCHRYSINE, NATURETIN, NEORAL, phenytoin, prazosin, probenecid, propranolol, RHEUMATREX DOSE PACK, SANDIMMUNE, timolol, TIMOPTIC, TORADOL, warfarin.

Adverse Effects

Call your doctor immediately if you experience:

• abdominal pain or swelling
• appetite loss
• bloody or black, tarry stools
• increase or decrease in blood pressure
• difficulty breathing
• unusual bruising
• chest pains
• chills
• confusion
• cough or hoarseness
• depression
• drowsiness
• facial skin color changes
• fever
• gastrointestinal pain, cramping or burning
• swollen glands
• headache
• hearing change or ringing or buzzing
• heartburn
• hives on face, eyelids or tongue

- indigestion
- lower back, neck or side pain
- unusually heavy menstrual bleeding
- muscle cramps or pain
- nausea, vomiting
- numbness, tingling, pain or weakness in hands or feet
- pinpoint red spots on skin
- rectal bleeding
- skin rash, hives, itching, scaling or changing of skin color
- sore throat
- sores, ulcers, or white spots on lips or in mouth
- spitting blood
- swelling of face, lips, tongue, fingers, lower legs or feet
- continuous thirst
- unusual tiredness or weakness
- difficulty urinating
- bloody or cloudy urine
- vision change
- vomiting blood or material that looks like coffee grounds
- rapid weight gain
- yellow eyes or skin

Call your doctor if these symptoms continue:

- constipation, diarrhea
- dizziness
- drowsiness
- irregular heartbeat
- insomnia
- lightheadedness
- muscle weakness
- sunburn
- sweating
- weakness

Periodic Tests

Ask your doctor which of these tests should be done periodically while you are taking this drug:

- kidney function tests

- liver function tests
- stool tests for possible blood loss
- hematocrit and/or hemoglobin test
- blood concentrations of creatinine, potassium, and urea nitrogen
- white blood cell count
- upper GI diagnostic tests
- ophthalmologic exams

 Do Not Use

ALTERNATIVE TREATMENT:
Rest, exercise, physical therapy, and an anti-inflammatory drug such as aspirin.

Orphenadrine, Aspirin, and Caffeine
NORGESIC FORTE (3M)

FAMILY: Muscle Relaxants
Painkillers

This combination of orphenadrine (or *fen* a dreen), aspirin (see p. 275), and caffeine is promoted to relieve the pain of muscle disorders. However, neither orphenadrine nor caffeine is effective for these conditions. Aspirin by itself may be helpful along with rest, exercise, physical therapy, or other treatment recommended by your doctor. When taking this product, you are in fact taking three drugs, each with its own cautions, adverse effects, and drug interactions. Like other fixed-combination products, this combination curtails the ability to vary doses of each drug.

Orphenadrine has not been shown to be any more effective than painkillers or anti-inflammatory drugs, such as aspirin alone, for relieving the pain of local muscle spasm. It has a higher risk of adverse effects than these painkillers. Since orphenadrine is similar to a family of drugs called antihistamines, which are used to relieve symptoms of hay fever and other allergies (see p. 405), it may cause some of the same adverse effects and dangerous drug interactions as antihistamines. Some people taking orphenadrine experience blurred vision, dry mouth, mild excitement, temporary dizziness, and lightheadedness. Many of these effects occur more often in older adults. Orphenadrine is particularly dangerous for people who have glaucoma, myasthenia gravis, heart problems, or an enlarged prostate.

Aspirin relieves mild to moderate pain, but does not treat the underlying problem (see p. 275). Regular use could mask a fever due to bacterial infection. You should not take aspirin if you have ulcers, a severely irritated stomach, gout, severe anemia, hemophilia or other bleeding problems, if you take an anticoagulant drug such as heparin or warfarin, or if you are allergic to aspirin or similar painkillers.

Caffeine has not proven effective in relieving pain. It can aggravate incontinence, produce insomnia, and lead to dependence, causing withdrawal headaches. It can also irritate the stomach, so people with ulcers should avoid it.

WARNING: SPECIAL MENTAL AND PHYSICAL ADVERSE EFFECTS

Older adults are especially sensitive to the harmful anticholinergic (see Glossary, p. 768) effects of orphenadrine because of its similarity to the antihistamines.

Mental Effects: confusion, delirium, short-term memory problems, disorientation, and impaired attention.

Physical Effects: dry mouth, constipation, difficulty urinating (especially for a man with an enlarged prostate), blurred vision, decreased sweating with increased body temperature, sexual dysfunction, and worsening of glaucoma.

ASPIRIN/REYE'S SYNDROME ALERT

Do not use this product for treating chicken pox, flu, or flu-like illness. It will increase the risk of contracting Reye's syndrome, a rare but often fatal disease.

Ketoprofen
ORUDIS (Wyeth-Ayerst)

GENERIC: available

FAMILY: Nonsteroidal Anti-inflammatory Drugs "NSAIDs" Arthritis Drugs (see p. 265)

Ketoprofen (keat oh *pro* fen) belongs to the family of drugs called nonsteroidal anti-inflammatory drugs, shortened to NSAIDs (*n* sayds), often used to treat arthritis in older adults. NSAIDs can cause serious harm, even fatalities, from bleeding in the stomach or intestines. Bleeding can occur at any time and without warning and older people are more likely to experience adverse effects from bleeding. Older adults are also more likely to have reduced liver and kidney function. Some doctors believe people over age 70 should be started with half the usual dose of drugs in this group.[105] Those underweight should also start with a low dose of ketoprofen.[106]

Ketoprofen relieves inflammation and pain. It is used to treat mild to moderate pain and symptoms of rheumatoid arthritis, osteoarthritis, and pain due to disease or injury. Improvement starts within a couple of weeks, while maximum improvement takes several weeks. **In general, if you are over 60, you should take less than the usual adult dose, especially if you have decreased kidney function.**

Women also appear to be more susceptible to the adverse effects of ketoprofen.[107]

Aspirin (see p. 275) is just as effective and less costly than other NSAIDs and is the drug of choice to treat pain, fever, and inflammation in people who do not have ulcers, gastritis (inflammation of the stomach, or an allergy to aspirin. Some rheumatologists (arthritis specialists) prefer aspirin to other NSAIDs for rheumatoid arthritis.[108]

Before You Use This Drug

Do not use if you have or have had:

- an allergic reaction to aspirin, any other NSAID or iodides[109]
- alcohol dependence
- peptic ulcers
- nasal polyps

Tell your doctor if you have or have had:

- allergies to drugs
- heart, kidney or liver problems
- hemophilia or other bleeding problems
- high blood pressure
- anemia
- asthma
- diabetes
- tuberculosis[110]
- stomach or intestinal problems
- tobacco use

Tell your doctor about any other drugs you take, including aspirin, herbs, vitamins, and other nonprescription products.

When You Use This Drug

- Do not drink alcohol. It irritates the stomach lining and increases the risk of stomach bleeding.
- Call your doctor immediately if you have flu-like symptoms (chills, fever, muscle aches or pains) shortly before or with a skin rash. This may indicate a serious reaction to ketoprofen.

- You may feel dizzy when rising from a lying or sitting position. If you are lying down, hang your legs over the side of the bed for a few minutes, then get up slowly. When getting up from a chair, stay by the chair until you are sure that that you are not dizzy. (See p. 16.)
- Avoid driving or other activities that require alertness because this drug may make you drowsy, dizzy, or lightheaded.
- If you plan to have any surgery, including dental, tell your doctor that you take this drug.

How to Use This Drug

- Take with food, milk or an antacid to reduce stomach irritation. The antacid may delay time the drug takes to work.[111]
- Take with **a full glass (eight ounces) of water.** Do not lie down for 30 minutes afterwards.
- If you miss a dose, take it as soon as possible, but skip it if it is almost time for the next dose. **Do not take double doses.**
- Store capsules at room temperature with cap on tightly. Do not expose to heat.

Interactions with Other Drugs

The following drugs are listed in the *Evaluations of Drug Interactions* 1997 as causing "highly clinically significant" or "clinically significant" interactions when used together with this drug. We have also included potentially serious interactions listed in the drug's FDA-approved professional product labeling or package insert. New scientific techniques have allowed researchers to predict some drug interactions before they have been documented in people. There may be other drugs, especially those in the families of drugs listed below, that also will react with this drug to cause severe adverse effects. The number of new drugs approved for marketing increases the chance of drug interactions, and new drug interactions are being identified with old drugs. Be vigilant. Make sure to tell your doctor and pharmacist the drugs you are taking and tell your doctor if you are taking any of these interacting drugs:

> bendroflumethiazide, BENEMID, CAPOTEN, captopril, COUMADIN, cyclosporine, DEXATRIM, digoxin, DILANTIN, DYAZIDE, DYRENIUM, GARAMYCIN, gentamicin, gold sodium thiomolate, INDERAL, INDERAL LA, ketoprofen, LANOXICAPS, LANOXIN, lithium, LITHOBID, LITHONATE, MAXZIDE, methotrexate, MINIPRESS, MYOCHRYSINE, NATURETIN, NEORAL, ORUDIS, phenylpropanolamine, phenytoin, prazosin, probenecid, propranolol, RHEUMATREX DOSE PACK, SANDIMMUNE, TORADOL, triamterene, triamterene and hydrochlorothiazide, warfarin.

Adverse Effects

Call your doctor immmediately if you experience:

- abdominal pain or swelling
- appetite loss
- bloody or black, tarry stools
- increase or decrease in blood pressure
- difficulty breathing
- unusual bruising
- chest pain
- chills
- confusion
- convulsions
- depression
- pain, dryness, redness, irritation or swelling of the eyes
- facial skin color changes
- fever
- forgetfulness
- gastrointestinal pain, cramping or burning

- swollen glands
- headache
- hearing change or ringing or buzzing
- heartburn
- indigestion
- unusually heavy menstrual bleeding
- muscle cramps or pain
- nails loosening or splitting
- nausea, vomiting
- nosebleeds, runny nose or sneezing
- numbness, tingling, pain or weakness in hands or feet
- pinpoint red spots on skin
- rectal bleeding
- skin rash, blisters, hives, itching, scaling
- sore throat
- sores, ulcers, or white spots on lips or in mouth
- difficulty speaking
- spitting blood
- swelling of face, lips, tongue, fingers, lower legs or feet
- continuing thirst
- unusual tiredness or weakness
- difficulty urinating
- bloody or cloudy urine
- vision change
- vomiting blood or material that looks like coffee grounds
- rapid weight gain
- yellow eyes or skin

Call your doctor if these symptoms continue:

- constipation, diarrhea, gas
- dizziness
- drowsiness
- irregular heartbeat
- insomnia
- lightheadedness
- irritated or dry mouth
- nervousness, irritability
- rectal irritation
- sunburn

- sweating
- bitter taste
- weight loss

Periodic Tests

Ask your doctor which of these tests should be done periodically while you are taking this drug:

- kidney function tests
- liver function tests
- stool tests for possible blood loss
- hematocrit and/or hemoglobin test
- blood concentrations of creatinine, potassium, and urea nitrogen
- white blood cell count
- upper GI diagnostic tests
- ophthalmologic exams

Acetaminophen and Oxycodone
PERCOCET (Endo)
TYLOX (Ortho-McNeil Pharmaceutical)

GENERIC: available
FAMILY: Painkillers
Fever Reducers
Narcotics (see p. 264)

Acetaminophen (see p. 338) and oxycodone (oxi *koe* done) are both painkillers. Acetaminophen also reduces fever, but it does not relieve the redness, stiffness, or swelling of rheumatoid arthritis or other conditions that cause inflammation. Oxycodone works similarly to narcotic drugs like morphine and has similar pain-killing and addictive effects.

Together, these two drugs produce a rational combination that relieves pain better than acetaminophen alone but has less risk of adverse effects than the larger dose of oxycodone that would be needed if oxycodone were used alone. This combination is available in tablets and capsules.

Although this combination is the best choice in some situations, it is overused. Many people who are prescribed this combination would get pain relief from acetaminophen alone, and would avoid the danger of becoming addicted to oxycodone. So before taking this drug, ask your doctor about trying plain acetaminophen first.

One hazard of taking oxycodone continuously for longer than several weeks is drug-induced dependence. **Do not stop taking your drug suddenly.** With the help of your doctor, work out a schedule for slowly decreasing the amount of the drug you take by about 5 to 10% each day. Keep a written record of the dosage reduction schedule with you. These steps will make it much easier to become drug free without developing distressing symptoms of drug withdrawal.

WARNING

There have been a number of case reports of liver damage involving a possible drug interaction between isoniazid, a medication used to prevent and treat tuberculosis, and acetaminophen, an over-the-counter painkiller and the active ingredient in Tylenol. Isoniazid alone, especially as people get older, has been documented to cause liver damage. Acetaminophen, alone in large doses or probably in combination with alcohol, also increases the risk of liver damage. The combination of acetaminophen with isoniazid, according to the authors of these case reports, may also be dangerous.[112]

If you are taking isoniazid for tuberculosis or have a positive TB skin test and are using the drug, consult your physician before using acetaminophen or any combination product containing acetaminophen. Discuss alternatives to acetaminophen with your physician.[113]

DRUG INTERACTION WARNING

INCREASED RISK OF BLEEDING WHEN ACETAMINOPHEN AND WARFARIN (COUMADIN) ARE TAKEN TOGETHER

Acetaminophen may interact with warfarin to increase the risk of bleeding. This risk increases with increasing doses of acetaminophen. The risk of bleeding has been found to increase tenfold in people who were taking 28 or more regular strength acetaminophen tablets per week, or the equivalent of 18 or more extra-strength tablets per week compared to those taking warfarin and no acetaminophen.[114] A regular strength tablet contains 325 milligrams of acetaminophen and extra-strength tablets contain 500 milligrams each of the drug.

Warfarin is a drug of considerable benefit after heart valve replacement and in preventing blood clots from a type of heart rhythm disturbance known as atrial fibrillation. It also reduces the risk of death, recurrent heart attacks, and stroke after a heart attack.

Based on this new evidence, if you are taking warfarin, you should notify your doctor before taking any product containing acetaminophen.

PREGNANCY WARNING

This drug caused harm to developing fetuses in animal studies, or such studies were not done. Use during pregnancy only for clear medical reasons. Tell your doctor if you are pregnant or thinking of becoming pregnant before you take this drug.

Aspirin and Oxycodone
PERCODAN, PERCODAN-DEMI (Endo)

GENERIC: available
FAMILY: Painkillers
Fever Reducers
Narcotics (see p. 264)

Aspirin (see p. 275) and oxycodone (ox i *koe* done) are painkillers. Oxycodone works similarly to narcotic drugs like morphine and has similar painkilling and addictive effects. Together, aspirin and oxycodone produce a rational combination drug that relieves pain better than aspirin alone but has less risk of adverse effects than the larger dose of oxycodone that would be needed if oxycodone were used alone.

Although this combination is the best choice in some situations, it is overused. Many people who are prescribed this combination would get pain relief from aspirin alone and would avoid the danger of becoming addicted to oxycodone. So before taking this drug, ask your doctor about trying plain aspirin first.

One hazard of taking oxycodone continuously for longer than several weeks is drug-induced dependence. **Do not stop taking your drug suddenly**. With the help of your doctor, work out a schedule for slowly decreasing the amount of the drug you take by about 5 to 10% each day. Keep a written record of the dosage reduction schedule with you. These steps will make it much easier to become drug free without developing distressing symptoms of drug withdrawal.

ASPIRIN/REYE'S SYNDROME ALERT

Do not use this product for treating chicken pox, flu, or flu-like illness. It will increase the risk of contracting Reye's syndrome, a rare but often fatal disease.

Limited Use

Hydroxychloroquine
PLAQUENIL (Sanofi)

GENERIC: available
FAMILY: Antiarthritis Drugs (see p. 265)

Hydroxychloroquine (hye drox ee *klor* oh kwin) is used to treat malaria, rheumatoid arthritis, and lupus erythematosus. Like other anti-arthritis drugs, it reduces symptoms caused by inflammation. Because hydroxychloroquine has serious adverse effects, you should not be taking it for rheumatoid arthritis unless you have already tried other drugs that reduce inflammation and they have not worked.

Hydroxychloroquine takes time to produce results, and you may not notice improvement in your condition for weeks or months. Continue to take the drug as directed by your doctor, and use a nonsteroidal anti-inflammatory drug such as aspirin at the same time to relieve your symptoms until the hydroxychloroquine works. If the drug doesn't begin to work after six months, it should be discontinued.

Hydroxychloroquine can cause serious adverse effects, some of which may occur months after you have stopped using it. The drug can collect in your eyes and cause vision problems, so an eye specialist should check your eyes before and during your treatment with hydroxychloroquine. If you develop blurred vision, difficulty reading, or any other change in your vision, stop taking the drug and call your doctor. Hydroxychloroquine has also caused some cases of rash, hearing loss, muscle weakness, and blood disorders. You should not take a dose greater than 400 milligrams per day, since taking such a large dose for a long time increases your risk of adverse effects.

Keep this drug out of the reach of children. Children are especially sensitive to the effects of hydroxychloroquine, and some have died after taking as few as three or four tablets.

Before You Use This Drug

Tell your doctor if you have or have had:

- allergies to drugs
- alcohol dependence
- liver problems
- severe blood disorders
- gastrointestinal disease
- glucose-6-phosphate dehydrogenase deficiency
- disorders of the nervous system or seizures

- psoriasis
- eye disease
- porphyria

Tell your doctor about any other drugs you take, including aspirin, herbs, vitamins, and other nonprescription products.

When You Use This Drug

- Do not drink alcohol.
- Until you know how you react to this drug, do not drive or perform other activities requiring alertness. Hydroxychloroquine causes lightheadedness and drowsiness.

How to Use This Drug

- Take with meals to reduce stomach upset.
- Do not store in the bathroom. Do not expose to heat or direct light.
- *If you miss a dose, use the following guidelines:* If you take the drug once a week, take the missed dose as soon as you remember and resume your regular schedule.

If you take the drug once a day, take the missed dose as soon as you remember, but skip it if you don't remember until the next day.

If you take the drug more than once a day, take the missed dose if you remember less than an hour after you were supposed to take it. If more than an hour has passed since you were supposed to take it, skip it. Continue to follow your regular schedule.

Do not take double doses.

Interactions with Other Drugs

The following drugs are listed in the *Evaluations of Drug Interactions* 1997 as causing "highly clinically significant" or "clinically significant" interactions when used together with this drug. We have also included potentially serious interactions listed in the drug's FDA-approved professional product labeling or package insert. New scientific techniques have allowed researchers to predict some drug interactions before they have been documented in people. There may be other drugs, especially those in the families of drugs listed below, that also will react with this drug to cause severe adverse effects. The number of new drugs approved for marketing increases the chance of drug interactions, and new drug interactions are being identified with old drugs. Be vigilant. Make sure to tell your doctor and pharmacist the drugs you are taking and tell your doctor if you are taking any of these interacting drugs:

digoxin, FLAGYL, LANOXICAPS, LANOXIN, metronidazole.

Adverse Effects

Call your doctor immediately if you experience:

- **signs of overdose:** difficulty breathing, drowsiness, fainting
- changes in vision
- seizures
- mood or mental changes
- hearing loss, ringing in ears
- unusual bleeding or bruising
- unusual muscle weakness
- sore throat and fever
- fatigue, weakness

Call your doctor if these symptoms continue:

- diarrhea
- headache
- nausea, vomiting
- stomach cramps or pain
- lightening of hair color or hair loss
- dark discoloration of skin, nails, or inside of mouth
- skin rash or itching
- dizziness or lightheadedness
- nervousness or restlessness

Call your doctor if these symptoms continue after you stop taking this drug:

- vision changes

Periodic Tests

Ask your doctor which of these tests should be done periodically while you are taking this drug:

- eye exams (before use, and at least annually during long-term use)
- complete blood count
- neuromuscular exams

Limited Use

Methotrexate
RHEUMATREX DOSE PACK (Lederle)

GENERIC: available
FAMILY: Arthritis Drugs (see p. 265)
Anticancer Drugs

Methotrexate (meth o *trex* ate) is used to treat rheumatoid arthritis and a few types of cancer.

For rheumatoid arthritis, methotrexate should be used only for the most severe cases that have not responded to treatment with other drugs. Before prescribing methotrexate, your doctor should try anti-inflammatory drugs such as aspirin (see p. 275) or ibuprofen (see p. 311) and other antiarthritis drugs such as gold salts (see p. 329) or penicillamine. You should only use methotrexate if these other drugs are not effective.

Methotrexate takes time to relieve the symptoms of arthritis, and you may not see improvement for weeks or months. Continue to take the drug as directed by your doctor, and also use a nonsteroidal anti-inflammatory drug other than aspirin until the methotrexate begins to work.

If you are using methotrexate for cancer, you may have to take it despite side effects such as sore mouth, stomach upset, nausea, vomiting, and loss of appetite. If a side effect is causing you problems, ask your doctor or other health professional to suggest ways to avoid or decrease the problem. Be aware, however, that some side effects are unavoidable. In fact, doctors use some side effects to tell whether the drug is working. Methotrexate can also cause liver and blood problems. For example, it can damage your bone marrow, disrupting the bone marrow's production of blood cells.

Drugs used to treat cancer often cause severe nausea and vomiting, either immediately after the drug is taken or several hours later. You can treat this kind of nausea and vomiting by changing your diet or by taking an antinausea drug. You should always try dietary changes first:[115]
- Eat small, frequent meals so your stomach is never empty.
- When you get up from sleeping or resting, eat some dry crackers or toast before you start being active.
- Drink carbonated drinks or other clear liquids such as soups and gelatin.
- Eat tart foods such as lemons and pickles.
- Do not eat foods with strong smells.

Before You Use This Drug

Do not use if you have or have had:

- recent chicken pox exposure or infection
- shingles (herpes zoster)

Tell your doctor if you have or have had:

- allergies to drugs
- alcohol dependence
- bone marrow depression
- gout
- kidney stones
- recent infection
- kidney or liver problems
- colitis

- stomach ulcers
- intestinal obstruction
- mouth sores or inflammation

Tell your doctor about any other drugs you take, including aspirin, herbs, vitamins, and other nonprescription products.

When You Use This Drug

- **Do not use more or less often or in a higher or lower dose than prescribed.** Check with your doctor before you stop using this drug.
- **Do not drink alcohol. It increases your chances of liver damage.**
- Try to stay out of the sun. Methotrexate makes your skin more sensitive to sunlight.
- **Do not get immunizations without your doctor's approval, and avoid exposure to people who have colds or other infections or who have recently been immunized.** Because methotrexate decreases the number of white blood cells, which fight infection, you are more likely to get an infecction while you are taking it.
- Schedule regular visits with your doctor to check your blood counts, liver function, and progress on the drug.
- If you plan to have any surgery, including dental, tell your doctor that you take this drug.

How to Use This Drug

- Do not store in the bathroom. Do not expose to heat, moisture, or strong light.
- Call your doctor if you miss a dose or vomit shortly after taking the drug.

Interactions with Other Drugs

The following drugs are listed in *Evaluations of Drug Interactions* 1997 as causing "highly clinically significant" or "clinically significant" interactions when used together with this drug. We have also included potentially serious interactions listed in the drug's FDA-approved professional product labeling or package insert. New scientific techniques have allowed researchers to predict some drug interactions before they have been documented in people. There may be other drugs, especially those in the families of drugs listed below, that also will react with this drug to cause severe adverse effects, The number of new drugs approved for marketing increases the chance of drug interactions, and new drug interactions are being identified with old drugs. Be vigilant. Make sure to tell your doctor and pharmacist the drugs you are taking and tell your doctor if you are taking any of these interacting drugs:

aspirin, BACTRIM, GENUINE BAYER ASPIRIN, BENEMID, cisplatin, COTRIM, DILANTIN, ECOTRIN, EMPIRIN, etretinate, ketoprofen, leucovorin, MATULANE, neomycin, ORUDIS, phenytoin, PLATINOL, probenecid, procarbazine, SEPTRA, TEGISON, trimethoprim/sulfamethoxazole, WELLCOVORIN.

Adverse Effects

Call your doctor immediately if you experience:

- black, tarry stools
- stomach pain
- diarrhea
- bloody vomit
- fever, chills, or sore throat
- unusual bleeding or bruising
- sores in mouth or on lips
- blood in urine
- swelling of feet or lower legs
- joint pain
- cough, shortness of breath
- dark urine, yellow eyes or skin

Call your doctor if these symptoms continue:

- nausea, vomiting, loss of appetite
- hair loss

- rash, hives, or itching
- acne or boils
- pale or reddened skin

Periodic Tests

Ask your doctor which of these tests should be done periodically while you are taking this drug:

- kidney function tests
- monthly liver function tests
- blood levels of uric acid
- monthly complete blood tests (including hematocrit, platelet count, white blood cell count)
- examination for mouth ulcers

_____

Limited Use

Aurothioglucose
SOLGANAL (Schering)

Gold Sodium Thiomalate
MYOCHRYSINE (Merck)

GENERIC: available for gold sodium thiomolate

FAMILY: Gold Compound
Arthritis Drugs (see p. 265)

Aurothioglucose (aur oh thye oh *gloo* kose) and gold sodium thiomalate (thye oh *mah* late) are gold salts used to treat rheumatoid arthritis. These drugs have severe adverse effects. A large proportion of users show signs of toxicity from these drugs, and some adverse effects may occur many months after you stop taking the drug (see Adverse Effects). Because of the danger of adverse effects, you should only be taking gold salts for rheumatoid arthritis if you have already tried anti-inflammatory drugs without success.

Aurothioglucose and gold sodium thiomalate are injected into the muscle, and you may have joint pain for one or two days afterward.

These drugs cause gradual improvement, and you may not notice the improvement until you have been injected with a total of approximately 1,000 milligrams. Until the gold therapy begins to work, you should take a nonsteroidal anti-inflammatory drug such as aspirin at the same time to relieve your arthritis symptoms. If the cumulative dose of gold salts reaches 1,000 milligrams and you still do not notice any improvement, the drug should be discontinued.[116]

If you cannot tolerate the adverse effects of the injections, you may better tolerate auranofin, a recently approved gold salt that can be taken by mouth. It appears to have effects comparable to those of the gold injections. It is almost as effective and less toxic, although it commonly causes diarrhea.

Before You Use This Drug

Do not use if you have or have had:

- severe adverse effects from previous gold treatments (bone marrow disease, low blood platelet count, severe skin rashes or intestinal diseases, formation of fibrous tissue in the lungs, protein in the urine)

Tell your doctor if you have or have had:

- allergies to drugs
- bone marrow depression or blood cell diseases
- decreased circulation to the heart or brain
- extreme weakness
- kidney disease
- skin rash, hives, or eczema
- lupus erythematosus
- Sjogren's syndrome, *for aurothioglucose*
- colitis
- blood or blood vessel disease

Tell your doctor about any other drugs you take, including aspirin, herbs, vitamins, and other nonprescription products.

When You Use This Drug

• Because you may lose consciousness and/or suffer allergic shock after an injection, take this drug in the presence of a friend or family member.

Interactions with Other Drugs

The following drugs are listed in the *Evaluations of Drug Interactions* 1997 as causing "highly clinically significant" or "clinically significant" interactions when used together with this drug. We have also included potentially serious interactions listed in the drug's FDA-approved professional product labeling or package insert. New scientific techniques have allowed researchers to predict some drug interactions before they have been documented in people. There may be other drugs, especially those in the families of drugs listed below, that also will react with this drug to cause severe adverse effects. The number of new drugs approved for marketing increases the chance of drug interactions, and new drug interactions are being identified with old drugs. Be vigilant. Make sure to tell your doctor and pharmacist the drugs you are taking and tell your doctor if you are taking any of these interacting drugs:

ANAPROX, ALEVE, nabumetone, NAPROSYN, naproxen, RELAFEN.

Adverse Effects

Call your doctor immediately, even if these occur many months after you stop taking the drug:

• skin rash, hives, itching or scaling
• bloody or cloudy urine
• coughing or trouble breathing
• diarrhea or stomach pain
• swelling of face, eyes, fingers, ankles, lower legs
• irritation or soreness of tongue or gums
• numbness or tingling in hands, arms or feet
• metallic taste in mouth
• sore throat and fever
• ulcers, sores or white spots in mouth or throat
• unusual bleeding or bruising
• unusual tiredness or weakness
• yellow eyes or skin
• hallucinations
• confusion
• changes in facial skin color
• decrease in blood pressure
• fainting

Call your doctor if these symptoms continue:

• dizziness, faintness
• flushing or redness of face
• nausea, vomiting
• gas, bloated feeling
• abdominal cramps or pain
• loss of appetite
• fever
• chills
• swollen glands

Periodic Tests

Ask your doctor which of these tests should be done periodically while you are taking this drug:

• white blood cell count*
• platelet count*
• hemoglobin or hematocrit*
• liver function tests
• kidney function tests
• urinary protein (before each injection)

Before each injection for the first six months, then less often as dosage decreases.

Do Not Use

ALTERNATIVE TREATMENT:
Oral (by mouth) narcotic painkillers.

Butorphanol
STADOL, STADOL NS (Bristol-Myers Squibb)

FAMILY: Narcotics (see p. 264)

Butorphanol (byoo *tor* fa nole) is a strong pain reliever chemically related to morphine, and milligram for milligram, about 25 to 50 times more potent. In 1978, the Food and Drug Administration ignored the advice of its own advisory committee, that had voted 12 to 2 to classify the injectable form of butorphanol as a controlled substance, and allowed the drug to be marketed as a non-narcotic.

The scope of distribution of butorphanol changed dramatically when, in 1992, Bristol-Myers Squibb sought and received approval for butorphanol nasal spray. Once this dosage form was approved, the company embarked on a major promotional campaign for butorphanol nasal spray. Advertising to doctors minimized the drug's adverse effects and addictive potential. During the first three years after the appearance of butorphanol nasal spray, the number of adverse drug reaction reports to the FDA increased from 60 to about 400 per year. Dependence and/or addiction was by far the most common adverse reaction.[117]

After 19 years on the market with countless unsuspecting consumers having become addicted to butorphanol, the Drug Enforcement Administration finally decided—in July 1997—to classify this drug as a controlled substance.

Though more potent, butorphanol is no more effective a pain reliever than morphine or other morphine-like drugs and is more expensive, particularly the nasal spray. There is no medical reason why you should be using butorphanol rather than morphine or other morphine-like drugs to control severe pain.

One hazard of taking butorphanol continuously for longer than several weeks is drug-induced dependence. **Do not stop taking your drug suddenly**. With the help of your doctor, work out a schedule for slowly decreasing the amount of the drug you take by about 5 to 10% each day. Keep a written record of the dosage reduction schedule with you. These steps will make it much easier to become drug free without developing distressing symptoms of drug withdrawal.

 Do Not Use

ALTERNATIVE TREATMENT:
See Aspirin, p. 275, and Aspirin with Codeine, p. 273.

Dihydrocodeine, Aspirin, and Caffeine
SYNALGOS-DC (Wyeth-Ayerst)

FAMILY: Painkillers
Fever Reducers
Narcotics (see p. 264)

This is a combination drug composed of aspirin (see p. 275), caffeine (ka *feen*) and dihydrocodeine (dye hye droe *koe* deen). However, it is an *irrational* combination because it includes caffeine. There is no acceptable scientific evidence that caffeine helps to relieve pain. Another problem with this combination is that it includes dihy-drocodeine, which is related to codeine (see p. 284) and is addictive. Rather than taking this drug, ask your doctor about taking plain aspirin (see p. 275) or, if necessary, aspirin with codeine (see p. 273).

ASPIRIN/REYES SYNDROME

Do not use this product for treating chicken pox, flu, or flu-like illness. It will increase the risk of contracting Reye's syndrome, a rare but often fatal disease.

One hazard of taking dihydrocodeine continuously for longer than several weeks is drug-induced dependence. **Do not stop taking your drug suddenly.** With the help of your doctor, work out a schedule for slowly decreasing the amount of the drug you take by about 5 to 10% each day. Keep a written record of the dosage reduction schedule with you. These steps will make it much easier to become drug free without developing distressing symptoms of drug withdrawal.

Do Not Use

ALTERNATIVE TREATMENT:
See Aspirin, p. 275, and Aspirin with Codeine, p. 273.

Pentazocine
TALWIN (Sanofi)

Pentazocine and Naloxone
TALWIN-NX (Sanofi)

FAMILY: Narcotics (see p. 264)

Pentazocine (pen *taz* oh seen) relieves moderate to severe pain. **Older adults should not use this drug, either alone or in combination with naloxone, because of the high risk of adverse effects, especially confusion.** The risk is so high that the World Health Organization recommends that this drug not be used if possible.[118] Pentazocine is also addictive.

One hazard of taking pentazocine continuously for longer than several weeks is drug-induced dependence. **Do not stop taking your drug suddenly.** With the help of your doctor, work out a schedule for slowly decreasing the amount of the drug you take by about 5 to 10% each day. Keep a written record of the dosage reduction schedule with you. These steps will make it much easier to become drug free without developing distressing symptoms of drug withdrawal.

Limited Use

Tolmetin
TOLECTIN (Ortho-McNeil Pharmaceutical)

GENERIC: available
FAMILY: Nonsteroidal Anti-inflammatory Drugs "NSAIDs" Arthritis Drugs (see p. 265)

Tolmetin (*tole* met in) belongs to the family of drugs called nonsteroidal anti-inflammatory drugs, shortened to NSAIDs (*n* sayds), often used to treat arthritis in older adults. NSAIDs can cause serious harm, even fatalities, from bleeding in the stomach or intestines. Bleeding can occur at any time and without warning and older people are more likely to experience adverse effects from bleeding. Older adults are also more likely to have reduced liver and kidney function. So, some doctors believe people over age 70 should be started with half the usual dose of drugs in this group.[119]

Tolmetin is used mainly to relieve the pain and inflammation of two kinds of arthritis, rheumatoid arthritis and osteoarthritis. **In general, if you are over 60, you should** take less than the usual adult dose, especially if you have decreased kidney function. Tolmetin has been reported to cause severe allergic reactions.[120] **You should never use tolmetin intermittently (on-and-off) because this greatly increases the risk of allergic reactions, which can be fatal.**

Aspirin (see p. 275) is just as effective and less costly than other NSAIDs and is the drug of choice for treating pain, fever, and inflammation in people who do not have ulcers, gastritis (inflammation of the stomach), or an allergy to aspirin. Some rheumatologists (arthritis specialists) prefer aspirin to other NSAIDs for treating rheumatoid arthritis.[121]

If you are taking tolmetin, ask your doctor if you can switch to taking enteric-coated aspirin (aspirin coated so it won't dissolve in the stomach) twice a day. If you cannot take aspirin and are having trouble with adverse effects on tolmetin, ask about switching to another NSAID such as ibuprofen (see p. 311) or naproxen (see p. 317). Each person responds differently to different NSAIDs.

WARNING

NONSTEROIDAL ANTI-INFLAMMATORY DRUG (NSAID) INDUCED GASTROINTESTINAL TOXICITY

All members of the NSAID family of drugs can cause gastrointestinal toxicity that can lead to gastrointestinal bleeding and hospitalization or death. The risk of gastrointestinal toxicity from these drugs increases with increasing doses and the length of treatment.

If the following symptoms develop while you are taking an NSAID, stop the drug immediately and contact your doctor: severe abdominal or stomach pain, cramping, or burning, severe and continuing nausea, heartburn, or indigestion, bloody or black, tarry stools, vomiting blood or material that looks like coffee grounds, or spitting up blood.

Before You Use This Drug

Do not use if you have or have had:

- an allergic reaction to aspirin, any other NSAID or iodides[122]
- peptic ulcers
- alcohol dependence
- nasal polyps or asthma

Tell your doctor if you have or have had:

- allergies to drugs
- heart, kidney, or liver problems
- hemophilia or other bleeding problems
- high blood pressure
- anemia
- asthma
- diabetes
- stomach or intestinal problems
- tobacco use
- epilepsy (seizures)
- mental depression or other psychiatric conditions
- Parkinson's disease
- lupus erythematosus

Tell your doctor about any other drugs you take, including aspirin, herbs, vitamins, and other nonprescription products.

When You Use This Drug

- Do not drink alcohol. It irritates the stomach lining and increases the risk of stomach bleeding.
- Call your doctor immediately if you have flu-like symptoms (chills, fever, muscle aches or pains) shortly before or with a skin rash. This may indicate a serious reaction to tolmetin.
- You may feel dizzy when rising from a lying or sitting position. If you are lying down, hang your legs over the side of the bed for a few minutes, then get up slowly. When getting up from a chair, stay by the chair until you are sure that you are not dizzy. (See p. 16.)
- If you plan to have any surgery, including dental, tell your doctor that you take this drug.

How to Use This Drug

• Take with food to reduce stomach irritation.

• Take with **a full glass (eight ounces) of water.** Do not lie down within 30 minutes afterward.

• If you miss a dose, take it as soon as possible, but skip it if it is almost time for the next dose. **Do not take double doses.**

• Store at room temperature, with lid on tightly. Do not store in the bathroom. Do not expose to moisture or heat.

Interactions with Other Drugs

The following drugs are listed in the *Evaluations of Drug Interactions* 1997 as causing "highly clinically significant" or "clinically significant" interactions when used together with this drug. We have also included potentially serious interactions listed in the drug's FDA-approved professional product labeling or package insert. New scientific techniques have allowed researchers to predict some drug interactions before they have been documented in people. There may be other drugs, especially those in the families of drugs listed below, that also will react with this drug to cause severe adverse effects. The number of new drugs approved for marketing increases the chance of drug interactions, and new drug interactions are being identified with old drugs. Be vigilant. Make sure to tell your doctor and pharmacist the drugs you are taking and tell your doctor if you are taking any of these interacting drugs:

bendroflumethiazide, BENEMID, CAPOTEN, captopril, COUMADIN, cyclosporine, digoxin, DILANTIN, GARAMYCIN, gentamicin, gold sodium thiomalate, INDERAL, INDERAL LA, ketorolac, LANOXICAPS, LANOXIN, lithium, LITHOBID, LITHONATE, methotrexate, MINIPRESS, MYOCHRYSINE, NATURETIN, NEORAL, phenytoin, prazosin, probenecid, propranolol, RHEUMATREX DOSE PACK, SANDIMMUNE, TORADOL, warfarin.

Adverse Effects

Call your doctor immediately if you experience:

• abdominal pain or swelling
• appetite loss
• bloody or black tarry stools
• increase or decrease in blood pressure
• difficulty breathing
• unusual bruising
• chest pains
• chills
• confusion
• depression
• drowsiness
• color changes in facial skin
• fever
• gastrointestinal pain, cramping or burning
• swollen glands
• headache
• hearing change or ringing or buzzing
• heartburn
• indigestion
• lower back, neck or side pain or stiffness
• muscle cramps or pain
• nausea, vomiting
• nosebleeds
• pinpoint red spots on skin
• skin rash, hives, itching
• sore throat
• sores, ulcers, or white spots on lips or in mouth
• swelling of face, lips, tongue, fingers, lower legs or feet
• continuous thirst
• irritated tongue
• unusual tiredness or weakness

- difficulty urinating
- bloody or cloudy urine
- vision change
- vomiting blood or material that looks like coffee grounds
- rapid weight gain
- yellow eyes or skin

Call your doctor if these symptoms continue:

- constipation, diarrhea, gas
- dizziness
- insomnia
- irritated or dry mouth
- muscle weakness
- nervousness, irritability
- weakness
- weight loss

Periodic Tests

Ask your doctor which of these tests should be done periodically while you are taking this drug:

- kidney function tests
- liver function tests
- stool tests for possible blood loss
- hematocrit and/or hemoglobin test
- blood concentrations of creatinine, potassium, and urea nitrogen
- white blood cell count
- upper GI diagnostic tests
- ophthalmologic exams

PREGNANCY WARNING

This drug caused harm to developing fetuses in animal studies, or such studies were not done. Use during pregnancy only for clear medical reasons. Tell your doctor if you are pregnant or thinking of becoming pregnant before you take this drug.

 Do Not Use

ALTERNATIVE TREATMENT:
Narcotic pain relievers.

Ketorolac
TORADOL (Roche)

FAMILY: Nonsteroidal Anti-inflammatory Drugs "NSAIDs"
Arthritis Drugs (see p. 265)

Ketorolac (kee *toe* role ak) belongs to the family of drugs called nonsteroidal anti-inflammatory drugs, shortened to NSAIDs (*n* sayds), often used to treat arthritis in older adults. NSAIDs can cause serious harm, even fatalities, from bleeding in the stomach or intestines. Bleeding can occur at any time and without warning and older people are more likely to experience adverse effects from bleeding. Older adults are also more likely to have reduced liver and kidney function. Some doctors believe people over age 70 should be started with half the usual dose of drugs in this group.[123]

Ketorolac is only approved for short-term use, five days or less, in the treatment of acute pain. This drug is available in both oral (by mouth) and injectable forms.

The professional product labeling, or package insert, for ketorolac warns about the risks of gastrointestinal bleeding, kidney and liver damage, against the use of the drug in labor and delivery, against the drug being used by nursing mothers, that it should not be used before or during surgery, and using anything but the lowest dose in small or older adults.

Other available pain relieving drugs are just as effective as ketorolac—or more so—without the risks. This drug should not be used.

Aspirin (see p. 275) is just as effective and less costly than other NSAIDs and is the drug of choice for treating pain, fever, and inflammation in people who do not have ulcers, gastritis (inflammation of the stomach), or an allergy to aspirin. Some rheumatologists (arthritis specialists) prefer aspirin to other NSAIDs for treating rheumatoid arthritis.[124]

If you are taking ketorolac ask your doctor if you can switch to taking enteric-coated aspirin (aspirin coated so it won't dissolve in the stomach) twice a day. If you cannot take aspirin, ask about switching to another drug in this family such as ibuprofen (see p. 311). Each person responds differently to different NSAIDs.

WARNING

NONSTEROIDAL ANTI-INFLAMMATORY DRUG (NSAID) INDUCED GASTROINTESTINAL TOXICITY

All members of the NSAID family of drugs can cause gastrointestinal toxicity that can lead to gastrointestinal bleeding and hospitalization or death. The risk of gastrointestinal toxicity from these drugs increases with increasing doses and the length of treatment.

If the following symptoms develop while you are taking an NSAID, stop the drug immediately and contact your doctor: severe abdominal or stomach pain, cramping, or burning, severe and continuing nausea, heartburn, or indigestion, bloody or black, tarry stools, vomiting blood or material that looks like coffee grounds, or spitting up blood.

Limited Use

Choline and Magnesium Salicylates
TRILISATE (Purdue Frederick)

Choline Salicylate
ARTHROPAN (Purdue Frederick)

Magnesium Salicylate
DOAN'S PILLS (Novartis)

GENERIC: available
FAMILY: Salicylates (see p. 261)

Choline (*koe* leen) and magnesium salicylates (mag *nee* zee um sa *li* si lates), alone or combined, relieve pain and reduce fever. They offer few advantages over aspirin (see p. 275). If you are allergic to aspirin, you may be able to use choline and magnesium salicylates. These drugs may cause fewer stomach problems than plain aspirin but are more expensive, may not be as effective, and have the same potential adverse effects.[125] For the vast majority of people, aspirin is the drug of choice. For long-term use, enteric-coated aspirin is best because it helps prevent stomach bleeding.

If you are taking choline or magnesium salicylates and you are over 60 years old, you should probably take less than the usual adult dose because of the risk of harmful adverse effects.

ASPIRIN/REYE'S SYNDROME ALERT

Do not use this product for treating chicken pox, flu, or flu-like illness. It will increase the risk of contracting Reye's syndrome, a rare but often fatal disease.

Before You Use This Drug

Tell your doctor if you have or have had:

- allergies to drugs
- a reaction to aspirin, other salicylates, or nonsteroidal anti-inflammatory drugs such as ibuprofen or naproxen
  - bleeding problems
  - ulcer or other stomach problems
  - anemia

- heart, kidney or liver problems
- gout
- overactive thyroid
- asthma
- nasal polyps
- glucose-6-phosphate dehydrogenase deficiency

Tell your doctor about any other drugs you take, including aspirin, herbs, vitamins, and other nonprescription products.

When You Use This Drug

- Do not drink alcohol. This combination increases the risk of stomach or intestinal bleeding.
- Never take more than the amount prescribed by your doctor or recommended on the package label.
- **Caution diabetics:** see p. 550.
- Do not take for five days before any surgery, unless your doctor or dentist tells you otherwise. These drugs interfere with your body's ability to stop bleeding.
- If you are on long-term or high-dose treatment, you should have regular checkups.
- Never place this drug directly on teeth or gums because it is irritating to these tissues.
- Do not chew this drug within one week after you have any type of mouth surgery.

How to Use This Drug

- Take tablets and capsules with **a full glass (eight ounces) of water.** Oral solutions may be mixed with fruit juice just before taking. Take after meals or with food to help protect your stomach. Do not lie down for 30 minutes.
- Do not store in the bathroom. Do not expose to heat, moisture, or strong light.
- If you miss a dose, take it as soon as you remember, but skip it if it is almost time for the next dose. **Do not take double doses.**

Interactions with Other Drugs

The following drugs are listed in the *Evaluations of Drug Interactions* 1997 as causing "highly clinically significant" or "clinically significant" interactions when used together with this drug. We have also included potentially serious interactions listed in the drug's FDA-approved professional product labeling or package insert. New scientific techniques have allowed researchers to predict some drug interactions before they have been documented in people. There may be other drugs, especially those in the families of drugs listed below, that also will react with this drug to cause severe adverse effects. The number of new drugs approved for marketing increases the chance of drug interactions, and new drug interactions are being identified with old drugs. Be vigilant. Make sure to tell your doctor and pharmacist the drugs you are taking and tell your doctor if you are taking any of these interacting drugs:

acetazolamide, aluminum hydroxide, AMPHOJEL, ANTURANE, CAPOTEN, captopril, chlorpropamide, COUMADIN, DEPAKENE/DEPAKOTE, DIABINESE, DIAMOX, ketorolac, magnesium hydroxide, MEDROL, methotrexate, methylprednisolone, PHILLIPS' MILK OF MAGNESIA, RHEUMATREX DOSE PACK, sulfinpyrazone, TORADOL, valproic acid, warfarin.

Adverse Effects

Call your doctor immediately if you experience:

- **signs of overdose:** mild to severe or persistent headache, ringing or buzzing in ears, loss of hearing, severe or continuing diarrhea, dizziness or lightheadedness, extreme drowsiness, confusion, nausea or vomiting, stomach pain, abnormal increase in sweating, abnormally fast or deep breathing, abnormal thirst, abnormal or uncontrolled flapping of the hands, vision problems, bloody urine, seizures, hallucinations, nervousness or excitement, trouble breathing, unexplained fever, difficulty swallowing, drowsiness, flushing, redness or change in skin color, sweating, nausea or vomiting, stomach pain, swelling of eyelids, face or lips

- vomiting material that looks bloody or like coffee grounds
- bloody or black, tarry stools
- wheezing, tightness in chest, or trouble breathing
- skin rash, hives, or itching
- fainting or dizzy spells

Call your doctor if these symptoms continue:

- heartburn or indigestion
- abnormal tiredness or weakness

Periodic Tests

Ask your doctor which of these tests should be done periodically while you are taking this drug:

- liver function tests
- salicylate and magnesium concentrations
- hematocrit detection

PREGNANCY WARNING

Magnesium salicylates caused harm to developing fetuses in animal studies, or such studies were not done. Use during pregnancy only for clear medical reasons. You should always tell your doctor if you are pregnant or thinking of becoming pregnant before you take this drug.

Acetaminophen
TYLENOL (Ortho-McNeil Consumer Products)

GENERIC: available
FAMILY: Painkillers
          Fever Reducers

Acetaminophen (a seat a *mee* noe fen), like aspirin, kills pain and reduces fever, but unlike aspirin does *not* help the redness, stiffness, or swelling of inflammation. Because of this, aspirin (see p. 275) is much more effective for treating the inflammation of arthritis.[126]

In general, you should not take anything to reduce a fever until the cause of the fever is known. It is rarely *necessary* to treat a fever. However, if a fever is having damaging effects

---

WARNING

There have been a number of case reports of liver damage involving a possible drug interaction between isoniazid, a medication used to prevent and treat tuberculosis, and acetaminophen, an over-the-counter painkiller and the active ingredient in Tylenol. Isoniazid alone, especially as people get older, has been documented to cause liver damage. Acetaminophen, alone in large doses or probably in combination with alcohol, also increases the risk of liver damage. The combination of acetaminophen with isoniazid, according to the authors of these case reports, may also be dangerous.[127]

If you are taking isoniazid for tuberculosis or have a positive TB skin test and are using the drug, consult your physician before using acetaminophen or any combination product containing acetaminophen. Discuss alternatives to acetaminophen with your physician.[128]

---

or is making you extremely uncomfortable, it can be reduced with acetaminophen. When you are taking acetaminophen to reduce a fever, you should take it regularly every three or four hours, and stop taking it when the underlying problem is gone or has been controlled through other treatment.

One advantage of acetaminophen over aspirin is that acetaminophen does not cause the stomach bleeding that aspirin can cause. For this reason, doctors often prescribe or recommend acetaminophen to people who are likely to suffer from bleeding when they take aspirin. This includes people taking blood-thinning drugs like warfarin or heparin and people who have ulcers, gout, or bleeding problems such as hemophilia. Also, people who are allergic to aspirin can often take acetaminophen.

On the other hand, for most people, aspirin is not likely to cause harmful stomach effects if taken in small amounts for a short time.[129] And acetaminophen has its own harmful effects—it can cause liver damage, especially in older adults, if you take more than the recommended dose or if you take it continuously for more than 10 days.[130]

Before You Use This Drug

Tell your doctor if you have or have had:

- allergies to drugs
- a reaction to acetaminophen
- alcohol dependence
- a viral infection
- kidney or liver problems
- phenylketonuria

Tell your doctor about any other drugs you take, including aspirin, herbs, vitamins, and other nonprescription products.

DRUG INTERACTION WARNING

INCREASED RISK OF BLEEDING WHEN ACETAMINOPHEN AND WARFARIN (COUMADIN) ARE TAKEN TOGETHER

Acetaminophen may interact with warfarin to increase the risk of bleeding. This risk increases with increasing doses of acetaminophen. The risk of bleeding has been found to increase tenfold in people who were taking 28 or more regular strength acetaminophen tablets per week, or the equivalent of 18 or more extra-strength tablets per week compared to those taking warfarin and no acetaminophen.[131] A regular strength tablet contains 325 milligrams of acetaminophen and extra-strength tablets contain 500 milligrams each of the drug.

Warfarin is a drug of considerable benefit after heart valve replacement and in preventing blood clots from a type of heart rhythm disturbance known as atrial fibrillation. It also reduces the risk of death, recurrent heart attacks, and stroke after a heart attack.

Based on this new evidence, if you are taking warfarin, you should notify your doctor before taking any product containing acetaminophen.

When You Use This Drug

- If you are treating yourself with acetaminophen, call your doctor if you have a fever that lasts for more than three days or if your symptoms do not improve.
- Do not take more than is recommended on the package or prescribed by your doctor.

- **Do not take for more than 10 days.**
- Do not drink alcohol. This combination increases the risk of liver damage.
- Acetaminophen may affect the results of lab tests for blood sugar or uric acid.

How to Use This Drug

- Do not store in the bathroom. Do not expose to heat, moisture, or strong light.
- Tablets may be crushed.
- Avoid buffered (sodium-containing) acetaminophen and acetaminophen products that include other ingredients such as caffeine. They increase the likelihood of harmful drug interactions and adverse effects.

Interactions with Other Drugs

The following drugs are listed in the *Evaluations of Drug Interactions* 1997 as causing "highly clinically significant" or "clinically significant" interactions when used together with this drug. We have also included potentially serious interactions listed in the drug's FDA-approved professional product labeling or package insert. New scientific techniques have allowed researchers to predict some drug interactions before they have been documented in people. There may be other drugs, especially those in the families of drugs listed below, that also will react with this drug to cause severe adverse effects. The number of new drugs approved for marketing increases the chance of drug interactions, and new drug interactions are being identified with old drugs. Be vigilant. Make sure to tell your doctor and pharmacist the drugs you are taking and tell your doctor if you are taking any of these interacting drugs:

INH, isoniazid.

Adverse Effects

Call your doctor immediately if you experience:

- **signs of overdose:** diarrhea, loss of appetite, nausea or vomiting, pain or cramps in stomach, sore or swollen upper abdomen, abnormal increase in sweating
  - yellow eyes or skin
  - bloody or cloudy urine
  - trouble urinating, painful urination, or sudden decrease in amount of urine
  - skin rash, hives, or itching
  - unexplained fever or sore throat
  - unusual bleeding or bruising
  - unusual tiredness or weakness
  - bloody or black, tarry stools
  - lower back or side pain
  - pinpoint red spots on skin
  - sores, ulcers or white spots on lips or in mouth

Periodic Tests

Ask your doctor which of these tests should be done periodically while you are taking this drug:

- liver function tests, for long-term or high-dose therapy

Acetaminophen and Codeine
TYLENOL NO. 3 (Ortho-McNeil Pharmaceutical)

GENERIC: available
FAMILY: Painkillers
Fever Reducers
Narcotics (see p. 264)

Acetaminophen (see p. 338) and codeine (see p. 284) are both effective painkillers. Together, they produce a rational combination drug that relieves pain better than acetaminophen alone but has less risk of adverse effects than the larger amount of codeine that would be needed if codeine were used alone. This combination is similar in effect to aspirin and codeine (see p. 273), except that acetaminophen, unlike aspirin, will not help the redness, stiffness, or swelling caused by rheumatoid arthritis or other types of inflammation. This combination is available in capsules and tablets and as a liquid.

Although this drug is the best choice in some situations, it is overused. Many people who are prescribed this combination would get pain relief from acetaminophen alone, and would avoid the harmful adverse effects that codeine can cause—addiction and constipation. So before taking this drug, ask your doctor about trying plain acetaminophen first.

WARNING

There have been a number of case reports of liver damage involving a possible drug interaction between isoniazid, a medication used to prevent and treat tuberculosis, and acetaminophen, an over-the-counter painkiller and the active ingredient in Tylenol. Isoniazid alone, especially as people get older, has been documented to cause liver damage. Acetaminophen, alone in large doses or probably in combination with alcohol, also increases the risk of liver damage. The combination of acetaminophen with isoniazid, according to the authors of these case reports, may also be dangerous.[132]

If you are taking isoniazid for tuberculosis or have a positive TB skin test and are using the drug, consult your physician before using acetaminophen or any combination product containing acetaminophen. Discuss alternatives to acetaminophen with your physician.[133]

DRUG INTERACTION WARNING

INCREASED RISK OF BLEEDING WHEN ACETAMINOPHEN AND WARFARIN (COUMADIN) ARE TAKEN TOGETHER

Acetaminophen may interact with warfarin to increase the risk of bleeding. This risk increases with increasing doses of acetaminophen. The risk of bleeding has been found to increase tenfold in people who were taking 28 or more regular strength acetaminophen tablets per week, or the equivalent of 18 or more extra-strength tablets per week compared to those taking warfarin and no acetaminophen.[134] A regular strength tablet contains 325 milligrams of acetaminophen and extra-strength tablets contain 500 milligrams each of the drug.

Warfarin is a drug of considerable benefit after heart value replacement and in preventing blood clots from a type of heart rhythm disturbance known as atrial fibrillation. It also reduces the risk of death, recurrent heart attacks, and stroke after a heart attack.

Based on this new evidence, if you are taking warfarin, you should notify your doctor before taking any product containing acetaminophen.

One hazard of taking codeine continuously for longer than several weeks is drug-induced dependence. **Do not stop taking your drug suddenly.** With the help of your doctor, work out a schedule for slowly decreasing the amount of the drug you take by about 5 to 10% each day. Keep a written record of the dosage reduction schedule with you. These steps will make it much easier to become drug free without developing distressing symptoms of drug withdrawal.

This drug can increase the risk of hip fracture.[135]

PREGNANCY WARNING

This drug caused harm to developing fetuses in animal studies, or such studies were not done. Use during pregnancy only for clear medical reasons. Tell your doctor if you are pregnant or thinking of becoming pregnant before you take this drug.

Do Not Use

ALTERNATIVE TREATMENT:
Ibuprofen or combination painkillers containing a narcotic with acetaminophen.

Tramadol
ULTRAM (Oortho-McNeil)
FAMILY: Narcotics (see p. 264)

Tramadol (tra *ma* dole) is an old German painkiller first marketed in 1977, but not sold in the U.S. until 1995. It is heavily promoted to doctors as being equivalent to acetaminophen with codeine (TYLENOL WITH CODEINE), and having a low potential to cause addiction. Tramadol was approved without being classified as a controlled substance, even though it has many chemical similarities to narcotic drugs like morphine and codeine. After being on the market for only one year in this country, serious adverse reactions were reported with tramadol, even after the first dose, including seizures, dependence, and severe allergic reactions.

Within the first year of marketing the Food and Drug Administration (FDA) had received 83 reports of seizures or convulsions among people using tramadol.[136] During its second year on the market, the FDA received more than 200 reports of seizures. Many of these reports noting seizures occurred within one day of starting tramadol. Most of these people were healthy and between the ages of 20 and 39 years, and most had no previous history of seizures. This adverse reaction can occur at recommended dosages, although an overdose may increase the risk of tramadol related seizures. Taking tramadol with antidepressant drugs, including the new selective serotonin reuptake inhibitors and older tricyclic antidepressants, increases the risk of seizures.[137] The FDA conservatively estimates that for every report of an adverse drug reaction, ten go unreported.

Tramadol has effects similar to the narcotic pain relievers morphine and codeine including the potential to cause addiction, but it was not classified as a controlled substance at the time of its approval. Ortho-McNeil Pharmaceutical of Raritan NJ, the producer of the drug, advertised heavily to doctors that tramadol had a low potential for abuse. Within the drug's first year on the market, the FDA had received 115 reports of adverse events described as drug abuse, dependence, withdrawal, or intentional overdose associated with the use of tramadol.[138] Countless consumers who were not told that tramadol was addicting may have unknowingly become dependent on this drug.

Tramadol appears to be no more and sometimes less effective than combinations of codeine with aspirin or acetaminophen.[139] It is more dangerous, less effective, and more expensive than other comparable pain relievers and the FDA should take steps immediately to begin procedures to withdraw tramadol from the market.

Limited Use

Diclofenac
VOLTAREN (Novartis)

GENERIC: available

FAMILY: Nonsteroidal Anti-inflammatory Drugs "NSAIDs"
Arthritis Drugs (see p. 265)

Diclofenac (dick *low* fen ak) belongs to the family of drugs called nonsteroidal anti-inflammatory drugs, shortened to NSAIDs (*n* sayds), often used to treat arthritis in older adults. NSAIDs can cause serious harm, even fatalities, from bleeding in the stomach or intestines. Bleeding can occur at any time and without warning and older people are more likely to experience adverse effects from bleeding. Older adults are also more likely to have reduced liver and kidney function. Some doctors believe people over age 70 should be started with half the usual dose of drugs in this group.[140] Like other NSAIDs, diclofenac relieves symptoms but does not cure any condition.

Diclofenac is used to treat mild to moderate pain and symptoms of rheumatoid arthritis, osteoarthritis, and spondylitis. **In general, if you are over 60, you should take less than the usual adult dose, especially if you have decreased kidney function.**

According to the International Agranulocytosis and Aplastic Anemia Study of 1986, toxic effects to the bone marrow and killing of white blood cells happen with diclofenac at a rate as high as with phenylbutazone[141] (see p. 281). There have also been a number of cases of severe hepatitis in patients using diclofenac.[142]

Aspirin (see p. 275) is just as effective and less costly than other NSAIDs and is the drug of choice to treat pain, fever, and inflammation in people who do not have ulcers, gastritis (inflammation of the stomach), or an allergy to aspirin. Some rheumatologists (arthritis specialists) prefer aspirin to other NSAIDs for rheumatoid arthritis.[143]

If you are taking diclofenac ask your doctor if you can switch to taking enteric-coated aspirin (aspirin coated so it won't dissolve in your stomach) twice a day. If you cannot take aspirin, ask about switching to another drug in this family such as ibuprofen (see p. 311). Each person responds differently to different NSAIDs.

WARNING

NONSTEROIDAL ANTI-INFLAMMATORY DRUG (NSAID) INDUCED GASTROINTESTINAL TOXICITY

All members of the NSAID family of drugs can cause gastrointestinal toxicity that can lead to gastrointestinal bleeding and hospitalization or death. The risk of gastrointestinal toxicity from these drugs increases with increasing doses and the length of treatment.

If the following symptoms develop while you are taking an NSAID, stop the drug immediately and contact your doctor: severe abdominal or stomach pain, cramping, or burning, severe and continuing nausea, heartburn, or indigestion, bloody or black, tarry stools, vomiting blood or material that looks like coffee grounds, or spitting up blood.

Before You Use This Drug

Do not use if you have or have had:

- an allergic reaction to aspirin, any other NSAID or iodides[144]
- peptic ulcers
- alcohol dependence
- nasal polyps

Tell your doctor if you have or have had:

- allergies to drugs
- heart, kidney or liver problems
- hemophilia or other bleeding problems
- high blood pressure
- blood transfusion[145]
- hemorrhoids[146]
- occupational exposure to chemicals[147]
- psoriasis[148]
- salt-restricted diet[149]
- seizures[150]
- anemia
- asthma
- diabetes
- stomach or intestinal problems
- tobacco use

Tell your doctor about any other drugs you take, including aspirin, herbs, vitamins, and other nonprescription products.

When You Use This Drug

- Do not drink alcohol. It irritates the stomach lining and increases the risk of stomach bleeding.
- Call your doctor immediately if you have flu-like symptoms (chills, fever, muscle aches or pains) shortly before or with a skin rash. This may indicate a serious reaction to diclofenac.
- You may feel dizzy when rising from a lying or sitting position. If you are lying down, hang your legs over the side of the bed for a few minutes, then get up slowly. When getting up from a chair, stay by the chair until you are sure that you are not dizzy. (See p. 16.)

- Do not drive or perform other activities that require alertness because this drug may make you drowsy, dizzy, or lightheaded.
- If you plan to have any surgery, including dental, tell your doctor that you take this drug.

How to Use This Drug

- Take with food to reduce stomach irritation.
- Take with **a full glass (eight ounces) of water.** Do not lie down for 30 minutes afterwards.
- If you miss a dose, take it as soon as possible, but skip it if is almost time for the next dose. **Do not take double doses.**
- Store at room temperature, with lid on tightly. Do not store in the bathroom. Do not expose to moisture or heat.

Interactions with Other Drugs

The following drugs are listed in the *Evaluations of Drug Interactions* 1997 as causing "highly clinically significant" or "clinically significant" interactions when used together with this drug. We have also included potentially serious interactions listed in the drug's FDA-approved professional product labeling or package insert. New scientific techniques have allowed researchers to predict some drug interactions before they have been documented in people. There may be other drugs, especially those in the families of drugs listed below, that also will react with this drug to cause severe adverse effects. The number of new drugs approved for marketing increases the chance of drug interactions, and new drug interactions are being identified with old drugs. Be vigilant. Make sure to tell your doctor and pharmacist the drugs you are taking and tell your doctor if you are taking any of these interacting drugs:

bendroflumethiazide, CAPOTEN, captopril, COUMADIN, cyclosporine, DEXATRIM, digoxin, DILANTIN, DYAZIDE, DYRENIUM,

GARAMYCIN, gentamicin, gold sodium thiomalate, INDERAL, INDERAL LA, ketorolac, LANOXICAPS, LANOXIN, lithium, LITHOBID, LITHONATE, MAXZIDE, methotrexate, MINIPRESS, MYOCHRYSINE, NATURETIN, NEORAL, phenylpropanolamine, phenytoin, prazosin, propranolol, RHEUMATREX DOSE PACK, SANDIMMUNE, TORADOL, triamterene, triamterene and hydrochlorothiazide, warfarin.

Adverse Effects

Call your doctor immediately if you experience:

- abdominal pain or swelling
- appetite loss
- bloody or black, tarry stools
- increase or decrease in blood pressure
- difficulty breathing
- unusual bruising
- chest pains
- chills
- confusion
- convulsions
- cough or hoarseness
- depression
- drowsiness
- color changes in facial skin
- fever
- forgetfulness
- gastrointestinal pain, cramping or burning
- swollen glands
- headache
- hearing change or ringing or buzzing
- heartburn
- hives on face, eyelids or tongue
- indigestion
- lower back, neck or side pain
- unusually heavy menstrual bleeding
- muscle cramps or pain
- nausea, vomiting
- nosebleeds
- numbness, tingling, pain or weakness in hands or feet
- pinpoint red spots on skin
- psychotic reaction
- rectal bleeding
- skin rash, blisters, hives, itching, scaling
- sore throat
- sores, ulcers, or white spots on lips or in mouth
- swelling of face, lips, tongue, fingers, lower legs or feet
- unusual tiredness or weakness
- difficulty urinating
- bloody or cloudy urine
- vision change
- vomiting blood or material that looks like coffee grounds
- rapid weight gain
- yellow eyes and skin

Call your doctor if these symptoms continue:

- constipation, diarrhea, gas
- dizziness
- flushing or hot flashes
- irregular heartbeat
- insomnia
- irritated or dry mouth
- nervousness, irritability
- sunburn
- sweating
- bitter taste
- trembling
- weakness
- weight loss
- hair loss or changes in nails[151]

Periodic Tests

Ask your doctor which of these tests should be done periodically while you are taking this drug:

- kidney function tests
- liver function tests
- stool tests for possible blood loss

- hematocrit and/or hemoglobin test
- blood concentrations of creatinine, potassium, and urea nitrogen
- white blood cell count
- upper GI diagnostic tests
- ophthalmologic exams

Lidocaine
XYLOCAINE (Astra)

GENERIC: available

FAMILY: Anesthetics
Antiarrhythmics

Lidocaine (*lye* doe kane) is used to treat disturbances in heartbeats (arrhythmias) and as a local anesthetic. This page does not discuss its use for irregular heartbeats, since this use occurs mostly in the hospital. As a local anesthetic, a lidocaine injection or ointment is used for minor surgical procedures and for pain relief.

Before You Use This Drug

Do not use if you have or have had:

- Adams-Stokes syndrome (fainting episodes due to brief failure of the heart to pump)
- complete heart block
- allergies to novocaine

Tell your doctor if you have or have had:

- allergies to drugs
- heart, kidney or liver problems
- congestive heart failure
- low blood pressure or shock due to fluid loss

Tell your doctor about any other drugs you take, including aspirin, herbs, vitamins, and other nonprescription products.

When You Use This Drug

- The ointment form of this drug (used as an anesthetic) should not be used for a long time.

How to Use This Drug

- Do not apply ointment to large areas of your body. Use the smallest amount that is effective, to avoid absorbing large amounts of the drug into your bloodstream.
- If you use this drug in your mouth or throat, do not eat or chew gum for one hour afterward. The drug's anesthetic effect may make it hard for you to swallow and increase your risk of badly biting your tongue or cheek.

Interactions with Other Drugs

The following drugs are listed in the *Evaluations of Drug Interactions* 1997 as causing "highly clinically significant" or "clinically significant" interactions when used together with this drug. We have also included potentially serious interactions listed in the drug's FDA-approved professional product labeling or package insert. New scientific techniques have allowed researchers to predict some drug interactions before they have been documented in people. There may be other drugs, especially those in the families of drugs listed below, that also will react with this drug to cause severe adverse effects. The number of new drugs approved for marketing increases the chance of drug interactions, and new drug interactions are being identified with old drugs. Be vigilant. Make sure to tell your doctor and pharmacist the drugs you are taking and tell your doctor if you are taking any of these interacting drugs:

amiodarone, ANECTINE, cimetidine, CORDARONE, INDERAL, INDERAL LA, propranolol, ritodrine, succinylcholine, TAGAMET, YUTOPAR.

Adverse Effects

Call your doctor immediately if you experience:

- **signs of overdose:** blurred or double vision, nausea or vomiting, ringing in ears, tremors or

twitching, convulsions, difficulty breathing, dizziness or fainting, unusually slow heartbeat
- itching or skin rash
- unusual swelling of skin (allergic reaction)

Call your doctor if these symptoms continue:
- pain at the site of injection
- anxiety, nervousness
- drowsiness
- feelings of coldness, heat, or numbness

Periodic Tests

Ask your doctor which of these tests should be done periodically while you are taking this drug:
- heart function tests, such as electrocardiogram (ECG, EKG)
- blood pressure
- blood levels of lidocaine and electrolytes

Limited Use

Allopurinol
ZYLOPRIM (Glaxo Wellcome)

GENERIC: available

FAMILY: Antigout Drugs (see p. 265)

Allopurinol (al oh *pure* i nole) helps to prevent gout attacks. Gout occurs in people who have high levels of uric acid in their body, and an attack occurs when crystals of uric acid form in your joints and your body releases chemicals in response to the crystals. This causes pain and inflammation. Allopurinol works by decreasing your body's production of uric acid and thereby lowering the level of uric acid in your blood.

Allopurinol will not relieve a gout attack that has already started. If you are taking allopurinol, keep taking it during an attack, even if another drug is prescribed to treat the attack.

After you start using allopurinol, your gout attacks may become more frequent for a while.

Keep taking the drug. If you take it regularly, the attacks gradually will become less frequent and less painful, and they may stop completely after several months.

Allopurinol can cause skin rashes, allergic reactions and kidney stones. **Stop taking allopurinol and call your doctor at the first sign of skin rash or allergic reaction.** To help prevent kidney stones while taking allopurinol, drink at least 10 to 12 full glasses (eight ounces each) of fluid each day, unless your doctor tells you otherwise. Too much vitamin C (see p. 614) also increases your risk of forming kidney stones, so do not take vitamin C supplements while you are taking allopurinol unless you have checked with your doctor first.

Before You Use This Drug

Tell your doctor if you have or have had:
- allergies to drugs
- kidney function impairment
- diabetes
- heart disease or high blood pressure

Tell your doctor about any other drugs you take, including aspirin, herbs, vitamins, and other nonprescription products.

When You Use This Drug
- Do not drink alcohol. Alcohol increases the amount of uric acid in your blood and may make your gout attacks more frequent and more difficult to control. It also increases your risk of stomach problems.
- Until you know how you react to this drug, do not drive or perform other activities requiring alertness. Allopurinol can cause drowsiness.

How to Use This Drug
- Take with food to decrease stomach upset. If this does not work and your stomach continues to be upset, check with your doctor.

- Do not store in the bathroom. Do not expose to heat, moisture, or strong light.
- If you miss a dose, take it as soon as you remember, but skip it if you don't remember until the next day. **Do not take double doses.**

Interactions with Other Drugs

The following drugs are listed in the *Evaluations of Drug Interactions* 1997 as causing "highly clinically significant" or "clinically significant" interactions when used together with this drug. We have also included potentially serious interactions listed in the drug's FDA-approved professional product labeling or package insert. New scientific techniques have allowed researchers to predict some drug interactions before they have been documented in people. There may be other drugs, especially those in the families of drugs listed below, that also will react with this drug to cause severe adverse effects. The number of new drugs approved for marketing increases the chance of drug interactions, and new drug interactions are being identified with old drugs. Be vigilant. Make sure to tell your doctor and pharmacist the drugs you are taking and tell your doctor if you are taking any of these interacting drugs:

> ARA-A, ARABINOSIDE, cyclophosphamide, CYTOXAN, dicumarol, DILANTIN, ELIXO-PHYLLIN, mercaptopurine, phenytoin, PURINETHOL, SLO-BID, THEO-24, theophylline, vidarabine, VIRA-A.

Adverse Effects

Call your doctor immediately if you experience:

- skin rash, hives, itching
- bloody or cloudy urine
- difficult or painful urination
- lower back or side pain
- chills, fever, or muscle aches
- nausea or vomiting along with chills or fever
- numbness or tingling of hands or feet
- red, thick, tender, burning or scaly skin
- sore throat and fever
- unusual bleeding or bruising
- unusual tiredness or weakness
- decrease in amount of urine
- yellow eyes or skin
- loosening of fingernails
- weight gain
- difficulty breathing
- nosebleeds
- bloody or black, tarry stools
- bleeding sores on lips
- pinpoint red spots on skin
- sores, ulcers or white spots in mouth or on lips
- swelling in stomach area
- swelling of face, fingers, feet or lower legs
- swollen glands

Call your doctor if these symptoms continue:

- diarrhea
- drowsiness
- nausea, vomiting, or stomach pain
- headache
- hair loss

Periodic Tests

Ask your doctor which of these tests should be done periodically while you are taking this drug:

- complete blood count
- liver function tests
- kidney function tests
- blood levels of uric acid

PREGNANCY WARNING

This drug caused harm to developing fetuses in animal studies, or such studies were not done. Use during pregnancy only for clear medical reasons. Tell your doctor if you are pregnant or thinking of becoming pregnant before you take this drug.

NOTES FOR PAINKILLERS AND ARTHRITIS DRUGS

1. 42 *Federal Register* 35390. July 8, 1977.
2. *The Medical Letter on Drugs and Therapeutics.* New York: The Medical Letter Inc., 1991; 33:66.
3. Plotz P. Aspirin and Salicylates. In *Textbook of Rheumatology,* W. Kelley, ed., Philadelphia: Saunders, 1985.
4. *The Medical Letter on Drugs and Therapeutics.* New York: The Medical Letter Inc., 1976; 18:119.
5. Orland MJ, Saltman RJ, eds. *Manual of Medical Therapeutics.* 25th ed. Boston: Little, Brown and Company, 1986:373.
6. Herxheimer A. Many NSAID users who bleed don't know when to stop. *British Medical Journal* 1998; 316:492 [editorial].
7. Wynne HA, Long A. Patient awareness of the adverse effects of nonsteroidal anti-inflammatory drugs (NSAIDs). *British Journal of Clinical Pharmacology* 1996; 42:253–6.
8. Gilman AG, Goodman LS, Rall TW, Murad F, eds. *The Pharmacological Basis of Therapeutics.* 7th ed. New York: Macmillan, 1985.
9. Angell M. The quality of mercy. *New England Journal of Medicine* 1982; 306:98–9.
10. Simonson W. *Medications and the Elderly.* Rockville, MD: Aspen Systems Corporation, 1984:116.
11. *The Medical Letter on Drugs and Therapeutics.* New York: The Medical Letter Inc., 1982; 24:96.
12. AMA Department of Drugs. *AMA Drug Evaluations.* 5th ed. Chicago: American Medical Association, 1983:70.
13. Vestal RE, ed. *Drug Treatment in the Elderly.* Sydney, Australia: ADIS Health Science Press, 1984.179.
14. Plotz, op. cit.
15. *USP DI, Drug Information for the Health Care Professional.* 12th ed. Rockville MD: The United States Pharmacopeial Convention Inc., 1992:460–70.
16. *The Medical Letter on Drugs and Therapeutics.* New York: The Medical Letter Inc., 1980; 22:29–31.
17. Olin BR, ed. *Facts and Comparisons.* St. Louis: J.B. Lippincott Co., September 1992:251b.
18. American Society of Hospital Pharmacists. *American Hospital Formulary Service Drug Information,* Bethesda, MD, 1992:1698–9.
19. *USP DI,* op. cit.
20. Kaufhold J, Wilkowski M, McCabe K. Flurbiprofen-associated acute tubulointerstitial nephritis. *American Journal of Nephrology* 1991; 11:144–6.
21. Shorr RI. Opioid analgesics and the risk of hip fracture in the elderly: codeine and propoxyphene. *Journal of Gerontology* 1992; 47:M111–5.
22. Hylek EM, Heiman H, Skates SJ, Sheehan MA, Singer DE. Acetaminophen and other risk factors for excessive warfarin anticoagulation. *Journal of the American Medical Association* 1998; 279:657–62.
23. Murphy R, Swartz R, Watkins PB. Severe acetaminophen toxicity in a patient receiving isoniazid. *Annals of Internal Medicine* 1990; 113:799–800.
24. Moulding TS, Redeker AG, Konel GC. Acetaminophen, isoniazid, and hepatic toxicity. *Annals of Internal Medicine* 1991; 114:431.
25. *USP DI,* op. cit.
26. Orland, op. cit., p. 2.
27. 42 *Federal Register* 35480, July 8, 1977.
28. *USP DI,* op. cit.
29. *Drugs for the Elderly.* 2nd ed. Copenhagen, Denmark: World Health Organization, 1997:95
30. *The Medical Letter on Drugs and Therapeutics,* 1980, op. cit.
31. *USP DI,* op. cit.
32. Patrono C, Dunn MJ. The clinical significance of inhibition of renal prostaglandin synthesis. *Kidney International* 1987; 32:42.
33. *The Medical Letter on Drugs and Therapeutics,* 1980, op. cit.
34. Olin, op. cit.
35. Shorr, op. cit.
36. Wallace SL, Singer JZ, Duncan GJ, Wigley FM, Kuncl RW. Renal function predicts colchicine toxicity: guidelines for the prophylactic use of colchicine in gout. *Journal of Rheumatology* 1991; 18:264–9.
37. Miller RR, Feingold A, Paxinos J. Propoxyphene hydrochloride: a critical review. *Journal of the American Medical Association* 1970; 213: 996–1006.
38. Moertel CG, Ahmann DL, Taylor WF, Schwartan N. A comparative evaluation of marketed analgesic drugs. *New England Journal of Medicine* 1972; 286:813–5.
39. Avorn JL, Lamy PP, Vestal RE. Prescribing for the elderly—safely. *Patient Care* 1982; 16:14–62.
40. Ibid.
41. Shorr, op. cit.
42. Murphy, op. cit.
43. Moulding, op. cit.
44. Orland, op. cit., p. 373.
45. Plotz, op. cit.
46. *USP DI,* op. cit.
47. Plotz, op. cit.
48. *The Medical Letter on Drugs and Therapeutics,* 1980, op. cit.
49. *USP DI,* op. cit.
50. Dear Health Care Professional Letter from Phillip J. de Vane, MD, Vice President Clinical Affairs, Wyeth-Ayerst Laboratories, dated February 1998.
51. *The Medical Letter on Drugs and Therapeutics.* New York: The Medical Letter Inc., 1997; 39:93–4.
52. *The Medical Letter on Drugs and Therapeutics,* 1980, op. cit.
53. *USP DI, Drug Information for the Health Care Professional.* 16th ed. Rockville MD: The United States Pharmacopeial Convention Inc., 1996: 1448–54.
54. Ibid.
55. American Society of Health System Pharmacists. *American Hospital Formulary Service Drug Information,* Bethesda, MD, 1996.
56. *USP DI,* 1996, op. cit.
57. Ibid.
58. Murphy, op. cit.
59. Moulding, op. cit.
60. *USP DI,* 1992, op. cit.
61. Wolfe S. The safety of piroxicam. *the Lancet* 1986; 2:808–9.
62. Armstrong CP, Blower AL. Ulcerogenicity of piroxicam. *British Medical Journal* 1987; 294:772.
63. *The Medical Letter on Drugs and Therapeutics,* 1980, op. cit.
64. *Drugs for the Elderly,* op. cit.
65. Shorr, op. cit.
66. Younger IR, Harris DWS, Colver GB. Azathioprine in dermatology. *Journal of the American Academy of Dermatology* 1991; 25:281–6.
67. Yudkin PL, Ellison GW, Ghezzi A, Goodkin DE, Hughes RAC, McPherson K, Mertin J, Milanese C. Overview of azathioprine treatment in multiple sclerosis. *The Lancet* 1991; 338:1051–5.
68. American Society of Hospital Pharmacists, op. cit., p. 2252–5.
69. Singh G, Fries JF, Williams CA, Zatarain E, Spitz P, Block DA. Toxicity profiles of disease modifying antirheumatic drugs in rheumatoid arthritis. *The Journal of Rheumatology* 1991; 18:188–94.

70. Callen JP, Spencer LV, Burruss JB, Holtman J. Azathioprine: An effective, corticosteroid-sparing therapy for patients with recalcitrant cutaneous lupus erythematosus or with recalcitrant cutaneous leukocytoclastic vasculitis. *Archives of Dermatology* 1991; 127:515–22.

71. Singh, op. cit.

72. *USP DI,* 1992, op. cit.

73. Orland, op. cit., p. 373.

74. *Physicians' Desk Reference.* 40th ed. Oradell NJ: Medical Economics Company, 1986:1187.

75. *USP DI, Drug Information for the Health Care Provider.* 6th ed. Rockville MD: The United States Pharmacopeial Convention, Inc., 1986:871.

76. Kastrup EK, ed. *Facts and Comparisons.* St. Louis: J.B. Lippincott Co., July 1987:732b.

77. *The Medical Letter on Drugs and Therapeutics,* 1980, op. cit.

78. *USP DI,* 1992, op. cit.

79. Nabumetone (Relafen) Warning Letter to Howard Pien, President, North America, SmithKline Beecham Pharmaceuticals from Minnie Baylor-Henry, R.Ph., J.D., Director, Division of Drug Marketing, Advertising, and Communications, Food and Drug Administration, dated March 13, 1998.

80. Balfour JA, Buckley MMT. Etodolac a reappraisal of its pharmacology and therapeutic use in rheumatic diseases and pain states. *Drugs* 1991; 42(2):274–99.

81. Bem JL, Breckenridge AM, Mann RD, Rawlins MD. Review of yellow cards (1986): Report to the Committee on the Safety of Medicines. *British Journal of Clinical Pharmacology* 1988; 26:679–89.

82. Hughes G. Therapeutic choices for rheumatic disorders. *Gerontology* 1988; 34 (Suppl. 1):27–32.

83. *The Medical Letter on Drugs and Therapeutics,* 1991, op. cit., p. 79–80.

84. Olin, op. cit.

85. Taha AS, McLaughlin S, Sturrock RD, Russell RI. Evaluation of the efficacy and comparative effects on gastric and duodenal mucosa of etodolac and naproxen in patients with rheumatoid arthritis using endoscopy. *British Journal of Rheumatology* 1989; 28:329–32.

86. *USP DI,* 1992, op. cit.

87. Gilman, op. cit.

88. Ibid.

89. *The Medical Letter on Drugs and Therapeutics,* 1980, op. cit.

90. AMA, op. cit., p. 123.

91. Olin, op. cit.

92. Tilley BC, Alarcón GS, Heyse ST, Trentham DE, Neuner R, Kaplan DA, et al. Minocycline in rheumatoid arthritis: a 48-week, double-blind, placebo-controlled trial. *Annals of Internal Medicine* 1995; 122:81–9.

93. *USP DI,* 1992, op. cit.

94. *The Medical Letter on Drugs and Therapeutics,* 1980, op. cit.

95. Olin, op. cit

96. *USP DI,* 1992, op. cit.

97. George Washington University. *Drug Information Bulletin,* January/February 1987; 12(1).

98. Kastrup, op. cit, p. 251a-c

99. Ibid.

100. *The Medical Letter on Drugs and Therapeutics,* 1980, op. cit.

101. Olin, op. cit.

102. *USP DI,* 1992, op. cit.

103. *The Medical Letter on Drugs and Therapeutics,* 1980, op. cit.

104. Olin, op. cit.

105. *USP DI,* 1992, op. cit.

106. Veys EM. 20 years' experience with ketoprofen. *Scandinavian Journal of Rheumatology* 1991; Suppl. 90:3–44.

107. Ibid.

108. *The Medical Letter on Drugs and Therapeutics,* 1980, op. cit.

109. Olin, op. cit.

110. *USP DI,* 1992, op. cit.

111. Neuvonen PJ. The effect of magnesium hydroxide on the oral absorption of ibuprofen, ketoprofen and diclofenac. *British Journal of Clinical Pharmacology* 1991; 31:263–6.

112. Murphy, op. cit.

113. Moulding, op. cit.

114. Hylek, op. cit.

115. Fong NL. Chemotherapy and nutritional management. In *Nutritional Management of the Cancer Patient,* edited by Walford. New York: Raven Press, 1979.

116. Orland, op. cit., p. 375.

117. Fisher MA, Glass S. Butorphanol (Stadol): a study in problems of current drug information and control. *Neurology* 1997; 48:1156–60.

118. *Drugs for the Elderly,* op. cit.

119. *USP DI,* 1992, op. cit.

120. Kastrup, op. cit., p. 251a-c.

121. *The Medical Letter on Drugs and Therapeutics,* 1980, op. cit.

122. Olin, op. cit.

123. *USP DI,* 1992, op. cit.

124. *The Medical Letter on Drugs and Therapeutics,* 1980, op. cit.

125. Orland, op. cit., p. 373.

126. *The Medical Letter on Drugs and Therapeutics,* 1976, op. cit., p. 73.

127. Murphy, op. cit.

128. Moulding, op. cit.

129. Orland, op. cit., p. 2.

130. 42 *Federal Register,* 35480, July 8, 1977.

131. Hylek, op. cit.

132. Murphy, op. cit.

133. Moulding, op. cit.

134. Hylek, op. cit.

135. Shorr, op. cit.

136. Dear Health Care Professional Letter from Thomas Gibson MD, Executive Director for Medical Affairs, Ortho-McNeil Pharmaceutical, dated March 20, 1996.

137. Kahn LH, Alderfer RJ, Graham DJ. Seizures reported with tramadol. *Journal of the American Medical Association* 1997; 278:1661[letter].

138. Gibson letter, op. cit.

139. *The Medical Letter on Drugs and Therapeutics.* New York. The Medical Letter, Inc; 1995; 37:59–60.

140. *USP DI,* 1992, op. cit.

141. AMA Department of Drugs. *AMA Drug Evaluations.* 8th ed. Chicago: American Medical Association, 1991:1706–7.

142. Helfgott SM, Sandberg-Cook J, Zakim D, Nestler J. Diclofenac-associated hepatotoxicity. *Journal of the American Medical Association* 1990; 264:2660–2.

143. *The Medical Letter on Drugs and Therapeutics,* 1980, op. cit.

144. Olin, op. cit.

145. Gay GR. Another side effect of NSAIDs. *Journal of the American Medical Association* 1990; 264:2677–8.

146. Stadler P, Armstrong D, Margalith D, Saraga E, Stolte M, Lualdi P, et al. Diclofenac delays healing of gastroduodenal mucosal lesions. *Digestive Diseases and Sciences* 1991; 36:594–600.

147. Gay, op. cit.

148. Dukes MNG, Beeley L. *Side Effects of Drugs Annual* 13, Amsterdam: Elsevier, 1989:80.

149. *USP DI,* 1992, op. cit.

150. Heim M, Nadvorna H, Azaria M. Grand mal seizures following treatment with diclofenac and pentazocine. *South African Medical Journal* 1990; 78:700–1.

151. Dukes, op. cit., p. 74.

Gastrointestinal Drugs

Diarrhea		**352**
Constipation		**354**
Gas		**354**

DRUG LISTINGS

ULCER DRUGS

Antibiotic Treatment for Ulcer Disease		354
AXID		383
CARAFATE	Limited Use	363
cimetidine		395
CYTOTEC	Limited Use	369
famotidine		383
lansoprazole	Do Not Use Until Five Years After Release	389
misoprostol	Limited Use	369
nizatidine		383
omeprazole	Limited Use	389
PEPCID		383
PREVACID	Do Not Use Until Five Years After Release	389
PRILOSEC	Limited Use	389
ranitidine		383
sucralfate	Limited Use	363
TAGAMET		395
ZANTAC		383

ANTACIDS AND COATING AGENTS

aluminum hydroxide	Limited Use	358
aluminum hydroxide and magnesium carbonate		373
aluminum hydroxide and magnesium hydroxide		378
AMPHOJEL	Limited Use	358
GAVISCON		373
GAVISCON-2		373
MAALOX		378
MAALOX TC		378
magaldrate		378
magnesium hydroxide	Limited Use	388
magnesium hydroxide, aluminum hydroxide, and simethicone	Ⓧ Do Not Use	381
M.O.M.	Limited Use	388
MYLANTA	Ⓧ Do Not Use	381
MYLANTA-II	Ⓧ Do Not Use	381
MYLICON	Ⓧ Do Not Use	382
PHAZYME	Ⓧ Do Not Use	382
PHILLIPS' MILK OF MAGNESIA	Limited Use	388
RIOPAN		378
simethicone	Ⓧ Do Not Use	382

ANTINAUSEA DRUGS

ANTIVERT	Limited Use	359
cisapride	Ⓧ Do Not Use	392
COMPAZINE	Limited Use	366

meclizine	Limited Use	359
metoclopramide	Limited Use	393
PHENERGAN	Limited Use	385
prochlorperazine	Limited Use	366
promethazine	Limited Use	385
PROPULSID	⊘ Do Not Use	392
REGLAN	Limited Use	393
TIGAN	⊘ Do Not Use	397
trimetho-benzamide	⊘ Do Not Use	397

LAXATIVES

bisacodyl	⊘ Do Not Use	373
COLACE	⊘ Do Not Use	365
DIALOSE PLUS	⊘ Do Not Use	371
docusate	⊘ Do Not Use	365
docusate and casanthranol	⊘ Do Not Use	371
DULCOLAX	⊘ Do Not Use	373
METAMUCIL		380
PERDIEM		380
PERI-COLACE	⊘ Do Not Use	371
psyllium		380
SURFAK	⊘ Do Not Use	365

ANTISPASMODICS AND OTHER GASTROINTESTINAL DRUGS

atropine	⊘ Do Not Use	361
atropine, hyoscyamine, scopolamine and phenobarbital	⊘ Do Not Use	372
AZULFIDINE		361
BENTYL	⊘ Do Not Use	363
chlordiazepoxide and clidinium	⊘ Do Not Use	377
dicyclomine	⊘ Do Not Use	363
diphenoxylate and atropine	⊘ Do Not Use	378
DONNATAL	⊘ Do Not Use	372

IMODIUM	Limited Use	375
LIBRAX	⊘ Do Not Use	377
LOMOTIL	⊘ Do Not Use	378
loperamide	Limited Use	375
sulfasalazine		361

DIARRHEA

Diarrhea is a change in the frequency and consistency of bowel movements, characterized by abnormally frequent passage of loose or watery stools. Diarrhea is common in older people and can be associated with underlying disease, complications of therapy (see Common Causes of Acute Simple Diarrhea below) or can be infectious in origin, usually due to a virus in the intestinal tract. Acute or sudden simple diarrhea lasts only a few days and typically improves with or without medication.

When older adults get diarrhea, they have a greater risk of complications from the loss of fluid, sodium and potassium chloride and other electrolytes than younger adults do.

According to a study by the federal Centers for Disease Control and Prevention, there were 28,538 Americans who died during a nine year period for whom diarrhea was listed as an immediate or underlying cause of death. A disproportionate fraction of these deaths (51%) were in people older than 74, with a diarrhea death rate 10 times that of the total population. People 55 to 74 made up an additional 27% of diarrheal deaths so that 78% of deaths caused by diarrhea were in people 55 or older[1] even though this group makes up only 21% of the population.

Despite the heavy promotion and frequent use of ineffective and/or dangerous prescription or over-the-counter drugs, the world standard for hydrating patients with diarrhea is oral rehydration therapy. Many of the deaths in older adults described above might have been prevented if the patients had been given oral rehydration solution (ORS) (see box on this page).

Common Causes of Acute Simple Diarrhea

Acute diarrhea is often caused by a viral infection in the intestinal tract, food poisoning, anxiety, or a reaction to medication, food, or alcohol. Some drugs that commonly cause diarrhea include the following:

- Antibiotics taken for infections
- Antacids containing magnesium, such as Maalox and Mylanta
- Dietary supplements with magnesium[2]
- Drugs for high blood pressure
- All laxatives except the bulk-forming variety (those that contain psyllium, for example)
- Drugs for irregular heartbeat, such as quinidine (DURAQUIN, QUINAGLUTE DURA-TABS, QUINIDEX)

See Chapter 2, p. 33, for a longer list of drugs that can cause diarrhea.

How to Treat Acute Simple Diarrhea

- Do not eat or drink milk and dairy products, fresh fruits and vegetables, coffee, spicy foods, and other food you do not tolerate well.
- Do not consume drinks with a high sugar content like grape or apple juice, soft drinks including cola, ginger ale and sports drinks, or eat highly sweetened foods such as candy, ice cream or Jell-O because they have too much sugar which can make the diarrhea worse.[3]
- Drink plenty of oral rehydration solution (ORS)—the formula for which is shown in the box to the right. Once you have noticed watery diarrhea in the toilet bowl, you are probably already a liter (slightly more than a quart) dehydrated. This means you should try to catch up with the fluids you have already lost by drinking three to four eight-ounce glasses of ORS over the next several hours. Once you have caught up—this will be apparent because you will be well enough hydrated to pass urine—you should drink at least four additional eight-ounce glasses of ORS every 12 hours until the diarrhea stops. Patients on a fluid or salt restricted diet should consult their physicians concerning the use of ORS.

- Do not eat salty foods like salty soup, potato chips or peanuts.
- Do not take medication not prescribed or directed by your doctor or other health professional.
- Take your temperature once a day.

When to Seek Help from a Health Professional
Get assistance when:

- severe diarrhea occurs in an older adult, particularly one who is very weak.
- fever is above 101°F (38.3°C).
- there is evidence of blood in the stools or black, tarry stools.
- diarrhea persists for more than three days.
- you suspect that a drug taken under the direction of a doctor may be the cause of the diarrhea.
- diarrhea is accompanied by severe, incapacitating abdominal pain.
- diarrhea results in a severe loss of water (dehydration) characterized by dizziness while standing, confusion, or unresponsiveness.

How to Make Oral Rehydration Solution[4]
   To one liter (slightly more than a quart) of clean water add:
- one-half of a level teaspoon of *salt*
- eight level teaspoons of *sugar*
   (Caution: Before adding the sugar, taste the drink and be sure it is less salty than tears.)
- If it is available, you can add a mashed ripe banana which also provides potassium.

CONSTIPATION

For a discussion of ways to avoid, and if necessary, treat constipation, see Psyllium (p. 380). Also see a list of drugs (p. 31) which can cause constipation.

GAS

One of the miracles of modern Madison Avenue marketing is that the public is still spending money for simethicone, alone or in combination with other drugs, for gas or infant colic.

Despite the millions spent on advertising to convince us otherwise, the feeling of bloating and pain after eating is not caused by gas. Evidence shows that there is no relation between these symptoms and the amount of gas in the intestinal tract. The use of anti-gas products to relieve this discomfort is inappropriate, as there is no need to expel gas from the body. Taking an antacid product is even more irrational, since the amount of acid in the stomach is not at fault and should not be interfered with needlessly.

Belching and passing flatus (gas passed by the rectum) are undoubtedly caused by gas. There are two major sources of gas in the gastrointestinal tract. The first is swallowed air that is either released in belching or continues through the intestines and must be passed as flatus. The other source is produced in the intestine and must eventually leave the body as flatus. Both of these processes are perfectly normal.

In 1975, *The Medical Letter on Drugs and Therapeutics,* one of the world's most respected sources of objective drug information, wrote: "There is no convincing evidence that simethicone, alone or in combination, is effective for the treatment of flatulence [gas] associated with functional disorders of the gastrointestinal tract."[5] Now, more than two decades later, more studies have confirmed that simethicone does not work. Included is a study of 83 infants between two and eight weeks of age with colic that found no significant difference between simethicone and placebo (a look-alike dummy drug). *The Medical Letter* reviewed simethicone again in 1996 and said: "There is no convincing evidence that simethicone, alone or in combination, is effective for treatment of eructation [belching], flatulence or any other signs or symptoms of excess gastrointestinal gas."[6]

DRUG PROFILES

Antibiotic Treatment for Ulcer Disease

Amoxicillin (see p. 476)
AMOXIL (SmithKline Beecham)

GENERIC: available

Bismuth Subsalicylate
PEPTO BISMOL (Procter & Gamble)

Bismuth Subsalicylate, Metronidazole, Tetracycline packaged together
HELIDAC (Procter & Gamble)

GENERIC: available for each ingredient

Clarithromycin (see p. 481)
BIAXIN (Abbott)

GENERIC: not available

Lansoprazole (see p. 389)
PREVACID (TAP Pharm)

GENERIC: not available

Metronidazole (see p. 500)
FLAGYL (Searle)

GENERIC: available

Omeprazole (see p. 389)
PRILOSEC (Astra Merck)

GENERIC: not available

Ranitidine (see p. 383)
ZANTAC (Glaxo Wellcome)

Ranitidine Bismuth Citrate
TRITEC (Glaxo Wellcome)

GENERIC: not available

Tetracycline (see p. 475)
ACHROMYCIN (Lederle)

GENERIC: available

All of the above antibiotics are used to treat ulcers. When the bacteria Helicobacter pylori (H. pylori), present in a large proportion of people with ulcers, is eradicated, ulcers can heal and the likelihood of reoccurrence is reduced. Generally, H. pylori are more easily eradicated in duodenal ulcers than in gastric ulcers. *If you have H. pylori, but do not have an ulcer, there is evidence that H. pylori may protect against the symptoms of esophagitis and you should not take medicine to eradicate H. pylori.*[7]

If only one drug is used, resistance is apt to develop and relapse to occur, particularly with metronidazole. Low doses also lead to resistance. Combining a single antibiotic (amoxicillin or clarithromycin) with a proton pump inhibitor (lansoprazole or omeprazole) results in less than 70% of H. pylori being eradicated. The American College of Gastroenterology recommends using two antibiotics with a proton pump inhibitor, which allow for shorter periods of therapy. Recently, combinations of omeprazole with clarithromycin and either amoxicillin or metronidazole have been shown to be over 90% effective in eradicating H. pylori after one week. People intolerant of clarithromycin can use omeprazole with amoxicillin and metronidazole. Another alternative is bismuth. When bismuth and metronidazole are combined with tetracycline and amoxicillin, the eradication ranges from 75% to 90%; if bismuth, metronidazole, and tetracycline are combined with omeprazole, eradication rises to 98%. Raniti-dine bismuth subcitrate has also been used with clarithromycin and either tetracycline or amoxicillin. To date, regimens with ranitidine require two weeks of therapy.

The choice of combinations will depend on your allergies, condition, other medications you take, as well as resistance and your likelihood of taking several drugs several times a day for one to four weeks. Some drugs must be taken with food, others on an empty stomach. The more drugs you take the more adverse reactions are possible. Prolonged use of antibiotics can cause superinfections. To simplify things, some companies have packaged drugs together and made new combination drugs. In this case, you are paying more for convenience, since equivalent drugs are usually available generically. Some of the individual drugs are available without a prescription. The latest recommendations suggest that after an initial course of antibiotics for at least one week, the proton pump inhibitor be continued for three weeks in duodenal ulcer, and five weeks in gastric ulcer. If ulcers previously bled or perforated, then the proton pump inhibitor is used long term.[8]

On p. 357 is a chart listing the drug treatments for H. pylori and a cost comparison. For more complete information, look up each drug separately.

Before You Use Any of These Drugs

Tell your doctor if you have or have had:

- allergies
- bleeding of the gastrointestinal tract
- colitis
- heart trouble
- heart, kidney or liver problems
- nerve diseases

Tell your doctor about any other drugs you take, including aspirin, herbs, vitamins, and other nonprescription products.

When You Use These Drugs for Treating Ulcers

• Do not drink alcohol while taking metronidazole and for two weeks after you complete taking it.

• Avoid taking NSAIDs (such as ADVIL, ALEVE, ANAPROX, ANSAID, aspirin, GENUINE BAYER ASPIRIN, CLINORIL, DAYPRO, diclofenac, ECOTRIN, etodolac, FELDENE, fenoprofen, flurbiprofen, ibuprofen, INDOCIN, indomethacin, ketoprofen, ketorolac, LODINE, MOTRIN, nabumetone, NALFON, NAPROSYN, naproxen, OCUFEN, ORUDIS, oxaprozin, piroxicam, PONSTEL, RELAFEN, sulindac, TOLECTIN, tolmetin, TORADOL, and VOLTAREN). These drugs often cause ulcers, especially gastric ulcers.

• Avoid smoking, which aggravates ulcers.

• Protect yourself from the sun and sunlamps (using sun screen, wearing long sleeves, hats) if you take tetracycline. A reaction to sunlight can happen for several days after you stop the tetracycline.

How to Use These Drugs

• Follow instructions for your individual regimen carefully. If you use liquid amoxicillin, bismuth, or clarithromycin shake it well. Bismuth tablets are to be chewed and swallowed. Swallow tetracycline whole with a full glass of water one hour before or two hours after meals. Swallow omeprazole whole before eating. Take metronidazole with food or milk to avoid nausea. Amoxicillin and clarithromycin may be taken without regard to food.

• If you miss a dose, take as soon as you remember but skip it if it is almost time for the next dose. **Do not take double doses.** If you miss four or more doses, contact your doctor.

• Store capsules or tablets of these medications at room temperature. Liquid amoxicillin or clarithromycin should be refrigerated.

Interactions with Other Drugs

The following drugs are listed in the *Evaluations of Drug Interactions* 1997 as causing "highly clinically significant" or "clinically significant" interactions when used together with this drug. We have also included potentially serious interactions listed in the drug's FDA-approved professional product labeling or package insert. New scientific techniques have allowed researchers to predict some drug interactions before they have been documented in people. There may be other drugs, especially those in the families of drugs listed below, that also will react with this drug to cause severe adverse effects. The number of new drugs approved for marketing increases the chance of drug interactions, and new drug interactions are being identified with old drugs. Be vigilant. Make sure to tell your doctor and pharmacist the drugs you are taking and tell your doctor if you are taking any of these interacting drugs:

Antibiotics can reduce effectiveness of oral contraceptives. Use a different form of contraception. Clarithromycin interacts dangerously with astemizole (HISMANAL) and terfenadine (SELDANE) to slow the heart rhythm. This can be fatal. Do not take these drugs while taking clarithromycin. Metronidazole interacts with alcohol. Do not drink alcohol while you take metronidazole and for several days afterwards. Tetracycline interacts with calcium and iron and may cause reactions when patients are exposed to sunlight. Do not take with dairy foods, calcium or iron or multiple mineral supplements. These reduce absorption of tetracycline. *See the individual drug profiles for a more complete listing of possible drug interactions.*

Adverse Effects

Call your doctor immediately if you experience:

• difficulty breathing

- confusion (brain dysfunction is an adverse effect of bismuth)
- diarrhea
- fever
- headache
- irregular menstrual bleeding
- numbness in hands or feet
- seizures
- skin itches or develops rash
- stomach pain
- difficulty urinating
- blurred vision

Call your doctor if these symptoms continue:

- decrease in appetite
- dark stools or tongue *(from bismuth)*

- dizziness
- nausea or vomiting
- ringing in ears *(from bismuth)*
- sunburn *(from tetracycline)*
- taste disturbance *(more likely with clarithromycin, metronidazole, and omeprazole)*

The table below describes various drug treatments used to eradicate H. pylori. The various drug combinations are grouped together, along with the daily dosages of the drugs and the duration of treatment for each of the drugs. The last column lists the cost of each individual drug and the total cost for each of the treatments. These costs were obtained in 1998 from a Washington, DC, pharmacy chain.

DRUG TREATMENTS USED TO ERADICATE H. PYLORI, AN ULCER-CAUSING BACTERIA

DRUGS	DAILY DOSE	DURATION	COST
bismuth subsalicylate (generic)	2 tablets - 525 milligrams four times a day	2 weeks	$5.29
+metronidazole (generic)	250 milligrams four times a day	2 weeks	$18.69
+tetracycline (generic)	500 milligrams four times a day	2 weeks	$9.19
+ranitidine (Zantac)	150 milligrams two times a day	2 weeks	$42.39
		TOTAL	$75.56
Helidac Therapy (supplied as 14 blister cards, each containing eight 262.4 milligram bismuth subsalicylate, four 250 milligram metronidazole tablets, and four 500 milligram tetracycline tablets)		2 weeks	$95.59
+ranitidine	150 milligrams two times a day	2 weeks	$42.39
		TOTAL	$137.98
clarithromycin (Biaxin)	500 milligrams three times a day.	2 weeks	$154.99
+omeprazole (Prilosec)	40 milligrams once daily	2 weeks	$119.99
followed by omeprazole	20 milligrams once daily	2 weeks	$60.99
		TOTAL	$335.97
clarithromycin	500 milligrams twice a day	10 days	$75.99
+omeprazole	20 milligrams two times a day	10 days	$85.59
+metronidazole	500 milligrams two times a day	10 days	$14.79
or amoxicillin	1.0 gram two times a day	10 days	$19.69
		TOTAL	$196.06
ranitidine bismuth citrate (Tritec)	400 milligrams two times a day	2 weeks	$70.99
+clarithromycin	500 milligrams three times a day	2 weeks	$154.99
followed by ranitidine bismuth citrate	400 milligrams two times a day	2 weeks	$70.99
		TOTAL	$296.97

Limited Use

Aluminum Hydroxide
AMPHOJEL (Wyeth-Ayerst)

GENERIC: available
FAMILY: Antacids

Aluminum hydroxide (a *loo* mi num hye *drox* ide) is used to treat ulcers and stomach upset caused by stomach acid and to prevent a certain type of kidney stones. Older adults with metabolic bone diseases should not take aluminum antacids,[9] and those with kidney disease should not use them for a long time.[10]

The aluminum in this drug can cause constipation. If you become constipated while using aluminum hydroxide, ask your doctor about switching to a product that contains both aluminum and magnesium hydroxide (see p. 378).

The liquid form of this drug is better than tablets because it is more effective and costs less. If you use tablets, chew them thoroughly. If you take large doses of this drug or take it for a long time, see your doctor for regular check-ups. If you are treating yourself with this drug, do not take it for longer than two weeks unless you check with your doctor.

Before You Use This Drug
Tell your doctor if you have or have had:

- allergies to drugs
- severe abdominal pain
- gastrointestinal or rectal bleeding
- constipation
- prolonged diarrhea
- hemorrhoids
- intestinal blockage
- kidney problems
- metabolic bone disease
- Alzheimer's disease
- appendicitis

Tell your doctor about any other drugs you take, including aspirin, herbs, vitamins, and other nonprescription products.

When You Use This Drug
- **Call your doctor immediately if you have black, tarry stools or you vomit material that looks like coffee grounds. These are signs of a bleeding ulcer.**
- If you are on a low-salt (low-sodium) diet, ask your doctor or pharmacist to help you choose an antacid. Many antacids contain sodium.

How to Use This Drug
- Take one to three hours after meals and at bedtime for maximum effectiveness. Drink plenty of fluids.
- Do not take any other drugs by mouth for at least one or two hours after taking aluminum hydroxide.
- Do not store in the bathroom. Do not expose to heat, moisture, or strong light. Do not let the liquid form freeze.
- If you miss a dose, take it as soon as you remember, but skip it if it is almost time for the next dose. **Do not take double doses.**

Interactions with Other Drugs
The following drugs are listed in the *Evaluations of Drug Interactions* 1997 as causing "highly clinically significant" or "clinically significant" interactions when used together with this drug. We have also included potentially

serious interactions listed in the drug's FDA-approved professional product labeling or package insert. New scientific techniques have allowed researchers to predict some drug interactions before they have been documented in people. There may be other drugs, especially those in the families of drugs listed below, that also will react with this drug to cause severe adverse effects. The number of new drugs approved for marketing increases the chance of drug interactions, and new drug interactions are being identified with old drugs. Be vigilant. Make sure to tell your doctor and pharmacist the drugs you are taking and tell your doctor if you are taking any of these interacting drugs:

ACHROMYCIN, aspirin, GENUINE BAYER ASPIRIN, CALCIFEROL, CHIBROXIN, CILOXAN, CIPRO, ciprofloxacin, digoxin, ECOTRIN, enoxacin, FLOXIN, grepafloxacin, KAYEXALATE, ketoconazole, LANOXICAPS, LANOXIN, LEVAQUIN, levofloxacin, lomefloxacin, MAXAQUIN, NIZORAL, norfloxacin, NOROXIN, OCUFLOX, ofloxacin, PANMYCIN, PENETREX, RAXAR, sodium polystyrene sulfonate, sparfloxacin, SUMYCIN, tetracycline, TORVAN, trovafloxacin, vitamin D, ZAGAM.

Adverse Effects

Call your doctor immediately if you experience:

- severe constipation
- bone pain, swelling of wrists, feet or lower legs
- loss of appetite, weight loss
- muscle weakness
- frequent urge to urinate
- headache
- nausea, vomiting
- continuing feeling of discomfort

- unusual tiredness or weakness
- mood or mental changes

Call your doctor if these symptoms continue:

- nausea, vomiting
- chalky taste
- constipation
- speckled or whitish stools
- stomach cramps

Periodic Tests

Ask your doctor which of these tests should be done periodically while you are taking this drug:

- blood aluminum, calcium, phosphate, and potassium levels
- kidney function tests

Limited Use

Meclizine
ANTIVERT (Pfizer)

GENERIC: available

FAMILY: Antinausea Drugs
Antihistamines (see p. 402)

Meclizine (*mek* li zeen) is used to prevent motion sickness. **It is also used to treat vertigo (dizziness), but it has not been proven effective for this purpose.**[11]

If you are taking meclizine to prevent motion sickness, take it at least one hour before traveling. Do not take more than is recommended.

If you have asthma, glaucoma, an obstructed intestine, or an enlarged prostate gland, meclizine can make your symptoms worse.[12] If you take meclizine regularly for some time and you are also taking high doses of aspirin or other drugs in the salicylate family, the meclizine may hide signs of an aspirin or salicylate overdose.[13]

WARNING: SPECIAL MENTAL AND PHYSICAL ADVERSE EFFECTS

Older adults are especially sensitive to the harmful anticholinergic (see Glossary p., 768) effects of meclizine. Drugs in this family should not be used unless absolutely necessary.

Mental Effects: confusion, delirium, short-term memory problems, disorientation, and impaired attention.

Physical Effects: dry mouth, constipation, difficulty urinating (especially for a man with an enlarged prostate), blurred vision, decreased sweating with increased body temperature, sexual dysfunction, and worsening of glaucoma.

Before You Use This Drug

Tell your doctor if you have or have had:

- allergies to drugs
- problems with urination
- glaucoma
- peptic ulcer or intestinal obstruction
- enlarged prostate
- asthma, bronchitis, emphysema or other chronic lung disease

Tell your doctor about any other drugs you take, including aspirin, herbs, vitamins, and other nonprescription products.

When You Use This Drug

- Do not drink alcohol or use other drugs that can cause drowsiness.
- Until you know how you react to this drug, do not drive or perform other activities requiring alertness.

How to Use This Drug

- Take with food or milk to decrease stomach upset.

- Do not store in the bathroom. Do not expose to heat, moisture, or strong light. Do not let the liquid form freeze.
- If you miss a dose, take it as soon as you remember, but skip it if it is almost time for the next dose. **Do not take double doses.**

Interactions with Other Drugs

The following drugs are listed in the *Evaluations of Drug Interactions* 1997 as causing "highly clinically significant" or "clinically significant" interactions when used together with this drug. We have also included potentially serious interactions listed in the drug's FDA-approved professional product labeling or package insert. New scientific techniques have allowed researchers to predict some drug interactions before they have been documented in people. There may be other drugs, especially those in the families of drugs listed below, that also will react with this drug to cause severe adverse effects. The number of new drugs approved for marketing increases the chance of drug interactions, and new drug interactions are being identified with old drugs. Be vigilant. Make sure to tell your doctor and pharmacist the drugs you are taking and tell your doctor if you are taking any of these interacting drugs:

alcohol.

Adverse Effects

Call your doctor if these symptoms continue:

- drowsiness
- blurred vision
- dry mouth, nose, or throat
- difficult or painful urination
- constipation, diarrhea
- dizziness
- irregular heartbeat
- headache
- loss of appetite
- nervousness, restlessness or trouble sleeping

- skin rash
- upset stomach

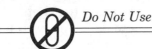

Do Not Use

ALTERNATIVE TREATMENT:
For diarrhea, see Diarrhea, p. 352. For spastic colon, see Psyllium, p. 380.

Atropine

FAMILY: Antispasmodics
Anticholinergics

Atropine (*a* tro peen) is used to relieve abdominal discomfort from cramping (spasms) and to control diarrhea. **It has such severe adverse effects that older adults should not use it.** Even if you are taking only the usual adult dose, you may suffer from excitement, restlessness, drowsiness, or confusion.[14] If you are taking atropine, ask your doctor to change your medication.

WARNING: SPECIAL MENTAL AND PHYSICAL ADVERSE EFFECTS

Older adults are especially sensitive to the harmful anticholinergic (see Glossary, p. 768) effects of a family of drugs known as belladonna alkaloids. Atropine is in this family. Drugs in this family should not be used unless absolutely necessary.

Mental Effects: confusion, delirium, short-term memory problems, disorientation, and impaired attention.

Physical Effects: dry mouth, constipation, difficulty urinating (especially for a man with an enlarged prostate), blurred vision, decreased sweating with increased body temperature, sexual dysfunction, and worsening of glaucoma.

Sulfasalazine
AZULFIDINE (Pharmacia & Upjohn)

GENERIC: available
FAMILY: Gastrointestinal Drugs

Sulfasalazine (sul fa *sal* a zeen) is used to treat two diseases of the intestines: ulcerative colitis and Crohn's disease. The drug is usually taken for a long time. If your disease improves enough, you may be able to lower your dose to a maintenance level. If your condition continues to improve, you may be able to stop using the drug for periods of time. Ask your doctor about this.

If you have impaired kidney function, you may need to take less than the usual adult dose.

Before You Use This Drug

Tell your doctor if you have or have had:

- allergies to drugs
- an unusual reaction to sulfa drugs, furosemide, thiazide diuretics (water pills), or diabetes or glaucoma drugs taken by mouth
  - blood problems
  - glucose-6-phosphate dehydrogenase deficiency
  - kidney or liver problems
  - porphyria
  - stomach or intestinal blockage

Tell your doctor about any other drugs you take, including aspirin, herbs, vitamins, and other nonprescription products.

When You Use This Drug

- **Check with your doctor to make certain your fluid intake is adequate and appropriate.**
- Call your doctor if your symptoms (including diarrhea) do not improve in a month or so, or if they get worse. Schedule regular visits to your doctor to check your progress.
- Your skin or urine may turn orange-yellow in color. This is no cause for alarm.

- **Take all the sulfasalazine your doctor prescribed, even if you begin to feel better. If you stop too soon, your symptoms could come back.**
- Do not give this drug to anyone else. Throw away outdated drugs.
- **Caution diabetics:** see p. 550.
- This drug makes you more sensitive to the sun. Stay out of the sun as much as possible, and call your doctor if you get a rash, hives, or any other skin reaction.
- You may need more folic acid than usual while taking sulfasalazine. Ask your doctor about how to get more folic acid in your diet.
- If you plan to have any surgery, including dental, tell your doctor that you take this drug.
- Until you know how you react to this drug, do not drive or perform other activities requiring alertness.

How to Use This Drug

- Take with **a full glass (eight ounces) of water.** Sulfasalazine can be taken right after meals or with food to lessen stomach upset. Swallow tablets whole.
- Do not store in the bathroom. Do not expose to heat, moisture, or strong light. Do not let the liquid form freeze.
- If you miss a dose, take it as soon as you remember, but skip it if it is almost time for the next dose. **Do not take double doses.**

Interactions with Other Drugs

The following drugs are listed in the *Evaluations of Drug Interactions* 1997 as causing "highly clinically significant" or "clinically significant" interactions when used together with this drug. We have also included potentially serious interactions listed in the drug's FDA-approved professional product labeling or package insert. New scientific techniques have allowed researchers to predict some drug inter-

actions before they have been documented in people. There may be other drugs, especially those in the families of drugs listed below, that also will react with this drug to cause severe adverse effects. The number of new drugs approved for marketing increases the chance of drug interactions, and new drug interactions are being identified with old drugs. Be vigilant. Make sure to tell your doctor and pharmacist the drugs you are taking and tell your doctor if you are taking any of these interacting drugs:

COUMADIN, digoxin, LANOXICAPS, LANOXIN, methotrexate, ORINASE, RHEUMATREX DOSE PACK, tolbutamide, warfarin.

Adverse Effects

Call your doctor immediately if you experience:

- itching or skin rash
- aching joints or muscles
- difficulty swallowing
- fever, pale skin, sore throat
- abnormal bleeding or bruising
- abnormal tiredness or weakness
- yellow eyes or skin
- continuing headache
- back, leg or stomach pain
- bloody diarrhea
- bluish fingernails, lips or skin
- chest pain
- cough or difficulty breathing
- general feeling of discomfort or illness
- loss of appetite
- redness, blistering, peeling or loosening of skin

Call your doctor if these symptoms continue:

- diarrhea
- dizziness or headache
- loss of appetite
- nausea or vomiting
- abdominal or stomach pain or upset

Periodic Tests

Ask your doctor which of these tests should be done periodically while you are taking this drug:

- complete blood count
- proctoscopy, sigmoidoscopy
- urine tests
- liver and kidney function tests, if you take this drug for a long time

 Do Not Use

ALTERNATIVE TREATMENT:
For diarrhea, see Diarrhea, p. 352. For spastic colon, see Psyllium, p. 380.

Dicyclomine
BENTYL (Hoechst Marion Roussel)

FAMILY: Antispasmodics
Anticholinergics

Dicyclomine (dye *sye* kloe meen) is used to relieve abdominal discomfort from cramping (spasms). **Although the effective and usual adult dose is 160 milligrams per day, older adults have an unacceptably high rate of adverse effects at this dose.** In addition to its anticholinergic effects (see box), dicyclomine may cause excitement or confusion.[15]

A respected drug reference book recommends that dicyclomine be discontinued if your condition does not improve after two weeks of treatment or if adverse effects force your doctor to lower your dose to below 80 milligrams per day. There is no documented data available on dicyclomine's safety at doses of 80 to 160 milligrams daily for periods longer than two weeks.[16]

We believe that older adults should not use dicyclomine because of the high rate

of serious adverse effects. If you use it, ask your doctor to change your medication.

WARNING: SPECIAL MENTAL AND PHYSICAL ADVERSE EFFECTS

Older adults are especially sensitive to the harmful anticholinergic (see Glossary, p. 768) effects of a family of drugs known as belladonna alkaloids. Dicyclomine is in this family. Drugs in this family should not be used unless absolutely necessary.

Mental Effects: confusion, delirium, short-term memory problems, disorientation, and impaired attention.

Physical Effects: dry mouth, constipation, difficulty urinating (especially for a man with an enlarged prostate), blurred vision, decreased sweating with increased body temperature, sexual dysfunction, and worsening of glaucoma.

Limited Use

Sucralfate
CARAFATE (Hoechst Marion Roussel)

GENERIC: available
FAMILY: Antiulcer Drugs

Sucralfate (soo *kral* fate) is used to treat ulcers. After you take it, it forms a gummy substance that sticks to the part of your stomach where the ulcer is. This protects the ulcer from stomach acid and prevents further damage to the ulcer and the stomach lining.

You should not take sucralfate for minor digestive problems. Do not take sucralfate for more than 12 weeks unless your doctor tells you to.

Sucralfate can cause constipation.

Before You Use This Drug

Tell your doctor if you have or have had:

- allergies to drugs
- intestinal obstruction
- kidney failure

Tell your doctor about any other drugs you take, including aspirin, herbs, vitamins, and other nonprescription products.

When You Use This Drug

• **Call your doctor immediately if you have black, tarry stools or you vomit material that looks like coffee grounds. These are signs of a bleeding ulcer.**

• Take antacids for ulcer pain, but not too close to the time you take sucralfate.

How to Use This Drug

• Do not chew tablets.

• Take on an empty stomach, at least one hour before or two hours after eating, and take a dose at bedtime.

• Do not store in the bathroom. Do not expose to heat, moisture, or strong light.

• If you miss a dose, take it as soon as you remember, but skip it if it is almost time for the next dose. **Do not take double doses.**

Interactions with Other Drugs

The following drugs are listed in the *Evaluations of Drug Interactions* 1997 as causing "highly clinically significant" or "clinically significant" interactions when used together with this drug. We have also included potentially serious interactions listed in the drug's FDA-approved professional product labeling or package insert. New scientific techniques have allowed researchers to predict some drug interactions before they have been documented in people. There may be other drugs, especially those in the families of drugs listed below, that also will react with this drug to cause severe adverse effects. The number of new drugs approved for marketing increases the chance of drug interactions, and new drug interactions are being identified with old drugs. Be vigilant. Make sure to tell your doctor and pharmacist the drugs you are taking and tell your doctor if you are taking any of these interacting drugs:

ACHROMYCIN, CHIBROXIN, CILOXAN, CIPRO, ciprofloxacin, DILANTIN, enoxacin, FLOXIN, grepafloxacin, LEVAQUIN, levofloxacin, lomefloxacin, MAXAQUIN, norfloxacin, NOROXIN, OCUFLOX, ofloxacin, PANMYCIN, PENETREX, phenytoin, RAXAR, sparfloxacin, SUMYCIN, tetracycline, TORVAN, trovafloxacin, ZAGAM.

Adverse Effects

Call your doctor immediately if you experience:

- seizures
- drowsiness

Call your doctor if these symptoms continue:

- constipation, diarrhea
- dizziness, lightheadedness
- backache
- dry mouth
- indigestion, nausea
- stomach cramps or pain
- skin rash, hives, itching

Periodic Tests

Ask your doctor which of these tests should be done periodically while you are taking this drug:

- blood levels of phosphate

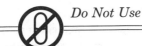 *Do Not Use*

ALTERNATIVE TREATMENT:
See Psyllium, p. 380.

Docusate
COLACE (Roberts)
SURFAK (Pharmacia & Upjohn)

FAMILY: Stool-softener Laxatives

Docusate (*dok* yoo sate) is a laxative that works by softening your stools. **You should not take it for simple constipation.** Docusate and other laxatives in its family can cause long-lasting damage to your intestine and can interfere with your body's use of nutrients. Docusate can also be dangerous if you are taking other drugs at the same time, since it can make your body absorb the other drugs at an increased rate. Since there are other laxatives that are safer than docusate, we do not recommend that you use it.

Many people take laxatives more often than they need to. This is dangerous for several reasons. First, some laxatives, such as docusate, can have harmful adverse effects. Second, all laxatives can be habit-forming. If you take them too often or for too long, your body will become less able to pass stools without them. This leads to a cycle of abuse in which you become dependent on laxatives and have to take them continuously. If you think you have become dependent on laxatives, talk to your doctor.

When do you really need to take a laxative? You should not take a laxative to "clean out your system" or to make your body act more "normally." Nor should you take a laxative just because you are having less than one bowel movement a day. It is untrue that everyone must have a bowel movement (stool) daily. Perfectly healthy people may have from two bowel movements per week to three bowel movements per day.

If the frequency of your bowel movements has decreased, if you are having bowel movements less than twice a week, or if you are having difficulty in passing stools, you are constipated, but this does not mean that you need a laxative. It is better to treat simple, occasional constipation without drugs, by eating a high-fiber diet that includes whole-grain breads and cereals, raw vegetables, raw and dried fruits, and beans, and by drinking plenty of nonalcoholic liquids (six to eight glasses per day). This type of diet will both prevent and treat constipation, and it is less costly than taking drugs. Regular exercise—at least 30 minutes per day of swimming, cycling, jogging, or brisk walking—will also help your body maintain regularity.

If you are constipated while traveling or at some other time when it is hard for you to eat properly, it may be appropriate to take a laxative for a short time. The only type of laxative you should use for self-medication is a bulk-forming laxative such as psyllium (see p. 380). This type usually takes effect in 12 hours to three days, compared with docusate which takes effect one or two days after the first dose, but may require three to five days of treatment. Even bulk-forming laxatives should only be used occasionally.

If you are on a special diet such as a low-salt or low-sugar diet, ask your doctor or pharmacist to help you choose a laxative without ingredients you are trying to avoid. Some laxatives contain sugar (up to half of the product), salt (up to 250 milligrams per dose), or the artificial sweetener NutraSweet®.

Limited Use

Prochlorperazine
COMPAZINE (SmithKline Beecham)

GENERIC: available

FAMILY: Antinausea Drugs
Antipsychotics (see p. 187)

Prochlorperazine (proe klor *pair* a zeen) is used to control nausea and vomiting, to treat serious mental illness (psychosis), and to manage behavior problems in mentally retarded people.

For severe nausea and vomiting, you should only be taking prochlorperazine if you have already tried making changes in your diet (see box below) and this has not worked. This drug has "questionable value" in treating psychosis[17] and has not been proven effective for managing behavior problems of mentally retarded people.

Prochlorperazine can cause serious adverse effects: drug-induced parkinsonism (see p. 193) and tardive dyskinesia (involuntary movements of parts of the body, which may last indefinitely). More information appears under Adverse Effects. **If you are over 60, you should generally be taking less than the usual adult dose.**

WARNING: SPECIAL MENTAL AND PHYSICAL ADVERSE EFFECTS

Older adults are especially sensitive to the harmful anticholinergic (see Glossary, p. 768) effects of antipsychotic drugs such as prochlorperazine. Drugs in this family should not be used unless absolutely necessary.

Mental Effects: confusion, delirium, short-term memory problems, disorientation, and impaired attention.

Physical Effects: dry mouth, constipation, difficulty urinating (especially for a man with an enlarged prostate), blurred vision, decreased sweating with increased body temperature, sexual dysfunction, and worsening of glaucoma.

Drugs used to treat cancer often cause severe nausea and vomiting, either immediately after the drug is taken or several hours later. You can treat this kind of nausea and vomiting by changing your diet or by taking an anti-nausea drug. You should always try dietary changes first.[18]

• Eat small, frequent meals so your stomach is never empty.

• When you get up from sleeping or resting, eat some dry crackers or toast before you start being active.

• Drink carbonated drinks or other clear liquids such as soups and gelatin.

• Eat tart foods such as lemons and pickles.

• Do not eat foods with strong smells.

Before You Use This Drug

Tell your doctor if you have or have had:

• allergies to drugs
• an unusual reaction to other antipsychotics (see p. 247 for examples)
• heart or blood vessel disease
• blood disease
• Reye's syndrome
• Parkinson's disease
• epilepsy, seizures
• enlarged prostate or difficulty urinating
• diabetes
• glaucoma
• liver disease
• bone marrow depression
• lung disease or breathing problems
• alcohol dependence
• breast cancer
• stomach ulcer

Tell your doctor about any other drugs you take, including aspirin, herbs, vitamins, and other nonprescription products.

When You Use This Drug

• **Do not stop taking this drug suddenly. Your doctor must give you a schedule to lower your dose gradually, to prevent withdrawal symptoms** such as nausea, vomiting, stomach upset, trembling, dizziness, and symptoms of Parkinson's disease.

• It may take two or three weeks before you can tell that this drug is working.

• Until you know how you react to this drug, do not drive or perform other activities requiring alertness. Prochlorperazine can cause blurred vision, drowsiness, and fainting.

• Do not drink alcohol or use other drugs that can cause drowsiness.

• You may feel dizzy when rising from a lying or sitting position. When getting out of bed, hang your legs over the side of the bed for a few minutes, then get up slowly. When getting up from a chair, stay by the chair until you are sure that you are not dizzy. (See p. 16.)

• If you plan to have any surgery, including dental, tell your doctor that you take this drug.

How to Use This Drug

• Take with food or **a full glass (eight ounces)** of milk or water to prevent stomach upset.

• Swallow extended-release capsules whole.

• If you take antacids or drugs for diarrhea, take them at least two hours apart from prochlorperazine.

• Do not store in the bathroom. Do not expose to heat, moisture, or strong light. Do not let the liquid form freeze.

• If you miss a dose, take it as soon as you remember, but skip it if it is almost time for the next dose. **Do not take double doses.**

Interactions with Other Drugs

The following drugs are listed in the *Evaluations of Drug Interactions* 1997 as causing "highly clinically significant" or "clinically significant" interactions when used together with this drug. We have also included potentially serious interactions listed in the drug's FDA-approved professional product labeling or package insert. New scientific techniques have allowed researchers to predict some drug interactions before they have been documented in people. There may be other drugs, especially those in the families of drugs listed below, that also will react with this drug to cause severe adverse effects. The number of new drugs approved for marketing increases the chance of drug interactions, and new drug interactions are being identified with old drugs. Be vigilant. Make sure to tell your doctor and pharmacist the drugs you are taking and tell your doctor if you are taking any of these interacting drugs:

AEROSPORIN, alcohol, amphetamines, ANECTINE, benztropine, bromocriptine, CAPOTEN, captopril, carbamazepine, COGENTIN, DEMEROL, desipramine, diazoxide, guanethidine, INDERAL, INDERAL LA, ISMELIN, lithium, LITHOBID, LITHONATE, meperidine, NORPRAMIN, PARLODEL, polymyxin B, PROGLYCEM, propranolol, succinylcholine, TEGRETOL.

Adverse Effects

Call your doctor immediately if you experience:

• **signs of tardive dyskinesia:** lip smacking, chewing movements, puffing of cheeks, rapid, darting tongue movements, uncontrolled movements of arms or legs

• **signs of parkinsonism:** difficulty speaking or swallowing, loss of balance, mask-like face, muscle spasms, stiffness of arms or legs, trembling and shaking, unusual twisting movements of body

- changed or blurred vision
- difficulty urinating
- **signs of neuroleptic malignant syndrome:** troubled or fast breathing, high or low blood pressure, increased sweating, loss of bladder control, muscle stiffness, seizures, unusual tiredness, weakness, fast heartbeat, irregular pulse, pale skin
  - fever
  - sore mouth, gums, or throat
  - abnormal bleeding or bruising
  - nightmares
  - fainting
  - skin rash, itching or sunburn
  - yellow eyes or skin
  - tanning or blue/gray discoloration of skin
  - prolonged, painful or inappropriate penile erection
  - confusion
  - restlessness or need to keep moving
  - inability to move eyes
  - weakness in arms, legs or muscles
  - difficulty urinating
  - abdominal or stomach pain
  - aching muscles and joints
  - fatigue
  - nausea, vomiting, diarrhea
  - difficulty breathing
  - hot, dry skin
  - inability to sweat

Call your doctor if these symptoms continue:

- constipation
- decreased sexual ability
- decreased sweating
- dizziness, lightheadedness
- drowsiness
- dry mouth
- increased skin sensitivity to sun
- nasal congestion
- swelling or pain in breasts
- unusual secretion of milk
- changes in menstrual period
- unusual weight gain

Call your doctor if these symptoms continue after the medication is discontinued:

- signs of tardive dyskinesia (listed above)
- dizziness
- nausea and vomiting
- stomach pain
- trembling of fingers and hands

Periodic Tests

Ask your doctor which of these tests should be done periodically while you are taking this drug:

- complete blood count
- glaucoma tests
- liver function tests
- urine tests for bile and bilirubin
- observation for early signs of tardive dyskinesia
- evaluation of continued need for prochlorperazine
- blood pressure
- ophthalmologic examinations

DECREASED SWEATING

Drugs such as chlorpromazine (Thorazine), fluphenazine (Prolixin), prochlorperazine (Compazine), thioridazine (Mellaril), and trifluoperazine (Stelazine) may make you sweat less, causing your body temperature to increase. Use extra care not to become overheated during exercise or hot weather while you are taking one of these medications, since overheating may result in heat stroke. Hot baths or saunas may make you feel dizzy or faint while you are taking this medicine.

SENSITIVITY TO COLD

Drugs such as chlorpromazine (Thorazine), fluphenazine (Prolixin), prochlorperazine (Compazine), thioridazine (Mellaril), and trifluoperazine (Stelazine) may make you more sensitive to cold temperatures. Dress warmly during cold weather. Be careful during prolonged exposure to cold, such as in winter sports or swimming in cold water.

Limited Use

Misoprostol
CYTOTEC (Searle)

GENERIC: not available
FAMILY: Ulcer Drugs

Misoprostol (mice o *prost* all) is used to prevent ulcers, specifically, gastric ulcers caused by aspirin, ibuprofen, and other nonsteroidal anti-inflammatory drugs (NSAIDs) commonly used to treat arthritis. NSAIDs can cause serious harm, even fatalities, from bleeding in the stomach or intestines. Misoprostol is a synthetic prostaglandin drug which may protect the lining of the stomach and modestly decreases gastric acid.

People with high risk of ulcers from NSAIDs include the elderly, people with another debilitating disease, and those who had an ulcer previously. **Misoprostol should only be used by those who had an ulcer previously. However, arthritis in such people should be severe to warrant treatment with both an NSAID and misoprostol.** Healing of ulcers may be slower in people who smoke.

The elderly, the target group at high risk from the complications of gastric ulcer, are also at high risk from the complications of misoprostol. Misoprostol has been shown to alter bone metabolism in animals, and to alter chemical markers of bone metabolism in humans. Though the drug is intended for lifelong use by older people with arthritic conditions, a group known to be at risk for osteoporosis (thinning and weakening of the bones), little information has been gathered by its manufacturer on misoprostol's long-term effect on the human skeleton.

Diarrhea is a common adverse effect of misoprostol, ranging from minor to severe enough to be life-threatening.[19,20,21] In older people loss of fluids and minerals from diarrhea can in turn worsen blood pressure, or cause heart, kidney, and mental problems. Misoprostol predictably causes diarrhea in a significant number of patients who may tolerate it poorly. In clinical trials the incidence of loose stools ranged from 14 to 40%.

Since too many people receive NSAIDs for too long for no reason, approach taking one drug to treat the adverse effects of another drug with great caution. Many of these patients have conditions which can be treated with more conservative measures, or with generic acetaminophen (which does not induce stomach ulcers) for pain relief. Of patients chronically taking NSAIDs, 2 to 5% will develop a serious complication requiring hospitalization, but there is no evidence that misoprostol prevents the serious, life-threatening gastrointestinal complications associated with NSAIDs.

WARNING

Misoprostol should not be used, because of the possibility of inducing an abortion, in women who are pregnant. Patients must be advised of the abortifacient property and warned not to give the drug to others.

Before deciding to take misoprostol along with an NSAID, ask your doctor why misoprostol was prescribed and how long you could expect to take it. Ask if a different arthritis drug with a lower incidence of adverse effects can be used. Also inquire if alternative therapy is possible.[22,23,24,25] If you develop a duodenal ulcer, instead of a gastric ulcer, one of the stomach blockers should be tried first.[26] Also, consider the expense, since the price of misoprostol in the United States usually exceeds the cost of the drug you are taking for arthritis[27,28,29] and taking both may double your treatment cost.

Before You Use This Drug

Do not use if you have or have had:[30]

- Crohn's disease
- inflammatory bowel disease
- ulcerative colitis

Tell your doctor if you have or have had:

- allergies to drugs
- cerebral vascular disease
- coronary artery disease
- heart or kidney problems
- epilepsy
- low blood pressure
- osteoporosis

Tell your doctor about any other drugs you take, including aspirin, herbs, vitamins, and other nonprescription products.

When You Use This Drug

- Restrict your use of alcohol and cigarettes, which aggravate ulcers.
- Limit your intake of foods which you know bother your stomach, or cause diarrhea.
- Use antacids and laxatives which do not contain magnesium.
- Drink liquids to replace fluids lost by diarrhea.

How to Use This Drug

- Swallow tablets whole or break in half. Take with or after meals to lessen chance of diarrhea.
- If you miss a dose, take it as soon as you remember, but skip it if it is almost time for the next dose. **Do not take double doses.**
- Do not store in the bathroom. Do not expose to heat, moisture, or strong light.

Interactions with Other Drugs

Some other drugs that you may be taking (either over-the-counter or prescription drugs) can interact with this one, causing adverse effects. Ask your doctor what these drugs are and let him or her know if you are taking any of them.

Adverse Effects

Call your doctor immediately if you experience:

- **signs of overdose:**[31] severe drowsiness, convulsions, muscle twitching, abdominal pain, fever, heartbeat slows or becomes more rapid, dizziness, shortness of breath
- severe diarrhea

Call your doctor if these symptoms continue:

- confusion[32]
- constipation or diarrhea
- cramps
- gas
- headache
- heartburn, indigestion
- nausea or vomiting
- urinary incontinence[33]
- vaginal bleeding

Do Not Use

ALTERNATIVE TREATMENT:
See Psyllium, p. 380.

Docusate and Casanthranol
DIALOSE PLUS (J & J Merck Consumer)
PERI-COLACE (Roberts)

FAMILY: Stool-softener Laxatives
        Stimulant Laxatives

The combination of docusate (see p. 365) and casanthranol (ka *san* thra nole) is a laxative which combines two drugs, one that works by softening your stools and the other that works as a stimulant. The two ingredients in this product can cause serious health problems. **You should not take this combination to treat simple constipation.**

Casanthranol is a stimulant laxative, a type that is not recommended to treat simple constipation. If you take this type of laxative for a long time, it gradually reduces your intestine's ability to work efficiently. This causes increasing constipation and a disease of the large intestine called cathartic colon, in which the intestine becomes enlarged and will not move without chemical stimulation. According to one pharmacology textbook, *"the medical importance of the stimulant laxatives stems more from their popularity and abuse than from their valid therapeutic applications."*[34]

Docusate is a stool-softener laxative. This type of laxative can cause lasting damage to the intestine and can interfere with your body's absorption of nutrients. Docusate may also make your body absorb other drugs at an increased rate, so the combination of docusate with some other drugs may be dangerous.

Many people take laxatives more often than they need to. When do you really need them? You should not take a laxative to "clean out your system" or to make your body act more "normally." Nor should you take a laxative just because you are having less than one bowel movement a day. It is untrue that everyone must have a bowel movement (stool) daily. Perfectly healthy people may have from two bowel movements per week to three bowel movements per day.

If the frequency of your bowel movements has decreased, if you are having bowel movements less than twice a week, or if you are having difficulty in passing stools, you are constipated, but this does not mean that you need a laxative. It is better to treat simple, occasional constipation without drugs, by eating a high-fiber diet that includes whole-grain breads and cereals, raw vegetables, raw and dried fruits, and beans, and by drinking plenty of nonalcoholic liquids (six to eight glasses per day). This type of diet will both prevent and treat constipation, and it is less costly than taking drugs. Regular exercise—at least 30 minutes per day of swimming, cycling, jogging, or brisk walking—will also help your body maintain regularity.

If you are constipated while traveling or at some other time when it is hard for you to eat properly, it may be appropriate to take a laxative for a short time. The only type of laxative you should use for self-medication is a bulk-forming laxative such as psyllium (see p. 380). This type usually takes effect in 12 hours to three days, compared with docusate which takes effect one or two days after the first dose, but may require three to five days. Even bulk-forming laxatives should only be used occasionally.

If you are on a special diet such as a low-salt or low-sugar diet, ask your doctor or pharmacist to help you choose a laxative without ingredients you are trying to avoid. Some laxatives contain sugar (up to half of the product), salt (up to 250 milligrams per dose), or the artificial sweetener NutraSweet®.

Do Not Use

ALTERNATIVE TREATMENT:
For spastic colon, see Psyllium, p. 380.

Atropine, Hyoscyamine, Scopolamine, and Phenobarbital
DONNATAL (Robins)

FAMILY: Antispasmodics
Anticholinergics
Barbiturates

This combination of atropine (see p. 361), hyoscyamine (hye oh *sye* a meen), scopolamine (skoe *pol* a meen), and phenobarbital (see p. 584) is used to relieve abdominal discomfort from cramps (spasms) and to reduce the amount of acid produced in the stomach. **It is an irrational mixture of drugs**[35] **that is dangerous for older adults to use.**

Atropine, hyoscyamine, and scopolamine, three of the four ingredients in this combination, have severe adverse effects that make them too dangerous for older adults to use (see below). Even if you are taking only the usual adult dose, you may suffer from excitement, restlessness, drowsiness, or confusion.[36]

Phenobarbital, the fourth drug in this combination, causes problems so serious that the World Health Organization has said older adults should not use it.[37] Epilepsy is the only reason to take this drug. You can easily become addicted to phenobarbital. If you stop taking this drug suddenly, you will probably suffer withdrawal symptoms such as anxiety, restlessness, muscle twitching, trembling hands, weakness, dizziness, vision problems, nausea, vomiting, trouble sleeping, faintness, and lightheadedness. Later, you will suffer more serious symptoms such as convulsions, seizures, and hallucinations. These may last for more than two weeks after you stop taking phenobarbital.

WARNING: SPECIAL MENTAL AND PHYSICAL ADVERSE EFFECTS

Older adults are especially sensitive to the harmful anticholinergic (see Glossary, p. 768) effects of a family of drugs called belladonna alkaloids. Atropine, hyoscyamine and scopolamine are all in this family. Drugs in this family should not be used unless absolutely necessary.

Mental Effects: confusion, delirium, short-term memory problems, disorientation, and impaired attention.

Physical Effects: dry mouth, constipation, difficulty urinating (especially for a man with an enlarged prostate), blurred vision, decreased sweating with increased body temperature, sexual dysfunction, and worsening of glaucoma.

One hazard of taking Donnatal continuously for longer than several weeks is drug-induced dependence. **Do not stop taking your drug suddenly.** With the help of your doctor, work out a schedule for slowly decreasing the amount of the drug you take by about 5 to 10% each day. Keep a written record of the dosage reduction schedule with you. These steps will make it much easier to become drug free without developing distressing symptoms of drug withdrawal.

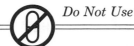

Do Not Use

ALTERNATIVE TREATMENT:
See Psyllium, p. 380.

Bisacodyl
DULCOLAX (Novartis)

FAMILY: Stimulant Laxatives

Bisacodyl (bis a *koe* dill) is a stimulant laxative. **We do not recommend taking it to treat constipation.** If you take stimulant laxatives for a long time, they gradually reduce your intestine's ability to work efficiently. This causes increasing constipation and a disease of the large intestine called cathartic colon, in which the intestine becomes enlarged and will not move without chemical stimulation. According to one pharmacology textbook, "the medical importance of the stimulant laxatives stems more from their popularity and abuse than from their valid therapeutic applications."[38]

Many people take laxatives more often than they need to. This is dangerous for several reasons. First, some laxatives, such as bisacodyl, can have harmful adverse effects. Second, all laxatives can be habit-forming. If you take them too often or for too long, your body will become less able to pass stools without them. This leads to a cycle of abuse in which you become dependent on laxatives and have to take them continuously. If you think you have become dependent on laxatives, talk to your doctor.

When do you need a laxative? You should not take a laxative to "clean out your system" or to make your body act more "normally." Nor should you take a laxative just because you are having less than one bowel movement a day. It is untrue that everyone must have a bowel movement (stool) daily. Perfectly healthy people may have from two bowel movements per week to three bowel movements per day.

If the frequency of your bowel movements has decreased, if you are having bowel movements less than twice a week, or if you are having difficulty in passing stools, you are constipated, but this does not mean that you need a laxative. It is better to treat simple, occasional constipation without drugs, by eating a high-fiber diet that includes whole-grain breads and cereals, raw vegetables, raw and dried fruits, and beans, and by drinking plenty of nonalcoholic liquids (six to eight glasses per day). This type of diet will both prevent and treat constipation, and it is less costly than taking drugs. Regular exercise—at least 30 minutes per day of swimming, cycling, jogging, or brisk walking—will also help your body maintain regularity.

If you are constipated while traveling or at some other time when it is hard for you to eat properly, it may be appropriate to take a laxative for a short time. The only type of laxative you should use for self-medication is a bulk-forming laxative such as psyllium (see p. 380). This type usually takes effect in 12 hours to three days, compared with docusate which takes effect one or two days after the first dose, but may require three to five days of treatment. Even bulk-forming laxatives should only be used occasionally.

If you are on a special diet such as a low-salt or low-sugar diet, ask your doctor or pharmacist to help you choose a laxative without ingredients you are trying to avoid. Some laxatives contain sugar (up to half of the product), salt (up to 250 milligrams per dose), or the artificial sweetener NutraSweet®.

Aluminum Hydroxide and Magnesium Carbonate
GAVISCON, GAVISCON-2 (SmithKline Beecham Consumer)

GENERIC: not available

FAMILY: Reflux Esophagitis Drugs

This combination of aluminum hydroxide (see p. 358) and magnesium carbonate (mag *nee* zee um car *bon* ate) is used to temporarily relieve heartburn caused by reflux esophagitis. In reflux esophagitis, acidic stomach contents flow backwards up into the esophagus (tube leading from the mouth to the stomach), causing a burning sensation under the breastbone.

You should not be taking Gaviscon and Gaviscon-2, two brand name products which contain this combination of drugs, for ulcers or serious stomach upset due to stomach acid. They do not contain enough aluminum hydroxide and magnesium carbonate to neutralize stomach acid. Instead, you should be taking a generic combination of aluminum hydroxide and magnesium hydroxide (see p. 378).

By combining aluminum with magnesium, this product reduces the problems that either substance alone can cause. Aluminum can cause constipation, and magnesium can cause diarrhea, but when the two are combined in one product, these effects are often balanced out. However, the combination may still cause either constipation or diarrhea.

If you take large doses of this drug or use it for a long time, see your doctor for regular checkups. If you are treating yourself with this drug, do not take it for more than two weeks unless you check with your doctor.

Older adults with metabolic bone diseases should not take aluminum antacids,[39] and those with kidney disease should not use them for a long time.[40] Taking magnesium carbonate for a long time or in large doses may cause kidney stones.[41] Anyone with severe kidney disease should not use magnesium antacids.[42]

Before You Use This Drug

Do not use if you have or have had:

- severely reduced kidney function
- metabolic bone disease

Tell your doctor if you have or have had:

- allergies to drugs
- constipation

- severe abdominal pain
- gastrointestinal or rectal bleeding
- prolonged diarrhea
- hemorrhoids
- intestinal blockage
- kidney problems
- Alzheimer's disease
- appendicitis

Tell your doctor about any other drugs you take, including aspirin, herbs, vitamins, and other nonprescription products.

When You Use This Drug

- **Call your doctor immediately if you have black, tarry stools or you vomit material that looks like coffee grounds. These are signs of a bleeding ulcer.**

How to Use This Drug

- Take each dose with **a full glass (eight ounces) of water.** The liquid form is better than tablets because it is more effective and costs less. If you use tablets, chew them thoroughly.
- Take immediately after meals and at bedtime for maximum effectiveness. Drink plenty of fluids.
- Do not take any other drugs by mouth for at least one or two hours after taking this drug.
- Do not store in the bathroom. Do not expose to heat, moisture, or strong light. Do not let the liquid form freeze.
- If you miss a dose, take it as soon as you remember, but skip it if it is almost time for the next dose. **Do not take double doses.**

Interactions with Other Drugs

The following drugs are listed in the *Evaluations of Drug Interactions* 1997 as causing "highly clinically significant" or "clinically significant" interactions when used together with this drug. We have also included potentially

serious interactions listed in the drug's FDA-approved professional product labeling or package insert. New scientific techniques have allowed researchers to predict some drug interactions before they have been documented in people. There may be other drugs, especially those in the families of drugs listed below, that also will react with this drug to cause severe adverse effects. The number of new drugs approved for marketing increases the chance of drug interactions, and new drug interactions are being identified with old drugs. Be vigilant. Make sure to tell your doctor and pharmacist the drugs you are taking and tell your doctor if you are taking any of these interacting drugs:

ACHROMYCIN, aspirin, GENUINE BAYER ASPIRIN, CALCIFEROL, CHIBROXIN, CILOXAN, CIPRO, ciprofloxacin, digoxin, ECOTRIN, enoxacin, FLOXIN, grepafloxacin, KAYEXALATE, ketoconazole, LANOXICAPS, LANOXIN, LEVAQUIN, levofloxacin, lomefloxacin, MAXAQUIN, NIZORAL, norfloxacin, NOROXIN, OCUFLOX, ofloxacin, PANMYCIN, PENETREX, RAXAR, sodium polystyrene sulfonate, sparfloxacin, SUMYCIN, tetracycline, TORVAN, trovafloxacin, vitamin D$_3$, ZAGAM.

Adverse Effects

Call your doctor immediately if you experience:

- difficult or painful urination
- irregular heartbeat
- mood or mental changes
- unusual tiredness or weakness
- severe constipation
- swelling of feet or lower legs
- bone pain, swelling of wrists or ankles
- loss of appetite, weight loss
- muscle weakness

- feeling of discomfort
- dizziness or lightheadedness

Call your doctor if these symptoms continue:

- nausea or vomiting
- speckled or whitish stools
- stomach cramps
- diarrhea or laxative effect
- chalky taste
- constipation

Periodic Tests

Ask your doctor which of these tests should be done periodically while you are taking this drug:

- blood aluminum, calcium, phosphate, and potassium levels
- kidney function tests

Limited Use

Loperamide
IMODIUM (Janssen)

GENERIC: available
FAMILY: Antispasmodics
Anticholinergics

Loperamide (loe *per* a mide) is used to treat severe diarrhea. When older adults get diarrhea, they have a greater risk than younger people of complications from the loss of fluid, sodium and potassium chloride, and other electrolytes.[43] If you occasionally have short-term diarrhea, it is best to treat it without drugs using oral rehydration solution (ORS) (see p. 353). If nondrug treatments do not control your diarrhea, ask your doctor if loperamide is appropriate for you.

If you use loperamide, do not take more than four 2-milligram capsules of loperamide per day (total of 8 milligrams).[44] An overdose can depress your breathing severely and can cause coma, permanent brain damage, and sometimes death.

If you still have diarrhea after using loperamide for two days, or if you develop a fever, stop taking the drug and call your doctor.[45]

WARNING: SPECIAL MENTAL AND PHYSICAL ADVERSE EFFECTS

Older adults are especially sensitive to the harmful anticholinergic (see Glossary, p. 768) effects of loperamide. Drugs in this family should not be used unless absolutely necessary.

Mental Effects: confusion, delirium, short-term memory problems, disorientation, and impaired attention.

Physical Effects: dry mouth, constipation, difficulty urinating (especially for a man with an enlarged prostate), blurred vision, decreased sweating with increased body temperature, sexual dysfunction, and worsening of glaucoma.

Before You Use This Drug

Do not use if you have or have had:

- severe inflammation of the colon
- diarrhea caused by antibiotics
- acute dysentery

Tell your doctor if you have or have had:

- allergies to drugs
- a condition in which constipation must be avoided
- dehydration
- infectious diarrhea
- liver problems

Tell your doctor about any other drugs you take, including aspirin, herbs, vitamins, and other nonprescription products.

When You Use This Drug

- **Call your doctor immediately if diarrhea continues past two days or if you get a fever.**
- To prevent severe constipation, stop taking this drug once your diarrhea stops.
- Until you know how you react to this drug, do not drive or perform other activities requiring alertness. Loperamide may cause drowsiness.
- Have regular checkups if you use loperamide for a long time.

How to Use This Drug

- Do not take more than prescribed.
- Do not store in the bathroom. Do not expose to heat or direct light. Do not let the liquid form freeze.
- If you miss a dose, skip the missed dose. **Do not take double doses.**

Interactions with Other Drugs

Some other drugs that you may be taking (either over-the-counter or prescription drugs) can interact with this one, causing adverse effects. Ask your doctor what these drugs are and let him or her know if you are taking any of them.

Adverse Effects

Call your doctor immediately if you experience:

- constipation
- skin rash
- loss of appetite
- stomach pain
- nausea or vomiting
- bloated feeling

Call your doctor if these symptoms continue:

- dry mouth
- drowsiness
- unexplained fever

Do Not Use

ALTERNATIVE TREATMENT:
For spastic colon, see Psyllium, p. 380.

Chlordiazepoxide and Clidinium
LIBRAX (Roche)

FAMILY: Ulcer and Irritable Bowel Drugs

This combination of chlordiazepoxide (see p. 222) and clidinium (kli *di* nee um) is used to treat ulcers and colitis. It is said to relieve the abdominal discomfort from cramping (spasms), reduce the amount of stomach acid, and relax the digestive system. **However, it is an *irrational* and ineffective mixture of drugs**[46] which older adults should not use.

One of the ingredients in this combination, chlordiazepoxide, is a tranquilizer. **Because of this ingredient, this product is *addictive*.** Chlordiazepoxide (sold by itself as LIBRIUM) belongs to a family of drugs called benzodiazepines (see p. 178) that can cause confusion, lack of muscle coordination leading to falls and hip fractures, and drowsiness in older adults. We believe that people 60 years of age and older should not use chlordiazepoxide. Other drugs in the benzodiazepine family are sometimes appropriate to treat anxiety or sleeping problems on a *short-term* basis, but because they are addictive, they should be used only as a last resort. They should not be used to treat digestive problems.

Clidinium has such severe adverse effects that older adults should not use it (see warning box). Even if you are taking only the usual adult dose, you may suffer excitement, restlessness, drowsiness, or confusion.[47] Clidinium can also reduce the amount of saliva. Since saliva fights bacteria in the mouth, a decrease in the amount of saliva leads to erosion of the gums and teeth, and later to dental or denture problems like tooth decay.

If you are taking this combination of chlordiazepoxide and clidinium, ask your doctor to prescribe another drug. If you have used the drug continuously for several weeks or longer, ask for a schedule that lowers your dose gradually.

One hazard of taking chlordiazepoxide continuously for longer than several weeks is drug-induced dependence. **Do not stop taking your drug suddenly.** With the help of your doctor, work out a schedule for slowly decreasing the amount of the drug you take by about 5 to 10% each day. Keep a written record of the dosage reduction schedule with you. These steps will make it much easier to become drug free without developing distressing symptoms of drug withdrawal.

WARNING: SPECIAL MENTAL AND PHYSICAL ADVERSE EFFECTS

Older adults are especially sensitive to the harmful anticholinergic (see Glossary, p. 768) effects of drugs such as clidinium. Drugs in this family should not be used unless absolutely necessary.

Mental Effects: confusion, delirium, short-term memory problems, disorientation, and impaired attention.

Physical Effects: dry mouth, constipation, difficulty urinating (especially for a man with an enlarged prostate), blurred vision, decreased sweating with increased body temperature, sexual dysfunction, and worsening of glaucoma.

The Food and Drug Administration has concluded that this drug lacks evidence of effectiveness.

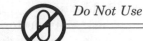

Do Not Use

ALTERNATIVE TREATMENT:
See Diarrhea—treating without drugs, p. 352.

Diphenoxylate and Atropine
LOMOTIL (Searle)

FAMILY: Antidiarrheals (see p. 352)

This combination of diphenoxylate (dye fen *ox* i late) and atropine (see p. 361) is used to treat severe diarrhea. Because of serious adverse effects, we recommend that older adults not use this product.

If you occasionally have short-term diarrhea, it is best to treat it without drugs using oral rehydration solution (ORS) (see p. 353). If non-drug treatments do not control your diarrhea, see your doctor. This combination of diphenoxylate and atropine should never be used to self-treat diarrhea. If you are using it, talk to your doctor about changing to a different drug.

Diphenoxylate can depress your breathing, causing severe shortness of breath or troubled breathing.[48] An overdose can cause severe respiratory depression and coma, possibly leading to permanent brain damage or death.[49]

WARNING: SPECIAL MENTAL AND PHYSICAL ADVERSE EFFECTS

Older adults are especially sensitive to the harmful anticholinergic (see Glossary, p. 768) effects of a family of drugs called belladonna alkaloids. Atropine is in this family. Drugs in this family should not be used unless absolutely necessary.

Mental Effects: confusion, delirium, short-term memory problems, disorientation, and impaired attention.

Physical Effects: dry mouth, constipation, difficulty urinating (especially for a man with an enlarged prostate), blurred vision, decreased sweating with increased body temperature, sexual dysfunction, and worsening of glaucoma.

Aluminum Hydroxide and Magnesium Hydroxide
MAALOX, MAALOX TC (Novartis)

Magaldrate
RIOPAN (Ayerst)

GENERIC: available
FAMILY: Antacids

The mixture of aluminum hydroxide (see p. 358) and magnesium hydroxide (see p. 388) neutralizes stomach acid and is used to treat ulcers and stomach upset caused by stomach acid. Magaldrate (*mag* al drate), a chemical combination of aluminum hydroxide and magnesium hydroxide, is used in the same way.

By combining aluminum with magnesium, these drugs reduce the problems that either substance alone can cause. Aluminum can cause constipation, and magnesium can cause diarrhea, but when the two are combined in one product, these effects are often balanced out. However, the combination may still cause either constipation or diarrhea.

If you take large doses of one of these drugs or use it for a long time, see your doctor for regular checkups. If you are treating yourself with this drug, do not take it for more than two weeks unless you check with your doctor.

Older adults with metabolic bone diseases should not take antacids that contain aluminum,[50] and those with kidney disease should not use them for a long time.[51] Anyone with severe kidney disease should not use magnesium antacids.[52]

Before You Use This Drug

Do not use if you have or have had:

- severely reduced kidney function
- metabolic bone disease
- intestinal obstruction

Tell your doctor if you have or have had:

- allergies to drugs

- severe abdominal pain
- gastrointestinal or rectal bleeding
- inflammation of the colon (colitis)
- diverticulitis
- prolonged diarrhea
- severe or prolonged constipation
- intestinal blockage
- kidney problems
- Alzheimer's disease
- appendicitis
- colostomy
- ileostomy

Tell your doctor about any other drugs you take, including aspirin, herbs, vitamins, and other nonprescription products.

When You Use This Drug

- **Call your doctor immediately if you have black, tarry stools or you vomit material that looks like coffee grounds. These are signs of a bleeding ulcer.**
- If you are on a low-salt (low-sodium) or low-phosphate diet, ask your doctor or pharmacist to help you choose an antacid. Many brands contain one of these substances.

How to Use This Drug

- Take each dose with **a full glass (eight ounces) of water.** The liquid form is better than tablets because it is more effective and costs less. If you use tablets, chew them thoroughly.
- Take one to three hours after meals and at bedtime for maximum effectiveness. Drink plenty of fluids.
- Do not take any other drugs by mouth for at least one to two hours after taking this drug.
- Do not store in the bathroom. Do not expose to heat, moisture, or strong light. Do not let liquid form freeze.
- If you miss a dose, take it as soon as you remember, but skip it if it is almost time for the next dose. **Do not take double doses.**

Interactions with Other Drugs

The following drugs are listed in the *Evaluations of Drug Interactions* 1997 as causing "highly clinically significant" or "clinically significant" interactions when used together with this drug. We have also included potentially serious interactions listed in the drug's FDA-approved professional product labeling or package insert. New scientific techniques have allowed researchers to predict some drug interactions before they have been documented in people. There may be other drugs, especially those in the families of drugs listed below, that also will react with this drug to cause severe adverse effects. The number of new drugs approved for marketing increases the chance of drug interactions, and new drug interactions are being identified with old drugs. Be vigilant. Make sure to tell your doctor and pharmacist the drugs you are taking and tell your doctor if you are taking any of these interacting drugs:

ACHROMYCIN, aspirin, GENUINE BAYER ASPIRIN, CALCIFEROL, CHIBROXIN, CILOXAN, CIPRO, ciprofloxacin, digoxin, ECOTRIN, enoxacin, FLOXIN, grepafloxacin, KAYEXALATE, ketoconazole, LANOXICAPS, LANOXIN, LEVAQUIN, levofloxacin, lomefloxacin, MAXAQUIN, NIZORAL, norfloxacin, NOROXIN, OCUFLOX, ofloxacin, PANMYCIN, PENETREX, RAXAR, sodium polystyrene sulfonate, sparfloxacin, SUMYCIN, tetracycline, TORVAN, trovafloxacin, vitamin D_3, ZAGAM.

Adverse Effects

Call your doctor immediately if you experience:

- severe constipation
- bone pain, swelling of wrists, feet or lower legs

- loss of appetite, weight loss
- muscle weakness
- frequent urge to urinate
- headache
- nausea, vomiting
- continuing feeling of discomfort
- unusual tiredness or weakness
- mood or mental changes

Call your doctor if these symptoms continue:

- stomach cramps
- diarrhea or laxative effect
- speckled or whitish stools
- chalky taste
- constipation

Periodic Tests

Ask your doctor which of these tests should be done periodically while you are taking this drug:

- blood aluminum, calcium, phosphate, and potassium levels
- kidney function tests

Psyllium
METAMUCIL (Procter & Gamble)
PERDIEM (Rorer)

GENERIC: available
FAMILY: Bulk-forming Laxatives
Cholesterol-lowering Drugs (see p. 54)

Psyllium (*sill* i yum) is a laxative that works by absorbing water and softening the stools in your intestine. Fiber that you get from food works exactly the same way. **Since a diet high in fiber, combined with plenty of nonalcoholic liquids, has the same effect as psyllium, this drug is usually not necessary.** Eating high-fiber foods is preferable to taking psyllium because these foods give you essential nutrients in addition to fiber.

When do you really need to take a laxative? You should not take a laxative to "clean out your system" or to make your body act more "normally." Nor should you take a laxative just because you are having less than one bowel movement a day. It is untrue that everyone must have a bowel movement (stool) daily. Perfectly healthy people may have from two bowel movements per week to three bowel movements per day.

If the frequency of your bowel movements has decreased, if you are having bowel movements less than twice a week, or if you are having difficulty in passing stools, you are constipated, but this does not mean that you need a laxative. It is better to treat simple, occasional constipation by eating a high-fiber diet that includes whole-grain breads and cereals, raw vegetables, raw and dried fruits, and beans, and by drinking plenty of nonalcoholic liquids (six to eight glasses per day). This type of diet will both prevent and treat constipation, and it is less costly than taking drugs. Regular exercise—at least 30 minutes per day of swimming, cycling, jogging, or brisk walking—will also help your body maintain regularity.

If you are constipated while you are traveling or at some other time when it is difficult for you to eat properly, using psyllium may be appropriate. Psyllium usually takes effect in 12 hours to three days.

If you are on a special diet such as a low-salt or low-sugar diet, ask your doctor or pharmacist to help you choose a laxative that does not contain ingredients you are trying to avoid. Some psyllium products contain sugar (up to half of the product) or salt (up to 250 milligrams per dose).

Before You Use This Drug

Tell your doctor if you have or have had:

- allergies to drugs
- severe abdominal pain
- rectal bleeding
- impacted bowel movement
- occupational exposure to psyllium

- obstruction of the intestine
- problems with swallowing
- appendicitis
- colostomy
- ileostomy
- heart disease or high blood pressure
- kidney problems

Tell your doctor about any other drugs you take, including aspirin, herbs, vitamins, and other nonprescription products.

When You Use This Drug

- **Check with your doctor to make certain your fluid intake is adequate and appropriate.** If you do not get enough fluids, the laxative will not work properly and may dry and harden, clogging the intestine.
- **Do not use for more than one week.** If you have used psyllium for a week, stop taking it to see if a high-fiber diet and liquids alone will work. If your constipation continues for longer than a week, call your doctor.

How to Use This Drug

- **Take each dose with a full glass (eight ounces) of water or juice.**
- If you take any other drugs, take them at least two hours before or after the time you take psyllium.
- Do not store in the bathroom. Do not expose to heat, moisture, or strong light.

Interactions with Other Drugs

Some other drugs that you may be taking (either over-the-counter or prescription drugs) can interact with this one, causing adverse effects. Ask your doctor what these drugs are and let him or her know if you are taking any of them.

Adverse Effects

Call your doctor immediately if you experience:

- trouble swallowing
- intestinal obstruction (cramping, bloating, nausea)
- skin rash or itching
- breathing difficulty

Periodic Tests

Ask your doctor which of these tests should be done periodically while you are taking this drug:

- blood glucose and potassium levels, if used for a long time

---

 Do Not Use

ALTERNATIVE TREATMENT:
See Aluminum Hydroxide and Magnesium Hydroxide, p. 378.

Magnesium Hydroxide, Aluminum Hydroxide, and Simethicone
MYLANTA, MYLANTA-II (J&J/Merck)

FAMILY: Antiflatulents (Anti-gas)
Antacids

This combination of magnesium hydroxide (see p. 388), aluminum hydroxide (see p. 358), and simethicone (see p. 382) is used both as an antacid and as an antiflatulent (anti-gas) drug. As an antacid, it is used to treat ulcers and serious stomach upset caused by stomach acid and to relieve heartburn. As an antiflatulent, it is used to relieve "excess gas."

We do not recommend this widely used drug because it contains an ineffective and unnecessary ingredient, simethicone. There is no convincing evidence that simethicone, alone or in combination with other drugs, is effective in treating so-called excess gas.[53] Since this drug has no benefit, there is no reason to take it. If you need an antacid, use a combination of aluminum hydroxide and magnesium hydroxide (see p. 378). **Do not waste your money on products that contain simethicone.**

If you think that you suffer from "excess gas," it may be that you actually have a bloated feeling from overeating or discomfort from eating the wrong food. In this case, no anti-gas drug will help you because the problem has nothing to do with gas. If you do have excess gas in your stomach, the best way to treat it is to reduce the amount of air that you swallow. You can do this by cutting down on smoking, carbonated drinks, and gum-chewing, which make you swallow air. A dry mouth (which may be due to anxiety or a drug you are taking) and badly fitting dentures also make you swallow more air, so correcting these problems will help.

Most gas in the large intestine is created when bacteria come into contact with carbohydrates, especially those found in cabbage, broccoli, and beans.[54] This bacterial action is normal, as is the passing of gas (flatus). Different people pass different amounts of gas, and passing gas is no cause for medical concern.

Older adults with metabolic bone disease should not take antacids that contain aluminum,[55] and those with kidney disease should not use them for a long time.[56] Anyone with severe kidney disease should not use magnesium antacids.[57]

 Do Not Use

ALTERNATIVE TREATMENT:
Reduce the causes of "excess gas" (see below).

Simethicone
MYLICON (J&J/Merck)
PHAZYME (Reed & Carnrick)

FAMILY: Antiflatulents (Anti-gas)

Simethicone (si *meth* i kone) is marketed as a drug to reduce the amount of "excess gas" and the discomfort that it causes. **There is no convincing evidence that this drug, alone or combined with others, is effective for this purpose.**[58] **Do not waste your money on products containing simethicone that claim to relieve "excess gas."**

If you think that you suffer from "excess gas," it may be that you actually have a bloated feeling from overeating or discomfort from eating the wrong food. In this case, no anti-gas drug will help you because the problem has nothing to do with gas. If you do have excess gas in your stomach, the best way to treat it is to reduce the amount of air that you swallow. You can do this by cutting down on smoking, carbonated drinks, and gum-chewing, which make you swallow air. A dry mouth (which may be due to anxiety or a drug you are taking) and badly fitting dentures also make you swallow more air, so correcting these problems will help.

Most gas in the large intestine is created when bacteria come into contact with carbohydrates, especially those found in cabbage, broccoli, and beans.[59] This bacterial action is normal, as is the passing of gas (flatus). Different people pass different amounts of gas, and passing gas is no cause for medical concern.

Famotidine
PEPCID (Merck)

Nizatidine
AXID (Lilly)

Ranitidine
ZANTAC (Glaxo Wellcome)

GENERIC: not available
FAMILY: Stomach Acid Blockers

Famotidine (fam *oat* id ine), nizatidine (ni *zat* id dean) and ranitidine (ra *nit* te deen) block the release of stomach acid and are used to treat ulcers and conditions caused by excess stomach acid. There is no valid scientific evidence that one of these stomach acid blockers is better than another. Cimetidine (TAGAMET) is similar to these drugs with some minor differences (see p. 395). All of the stomach acid blockers are now available in nonprescription strengths. You should not be using stomach acid blockers for minor digestive complaints such as occasional upset stomach, nausea, or heartburn.

Ulcers often come back after a few months. For frequent, severe recurrences, maintenance therapy is used. If your ulcer disease is resistant to treatment with stomach acid blockers talk to your doctor about the antibiotic combination treatments that are used to eradicate the bacterium Helicobactor pylori (see p. 354). This bacterium is present in a large number of people with ulcers. *The presence of this bacterium can be diagnosed with a blood test in people with a history of ulcer disease.*

A possible adverse effect of these drugs is confusion.[60] Elderly people are more likely to have reduced function of kidney and liver.[61,62] **If you have reduced kidney function, your doctor should start you on a low, or less frequent dose.**

If you are over 60, you should generally be taking less than the usual adult dose of these drugs, especially if you have reduced kidney or liver function. Your body will eliminate these drugs more slowly than younger people's bodies.[63] This means that more of the drug stays in your body for a longer time, which puts you at a higher risk of adverse effects, especially confusion. Famotidine, nizatidine and ranitidine are less likely than cimetidine to cause enlarged breasts, decreased sexual ability, dizziness and confusion.[64]

Cigarette smoking can delay healing of ulcers.[65] Some people find relief of reflux esophagitis by elevating the head of the bed. Liquid antacids of magnesium and aluminum in low doses are as effective at healing ulcers as stomach acid blockers, and less costly. However, long-term use of antacids has risks. Antacids with aluminum can cause bone damage, ones with magnesium can cause severe diarrhea. Too much calcium or sodium also causes serious problems. If ulcer symptoms worsen or bleeding occurs, medical help should be sought.

Before You Use This Drug

Tell your doctor if you have or have had:

- allergies to drugs
- kidney or liver problems
- a weakened immune system

Tell your doctor about any other drugs you take, including aspirin, herbs, vitamins, and other nonprescription products.

When You Use This Drug

- **Call your doctor immediately if you have black, tarry stools or if you vomit material that looks like coffee grounds. These are signs of a bleeding ulcer.**
- If you take an antacid, take it at least 30 minutes apart from these drugs. One source suggests taking stomach acid blockers two hours before antacids.[66]
- Avoid any food or drink that aggravates your ulcer.

• Check with your doctor before taking any aspirin, ibuprofen or other NSAIDs. These drugs can cause or aggravate ulcers.
• Do not drink alcohol or smoke.

How to Use This Drug

• Make sure that one of your doses is taken at bedtime.
• Do not store in the bathroom. Do not expose to heat, moisture, or strong light. Do not let the liquid form freeze.
• If you miss a dose, take it as soon as you remember, but skip it if it is almost time for the next dose. **Do not take double doses.**

Interactions with Other Drugs

The following drugs are listed in the *Evaluations of Drug Interactions* 1997 as causing "highly clinically significant" or "clinically significant" interactions when used together with this drug. We have also included potentially serious interactions listed in the drug's FDA-approved professional product labeling or package insert. New scientific techniques have allowed researchers to predict some drug interactions before they have been documented in people. There may be other drugs, especially those in the families of drugs listed below, that also will react with this drug to cause severe adverse effects. The number of new drugs approved for marketing increases the chance of drug interactions, and new drug interactions are being identified with old drugs. Be vigilant. Make sure to tell your doctor and pharmacist the drugs you are taking and tell your doctor if you are taking any of these interacting drugs:

COUMADIN, DURAQUIN, glipizide, GLUCOTROL, procainamide, PROCANBID, QUINAGLUTE DURA-TABS, QUINIDEX, quinidine, warfarin.

Adverse Effects

Call your doctor immediately if you experience:

• confusion
• hallucinations
• sore throat and fever
• unusual bleeding or bruising
• slow, fast, or irregular heartbeat
• unusual tiredness or weakness
• burning, redness, skin rash or swelling

Call your doctor if these symptoms continue:

• constipation, diarrhea
• dizziness or headache
• nausea or vomiting
• skin rash
• stomach pain
• loss of hair
• decreased sexual desire and ability
• swelling or soreness of breasts
• blurred vision
• drowsiness
• dryness of mouth or skin
• increased sweating
• joint or muscle pain
• loss of appetite
• ringing or buzzing in ears

Periodic Tests

Ask your doctor which of these tests should be done periodically while you are taking this drug:

• vitamin B_{12} concentrations

Limited Use

Promethazine
PHENERGAN (Wyeth-Ayerst)

GENERIC: available

FAMILY: Antinausea Drugs
Antipsychotics (see p. 187)
Antihistamines

Promethazine (proe *meth* a zeen) is most often used to treat severe nausea or vomiting, after the patient has already tried dietary changes without relief (see box below). It is also used to treat or prevent allergy symptoms and motion sickness and to promote sleep and sedation, but because of its serious adverse effects, it should *not* be used for these purposes.

Promethazine can cause serious adverse effects: drug-induced parkinsonism (see p. 193) and tardive dyskinesia (involuntary movements of parts of the body, which may last indefinitely). More information appears under Adverse Effects. Taking large doses of promethazine or taking it for a long time could increase your chance of experiencing these and other adverse effects. If you have used promethazine regularly for some time, ask your doctor if your drug can be changed in order to avoid developing serious adverse effects.

If you are over 60, you should generally be taking less than the usual adult dose.

WARNING: SPECIAL MENTAL AND PHYSICAL ADVERSE EFFECTS

Older adults are especially sensitive to the harmful anticholinergic (see Glossary, p. 768) effects of antipsychotics and antihistamines such as promethazine. Drugs in these families should not be used unless absolutely necessary.

Mental Effects: confusion, delirium, short-term memory problems, disorientation, and impaired attention.

Physical Effects: dry mouth, constipation, difficulty urinating (especially for a man with an enlarged prostate), blurred vision, decreased sweating with increased body temperature, sexual dysfunction, and worsening of glaucoma.

Drugs used to treat cancer often cause severe nausea and vomiting, either immediately after the drug is taken or several hours later. You can treat this kind of nausea and vomiting by changing your diet or by taking an antinausea drug. You should always try dietary changes first.[67]

• Eat small, frequent meals so your stomach is never empty.

• When you get up from sleeping or resting, eat some dry crackers or toast before you start being active.

• Drink carbonated drinks or other clear liquids such as soups and gelatin.

• Eat tart foods such as lemons and pickles.

• Do not eat foods with strong smells.

Before You Use This Drug

Tell your doctor if you have or have had:

• allergies to drugs
• an unusual reaction to other antipsychotics (see p. 247 for examples)

- heart or blood vessel disease
- Parkinson's disease
- epilepsy, seizures
- enlarged prostate or difficulty urinating
- diabetes
- glaucoma
- liver disease
- bone marrow depression
- lung disease or breathing problems
- alcohol dependence
- breast cancer
- stomach ulcer
- blood disease
- Reye's syndrome

Tell your doctor about any other drugs you take, including aspirin, herbs, vitamins, and other nonprescription products.

When You Use This Drug

- **Do not stop taking this drug suddenly. The dosage must be gradually decreased by your doctor to prevent withdrawal symptoms** such as nausea, vomiting, stomach upset, trembling, dizziness, and symptoms of Parkinson's disease.
- It may take two or three weeks before you can tell that this drug is working.
- Until you know how you react to this drug, do not drive or perform other activities requiring alertness. Promethazine may cause blurred vision, drowsiness, and fainting.
- Do not drink alcohol or take drugs that cause drowsiness.
- You may feel dizzy when rising from a lying or sitting position. When getting out of bed, hang your legs over the side of the bed for a few minutes, then get up slowly. When getting up from a chair, stay by the chair until you are sure that you are not dizzy. (See p. 16.)
- If you plan to have any surgery, including dental, tell your doctor that you take this drug.

How to Use This Drug

- Take with food or **a full glass (eight ounces) of milk or water** to prevent stomach upset.
- If you take antacids or drugs for diarrhea, take them at least two hours apart from promethazine.
- Do not store in the bathroom. Do not expose to heat, moisture, or strong light. Do not let the liquid form freeze.
- If you miss a dose, take it as soon as you remember, but skip it if it is almost time for the next dose. **Do not take double doses.**

Interactions with Other Drugs

The following drugs are listed in the *Evaluations of Drug Interactions* 1997 as causing "highly clinically significant" or "clinically significant" interactions when used together with this drug. We have also included potentially serious interactions listed in the drug's FDA-approved professional product labeling or package insert. New scientific techniques have allowed researchers to predict some drug interactions before they have been documented in people. There may be other drugs, especially those in the families of drugs listed below, that also will react with this drug to cause severe adverse effects. The number of new drugs approved for marketing increases the chance of drug interactions, and new drug interactions are being identified with old drugs. Be vigilant. Make sure to tell your doctor and pharmacist the drugs you are taking and tell your doctor if you are taking any of these interacting drugs:

AEROSPORIN, alcohol, ANECTINE, benztropine, bromocriptine, cabergoline, CAPOTEN, captopril, COGENTIN, DEMEROL, desipramine, diazoxide, DOSTINEX, INDERAL, INDERAL LA, meperidine, NORPRAMIN, PARLODEL, polymyxin B, PROGLYCEM, propranolol, succinylcholine.

Adverse Effects

Call your doctor immediately if you experience:

- **signs of tardive dyskinesia:** lip smacking, chewing movements, puffing of cheeks, rapid, darting tongue movements, uncontrolled movements of arms or legs
- **signs of parkinsonism:** difficulty speaking or swallowing, loss of balance, mask-like face, muscle spasms, stiffness of arms or legs, trembling and shaking, unusual twisting movements of body
  - changed or blurred vision
  - difficulty urinating
- **signs of neuroleptic malignant syndrome:** troubled or fast breathing, high or low blood pressure, increased sweating, loss of bladder control, muscle stiffness, seizures, unusual tiredness, weakness, fast heartbeat, irregular pulse, pale skin
  - fever
  - sore mouth, gums, or throat
  - abnormal bleeding or bruising
  - nightmares
  - fainting
  - skin rash
  - yellow eyes or skin
  - clumsiness or unsteadiness
  - dizziness

Call your doctor if these symptoms continue:

- constipation
- decreased sexual ability
- increased sweating
- dizziness, lightheadedness, faintness
- drowsiness
- dry mouth
- increased skin sensitivity to sun
- nasal congestion
- swelling or pain in breasts
- milk from breasts
- loss of appetite
- blurred vision
- burning or stinging of rectum

- confusion
- difficult or painful urination
- nightmares
- unusual excitement, nervousness, restlessness or irritability
- irregular heartbeat
- skin rash
- ringing or buzzing in ears

Periodic Tests

Ask your doctor which of these tests should be done periodically while you are taking this drug:

- complete blood count
- glaucoma test
- liver function tests
- urine tests for bile and bilirubin
- observation for tremors or jerking movements, early signs of tardive dyskinesia
- evaluation of continued need for promethazine

PREGNANCY WARNING

This drug caused harm to developing fetuses in animal studies, or such studies were not done. Use during pregnancy only for clear medical reasons. Tell your doctor if you are pregnant or thinking of becoming pregnant before you take this drug.

Limited Use

Magnesium Hydroxide
PHILLIPS' MILK OF MAGNESIA (Glenbrook)
M.O.M (Ulmer)

GENERIC: available
FAMILY: Antacids
             Laxatives

Magnesium hydroxide (mag *nee* zium hye *drox* ide) is both a laxative and an antacid. As a laxative, this drug may be used occasionally but should not be used regularly (see p. 380 for alternatives). As an antacid, this drug is stronger than aluminum hydroxide (see p. 358), but it tends to cause diarrhea. **Older adults who have severe kidney disease should not use magnesium antacids.**[68]

If you take large doses of magnesium hydroxide or use it for a long time, see your doctor for regular checkups. If you are treating yourself with this drug, do not take it for more than two weeks unless you check with your doctor.

Before You Use This Drug

Tell your doctor if you have or have had:

- allergies to drugs
- abdominal pain
- blood in stools
- inflammation of the colon (colitis) or bowel
- diverticulitis
- prolonged diarrhea
- intestinal blockage
- kidney disease
- appendicitis
- continuing diarrhea
- toxemia of pregnancy
- swelling of feet or lower legs
- difficulty swallowing
- colostomy
- ileostomy
- diabetes
- heart disease or high blood pressure
- bone fractures

Tell your doctor about any other drugs you take, including aspirin, herbs, vitamins, and other nonprescription products.

When You Use This Drug

- **Call your doctor immediately if you have black, tarry stools or you vomit material that looks like coffee grounds. These are signs of a bleeding ulcer.**
- If you are on a low-salt (low-sodium) diet, ask your doctor or pharmacist to help you choose an antacid or laxative. Many brands contain sodium.

How to Use This Drug

- Take each dose of magnesium hydroxide with **a full glass (eight ounces) of water.** The liquid form is better than tablets because it is more effective and costs less. If you use tablets, chew them thoroughly.
- If you are taking magnesium hydroxide as an antacid, take it one to three hours after meals and at bedtime for maximum effectiveness. Drink plenty of fluids.
- Do not take any other drugs by mouth for at least one or two hours after taking magnesium hydroxide.
- Do not store in the bathroom. Do not expose to heat, moisture, or strong light. Do not let the liquid form freeze.
- If you miss a dose, take it as soon as you remember, but skip it if it is almost time for the next dose. **Do not take double doses.**

Interactions with Other Drugs

The following drugs are listed in the *Evaluations of Drug Interactions* 1997 as causing "highly clinically significant" or "clinically significant" interactions when used together with this drug. We have also included potentially

serious interactions listed in the drug's FDA-approved professional product labeling or package insert. New scientific techniques have allowed researchers to predict some drug interactions before they have been documented in people. There may be other drugs, especially those in the families of drugs listed below, that also will react with this drug to cause severe adverse effects. The number of new drugs approved for marketing increases the chance of drug interactions, and new drug interactions are being identified with old drugs. Be vigilant. Make sure to tell your doctor and pharmacist the drugs you are taking and tell your doctor if you are taking any of these interacting drugs:

ACHROMYCIN, aspirin, GENUINE BAYER ASPIRIN, CHIBROXIN, CILOXAN, CIPRO, ciprofloxacin, digoxin, ECOTRIN, enoxacin, FLOXIN, grepafloxacin, KAYEXALATE, ketoconazole, LANOXICAPS, LANOXIN, LEVAQUIN, levofloxacin, lomefloxacin, MAXAQUIN, NIZORAL, norfloxacin, NOROXIN, OCUFLOX, ofloxacin, PANMYCIN, PENETREX, RAXAR, sodium polystyrene sulfonate, sparfloxacin, SUMYCIN, tetracycline, TORVAN, trovafloxacin, ZAGAM.

Adverse Effects

Call your doctor immediately if you experience:

- difficult or painful urination
- dizziness, lightheadedness
- irregular heartbeat
- mood or mental changes
- unusual tiredness or weakness
- feeling of discomfort
- confusion
- continuing loss of appetite
- muscle cramps or weakness
- weight loss

Call your doctor if these symptoms continue:

- diarrhea or laxative effect
- nausea, vomiting
- stomach cramps
- chalky taste
- mild constipation
- increased thirst
- speckled or whitish stools
- gas

Periodic Tests

Ask your doctor which of these tests should be done periodically while you are taking this drug:

- potassium concentrations
- kidney function tests

Limited Use

Omeprazole
PRILOSEC (Astra Merck)

Do Not Use Until Five Years After Release

Lansoprazole (Do Not Use Until 2001)
PREVACID (Tap)

GENERIC: not available
FAMILY: Ulcer Drugs

Omeprazole (o *mep* ra zole) and lansoprazole (lan *soe* pra zole) are close chemical relatives. Both drugs are approved for short-term treatment of gastroesophageal reflux as well as duodenal and gastric ulcers resistant to treatment with acid blockers and antacids. Also, both drugs are used in combination with antibiotics to treat

You should wait at least five years from the date of release to take any new drug unless it is one of those rare "breakthrough" drugs that offers you a documented therapeutic advantage over older proven drugs. New drugs are tested in a relatively small number of people before being approved, and serious adverse effects or life-threatening drug interactions may not be detected until the new drug has been taken by hundreds of thousands of people. A number of new drugs have been withdrawn within their first five years after release. Also, serious new adverse reaction warnings have been added to the labeling of a number of drugs, or new drug interactions have been detected, usually within five years after a drug's release.

ulcer disease caused by the bacterium Helicobacter pylori (H. pylori, see p. 354). Omeprazole is the drug of choice for long-term treatment of Zollinger-Ellison syndrome, although it does not alter the course of the disease. Lansoprazole is also approved for Zollinger-Ellison syndrome.

WARNING

In long-term (two-year) studies in rats, omeprazole and lansoprazole caused an increase in carcinoid tumors of the stomach. Although such tumors have not yet been demonstrated in humans, using these drugs for long-term therapy is not advisable, except for the treatment of Zollinger-Ellison syndrome.

Omeprazole and lansoprazole inhibit secretion of the gastric acid, whereas stomach acid blockers, such as cimetidine (TAGAMET), prevent production of the acid. Compared to stomach acid blockers, omeprazole relieves pain more quickly during the first two weeks,[69] and generally has fewer adverse effects short-term. Preventing the need for surgery is especially desirable in the elderly.[70,71,72] For ulcers, treatment takes a few weeks; for Zollinger-Ellison syndrome, a few years. To maintain effectiveness in treating Zollinger-Ellison syndrome, the dose may need to be increased annually.[73] Individual response to omeprazole varies considerably. In older people, decreased liver function may affect the response. Relapse of acid reflux is common. Long-term suppression of acid can lead to intestinal infections.[74,75] It is uncertain whether long-term suppression of stomach acid may also cause stomach cancer.[76,77,78,79,80,81,82,83]

For now, omeprazole and lansoprazole are recommended for short-term treatment of severe refractory reflux esophagitis or peptic ulcers only when other agents such as H_2 antagonists (stomach acid blockers, such as cimetidine (TAGAMET) or antacids do not work. Omeprazole and lansoprazole are more costly than stomach acid blockers, but less costly than surgery. For all these conditions try to avoid foods which trigger your condition, and avoid alcohol and smoking. Also, avoid drugs known to aggravate ulcers, especially aspirin, ibuprofen, and other nonsteroidal anti-inflammatory drugs (NSAIDs) (see p. 261). Ask your doctor if acetaminophen could be substituted. If these practices are not enough, try liquid antacids next. Long-term use of antacids also has risks. Aluminum can cause bone damage, magnesium severe diarrhea. Too much calcium and sodium also causes problems.

If you have gastric reflux or Zollinger-Ellison syndrome, try raising the head of your bed six inches.[84] If you have reflux esophagitis, try eating smaller, low-fat meals, more frequently, but do not eat for at least two hours before bedtime. Check with your doctor about other medications that aggravate the esophagus. If symptoms worsen or bleeding occurs, call your doctor.

Before You Use This Drug

Tell your doctor if you have or have had:

- allergies to drugs
- heart problems[85]
- liver problems[86]
- pernicious anemia[87,88]

Tell your doctor about any other drugs you take, including aspirin, herbs, vitamins, and other nonprescription products.

When You Use This Drug

- Try to stop smoking, since smoking may delay healing, especially of large ulcers.[89,90]
- Follow a diet recommended by your doctor.

How to Use This Drug

- Swallow capsule whole. Do not crush, chew, or open the capsule.
- Take these drugs before a meal. If you take it once a day, schedule it in the morning. You may take with or without antacids.
- Take for the full amount of time prescribed by your doctor, even if you are feeling better.
- Do not store in the bathroom. Do not expose to heat, moisture, or strong light. Do not let the liquid form freeze.
- If you miss a dose, take it as soon as you remember, but skip it if it is almost time for the next dose. **Do not take double doses.**

Interactions with Other Drugs

The following drugs are listed in the *Evaluations of Drug Interactions* 1997 as causing "highly clinically significant" or "clinically significant" interactions when used together with this drug. We have also included potentially serious interactions listed in the drug's FDA-approved professional product labeling or package insert. New scientific techniques have allowed researchers to predict some drug inter-actions before they have been documented in people. There may be other drugs, especially those in the families of drugs listed below, that also will react with this drug to cause severe adverse effects. The number of new drugs approved for marketing increases the chance of drug interactions, and new drug interactions are being identified with old drugs. Be vigilant. Make sure to tell your doctor and pharmacist the drugs you are taking and tell your doctor if you are taking any of these interacting drugs:

COUMADIN, cyclosporine, diazepam, DILANTIN, NEORAL, phenytoin, SANDIMMUNE, VALIUM, warfarin.

Adverse Effects

Call your doctor immediately if you experience:

- unusual bleeding or bruising
- diarrhea
- skin rash or itching
- abdominal or stomach pain
- increased or decreased appetite
- nausea
- anxiety
- cold or flu-like symptoms
- constipation
- increased cough
- depression
- muscle pain
- rectal bleeding

Call your doctor if these symptoms continue:

- breast enlargement in men[91,92]
- chest pain
- dizziness
- unusual drowsiness or tiredness
- painful erections
- gas
- headache
- heartburn
- vomiting
- numbness[93]

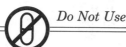

Do Not Use

ALTERNATIVE TREATMENT:
Nondrug treatment of nighttime heartburn; Maalox (see p. 378); histamine-2 blockers (see p. 383); omeprazole (see p. 389); metoclopramide (see p. 393).

Cisapride
PROPULSID (Janssen)

FAMILY: Antinausea Drugs

WARNING: POTENTIALLY LIFE-THREATENING DRUG INTERACTIONS WITH CISAPRIDE

Antipsychotic medications, astemizole (Hismanal), bepridil (Vascor), clarithromycin (Biaxin), disopyramide (Norpace), erythromycin (Erythrocin, EES), fluconazole (Diflucan), grepafloxacin (Raxar), indinavir (Crixivan), itraconazole (Sporanox), ketoconazole (Nizoral), mexiletine (Mexitil), nefazodone (Serzone), procainamide (Procanbid), quinidine (Duraquin, Quinaglute Dura-Tabs, Quinidex), ritonavir (Norvir), sparfloxacin (Zagam), tetracyclic antidepressants, tocainide (Tonocard), tricyclic antidepressants, troleandomycin (TAO). The use of cisapride with these drugs can lead to heart rhythm disturbance that can be fatal.

Cisapride (*sis* a pride) is used to control symptoms of daytime and nighttime heartburn, esophagitis due to GERD (gastroesophageal reflux disease), and delayed emptying of the stomach. Cisapride reduces exposure of the esophagus to stomach acid, and decreases the amount of time food stays in the stomach and upper and lower gastrointestinal tract. It is sometimes prescribed for constipation.

In June 1998 the Food and Drug Administration (FDA) announced new warnings for cisapride. The FDA has received 38 reports of deaths in people taking the drug since it was first sold in the U.S. in September 1993. People taking cisapride alone or in combination with a number of interacting drugs have experienced serious heart rhythm disturbances in some cases resulting in death.[94] Adverse reactions, including death, have also been reported in infants and children treated with the drug.

The new warnings caution that cisapride should not be taken by people with a type of electrical disturbance of the heart called prolonged QT syndrome, kidney failure, a history of rhythm disturbances of the large chambers of the heart known as the ventricles, heart disease, and congestive heart failure, low potassium or magnesium levels in the blood, or respiratory failure.

A number of other new adverse reactions that have been reported in adults since cisapride was cleared for marketing are now listed in the new warnings for this drug. These adverse reactions were included in the package insert due to a combination of their seriousness, frequency of reporting, or potential causal connection to cisapride. These are: allergic reactions, including bronchospasm, skin rash, and hives, possible worsening of asthma, psychiatric events, including confusion, depression, suicide attempt, and hallucinations, breast enlargement in men and women, urinary incontinence, high blood levels of the hormone prolactin and a white discharge from the nipple that looks like milk in women who are not nursing.

Serious events, including death, have been reported in infants and children treated with cisapride. These deaths have been associated with heart rhythm disturbances and seizures and there has been at least one case report of "sudden unexplained death" in a three-month-old infant. Other potentially serious adverse reactions reported in children taking cisapride include: a breakdown of red blood cells, high blood sugar (hyperglycemia), low blood sugar (hypoglycemia), unexplained stoppage in breathing, confusion, impaired concentration, depression, apathy, visual changes accompanied by amnesia, and severe sensitivity to the sun.

According to the editors of the highly respected independent source of drug information written for doctors and pharmacists, *The Medical Letter on Drugs and Therapeutics,* standard nonpharmacological treatment of nocturnal heartburn includes avoidance of food and alcohol near bedtime and elevating the head of the bed or sleeping with extra pillows. Antacids should also be tried. These methods should always be tried before starting treatment with other drugs for nocturnal heartburn.[95]

Limited Use

Metoclopramide
REGLAN (Robins)

GENERIC: available

FAMILY: Antinausea Drugs
Antipsychotics (see p. 187)

Metoclopramide (met oh *kloe* pra mide) has several uses. For people who have a condition in which the stomach takes too long to empty, it relieves symptoms such as nausea, vomiting, loss of appetite, heartburn, and a feeling of fullness. It also controls reflux esophagitis, a condition in which the stomach contents flow backwards into the esophagus (the tube connecting the mouth to the stomach), causing heartburn. It prevents nausea and vomiting caused by chemotherapy for cancer. This drug should not be used to treat motion sickness or vertigo (dizziness).[96]

If you are suffering nausea and vomiting from cancer chemotherapy, you should try changing your diet to relieve these effects before taking a drug such as metoclopramide (see box below).

Metoclopramide can cause serious adverse effects: severe drowsiness,[97] drug-induced parkinsonism (see p. 193),[98] and tardive dyskinesia (involuntary movements of parts of the body, which may last indefinitely). The latter two conditions can occur when the drug is used over a long period of time,[99] especially in people with impaired kidney function.[100] More information appears under Adverse Effects.

If you are over 60, you should generally be taking less than the usual adult dose because older adults often do not tolerate metoclopramide well.

Drugs used to treat cancer often cause severe nausea and vomiting, either immediately after the drug is taken or several hours later. You can treat this kind of nausea and vomiting by changing your diet or by taking an antinausea drug. You should always try dietary changes first.[101]

• Eat small, frequent meals so your stomach is never empty.

• When you get up from sleeping or resting, eat some dry crackers or toast before you start being active.

• Drink carbonated drinks or other clear liquids such as soups and gelatin.

• Eat tart foods such as lemons and pickles.

• Do not eat foods with strong smells.

Before You Use This Drug

Do not use if you have or have had:

• seizures

- bleeding, obstruction, or perforation of the stomach or intestine

Tell your doctor if you have or have had:

- allergies to drugs
- kidney or liver problems
- Parkinson's disease
- asthma
- high blood pressure

Tell your doctor about any other drugs you take, including aspirin, herbs, vitamins, and other nonprescription products.

When You Use This Drug

- Do not drink alcohol or use other drugs that can cause drowsiness.
- Until you know how you react to this drug, do not drive or perform other activities requiring alertness. Metoclopramide can cause drowsiness.

How to Use This Drug

- Take 30 minutes before meals and at bedtime for maximum effectiveness. Do not take more than prescribed.
- Do not store in the bathroom. Do not expose to heat, moisture, or strong light. Do not let the liquid form freeze.
- If you miss a dose, take it as soon as you remember, but skip it if it is almost time for the next dose. **Do not take double doses.**

Interactions with Other Drugs

The following drugs are listed in the *Evaluations of Drug Interactions* 1997 as causing "highly clinically significant" or "clinically significant" interactions when used together with this drug. We have also included potentially serious interactions listed in the drug's FDA-approved professional product labeling or package insert. New scientific techniques have allowed researchers to predict some drug interactions before they have been documented in people. There may be other drugs, especially those in the families of drugs listed below, that also will react with this drug to cause severe adverse effects. The number of new drugs approved for marketing increases the chance of drug interactions, and new drug interactions are being identified with old drugs. Be vigilant. Make sure to tell your doctor and pharmacist the drugs you are taking and tell your doctor if you are taking any of these interacting drugs:

cyclosporine, digoxin, LANOXICAPS, LANOXIN, NEORAL, SANDIMMUNE.

Adverse Effects

Call your doctor immediately if you experience:

- **signs of overdose:** confusion, severe drowsiness, muscle spasms, tic-like, jerky movements of head and face, shaking, trembling hands
- **signs of tardive dyskinesia:** lip smacking, chewing movements, puffing of cheeks, rapid, darting tongue movements, uncontrolled movements of arms or legs
- **signs of parkinsonism:** difficulty speaking or swallowing, loss of balance, mask-like face, muscle spasms, stiffness of arms or legs, trembling and shaking, unusual twisting movements of body
  - difficulty speaking or swallowing
  - chills
  - fever
  - sore throat
  - general feeling of tiredness or weakness
  - severe or continued headache
  - dizziness or fainting
  - increase in blood pressure
  - irregular heartbeat
  - aching, discomfort or sensation of crawling in legs
  - panic-like sensation
  - unusual nervousness, restlessness or irritability

Call your doctor if these symptoms continue:

- drowsiness
- restlessness, trouble sleeping
- breast tenderness and swelling
- constipation or diarrhea
- depression, irritability
- headache
- nausea
- skin rash
- dry mouth
- menstruation changes
- increased flow of breast milk

Periodic Tests

Ask your doctor which of these tests should be done periodically while you are taking this drug:

- clinical exams for tremors and jerky movements

Cimetidine
TAGAMET (SmithKline Beecham)

GENERIC: available

FAMILY: Stomach Acid Blockers

Cimetidine (sye *met* i deen) blocks the release of stomach acid and is used to treat ulcers and conditions caused by excess stomach acid. Similar drugs in this family include ranitidine (ZANTAC), nizatidine (AXID) and famotidine (PEPCID). You should not be taking cimetidine for minor digestive complaints such as occasional upset stomach, nausea, or heartburn, as there is no evidence that it is effective for treating these problems.

Ulcers often come back after a few months. For frequent, severe recurrences, maintenance therapy is used. If your ulcer disease is resistant to treatment with stomach acid blockers, talk to your doctor about the antibi-otic combination treatments that are used to eradicate the bacterium Helicobacter pylori (see p. 354). This bacterium is present in a large number of people with ulcers. *The presence of this bacterium can be diagnosed with a blood test in people with a history of ulcer disease.*

A possible adverse effect with this drug is confusion, but this also occurs with other drugs in this family.[102] Elderly people are more likely to have reduced function of kidney and liver.[103] **If you have reduced kidney function, your doctor should start you on a low or less frequent dose.**

If you are over 60, you should generally be taking less than the usual adult dose of cimetidine, especially if you have reduced kidney or liver function. Your body eliminates cimetidine more slowly than younger people's bodies.[104] This means that more of the drug stays in your body for a longer time, which puts you at a higher risk of adverse effects, particularly dizziness and confusion.[105] Rarely, people taking cimetidine have developed bone marrow depression, a serious adverse effect in which your bone marrow is unable to normally produce blood cells. Cimetidine has been shown to cause benign tumors in the testicles of rats,[106] and it can reduce men's sperm count (and therefore their ability to father children) if it is taken regularly for at least nine weeks.[107]

Cigarette smoking can delay healing of ulcers.[108] Some people find relief of reflux esophagitis by elevating the head of the bed. Liquid antacids of magnesium and aluminum in low doses are as effective at healing ulcers as stomach acid blockers, and less costly. However, long-term use of antacids has risks. Antacids with aluminum can cause bone damage, ones with magnesium can cause severe diarrhea. Too much calcium or sodium also causes serious problems. If ulcer symptoms worsen or bleeding occurs, medical help should be sought.

Before You Use This Drug

Tell your doctor if you have or have had:

- allergies to drugs
- kidney or liver problems
- weakened immune system

Tell your doctor about any other drugs you take, including aspirin, herbs, vitamins, and other nonprescription products.

When You Use This Drug

- **Call your doctor immediately if you have black, tarry stools or if you vomit material that looks like coffee grounds. These are signs of a bleeding ulcer.**
- If you take an antacid, take it at least 30 minutes apart from cimetidine. One source suggests taking stomach acid blockers two hours before antacids.[109]
- Do not drink alcohol or smoke.
- Avoid any food or drink that triggers your ulcer.
- Check with your doctor before taking any aspirin, ibuprofen or other NSAIDs. These drugs can cause or aggravate ulcers.
- Do not expose yourself to organophosphate pesticides, such as Diazinon.[110]

How to Use This Drug

- Take with meals. Make sure that one of your doses is taken at bedtime.
- Tablets have an odor. This is normal and no cause for concern.
- Do not store in the bathroom. Do not expose to heat, moisture, or strong light. Do not let the liquid form freeze.
- If you miss a dose, take it as soon as you remember, but skip it if it is almost time for the next dose. **Do not take double doses.**

Interactions with Other Drugs

The following drugs are listed in the *Evaluations of Drug Interactions* 1997 as causing "highly clinically significant" or "clinically significant" interactions when used together with this drug. We have also included potentially serious interactions listed in the drug's FDA-approved professional product labeling or package insert. New scientific techniques have allowed researchers to predict some drug interactions before they have been documented in people. There may be other drugs, especially those in the families of drugs listed below, that also will react with this drug to cause severe adverse effects. The number of new drugs approved for marketing increases the chance of drug interactions, and new drug interactions are being identified with old drugs. Be vigilant. Make sure to tell your doctor and pharmacist the drugs you are taking and tell your doctor if you are taking any of these interacting drugs:

ADALAT, ADALAT CC, ANECTINE, BICNU, carbamazepine, carmustine, clozapine, CLOZARIL, COUMADIN, diazepam, DILANTIN, DURAQUIN, ELIXOPHYLLIN, flecainide, glipizide, GLUCOTROL, imipramine, INDERAL, INDERAL LA, ketoconazole, lidocaine, M S CONTIN, morphine, nifedipine, NIZORAL, phenytoin, procainamide, PROCANBID, PROCARDIA, PROCARDIA XL, propranolol, QUINAGLUTE DURATABS, QUINIDEX, quinidine, ROXANOL, SLO-BID, succinylcholine, TAMBOCOR, TEGRETOL, THEO-24, theophylline, TOFRANIL, VALIUM, warfarin, XYLOCAINE.

Adverse Effects

Call your doctor immediately if you experience:

- confusion
- hallucinations
- sore throat and fever
- unusual bleeding or bruising
- slow, fast, or irregular heartbeat
- unusual tiredness or weakness

Call your doctor if these symptoms continue:

- decreased sexual ability or desire
- diarrhea
- dizziness or headache
- muscle cramps or pain
- skin rash
- enlarged or sore breasts
- burning, redness, skin rash or swelling
- drowsiness
- loss of hair
- nausea or vomiting

 Do Not Use

ALTERNATIVE TREATMENT:
Dietary modifications, see p. 366.

Trimethobenzamide
TIGAN (Roberts)

FAMILY: Antinausea Drugs
Anticholinergics

Trimethobenzamide (trye meth oh *ben* za mide) is used to relieve nausea and vomiting, but **there is no convincing proof that it is effective.**[111] It has little or no value for preventing or treating vertigo (dizziness) or motion sickness.[112]

If you have been taking trimethobenzamide regularly for some time and you have also been taking high doses of aspirin or other similar drugs (salicylates), the trimethobenzamide can hide the signs of an aspirin or salicylate overdose.[113] Rarely, trimethobenzamide causes convulsions, and this is more common among older users of the drug.[114]

WARNING: SPECIAL MENTAL AND PHYSICAL ADVERSE EFFECTS

Older adults are especially sensitive to the harmful anticholinergic (see Glossary, p. 768) effects of trimethobenzamide. Drugs in this family should not be used unless absolutely necessary.

Mental Effects: confusion, delirium, short-term memory problems, disorientation, and impaired attention.

Physical Effects: dry mouth, constipation, difficulty urinating (especially for a man with an enlarged prostate), blurred vision, decreased sweating with increased body temperature, sexual dysfunction, and worsening of glaucoma.

NOTES FOR GASTROINTESTINAL DRUGS

1. Lew JF, Glass RI, Gangarosa RE, Cohen IP, Bern C, Moe CL. Diarrheal deaths in the United States, 1979 through 1987: A special problem for the elderly. *Journal of the American Medical Association* 1991; 265:3280–4.

2. Fine KD, Santa Ana CA, Fordtran JS. Diagnosis of magnesium-induced diarrhea. *New England Journal of Medicine* 1991; 324:1012–7.

3. *Training Manual for Treatment and Prevention of Childhood Diarrhea with Oral Rehydration Therapy, Proper Nutrition and Hygiene* 1992. International Child Health Foundation, P.O. Box 1205, 10227 Wincopa Circle, Columbia Md 21044.

4. Recipe for Oral Rehydration Solution. From Werner D, Thuman C, Maxell J. *Where There Is No Doctor: A Village Health Care Handbook* 1992. The Hesperian Foundation, P.O. Box 1692, Palo Alto, CA 94302.

5. *The Medical Letter on Drugs and Therapeutics.* New York: The Medical Letter Inc., 1975; 17:80.

6. *The Medical Letter on Drugs and Therapeutics* New York: The Medical Letter Inc., 1996; 38:57–8.

7. Labenz J, Malfertheiner P. Helicobacter pylori in gastro-oesophageal reflux disease: causal agent, independent or protective factor? *Gut* 1997; 41:277–80.

8. New treatments for gastric and duodenal ulcers. *Prescrire International* 1997; 6:50–6.

9. *USP DI, Drug Information for the Health Care Provider.* 6th ed. Rockville MD: The United States Pharmacopeial Convention, Inc., 1986:190.

10. *The Medical Letter on Drugs and Therapeutics.* New York: The Medical Letter Inc., 1982; 24:61.

11. *Physicians' Desk Reference.* 40th ed. Oradell, NJ: Medical Economics Company, 1986:1520.

12. Kastrup EK, ed. *Facts and Comparisons.* St. Louis: J.B. Lippincott Co., July 1987:258–2591.

13. *USP DI,* op. cit., p. 979.

14. *USP DI, Drug Information for the Health Care Provider.* 7th ed. Rockville MD: The United States Pharmacopeial Convention Inc., 1987:366.

15. Ibid., p. 766.

16. *Physicians' Desk Reference.* 41st ed. Oradell, NJ: Medical Economics Company, 1987:1068.

17. Gilman AG, Goodman LS, Rall TW, Murad F, eds. *The Pharmacological Basis of Therapeutics.* 7th ed. New York: Macmillan, 1985:402.

18. Fong NL. Chemotherapy and Nutritional Management. In *Nutritional Management of the Cancer Patient.* New York: Raven Press, 1979.

19. Gabriel SE. Is misoprostol prophylaxis indicated for NSAID-induced adverse gastrointestinal events? An epidemiologic opinion. *The Journal of Rheumatology* 1991; 18:958–60.

20. Koretz RL. Prevention of NSAID-induced gastric ulcer. *Annals of Internal Medicine* 1991; 115:911–2.

21. Kornbluth A, Gupta R, Gerson CD. Life-threatening diarrhea after short-term misoprostol use in a patient with Crohn ileocolitis. *Annals of Internal Medicine* 1990; 113:474–5.

22. Clearfield HR. Management of NSAID-induced ulcer disease. *American Family Physician* 1992; 45:255–8.

23. Mazzuca SA, Brandt KD, Anderson SL, Musick BS, Katz BP. The therapeutic approaches of community based primary care practitioners to osteoarthritis of the hip in an elderly patient. *The Journal of Rheumatology* 1991; 18:1593–1600.

24. Rubin W. Medical treatment of peptic ulcer disease. *Medical Clinics of North America* 1991; 75:981–98.

25. Dukes MNG, Beeley L. *Side Effects of Drugs Annual 14,* Amsterdam: Elsevier, 1990:317.

26. Rubin, op. cit.

27. Gabriel, op. cit.

28. Renfrew RA. Prevention of NSAID-induced gastric ulcer (letter). *Annals of Internal Medicine* 1991; 115:912–3.

29. Mazzuca, op. cit.

30. Kornbluth, op. cit.

31. Graber DJ, Meier KH. Acute misoprostol toxicity. *Annals of Emergency Medicine* 1991; 20:549–51.

32. Morton MR, Robbins ME. Delirium in an elderly woman possibly associated with administration of misoprostol. *DICP, The Annals of Pharmacotherapy* 1991; 25:133–4.

33. Fossaluzza V, Di Benedetto P, Zampa A, De Vita S. Misoprostol-induced urinary incontinence. *Journal of Internal Medicine* 1991; 230:463–4.

34. Gilman, op. cit., p. 999.

35. AMA Department of Drugs. *AMA Drug Evaluations.* 1st ed. Chicago: American Medical Association, 1971:594.

36. *USP DI,* 1987, op. cit., p. 366.

37. *Drugs for the Elderly.* 2nd ed. Copenhagen, Denmark: World Health Organization, 1997:29.

38. Gilman, op. cit., p. 999.

39. *USP DI,* 1986, op. cit., p. 190.

40. *The Medical Letter on Drugs and Therapeutics,* 1982, op. cit.

41. *USP DI,* 1986, op. cit., p. 192.

42. *The Medical Letter on Drugs and Therapeutics,* 1982, op. cit.

43. *USP DI,* 1986, op. cit., p. 956.

44. Phone conversation with James Butt, M.D., Professor of Medicine, University of Missouri, School of Medicine, Columbia MO, January 5, 1987.

45. Kastrup, op. cit., p. 324C.

46. AMA, op. cit.

47. *USP DI,* 1987, op. cit., p. 587.

48. *USP DI,* 1986, op. cit., p. 693.

49. *Physicians' Desk Reference,* 1986, op. cit., p. 1690.

50. *USP DI,* 1986, op. cit., p. 190.

51. *The Medical Letter on Drugs and Therapeutics,* 1982, op. cit.

52. Ibid.

53. *The Medical Letter on Drugs and Therapeutics,* 1996, op. cit.

54. Ibid.

55. *USP DI,* 1986, op. cit., p. 190.

56. *The Medical Letter on Drugs and Therapeutics,* 1982, op. cit.

57. Ibid.

58. *The Medical Letter on Drugs and Therapeutics,* 1996, op. cit.

59. Ibid.

60. Karlstadt RG, Palmer RH. Unrecognized drug interactions with famotidine and nizatidine. *Archives of Internal Medicine* 1991; 151:810.

61. Gilman AG, Rall TW, Nies AS, Taylor P, eds. *The Pharmacological Basis of Therapeutics.* 8th ed. New York: Pergamon Press, 1990:899–902.

62. Dukes, op. cit.

63. Vestal RE, ed. *Drug Treatment in the Elderly.* Sydney, Australia: ADIS Health Science Press, 1984:250.

64. *USP DI,* 1986, op. cit., p. 1323.

65. Sontag SJ. The medical management of reflux esophagitis; role of antacids and acid inhibition. *Gastroenterology Clinics of North America* 1990; 19:683–712.

66. Lipsy RJ, Fennerty B, Fagan TC. Clinical review of histamine 2 receptor antagonists. *Archives of Internal Medicine* 1990; 150:745–51.

67. Fong, op. cit.

68. *The Medical Letter on Drugs and Therapeutics,* 1982, op. cit.

69. Lampkin TA, Ouellet D, Hak LJ, Dukes GE. Omeprazole: A novel antisecretory agent for the treatment of acid-peptic disorders. *DICP, The Annals of Pharmacotherapy* 1990; 24:393–402.

70. Langman M. Omeprazole. *British Medical Journal* 1991; 303:481–2.

71. Lind T, Cederberg C, Olausson M, Olbe L. Omeprazole in elderly duodenal ulcer patients: relationship between reduction in gastric acid secretion and fasting plasma gastrin. *European Journal of Clinical Pharmacology* 1991; 40:557–60.

72. Richter JE. Gastroesophageal reflux: diagnosis and management. *Hospital Practice* 1992; 27:59–66.

73. Maton PN, Vinayek R, Frucht H, McArthur KA, Miller LS, Saeed ZA, et al. Long-term efficacy and safety of omeprazole in patients with Zollinger-Ellison syndrome: a prospective study. *Gastroenterology* 1989; 97:827–36.

74. Dukes MNG, Beeley L. *Side Effects of Drugs Annual* 15, Amsterdam: Elsevier, 1991: 397.

75. Sontag, op. cit.

76. Omeprazole. *British Medical Journal* 1991; 303:1200–1 (letters).

77. Lampkin, op. cit.

78. Langman, op. cit.

79. Maton, op. cit.

80. Parkinson A, Hurwitz A. Omeprazole and the induction of human cytochrome P-450: a response to concerns about potential adverse effects. *Gastroenterology* 1991; 100:1157–64.

81. Misiewicz JJ, Poynter D. Omeprazole and genotoxicity (letters). *The Lancet* 1990; 335:611.

82. Sachs G, Scott D, Reuben M. Omeprazole and the gastric mucosa (abstract). *Digestion* 1990; 47 (Supp. 1):35.

83. Wright NA, Goodlad RA, Diaz de Rojas F. Omeprazole and genotoxicity (letters). *The Lancet* 1990; 335:909–10.

84. Richter, op. cit.

85. Langman, op. cit.

86. Walker S, Klotz U, Sarem-Aslani A, Treiber G, Bode JC. Effect of omeprazole on nocturnal intragastric pH in cirrhotics with inadequate antisecretory response to ranitidine. *Digestion* 1991; 48:179–84.

87. Langman, op. cit.

88. Lind, op. cit

89. Lysy J, Karmeli F, Wengrower D, Rachmilewitz D. Effect of duodenal ulcer healing by omeprazole and ranitidine on the generation of gastroduodenal eicosanoids, platelet-activating factor, pepsinogen A, and gastrin in duodenal ulcer patients. *Scandinavian Journal of Gastroenterology* 1992; 27:13–9.

90. McTavish D, Buckley MMT, Heel RC. Omeprazole: An updated review of its pharmacology and therapeutic use in acid-related disorders. *Drugs* 1991; 42(1):138–70.

91. Convens C, Verhelst J, Mahler C. Painful gynaecomastia during omeprazole therapy. *The Lancet* 1991; 338:1153.

92. Santucci L, Farroni F, Fiorucci S, Morelli A. Gynecomastia during omeprazole therapy. *New England Journal of Medicine* 1991; 324:635.

93. Sontag, op. cit.

94. FDA Strengthens Warning Label for Propulsid, FDA Talk Paper, June 29, 1998.

95. *The Medical Letter on Drugs and Therapeutics.* New York: The Medical Letter Inc., 1994; 38:11–3.

96. Kastrup, op. cit, p. 258–259l.

97. AMA Department of Drugs. *AMA Drug Evaluations.* 5th ed. Chicago: American Medical Association, 1983:536–7.

98. Bateman DN, Rawlins MD, Simpson JM. Extrapyramidal reactions with metoclopramide. *British Medical Journal* 1985; 291:930–2.

99. *USP DI,* 1986, op. cit., p. 1025.

100. AMA, 1983, op. cit.

101. Fong, op. cit.

102. Karlstadt, op. cit.

103. Gilman, 1990, op. cit.

104. Vestal, op cit.

105. *USP DI,* 1986, op. cit., p. 525.

106. Vestal, op. cit.

107. Van Thiel DH, Gavaler JS, Smith WI, Paul G. Hypothalmic-pituitary-gonadal dysfunction in men using cimetidine. *The New England Journal of Medicine* 1979; 300:1012.

108. Sontag, op. cit.

109. Lipsy, op. cit.

110. According to University of Texas (Dallas) expert on drug toxicity Dr. Thomas L. Kurt, MD, MPH, cimetidine can interfere with the body's clearance of organophosphate pesticides, since it inhibits the liver enzyme which breaks them down. As a result, there can be increased levels of pesticides in the body and increased pesticide toxicity.

111. *The Medical Letter on Drugs and Therapeutics,* 1974, op. cit., p. 48.

112. AMA, 1983, op. cit.

113. *USP DI,* 1986, op. cit., p. 1505.

114. AMA, 1983, op. cit.

Cold, Cough, Allergy, and Asthma Drugs

Cold	**402**
Allergy and Hay Fever	**405**
Asthma, Chronic Bronchitis, and Emphysema	**408**

DRUG LISTINGS

ANTIHISTAMINES AND DECONGESTANTS

ACTIFED	⊘ Do Not Use	412
ALERMINE		413
ALLEGRA	Do Not Use Until Five Years After Release	415
astemizole	⊘ Do Not Use	439
ATARAX		420
azatadine and pseudoephedrine	⊘ Do Not Use	458
BENADRYL		424
brompheniramine and phenylpropanolamine	⊘ Do Not Use	433
cetirizine	Do Not Use Until Five Years After Release	462
chlorpheniramine		413
chlorpheniramine and phenylpropanolamine	⊘ Do Not Use	446
chlorpheniramine, phenyltoloxamine, phenylpropanolamine, and phenylephrine	⊘ Do Not Use	443
chlorpheniramine and pseudoephedrine	⊘ Do Not Use	429
CHLOR-TRIMETON		413
CHLOR-TRIMETON 12 HOUR	⊘ Do Not Use	429
CLARITIN	Limited Use	431
clemastine	Limited Use	454
clemastine and phenylpropanolamine	⊘ Do Not Use	456
cyproheptadine		447
DIMETAPP	⊘ Do Not Use	433
diphenhydramine		424
fexofenadine	Do Not Use Until Five Years After Release	415
HISMANAL	⊘ Do Not Use	439
hydroxyzine		420
HY-PAM		420
loratadine	Limited Use	431
NALDECON	⊘ Do Not Use	443
ORNADE	⊘ Do Not Use	446
PERIACTIN		447
SELDANE	⊘ Do Not Use	453
SELDANE-D	⊘ Do Not Use	453
SOMINEX FORMULA		424
TAVIST	Limited Use	454
TAVIST-1	Limited Use	454
TAVIST-D	⊘ Do Not Use	456
terfenadine	⊘ Do Not Use	453
terfenadine and pseudoephedrine	⊘ Do Not Use	453

TRINALIN	Ⓧ Do Not Use	458
triprolidine and pseudoephedrine	Ⓧ Do Not Use	412
VISTARIL		420
ZYRTEC	Do Not Use Until Five Years After Release	462

COUGH AND COLD DRUGS

benzonatate	Limited Use	457
codeine and pseudoephedrine	Ⓧ Do Not Use	444
codeine, pseudo-ephedrine, guaifenesin and alcohol	Ⓧ Do Not Use	444
ENTEX	Ⓧ Do Not Use	434
ENTEX LA	Ⓧ Do Not Use	436
guaifenesin	Ⓧ Do Not Use	452
guaifenesin and dex-tromethorphan	Ⓧ Do Not Use	453
guaifenesin and phenyl-propanolamine	Ⓧ Do Not Use	436
guaifenesin, phenyl-propanolamine, and phenyl-ephrine	Ⓧ Do Not Use	434
hydrocodone and phenyltoloxamine	Ⓧ Do Not Use	460
NUCOFED (capsules and syrup)	Ⓧ Do Not Use	444
NUCOFED (expectorant syrup)	Ⓧ Do Not Use	444
ROBITUSSIN	Ⓧ Do Not Use	452
ROBITUSSIN DAC	Ⓧ Do Not Use	444
ROBITUSSIN-DM	Ⓧ Do Not Use	453
TESSALON	Limited Use	457
TUSSIONEX	Ⓧ Do Not Use	460

ASTHMA DRUGS

ACCOLATE	Do Not Use Until Five Years After Release	410
albuterol		449
aminophylline	Limited Use	417
AMOLINE	Limited Use	417
BETA-2	Ⓧ Do Not Use	426
BRETHAIRE		449
BRETHINE		449
BRICANYL		449
BRONKODYL		426
BRONKOMETER	Ⓧ Do Not Use	426
BRONKOSOL	Ⓧ Do Not Use	426
CHOLEDYL	Ⓧ Do Not Use	430
CONSTANT-T		426
cromolyn		437
ELIXOPHYLLIN		426
GASTROCOM		437
guaifenesin and theophylline	Ⓧ Do Not Use	451
INTAL		437
isoetharine	Ⓧ Do Not Use	426
MAXAIR		440
NASALCROM		437
oxtriphylline	Ⓧ Do Not Use	430
pirbuterol		440
PROVENTIL		449
QUIBRON	Ⓧ Do Not Use	451
QUIBRON-T-SR		426
SLO-BID		426
SLO-PHYLLIN		426
SOMOPHYLLIN	Limited Use	417
SOMOPHYLLIN-CRT		426
SOMOPHYLLIN-DF	Limited Use	417
SOMOPHYLLIN-T		426
SUSTAIRE		426
terbutaline		449
THEO-24		426
THEO-DUR		426
THEOLAIR		426
theophylline		426
VENTOLIN		449

zafirlukast   Do Not Use Until
                       Five Years After Release   410
zileuton   Do Not Use Until
                       Five Years After Release   461
ZYFLO   Do Not Use Until
                       Five Years After Release   461

DRUGS TO TREAT LUNG DISEASE

ATROVENT   422
ipratropium   422

WARNING: TERFENADINE (SELDANE) WITHDRAWN FROM THE MARKET

Effective February 1, 1998, this once widely prescribed antihistamine is no longer being sold in the United States. Terfenadine is associated with a number of potentially life-threatening drug interactions and should not be used. See p. 453 for these interactions.

You should check your medicine cabinet for old prescriptions of terfenadine. If you do have any, take them to your pharmacist for disposal or destroy them yourself.

Caution: Terfenadine is still available in foreign countries. If you are traveling outside the United States and need an antihistamine, make sure that you check the generic name of the product. For example, terfenadine is sold under the brand name Teldane in many European countries.

DO NOT USE: ASTEMIZOLE (HISMANAL)

The antihistamine astemizole is at least as dangerous as terfenadine in its potential to cause life-threatening drug reactions. Alone, in higher doses, or in combination with other drugs, it can cause fatal heart rhythm disturbances. This drug should not be used. See p. 439 for a listing of these interactions.

COLD

The viral infection we call "the common cold" can usually be treated without any professional help by rest and plenty of liquids, occasionally aided by the use of simple over-the-counter (nonprescription) remedies for relief of certain symptoms. There are no drugs that can kill the viruses that cause colds.

A cold cannot be "cured," except by time, but you are less likely to catch a cold if you do not smoke, since smoking paralyzes the hair-like cells (cilia) that clean out the body's airways. Colds are usually spread by hand more often than they are spread through the air. It's a good idea to prevent the spread of viruses by trying not to touch your eyes, mouth, and nose, and by washing your hands frequently when you are ill or with an ill person.

Certain other illnesses appear similar to colds, but warrant medical advice. If you have a high fever (above 101°F or 38.3°C) accompanied by chills and you are coughing up thick phlegm, or if coughing or breathing deeply causes sharp chest pain, you may have pneumonia. You should call your doctor for diagnosis and appropriate treatment.

The safest, best, and least expensive way to care for a cold is to not take anything at all and let the illness run its short, usually self-limiting course. If necessary, purchase single-ingredient products to treat the individual symptoms that you have.

What Is the Common Cold?

The common cold is a viral infection of the upper respiratory tract (nose, throat, and upper airways), resulting in inflammation of the mucous membrane lining of those areas. The most common symptoms are runny nose, sneezing, and a sore throat.

How to Treat a Cold

Nondrug Measures

A cold is best treated without drugs by drinking plenty—at least 8 to 10 full (eight-ounce) glasses per day—of nonalcoholic liquids (especially warm or hot liquids), getting enough rest, and not smoking.

Drugs to Use

If symptoms do not respond to these nondrug measures and interfere with normal activities, the following products are safe and effective. Please note that all of the drug products we recommend for treating various cold symptoms—stuffy nose, fever, nonproductive cough—are available without a prescription (over-the-counter, OTC). None of the prescription cough or cold drugs among the 456 most-prescribed drugs for older adults is recommended; 14 of the 15 drugs are classified as **Do Not Use.**

For a runny nose: No OTC or prescription drug is appropriate. A runny nose promotes drainage and should not be treated with medication. If it lasts longer than a week, call your doctor.

For a stuffy nose: If your nose is blocked, especially if you can't breathe through it, use nose drops or spray containing oxymetazoline hydrochloride (AFRIN, for example), xylometazoline hydrochloride (OTRIVIN NASAL SPRAY, for example), or phenylephrine hydrochloride (NEO-SYNEPHRINE nose drops and nasal spray, for example). Buy a less expensive generic or store brand product of any of these if it is available. Do not use these drugs for more than three days.

For fever, headaches and body aches: Use aspirin or acetaminophen, if needed (see pp. 275 and 338). (Also see Reye's Syndrome Warning, p. 263.)

For a cough: A productive cough (when you are coughing something up) should not be treated. If you have an unproductive (dry) cough that keeps you from sleeping, use dextromethorphan, available in Hold, St. Joseph's Cough Syrup for Children, or Sucrets Cough Control Formula.

Buy a less expensive generic or store brand dextromethorphan product if it is available.

Cold Remedies (Not to Use)

Oral nasal decongestants (pills or syrup): We do not recommend the use of any nasal decongestants that are taken by mouth for treatment of a cold, although a Food and Drug Administration (FDA) panel has found three ingredients safe and effective. These ingredients are in the OTC drugs Afrinol, Actifed and Sudafed, and 12 of the 18 prescription cough and cold drugs presented in this book. The reason we do not recommend them is that they all contain large amounts of amphetamine-like drugs which can increase your heart rate and blood pressure. In addition, they can make you jittery and keep you awake. By using nose drops or spray, for one to three days (no more), you get less than $\frac{1}{25}$th as much of these drugs—and just in your nose where they are needed, instead of throughout your system as you do when you take these drugs by mouth.

Antihistamines: Although the FDA has tentatively approved these drugs, we do not recommend the use of the following for treatment of a cold, largely because they are ineffective for this purpose: Chlor-Trimeton and Dimetane (OTC) or any of the prescription antihistamines (see p. 400).

The most widely read book on drugs, a standard reference for doctors called *The Pharmacological Basis of Therapeutics,* says this about the use of antihistamines for treating the common cold: "Despite early claims and persistent popular belief, histamine-blocking drugs [antihistamines] are without value in combating the common cold." Antihistamines also have a sedative effect.

Another reason to avoid unnecessary use of antihistamines is that older adults are more sensitive to their adverse effects. (See Chapter 2: Adverse Drug Reactions, p. 9.)

Eight of the 15 prescription cough and cold drugs that are in this book contain an antihistamine and are therefore classified as **"Do Not**

Use." They include Chlor-Trimeton 12 Hour, Ornade, Trinalin, Actifed*, Dimetapp*, Tavist-D, Naldecon, and Tussionex. These eight also contain an oral decongestant.

Commonly used oral OTC cold remedies that contain an antihistamine, and a decongestant, a combination that we label **Do Not Use** include Alka-Seltzer Plus, Chlor-Trimeton Decongestant, Comtrex, Contac, Contac Severe Cold Formula, Coricidin, Coricidin-D, CoTylenol, Dimetane Decongestant, Dristan Advanced Formula, Drixoral, Maximum Strength Tylenol Sinus Medication, Nyquil, Pyrroxate, Sinarest, Sine-Aid, Sine-Off, Sinutab, Sudafed Plus, Triaminic Syrup, Triaminicin Tablets, and Vicks Formula 44D.

Cough: A Necessary Evil

Your lungs clean themselves constantly in order to maintain efficient breathing. Mucus normally lines the walls of the lungs and captures foreign particles, such as inhaled smoke and infecting virus particles. Hair-like cells (cilia) push this out of the lungs. Coughing adds an additional, rapid-fire means of removing unwanted material from the lungs.

A cough is beneficial as long as it is bringing up material, such as sputum (phlegm), from your airways and lungs. This is called a productive cough and is often seen with colds, bronchitis, and pneumonia. A dry, hacking, nonproductive cough, on the other hand, can be irritating and keep you awake at night. Cough can also be part of a chronic condition, such as asthma or emphysema, or it may be caused by cigarette smoking.

Cough resulting from a chronic condition should be evaluated by your doctor. You should also seek medical advice if your sputum (phlegm) becomes greenish, yellowish, or foul smelling, if your cough is accompanied by a high fever lasting several days, if coughing or breathing deeply causes sharp chest pain, or if you develop shortness of breath. Any of the

* available OTC as well

symptoms may indicate pneumonia. Anyone who coughs up blood should call a doctor.

Types of Coughs

A *productive cough* is useful in helping you to recover from a cold or flu. You should do what you can to encourage the clearance of material from your lungs by "loosening up" the mucus. This is the purpose of an expectorant, which thins secretions so that they can be removed more easily by coughing (or "expectoration"). The best expectorant is water, especially in warm liquids such as soup, which thins the mucus and increases the amount of fluid in the respiratory tract. A moist environment also helps this effort. You should drink plenty of liquids and if you can, moisten the air in your home with a humidifier or plain water steamed by a vaporizer. A pan of water on the radiator can help in the winter.

A *nonproductive cough,* a dry cough bringing up no mucus, may be treated with a cough suppressant, also called an antitussive. A cough that keeps you up at night or is extremely exhausting may also call for the use of one of these agents. Cough suppressants should be used in a single-ingredient product. Rest and plenty of fluids are also in order.

Cough Remedies (Not to Use)

As mentioned above, the only time a cough medicine should be used is to suppress a nonproductive cough preventing sleep or other activities. The only drug recommended is single-ingredient dextromethorphan. Codeine, present in many prescription cough medicines, is not recommended for coughs. It is addictive and likely to cause constipation, especially in older adults.

Another ingredient in prescription (and OTC) cough products that we recommend against using is the expectorant guaifenesin (in all Robitussin products). We believe guaifenesin lacks evidence of effectiveness in loosening secretions (see Entex, Entex LA, and Robitussin).

Fever, Headache, and Muscle Aches

Fever, headache, and muscle aches are sometimes companions of the common cold. They are best treated without drugs, with rest and adequate fluids or with plain aspirin or acetaminophen. (A generic or store brand is as effective as heavily advertised brand names like Genuine Bayer, Datril, and Tylenol and generally costs less.)

Never give aspirin to a feverish person under 40 years old: he or she may have influenza rather than a cold. There is strong evidence that young people who take aspirin when they have flu (or chicken pox) have a greatly increased risk of later getting Reye's syndrome. This is a rather rare but potentially fatal disease that often leaves its victims impaired for life, if they survive.

Call your doctor if a fever climbs above 103°F (39.4°C), or if a fever at or above 100°F (38°C) lasts for more than four days. Under either of these circumstances, the patient probably does not have a cold.

Seek Medical Help When Any of the Following Occur:

• A fever greater than 101°F (38.3°C) accompanied by chills and coughing up thick phlegm (especially if greenish or foul smelling)
• Sharp chest pain when taking a deep breath
• Cold-like symptoms that do not improve after seven days
• Any fever greater than 103°F or 39.4°C
• Coughing up blood
• A painful throat with any of the following
   1) Pus (yellowish-white spots) on the tonsils or the throat
   2) Fever greater than 101°F (38.3°C)
   3) Swollen or tender glands or bumps in the front of the neck
   4) Exposure to someone who has a documented case of "strep" throat
   5) A rash that came during or after a sore throat

6) A history of rheumatic fever, rheumatic heart disease, kidney disease, or chronic lung disease such as emphysema or chronic bronchitis

ALLERGY AND HAY FEVER

If you suffer from an itchy and runny nose, watery eyes, sneezing, and a tickle in the back of your throat, then you probably have an allergy. An allergy means a "hypersensitivity" to a particular substance called an "allergen."

Hypersensitivity means that the body's immune system, which defends against infection, disease, and foreign bodies, reacts inappropriately to the allergen. Examples of common allergens are pollen, mold, ragweed, dust, feathers, cat hair, makeup, walnuts, aspirin, shellfish, poison ivy, and chocolate.

There are four common types of allergic responses, although many substances can cause more than one type of response in a given person:

• Itchy and runny nose, watery eyes, sneezing, and a tickle in the back of your throat. This type of allergy is sometimes called *allergic rhinitis* and is commonly caused by exposure to allergens in the air, such as pollen, dust, and animal feathers or hair. It is called "hay fever" when it occurs seasonally, such as in response to ragweed in the fall.
• Hives or other skin reactions. These commonly result from something you eat or from skin exposure to an allergenic substance, such as poison ivy or chemicals. Allergic skin reactions may also follow insect bites or an emotional disturbance.
• Asthma (see p. 408).
• Sudden, generalized itching, rapidly followed by difficulty breathing, and possible shock (extremely low blood pressure) or death. This rare and serious allergic response, called anaphylaxis, usually occurs as a response to certain injections (including allergy shots), drugs (including antibiotics such as penicillin

and many arthritis drugs especially tolmetin (TOLECTIN), and insect bites as from a bee or wasp. This reaction may become increasingly severe with repeated exposures. Anaphylaxis is a medical emergency requiring an immediate trip to an emergency room, clinic, or doctor's office. If you are likely to have an anaphylactic response to an allergen, such as a bee sting, in a locale where medical attention may be out of reach, you should obtain a prescription from a doctor for an emergency kit containing injectable epinephrine to keep with you, and learn how to use it.

How to Treat Allergic Symptoms

The best way to treat an allergy is to discover its cause and, if possible, to avoid the substance. Sometimes this is easy, but in many cases it is not. If, for example, your eyes swell, your nose runs, and you break out in hives each time you are around cats, avoid cats and you have solved your problem.

If, however, you sneeze during one particular season (typically, late spring, summer, or fall) each year or all year round, there is not too much you can do to avoid the pollens, dust or grass particles in the air. Some people find relief in an indoor retreat where it is cooler, closed, and less dusty, but this is not always possible.

If you can't seem to figure out the cause of your allergy, have tried eliminating most of the common allergens from your environment, and are still suffering significant discomfort, you may have to see your doctor or another health professional. It is possible that you may be an appropriate candidate for skin testing, and may be referred to a doctor specializing in allergies.

Beware of the allergist who sends you home with a long list of substances to avoid because they gave positive patch tests. Even if you avoid all of them, you may be left with your allergy if none of the substances on the list is the particular one responsible for your symptoms.

When identifying the cause of your allergy is not possible, you may choose to treat the symptoms. Allergy symptoms are caused primarily by the release of a chemical in your body called histamine, and a class of drugs known as the antihistamines is the most effective initial treatment available. We recommend that you use antihistamines in a single-ingredient preparation to treat your symptoms.

Allergic rhinitis should not be treated with topical nasal decongestants (drops, sprays, and inhalers) that are recommended for treating the temporary stuffy nose of a cold. Allergies are long-term conditions, lasting for weeks, months, or years, and use of these topical decongestants for more than a few days can lead to rebound congestion (an increase in nasal stuffiness after the medication wears off) and sometimes permanent damage to the membranes lining the nose. If you think your congestion is caused by allergies, don't use an OTC nasal spray, or you may eventually find that you can't breathe through your nose without it.

Drugs for Allergy
Antihistamines: Of all of the products sold for allergy, we recommend that you use a single-ingredient product containing only an antihistamine. Antihistamines are the most effective ingredients you can buy for treating an allergy, and you will minimize the adverse effects by buying the single-ingredient formulation.

A major adverse effect of antihistamines is drowsiness. If they make you drowsy, you should avoid driving a motor vehicle or operating heavy machinery while taking these drugs. Even if they don't make you drowsy, they may still slow your reaction time. Additionally, keep in mind that drowsiness is increased dramatically by adding other sedatives, including alcoholic beverages.

The amount of drowsiness produced by an antihistamine differs depending on the person who takes it and the antihistamine that is used. Of antihistamines classified by the FDA as safe and effective for OTC use, those causing the least drowsiness are chlorpheniramine maleate, brompheniramine maleate, pheniramine maleate and clemastine. For daytime use, we urge you to use one of these.

Other FDA-approved antihistamines, causing somewhat more sedation, are pyrilamine maleate and thonzylamine maleate. Those causing a great deal of drowsiness include diphenhydramine hydrochloride and doxylamine succinate, which are the ingredients in currently available OTC sleep aids.

The advent of the less sedating but, as it turns out, potentially more dangerous prescription antihistamines such as astemizole and terfenadine (see the warning about these two drugs, p. 402) has lessened the tendency of physicians and patients to use the lowest possible dose of the older, less expensive and safer antihistamines such as chlorpheniramine maleate, the active ingredient in Chlor-Trimeton and dozens of other prescription and over-the-counter allergy medicines. By trying a lower dose, you may find that you significantly reduce the sedating effects.

Another common adverse effect of antihistamines is dryness of the mouth, nose, and throat. Other less common adverse effects include blurred vision, dizziness, loss of appetite, nausea, upset stomach, low blood pressure, headache, and loss of coordination. Difficulty in urinating is often a problem in older men with enlarged prostate glands. Antihistamines occasionally cause nervousness, restlessness, or insomnia, especially in children.

For antihistamine treatment of allergies, your first choice should be a low dose of chlorpheniramine maleate or brompheniramine maleate, available in OTC single-ingredient products such as Chlor-Trimeton or Dimetane or generically. Check the label and be sure that nothing else is in the product. Chlor-Trimeton Decongestant or Dimetane Decongestant both

contain additional ingredients which are not necessary for the treatment of allergy. Less expensive store brand or generic equivalents are often available and should be purchased if possible. If you can't find them, ask the pharmacist; he or she should have them behind the counter if they are not on display.

You should not use antihistamines for self-medication if you have asthma, glaucoma, or difficulty urinating due to enlargement of the prostate gland.

ANTIHISTAMINE COSTS FOR ONE MONTH TREATMENT OBTAINED FROM DRUG STORES IN WASHINGTON, D.C.

brompheniramine/phenylpropanolamine		
generic	12 mg 75 mg	$18.95
Dimetapp	12 mg 75 mg	$21.95
chlorpheniramine		
generic	4 mg	$22.33
Chlor-Trimeton	4 mg	$38.29
clemastine		
generic	1 mg	$19.96
Tavist-1	1 mg	$29.96
diphenhydramine		
generic	25 mg	$44.85
Benadryl	25 mg	$58.35
astemizole		
Hismanal	10 mg	$78.59
cetirizine		
Zyrtec	10 mg	$66.99
fexofenadine		
Allegra	120 mg	$35.79
loratadine		
Claritin	10 mg	$72.99

Nasal decongestants: Many over-the-counter products sold for allergies contain amphetamine-like nasal decongestants, such as pseudoephedrine hydrochloride or ingredients found in many oral cold preparations (see earlier discussion on oral decongestants for colds).

Some of these adverse effects and adverse reactions (such as jitteriness, sleeplessness, and potential heart problems) occur even more frequently when they are used to treat allergies, because allergy medication is usually taken for a longer period of time than a cold remedy is.

More to the point, nasal decongestants do not treat the symptoms most frequently experienced by allergy sufferers: the runny nose, itchy and watery eyes, sneezing, cough, and the tickle in the back of the throat. They treat only a stuffy nose, which is not the major problem for most allergy sufferers.

Examples of OTC nasal decongestants that are labeled to treat allergy symptoms "without drowsiness" (since they do not contain antihistamines) include Afrinol and Sudafed. **We do not recommend** the use of these products for allergies.

Combination allergy products: As usual in the OTC market (particularly in the cold and allergy area), most products available are fixed-combination products, using a "shotgun" approach to your ailment. The majority of allergy combination products contain antihistamines and nasal decongestants; some also contain pain relievers. We do not recommend any of these for self-treatment.

It is our opinion that nasal decongestants should not be used for allergy symptoms that are appropriate for self-treatment. The likelihood of adverse effects is increased by taking a combination product, and decongestants are seldom useful for allergy symptoms.

Examples of OTC combination drugs for allergy, which we cannot recommend, are Actifed, A.R.M., Allerest, Chlor-Trimeton Decongestant, Dimetane Decongestant, Drixoral, and Sudafed Plus. **Many of the combination cold products that we urge you not to use are also marketed for allergic symptoms and hay fever. We do not recommend using any of these products for allergies either.**

ASTHMA, CHRONIC BRONCHITIS, AND EMPHYSEMA

Asthma, chronic bronchitis, and emphysema all occur commonly, may occur together, and may have similar treatments.

Asthma is a disease in which the smaller air passages in the lungs are hyperirritable. Attacks, which may be initiated by various influences, lead to narrowing of the airways and difficulty breathing. Wheezing, chest tightness, and an unproductive cough usually accompany the sensation of shortness of breath. Most asthmatics have only occasional trouble breathing.

Asthma attacks are commonly caused by exposure to specific allergens, air pollutants, industrial chemicals, or infection. They can be caused by exercise (especially in cold air). Asthma can be worsened by emotional factors, and the disease often runs in families. Other ailments common to many asthma sufferers, or their family members, are hay fever and an allergic skin condition called eczema.

Chronic bronchitis is a disease in which the cells lining the lungs secrete excess mucus, leading to a chronic cough, usually accompanied by phlegm.

Emphysema is due to destruction of the walls of lung air sacs and is characterized by shortness of breath, with or without a cough. There is a fair degree of overlap between chronic bronchitis and emphysema, and the two are sometimes lumped together into "chronic obstructive pulmonary disease" or COPD. Wheezing may occur with chronic bronchitis or emphysema.

Chronic bronchitis or emphysema is most commonly the end result of many years of cigarette smoking. Other causes include occupational or environmental air pollution, chronic lung infections, and hereditary factors.

Asthma, chronic bronchitis, and emphysema may be occupational illnesses (a problem related to the workplace). Asthma frequently occurs among meat wrappers, bakers, woodworkers, and farmers, and among workers exposed to specific chemicals. Chronic bronchitis frequently is the result of exposure to dusts and noxious gases.

Asthma, bronchitis, or emphysema may be mild. For some people, however, these diseases can become life-threatening or can cause restriction in lifestyle. For all people afflicted with these problems, the types of drugs prescribed to treat or prevent the attacks are quite strong. If used incorrectly, they may have an immediate and dangerous effect on the health of the user.

Do not try to diagnose or treat yourself. Asthma, chronic bronchitis, and emphysema must be diagnosed and treated by a doctor or other health professional. Two other common conditions that cause breathing difficulties, congestive heart failure and pneumonia have similar symptoms and many of the drugs used to treat asthma or COPD may worsen these conditions. Therefore it is extremely important that you have your condition properly diagnosed before starting any medication.

Treatment

Like its diagnosis, the treatment of asthma or COPD should be determined by a doctor. Attacks can be very frightening, and sufferers often over-treat themselves, especially when the desired relief has not been provided by the recommended dosage. Do not use more or less than the prescribed dose of any asthma or bronchitis medication without first consulting your doctor.

All medications for the treatment of these disorders, including those available without a prescription, should be chosen by you and your doctor together. A doctor is likely to prescribe one or more prescription drugs for the asthmatic. The currently available nonpre-

scription (over-the-counter) drugs are not the best drugs even for the treatment of minor or infrequent asthmatic episodes. The drug of choice for treatment of occasional acute symptoms of asthma is an inhaled beta2-agonist, such as albuterol (PROVENTIL, VENTOLIN), pirbuterol (MAXAIR) or terbutaline (BRETHAIRE, BRETHINE, BRICANYL).[1] These drugs are also commonly used for chronic bronchitis or emphysema.

Corticosteroids such as oral prednisone (DELTASONE, METICORTEN), or inhaled beclomethasone (BECLOVENT, VANCENASE, VANCERIL), flunisolide (AEROBID, NASALIDE), and triamcinolone (AZMACORT) are commonly used when severe acute symptoms of asthma do not improve after treatment with inhaled albuterol or terbutaline.[2] These are not used in COPD unless there is a component of asthma on top of the COPD.

Theophylline and aminophylline are commonly used for suppressing the symptoms of chronic asthma, bronchitis, or emphysema. Aminophylline is identical to theophylline except that aminophylline contains a salt called ethylenediamine, which has caused rashes and hives in some people. Oxtryphylline (CHOLEDYL) is not recommended because it is no more effective than theophylline, but costs more. These drugs must be taken exactly as prescribed, and the level of drug in the bloodstream must be monitored by a doctor. These measures will prevent adverse effects and ensure the optimal dose.

Zafirlukast and zileuton are members of a new family of asthma drugs called leukotriene antagonists. Both of these drugs are approved only to prevent asthma attacks in people with chronic asthma, not to treat acute attacks of asthma. Zafirlukast and zileuton both cause liver toxicity and are associated with a number of potentially serious drug interactions. The role of these drugs in the treatment of asthma has yet to be determined.

Proper Use of Inhalers

To receive the most benefit from your inhaler, follow the directions below[3] even though they may not agree with the directions on the drug manufacturer's packaging. Always shake well before taking each dose. Remove the plastic cap that covers the mouthpiece. Hold the inhaler upright, approximately 1 to 1½ inches from your lips. Open your mouth widely. Breathe out as fully as you comfortably can. Breathe in deeply as you press down on the can with your index finger. When you have finished breathing in, hold your breath as long as you comfortably can (try to hold it for 10 seconds). This allows time for the medication to treat your lungs before you breathe it out. If you have difficulty with hand-breath coordination, as many people do, ask your doctor for an "add-on" device that attaches to your inhaler. It allows you to close your lips around the inhaler, yet still receive the full therapeutic benefit from that dose.

If your doctor has told you to take more than one puff at each treatment, wait one minute, shake the can again, and repeat. If you also take a bronchodilator, in addition to the corticosteroids, you should inhale the bronchodilator first. Wait 15 minutes before inhaling the corticosteroids. This allows more corticosteroid to be absorbed in the lungs.

Your inhaler should be cleaned every day. To do this properly, remove the can from the plastic case. Rinse the plastic case and cap under warm running water. Dry thoroughly. Using a gentle, twisting motion, replace the metal can into the case. Put the cap on the mouthpiece.

Inhaled steroids for asthma have been available in the U.S. mainly in pressurized metered-dose inhalers, which require a propellant. The chlorofluorocarbon (CFC) propellants in these formulations are being changed for environmental reasons. Dry-powder inhalers, which are activated by inhalation, do not require a propellant, and people who have difficulty with hand-breath coordination find them easier to use.

If you have difficulty with hand-breath coordination, talk to your doctor about a dry powder inhaler.

DRUG PROFILES

Do Not Use Until Five Years After Release

Zafirlukast (Do Not Use Until 2002) ACCOLATE (Zeneca)

GENERIC: not available
FAMILY: Asthma Drugs (see p. 408)

You should wait at least five years from the date of release to take any new drug unless it is one of those rare "breakthrough" drugs that offers you a documented therapeutic advantage over older proven drugs. New drugs are tested in a relatively small number of people before being approved, and serious adverse effects or life-threatening drug interactions may not be detected until the new drug has been taken by hundreds of thousands of people. A number of new drugs have been withdrawn within their first five years after release. Also, serious new adverse reaction warnings have been added to the labeling of a number of drugs, or new drug interactions have been detected, usually within the first five years after a drug's release.

Zafirlukast (za *fir* loo kast) is used to prevent mild to moderate asthma. It belongs to a new group of drugs called leukotriene inhibitors, in the same family as zileuton. These drugs are not bronchodilators and are not useful for acute asthma attacks. The usual dose of zafirlukast is 20 mg twice daily for adults and children over age 12. People with liver problems may need to take a lower dose. Older people taking zafirlukast had more respiratory infections than younger people. Zafirlukast may remain in the body of older people twice as long.[4] Shortly after zafirlukast was approved for marketing it was found to cause a serious, even fatal, inflammation of the blood vessels called Churg-Strauss syndrome. Do not take if you are breast-feeding. In animals, zafirlukast increased liver tumors and bladder cancer. Information about the long-term effects of zafirlukast in humans is not yet known.

ADDITIONAL PRECAUTIONS

Avoid exposure to things which trigger your allergies or asthma, such as animals, bedding, chemicals, cosmetics, drugs, dust, mold, foods, pollens or smoke. Wearing a mask reduces inhalation of drugs, pollens and smoke.

Aspirin can trigger asthma in people who are aspirin-allergic, as can beta-blockers. Infections aggravate lung problems. During epidemics of respiratory illnesses, avoid crowded places and wash your hands frequently to help prevent infection. If you have asthma, get a flu vaccination.

Note: The information in this profile addresses the care of asthma that is not serious enough to need emergency treatment.

Before You Use This Drug

Tell your doctor if you have or have had:

- allergies, including lactose and iodine
- liver problems
- pregnant or nursing

Tell your doctor about any other drugs you take, including aspirin, herbs, vitamins, and other nonprescription products.

When You Use This Drug

- Keep short-acting bronchodilators on hand for acute asthma attacks.
- Do not decrease your dose of other asthma medication you take, especially steroids, unless your doctor tells you to.
- If you plan to have any surgery, including dental, tell your doctor that you take this drug.

How to Use This Drug

- Swallow tablets whole. Take at regular intervals on an empty stomach, one hour before or two hours after meals.
- Take regularly even if you do not have symptoms of asthma.
- If you miss a dose, take as soon as you remember, but skip it if it is almost time for the next dose. **Do not take double doses.**
- Do not store in the bathroom. Do not expose to heat, moisture, or strong light.

Interactions with Other Drugs

The following drugs are listed in the *Evaluations of Drug Interactions* 1997 as causing "highly clinically significant" or "clinically significant" interactions when used together with this drug. We have also included potentially serious interactions listed in the drug's FDA-approved professional product labeling or package insert. New scientific techniques have allowed researchers to predict some drug interactions before they have been documented in people. There may be other drugs, especially those in the families of drugs listed below, that also will react with this drug to cause severe adverse effects. The number of new drugs approved for marketing increases the chance of drug interactions, and new drug interactions are being identified with old drugs. Be vigilant. Make sure to tell your doctor and pharmacist the drugs you are taking and tell your doctor if you are taking any of these interacting drugs:

ADALAT, ADALAT CC, astemizole, carbamazepine, CARDENE, CARDENE SR, cisapride, COUMADIN, cyclosporine, DILANTIN, DYNACIRC, DYNACIRC CR, felodipine, HISMANAL, isradipine, NEORAL, nicardipine, nifedipine, nimodipine, NIMOTOP, ORINASE, phenytoin, PLENDIL, PROCARDIA, PROCARDIA XL, PROPULSID, SANDIMMUNE, TEGRETOL, tolbutamide, warfarin.

Adjustments in dosage may be made, or the drug discontinued.

Adverse Effects

Call your doctor immediately if you experience:

- flu-like symptoms, such as fever, muscle aches and pains
- weight loss

Call your doctor if these symptoms continue:

- cough
- dizziness
- headache
- nasal congestion
- nausea or vomiting
- stomach upset

Do Not Use

ALTERNATIVE TREATMENT:
See Cold, p. 402, and Allergy and Hay Fever, p. 405.

Triprolidine and Pseudoephedrine
ACTIFED (Warner-Lambert Consumer Products)

FAMILY: Cold and Allergy Drugs (see p. 402)

This combination of triprolidine (trye *proe* li deen) and pseudoephedrine (soo doe e *fed* rin) is marketed as a drug that relieves congestion and other problems caused by allergies and the common cold. Actifed, a brand-name product, is advertised as a remedy for sneezing, runny nose, and other symptoms of nasal congestion. You should not use it. Fixed-combination products containing an antihistamine (triprolidine) and a decongestant (pseudoephedrine) exemplify the "shotgun" approach to treating cold and allergy symptoms, which are better treated with individual drugs for individual symptoms. In our view, the combination lacks clinical evidence of effectiveness.

If you want to treat congestion caused by an allergy, the best treatment is an antihistamine such as triprolidine. If you want to treat congestion caused by a cold, the best treatment is a decongestant nose spray or nose drops. There is no reason to combine an antihistamine and a decongestant in one product.

Triprolidine is an effective antihistamine for treating hay fever and other allergies. If you have congestion caused by an allergy, taking triprolidine or another antihistamine alone will help. There is no satisfactory evidence that allergy patients benefit from adding a decongestant such as pseudoephedrine to an antihistamine. Triprolidine can cause drowsiness, loss of coordination, mental inattention, and dizziness.[5]

ADDITIONAL PRECAUTIONS

Avoid exposure to things which trigger your allergies or asthma, such as animals, bedding, chemicals, cosmetics, drugs, dust, mold, foods, pollens or smoke. Wearing a mask reduces inhalation of drugs, pollens and smoke. Many people with mildly red, itching eyes require no treatment. Cold compresses to the eyes may prove helpful. Using eye drops with vasoconstrictors whitens eyes for a while, but rebound redness can occur. Misuse of vasoconstrictors sets up a vicious cycle.

If your congestion is caused by a cold rather than an allergy, you can use decongestant nasal sprays or drops such as phenylephrine, oxymetazoline, or xylometazoline, all available without a prescription. Any of these is a better choice than a drug like pseudoephedrine, which can have dangerous adverse effects because it is taken by mouth and it affects your whole system. Do not use decongestant nasal sprays or drops longer than three days (see p. 403).

WARNING

Pseudoephedrine can cause or worsen high blood pressure. It is especially dangerous for people who have high blood pressure, heart disease, diabetes, or thyroid disease. People over 60 are more likely than younger people to experience effects on the heart and blood pressure, restlessness, nervousness, and confusion. Do not use pseudoephedrine during or within 14 days following administration of monoamine oxidase (MAO) inhibitors.

WARNING: SPECIAL MENTAL AND PHYSICAL ADVERSE EFFECTS

Older adults are especially sensitive to the harmful anticholinergic (see Glossary, p. 768) effects of antihistamines such as triprolidine. Drugs in this family should not be used unless absolutely necessary.

Mental Effects: confusion, delirium, short-term memory problems, disorientation, and impaired attention.

Physical Effects: dry mouth, constipation, difficulty urinating (especially for a man with an enlarged prostate), blurred vision, decreased sweating with increased body temperature, sexual dysfunction, and worsening of glaucoma.

Chlorpheniramine
ALERMINE (Reid-Rowell)
CHLOR-TRIMETON (Schering-Plough)

GENERIC: available

FAMILY: Antihistamines (see p. 402)

Chlorpheniramine (klor fen *eer* a meen) relieves the symptoms of hay fever and other allergic reactions. Do not use it to treat a cold. Colds and allergies have different causes, and chlorpheniramine is not effective against either the cause of a cold or its symptoms. In fact, the drug can make a cold or cough worse by thickening nasal secretions and drying mucous membranes. Chlorpheniramine also causes drowsiness.

Chlorpheniramine can cause harmful adverse effects, more commonly in people over 60 than in younger people. These effects include: confusion, dizziness, fainting, difficult or painful urination, dry mouth, nose, or throat, nightmares, unusual excitement, nervousness, restlessness, or irritability. If you have any of these symptoms while taking chlorpheniramine, ask your doctor about changing or discontinuing this drug. Since older people can be more sensitive to the usual adult dose, start with a low dose. This may decrease adverse effects.

ADDITIONAL PRECAUTIONS

Avoid exposure to things which trigger your allergies or asthma, such as animals, bedding, chemicals, cosmetics, drugs, dust, mold, foods, pollens or smoke. Wearing a mask reduces inhalation of drugs, pollens and smoke. Many people with mildly red, itching eyes require no treatment. Cold compresses to the eyes may prove helpful. Using eye drops with vasoconstrictors whitens eyes for a while, but rebound redness can occur. Misuse of vasoconstrictors sets up a vicious cycle.

WARNING: SPECIAL MENTAL AND PHYSICAL ADVERSE EFFECTS

Older adults are especially sensitive to the harmful anticholinergic (see Glossary, p. 768) effects of antihistamines such as chlorpheniramine. Drugs in this family should not be used unless absolutely necessary.

Mental Effects: confusion, delirium, short-term memory problems, disorientation, and impaired attention.

Physical Effects: dry mouth, constipation, difficulty urinating (especially for a man with an enlarged prostate), blurred vision, decreased sweating with increased body temperature, sexual dysfunction, and worsening of glaucoma.

Before You Use This Drug

Tell your doctor if you have or have had:

- allergies to drugs
- asthma
- problems with urination
- glaucoma
- enlarged prostate

Tell your doctor about any other drugs you take, including aspirin, herbs, vitamins, and other nonprescription products.

When You Use This Drug

- Do not use more often or in a higher dose than prescribed. Overuse increases your risk of adverse effects.
- Do not drink alcohol or use other drugs that can cause drowsiness.
- Until you know how you react to this drug, do not drive or perform other activities requiring alertness.
- If you plan to have any surgery, including dental, tell your doctor that you take this drug.

How to Use This Drug

- Do not store in the bathroom. Do not expose to heat, moisture, or strong light. Do not allow liquid form to freeze.
- Take with food, water, or milk to avoid stomach upset.
- Swallow extended-release forms whole.
- If you miss a dose, take it as soon as you remember, but skip it if it is almost time for the next dose. **Do not take double doses.**

Interactions with Other Drugs

The following drugs are listed in the *Evaluations of Drug Interactions* 1997 as causing "highly clinically significant" or "clinically significant" interactions when used together with this drug. We have also included potentially serious interactions listed in the drug's FDA-approved professional product labeling or package insert. New scientific techniques have allowed researchers to predict some drug interactions before they have been documented in people. There may be other drugs, especially those in the families of drugs listed below, that also will react with this drug to cause severe adverse effects. The number of new drugs approved for marketing increases the chance of drug interactions, and new drug interactions are being identified with old drugs. Be vigilant. Make sure to tell your doctor and pharmacist the drugs you are taking and tell your doctor if you are taking any of these interacting drugs:

alcohol, DILANTIN, phenytoin.

Adverse Effects

Call your doctor immediately if you experience:

- **signs of overdose:** clumsiness or unsteadiness, dry mouth, nose, or throat, flushed or red face, shortness of breath, trouble breathing, seizures, hallucinations, trouble sleeping, severe drowsiness, faintness or lightheadedness
  - sore throat and fever
  - unusual bleeding or bruising
  - unusual tiredness or weakness

Call your doctor if these symptoms continue:

- thickening bronchial secretions
- change in vision
- confusion
- difficult or painful urination
- nightmares
- loss of appetite
- unusual excitement, nervousness, restlessness, or irritability
- ringing or buzzing in ears
- skin rash
- stomach upset or pain
- increased sweating
- unusually fast heartbeat

- increased sensitivity to sun (rash, hives, skin reactions)
- dizziness
- drowsiness
- thickening of mucus
- dryness of mouth, nose or throat

PREGNANCY WARNING

This drug caused harm to developing fetuses in animal studies, or such studies were not done. Use during pregnancy only for clear medical reasons. Tell your doctor if you are pregnant or thinking of becoming pregnant before you take this drug.

Do Not Use Until Five Years After Release

Fexofenadine (Do Not Use Until 2002)
ALLEGRA (Hoechst Marion Roussel)

GENERIC: not available
FAMILY: Antihistamines (see p. 402)

You should wait at least five years from the date of release to take any new drug unless it is one of those rare "breakthrough" drugs that offers you a documented therapeutic advantage over older proven drugs. New drugs are tested in a relatively small number of people before being approved, and serious adverse effects or life-threatening drug interactions may not be detected until the new drug has been taken by hundreds of thousands of people. A number of new drugs have been withdrawn within their first five years after release. Also, serious new adverse reaction warnings have been added to the labeling of a number of drugs, or new drug interactions have been detected, usually within the first five years after a drug's release.

Fexofenadine (fex oh *fen* a deen), an antihistamine, is the metabolic breakdown product of terfenadine (see p. 453). Fexofenadine apparently lacks the serious, sometimes fatal adverse effects on the heart that terfenadine (SELDANE) has. This information is based on small studies in healthy people. Although highly promoted, little information is published about fexofenadine.

Fexofenadine relieves symptoms of seasonal allergies, such as sneezing, itchy, watery eyes and red eyes, but does not cure allergies. Fexofenadine belongs to the family of "nonsedating" antihistamines, that are less apt to cause drowsiness than older antihistamines. People with impaired kidney function, and older adults, should use 60 mg once daily.

WARNING: SPECIAL MENTAL AND PHYSICAL ADVERSE EFFECTS

Older adults are especially sensitive to the harmful anticholinergic (see Glossary, p. 768) effects of antihistamines such as fexofenadine. Drugs in this family should not be used unless absolutely necessary.

Mental Effects: confusion, delirium, short-term memory problems, disorientation, and impaired attention.

Physical Effects: dry mouth, constipation, difficulty urinating (especially for a man with an enlarged prostate), blurred vision, decreased sweating with increased body temperature, sexual dysfunction, and worsening of glaucoma.

ADDITIONAL PRECAUTIONS

Avoid exposure to things which trigger your allergies or asthma, such as animals, bedding, chemicals, cosmetics, drugs, dust, mold, foods, pollens or smoke. Wearing a mask reduces inhalation of drugs, pollens and smoke. Many people with mildly red, itching eyes require no treatment. Cold compresses to the eyes may prove helpful. Using eye drops with vasoconstrictors whitens eyes for a while, but rebound redness can occur. Misuse of vasoconstrictors sets up a vicious cycle.

Before You Use This Drug

Tell your doctor if you have or have had:

- allergies, including lactose
- glaucoma
- kidney or liver problems
- enlarged prostate
- difficulty urinating

Tell your doctor about any other drugs you take, including aspirin, herbs, vitamins, and other nonprescription products.

When You Use This Drug

- Do not drink alcohol.
- Until you know how you react to this drug, do not drive or perform other activities that require alertness.
- Protect yourself from sunburn with sunscreen and/or protective clothing.
- If you plan to have any surgery, including dental, tell your doctor that you take this drug.

How to Use This Drug

• Swallow whole capsule. Take with or without food at regular intervals.

• If you miss a dose, take it as soon as you remember but skip it if it is almost time for the next dose. **Do not take double doses.**

• Store at room temperature below 78°F. Protect from moisture.

Interactions with Other Drugs

The following drugs are listed in the *Evaluations of Drug Interactions* 1997 as causing "highly clinically significant" or "clinically significant" interactions when used together with this drug. We have also included potentially serious interactions listed in the drug's FDA-approved professional product labeling or package insert. New scientific techniques have allowed researchers to predict some drug interactions before they have been documented in people. There may be other drugs, especially those in the families of drugs listed below, that also will react with this drug to cause severe adverse effects. The number of new drugs approved for marketing increases the chance of drug interactions, and new drug interactions are being identified with old drugs. Be vigilant. Make sure to tell your doctor and pharmacist the drugs you are taking and tell your doctor if you are taking any of these interacting drugs:

Central nervous system (CNS) depressant drugs including alcohol, antidepressants, antihistamines, antipsychotics, some blood pressure medications (reserpine, methyldopa, beta-blockers), motion sickness medications, muscle relaxants, narcotics, sedatives, sleeping pills, and tranquilizers.

Adverse Effects

Call your doctor immediately if you experience:

• bleeding or bruising

• rapid or irregular heartbeat
• sore throat or fever

Call your doctor if these symptoms continue:

• drowsiness
• dry mouth, nose, or throat
• indigestion
• painful menstruation
• rash
• ringing in ears
• sunburn
• sweating
• thickened mucus
• unusual tiredness or weakness
• difficulty urinating
• vision changes
• weight gain

PREGNANCY WARNING

This drug caused harm to developing fetuses in animal studies, or such studies were not done. Use during pregnancy only for clear medical reasons. Tell your doctor if you are pregnant or thinking of becoming pregnant before you take this drug.

Limited Use

Aminophylline
AMOLINE (Major)
SOMOPHYLLIN, SOMOPHYLLIN-DF (Fisons)

GENERIC: available
FAMILY: Asthma Drugs (see p. 408)

Aminophylline (am in *off* i lin) is used to treat symptoms of chronic asthma, bronchitis, and emphysema, including trouble breathing, wheezing, chest tightness, or shortness of breath. The drug opens airways in the lungs and increases the flow of air through them, making breathing easier.

Aminophylline is identical to theophylline (see p. 426), except that aminophylline contains a salt called ethylenediamine, which has caused rashes and hives in some people.[6] For this reason, theophylline is preferable to aminophylline if you need to take a drug in this family by mouth. (Both drugs are also available in an intravenous form for hospital use.)

You must take aminophylline exactly as prescribed. Because there is a narrow range between a helpful and harmful amount of this drug in your body, your doctor must monitor your dose and the level of the drug in your bloodstream. Too little aminophylline may bring on an asthma attack; too much can lead to an overdose. The more serious signs of an overdose include seizures, irregular heart rhythms and pounding heartbeat. Less severe signs may or may not appear before the serious ones.[7]

The preferred forms of aminophylline are the liquid and the uncoated, plain tablets. These forms are absorbed best by the body. The enteric-coated tablets and some sustained-release forms are unreliable. The elixir form contains alcohol.

ADDITIONAL PRECAUTIONS

Avoid exposure to things which trigger your allergies or asthma, such as animals, bedding, chemicals, cosmetics, drugs, dust, mold, foods, pollens or smoke. Wearing a mask reduces inhalation of drugs, pollens and smoke.

Aspirin can trigger asthma in people who are aspirin-allergic, as can beta-blockers. Infections aggravate lung problems. During epidemics of respiratory illnesses, avoid crowded places and wash your hands frequently to help prevent infection. If you have asthma, get a flu vaccination.

Note: The information in this profile addresses the care of asthma that is not serious enough to need emergency treatment.

WARNING

Extreme caution should be used when fluoro-quinolones such as ciprofloxacin (Ciloxan, Cipro), enoxacin (Penetrex), lomefloxacin (Maxaquin), norfloxacin (Chibroxin, Noroxin), and ofloxacin (Floxin, Ocuflox) are to be prescribed in conjunction with aminophylline or theophylline, particularly in elderly patients. Aminophylline doses should be adjusted, perhaps reduced by 30% to 50% at the start of fluoroquinolone therapy. The reduction in dose must be guided by the clinical conditions of the patient, the use of other medications and the baseline level of the aminophylline in the blood. In addition, blood aminophylline levels should be obtained following the initiation of a fluoro-quinolone no later than two days into therapy.[8]

Before You Use This Drug

Do not use if you have or have had:

• an allergy to caffeine or any other xanthine, such as theobromine (found in chocolate or theophylline)

Tell your doctor if you have or have had:

• allergies to drugs
• alcohol dependence
• irregular heartbeats
• heart failure
• diarrhea
• fibrocystic breast disease
• stomach inflammation
• ulcers
• prolonged fever
• respiratory infections
• seizures
• liver problems
• underactive thyroid
• a recent low-protein, high-carbohydrate or high-protein, low-carbohydrate diet
• regularly smoked marijuana or tobacco in the last two years

Tell your doctor about any other drugs you take, including aspirin, herbs, vitamins, and other nonprescription products.

When You Use This Drug

• Do not use more often or in a higher dose than prescribed by your doctor. Do not change brands or dosage forms without checking with your doctor or pharmacist first.

• Reduce your intake of charcoal-broiled foods and foods that contain caffeine, such as chocolate, cocoa, tea, coffee, and colas.

• Call your doctor immediately if you get a fever, diarrhea, or the flu while taking aminophylline, because these increase your chance of developing adverse effects from the drug.

• If you plan to have any surgery, including dental, tell your doctor that you take this drug.

How to Use This Drug

• Take on an empty stomach, at least one hour before or two hours after meals, to increase absorption. If the drug upsets your stomach, take with food instead.

• Do not store in the bathroom. Do not expose to heat, moisture, or strong light.

• If you miss a dose, take it as soon as you remember, but skip it if it is almost time for the next dose. **Do not take double doses.**

Interactions with Other Drugs

The following drugs are listed in the *Evaluations of Drug Interactions* 1997 as causing "highly clinically significant" or "clinically significant" interactions when used together with this drug. We have also included potentially serious interactions listed in the drug's FDA-approved professional product labeling or package insert. New scientific techniques have allowed researchers to predict some drug interactions before they have been documented in people. There may be other drugs, especially those in the families of drugs listed below, that also will react with this drug to cause severe adverse effects. The number of new drugs approved for marketing increases the chance of drug interactions, and new drug interactions are being identified with old drugs. Be vigilant. Make sure to tell your doctor and pharmacist the drugs you are taking and tell your doctor if you are taking any of these interacting drugs:

allopurinol, ANTABUSE, ANTIMINTH, CALAN SR, carbamazepine, CHIBROXIN, CILOXAN, cimetidine, CIPRO, ciprofloxacin, COGNEX, COVERA-HS, DILANTIN, disulfiram, EES, ERYTHROCIN, erythromycin, FLOXIN, FLUOTHANE, furosemide, halothane, imipenem/cilastatin, INDERAL, INDERAL LA, interferon alfa, INTRON A, ISOPTIN SR, LASIX, lithium, LITHOBID, LITHONATE, LUMINAL, mexiletine, MEXITIL, MINTEZOL, norfloxacin, NOROXIN, OCUFLOX, ofloxacin, pancuronium, PAVULON, phenobarbital, phenytoin, PRIMAXIN, propranolol, pyrantel, RIFADIN, rifampin, RIMACTANE, ROFERON-A, SOLFOTON, tacrine, TAGAMET, TEGRETOL, thiabendazole, tobacco, verapamil, VERELAN, ZYLOPRIM.

Adverse Effects

Call your doctor immediately if you experience:

• **signs of overdose:** bloody or black, tarry stools, confusion or change in behavior, seizures, diarrhea, dizziness or lightheadedness, flushed or red face, headache, increased urination, irritability, loss of appetite, muscle twitching, continued or severe nausea, stomach cramps or pain, trembling, trouble sleeping, unusually fast breathing, pounding or irregular heartbeat, abnormal tiredness or weakness, vomiting blood or material that looks like coffee grounds

- heartburn and/or vomiting
- skin rash or hives
- chest pain
- decrease in blood pressure
- chills or fever

Call your doctor if these symptoms continue:

- headache
- fast heartbeat
- increased urination
- nausea
- nervousness
- trembling

Periodic Tests

Ask your doctor which of these tests should be done periodically while you are taking this drug:

- blood levels of aminophylline
- lung function tests
- caffeine concentrations

PREGNANCY WARNING

This drug caused harm to developing fetuses in animal studies, or such studies were not done. Use during pregnancy only for clear medical reasons. Tell your doctor if you are pregnant or thinking of becoming pregnant before you take this drug.

Hydroxyzine
ATARAX (Pfizer)
HY-PAM (Lemmon)
VISTARIL (Pfizer)

GENERIC: available
FAMILY: Antihistamines (see p. 402)

Hydroxyzine (hy *drox* i zeen) is used to treat itching and hives caused by allergic reactions and to relieve drug withdrawal symptoms, nausea, and anxiety. It also promotes sleep and is commonly found in nonprescription sleeping pills. If you need a sleeping pill, an antihistamine such as hydroxyzine is preferable to the overprescribed and addictive benzodiazepine sleeping pills and tranquilizers such as Valium, Librium, and Dalmane (see p. 178).

Do not use hydroxyzine to treat a cold. Colds and allergies have different causes, and hydroxyzine is not effective against either the cause of a cold or its symptoms. In fact, it can make a cold or cough worse by thickening nasal secretions and drying mucous membranes. It also causes drowsiness.

Hydroxyzine can cause harmful adverse effects, most commonly in people over 60. These effects include: confusion, dizziness, fainting, difficult or painful urination, dry mouth, nose, or throat, nightmares, unusual excitement, nervousness, restlessness, or irritability. If you have any of these while taking hydroxyzine, ask your doctor about changing or discontinuing this drug. Since older people can be more sensitive to the usual adult dose, start with a low dose. This may decrease adverse effects.

ADDITIONAL PRECAUTIONS

Avoid exposure to things which trigger your allergies or asthma, such as animals, bedding, chemicals, cosmetics, drugs, dust, mold, foods, pollens or smoke. Wearing a mask reduces inhalation of drugs, pollens and smoke. Many people with mildly red, itching eyes require no treatment. Cold compresses to the eyes may prove helpful. Using eye drops with vasoconstrictors whitens eyes for a while, but rebound redness can occur. Misuse of vasoconstrictors sets up a vicious cycle.

WARNING: SPECIAL MENTAL AND PHYSICAL ADVERSE EFFECTS

Older adults are especially sensitive to the harmful anticholinergic (see Glossary, p. 768) effects of antihistamines such as hydroxyzine. Drugs in this family should not be used unless absolutely necessary.

Mental Effects: confusion, delirium, short-term memory problems, disorientation, and impaired attention.

Physical Effects: dry mouth, constipation, difficulty urinating (especially for a man with an enlarged prostate), blurred vision, decreased sweating with increased body temperature, sexual dysfunction, and worsening of glaucoma.

Before You Use This Drug

Tell your doctor if you have or have had:

- allergies to drugs
- asthma
- problems with urination
- glaucoma
- enlarged prostate
- heart rhythm problems
- low potassium levels
- liver problems

Tell your doctor about any other drugs you take, including aspirin, herbs, vitamins, and other nonprescription products.

When You Use This Drug

- Do not use more often or in a higher dose than prescribed. Overuse increases your risk of adverse effects.
- Do not drink alcohol or use other drugs that can cause drowsiness.
- Until you know how you react to this drug, do not drive or perform other activities requiring alertness.

- If you plan to have any surgery, including dental, tell your doctor that you take this drug.

How to Use This Drug

- Do not store in the bathroom. Do not expose to heat, moisture, or strong light. Do not allow liquid form to freeze.
- Take with food, water, or milk to decrease stomach upset.
- If you miss a dose, take it as soon as you remember, but skip it if it is almost time for the next dose. **Do not take double doses.**

Interactions with Other Drugs

Some other drugs that you may be taking (either over-the-counter or prescription drugs) can interact with this one, causing adverse effects. Ask your doctor what these drugs are and let him or her know if you are taking any of them.

Adverse Effects

Call your doctor immediately if you experience:

- **signs of overdose:** clumsiness or unsteadiness, dry mouth, nose or throat, flushed or red face, shortness of breath, trouble breathing, seizures, hallucinations, trouble sleeping, severe drowsiness, faintness
  - seizures
  - trembling or shakiness
  - skin rash
  - sore throat and fever
  - unusual bleeding or bruising
  - unusual tiredness or weakness

Call your doctor if these symptoms continue:

- thickening bronchial secretions
- change in vision
- confusion
- difficult or painful urination
- nightmares

- loss of appetite
- unusual excitement, nervousness, restlessness, or irritability
- ringing or buzzing in ears
- stomach upset or pain
- increased sweating
- unusually fast heartbeat
- increased sensitivity to sun (rash, hives, skin reactions)
- dizziness
- drowsiness
- thickening of mucus
- dryness of mouth, nose or throat

Ipratropium
ATROVENT (Boehringer Ingelheim)

GENERIC: not available

FAMILY: Drugs to treat Bronchitis and Lung Disease

Ipratropium (ip ra *trop* ee um) prevents and relieves difficult breathing, coughing, and wheezing from lung diseases, such as bronchitis and emphysema. It is not approved for the treatment of asthma. It is an anticholinergic drug in the same family as atropine. Ipratropium takes about 15 minutes to work and lasts about three to six hours. So while effective for maintenance therapy, it is not useful by itself to treat asthma attacks because of its delayed onset of action. However, ipratropium may be useful in combination with other drugs. It offers an alternative to theophylline in people with chronic obstructive lung disease.

Ipratropium enlarges the bronchial tubes, but may also enlarge the intestines.[9] It does not control symptoms nor reduce inflammation, a drawback for treating asthma according to a report of the International Asthma Management Project.[10] Ipratropium may thicken secretions in the lungs, cause retention of urine, and cause or worsen narrow angle glaucoma. It does not relieve nasal congestion or sneezing. While ipratropium is often preferred for use in people over age 60, it should be used cautiously in older men with prostate problems.[11]

WARNING: SPECIAL MENTAL AND PHYSICAL ADVERSE EFFECTS

Older adults are especially sensitive to the harmful anticholinergic (see Glossary, p. 768) effects of drugs such as ipratropium. Drugs in this family should not be used unless absolutely necessary.

Mental Effects: confusion, delirium, short-term memory problems, disorientation, and impaired attention.

Physical Effects: dry mouth, constipation, difficulty urinating (especially for a man with an enlarged prostate), blurred vision, decreased sweating with increased body temperature, sexual dysfunction, and worsening of glaucoma.

Before You Use This Drug

Tell your doctor if you have or have had:

- allergies to drugs
- narrow angle glaucoma
- prostate problems
- difficulty urinating

Tell your doctor about any other drugs you take, including aspirin, herbs, vitamins, and other nonprescription products.

When You Use This Drug

- Check with your doctor if symptoms do not improve 30 minutes after using ipratropium.
- If you plan to have any surgery, including dental, tell your doctor that you take this drug.

How to Use This Drug

- If you also use a beta-agonist (ALUPENT, BRETHAIRE, BRETHINE, BRICANYL,

BRONKOSOL, MAXAIR, METAPREL, PRO-VENTIL, VENTOLIN), use it five minutes before using ipratropium.

• If you also use a corticosteroid (AZMA-CORT, BECLOVENT, VANCERIL) or cromolyn (INTAL) inhaler, use ipratropium five minutes before using those inhalers.

• Avoid getting ipratropium in your eyes. Use a well-fitting mask, goggles, T-piece extension, or at least close your eyes.[12,13,14]

• Shake canister well before using. Dilute solutions before using, according to instructions.

• Inhale through the mouth according to instructions for the inhaler. If you use more than one inhalation, wait one minute between inhalations. Do not use more than 12 inhalations in 24 hours.

• If you use a spacer device or nebulizer, be sure you understand the instructions for use. Ask questions and practice until you are comfortable using the device. Ask your doctor if a paper bag can be substituted.[15]

• If you miss a dose, take it as soon as you remember, and evenly space the remaining doses for that day.

• Do not store in the bathroom. Do not expose to heat, moisture, or strong light. Store metered dose inhaler at room temperature. Store solutions according to instructions on the label.

• Discard solutions of ipratropium without a preservative within 24 hours at room temperature, or 48 hours of refrigeration.

• Discard solutions with preservative stored at room temperature after seven days.

• Discard mixtures of ipratropium and albuterol or metaproterenol, with a preservative, after seven days at room temperature.

• Discard canisters with fluorocarbon propellants according to local waste disposal laws.

Interactions with Other Drugs

The following drugs are listed in the *Evaluations of Drug Interactions* 1997 as causing "highly clinically significant" or "clinically significant" interactions when used together with this drug. We have also included potentially serious interactions listed in the drug's FDA-approved professional product labeling or package insert. New scientific techniques have allowed researchers to predict some drug interactions before they have been documented in people. There may be other drugs, especially those in the families of drugs listed below, that also will react with this drug to cause severe adverse effects. The number of new drugs approved for marketing increases the chance of drug interactions, and new drug interactions are being identified with old drugs. Be vigilant. Make sure to tell your doctor and pharmacist the drugs you are taking and tell your doctor if you are taking any of these interacting drugs:

cromolyn solution (*If mixed with ipratropium a cloudy sludge will form. Do not use such mixtures.*) GASTROCOM, INTAL, NASALCROM.

Adverse Effects

Call your doctor immediately if you experience:

• constipation, or lower abdominal pain or bloating
• difficulty breathing
• severe eye pain
• swelling of face, lips or eyelids
• dizziness
• unusually fast heartbeat
• skin rash or hives
• large pupils
• sores or ulcers on lips or in mouth
• tremor

Call your doctor if these symptoms continue:

• cough
• dry mouth, hoarseness
• headache

- nausea
- nasal congestion
- nervousness
- metallic taste
- unusual tiredness or weakness
- difficulty urinating
- blurred vision, eye pain or burning
- pounding heartbeat
- sweating
- trembling

Diphenhydramine
BENADRYL (Parke-Davis)
SOMINEX FORMULA (Beecham Products)

GENERIC: available
FAMILY: Antihistamines (see p. 402)

Diphenhydramine (di fen *hye* dra meen) is used to treat allergic reactions, coughing, insomnia, motion sickness, and Parkinson's disease. Do not use it to treat a cold. Colds and allergies have different causes, and diphenhydramine is not effective against either the cause of a cold or its symptoms. In fact, it can make a cold worse by thickening nasal secretions and drying mucous membranes. Diphenhydramine also causes drowsiness.

Diphenhydramine can cause harmful adverse effects, more commonly in people over 60 than in younger people. These effects include: confusion, dizziness, fainting, difficult or painful urination, dry mouth, nose, or throat, nightmares, unusual excitement, nervousness, restlessness, or irritability. If you have any of these symptoms while taking diphenhydramine, ask your doctor about changing or discontinuing this drug. Since older people can be more sensitive to the usual adult dose, start with a low dose. This may decrease adverse effects.

ADDITIONAL PRECAUTIONS

Avoid exposure to things which trigger your allergies or asthma, such as animals, bedding, chemicals, cosmetics, drugs, dust, mold, foods, pollens or smoke. Wearing a mask reduces inhalation of drugs, pollens and smoke. Many people with mildly red, itching eyes require no treatment. Cold compresses to the eyes may prove helpful. Using eye drops with vasoconstrictors whitens eyes for a while, but rebound redness can occur. Misuse of vasoconstrictors sets up a vicious cycle.

WARNING: SPECIAL MENTAL AND PHYSICAL ADVERSE EFFECTS

Older adults are especially sensitive to the harmful anticholinergic (see Glossary, p. 768) effects of antihistamines such as diphenhydramine. Drugs in this family should not be used unless absolutely necessary.

Mental Effects: confusion, delirium, short-term memory problems, disorientation, and impaired attention.

Physical Effects: dry mouth, constipation, difficulty urinating (especially for a man with an enlarged prostate), blurred vision, decreased sweating with increased body temperature, sexual dysfunction, and worsening of glaucoma.

Before You Use This Drug

Tell your doctor if you have or have had:

- allergies to drugs
- asthma
- problems with urination
- glaucoma
- enlarged prostate

Tell your doctor about any other drugs you take, including aspirin, herbs, vitamins, and other nonprescription products.

When You Use This Drug

• Do not use more often or in a higher dose than prescribed. This will increase the risk of adverse effects and will not increase the effectiveness of the drug.

• Do not drink alcohol or use other drugs that can cause drowsiness.

• Until you know how you react to this drug, do not drive or perform other activities requiring alertness.

• If you plan to have any surgery, including dental, tell your doctor that you take this drug.

How to Use This Drug

• Do not store in the bathroom. Do not expose to heat, moisture, or strong light. Do not allow liquid form to freeze.

• Take with food, water, or milk to decrease stomach irritation.

• Swallow extended-release forms whole.

• If you miss a dose, take it as soon as you remember, but skip it if it is almost time for the next dose. **Do not take double doses.**

Interactions with Other Drugs

The following drugs are listed in the *Evaluations of Drug Interactions* 1997 as causing "highly clinically significant" or "clinically significant" interactions when used together with this drug. We have also included potentially serious interactions listed in the drug's FDA-approved professional product labeling or package insert. New scientific techniques have allowed researchers to predict some drug interactions before they have been documented in people. There may be other drugs, especially those in the families of drugs listed below, that also will react with this drug to cause severe adverse effects. The number of new drugs approved for marketing increases the chance of drug interactions, and new drug interactions are being identified with old drugs. Be vigilant. Make sure to tell your doctor and pharmacist the drugs you are taking and tell your doctor if you are taking any of these interacting drugs:

alcohol, DILANTIN, phenytoin, RESTORIL, temazepam.

Adverse Effects

Call your doctor immediately if you experience:

• **signs of overdose:** clumsiness or unsteadiness, dry mouth, nose, or throat, flushed or red face, shortness of breath, trouble breathing, seizures, hallucinations, trouble sleeping, severe drowsiness, faintness or lightheadedness

• sore throat and fever

• unusual bleeding or bruising

• unusual tiredness or weakness

Call your doctor if these symptoms continue:

• thickening bronchial secretions

• change in vision

• confusion

• difficult or painful urination

• nightmares

• loss of appetite

• unusual excitement, nervousness, restlessness, or irritability

• ringing or buzzing in ears

• skin rash

• stomach upset or pain

• increased sweating

• unusually fast heartbeat

• increased sensitivity to sun (rash, hives, skin reactions)

• dizziness

• drowsiness

• thickening of mucus

• dryness of mouth, nose or throat

Do Not Use

ALTERNATIVE TREATMENT:
See Albuterol and Terbutaline, p. 449.

Isoetharine
BETA-2 (Nephron)
BRONKOSOL, BRONKOMETER (Sanofi)

FAMILY: Asthma Drugs (see p. 408)

Isoetharine (eye soe *eth* a reen) is used to treat mild asthma, chronic bronchitis, emphysema, or occasional spasms of the airways called bronchospasm. If you have any of these conditions, the best drug to use is either albuterol or terbutaline (see p. 449), rather than isoetharine.

Isoetharine is an older inhaled drug that lasts for a shorter time than albuterol.[16] It is more likely to cause high blood pressure and an increase in your heart rate than the similar drugs albuterol, metaproterenol, and terbutaline.[17] If you are using isoetharine and have adverse effects, ask your doctor to change your inhalant to albuterol or terbutaline.

Whichever drug you take, use only the inhaled forms. Do not use the tablets, capsules, or liquids. Because these forms are swallowed, the drug is distributed throughout the body, increasing the risk of adverse effects. An inhaler deposits most of the drug in the lungs, where it is needed.

ADDITIONAL PRECAUTIONS

Avoid exposure to things which trigger your allergies or asthma, such as animals, bedding, chemicals, cosmetics, drugs, dust, mold, foods, pollens or smoke. Wearing a mask reduces inhalation of drugs, pollens and smoke.

Aspirin can trigger asthma in people who are aspirin-allergic, as can beta-blockers. Infections aggravate lung problems. During epidemics of respiratory illnesses, avoid crowded places and wash your hands frequently to help prevent infection. If you have asthma, get a flu vaccination.

Note: The information in this profile addresses the care of asthma that is not serious enough to need emergency treatment.

Theophylline
BRONKODYL (Winthrop-Breon)
SUSTAIRE (Pfizer)
SLO-BID (Rhone-Poulenc Rorer)
THEO-DUR (Key)
THEOLAIR (3M)
THEO-24 (UCB)
CONSTANT-T (Geigy)
ELIXOPHYLLIN (Forest)
QUIBRON-T-SR (Bristol)
SLO-PHYLLIN (Rhone-Poulenc Rorer)
SOMOPHYLLIN-CRT (Fisons)
SOMOPHYLLIN-T (Fisons)

GENERIC: available
FAMILY: Asthma Drugs (see p. 408)

Theophylline (thee *off* i lin) is used to treat symptoms of chronic asthma, bronchitis, and emphysema, including trouble breathing, wheezing, chest tightness, or shortness of breath. The drug opens airways in the lungs and increases the flow of air through them, making breathing easier. If you are over 60, you will generally need to take less than the usual adult dose.

Theophylline does not take effect right away, so a faster-acting drug must be used in situations where immediate action is necessary. In these situations, such as for occasional acute asthma, the best drug to use is inhaled albuterol or terbutaline (see p. 449).

You must take theophylline exactly as prescribed. Because there is a narrow range between a helpful and harmful amount of this drug in your body, your doctor must monitor your dose and the level of this drug in your bloodstream. Too little theophylline may bring on an asthma attack; too much can lead to an overdose. The more serious signs of an overdose include seizures, irregular heart rhythms, and pounding heartbeat. Less severe signs may or may not appear before the serious ones.[18]

The preferred forms of theophylline are the liquid and the plain, uncoated tablets. These forms are absorbed best by the body. The sustained-release forms that you take once a day are unreliable. The elixir form contains alcohol. The suppository form is absorbed erratically by your body and should not be used.

ADDITIONAL PRECAUTIONS

Avoid exposure to things which trigger your allergies or asthma, such as animals, bedding, chemicals, cosmetics, drugs, dust, mold, foods, pollens or smoke. Wearing a mask reduces inhalation of drugs, pollens and smoke.

Aspirin can trigger asthma in people who are aspirin-allergic, as can beta-blockers. Infections aggravate lung problems. During epidemics or respiratory illnesses, avoid crowded places and wash your hands frequently to help prevent infection. If you have asthma, get a flu vaccination.

Note: The information in this profile addresses the care of asthma that is not serious enough to need emergency treatment.

WARNING

Extreme caution should be used when fluoroquinolones such as ciprofloxacin (Ciloxan, Cipro), enoxacin (Penetrex), lomefloxacin (Maxaquin), norfloxacin (Chibroxin, Noroxin), and ofloxacin (Floxin, Ocuflox) are to be prescribed in conjunction with aminophylline or theophylline, particularly in elderly patients. Theophylline doses should be adjusted, perhaps reduced by 30% to 50% at the start of fluoroquinolone therapy. The reduction in dose must be guided by the clinical conditions of the patient, the use of other medications, and the baseline level of the theophylline in the blood. In addition, blood theophylline levels should be obtained following the initiation of a fluoroquinolone no later than two days into therapy.[19]

Before You Use This Drug

Do not use if you have or have had:
- an allergy to caffeine or another xanthine, such as theobromine (found in chocolate)

Tell your doctor if you have or have had:
- allergies to drugs
- alcohol dependence
- irregular heartbeats
- heart failure
- diarrhea
- fibrocystic breast disease
- stomach inflammation
- ulcers
- prolonged fever
- respiratory infections
- liver disease
- underactive thyroid
- a recent low-protein, high-carbohydrate or high-protein, low-carbohydrate diet
- regularly smoked marijuana or tobacco in the last two years

Tell your doctor about any other drugs you take, including aspirin, herbs, vitamins, and other nonprescription products.

When You Use This Drug

- Do not use more often or in a higher dose than prescribed by your doctor. Do not change brands or dosage forms without checking with your doctor or pharmacist first.
- Reduce your intake of charcoal-broiled foods and foods that contain caffeine, such as chocolate, cocoa, tea, coffee, and colas.
- Call your doctor immediately if you get a fever, diarrhea, or the flu while taking theophylline, because these increase your chance of developing adverse effects from the drug.
- If you plan to have any surgery, including dental, tell your doctor that you take this drug.

How to Use This Drug

- Swallow the coated or sustained-release tablets whole. Do not crush, break, or chew them.
- Take on an empty stomach (at least one hour before or two hours after meals) with **a full glass (eight ounces) of water.** Take your last dose of the day with a full glass of water at least an hour before bedtime to improve your body's absorption of the drug. If the drug upsets your stomach, take with food instead.
- Do not store in the bathroom. Do not expose to heat, moisture, or strong light.
- If you miss a dose, take it as soon as you remember, but skip it if it is almost time for the next dose. **Do not take double doses.**

Interactions with Other Drugs

The following drugs are listed in the *Evaluations of Drug Interactions* 1997 as causing "highly clinically significant" or "clinically significant" interactions when used together with this drug. We have also included potentially serious interactions listed in the drug's FDA-approved professional product labeling or package insert. New scientific techniques have allowed researchers to predict some drug interactions before they have been documented in people. There may be other drugs, especially those in the families of drugs listed below, that also will react with this drug to cause severe adverse effects. The number of new drugs approved for marketing increases the chance of drug interactions, and new drug interactions are being identified with old drugs. Be vigilant. Make sure to tell your doctor and pharmacist the drugs you are taking and tell your doctor if you are taking any of these interacting drugs:

allopurinol, ANTABUSE, ANTIMINTH, CALAN SR, carbamazepine, charcoal, CHIBROXIN, CILOXAN, cimetidine, CIPRO, ciprofloxacin, COVERA-HS, DILANTIN, disulfiram, EES, enoxacin, ERYTHROCIN, erythromycin, erythromycin estolate, ETHMOZINE, FLOXIN, flu vaccine, furosemide, grepafloxacin, ILOSONE, INDERAL, INDERAL LA, interferon, INTRON A, ISOPTIN SR, LASIX, LEVAQUIN, levofloxacin, lithium, LITHOBID, LITHONATE, lomefloxacin, LUMINAL, MAXAQUIN, mexiletine, MEXITIL, moricizine, norfloxacin, NOROXIN, OCUFLOX, ofloxacin, PENETREX, phenobarbital, phenytoin, propafenone, propranolol, pyrantel, RAXAR, RIFADIN, rifampin, RIMACTANE, ROFERON-A, RYTHMOL, SOLFOTON, sparfloxacin, TAGAMET, TEGRETOL, tobacco, verapamil, VERELAN, ZAGAM, ZYLOPRIM.

Adverse Effects

Call your doctor immediately if you experience:

- **signs of overdose:** bloody or black, tarry stools, confusion or change in behavior, seizures, diarrhea, dizziness or lightheadedness, flushed or red face, headache, increased urination, irritability, loss of appetite, muscle twitching, continued or severe nausea, stomach cramps or pain, trembling, trouble sleeping, unusually fast breathing, pounding or irregular heartbeat, abnormal tiredness or weakness, vomiting blood or material that looks like coffee grounds

- heartburn and/or vomiting
- skin rash or hives
- chest pain
- decrease in blood pressure
- chills or fever

Call your doctor if these symptoms continue:

- headache
- fast heartbeat
- increased urination
- nausea
- nervousness
- trembling
- trouble sleeping

Periodic Tests

Ask your doctor which of these tests should be done periodically while you are taking this drug:

- blood levels of theophylline
- lung function tests
- caffeine concentrations

PREGNANCY WARNING

This drug caused harm to developing fetuses in animal studies, or such studies were not done. Use during pregnancy only for clear medical reasons. Tell your doctor if you are pregnant or thinking of becoming pregnant before you take this drug.

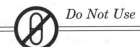 *Do Not Use*

ALTERNATIVE TREATMENT:
See Cold, p. 402, and Allergy and Hay Fever, p. 405.

Chlorpheniramine and Pseudoephedrine
CHLOR-TRIMETON 12 HOUR
(Schering-Plough)

FAMILY: Cold and Allergy Drugs (see p. 402)

This combination of chlorpheniramine (see p. 413) and pseudoephedrine (soo doe e *fed* rin) is marketed as a drug that relieves congestion and other problems caused by allergies and the common cold. Chlor-Trimeton 12 Hour is a brand name product, advertised as a remedy for sneezing, runny nose, and other symptoms of nasal congestion. You should not use them. Fixed-combination products containing an antihistamine (chlorpheniramine) and a decongestant (pseudoephedrine) exemplify the "shotgun" approach to treating cold and allergy symptoms, which are better treated with individual drugs for individual symptoms. The combination of drugs lacks clinical evidence of effectiveness.

If you want to treat congestion caused by an allergy, the best treatment is an antihistamine such as chlorpheniramine. If you want to treat congestion caused by a cold, the best treatment is a decongestant nose spray or nose drops. There is no reason to combine an antihistamine and a decongestant in one product.

Chlorpheniramine is an effective antihistamine for treating hay fever and other allergies. If you have congestion caused by an allergy, taking chlorpheniramine or another antihistamine alone will help. There is no satisfactory evidence that allergy patients benefit from adding a decongestant such as pseudoephedrine to an antihistamine. Chlorpheniramine can cause drowsiness, loss of coordination, mental inattention, and dizziness.

If your congestion is caused by a cold rather than an allergy, you can use decongestant nasal sprays or drops such as phenylephrine, oxymetazoline, or xylometazoline, all available without a prescription. Any of these is a better choice than a drug like pseudoephedrine, which can have dangerous adverse effects because it is taken by mouth and affects your whole system. Do not use decongestant nasal sprays or drops longer than three days (see p. 403).

WARNING

Pseudoephedrine can cause or worsen high blood pressure. It is especially dangerous for people who have high blood pressure, heart disease, diabetes, or thyroid disease. People over 60 are more likely than younger people to experience effects on the heart and blood pressure, restlessness, nervousness, and confusion. Do not use pseudoephedrine during or within 14 days following administration of monoamine oxidase (MAO) inhibitors.

WARNING: SPECIAL MENTAL AND PHYSICAL ADVERSE EFFECTS

Older adults are especially sensitive to the harmful anticholinergic (see Glossary, p. 768) effects of antihistamines such as chlorpheniramine. Drugs in this family should not be used unless absolutely necessary.

Mental Effects: confusion, delirium, short-term memory problems, disorientation, and impaired attention.

Physical Effects: dry mouth, constipation, difficulty urinating (especially for a man with an enlarged prostate), blurred vision, decreased sweating with increased body temperature, sexual dysfunction, and worsening of glaucoma.

ADDITIONAL PRECAUTIONS

Avoid exposure to things which trigger your allergies or asthma, such as animals, bedding, chemicals, cosmetics, drugs, dust, mold, foods, pollens or smoke. Wearing a mask reduces inhalation of drugs, pollens and smoke. Many people with mildly red, itching eyes require no treatment. Cold compresses to the eyes may prove helpful. Using eye drops with vasoconstrictors whitens eyes for a while, but rebound redness can occur. Misuse of vasoconstrictors sets up a vicious cycle.

 Do Not Use

ALTERNATIVE TREATMENT:
See Theophylline, p. 426.

Oxtriphylline
CHOLEDYL (Warner-Chilcott)

FAMILY: Asthma Drugs (see p. 408)

Oxtriphylline (ox *trye* fi lin) is used to treat symptoms of chronic asthma, bronchitis, and emphysema. It opens airways in the lungs and increases the flow of air through them, making breathing easier. Oxtriphylline is identical to theophylline, except that it contains a salt not found in theophylline. It is no more effective than theophylline (see p. 426), yet it costs more.[20] If you take oxtriphylline, ask your doctor to change your prescription to theophylline.

If you continue to use oxtriphylline, take it exactly as prescribed. Because there is a narrow range between a helpful and a harmful amount of this drug in your body, your doctor must monitor your dose and the level of the drug in your bloodstream. Too little oxtriphylline may bring on an asthma attack; too much can lead to an overdose. The more serious signs of an overdose include seizures, irregular heart rhythms, and pounding heartbeat. Less severe signs may or may not appear before the serious ones.[21]

ADDITIONAL PRECAUTIONS

Avoid exposure to things which trigger your allergies or asthma, such as animals, bedding, chemicals, cosmetics, drugs, dust, mold, foods, pollens or smoke. Wearing a mask reduces inhalation of drugs, pollens and smoke.

Aspirin can trigger asthma in people who are aspirin-allergic, as can beta-blockers. Infections aggravate lung problems. During epidemics of respiratory illnesses, avoid crowded places, and wash your hands frequently to help prevent infection. If you have asthma, get a flu vaccination.

Note: The information in this profile addresses the care of asthma that is not serious enough to need emergency treatment.

---

tamines that causes less drowsiness than older antihistamines. High doses increase the risk of adverse effects with loratadine. People with impaired kidney or liver function should only take 10 mg of the drug every other day. Older people may be more prone to adverse effects, such as dizziness and dry mouth. A dry mouth for a prolonged time can lead to dental problems. Men are more apt to experience urinary retention. Loratadine passes into the breast milk and should not be used when nursing. Do not use in the third trimester of pregnancy. Over eight years experience with loratadine suggests it lacks the serious, sometimes, fatal, slowing of the heart and drug interactions that terfenadine (SELDANE) and astemizole (HISMANAL) have.

Loratadine also comes in combinations with pseudoephedrine, a decongestant in Claritin-D. The decongestant acts immediately, while the loratadine is released over 24 hours. Fixed-dose combination drugs generally cost more, are inflexible for dosing, and increase adverse effects. A fixed-dose combination drug is not recommended for children under age 12. People who take Claritin-D should also check the possible adverse effects of pseudoephedrine. (See p. 430.)

Limited Use

Loratadine
CLARITIN (Schering)

GENERIC: not available
FAMILY: Antihistamines (see p. 402)

Loratadine (lor *at* a deen) is an antihistamine. Loratadine relieves symptoms of seasonal allergies, chronic itching, and supplements asthma therapy, but does not cure any condition. It decreases exercise-induced bronchospasm, and is a mild bronchodilator. Loratadine is one of the "nonsedating" antihis-

---

ADDITIONAL PRECAUTIONS

Avoid exposure to things which trigger your allergies or asthma, such as animals, bedding, chemicals, cosmetics, drugs, dust, mold, foods, pollens or smoke. Wearing a mask reduces inhalation of drugs, pollens and smoke. Many people with mildly red, itching eyes require no treatment. Cold compresses to the eyes may prove helpful. Using eye drops with vasoconstrictors whitens eyes for a while, but rebound redness can occur. Misuse of vasoconstrictors sets up a vicious cycle.

WARNING: SPECIAL MENTAL AND PHYSICAL ADVERSE EFFECTS

Older adults are especially sensitive to the harmful anticholinergic (see Glossary, p. 768) effects of antihistamines such as loratadine. Drugs in this family should not be used unless absolutely necessary.

Mental Effects: confusion, delirium, short-term memory problems, disorientation, and impaired attention.

Physical Effects: dry mouth, constipation, difficulty urinating (especially for a man with an enlarged prostate), blurred vision, decreased sweating with increased body temperature, sexual dysfunction, and worsening of glaucoma.

Before You Use This Drug

Tell your doctor if you have or have had:

- allergies, including lactose
- glaucoma
- kidney or liver problems
- pregnant or nursing
- prostate problems
- sleep apnea, snoring
- urinary retention

Tell your doctor about any other drugs you take, including aspirin, herbs, vitamins, and other nonprescription products.

When You Use This Drug

- Do not drink alcohol.
- Until you know how you react to this drug, do not drive or perform other activities that require alertness.
- Protect yourself from sunburn, using sunscreen or wearing protective clothing.
- Use sugarless gum, ice, or saliva substitute if dry mouth develops.
- If you plan to have any surgery, including dental, tell your doctor that you take this drug.

How to Use This Drug

- Swallow whole or half tablet on an empty stomach. In Canada and countries where a liquid form is available, measure dose with a calibrated teaspoon. Do not break or chew the Claritin-D. The combination may be taken with or without food.
- If you miss a dose, take it as soon as you remember, but skip it if it is almost time for the next dose. **Do not take double doses.**
- Store at room temperature.

Interactions with Other Drugs

The following drugs are listed in the *Evaluations of Drug Interactions* 1997 as causing "highly clinically significant" or "clinically significant" interactions when used together with this drug. We have also included potentially serious interactions listed in the drug's FDA-approved professional product labeling or package insert. New scientific techniques have allowed researchers to predict some drug interactions before they have been documented in people. There may be other drugs, especially those in the families of drugs listed below, that also will react with this drug to cause severe adverse effects. The number of new drugs approved for marketing increases the chance of drug interactions, and new drug interactions are being identified with old drugs. Be vigilant. Make sure to tell your doctor and pharmacist the drugs you are taking and tell your doctor if you are taking any of these interacting drugs:

Central nervous system (CNS) depressant drugs including alcohol, antidepressants, antihistamines, antipsychotics, some blood pressure medications (reserpine, methyldopa, beta-blockers), motion sickness medications, muscle relaxants, narcotics, sedatives, sleeping pills and tranquilizers.

Adverse Effects

Call your doctor immediately if you experience:

- **signs of overdose:** clumsiness or unsteadiness, dry mouth, nose, or throat, flushed or red face, shortness of breath, trouble breathing, seizures, hallucinations, trouble sleeping, severe drowsiness, faintness or lightheadedness
  - unusual bleeding or bruising
  - rapid or irregular heartbeat
  - sore throat and fever
  - unusual tiredness or weakness

Call your doctor if these symptoms continue:

- appetite increase, weight gain
- dizziness
- drowsiness
- dryness of mouth, nose, or throat
- unusual excitement, nervousness, restlessness, or irritability
- nightmares
- skin rash
- ringing or buzzing in ears
- stomach upset or pain
- increased sensitivity to sun (rash, hives, skin reactions)
- increased sweating
- thickening of bronchial secretions
- difficult or painful urination
- change in vision
- confusion
- loss of appetite
- unusually fast heartbeat

Do Not Use

ALTERNATIVE TREATMENT:
See Cold, p. 402, and Allergy and Hay Fever, p. 405.

Brompheniramine and Phenylpropanolamine
DIMETAPP (Robins)

FAMILY: Cold and Allergy Drugs (see p. 402)

This combination of brompheniramine (brome fen *eer* a meen) and phenylpropanolamine (fen ill proe pa *nole* a meen) is marketed as a drug that relieves congestion and other problems caused by allergies and the common cold. Dimetapp, a brand-name product, is advertised as a remedy for sneezing, runny nose, and other symptoms of nasal congestion. You should not use it, for two reasons.

First, the long-lasting tablet form of this drug is unacceptable because your body does not absorb it gradually at an even rate. This means that levels of the drug in your body may vary significantly over time rather than staying constant. Second, fixed-combination products containing an antihistamine (brompheniramine) and a decongestant phenylpropanolamine) exemplify the "shotgun" approach to treating cold and allergy symptoms, which are better treated with individual drugs for individual symptoms. The combination lacks clinical evidence of effectiveness.

If you want to treat congestion caused by an allergy, the best treatment is an antihistamine such as brompheniramine. If you want to treat congestion caused by a cold, the best treatment is a decongestant nose spray or nose drops. There is no reason to combine an antihistamine and a decongestant in one product.

Brompheniramine is an effective antihistamine for treating hay fever and other allergies. If you have congestion caused by an allergy, taking brompheniramine or another antihistamine alone will help. There is no satisfactory evidence that allergy patients benefit from adding a decongestant such as phenylpropanolamine to an antihistamine. Brompheniramine can cause drowsiness, loss of coordination, mental inattention, and dizziness.

If your congestion is caused by a cold rather than an allergy, you can use decongestant nasal sprays or drops such as phenylephrine, oxymetazoline, or xylometazoline, all available without a prescription. Any of these is a better choice than a drug like phenylpropanolamine, which can have dangerous adverse effects because you take it by mouth and it affects your whole system. Do not use decongestant nasal sprays or drops longer than three days (see p. 403).

ADDITIONAL PRECAUTIONS

Avoid exposure to things which trigger your allergies or asthma, such as animals, bedding, chemicals, cosmetics, drugs, dust, mold, foods, pollens or smoke. Wearing a mask reduces inhalation of drugs, pollens and smoke. Many people with mildly red, itching eyes require no treatment. Cold compresses to the eyes may prove helpful. Using eye drops with vasoconstrictors whitens eyes for a while, but rebound redness can occur. Misuse of vasoconstrictors sets up a vicious cycle.

WARNING

Phenylpropanolamine (PPA) can cause or worsen high blood pressure. It is especially dangerous for people who have high blood pressure, heart disease, diabetes, or thyroid disease. People over 60 are more likely than younger people to experience effects on the heart and blood pressure, restlessness, nervousness, and confusion.

WARNING: SPECIAL MENTAL AND PHYSICAL ADVERSE EFFECTS

Older adults are especially sensitive to the harmful anticholinergic (see Glossary, p. 768) effects of antihistamines such as brompheniramine. Drugs in this family should not be used unless absolutely necessary.

Mental Effects: confusion, delirium, short-term memory problems, disorientation, and impaired attention.

Physical Effects: dry mouth, constipation, difficulty urinating (especially for a man with an enlarged prostate), blurred vision, decreased sweating with increased body temperature, sexual dysfunction, and worsening of glaucoma.

 Do Not Use

ALTERNATIVE TREATMENT:
See Cold, p. 402, and Allergy and Hay Fever, p. 405.

Guaifenesin, Phenylpropanolamine, and Phenylephrine
ENTEX (Dura)

FAMILY: Cold and Allergy Drugs (see p. 402)

This combination of guaifenesin (see p. 452), phenylpropanolamine (fen ill proe pa *nole* a meen), and phenylephrine (fen ill *ef* rin) is marketed as a drug that relieves the symptoms of nasal and airway congestion. It contains two decongestants (phenylpropanolamine and phenylephrine) and a drug that is supposed to work as an expectorant, thinning mucus in the airways so that it can be coughed up more easily (guaifenesin). Entex, a brand-name product, is prescribed for sneezing, runny nose, and other symptoms of nasal congestion. You should not use it, for several reasons.

First, guaifenesin, the most widely used expectorant, has not been proven effective. No well-designed study has shown that it works, despite the efforts of drug manufacturers to convince people that it does.

Second, fixed-combination products containing an expectorant and decongestants exemplify the "shotgun" approach to treating cold symptoms, which are better treated with individual drugs for individual symptoms. The combination lacks clinical evidence of effectiveness.

Third, this product contains duplicates from a class of drugs. There is no reason to believe that two nasal decongestants in a product make it any more effective than an adequate amount of one. Increasing the number of drugs raises the risk of unwanted adverse effects without increasing the benefits.

Fourth, phenylpropanolamine, one of the decongestants in this product, may have major harmful effects on blood pressure and the heart (see box below).

choice than a drug like phenylpropanolamine, which can have dangerous adverse effects because it is taken by mouth and affects your whole system. Do not use decongestant nasal sprays or drops longer than three days (see p. 403).

If you have a cough, it is not necessarily a good idea to take a cough suppressant. Coughing clears mucous plugs and thick secretions from your airways and opens collapsed segments of your lungs. Drinking lots of liquids, especially soup and other hot drinks, and inhaling steam from hot showers and warm baths will help to loosen secretions and clean and soothe mucous membranes.

If you have a dry, irritating cough that is not producing mucus and that interferes with your sleep, you may benefit from a cough suppressant. The best nonnarcotic treatment is generic dextromethorphan, which you can get without a prescription. If your cough persists, you should see a doctor or other health professional, especially if you are a smoker.

ADDITIONAL PRECAUTIONS

Avoid exposure to things which trigger your allergies or asthma, such as animals, bedding, chemicals, cosmetics, drugs, dust, mold, foods, pollens or smoke. Wearing a mask reduces inhalation of drugs, pollens and smoke. Many people with mildly red, itching eyes require no treatment. Cold compresses to the eyes may prove helpful. Using eye drops with vasoconstrictors whitens eyes for a while, but rebound redness can occur. Misuse of vasoconstrictors sets up a vicious cycle.

WARNING

Phenylpropanolamine (PPA) can cause or worsen high blood pressure. It is especially dangerous for people who have high blood pressure, heart disease, diabetes, or thyroid disease. People over 60 are more likely than younger people to experience effects on the heart and blood pressure, restlessness, nervousness, and confusion.

A Food and Drug Administration advisory panel review of expectorants found that all nonprescription expectorants on the market lack evidence of effectiveness.

If you want to treat a stuffy nose caused by a cold (not an allergy), you can use decongestant nasal sprays or drops such as phenylephrine, oxymetazoline, or xylometazoline, all available without a prescription. Any of these is a better

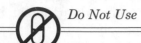

Do Not Use

ALTERNATIVE TREATMENT:
See Cold, p. 402, and Allergy and Hay Fever, p. 405.

Guaifenesin and Phenylpropanolamine
ENTEX LA (Dura)

FAMILY: Cold and Allergy Drugs (see p. 402)

This combination of guaifenesin (see p. 452) and phenylpropanolamine (fen ill proe pa *nole* a meen) is marketed as a drug that relieves symptoms of nasal and airway congestion. It contains a decongestant (phenylpropanolamine) and a drug that is supposed to work as an expectorant, thinning mucus in the airways so that it can be coughed up more easily (guaifenesin). Entex LA, a brand name product, is prescribed for sneezing, runny nose, and other symptoms of nasal congestion. You should not use it, for several reasons.

First, guaifenesin, the most widely used expectorant, has not been proven effective. No well-designed study has shown that it works, despite the efforts of drug manufacturers to convince people that it does.

Second, fixed-combination products containing an expectorant and a decongestant exemplify the "shotgun" approach to treating cold symptoms, which are better treated with individual drugs for individual symptoms. The combination lacks clinical evidence of effectiveness.

Third, phenylpropanolamine may have major effects on blood pressure and the heart (see below). And fourth, the long-lasting tablet form of this product is unacceptable because your body does not absorb it gradually at an even rate. This means that levels of the drug in your body may vary significantly over time rather than staying constant.

ADDITIONAL PRECAUTIONS

Avoid exposure to things which trigger your allergies or asthma, such as animals, bedding, chemicals, cosmetics, drugs, dust, mold, foods, pollens or smoke. Wearing a mask reduces inhalation of drugs, pollens and smoke. Many people with mildly red, itching eyes require no treatment. Cold compresses to the eyes may prove helpful. Using eye drops with vasoconstrictors whitens eyes for a while, but rebound redness can occur. Misuse of vasoconstrictors sets up a vicious cycle.

If you want to treat a stuffy nose caused by a cold (not an allergy), you can use decongestant nasal sprays or drops such as phenylephrine, oxymetazoline, or xylometazoline, all available without a prescription. Any of these is a better choice than a drug like phenylpropanolamine, which can have dangerous adverse effects because you take it by mouth and it affects your whole system. Do not use decongestant nasal sprays or drops longer than three days (see p. 403).

If you have a cough, it is not necessarily a good idea to take a cough suppressant. Coughing clears mucous plugs and thick secretions from your airways and opens collapsed segments of your lungs. Drinking lots of liquids, especially soup and other hot drinks, and inhaling steam from hot showers and warm baths will help to loosen secretions and clean and soothe mucous membranes.

If you have a dry, irritating cough that is not producing mucus and that interferes with your sleep, you may benefit from a cough suppressant. The best nonnarcotic treatment is generic dextromethorphan, which you can get without a prescription. If your cough persists, you should see a doctor or other health professional, especially if you are a smoker.

A Food and Drug Administration advisory panel review of expectorants found that all nonprescription expectorants on the market lack evidence of effectiveness.

Cromolyn
GASTROCROM Capsules (Mediva)
INTAL Capsules/Inhaler
(Rhone-Poulenc Rorer)
NASALCROM Nasal Solution (McNeil)

GENERIC: available

FAMILY: Allergy and Asthma Drugs (see p. 405)

Cromolyn (*chrome* o lynn) is used by inhalation to reduce the frequency and severity of bronchial asthma and bronchospasm. It is of no value in treating an asthma attack. Cromolyn is also used nasally to prevent severe symptoms of allergies. It is effective for nasal congestion only when congestion is due to an allergy.[22] Use of cromolyn often reduces or eliminates the use of antihistamines, decongestants, or steroids. The International Asthma Management Project released a report urging the treatment of inflammation in asthma with cromolyn or steroids.[23] Concerns about systemic steroid use include suppressing the adrenals, and causing glaucoma and cataracts.[24,25,26]

While cromolyn is relatively safe,[27,28,29,30,31] older people are more likely to have reduced kidney and liver function, so a lower dose of cromolyn may be required. Response to the cromolyn is unpredictable and it may take a month for benefits to be noticeable.

Oral cromolyn is also used to relieve symptoms of mastocytosis (abdominal pain, diarrhea, headache, itching).

ADDITIONAL PRECAUTIONS

Avoid exposure to things which trigger your allergies or asthma, such as animals, bedding, chemicals, cosmetics, drugs, dust, mold, foods, pollens or smoke. Wearing a mask reduces inhalation of drugs, pollens and smoke. Many people with mildly red, itching eyes require no treatment. Cold compresses to the eyes may prove helpful. Using eye drops with vasoconstrictors whitens eyes for a while, but rebound redness can occur. Misuse of vasoconstrictors sets up a vicious cycle.

Aspirin can trigger asthma in people who are aspirin-allergic, as can beta-blockers. Infections aggravate lung problems. During epidemics of respiratory illnesses, avoid crowded places, and wash your hands frequently to help prevent infection. If you have asthma, get a flu vaccination.

Note: The information in this profile addresses the care of asthma that is not serious enough to need emergency treatment.

Before You Use This Drug

Tell your doctor if you have or have had:

- allergies to drugs
- glaucoma
- heart, kidney or liver problems
- high blood pressure
- nasal polyps
- severe or constant coughing or wheezing[32]

Tell your doctor about any other drugs you take, including aspirin, herbs, vitamins, and other nonprescription products.

When You Use This Drug

• Do not use cromolyn during an asthma attack. It may worsen the attack.

• Rinsing the mouth and gargling with water before and/or after your treatment may prevent irritation of the mouth, nose, and throat, and prevent hoarseness.

• If you also take steroid drugs, your doctor may gradually reduce your dose after you are taking cromolyn.

• Avoid drugs that may trigger asthma. Check with your doctor about using aspirin. If you use beta-blockers orally or in the eye, or ACE inhibitors, check with your doctor about changing drugs, or reviewing your dose.[33,34]

• If you plan to have any surgery, including dental, tell your doctor that you take this drug.

How to Use This Drug

• Ask for a demonstration of any device you are expected to use. Do not hesitate to ask or repeat questions until you feel comfortable using any inhaler device. When used for seasonal allergy begin at least one week before the season. For exercise or environmentally induced asthma, start no more than one hour before anticipated exercise or exposure.

For the aerosol for oral inhalation:

• Invert the can, then shake well.

• Exhale as completely as possible.

• Place mouthpiece into the mouth. Close lips loosely around it. Tilt inhaler upward and head backward, then inhale deeply while actuating the inhaler. (Some physicians recommend placing inhaler about two inches from the front of the open mouth.) Remove inhaler from mouth. Hold breath a few seconds, then exhale slowly.

• Avoid contact with the eyes.

• Clean the inhaler and plastic mouthpiece with warm water.

• Do not puncture, burn, or incinerate the container. It contains fluorocarbons.

For the capsules for oral inhalation:

• Do not swallow the capsules.

• Load capsule in the Spinhaler according to instructions.

• Exhale as completely as possible, then place mouthpiece between the lips, tilt inhaler upward, head backward, and inhale deeply and rapidly with an even breath. Remove inhaler for a few seconds, then exhale. Repeat the process until all the powder is inhaled. A light dusting of powder remaining in the capsule is normal.

• Do not exhale into the device, since moisture from breath interferes with the operation.

• Be aware of adverse effects due to lactose in the Spinhaler powder (cough, wheezing, bronchospasm, irritation of the throat and lungs).

• Dismantle Spinhaler weekly and clean in warm water. Dry thoroughly.

• To improve distribution of cromolyn in the lungs, a bronchodilator is sometimes used five minutes prior to the cromolyn.[35,36]

For the solution for oral inhalation:

• If specified, mix with other drug solutions no more than 90 minutes before use. If mixture changes color, or contains particles, do not use it.[37]

• Use with power-operated nebulizer with a flow rate of six to eight liters per minute, and equipped with face mask or mouthpiece. Do not use hand-operated nebulizers, which deliver too small a volume.

For the solution for nasal inhalation:

• Clear your nasal passages first.

• Prime metered spray device prior to initial use.

• Spray in each nostril, while inhaling.

• Replace spray device every six months. Do not clean it.

For the oral capsules for dilution to swallow:

• Do not use these capsules in Spinhaler.

• Capsules are intentionally oversized to prevent spilling powder when capsule is opened.

• A half hour before meals, open the capsule(s) and stir in four ounces of hot water until dissolved, then add four ounces of cold water. Do not mix with fruit juice, milk, or foods. Drink the entire eight ounces.

For all forms:

• Read instructions for using the devices carefully. An instruction sheet should come with each package.

• Check with your doctor if there is no improvement.

• Do not stop taking because of an attack, but do not take during an attack.

• To be effective, cromolyn must be taken regularly. **If you miss a dose, take it as soon as you remember,** then space remaining doses for the day at regular intervals. Do not take more often than prescribed.

• Do not store in the bathroom. Do not expose to heat, moisture, or strong light.

Interactions with Other Drugs

Some other drugs that you may be taking (either over-the-counter or prescription drugs) can interact with this one, causing adverse effects. Ask your doctor what these drugs are and let him or her know if you are taking any of them.

Adverse Effects

Call your doctor immediately if you experience:

• difficulty breathing or swallowing
• chest pain
• chills
• dizziness
• severe headache
• muscle pain
• nausea or vomiting
• skin rash, hives or itching
• increased sweating
• swelling of face, lips, eyes, mouth, joints, hands, feet
• urge to urinate frequently, or pain on urination
• severe wheezing
• coughing
• nosebleeds
• redness or irritation of the eye

Call your doctor if these symptoms continue:

• cough

• diarrhea
• drowsiness
• dryness or irritation of mouth, throat or eye
• headache
• hoarseness
• nosebleed, or severe nasal congestion
• sneezing
• unpleasant taste
• watering eyes
• abdominal pain
• irritability
• joint pain
• nausea
• trouble sleeping

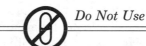

Do Not Use

ALTERNATIVE TREATMENT:
Chlorpheniramine (Chlor-Trimeton and many generics) p. 413, or loratadine (Claritin), p. 431.

Astemizole
HISMANAL (Janssen)

GENERIC: not available
FAMILY: Antihistamines (see p. 402)

Astemizole is a drug that we have long classified as a **Do Not Use** drug because of its potentially life-threatening drug interactions, and the fact that there are equally effective and safer antihistamines on the market. More warnings about the serious risks of astemizole were announced in February 1998.[38,39]

Astemizole was known to interact with ketoconazole (NIZORAL), itraconazole (SPORANOX), erythromycin (ERYTHROCIN, EES and generics), and quinine to cause potentially life-threatening irregular heart rhythms. The new FDA warning adds the following drugs to this list of drugs that can interact with astemizole to cause heart rhythm disturbances: the high blood pressure drug mibefradil (POSICOR—

now withdrawn from the market), and the antibiotics clarithromycin (BIAXIN) and trole-andomycin (TAO), the AIDS drugs nelfinavir (VIRACEPT), indinavir (CRIXIVAN), ritonavir (NORVIR), and saquinavir (INVIRASE), the serotonin reuptake inhibitor antidepressants such as fluoxetine (PROZAC), fluvoxamine (LUVOX), sertraline (ZOLOFT), nefazodone (SERZONE) and paroxetine (PAXIL), and the anti-asthma medication zileuton (ZYFLO). Additionally, the new warnings now recommend that astemizole should not be taken with grapefruit juice. This recommendation is based on the potential of these drugs and grapefruit juice to interfere with the body's handling and breakdown of astemizole.

Astemizole can also cause heart rhythm disturbances when used at higher than the recommended dose. The new warning emphasizes that people with liver disorders should not take astemizole. In addition, astemizole is not an antihistamine that should ever be used on an as-needed basis for immediate relief of allergic symptoms.

There is no medical reason that you should be taking astemizole. If you are taking astemizole, you should ask your doctor about switching to one of the less toxic antihistamines, such as nonprescription chlorpheniramine (CHLOR-TRIMETON and many generics) or loratadine (CLARITIN).

ADDITIONAL PRECAUTIONS

Avoid exposure to things which trigger your allergies or asthma, such as animals, bedding, chemicals, cosmetics, drugs, dust, mold, foods, pollens or smoke. Wearing a mask reduces inhalation of drugs, pollens and smoke. Many people with mildly red, itching eyes require no treatment. Cold compresses to the eyes may prove helpful. Using eye drops with vasoconstrictors whitens eyes for a while, but rebound redness can occur. Misuse of vasoconstrictors sets up a vicious cycle.

WARNING: SPECIAL MENTAL AND PHYSICAL ADVERSE EFFECTS

Older adults are especially sensitive to the harmful anticholinergic (see Glossary, p. 768) effects of antihistamines such as astemizole. Drugs in this family should not be used unless absolutely necessary.

Mental Effects: confusion, delirium, short-term memory problems, disorientation, and impaired attention.

Physical Effects: dry mouth, constipation, difficulty urinating (especially for a man with an enlarged prostate), blurred vision, decreased sweating with increased body temperature, sexual dysfunction, and worsening of glaucoma.

Pirbuterol
MAXAIR (3M)

GENERIC: not available

FAMILY: Asthma Drugs (see p. 408)

Pirbuterol (per *butte* er all) is used to prevent and treat asthma, as well as to treat bronchitis and emphysema. Within five minutes it begins to subdue wheezing and improve breathing. Pirbuterol controls symptoms, but does not cure any condition. It belongs to the same family as albuterol (PROVENTIL) and terbutaline (BRETHAIRE, BRETHINE) (see p. 449). According to Goodman and Gilman's *The Pharmacological Basis of Therapeutics,* there is little basis to choose one of this drug family over another.[40] As with all bronchodilators, it should be used cautiously by the elderly.[41] If you are over 60, you will generally need to take less than the usual adult dose of this drug, especially if you have heart disease.

Whichever of these drugs you take, use only the inhaled form. Do not take the tablets, capsules, or liquids. Because these forms are swallowed, the drug is distributed throughout your system, increasing the risk of adverse effects. An inhaler deposits most of the drug in the lungs, where it is needed.

Sometimes tolerance to pirbuterol develops. It can produce changes in your blood pressure, heart rate, pulse, and impede the flow of bile.[42] Fatal, paradoxical bronchospasms can occur. In fact, related drugs caused epidemics of asthma deaths in other countries several years ago.[43]

Since pirbuterol does not relieve inflammation of the lungs, The International Asthma Management Project recommends the use of bronchodilators, such as pirbuterol, be kept to a minimum in the treatment of asthma.[44] Sometimes pirbuterol is used along with corticosteroids or theophylline.

ADDITIONAL PRECAUTIONS

Avoid exposure to things which trigger your allergies or asthma, such as animals, bedding, chemicals, cosmetics, drugs, dust, mold, foods, pollens or smoke. Wearing a mask reduces inhalation of drugs, pollens and smoke.

Aspirin can trigger asthma in people who are aspirin-allergic, as can beta-blockers. Infections aggravate lung problems. During epidemics of respiratory illnesses, avoid crowded places and wash your hands frequently to help prevent infection. If you have asthma, get a flu vaccination.

Note: The information in this profile addresses the care of asthma that is not serious enough to need emergency treatment.

WARNING

Pirbuterol can cause or worsen high blood pressure. It is especially dangerous for people who have high blood pressure, heart disease, diabetes, or thyroid disease. People over 60 are more likely than younger people to experience effects on the heart and blood pressure, restlessness, nervousness, and confusion.

Before You Use This Drug

Tell your doctor if you have or have had:

- allergies to drugs
- convulsions
- diabetes
- heart problems including angina, and coronary artery disease
- stroke
- high blood pressure
- smoked
- thyroid problems

Tell your doctor about any other drugs you take, including aspirin, herbs, vitamins, and other nonprescription products.

When You Use This Drug

- Do not use more often or in a higher dose than that prescribed by your doctor. If your condition does not improve, or worsens, call your doctor.
- Avoid exercises that trigger asthma attacks. Ask your doctor to recommend appropriate exercises.

How to Use This Drug

For the aerosol for oral inhalation:

- Invert the can, then shake well.
- Exhale as completely as possible.
- Place mouthpiece into the mouth. Close lips loosely around it. Tilt inhaler upward and head backward, then inhale slowly and deeply while actuating the inhaler. (Some physicians recommend placing inhaler about two inches from the front of the open mouth.) Remove inhaler from mouth. Hold breath a few seconds, then exhale slowly.
- Avoid contact with the eyes.
- Clean the inhaler and plastic mouthpiece with warm water.
- Do not puncture, burn, or incinerate the container. It contains fluorocarbons.
- If your dose is more than one inhalation, wait a full minute between inhalations.

• Use your pirbuterol inhaler five minutes before using any corticosteroid or ipratropium inhaler.

• If you miss a dose, take it as soon as you remember, then space remaining doses for the day at regular intervals. Do not take more often than prescribed.

• Do not store in the bathroom. Do not expose to heat, moisture, or strong light. The canister can burst at 120°F.

• When discarded, do not burn in fire or incinerator.

Interactions with Other Drugs

The following drugs are listed in the *Evaluations of Drug Interactions* 1997 as causing "highly clinically significant" or "clinically significant" interactions when used together with this drug. We have also included potentially serious interactions listed in the drug's FDA-approved professional product labeling or package insert. New scientific techniques have allowed researchers to predict some drug interactions before they have been documented in people. There may be other drugs, especially those in the families of drugs listed below, that also will react with this drug to cause severe adverse effects. The number of new drugs approved for marketing increases the chance of drug interactions, and new drug interactions are being identified with old drugs. Be vigilant. Make sure to tell your doctor and pharmacist the drugs you are taking and tell your doctor if you are taking any of these interacting drugs:

FLUOTHANE, guanethidine, halothane, imipramine, INDERAL, INDERAL LA, ISMELIN, propranolol, timolol, TIMOPTIC, TOFRANIL.

Adverse Effects

Call your doctor immediately if you experience:

• severe dizziness
• chest pain
• feeling of choking
• irritation or swelling in the throat
• flushing or redness of skin
• hives
• increased shortness of breath
• skin rash
• swelling of face, lips, or eyelids
• tightness in chest or wheezing
• trouble breathing

Call your doctor if these symptoms continue:

• fast heartbeat
• headache
• nervousness
• trembling
• coughing or other bronchial irritation
• dizziness or lightheadedness
• dryness or irritation of mouth or throat
• chest discomfort or pain
• drowsiness or weakness
• muscle cramps or twitching
• nausea, vomiting
• nervousness, trembling
• restlessness
• trouble sleeping

Periodic Tests

Ask your doctor which of these tests should be done periodically while you are taking this drug:

• pulmonary function tests

PREGNANCY WARNING

This drug caused harm to developing fetuses in animal studies, or such studies were not done. Use during pregnancy only for clear medical reasons. Tell your doctor if you are pregnant or thinking of becoming pregnant before you take this drug.

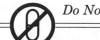 *Do Not Use*

ALTERNATIVE TREATMENT:
See Cold, p. 402, and Allergy and Hay Fever, p. 405.

Chlorpheniramine, Phenyltoloxamine, Phenylpropanolamine, and Phenylephrine
NALDECON (Apothecon)

FAMILY: Cold and Allergy Drugs (see p. 402)

This combination of chlorpheniramine (see p. 413), phenyltoloxamine (fen ill tole *ox* a meen), phenylpropanolamine (fen ill proe pa *nole* a meen), and phenylephrine (fen ill *ef* rin) is marketed as a drug that relieves congestion and other problems caused by allergies and the common cold. Naldecon, a brand-name product, is advertised as a remedy for sneezing, runny nose, and other symptoms of nasal congestion. You should not use it, for two reasons.

First, fixed-combination products containing antihistamines (chlorpheniramine and phenyltoloxamine) and decongestants (phenylpropanolamine and phenylephrine) exemplify the "shotgun" approach to treating cold and allergy symptoms, which are better treated with individual drugs for individual symptoms. The combination lacks clinical evidence of effectiveness.

Second, this product contains duplicates from each class of drugs. There is no reason to believe that two nasal decongestants or two antihistamines in a product make it any more effective than an adequate amount of one. Increasing the number of drugs increases the chance of unwanted adverse effects, without increasing the effectiveness.

If you want to treat congestion caused by an allergy, the best treatment is an antihistamine such as chlorpheniramine or phenyltoloxamine. If you want to treat congestion caused by a cold, the best treatment is a decongestant nose spray or nose drops. There is no reason to combine an antihistamine and a decongestant in one product.

Either chlorpheniramine or phenyltoloxamine is an effective antihistamine for treating hay fever and other allergies, although only chlorpheniramine is available as a single-drug product. If you have congestion caused by an allergy, taking chlorpheniramine or another antihistamine alone will help. Chlorpheniramine and phenyltoloxamine can cause drowsiness, loss of coordination, mental inattention, and dizziness. There is no satisfactory evidence that allergy patients benefit from adding a decongestant such as phenylpropanolamine or phenylephrine to an antihistamine.

If your congestion is caused by a cold rather than an allergy, you can use decongestant nasal sprays or drops such as phenylephrine, oxymetazoline, or xylometazoline, all available without a prescription. Any of these is a better choice than a drug like phenylpropanolamine, which can have dangerous adverse effects because it is taken by mouth and affects your whole system. Do not use decongestant nasal sprays or drops longer than three days (see p. 403).

WARNING

Phenylpropanolamine (PPA) can cause or worsen high blood pressure. It is especially dangerous for people who have high blood pressure, heart disease, diabetes, or thyroid disease. People over 60 are more likely than younger people to experience effects on the heart and blood pressure, restlessness, nervousness, and confusion.

Do Not Use

ALTERNATIVE TREATMENT:
See Cold, p. 402, and Allergy and Hay Fever, p. 405.

Codeine and Pseudoephedrine
NUCOFED Capsules and Syrup (Roberts)

Codeine, Pseudoephedrine, Guaifenesin, and Alcohol

NUCOFED Expectorant Syrup (Roberts)
ROBITUSSIN DAC (Robins)

FAMILY: Cold and Allergy Drugs (see p. 402)
         Cough Suppressants

These combination products with codeine (see p. 284), pseudoephedrine (soo doe eh *fed* rin), guaifenesin (see p. 452), and alcohol are promoted to relieve cough and congestion due to respiratory illnesses. Taking the capsule or syrup form is taking two drugs, each with its own cautions, adverse effects, and drug interactions. Taking the expectorant syrup is taking four drugs, each with its own cautions, adverse effects, and drug interactions. Fixed-combination products curtail the ability to vary doses of each drug.

Codeine effectively suppresses a cough, allowing for more rest. Codeine is best reserved for dry coughs. Productive cough clears mucous plugs and thick secretions from your airways and opens collapsed segments of your lungs. Drinking lots of liquids, especially soup and other hot drinks, and inhaling steam from hot showers and warm baths helps loosen secretions and cleans and soothes mucous membranes.

Ordinarily, it is inadvisable for people with asthma or emphysema to take codeine. Do not use codeine if you have a history of serious constipation.

Guaifenesin is the most widely used expectorant. An expectorant thins mucus in the airways so it can be coughed up more easily. No well-designed study has shown that guaifenesin works, despite the efforts of drug manufacturers to convince people that it does.

Products combining both a cough suppressant and an expectorant offer no advantage over a product containing only one of these ingredients.

If you have a dry, irritating cough that is not producing mucus and that interferes with your sleep, you may benefit from a cough suppressant. The best non-narcotic treatment is dextromethorphan, which you can get without a prescription. If your cough persists, see your doctor or other health professional, especially if you are a smoker.

If your congestion is caused by a cold, rather than an allergy, you can use decongestant nasal sprays or drops such as phenylephrine, oxymetazoline, or xylometazoline, all available without prescription. Any of these is a better choice than a drug like pseudoephedrine, which can have dangerous adverse effects because you take it by mouth and it affects your whole system. Do not use decongestant nasal sprays or drops longer than three days (see p. 403).

WARNING

Pseudoephedrine can cause or worsen high blood pressure. It is especially dangerous for people who have high blood pressure, heart disease, diabetes, or thyroid disease. People over 60 are more likely than younger people to experience effects on the heart and blood pressure, restlessness, nervousness, and confusion. Do not use pseudoephedrine during or within 14 days following administration of monoamine oxidase (MAO) inhibitors.

Alcohol is present in Nucofed Expectorant Syrup at 12.5%, about the same as fortified wines. A limited amount of alcohol may help you rest. However, if you are taking other medications, alcohol might interact with these. In this formulation alcohol is one of three ingredients that depresses the central nervous system. Older people, especially, should avoid these "shotgun" preparations.

One hazard of taking codeine continuously for longer than several weeks is drug-induced dependence. Do not stop taking your drug suddenly. With the help of your doctor, work out a schedule for slowly decreasing the amount of the drug you take by about 5 to 10% each day. Keep a written record of the dosage reduction schedule with you. These steps will make it much easier to become drug free without developing distressing symptoms of drug withdrawal.

A Food and Drug Administration advisory panel review of expectorants found that all nonprescription expectorants on the market lack evidence of effectiveness.

ADDITIONAL PRECAUTIONS

Avoid exposure to things which trigger your allergies or asthma, such as animals, bedding, chemicals, cosmetics, drugs, dust, mold, foods, pollens or smoke. Wearing a mask reduces inhalation of drugs, pollens and smoke. Many people with mildly red, itching eyes require no treatment. Cold compresses to the eyes may prove helpful. Using eye drops with vasoconstrictors whitens eyes for a while, but rebound redness can occur. Misuse of vasoconstrictors sets up a vicious cycle.

Do Not Use

ALTERNATIVE TREATMENT:
See Cold, p. 402, and Allergy and Hay Fever, p. 405.

Chlorpheniramine and Phenylpropanolamine
ORNADE (SmithKline Beecham)

FAMILY: Cold and Allergy Drugs (see p. 402)

This combination of chlorpheniramine (see p. 413) and phenylpropanolamine (fen ill proe pa *nole* a meen) is marketed as a drug that relieves congestion and other problems caused by allergies and the common cold. Ornade, a brand-name product, is advertised as a remedy for sneezing, runny nose, and other symptoms of nasal congestion. You should not use it, for two reasons.

First, the long-lasting capsule form of this drug is unacceptable because your body does not absorb it gradually at an even rate. This means that levels of the drug in your body may vary significantly over time rather than staying constant.

Second, fixed-combination products containing an antihistamine (chlorpheniramine) and a decongestant (phenylpropanolamine) exemplify the "shotgun" approach to treating cold and allergy symptoms, which are better treated with individual drugs for individual symptoms. The combination lacks clinical evidence of effectiveness.

If you want to treat congestion caused by an allergy, the best treatment is an antihistamine such as chlorpheniramine. If you want to treat congestion caused by a cold, the best treatment is a decongestant nose spray or nose drops. There is no reason to combine an antihistamine and a decongestant in one product.

Chlorpheniramine is an effective antihistamine for treating hay fever and other allergies. If you have congestion caused by an allergy, taking chlorpheniramine or another antihistamine alone will help. There is no satisfactory evidence that allergy patients benefit from adding a decongestant such as phenyl-propanolamine to an antihistamine. Chlorpheniramine can cause drowsiness, loss of coordination, mental inattention, and dizziness.

If your congestion is caused by a cold rather than an allergy, you can use decongestant nasal sprays or drops such as phenylephrine, oxymetazoline, or xylometazoline, all available without a prescription. Any of these is a better choice than a drug like phenylpropanolamine, which can have dangerous adverse effects because you take it by mouth and it affects your whole system. Do not use decongestant nasal sprays or drops longer than three days (see p. 403).

ADDITIONAL PRECAUTIONS

Avoid exposure to things which trigger your allergies or asthma, such as animals, bedding, chemicals, cosmetics, drugs, dust, mold, foods, pollens or smoke. Wearing a mask reduces inhalation of drugs, pollens and smoke. Many people with mildly red, itching eyes require no treatment. Cold compresses to the eyes may prove helpful. Using eye drops with vasoconstrictors whitens eyes for a while, but rebound redness can occur. Misuse of vasoconstrictors sets up a vicious cycle.

WARNING

Phenylpropanolamine (PPA) can cause or worsen high blood pressure. It is especially dangerous for people who have high blood pressure, heart disease, diabetes, or thyroid disease. People over 60 are more likely than younger people to experience effects on the heart and blood pressure, restlessness, nervousness, and confusion.

WARNING: SPECIAL MENTAL AND PHYSICAL ADVERSE EFFECTS

Older adults are especially sensitive to the harmful anticholinergic (see Glossary, p. 768) effects of antihistamines such as chlorpheniramine. Drugs in this family should not be used unless absolutely necessary.

Mental Effects: confusion, delirium, short-term memory problems, disorientation, and impaired attention.

Physical Effects: dry mouth, constipation, difficulty urinating (especially for a man with an enlarged prostate), blurred vision, decreased sweating with increased body temperature, sexual dysfunction, and worsening of glaucoma.

Cyproheptadine
PERIACTIN (Merck)

GENERIC: available
FAMILY: Antihistamines (see p. 402)

Cyproheptadine (si proe *hep* ta deen) relieves the symptoms of hay fever and other allergies. Do not use it to stimulate appetite, and do not use it to treat a cold. Colds and allergies have different causes, and cyproheptadine is not effective against either the cause of a cold or its symptoms. In fact, the drug can make a cold or cough worse by thickening nasal secretions and drying mucous membranes. It also causes drowsiness.

Cyproheptadine can cause harmful adverse effects, more commonly in people over 60 than in younger people. These effects include confusion, dizziness, fainting, difficult or painful urination, dry mouth, nose, or throat, nightmares, unusual excitement, nervousness, restlessness, or irritability. If you have any of these while taking cyproheptadine, ask your doctor about changing or discontinuing this drug.

ADDITIONAL PRECAUTIONS

Avoid exposure to things which trigger your allergies or asthma, such as animals, bedding chemicals, cosmetics, drugs, dust, mold, foods, pollens or smoke. Wearing a mask reduces inhalation of drugs, pollens and smoke. Many people with mildly red, itching eyes require no treatment. Cold compresses to the eyes may prove helpful. Using eye drops with vasoconstrictors whitens eyes for a while, but rebound redness can occur. Misuse of vasoconstrictors sets up a vicious cycle.

WARNING: SPECIAL MENTAL AND PHYSICAL ADVERSE EFFECTS

Older adults are especially sensitive to the harmful anticholinergic (see Glossary, p. 768) effects of antihistamines such as cyproheptadine. Drugs in this family should not be used unless absolutely necessary.

Mental Effects: confusion, delirium, short-term memory problems, disorientation, and impaired attention.

Physical Effects: dry mouth, constipation, difficulty urinating (especially for a man with an enlarged prostate), blurred vision, decreased sweating with increased body temperature, sexual dysfunction, and worsening of glaucoma.

Before You Use This Drug

Tell your doctor if you have or have had:

- allergies to drugs
- asthma
- problems with urination
- glaucoma
- enlarged prostate
- liver problems

Tell your doctor about any other drugs you take, including aspirin, herbs, vitamins, and other nonprescription products.

When You Use This Drug

- Do not use more often or in a higher dose than prescribed. Overuse increases your risk of adverse effects.
- Do not drink alcohol or use other drugs that can cause drowsiness.
- Until you know how you react to this drug, do not drive or perform other activities requiring alertness.
- If you plan to have any surgery, including dental, tell your doctor that you take this drug.

How to Use This Drug

- Do not store in the bathroom. Do not expose to heat, moisture, or strong light. Do not allow liquid form to freeze.
- Take with food, water, or milk to avoid stomach upset.
- Swallow extended-release forms whole.
- If you miss a dose, take it as soon as you remember, but skip it if it is almost time for the next dose. **Do not take double doses.**

Interactions with Other Drugs

The following drugs are listed in the *Evaluations of Drug Interactions* 1997 as causing "highly clinically significant" or "clinically sig-

nificant" interactions when used together with this drug. We have also included potentially serious interactions listed in the drug's FDA-approved professional product labeling or package insert. New scientific techniques have allowed researchers to predict some drug interactions before they have been documented in people. There may be other drugs, especially those in the families of drugs listed below, that also will react with this drug to cause severe adverse effects. The number of new drugs approved for marketing increases the chance of drug interactions, and new drug interactions are being identified with old drugs. Be vigilant. Make sure to tell your doctor and pharmacist the drugs you are taking and tell your doctor if you are taking any of these interacting drugs:

DILANTIN, EFFEXOR, fluoxetine, fluvoxamine, LUVOX, nefazodone, paroxetine, PAXIL, phenytoin, PROZAC, SERZONE, venlafaxine.

Adverse Effects

Call your doctor immediately if you experience:

- **signs of overdose:** clumsiness or unsteadiness, dry mouth, nose, or throat, flushed or red face, shortness of breath, trouble breathing, seizures, hallucinations, trouble sleeping, severe drowsiness, faintness or light-headedness
- sore throat and fever
- unusual bleeding or bruising
- unusual tiredness or weakness

Call your doctor if these symptoms continue:

- thickening bronchial secretions
- change in vision
- confusion
- difficult or painful urination

- nightmares
- loss of appetite
- unusual excitement, nervousness, restlessness, or irritability
- ringing or buzzing in ears
- skin rash
- stomach upset or pain
- increased sweating
- unusually fast heartbeat
- increased sensitivity to sun (rash, hives, skin reactions)
- dizziness
- drowsiness
- thickening of mucus
- dryness of mouth, nose or throat
- weight gain

Albuterol
PROVENTIL (Schering)
VENTOLIN (Glaxo Wellcome)

Terbutaline
BRETHAIRE, BRETHINE (Novartis)
BRICANYL (Hoechst Marion Roussel)

GENERIC: available
FAMILY: Asthma Drugs (see p. 408)

Inhaled albuterol (al *byoo* ter ole) and terbutaline (ter *byoo* ta leen) are used to treat asthma, as well as chronic bronchitis and emphysema. Within five minutes they begin to subdue wheezing and improve breathing.

They belong to the same family as pirbuterol (MAXAIR). According to Goodman and Gilman's *The Pharmacological Basis of Therapeutics*, there is little basis to choose one of this drug family over another.[45]

Albuterol and terbutaline can cause tremors, jitters, and nervousness, especially in older adults.[46] Albuterol has also been found to cause benign tumors in the ligament surrounding the ovaries in rats.[47]

If you are taking one of these drugs and are suffering from adverse effects, ask your doctor to change your prescription to the other one. If you are over 60, you will generally need to take less than the usual adult dose of these drugs, especially if you have heart disease.

Whichever of these drugs you take, use only the inhaled form. Do not take the tablets, capsules, or liquids. Because these forms are swallowed, the drug is distributed throughout your body, increasing the risk of adverse effects. An inhaler deposits most of the drug in the lungs, where it is needed.

ADDITIONAL PRECAUTIONS

Avoid exposure to things which trigger your allergies or asthma, such as animals, bedding, chemicals, cosmetics, drugs, dust, mold, foods, pollens or smoke. Wearing a mask reduces inhalation of drugs, pollens and smoke.

Aspirin can trigger asthma in people who are aspirin-allergic, as can beta-blockers. Infections aggravate lung problems. During epidemics of respiratory illnesses, avoid crowded places and wash your hands frequently to help prevent infection. If you have asthma, get a flu vaccination.

Note: The information in this profile addresses the care of asthma that is not serious enough to need emergency treatment.

WARNING

Albuterol and terbutaline can cause or worsen high blood pressure. It is especially dangerous for people who have high blood pressure, heart disease, diabetes, or thyroid disease. People over 60 are more likely than younger people to experience effects on the heart and blood pressure, restlessness, nervousness, and confusion.

Before You Use This Drug

Do not use if you have or have had:

- an allergy to other sympathomimetic drugs such as the decongestants pseudoephedrine or phenylpropanolamine (PPA)

Tell your doctor if you have or have had:

- allergies to drugs
- heart or blood vessel disease
- high blood pressure
- diabetes
- enlarged prostate
- enlarged thyroid
- history of seizures, *(for terbutaline)*

Tell your doctor about any other drugs you take, including aspirin, herbs, vitamins, and other nonprescription products.

When You Use This Drug

- Do not use more often or in a higher dose than that prescribed by your doctor. Call your doctor if you do not feel better after taking the usual dose, if you still have trouble breathing one hour after a dose, if symptoms return within four hours, or if your condition worsens.
- If you plan to have any surgery, including dental, tell your doctor that you take an asthma drug.
- Do not take other drugs without talking to your doctor first, especially nonprescription drugs for appetite control, asthma, colds, coughs, hay fever, or sinus problems.

How to Use This Drug

- Do not store in the bathroom. Do not expose to heat, moisture, or strong light. Do not allow inhaled form to freeze.
- To prevent dryness of the mouth and throat, gargle and rinse your mouth out with water after each time you use the inhaled form.

- If you use more than one inhalant, use them at least 15 minutes apart. Aerosol inhalants contain chemicals called chlorofluorocarbons, which can be harmful to your health.
- Be careful not to get medicine in your eyes.
- If you miss a dose, take it as soon as you remember, then space remaining doses for the day at regular intervals. Do not take more often than prescribed.

For the aerosol for oral inhalation:

- Invert the can, then shake well.
- Exhale as completely as possible.
- Place mouthpiece into the mouth. Close lips loosely around it. Tilt inhaler upward and head backward, then inhale slowly and deeply while actuating the inhaler. (Some physicians recommend placing inhaler about two inches from the front of the open mouth.) Remove inhaler from mouth. Hold breath a few seconds, then exhale slowly.
- Avoid contact with the eyes.
- Clean the inhaler and plastic mouthpiece with warm water.
- Do not puncture, burn, or incinerate the container. It contains fluorocarbons.

Interactions with Other Drugs

The following drugs are listed in the *Evaluations of Drug Interactions* 1997 as causing "highly clinically significant" or "clinically significant" interactions when used together with this drug. We have also included potentially serious interactions listed in the drug's FDA-approved professional product labeling or package insert. New scientific techniques have allowed researchers to predict some drug interactions before they have been documented in people. There may be other drugs, especially those in the families of drugs listed below, that also will react with this drug to cause severe adverse effects. The number of

new drugs approved for marketing increases the chance of drug interactions, and new drug interactions are being identified with old drugs. Be vigilant. Make sure to tell your doctor and pharmacist the drugs you are taking and tell your doctor if you are taking any of these interacting drugs:

flecainide, FLUOTHANE, halothane, imipramine, INDERAL, INDERAL LA, propranolol, TAMBOCOR, TOFRANIL.

Adverse Effects

Call your doctor immediately if you experience:

- severe dizziness
- chest pain
- feeling of choking
- irritation or swelling in the throat
- flushing or redness of skin
- hives
- increased shortness of breath
- skin rash
- swelling of face, lips, or eyelids
- tightness in chest or wheezing
- trouble breathing

Call your doctor if these symptoms continue:

- fast heartbeat
- headache
- nervousness
- trembling
- coughing or other bronchial irritation
- dizziness or lightheadedness
- dryness or irritation of mouth or throat
- chest discomfort or pain
- drowsiness or weakness
- muscle cramps or twitching
- nausea, vomiting
- nervousness, trembling
- restlessness
- trouble sleeping

- *heartburn* and unusual taste in mouth *(for albuterol)*

PREGNANCY WARNING

Proventil and Ventolin caused harm to developing fetuses in animal studies, or such studies were not done. Use during pregnancy only for clear medical reasons. Tell your doctor if you are pregnant or thinking of becoming pregnant before you take this drug.

 Do Not Use

ALTERNATIVE TREATMENT:
See Theophylline, p. 426.

Guaifenesin and Theophylline
QUIBRON (Roberts)

FAMILY: Asthma Drugs (see p. 408)

This combination of guaifenesin (see p. 452) and theophylline (see p. 426) is used to treat spasms of the airways (bronchospasm) in people with asthma, bronchitis, and emphysema. Theophylline alone is effective for this purpose. We do not recommend this combination because it contains an ineffective ingredient, guaifenesin.

Guaifenesin is marketed as an expectorant, a drug which supposedly thins the mucus in the airways so that it can be coughed up more easily. Although guaifenesin is the most widely used expectorant, no well-designed study has shown that it works, despite the efforts of drug manufacturers to convince people that it does. The best expectorant is water. If you have a cough or lung congestion, drinking lots of liquid (especially soup and other hot drinks) and inhaling steam from hot showers and warm baths will help to loosen secretions and clean and soothe mucous membranes.

If you have bronchospasms caused by asthma, bronchitis, or emphysema, theophylline alone is effective and is less expensive than this combination. It opens airways narrowed by bronchospasm, increasing the flow of air through them and making breathing easier. Since there is a narrow range between a helpful and a harmful amount of theophylline in your body, your doctor should monitor your dose and the level of the drug in your bloodstream. Too little theophylline may not work, bringing on an asthma attack. Too much may produce headache, nervousness, nausea, rapid heartbeats, and other adverse effects.[48]

> A Food and Drug Administration advisory panel review of expectorants found that all nonprescription expectorants on the market lack evidence of effectiveness.

ADDITIONAL PRECAUTIONS

Avoid exposure to things which trigger your allergies or asthma, such as animals, bedding, chemicals, cosmetics, drugs, dust, mold, foods, pollens or smoke. Wearing a mask reduces inhalation of drugs, pollens and smoke.

Aspirin can trigger asthma in people who are aspirin-allergic, as can beta-blockers. Infections aggravate lung problems. During epidemics of respiratory illnesses, avoid crowded places, and wash your hands to help prevent getting infected. If you have asthma, get a flu vaccination.

Note: The information in this profile addresses the care of asthma that is not serious enough to need emergency treatment.

 Do Not Use

ALTERNATIVE TREATMENT:
See Cold, p. 402, and Allergy and Hay Fever, p. 405.

Guaifenesin
ROBITUSSIN (Whitehall-Robins)

FAMILY: Expectorants (see p. 402)

Guaifenesin (gwye *fen* e sin) is the most widely used expectorant. An expectorant thins mucus in the airways so it can be coughed up more easily. No well-designed study has shown that guaifenesin works, despite the efforts of drug manufacturers to convince people that it does.

If you have a cough, it is not necessarily a good idea to take a cough suppressant. Coughing clears mucous plugs and thick secretions from your airways and opens collapsed segments of your lungs. Drinking lots of liquids, especially soup and other hot drinks, and inhaling steam from hot showers and warm baths will help to loosen secretions and clean and soothe mucous membranes.

If you have a dry, irritating cough that is not producing mucus and that interferes with your sleep, you may benefit from a cough suppressant. The best nonnarcotic treatment is generic dextromethorphan, which you can get without a prescription. If your cough persists, you should see a doctor or other health professional, especially if you are a smoker.

> A Food and Drug Administration advisory panel review of expectorants found that all nonprescription expectorants on the market lack evidence of effectiveness.

Do Not Use

ALTERNATIVE TREATMENT:
See Cold, p. 402, and Allergy and Hay Fever, p. 405.

Guaifenesin and Dextromethorphan
ROBITUSSIN-DM (Whitehall-Robins)

FAMILY: Expectorants
Cough Suppressants (see p. 402)

This combination of guaifenesin (see p. 452) and dextromethorphan (dex troe meth *or* fan) is promoted as a cough suppressant and an expectorant. An expectorant thins mucus in the airways so that it may be coughed up more easily. Dextromethorphan is an effective cough suppressant, but there is no convincing evidence that adding guaifenesin increases the effectiveness of dextromethorphan in any way. No well-designed study has shown that guaifenesin works as an expectorant, despite the efforts of drug manufacturers to convince people that it does.

If you have a cough, it is not necessarily a good idea to take a cough suppressant. Coughing clears mucous plugs and thick secretions from your airways and opens collapsed segments of your lungs. Drinking lots of liquids, especially soup and other hot drinks, and inhaling steam from hot showers and warm baths will help to loosen secretions and clean and soothe mucous membranes.

If you have a dry, irritating cough that is not producing mucus and that interferes with your sleep, you may benefit from a cough suppressant. The best nonnarcotic treatment is generic dextromethorphan, which you can get without a prescription. If your cough persists, you should see a doctor or other health professional, especially if you are a smoker.

A Food and Drug Administration advisory panel review of expectorants found that all nonprescription expectorants on the market lack evidence of effectiveness.

Do Not Use

ALTERNATIVE TREATMENT:
Chlorpheniramine (Chlor-Trimeton and many generics), p. 413 or loratadine (Claritin), p. 431.

Terfenadine
SELDANE (Hoechst Marion Roussel)

Terfenadine and Pseudoephedrine
SELDANE D (Hoechst Marion Roussel)

FAMILY: Antihistamines (see p. 402)

Terfenadine (ter *fen* a deen) has been withdrawn from the market. In January 1997, the FDA proposed removing all terfenadine products from the marketplace because of the approval of a safer alternative drug: fexofenadine (see p. 415). Fexofenadine provides the benefits of terfenadine, but it does not cause a potentially fatal heart condition when taken with some other commonly prescribed medications.[49] Generic nonprescription chlorpheniramine is just as effective as fexofenadine and can be taken by many people without drowsiness.

Products containing terfenadine have long been associated with potentially lethal heart rhythm disturbances when taken with certain antibiotics and antifungal drugs. In September 1997, new warnings were issued by the FDA against simultaneously using terfenadine-containing products with the blood pressure lowering drug mibefradil (POSICOR, now withdrawn from the market); the AIDS drugs indinavir (CRIXIVAN), ritonavir (NORVIR), saquinavir (Invirase), and nelfinavir (VIRA-CEPT), and selective serotonin reuptake inhibitor (SSRI) antidepressants such as fluvoxamine (LUVOX), sertraline (ZOLOFT), nefazodone (SERZONE), along with the additional medications zileuton (ZYFLO) to prevent asthma attacks, cisapride (PROPULSID), a drug used for night time heartburn, and the fluoroquinolone antibiotic sparfloxacin (ZAGAM).[50]

You should check your medicine cabinet for old prescriptions of terfenadine-containing products. These should be destroyed. There is no medical reason that you should be taking terfenadine when less toxic antihistamines, such as nonprescription chlorpheniramine (CHLOR-TRIMETON and many generics) or loratadine (CLARITAN) are available.

ADDITIONAL PRECAUTIONS

Avoid exposure to things which trigger your allergies or asthma, such as animals, bedding chemicals, cosmetics, drugs, dust, mold, foods, pollens or smoke. Wearing a mask reduces inhalation of drugs, pollens and smoke. Many people with mildly red, itching eyes require no treatment. Cold compresses to the eyes may prove helpful. Using eye drops with vasoconstrictors whitens eyes for a while, but rebound redness can occur. Misuse of vasoconstrictors sets up a vicious cycle.

Limited Use

Clemastine
TAVIST, TAVIST-1 (Geneva)

GENERIC: available
FAMILY: Antihistamines (see p. 402)

Clemastine (clem *as* tine) is used to treat symptoms of allergies and hay fever, such as itching, nasal congestion, runny nose, sneezing, or watery eyes. It does not cure an allergy. Do not use it to treat a cold. In fact the drug can make a cold worse by thickening nasal secretions and drying mucous membranes. Clemastine also causes drowsiness.

Clemastine can cause other harmful adverse effects more commonly in people over 60 than in younger people. These effects include: confusion, dizziness, fainting, difficult or painful urination, dry mouth, nose, or throat, nightmares, unusual excitement, nervousness, restlessness, or irritability. If you have any of these symptoms while taking clemastine, ask your doctor about changing or discontinuing this drug.

Since older people can be more sensitive to the usual adult dose, start with a low dose. This may decrease adverse effects.

ADDITIONAL PRECAUTIONS

Avoid exposure to things which trigger your allergies or asthma, such as animals, bedding, chemicals, cosmetics, drugs, dust, mold, foods, pollens or smoke. Wearing a mask reduces inhalation of drugs, pollens and smoke. Many people with mildly red, itching eyes require no treatment. Cold compresses to the eyes may prove helpful. Using eye drops with vasoconstrictors whitens eyes for a while, but rebound redness can occur. Misuse of vasoconstrictors sets up a vicious cycle.

If you need an antihistamine, chlorpheniramine or diphenhydramine are available without a prescription. The adverse effects are similar to clemastine, but the price is less (see pp. 413, 424).

WARNING: SPECIAL MENTAL AND PHYSICAL ADVERSE EFFECTS

Older adults are especially sensitive to the harmful anticholinergic (see Glossary, p. 768) effects of antihistamines such as clemastine. Drugs in this family should not be used unless absolutely necessary.

Mental Effects: confusion, delirium, short-term memory problems, disorientation, and impaired attention.

Physical Effects: dry mouth, constipation, difficulty urinating (especially for a man with an enlarged prostate), blurred vision, decreased sweating with increased body temperature, sexual dysfunction, and worsening of glaucoma.

Before You Use This Drug

Tell your doctor if you have or have had:

- allergies to drugs
- asthma
- problems with urination
- glaucoma
- enlarged prostate
- heart rhythm problems

Tell your doctor about any other drugs you take, including aspirin, herbs, vitamins, and other nonprescription products.

When You Use This Drug

- Do not use more often or in a higher dose than prescribed. Overuse increases your risk of adverse effects.
- Until you know how you react to this drug, do not drive or perform other activities requiring alertness.
- If you plan to have any surgery, including dental, tell your doctor that you take this drug.

How to Use This Drug

- Swallow tablet whole, or break tablets in half to ease swallowing. Take with food, water or milk to decrease stomach upset.
- If clemastine causes you to be drowsy, schedule at least one dose at bedtime.
- If you miss a dose, take it as soon as you remember, but skip it if it is almost time for the next dose. **Do not take double doses.**

Interactions with Other Drugs

The following drugs are listed in the *Evaluations of Drug Interactions* 1997 as causing "highly clinically significant" or "clinically significant" interactions when used together with this drug. We have also included potentially serious interactions listed in the drug's FDA-approved professional product labeling or package insert. New scientific techniques have allowed researchers to predict some drug interactions before they have been documented in people. There may be other drugs, especially those in the families of drugs listed below, that also will react with this drug to cause severe adverse effects. The number of new drugs approved for marketing increases the chance of drug interactions, and new drug interactions are being identified with old drugs. Be vigilant. Make sure to tell your doctor and pharmacist the drugs you are taking and tell your doctor if you are taking any of these interacting drugs:

alcohol (note: clemastine syrup contains 5% alcohol), DILANTIN, phenytoin, RESTORIL, temazepam.

Adverse Effects

Call your doctor immediately if you experience:

- **signs of overdose:** clumsiness or unsteadiness, dry mouth, nose, or throat, flushed or red face, shortness of breath, trouble breathing, seizures, hallucinations, trouble sleeping, severe drowsiness, faintness or lightheadedness

- sore throat or fever
- unusual bleeding or bruising
- unusual tiredness, weakness
- chills

Call your doctor if these symptoms continue:

- change in vision
- confusion
- difficult or painful urination
- nightmares
- change in appetite
- unusual excitement, nervousness, restlessness or irritability
- ringing or buzzing in ears
- skin rash
- stomach upset or pain
- increased sweating
- unusually fast heartbeat
- increased sensitivity to sun (rash, hives, skin reactions)
- drowsiness
- headache
- nausea
- dizziness
- thickening of mucus or bronchial secretions
- dryness of mouth, nose or throat

Do Not Use

ALTERNATIVE TREATMENT:
See Cold, p. 402, and Allergy and Hay Fever, p. 405.

Clemastine and Phenylpropanolamine
TAVIST-D (Geneva)

FAMILY: Cold and Allergy Drugs (see p. 402)

This combination of clemastine (see p. 454) and phenylpropanolamine (fen ill proe pa

nole a meen) is marketed as a drug that relieves congestion and other problems caused by allergies and the common cold. Tavist-D, a brand-name product, is advertised as a remedy for sneezing, runny nose, and other symptoms of nasal congestion. You should not use it.

Fixed-combination products containing an antihistamine (clemastine) and a decongestant (phenylpropanolamine) exemplify the "shotgun" approach to treating cold and allergy symptoms, which are better treated with individual drugs for individual symptoms. The combination lacks clinical evidence of effectiveness.

If you want to treat congestion caused by an allergy, the best treatment is an antihistamine such as clemastine. If you want to treat congestion caused by a cold, the best treatment is a decongestant nose spray or nose drops. There is no reason to combine an antihistamine and a decongestant in one product.

Clemastine is an effective antihistamine for treating hay fever and other allergies. If you have congestion caused by an allergy, taking clemastine or another antihistamine alone will help. There is no satisfactory evidence that allergy patients benefit from adding a decongestant such as phenylpropanolamine to an antihistamine. Clemastine can cause drowsiness, loss of coordination, mental inattention, and dizziness.

If your congestion is caused by a cold rather than an allergy, you can use decongestant nasal sprays or drops such as phenylephrine, oxymetazoline, or xylometazoline, all available without a prescription. Any of these is a better choice than a drug like phenylpropanolamine, which can have dangerous adverse effects because you take it by mouth and it affects your whole body. Do not use decongestant nasal sprays or drops longer than three days (see p. 403).

ADDITIONAL PRECAUTIONS

Avoid exposure to things which trigger your allergies or asthma, such as animals, bedding, chemicals, cosmetics, drugs, dust, mold, foods, pollens or smoke. Wearing a mask reduces inhalation of drugs, pollens and smoke. Many people with mildly red, itching eyes require no treatment. Cold compresses to the eyes may prove helpful. Using eye drops with vasoconstrictors whitens eyes for a while, but rebound redness can occur. Misuse of vasoconstrictors sets up a vicious cycle.

WARNING: SPECIAL MENTAL AND PHYSICAL ADVERSE EFFECTS

Older adults are especially sensitive to the harmful anticholinergic (see Glossary, p. 768) effects of antihistamines such as clemastine. Drugs in this family should not be used unless absolutely necessary.

Mental Effects: confusion, delirium, short-term memory problems, disorientation, and impaired attention.

Physical Effects: dry mouth, constipation, difficulty urinating (especially for a man with an enlarged prostate), blurred vision, decreased sweating with increased body temperature, sexual dysfunction, and worsening of glaucoma.

WARNING

Phenylpropanolamine (PPA) can cause or worsen high blood pressure. It is especially dangerous for people who have high blood pressure, heart disease, diabetes, or thyroid disease. People over 60 are more likely than younger people to experience effects on the heart and blood pressure, restlessness, nervousness, and confusion.

Limited Use

Benzonatate
TESSALON (Forest)

GENERIC: not available
FAMILY: Cough Suppressants (see p. 402)

Benzonatate (ben *zone* a tate) is a cough suppressant. It may be used for short-term treatment (no more than one week) of an unproductive cough, a dry cough bringing up no mucus, or a cough that is preventing you from sleeping. However, dextromethorphan, a less expensive cough suppressant that is available without a prescription, is a better choice.

You should not use benzonatate or any other drug to treat a cough that is producing mucus, because this is the body's way of ridding itself of secretions and decreasing infection. If you have this kind of cough, drinking lots of liquids, especially soup and other hot drinks, and inhaling steam from hot showers and warm baths will help to loosen secretions and clean and soothe mucous membranes. For more information on treating coughs, see Cold, p. 402, and Allergy and Hay Fever, p. 405.

Before You Use This Drug

Tell your doctor if you have or have had:

- allergies to drugs

- asthma
- mucus or phlegm with cough

Tell your doctor about any other drugs you take, including aspirin, herbs, vitamins, and other nonprescription products.

When You Use This Drug

- Do not use more often or in a higher dose than prescribed. Call your doctor if your cough continues after taking this drug for one week, or if you get a high fever, skin rash, or persistent headache.

How to Use This Drug

- Swallow capsules whole. Do not chew or break them. If this drug is released in your mouth, it can temporarily numb your mouth and throat.
- Do not store in the bathroom. Do not expose to heat, moisture, or strong light.
- If you miss a dose, take it as soon as you remember, but skip it if it is almost time for the next dose. **Do not take double doses.**

Interactions with Other Drugs

Some other drugs that you may be taking (either over-the-counter or prescription drugs) can interact with this one, causing adverse effects. Ask your doctor what these drugs are and let him or her know if you are taking any of them.

Adverse Effects

Call your doctor immediately if you experience:

- skin rash, itching
- numbness in the chest
- burning sensation in the eyes

- seizures
- restlessness
- trembling

Call your doctor if these symptoms continue:

- drowsiness
- dizziness, lightheadedness
- nausea or vomiting
- stomach pain
- nasal congestion
- constipation
- headache
- skin rash

PREGNANCY WARNING

This drug caused harm to developing fetuses in animal studies, or such studies were not done. Use during pregnancy only for clear medical reasons. Tell your doctor if you are pregnant or thinking of becoming pregnant before you take this drug.

 Do Not Use

ALTERNATIVE TREATMENT:
See Cold, p. 402, and Allergy and Hay Fever, p. 405.

Azatadine and Pseudoephedrine
TRINALIN (Key Pharmaceuticals)

FAMILY: Cold and Allergy Drugs (see p. 402)

This combination of azatadine (a *zat* ah deen) and pseudoephedrine (soo doe e *fed* rin) is marketed as a drug to relieve congestion and other problems caused by allergies and the common cold. When taking this product you are taking two drugs, each with its own cautions, adverse effects, and drug interactions. Fixed-combinations of an antihistamine (azatadine) and a decongestant (pseudoephedrine) exemplify the "shotgun" approach to treating cold and allergy symptoms, which are better treated with individual drugs for individual symptoms.

If you want to treat congestion caused by an allergy, the best treatment is an antihistamine, whether azatadine (OPTIMINE), available by prescription, or chlorpheniramine, available as a nonprescription generic.

If you want to treat congestion caused by a cold, the best treatment is a decongestant nose spray or nose drops. There is no reason to combine an antihistamine and a decongestant in one product. For colds, the effectiveness of anticholinergics, such as azatadine, has not been established when used in combination products. In fact, fixed-combinations and long-acting forms curtail the ability to individualize doses and adjust doses in response to adverse effects.

Used separately, azatadine is an effective antihistamine, for hay fever and other allergies. If you have congestion caused by an allergy, taking azatadine or other antihistamines available without a prescription, will help. There is no satisfactory evidence that allergy patients benefit from adding a decongestant, such as pseudoephedrine to an antihistamine. Antihistamines can cause drowsiness, loss of concentration, mental inattention, and dizziness. If your congestion is caused by a cold, rather than an allergy, you can use decongestant nasal sprays or drops such as phenylephrine, oxymetazoline, or xylometazoline, all available without a prescription. Do not use decongestant nasal sprays or drops longer than three days. Any of these is a better choice than a drug like pseudoephedrine, which can have dangerous adverse effects because it is taken by mouth and affects your whole body.

ADDITIONAL PRECAUTIONS

Avoid exposure to things which trigger your allergies or asthma, such as animals, bedding, chemicals, cosmetics, drugs, dust, mold, foods, pollens or smoke. Wearing a mask reduces inhalation of drugs, pollens and smoke. Many people with mildly red, itching eyes require no treatment. Cold compresses to the eyes may prove helpful. Using eye drops with vasoconstrictors whitens eyes for a while, but rebound redness can occur. Misuse of vasoconstrictors sets up a vicious cycle.

WARNING

Pseudoephedrine can cause or worsen high blood pressure. It is especially dangerous for people who have high blood pressure, heart disease, diabetes, or thyroid disease. People over 60 are more likely than younger people to experience effects on the heart and blood pressure, restlessness, nervousness, and confusion. Do not use pseudoephedrine during or within 14 days following administration of monoamine oxidase (MAO) inhibitors.

WARNING: SPECIAL MENTAL AND PHYSICAL ADVERSE EFFECTS

Older adults are especially sensitive to the harmful anticholinergic (see Glossary, p. 768) effects of antihistamines such as azatadine. Drugs in this family should not be used unless absolutely necessary.

Mental Effects: confusion, delirium, short-term memory problems, disorientation, and impaired attention.

Physical Effects: dry mouth, constipation, difficulty urinating (especially for a man with an enlarged prostate), blurred vision, decreased sweating with increased body temperature, sexual dysfunction, and worsening of glaucoma.

 Do Not Use

ALTERNATIVE TREATMENT:
See Cold, p. 402, and Allergy and Hay Fever, p. 405.

Hydrocodone and Phenyltoloxamine
TUSSIONEX (Medeva)

FAMILY: Cough Suppressants (see p. 402)

This combination of hydrocodone (hye droe *koe* done) and phenyltoloxamine (fen ill tole *ox* a meen) is promoted as a cough suppressant. The narcotic hydrocodone is an effective cough suppressant, but there is no convincing evidence that adding the antihistamine phenyltoloxamine improves the cough-suppressing action of hydrocodone in any way. In fact, antihistamines thicken lung secretions and may actually create problems for people who produce mucus with their coughs or who have difficulty breathing.

Phenyltoloxamine can cause drowsiness, loss of coordination, mental inattention, and dizziness. Hydrocodone, which is similar to codeine, can be addictive. If you have a cough that needs to be treated with drugs (see p. 402), the best nonnarcotic treatment is generic dextromethorphan, which you can get without a prescription.

WARNING: SPECIAL MENTAL AND PHYSICAL ADVERSE EFFECTS

Older adults are especially sensitive to the harmful anticholinergic (see Glossary, p. 768) effects of antihistamines such as phenyltoloxamine. Drugs in this family should not be used unless absolutely necessary.

Mental Effects: confusion, delirium, short-term memory problems, disorientation, and impaired attention.

Physical Effects: dry mouth, constipation, difficulty urinating (especially for a man with an enlarged prostate), blurred vision, decreased sweating with increased body temperature, sexual dysfunction, and worsening of glaucoma.

Do Not Use Until Five Years After Release

Zileuton (Do Not Use Until 2003)
ZYFLO (Abbott)

GENERIC: not available

FAMILY: Asthma Drugs (see p. 408)

> You should wait at least five years from the date of release to take any new drug unless it is one of those rare "breakthrough" drugs that offers you a documented therapeutic advantage over older proven drugs. New drugs are tested in a relatively small number of people before being approved, and serious adverse effects or life-threatening drug interactions may not be detected until the new drug has been taken by hundreds of thousands of people. A number of new drugs have been withdrawn within their first five years after release. Also, serious new adverse reaction warnings have been added to the labeling of a number of drugs, or new drug interactions have been detected, usually within the first five years after a drug's release.

Zileuton (zye *loo* ton) is used to prevent and treat mild, persistent asthma. It belongs to a new family of drugs called leukotriene inhibitors, in the same family as zafirkulast. According to *The Medical Letter,* zileuton is "modestly effective."[51] Zileuton is not useful as a bronchodilator in acute asthma attacks. The usual dose for adults and children age 12 and over is 600 mg four times daily. Zileuton can damage your liver and lower your white blood cells, making you more prone to infections. Women over age 65 may be at increased risk for liver damage.[52] There is no information on human use during pregnancy or nursing. Long-term effects are yet to be determined.

ADDITIONAL PRECAUTIONS

Avoid exposure to things which trigger your allergies or asthma, such as animals, bedding, chemicals, cosmetics, drugs, dust, mold, foods, pollens or smoke. Wearing a mask reduces inhalation of drugs, pollens and smoke.

Aspirin can trigger asthma in people who are aspirin-allergic, as can beta-blockers. Infections aggravate lung problems. During epidemics of respiratory illnesses, avoid crowded places and wash your hands frequently to help prevent infection. If you have asthma, get a flu vaccination.

Note: The information in this profile addresses the care of asthma that is not serious enough to need emergency treatment.

Before You Use This Drug

Tell your doctor if you have or have had:

- allergies
- alcohol abuse
- liver problems
- pregnant or nursing

Tell your doctor about any other drugs you take, including aspirin, herbs, vitamins, and other nonprescription products.

When You Use This Drug

- Keep short-acting bronchodilators available for acute asthma attacks. Tell your doctor how frequently you use these bronchodilators.
- If you plan to have any surgery, including dental, tell your doctor that you take this drug.

How to Use This Drug

- Swallow whole tablets. Take at regular intervals with or without food.

- Take regularly, even when you do not have symptoms of asthma.
- If you miss a dose, take it as soon as you remember, but skip it if it is almost time for the next dose. **Do not take double doses.**
- Store at room temperature.

Interactions with Other Drugs

The following drugs are listed in the *Evaluations of Drug Interactions* 1997 as causing "highly clinically significant" or "clinically significant" interactions when used together with this drug. We have also included potentially serious interactions listed in the drug's FDA-approved professional product labeling or package insert. New scientific techniques have allowed researchers to predict some drug interactions before they have been documented in people. There may be other drugs, especially those in the families of drugs listed below, that also will react with this drug to cause severe adverse effects. The number of new drugs approved for marketing increases the chance of drug interactions, and new drug interactions are being identified with old drugs. Be vigilant. Make sure to tell your doctor and pharmacist the drugs you are taking and tell your doctor if you are taking any of these interacting drugs:

COUMADIN, ELIXOPHYLLIN, INDERAL, INDERAL LA, propranolol, SELDANE, SLO-BID, terfenadine, THEO-24, theophylline, warfarin.

Adverse Effects

Call your doctor immediately if you experience:

- flu-like symptoms, such as sore throat, fever
- itching
- nausea
- pain in the right upper quadrant of your abdomen
- tiredness
- yellowing of skin or eyes

Call your doctor if these symptoms continue:

- headache
- stomach upset

Periodic Tests

Ask your doctor which of these tests should be done periodically while you are taking this drug:

- liver function tests
- blood tests

Do Not Use Until Five Years After Release

Cetirizine (Do Not Use Until 2002)
ZYRTEC (Pfizer)

GENERIC: unavailable
FAMILY: Antihistamines (see p. 402)

> You should wait at least five years from the date of release to take any new drug unless it is one of those rare "breakthrough" drugs that offers you a documented therapeutic advantage over older proven drugs. New drugs are tested in a relatively small number of people before being approved, and serious adverse effects or life-threatening drug interactions may not be detected until the new drug has been taken by hundreds of thousands of people. A number of new drugs have been withdrawn within their first five years after release. Also, serious new adverse reaction warnings have been added to the labeling of a number of drugs, or new drug interactions have been detected, usually within the first five years after a drug's release.

Cetirizine (se *ti* ra zeen) is an antihistamine. Antihistamines relieve symptoms of seasonal allergies due to pollens, reduce sneezing, and tearing due to dust mites, dander, and molds, chronic hives and itching, but do not cure any condition.

Cetirizine is a mild bronchodilator. In higher doses it has been shown to be more effective than other antihistamines in reducing the symptoms of asthma induced by pollens.[53] Cetirizine is the metabolic breakdown product of the older antihistamine hydroxyzine (VISTARIL), see p. 420. Although cetirizine does not cause as much drowsiness as hydroxyzine, it may cause more drowsiness than newer "nonsedating" antihistamines. Small studies suggest cetirizine does not slow the heart, but studies on drug interactions are limited. People with kidney and liver impairment, and older adults, should take 5 mg a day. Older people are more apt to develop dry mouth, which can increase dental problems. Men are more apt to experience urinary retention. Cetirizine is not recommended in early pregnancy or during nursing.

ADDITIONAL PRECAUTIONS

Avoid exposure to things which trigger your allergies or asthma, such as animals, bedding, chemicals, cosmetics, drugs, dust, mold, foods, pollens or smoke. Wearing a mask reduces inhalation of drugs, pollens and smoke. Many people with mildly red, itching eyes require no treatment. Cold compresses to the eyes may prove helpful. Using eye drops with vasoconstrictors whitens eyes for a while, but rebound redness can occur. Misuse of vasoconstrictors sets up a vicious cycle.

Before You Use This Drug
Tell your doctor if you have or have had:

- allergies, including lactose and iodine
- glaucoma
- heart, kidney or liver problems
- pregnant or nursing
- prostate problems
- urinary retention
- asthma

Tell your doctor about any other drugs you take, including aspirin, herbs, vitamins, and other nonprescription products.

When You Use This Drug

- Do not drink alcohol or use other drugs that can cause drowsiness.
- Until you know how you react to this drug, do not drive or perform other activities that require alertness.
- Protect yourself from sunburn, using a sunscreen or wearing protective clothing.
- Use sugarless gum, ice, or saliva substitutes if dry mouth develops.
- If you plan to have any surgery, including dental, tell your doctor that you take this drug.

How to Use This Drug

- Swallow tablets whole. Take with or without food about the same time each day. If you become drowsy, take cetirizine at bedtime.
- If you miss a dose, take it as soon as you remember but skip it if it is almost time for the next dose. **Do not take double doses.**
- Store at room temperature.

Interactions with Other Drugs

The following drugs are listed in the *Evaluations of Drug Interactions* 1997 as causing "highly clinically significant" or "clinically significant" interactions when used together with this drug. We have also included potentially serious interactions listed in the drug's FDA-approved professional product labeling or package insert. New scientific techniques have allowed researchers to predict some drug interactions before they have been documented in people. There may be other drugs, especially those in the families of drugs listed below, that also will react with this drug to cause severe adverse effects. The number of new drugs approved for marketing increases the chance of drug interactions, and new drug interactions are being identified with old drugs. Be vigilant. Make sure to tell your doctor and pharmacist the drugs you are taking and tell your doctor if you are taking any of these interacting drugs:

Central nervous system (CNS) depressant drugs including alcohol, antidepressants, antihistamines, antipsychotics, some blood pressure medications (reserpine, methyldopa, beta-blockers), motion sickness medications, muscle relaxants, narcotics, sedatives, sleeping pills and tranquilizers.

Adverse Effects

Call your doctor immediately if you experience:

• **signs of overdose:** clumsiness or unsteadiness, dry mouth, nose, or throat, flushed or red face, shortness of breath, trouble breathing, seizures, hallucinations, trouble sleeping, severe drowsiness, faintness or light-headedness
• unusual bleeding or bruising
• faster or irregular heartbeat
• sore throat or fever
• unusual tiredness or weakness

Call your doctor if these symptoms continue:

• confusion
• dizziness
• drowsiness
• dry mouth, nose, or throat
• excitement (a paradoxical reaction more apt to occur in children and older people)
• headache
• ringing in ears
• upset or painful stomach
• sunburn
• thickening of mucus
• tiredness
• difficulty urinating
• changes in vision
• weight gain

NOTES FOR COLD, COUGH, ALLERGY, AND ASTHMA DRUGS

1. *The Medical Letter on Drugs and Therapeutics.* New York: The Medical Letter Inc., 1987; 29:11–6.

2. Ibid.

3. Newhouse MT, Dolovich MB. Control of asthma by aerosols. *New England Journal of Medicine* 1986; 315:870.

4. *The Medical Letter on Drugs and Therapeutics.* New York: The Medical Letter Inc., 1996; 38:111-2.

5. AMA Department of Drugs. *AMA Drug Evaluations.* 5th ed. Chicago: American Medical Association, 1983:1478.

6. Dukes MNG, ed. *Side Effects of Drugs Annual* 10. New York: Elsevier 1986:11.

7. *USP DI, Drug Information for the Health Care Provider.* 7th ed. Rockville MD.: The United States Pharmacopeial Convention Inc., 1987:1552.

8. Grasela TH, Dreis MW. An evaluation of the quinolone-theophylline interaction using the Food and Drug Administration Spontaneous Reporting System. *Archives of Internal Medicine* 1992; 152:617-21.

9. Dukes MNG, Beeley L, eds. *Side Effects of Drugs Annual* 15, Amsterdam: Elsevier, 1991:137.

10. Randall T. International consensus report urges sweeping reform in asthma treatment. *Journal of the American Medical Association* 1992; 267:2153-4.

11. Pras E, Stienlauf S, Pinkhas J, Sidi Y. Urinary retention associated with ipratropium bromide. DICP, *The Annals of Pharmacology* 1991; 25:939-40.

12. AMA Department of Drugs. *AMA Drug Evaluations Annual* 1992. Chicago: American Medical Association, 1992:489.

13. Humphreys DM. Acute angle closure glaucoma associated with nebulised ipratropium bromide and salbutamol (letter). *British Medical Journal* 1992; 304:320.

14. Shah P, Dhurjon L, Metcalfe T, Gibson JM. Acute angle closure glaucoma associated with nebulised ipratropium bromide and salbutamol. *British Medical Journal* 1992; 304:40-1.

15. Weinberg H. Asthma in primary care patients. Challenges and controversies. *Postgraduate Medicine* 1990; 88:107-10, 113-4.

16. Kastrup EK, ed. *Facts and Comparisons.* St. Louis: J.B. Lippincott Co., January 1986:173a.

17. AMA, 1983, op. cit., p. 580.

18. *USP DI,* op. cit.

19. Grasela, op. cit.

20. Kastrup EK, ed. *Facts and Comparisons.* St. Louis: J.B. Lippincott Co., July 1987:178e-179b.

21. *USP DI,* op. cit.

22. Orgel HA, Meltzer EO, Kemp JP, Ostrom NK, Welch MJ. Comparison of intranasal cromolyn sodium, 4%, and oral terfenadine for allergic rhinitis: symptoms, nasal cytology, nasal ciliary clearance, and rhinomanometry. *Annals of Allergy* 1991; 66:237–44.

23. Randall, op. cit.

24. Friedlaender MH. Current concepts in ocular allergy. *Annals of Allergy* 1991; 67:5-10.

25. Kalpaxis JG, Thayer TO. Double-blind trial of penigetide ophthalmic solution, 0.5%, compared with cromolyn sodium, 4%, ophthalmic solution for allergic conjunctivitis. *Annals of Allergy* 1991; 66:393-8.

26. Weinberg, op. cit.

27. AMA Department of Drugs. *AMA Drug Evaluations Annual* 1991. Chicago: American Medical Association, 1991:455-6.

28. Gilman AG, Rall TW, Nies AS, Taylor P, eds. *The Pharmacological Basis of Therapeutics.* 8th ed. New York: Pergamon Press, 1990:630-2.

29. Hoag JE, McFadden ER. Long-term effect of cromolyn sodium on nonspecific bronchial hyperresponsiveness: a review. *Annals of Allergy* 1991; 66:53-63.

30. Schuller DE, Selcow JE, Joos TH, Hannaway PJ, Hirsch SR, Schwartz HJ, et al. A multicenter trial of nedocromil sodium, 1% nasal solution, compared with cromolyn sodium and placebo in ragweed seasonal allergic rhinitis. *Journal of Allergy and Clinical Immunology* 1990; 85:554-61.

31. Weinberg, op. cit.

32. O'Connell EJ, Rojas AR, Sachs MI. Cough-type asthma: a review. *Annals of Allergy* 1991; 66:278-85.

33. Ibid.

34. Weinberg, op. cit.

35. AMA, 1991, op. cit.

36. Gilman, op. cit.

37. Emm T, Metcalf JE, Lesko LJ, Chai MF. Update on the physical-chemical compatibility of cromolyn sodium nebulizer solution: bronchodilator inhalant solution admixtures. *Annals of Allergy* 1991; 66:185-9.

38. Food and Drug Administration Talk Paper. Important New Safety Information About Hismanal, February 9, 1998.

39. Dear Doctor Letter from Mark A. Klausner, MD, Vice President, Medical Affairs, Janssen Pharmaceutica, dated February 1998.

40. Gilman, op. cit.

41. Olin BR, ed. *Facts and Comparisons.* St. Louis: J.B. Lippincott Co., September 1992:173b.

42. Neilly JB, Carter R, Tweddel A, Martin W, Hutton I, Banham SW, et al. Long term haemodynamic, pulmonary function and symptomatic effects of pirbuterol in COPD. *Respiratory Medicine* 1989; 83:59-65.

43. Windom H, Grainger J, Burgess C, Crane J, Pearce N, Beasley R. A comparison of the haemodynamic and hypokalaemic effects of inhaled pirbuterol and salbutamol. *New Zealand Medical Journal* 1990; 103:259-61.

44. Randall, op. cit.

45. Gilman, op. cit.

46. *The Medical Letter on Drugs and Therapeutics.* New York: The Medical Letter Inc., 1982; 24:84.

47. *Physicians' Desk Reference.* 41st ed. Oradell, NJ: Medical Economics Company, 1987;1948.

48. *USP DI,* op. cit.

49. Food and Drug Administration Talk Paper. Seldane and Generic Terfenadine Withdrawn From the Market. February 27, 1998.

50. Dear Health Professional Letter from Hoechst Marion Roussel, dated September 1997.

51. *The Medical Letter on Drugs and Therapeutics.* New York: The Medical Letter Inc., 1997; 39:18–9.

52. AHFS Drug Information 97 & Current Developments, American System of Health Care Pharmacists, Bethesda, MD, 1997:22-4.

53. Woosley RL. Cardiac actions of antihistamines. *Annual Reviews in Pharmacology and Toxicology* 1996; 36:233–52.

Drugs for Infections

Antibiotics	**468**
Penicillins and Cephalosporins	**470**
Fluoroquinolones	**472**
Tetracyclines	**474**

DRUG LISTINGS

ANTIBIOTICS

ACHROMYCIN	Limited Use	475
amoxicillin		476
amoxicillin and clavulanate		476
AMOXIL		476
ampicillin		522
atropine, hyoscyamine, methenamine, methylene blue, phenyl salicylate, and benzoic acid	⊘ Do Not Use	538
AUGMENTIN		476
azithromycin	Limited Use	543
BACTRIM		478
BACTROBAN	Limited Use	480
BIAXIN	Limited Use	481
CECLOR		482
cefaclor		482
cefadroxil		496
cefixime	Limited Use	534
cefprozil	Limited Use	484
CEFTIN	Limited Use	484
cefuroxime axetil	Limited Use	484
CEFZIL	Limited Use	484
cephalexin		510
cephradine		486
CHIBROXIN (eye drops)	Limited Use	519
chloramphenicol	⊘ Do Not Use Except in the Hospital	488
CHLOROMYCETIN	⊘ Do Not Use Except in the Hospital	488
CILOXAN EYE DROPS	Limited Use	489
CIPRO	Limited Use	489
ciprofloxacin	Limited Use	489
clarithromycin	Limited Use	481
CLEOCIN	Limited Use	491
clindamycin	Limited Use	491
cloxacillin		493
CORTISPORIN EAR DROPS (otic)	⊘ Do Not Use	494
COTRIM		478
dicloxacillin		493
doxycycline		541
DURICEF		496
DYCILL		493
DYNAPEN		493
EES		498
enoxacin	Limited Use	523
ERYTHROCIN		498
erythromycin		498
erythromycin estolate	⊘ Do Not Use	507
FLAGYL	Limited Use	500
FLOXIN	Limited Use	502
FURADANTIN	⊘ Do Not Use	513
GANTRISIN		505
grepafloxacin	⊘ Do Not Use	523
ILOSONE	⊘ Do Not Use	507
KEFLEX		510
LEVAQUIN	⊘ Do Not Use Except for Community-Acquired Bacterial Pneumonia	523

levofloxacin	Ⓧ Do Not Use Except for Community-Acquired Bacterial Pneumonia	523
LINCOCIN	Ⓧ Do Not Use	513
lincomycin	Ⓧ Do Not Use	513
lomefloxacin	Limited Use	523
LORABID	Limited Use	484
loracarbef	Limited Use	484
MACROBID	Ⓧ Do Not Use	513
MACRODANTIN	Ⓧ Do Not Use	513
MAXAQUIN	Limited Use	523
metronidazole	Limited Use	500
mupirocin	Limited Use	480
MYCITRACIN	Ⓧ Do Not Use	518
neomycin, polymyxin B and bacitracin	Ⓧ Do Not Use	518
neomycin, polymyxin B and hydrocortisone	Ⓧ Do Not Use	494
NEOSPORIN MAXIMUM STRENGTH OINTMENT	Ⓧ Do Not Use	518
nitrofurantoin	Ⓧ Do Not Use	513
norfloxacin	Limited Use	519
NOROXIN (tablets)	Limited Use	519
OCUFLOX EYE DROPS	Limited Use	502
ofloxacin	Limited Use	502
OMNIPEN		522
PANMYCIN	Limited Use	475
PENETREX	Limited Use	523
penicillin G		527
penicillin V		527
PEN VEE K		527
POLYCILLIN		522
PROLOPRIM		528
RAXAR	Ⓧ Do Not Use	523
SEPTRA		478
SILVADENE		532
silver sulfadiazine		532
sparfloxacin	Ⓧ Do Not Use	523
sulfisoxazole		505
SUPRAX	Limited Use	534
tetracycline	Limited Use	475

TORVAN	Do Not Use Until Five Years After Release	523
trimethoprim		528
trimethoprim and sulfamethoxazole		478
TRIMPEX		528
trovafloxacin	Do Not Use Until Five Years After Release	523
URISED	Ⓧ Do Not Use	538
VIBRAMYCIN		541
ZAGAM	Ⓧ Do Not Use	523
ZITHROMAX	Limited Use	543

For eye antibiotics, *see p. 621.*

ANTI-TUBERCULOSIS DRUGS

INH	507
isoniazid	507
RIFADIN	530
rifampin	530
RIMACTANE	530

ANTIFUNGAL DRUGS

clotrimazole		515
DIFLUCAN		495
fluconazole		495
GYNE-LOTRIMIN		515
itraconazole	Ⓧ Do Not Use Except for Serious Fungal Infection	533
LAMISIL	Ⓧ Do Not Use Except for Serious Fungal Infection	533
LOTRIMIN		515
miconazole		513
MONISTAT 7		513
MONISTAT-DERM		513
MYCELEX		515
MYCOBIOTIC II	Ⓧ Do Not Use	516
MYCOLOG II	Ⓧ Do Not Use	516
MYCOSTATIN		517
nystatin		517

nystatin and triamcinolone	Ⓧ Do Not Use	516
SPORANOX	Ⓧ Do Not Use Except for Serious Fungal Infection	533
TERAZOL 3 (cream or suppositories)	Ⓧ Do Not Use	537
TERAZOL 7 (cream)	Ⓧ Do Not Use	537
terbinafine	Ⓧ Do Not Use Except for Serious Fungal Infection	533
terconazole	Ⓧ Do Not Use	537

ANTIVIRAL DRUGS

acyclovir	544
amantadine	536
SYMMETREL	536
ZOVIRAX	544

ANTIPARASITE DRUGS

KWELL	Ⓧ Do Not Use	512
lindane	Ⓧ Do Not Use	512
mebendazole	539
VERMOX	539

ANTIBIOTICS

Antibiotics (drugs used to treat bacterial infections) are overwhelmingly misprescribed in the United States. After congressional hearings and numerous academic studies on this issue, it has become the general consensus that 40 to 60% of all antibiotics in this country are misprescribed. New studies continue to confirm the fact that a large proportion of antibiotic prescribing for both children and adults continues to be inappropriate.[1,2] To put it simply, most antibiotics are prescribed in situations in which the infection cannot be treated by *any* antibiotic, or another, more effective and appropriate antibiotic should be used instead. This should be a major concern, since the misprescribing of antibiotics poses some real dangers to the population at large, as well as to the individuals taking them, especially older adults.

Problems from Misuse of Antibiotics

The problems resulting from misuse are adverse effects from the drugs, exposure to additional complications from ineffective treatment of an infection, and bacterial resistance to antibiotics. In addition, misprescribing is a waste of money.

Adverse Effects

Although the numbers of adverse effects and problems with antibiotics are often low compared with other drugs, there are still some serious adverse effects that can occur. For example, an allergic reaction to penicillin can cause death, although this is uncommon. Use of antibiotics taken by mouth can cause stomach irritation and diarrhea, which can progress to a more severe condition caused by intestinal bacteria that are difficult to kill.

Other antibiotics can cause problems with the liver and kidneys, which is a real concern when prescribing for older adults. The best way to avoid these adverse effects is not to use antibiotics unless they are indicated and to avoid especially dangerous ones whenever possible. This is not the current practice, however.

Chloramphenicol (see p. 488), for example, is one antibiotic that has a particular danger. In rare instances, this drug can cause irreversible bone marrow depression, which can be fatal. In 1983, 49% of all prescriptions of chloramphenicol were for conditions in which the drug was clearly not indicated, such as tonsillitis and infection prevention after surgery. This meant that half the prescriptions for chloramphenicol unnecessarily exposed people to a serious danger.

Exposure to Additional Complications

Antibiotics are often misused to treat the common cold or flu. In 1983, more than 51%

of the more than 3 million patients who saw doctors for treatment of the common cold were given an unnecessary prescription for an antibiotic.[3] Since both the cold and the flu are caused by viruses, there is absolutely no possible way antibiotics can help cure these diseases or speed up the natural cure. They can, however, make a person more susceptible to a dangerous bacterial superinfection, such as a pneumonia, which could be resistant to the antibiotic the person is taking. Patients should not insist that their doctors prescribe antibiotics for trivial conditions such as colds.

Germs that are not killed by the antibiotics can cause an infection, such as candidiasis, a fungal infection. Oral candidiasis is fairly common in older adults who wear dentures. A sore mouth or tongue or soreness of the vagina are possible symptoms.

Bacterial Resistance

This is becoming an ever-expanding problem. After antibiotics are used for a period of time, certain bacteria develop methods that enable them to become resistant to some antibiotics. The resistant bacteria are the ones that survive after antibiotic treatment, and after time they become the dominant force via a process of natural selection. For example, the staphylococcus, a common bacterium causing skin infections, used to be exquisitely sensitive to penicillin when the drug was first introduced. Twenty years later, penicillin was no longer anywhere near as effective against the staphylococcus. A new drug, called methicillin, was designed to combat the "staph bug," and it was widely used. Over time, strains of methicillin-resistant "super-staph" have also emerged. This illustrates that newer, improved antibiotics are not the final answer to bacterial resistance. If new antibiotics are developed but then overused, bacteria will find new ways to develop resistance, rendering those drugs ineffective.

Many bacteria in the hospital setting have now become resistant to multiple antibiotics,

and, as a result, infections with these bacteria have become a very dangerous occurrence. The only way to help stop the development of bacterial resistance is by discouraging the gross misuse and overuse of antibiotics. It makes sense to use these "magic bullets," especially the newer ones, only when necessary so that their power will still be effective when it is truly needed.

Thus, there are both dangers and benefits to antibiotics. When you have an infection that can be cured with the proper antibiotic, the benefit of taking the drug is much, much greater than its dangers. But since there are dangers, there are compelling reasons to avoid unnecessary use of antibiotics and to select the safest and most effective ones.

Avoiding Unnecessary Use of Antibiotics

There are several basic principles that should be followed in determining the correct antibiotic:

1. Establish that an antibiotic is necessary. This means that your infection has to be the type that can be effectively treated by an antibiotic. Antibiotics are used to specifically treat bacterial infections. Antibiotics do *not* treat viral infections, such as the common cold. (Although there has been some heartening progress in the development of specific antiviral agents such as amantadine and acyclovir, ribavirin, AZT and other drugs for HIV infections, viral infections, for the most part, cannot be treated with drugs.)

2. Choose the correct antibiotic. It must be effective against the most likely organisms that can cause your infection. In our drug pages on individual antibiotics, we state the types of infections for which each antibiotic is best suited.

3. Take a culture before using an antibiotic. A culture should be taken from where you have an infection, such as your throat, urine, or blood, and then grown to determine the specific organism that is causing your infection and whether it is susceptible to the preferred antibiotic. For example, if you have a urinary tract infection, the doctor should take a urine specimen and send it for culture before treating your infection. This does not mean that your infection cannot be treated right away, only that a culture is sent before you start antibiotics. In this way, if your infection persists, your doctor can determine which alternative antibiotic can be used against the bacteria. Your doctor may find out that you do not have an infection and do not require antibiotics.

4. Consider the cost of the antibiotic. This should be done when everything else is equal. If several antibiotics are equally effective, their cost should be taken into consideration when selecting a drug to use. Newer drugs on patent are much more expensive than older antibiotics that have been on the market for some time. For example, the oral cephalosporin cefuroxime (CEFTIN) is often used to treat urinary tract infections. There is no advantage between using this drug and using a generic drug such as trimethoprim and sulfamethoxazole. Cefuroxime, however, costs 12 times as much for two weeks of treatment.[4] Clearly, in the case of a simple infection, the less expensive drug is preferred as an initial choice.

The Importance of Completing a Full Course of Therapy

It is important with any antibiotic to take the entire amount of the drug that your doctor prescribes. Often, after the first few days of taking antibiotics, you will begin to feel better. Perhaps you think that you do not have to finish your course of treatment, since you are, after all, feeling healthy. This is not the case, however. The length of the regimen that your doctor prescribes for you is designed to eliminate *all* of the bacteria that are causing

your illness. If you do not take all of your medication, the bacteria will not be completely eliminated and can quickly multiply, causing another infection. This infection may then be resistant to the original antibiotic.

In general, antibiotics taken by mouth are preferred if you do not require hospitalization and can take the pills without any problem. There is no advantage to having an injection of an antibiotic.

Newer Versus Older Antibiotics

Remember, newer antibiotics are more expensive than the older ones. They should be used only when an advantage can be shown over older antibiotics—for example, if the new antibiotic is more active against resistant bacteria.

In summary, antibiotics can make a world of difference when the right antibiotic is chosen for the right situation. Unfortunately, in the United States today, this is only being done a minority of the time. Questioning your doctor about why he or she is prescribing an antibiotic is a step in the right direction toward safer and better antibiotic use.

PENICILLINS AND CEPHALOSPORINS

Penicillins are a group of antibiotics used to kill bacteria or prevent infections. They are probably the least toxic of all the antibiotics. The penicillins are some of the most commonly prescribed antibiotics and are often the drugs of choice for people who are not allergic to them.

Cephalosporins are relatives of the penicillins and have a similar, if slightly expanded, range of action. They have a good safety record,[5] but certain problems can occur with their use. Diarrhea is the most common adverse effect, and it may become so bad that treatment must be stopped.

Following is a list of the penicillins and cephalosporins that are discussed in this book. It does not identify the ones that are given mainly as injections or intravenously, most of which are used primarily in the hospital.

Penicillins (oral)
    Amoxicillin/AMOXIL
    Amoxicillin and Clavulanate/AUGMENTIN
    Ampicillin/OMNIPEN, POLYCILLIN
    Cloxacillin
    Dicloxacillin/DYCILL, DYNAPEN
    Penicillin G
    Penicillin V/PEN VEE K

Cephalosporins (oral)
    Cefaclor/CECLOR
    Cefadroxil/DURICEF
    Cefixime/SUPRAX
    Cefprozil/CEFZIL
    Cefuroxime/CEFTIN
    Cephalexin/KEFLEX
    Cephradine
    Loracarbef/LORABID

Types of Allergic Reactions

Allergic reactions are the most common adverse effects observed with penicillins. Between 5 and 10% of the general public are allergic to them. If you are allergic to penicillins you should carry a card or wear an ID bracelet stating that you are allergic. Make sure to tell your doctor if you think you have an allergy to penicillins so that the information will be recorded.

There are three kinds of allergic reactions to penicillins: immediate, accelerated, and delayed.

Immediate reactions, also known as anaphylaxis, usually happen within 20 minutes of receiving the drug. Symptoms range from skin rash and itching to swelling, difficulty breathing, and even death. Immediate anaphylactic reactions are very rare, occurring in less than 1% of the people who are allergic to penicillins.[6]

Accelerated reactions usually happen between 20 minutes and two days after taking penicillins. Itching, rash, and fever are some of the symptoms.

Delayed reactions usually happen at least two days to one month after taking penicillins. Symptoms can include fever, feeling sick or uncomfortable, skin rash, muscle or joint pain, or pain in the abdomen.

Similar allergies can occur in people who take cephalosporins since the drugs are related to penicillins. If you experience any of the above symptoms, call your doctor immediately. Although penicillin and cephalosporin allergies are more common in people who have had such a reaction previously, they also can occur in people who have repeatedly taken penicillins without prior incident.

Some people who are allergic to a penicillin may also be allergic to a cephalosporin; this occurs about 5% of the time. Cephalosporins should *not* be used for people who have had immediate reactions to penicillins. People who have had delayed reactions, such as a rash, should discuss with their doctors whether they should take a cephalosporin.

In older adults, caution must be used with high doses of penicillins and cephalosporins to prevent damage to the nervous system resulting in seizures, drowsiness, and confusion.[7] The dose of most penicillins and cephalosporins must be reduced when the kidneys do not function normally in order to prevent other complications. For example, a normal dose of 20 million units of penicillin G potassium injection in someone with kidney problems could lead to a severe or even fatal increase of potassium (hyperkalemia). Older adults and people with decreased kidney function are more likely to have damage to the kidney when a cephalosporin and an aminoglycoside antibiotic (gentamicin, tobramycin, and neomycin, for example) are used at the same time.

Almost any antibiotic can cause antibiotic-associated colitis (inflammation of the colon). Clindamycin, lincomycin and ampicillin are thought to cause this disease most frequently. Other penicillins and cephalosporins are implicated less often but this reaction is still common. Risk of this disease seems to increase with the age of the user.

Dosage Forms, Effects, and Uses

Oral forms of cefaclor, a cephalosporin, and most penicillins should be taken on an empty stomach (one hour before or two hours after meals) with a full glass (eight ounces) of water. Most other cephalosporins and amoxicillin can be taken on a full stomach. Try to take your doses at evenly spaced times during the day and night so that the amount of drug in your body will stay constant. Store liquid forms in the refrigerator, but do not allow them to freeze. Capsules may be opened to facilitate swallowing. Oral penicillins and cephalosporins may cause nausea, vomiting, or diarrhea.

Injectable forms of penicillins and cephalosporins can cause pain and swelling at the site of injection. Diabetics may not absorb these drugs well when they are given in the muscle. Tell your doctor if you are on a salt restricted (sodium) diet because injected penicillins and cephalosporins contain sodium. People who have congestive heart failure may have a hard time getting rid of extra sodium.[8]

People who are elderly, have poor nutrition, or are alcoholic may have a greater risk of developing bleeding problems (blood takes longer to clot, for example) that are associated with some of the cephalosporins.[9] Vitamin K supplements, as pills or injections, may prevent this complication.

Cephalosporins are often used to prevent infections caused by surgery. In most operations where an artificial part is used, such as open heart surgery, and in gynecologic and gastrointestinal surgery, the use of cephalosporins before surgery is generally justified.[10] For many operations, an older cephalosporin, such as cephalexin (KEFLEX) is preferred. An exception to this is pelvic and gastrointestinal surgery, for which cefoxitin (MEFOXIN) may be a better choice.[11]

Loracarbef is another expensive alternative for treatment of respiratory, urinary tract, and skin infections. For acute pharyngitis, penicillin remains the drug of choice. For skin or soft tissue infections, there is no reason to use loracarbef rather than dicloxacillin, cephalexin, or cephradine.[12] Cefprozil may be used as an alternative to cefaclor and cefuroxime axetil for treatment of otitis media or bronchitis. The same can be said for cefprozil as for loracarbef. For acute pharyngitis and skin infections, there is no reason to use cefprozil rather than dicloxacillin, cephalexin or cephradine.[13]

Cephalosporins are widely overused in the United States. They are not the first-choice drugs to treat most infections. Usually when a cephalosporin is chosen to treat an infection, an equally effective and less expensive antibiotic is available. The newer cephalosporins are relatively expensive, but some of them have become the drugs of choice for some serious infections.[14]

FLUOROQUINOLONES

The following list of fluoroquinolones are discussed in this book:

Ciprofloxacin/CIPRO, CILOXAN
Enoxacin/PENETREX
Grepafloxacin/RAXAR
Levofloxacin/LEVAQUIN
Lomefloxacin/MAXAQUIN
Norfloxacin/NOROXIN, CHIBROXIN
Ofloxacin/FLOXIN, OCUFLOX
Sparfloxacin/ZAGAM
Trovafloxacin/TORVAN

One of the biggest selling and most overprescribed new classes of drugs in the United States is the family called fluoroquinolones. One clue that a drug your doctor wants to give you is in this class is the fact that the generic names of all such drugs approved in the United States include the sequence *floxacin*. These drugs have been alternatives for individuals allergic to, or with infections resistant to, other antibiotics. Fluoroquinolones are commonly misprescribed for colds, sore throats or community-acquired (as opposed to hospital-acquired) pneumonia. No antibiotic should be prescribed for the common cold, and penicillin or—if allergic—erythromycin is the drug of choice for a strep throat. In the past no fluoroquinolone has been the drug of choice for treatment of bronchitis or pneumonia that could be caused by pneumococcal bacteria, the most common cause of community-acquired pneumonia. Unfortunately, due to the inappropriate overuse of older, safer, and less expensive antibiotics and depending on the resistance of the pneumococcal bacteria in the area in which you live, your physician may be forced to prescribe one of the newer fluoroquinolones if you have community acquired pneumonia.

With very few exceptions, fluoroquinolones are not the drug of choice for other infections. A seven-day course of treatment with one of the fluoroquinolone drugs can be 7 to 21 times more expensive than equally effective (for most infections) treatment with other drugs, for example generic ampicillin or trimethoprim/sulfamethoxazole (the generic version of BACTRIM/SEPTRA). Both resistance and allergy to one drug in this family usually cross to the rest of the fluoroquinolones and sometimes even occur during therapy.[15,16] Overgrowth of normal bacteria may cause yeast infections, especially when antibiotics are used for long periods. The fluoroquinolones can cause central nervous system problems and psychosis.[17] Severe, even fatal, allergic reactions have happened after just one dose. Collapse of the circulatory system has occurred. As a group, the fluoroquinolones are expensive, resistance is increasing, and many effective alternatives are available.[18]

WARNING

In mid-1992, only a few months after it was initially approved for release in the U.S., Abbott's Omniflox, generic name temafloxacin, was pulled off the market worldwide because of an unacceptably high number of cases of serious anemia, kidney failure and life-threatening anaphylactic (allergic) shock resulting in a number of deaths.

WARNING

INCREASED RISK OF TENDINITIS AND TENDON RUPTURE WITH ALL FLUOROQUINOLONE ANTIBIOTICS

Public Citizen's Health Research Group petitioned the Food and Drug Administration (FDA) to add a warning for doctors to the labeling, or package, for all fluoroquinolone antibiotics about the risk of tendinitis, including the possibility of complete tendon rupture.

This adverse reaction most frequently involves the Achilles tendon, the tendon that runs from the back of the heel to the calf. Rupture of the Achilles tendon may require surgical repair. Tendons in the rotator cuff (the shoulder), the hand, the biceps, and the thumb have also been involved. This reaction appears to be more common in those taking steroid drugs, in older patients, and in kidney transplant recipients but cases have occurred in people without any of these risk factors. The onset of symptoms is sudden and has occurred as soon as 24 hours after starting treatment with a fluoroquinolone. Most people have recovered completely after one to two months.

If you experience unexpected tendon pain while taking a fluoroquinolone antibiotic, stop the drug immediately, call your doctor, and rest.

TETRACYCLINES

Tetracyclines are rarely the antibiotics of choice to treat bacterial infections that are common in older adults. In general, tetracyclines are used to treat such infections as urethritis (inflammation of the urinary tract), prostate infections, pelvic inflammatory disease, acne, Rocky Mountain spotted fever, acute bronchitis in people with chronic lung disease, "walking" pneumonia and other miscellaneous infections.[19]

Considerations When Prescribing for Older Adults

Since a decrease in kidney function is one of the normal changes associated with the aging process, tetracyclines must be used with this in mind. With the exception of doxycycline, these drugs should *not* be used for someone with impaired kidney function, as they can damage the kidneys further. Tetracyclines also can cause liver damage. This is more likely to happen when they are injected into the blood (intravenously) in people who already have liver or kidney impairment.[20]

Dosage Forms, Uses, and Effects

The oral forms—tablet, capsule, suspension—should be taken **with a full glass (eight ounces) of water.** The last dose of the day should be taken at least an hour before bedtime.[21] **Esophageal ulcers (irritation of the esophagus, the tube leading from the throat to the stomach) have occurred in people who have taken doxycycline at bedtime with insufficient water to wash it down.** Liquid forms should be shaken well before use. Do not freeze them. Try to take your doses at evenly spaced times during the day and night so that the amount of drug in your body will stay constant. If you miss a dose, take it as soon as possible. If it is almost time for the next dose and you are supposed to take your medicine:

- *once a day:* space missed dose and next dose about 12 hours apart.
- *twice a day:* space missed dose and next dose about six hours apart.
- *three or more times a day:* space missed dose and next dose about three hours apart or double the next dose.
- Then go back to your regular schedule.

The injected forms should only be used when the oral forms are not adequate or not tolerated as they are very painful. The intravenous forms should be used only when the oral forms are not appropriate, as severe vein inflammation or clotting commonly occurs.[22]

Tetracyclines applied externally as ointments or creams are of little value except for treatment of some eye infections and possibly some skin conditions. Two types of eye (ophthalmic) preparations are available—ointment and drops. (See p. 622 for directions on applying eye preparations.)

Sometimes when tetracyclines are used, microbes that are not killed by these drugs cause infection. An example is candidiasis, a fungal infection. (Some of its symptoms are sore mouth and tongue and itching in the genital or rectal area.) Candidiasis in the mouth is fairly common in older adults who wear dentures.

Tell your doctor that you take a tetracycline before you have any tests done. These drugs may interfere with your urine test results. Talk to your doctor before you change your diet or any medication.

DRUG PROFILES

Limited Use

Tetracycline
ACHROMYCIN (Lederle)
PANMYCIN (Pharmacia & Upjohn)

GENERIC: available
FAMILY: Antibiotics (see p. 468)
          Tetracyclines (see p. 474)

WARNING

The use of tetracyclines during tooth development (last half of pregnancy, infancy, and childhood to the age of eight years) may cause permanent discoloration (yellow-gray-brown) of the teeth.

Tetracycline (te tra *sye* kleen) is used to treat chronic (long-term) infections of the prostate gland, urinary tract infections, pelvic inflammatory disease, and acute bronchitis (in people with chronic lung disease). **Tetracycline will not help a cold or the flu.**

Tetracycline is sometimes used to treat bacterial infections that are common in older adults, but it is rarely the best antibiotic for this purpose.[23] Penicillin (see p. 527) would be a better choice. **Also, tetracycline can worsen existing kidney damage, so you should not take it if you have significant kidney impairment.** If you have kidney damage and you do need to take a drug in this family (tetracyclines), doxycycline (see p. 541) is preferred.[24]

Practice measures to prevent urinary tract infections. Drink plenty of fluids, especially water. While cranberry juice is unreliable as a cure for urinary tract infections, the juice may reduce odor from incontinence.[25] Practice meticulous hygiene. After using the toilet, wipe backwards, not forwards, then wash your hands. Prepare and store foods properly, especially when traveling, to prevent diarrhea. Restrict caffeine, which widens the urethra. Indwelling catheters invite urinary tract infections. However, unless there are symptoms of urinary infection, it is not always necessary to take medication just because bacteria are found in a urine test.[26] Women are particularly prone to repeated urinary tract infections. If urinary tract symptoms occur often, ask your doctor about keeping a supply of medication on hand. Ideally, the antibiotic you use should be the most effective, least toxic, and least costly.[27,28]

People with liver disease may need to take less than the usual adult dose of tetracycline.

Before You Use This Drug

Tell your doctor if you have or have had:

- allergies to drugs
- an unusual reaction to tetracycline or another drug in its family, such as doxycycline
- kidney or liver problems
- diabetes insipidus

Tell your doctor about any other drugs you take, including aspirin, herbs, vitamins, and other nonprescription products.

When You Use This Drug

- Stay out of the sun as much as possible, and call your doctor if you get a rash, hives, or any other skin reaction. Tetracycline makes you more sensitive to the sun.
- Do not eat or drink milk or other dairy products, and do not take antacids or iron, vitamin, or mineral supplements for a few hours before and after you take each dose of tetracycline. These substances can keep your body from absorbing the drug, which makes it less effective.

• Call your doctor if your symptoms do not improve in two or three days or if you get diarrhea. Do not treat the diarrhea yourself.

• **Take all the tetracycline your doctor prescribed, even if you feel better before you run out. If you stop too soon, your symptoms could come back.**

• Do not give the drug to anyone else. Throw away outdated drugs.

• If you plan to have any surgery, including dental, tell your doctor that you take this drug.

How to Use This Drug

• Take on an empty stomach (at least one hour before or two hours after a meal) with **a full glass (eight ounces) of water.** Take your last dose of the day at least an hour before bedtime.

• Keep the container closed tightly and in a dry place. Do not store in the bathroom. Do not expose to heat, moisture, or strong light. **Do not use if the appearance or taste has changed.**

• Take tetracycline at least two hours apart from any other drug you are taking.

• If you miss a dose, take it as soon as you remember, but skip it if it is almost time for your next dose. **Do not take double doses unless you are taking it three or more times a day.**

Interactions with Other Drugs

The following drugs are listed in the *Evaluations of Drug Interactions* 1997 as causing "highly clinically significant" or "clinically significant" interactions when used together with this drug. We have also included potentially serious interactions listed in the drug's FDA-approved professional product labeling or package insert. New scientific techniques have allowed researchers to predict some drug interactions before they have been documented in people. There may be other drugs, especially those in the families of drugs listed below, that also will react with this drug to cause severe adverse effects. The number of new drugs approved for marketing increases the chance of drug interactions, and new drug interactions are being identified with old drugs. Be vigilant. Make sure to tell your doctor and pharmacist the drugs you are taking and tell your doctor if you are taking any of these interacting drugs:

aluminum hydroxide, AMPHOJEL, digoxin, ether, FEOSOL, ferrous sulfate, insulin, HUMALOG, HUMULIN, LANOXICAPS, LANOXIN, lithium, LITHOBID, LITHONATE, methoxyflurane, oral contraceptives, penicillin G, PENTHRANE, SLOW FE.

Adverse Effects

Call your doctor immediately if you experience:
• abdominal pain
• change in soft spot on the head (infants)
• changes in vision
• yellowing skin
• headache
• loss of appetite
• skin rash, increased sensitivity of skin to sun (increased sunburn)
• nausea or vomiting

Call your doctor if these symptoms continue:
• stomach cramps or burning sensation in the stomach
• diarrhea
• sore or discolored mouth or tongue
• itching in the genital or rectal area
• dizziness or clumsiness

––––––––––

Amoxicillin
AMOXIL (SmithKline Beecham)

Amoxicillin and Clavulanate
AUGMENTIN (SmithKline Beecham)

GENERIC: available for Amoxicillin
not available for Amoxicillin and Clavulanate

FAMILY: Antibiotics (see p. 468)
Penicillins (see p. 470)

Amoxicillin (a mox i *sill* in) is used to treat certain infections caused by bacteria, such as ear, sinus, and bladder infections. It is also prescribed for bronchitis in people with chronic lung disease and for gonorrhea. A second drug, clavulanate, is sometimes combined with amoxicillin. It helps amoxicillin work better by preventing bacteria from resisting the drug. **Amoxicillin will not help a cold or the flu.**

If you have kidney disease, you may need to take less than the usual adult dose of amoxicillin. In rare instances older people may develop hepatitis if taking the combination of amoxicillin and clavulanate. This is reversible but the hepatitis often does not occur until after the drug is stopped.[29,30]

Before You Use This Drug

Tell your doctor if you have or have had:

- allergics to drugs
- a reaction to any penicillin or cephalosporin (see p. 471 for examples)
- other allergies
- stomach or intestinal disease
- kidney disease
- liver disease *(for amoxicillin and clavulanate)*
- infectious mononucleosis
- a salt (sodium)-restricted diet (the injected form of amoxicillin contains sodium)

Tell your doctor about any other drugs you take, including aspirin, herbs, vitamins, and other nonprescription products.

When You Use This Drug

- Call your doctor if your symptoms do not improve in two or three days or if you get diarrhea. Do not treat the diarrhea yourself.
- **Take all the amoxicillin your doctor prescribed, even if you feel better before you run out. If you stop too soon, your symptoms could come back.**

- Do not give this drug to anyone else. Throw away outdated drugs.
- If you plan to have any surgery, including dental, tell your doctor that you take this drug.

How to Use This Drug

- Taking amoxicillin with food may help prevent stomach upset. Capsules may be opened and mixed with water or food.
- Store liquid form in the refrigerator but do not freeze. Shake well before using.
- Do not store capsules in the bathroom. Do not expose to heat, moisture, or strong light.
- If you miss a dose, take it as soon as you remember, but skip it if it is almost time for the next dose. **Do not take double doses.**

Interactions with Other Drugs

The following drugs are listed in the *Evaluations of Drug Interactions* 1997 as causing "highly clinically significant" or "clinically significant" interactions when used together with this drug. We have also included potentially serious interactions listed in the drug's FDA-approved professional product labeling or package insert. New scientific techniques have allowed researchers to predict some drug interactions before they have been documented in people. There may be other drugs, especially those in the families of drugs listed below, that also will react with this drug to cause severe adverse effects. The number of new drugs approved for marketing increases the chance of drug interactions, and new drug interactions are being identified with old drugs. Be vigilant. Make sure to tell your doctor and pharmacist the drugs you are taking and tell your doctor if you are taking any of these interacting drugs:

COUMADIN, GARAMYCIN, gentamicin, heparin, oral contraceptives, warfarin.

Adverse Effects

Call your doctor immediately if you experience:

• **signs of severe allergic reaction (anaphylactic shock):** severe asthma (wheezing), extreme weakness, abdominal pain, nausea or vomiting, diarrhea, rash

Call your doctor immediately, even if it has been a month since you stopped taking amoxicillin, if you experience:

• pain, cramps, or bloating in abdomen or stomach
• severe, watery diarrhea (may contain blood)
• fever
• increased thirst
• abnormal tiredness
• abnormal weight loss
• skin rash, hives, itching, blistering, peeling or loosening
• dark urine
• yellow eyes or skin
• light-colored stools
• loss of appetite
• dizziness or headache
• joint pain
• swelling at place of injection
• unusual bleeding or bruising
• seizures
• decrease in urine

Call your doctor if these symptoms continue:

• mild diarrhea
• sore mouth or tongue
• darkened or discolored tongue
• mild stomach pain
• itching of the genital or rectal area

Periodic Tests
Ask your doctor which of these tests should be done periodically while you are taking this drug:

• bleeding time

• prothrombin time
• stool exam

────────

Trimethoprim and Sulfamethoxazole
BACTRIM (Roche)
SEPTRA (Glaxo Wellcome)
COTRIM (Lemmon)

GENERIC: available
FAMILY: Antibiotics (see p. 468)

Trimethoprim (see p. 528) and sulfamethoxazole (sulfa meth *ox* a zole) are antibiotics that can be used separately to treat various infections. This combination of trimethoprim and sulfamethoxazole is a rational combination that offers more benefit than either drug alone. The combination is used to treat ear, prostate, intestinal, and urinary tract infections, and acute bronchitis in people with chronic lung disease. **Trimethoprim and sulfamethoxazole will not help a cold or the flu.** Rarely, this drug may cause severe blood disorders, especially in older adults.[31]

If you have either liver or kidney impairment, you might need to take less than the usual adult dose of this drug.

Practice measures to prevent urinary tract infections. Drink plenty of fluids, especially water. While cranberry juice is unreliable as a cure for urinary tract infections, the juice may reduce odor from incontinence.[32] Practice meticulous hygiene. After using the toilet, wipe backward, not forward, then wash your hands. Prepare and store foods properly, especially when traveling, to prevent diarrhea. Restrict caffeine, which widens the urethra. Indwelling catheters invite urinary tract infections. However, unless there are symptoms of urinary infection, it is not always necessary to take medication just because bacteria are found in a urine test.[33] Women are particularly prone to repeated urinary tract infections. If urinary tract symptoms occur often, ask your doctor about keeping a supply of medication on hand. Ideally, the antibiotic you use should be the most effective, least toxic, and least costly.[34,35]

Before You Use This Drug

Tell your doctor if you have or have had:

- allergies to drugs
- an unusual reaction to other sulfonamides (sulfa drugs), furosemide, thiazide diuretics, or diabetes or glaucoma drugs taken by mouth
  - glucose-6-phosphate dehydrogenase deficiency
  - kidney or liver problems
  - porphyria
  - anemia or other blood problems

Tell your doctor about any other drugs you take, including aspirin, herbs, vitamins, and other nonprescription products.

When You Use This Drug

- **Drink a full glass (eight ounces) of water with each dose, and drink several additional glasses of water every day, unless your doctor tells you differently.**
- Call your doctor if your symptoms do not get better in two or three days.
- **Take all the medication your doctor prescribed, even if you feel better before you run out. If you stop too soon, your symptoms could come back.**
- Do not give the drug to anyone else. Throw away outdated drugs.
- **Caution diabetics:** see p. 550.
- Stay out of the sun as much as possible, and call your doctor if rash, hives, or skin reaction develops. This drug makes you more sensitive to the sun.
- Ask your doctor if you need to get more vitamin K than usual.
- If you plan to have any surgery, including dental, tell your doctor that you take this drug.
- Until you know how you react to this drug, do not drive or perform other activities requiring alertness.

How to Use This Drug

- Take with **a full glass of water (eight ounces) on an empty stomach** (at least one hour before or two hours after meals). Tablets may be crushed and mixed with the water. Shake liquid form before using.
- Do not store in the bathroom. Do not expose to heat, moisture, or strong light. Do not let the liquid form freeze.
- If you miss a dose, take it as soon as you remember. If you are taking two doses a day of this drug, take the dose you missed and then wait at least five or six hours before taking the next one. If you are taking this drug three or more times a day, you can take the missed dose and the next one at the same time.

Interactions with Other Drugs

The following drugs are listed in the *Evaluations of Drug Interactions* 1997 as causing "highly clinically significant" or "clinically significant" interactions when used together with this drug. We have also included potentially serious interactions listed in the drug's FDA-approved professional product labeling or package insert. New scientific techniques have allowed researchers to predict some drug interactions before they have been documented in people. There may be other drugs, especially those in the families of drugs listed below, that also will react with this drug to cause severe adverse effects. The number of new drugs approved for marketing increases the chance of drug interactions, and new drug interactions are being identified with old drugs. Be vigilant. Make sure to tell your doctor and pharmacist the drugs you are taking and tell your doctor if you are taking any of these interacting drugs:

COUMADIN, DILANTIN, methotrexate, ORINASE, PENTOTHAL, phenytoin, RHEUMATREX DOSE PACK, thiopental, tolbutamide, warfarin.

Adverse Effects

Call your doctor immediately if you experience:

- increased sensitivity of skin to sun
- skin rash or itching
- aching joints or muscles
- difficulty swallowing or breathing
- fever
- pale skin
- sore throat
- abnormal bleeding or bruising
- abnormal tiredness or weakness
- yellow eyes or skin
- redness, blistering, peeling or loosening of skin
- abdominal cramps, pain or tenderness
- anxiety
- bloody urine
- bluish fingernails, lips or skin
- confusion
- watery and severe diarrhea
- problems urinating
- hallucinations
- severe headache
- increased thirst
- lower back or neck pain or stiffness
- depression
- nausea
- nervousness
- pain at injection site
- swelling of neck

Call your doctor if these symptoms continue:

- dizziness or headache
- loss of appetite
- vomiting

Periodic Tests

Ask your doctor which of these tests should be done periodically while you are taking this drug:

- complete blood count during long-term therapy

Limited Use

Mupirocin
BACTROBAN (SmithKline Beecham)

GENERIC: not available
FAMILY: Antibiotics (see p. 468)

Mupirocin (mu *pir* o sin) is an ointment used to treat impetigo and other skin infections. A review concluded that penicillin or erythromycin should be used to treat non-bullous (simple) impetigo,[36] and some doctors prefer to use oral antibiotics to treat it. If the impetigo affects only a small skin area and you prefer not to take oral therapy, consider mupirocin.

Resistance and secondary infection with mupirocin can occur with prolonged use.[37,38] Mupirocin is for external use, so do not use if your skin is broken or you have a burn, since you could absorb the drug internally and cause kidney problems.[39]

Before You Use This Drug

Tell your doctor if you have or have had:

- allergies to drugs or polyethylene glycol (PEG)

When You Use This Drug

- Call your doctor if no improvement occurs within three to five days.
- **Use all the mupirocin your doctor prescribed, even if you feel better before**

you run out. If you stop too soon, your symptoms could come back.

How to Use This Drug

• Wash the affected area with soap and water, then dry.

• Rub a small amount gently onto the skin. To avoid rubbing ointment off the skin and to protect your clothing, you may cover the site with a gauze dressing.

• If you miss a dose, apply it as soon as you remember, but skip it if it is almost time for the next application.

• Do not use in the eyes.

• Recap the tube. Store at room temperature. Do not store at high temperatures or freezing temperatures.

Interactions with Other Drugs

Some other drugs that you may be taking (either over-the-counter or prescription drugs) can interact with this one, causing adverse effects. Ask your doctor what these drugs are and let him or her know if you are taking any of them.

When using topical products it is advisable not to apply other topical preparations, including cosmetics, to the same site. This prevents interactions that could irritate your skin.

Adverse Reactions

Call your doctor if these symptoms continue:

• dry skin
• nausea
• skin rash, swelling, burning, itching, or pain

Limited Use

Clarithromycin
BIAXIN (Abbott)

GENERIC: not available
FAMILY: Antibiotics (see p. 468)

Clarithromycin (clare *ith* row mycin) is approved to treat infections, such as Legionnaire's disease, pneumonia, skin and soft tissue infections. **Clarithromycin will not help a cold,** but may be effective in treating bronchitis or sinusitis.[40,41]

If you are allergic to penicillin, your doctor may prescribe clarithromycin for other infections.

Clarithromycin belongs to the same family of antibiotics as erythromycin. For most infections, clarithromycin is similar in effectiveness to amoxicillin, erythromycin, cloxacillin, or penicillin. Clarithromycin, however, costs much more than these alternative antibiotics. Some experts recommend that it be reserved, in most instances, to treat AIDS-related infections.

If you have kidney disease you may require less than the usual adult dose of clarithromycin.

WARNING

If you are using clarithromycin do not use Propulsid, Seldane, Seldane-D or Hismanal. These drugs, when used in combination with clarithromycin can accumulate to dangerous levels in the body and can cause life-threatening, sometimes fatal heart arrhythmias.[42]

Before You Use This Drug

Tell your doctor if you have or have had:

• allergies to drugs
• liver or kidney problems

Tell your doctor about any other drugs you take, including aspirin, herbs, vitamins, and other nonprescription products.

When You Use This Drug

• Call your doctor if your symptoms do not improve in two or three days or if you get diarrhea. Do not treat the diarrhea yourself.

• **Take all the clarithromycin your doctor prescribed, even if you feel better before you run out. If you stop too soon, your symptoms could come back.**

• If you plan to have any surgery, including dental, tell your doctor that you take this drug.

How to Use This Drug

• Take tablets with **a full glass (eight ounces) of water.**

• Do not store tablets in the bathroom. Do not expose to heat, moisture, or strong light.

• If you miss a dose, take it as soon as you remember, but skip it if it is almost time for the next dose. **Do not take double doses.**

Interactions with Other Drugs

The following drugs are listed in the *Evaluations of Drug Interactions* 1997 as causing "highly clinically significant" or "clinically significant" interactions when used together with this drug. We have also included potentially serious interactions listed in the drug's FDA-approved professional product labeling or package insert. New scientific techniques have allowed researchers to predict some drug interactions before they have been documented in people. There may be other drugs, especially those in the families of drugs listed below, that also will react with this drug to cause severe adverse effects. The number of new drugs approved for marketing increases the chance of drug interactions, and new drug interactions are being identified with old drugs. Be vigilant. Make sure to tell your doctor and pharmacist the drugs you are taking and tell your doctor if you are taking any of these interacting drugs:

ALFENTA, alfentanil, astemizole, carbamazepine, cisapride, COUMADIN, cyclosporine, digoxin, disopyramide, ELIXOPHYLLIN, ERGOMAR, ERGOSTAT, ergotamine, HISMANAL, LANOXICAPS, LANOXIN, MEDROL, methylprednisolone, NEORAL, NORPACE, ORAP, pimozide, PROPULSID, RETROVIR, SANDIMMUNE, SELDANE, SLO-BID, TEGRETOL, terfenadine, THEO-24, theophylline, warfarin, zidovudine (AZT).

Adverse Effects

Call your doctor immediately if you experience:

• severe and watery diarrhea
• skin rash, itching
• abdominal tenderness
• fever
• nausea, vomiting
• severe abdominal or stomach cramps
• difficulty breathing
• unusual bleeding or bruising
• yellow eyes or skin

Call your doctor if these symptoms continue:

• dizziness
• headache
• taste change

PREGNANCY WARNING

This drug caused harm to developing fetuses in animal studies, or such studies were not done. Use during pregnancy only for clear medical reasons. Tell your doctor if you are pregnant or thinking of becoming pregnant before you take this drug.

Cefaclor
CECLOR (Lilly)

GENERIC: available
FAMILY: Antibiotics (see p. 468)
         Cephalosporins (see p. 470)

Cefaclor (*sef* a clor) is used to treat some infections caused by bacteria, such as infections of the ear or soft tissues (puncture wounds or deep cuts). For most of these infections, though, you could take an antibiotic from a different family that would be just as effective as cefaclor and much less expensive.[43]

For example, if you have an ear infection, taking cefaclor for 10 days will be four times as expensive as taking another antibiotic, amoxicillin (see p. 476), for 10 days.[44] **Cefaclor will not help a cold or the flu.**

Sometimes doctors prescribe cefaclor or another drug in its family because the person taking the drug is allergic to penicillin. However, there is a chance that someone allergic to penicillin will also be allergic to drugs in this family (cephalosporins).

If you have kidney disease, you may need to take less than the usual adult dose of cefaclor.

Before You Use This Drug

Tell your doctor if you have or have had:

- allergies to drugs
- a reaction to any penicillin or cephalosporin (see p. 471 for examples)
- other allergies
- stomach or intestinal disease
- kidney or liver disease
- a salt (sodium)-restricted diet (the injected form of cefaclor contains sodium)

Tell your doctor about any other drugs you take, including aspirin, herbs, vitamins, and other nonprescription products.

When You Use This Drug

- Call your doctor if your symptoms do not improve in two or three days or if you get diarrhea. Do not treat the diarrhea yourself.
- **Take all the cefaclor your doctor prescribed, even if you feel better before you run out. If you stop too soon, your symptoms could come back.**

- **Caution diabetics:** see p. 550.
- Do not give the drug to anyone else. Throw away outdated drugs.
- If you plan to have any surgery, including dental, tell your doctor that you take this drug.

How to Use This Drug

- Taking cefaclor with food may help prevent stomach upset.
- Store liquid form in the refrigerator but do not freeze. Shake well before using.
- Do not store capsules in the bathroom. Do not expose to heat, moisture, or strong light.
- Capsules may be opened and mixed with food or water.
- If you miss a dose, take it as soon as you remember, but skip it if it is almost time for the next dose. **Do not take double doses.**

Interactions with Other Drugs

The following drugs are listed in the *Evaluations of Drug Interactions* 1997 as causing "highly clinically significant" or "clinically significant" interactions when used together with this drug. We have also included potentially serious interactions listed in the drug's FDA-approved professional product labeling or package insert. New scientific techniques have allowed researchers to predict some drug interactions before they have been documented in people. There may be other drugs, especially those in the families of drugs listed below, that also will react with this drug to cause severe adverse effects. The number of new drugs approved for marketing increases the chance of drug interactions, and new drug interactions are being identified with old drugs. Be vigilant. Make sure to tell your doctor and pharmacist the drugs you are taking and tell your doctor if you are taking any of these interacting drugs:

BENEMID, COUMADIN, GARAMYCIN, gentamicin, probenecid, warfarin.

Adverse Effects

Call your doctor immediately if you experience:

- **signs of severe allergic reaction (anaphylactic shock):** severe asthma (wheezing), extreme weakness, abdominal pain, nausea or vomiting, diarrhea, rash

Call your doctor immediately, even if it has been a month since you stopped taking cefaclor, if you experience:

- pain, cramps, or bloating in the abdomen or stomach
- severe, watery diarrhea (may contain blood)
- fever
- nausea or vomiting
- increased thirst
- abnormal tiredness
- abnormal weight loss or loss of appetite
- dizziness or headache
- joint pain
- skin rash, hives, itching, blistering, peeling or loosening
- swelling at place of injection
- unusual bleeding or bruising
- seizures
- urine decrease
- yellowing of eyes and skin

Call your doctor if these symptoms continue:

- mild diarrhea
- sore mouth or tongue
- mild stomach pain
- itching of genital or rectal area

Periodic Tests

Ask your doctor which of these tests should be done periodically while you are taking this drug:

- bleeding time
- prothrombin time
- stool exam

Limited Use

Cefuroxime Axetil
CEFTIN (Glaxo Wellcome)

Cefprozil
CEFZIL (Bristol-Myers Squibb)

Loracarbef
LORABID (Lilly)

GENERIC: available for cefuroxime, not for cefprozil and loracarbef

FAMILY: Antibiotics (see p. 468)
Cephalosporins (see p. 470)

Cefuroxime (se *fyoor* ox eem), cefprozil (sef *proe* zil), and loracarbef (loe ra *kar* bef) are antibiotics, belonging to the family of second generation cephalosporins, used to cure infections caused by susceptible bacteria. The oral forms of these are used to treat bronchitis, and ear, urinary tract and skin infections. *The Medical Letter* rarely lists these as drugs of choice for any infection.[45]

Like all antibiotics, these do not help a cold. A sensitivity test should justify use of cefuroxime, cefprozil, and loracarbef. Otherwise, other antibiotics, including less costly cephalosporins, are likely to be as effective.

Sometimes doctors prescribe these or another drug in the cephalosporin family because the person taking the drug is allergic to penicillin. However, there is a chance that someone allergic to penicillin will also be allergic to drugs in this family (cephalosporins).

If you have kidney disease, you may need to take less than the usual adult dose of these drugs. Cefuroxime, cefprozil, and loracarbef may lower your vitamin K, especially if you are malnourished, prolonging bleeding.

Practice measures to prevent urinary tract infections. Drink plenty of fluids, especially water. While cranberry juice is unreliable as a cure for urinary tract infections, the juice may reduce odor from incontinence.[46] Practice meticulous hygiene. After using the toilet, wipe backward, not forward, then wash your hands. Prepare and store foods properly, especially when traveling, to prevent diarrhea. Restrict caffeine, which widens the urethra. Indwelling catheters invite urinary tract infections. However, unless there are symptoms of urinary infection, it is not always necessary to take medication just because bacteria are found in a urine test.[47] Women are particularly prone to repeated urinary tract infections. If urinary tract symptoms occur often, ask your doctor about keeping a supply of medication on hand. Ideally, the antibiotic you use should be the most effective, least toxic, and least costly.[48,49]

Before You Use This Drug

Tell your doctor if you have or have had:

- allergies to drugs
- a reaction to any penicillin or cephalosporin (see p. 471 for examples)
- allergy or rash after taking any paraben-containing products such as sun screens
- kidney or liver problems
- phenylketonuria
- a salt (sodium)-restricted diet (injected form of cefuroxime contains sodium)

Tell your doctor about any other drugs you take, including aspirin, herbs, vitamins, and other nonprescription products.

When You Use This Drug

- Call your doctor if your symptoms do not improve in two or three days or if you get diarrhea. Do not treat the diarrhea yourself.
- **Take all the cefuroxime, cefprozil or loracarbef your doctor prescribed, even if you feel better before you run out. If you stop too soon, your symptoms could come back.**
- **Caution diabetics:** see p. 550.

- Do not give the drug to anyone else. Throw away outdated drugs.
- If you plan to have any surgery, including dental, tell your doctor that you take this drug.

How to Use This Drug

- Swallow tablets whole. Take with food or milk. You may crush tablets and mix with food such as applesauce, chocolate milk, ice cream, or milk to mask the bitter taste. Or, pour two to three ounces of apple juice, or grape juice, and let it warm to room temperature. Then add your dose to the juice. After the tablets disintegrate, stir, then swallow immediately. Follow with more juice without the drug.
- If you miss a dose, take it as soon as possible. If it is almost time for the next dose, adjust your schedule. If you take one dose a day, take the missed dose, then the next dose 10 to 12 hours later. If you take two doses a day, take the missed dose, then the next dose five to six hours later. If you take three or more doses a day, take the missed dose and the next dose, two to four hours later.
- Do not store in the bathroom. Do not expose to heat, moisture, or strong light.

Interactions with Other Drugs

The following drugs are listed in the *Evaluations of Drug Interactions* 1997 as causing "highly clinically significant" or "clinically significant" interactions when used together with this drug. We have also included potentially serious interactions listed in the drug's FDA-approved professional product labeling or package insert. New scientific techniques have allowed researchers to predict some drug interactions before they have been documented in people. There may be other drugs, especially those in the families of drugs listed below, that also will react with this drug to cause severe adverse effects. The number of

new drugs approved for marketing increases the chance of drug interactions, and new drug interactions are being identified with old drugs. Be vigilant. Make sure to tell your doctor and pharmacist the drugs you are taking and tell your doctor if you are taking any of these interacting drugs:

BENEMID, COUMADIN, GARAMYCIN, gentamicin, probenecid, warfarin.

Adverse Effects

Call your doctor immediately if you experience:

- **signs of severe allergic reaction (anaphylactic shock):** severe asthma (wheezing), extreme weakness, abdominal pain, nausea or vomiting, diarrhea, rash
  - pain, cramps or bloating in the abdomen or stomach
  - difficulty breathing
  - seizures
  - severe, watery diarrhea (may contain blood)
  - fever
  - joint pain
  - low blood pressure
  - skin rash, hives, itching, blistering, peeling, or loosening
  - unusual bleeding or bruising
  - decreased urine
  - increased thirst
  - abnormal tiredness
  - abnormal weight loss or loss of appetite
  - dizziness or headache
  - swelling at place of injection
  - yellowing of eyes or skin

Call your doctor if these symptoms continue:

- mild diarrhea
- sore mouth or tongue
- mild stomach pain
- itching of the genital or rectal area

Periodic Tests

Ask your doctor which of these tests should be done periodically while you are taking this drug:

- bleeding or prothrombin time
- stool exam

Cephradine

GENERIC: available
FAMILY: Antibiotics (see p. 468)
Cephalosporins (see p. 470)

Cephradine (*sef* ra deen) is used to treat certain infections caused by bacteria, such as infections of the bladder and soft tissues (puncture wounds or deep cuts). For most of these infections, though, you could take an antibiotic from a different family that would be just as effective as cephradine and much less expensive.[50] Oral cephradine (taken by mouth) is also used to help prevent infection after some types of surgery.[51] **Cephradine will not help a cold or the flu.**

Sometimes doctors prescribe cephradine or another drug in its family because the person taking the drug is allergic to penicillin. However, there is a chance that someone allergic to penicillin will also be allergic to drugs in this family (cephalosporins).

If you have kidney disease, you may need to take less than the usual adult dose of cephradine.

Practice measures to prevent urinary tract infections. Drink plenty of fluids, especially water. While cranberry juice is unreliable as a cure for urinary tract infections, the juice may reduce odor from incontinence.[52] Practice meticulous hygiene. After using the toilet, wipe backward, not forward, then wash your hands. Prepare and store foods properly, especially when traveling, to prevent diarrhea. Restrict caffeine, which widens the urethra. Indwelling catheters invite urinary tract infections. However, unless there are symptoms of urinary infection, it is not always necessary to take medication just because bacteria are found in a urine test.[53] Women are particularly prone to repeated urinary tract infections. If urinary tract symptoms occur often, ask your doctor about keeping a supply of medication on hand. Ideally, the antibiotic you use should be the most effective, least toxic, and least costly.[54,55]

Before You Use This Drug

Tell your doctor if you have or have had:

- allergies to drugs
- a reaction to any penicillin or cephalosporin (see p. 471 for examples)
- other allergies
- stomach or intestinal disease
- kidney or liver disease
- a salt (sodium)-restricted diet (the injected form of cephradine contains sodium)

Tell your doctor about any other drugs you take, including aspirin, herbs, vitamins, and other nonprescription products.

When You Use This Drug

- Call your doctor if your symptoms do not improve in two or three days or if you get diarrhea. Do not treat the diarrhea yourself.
- **Take all the cephradine your doctor prescribed, even if you feel better before you run out. If you stop too soon, your symptoms could come back.**
- **Caution diabetics:** see p. 550.
- Do not give the drug to anyone else. Throw away outdated drugs.

- If you plan to have any surgery, including dental, tell your doctor that you take this drug.

How to Use This Drug

- Taking cephradine with food may help prevent stomach upset.
- Store liquid form in the refrigerator but do not freeze. Shake well before using.
- Do not store capsules in the bathroom. Do not expose to heat, moisture, or strong light.
- Capsules may be opened and mixed with food or water.
- If you miss a dose, take it as soon as you remember, but skip it if it is almost time for the next dose. **Do not take double doses.**

Interactions with Other Drugs

The following drugs are listed in the *Evaluations of Drug Interactions* 1997 as causing "highly clinically significant" or "clinically significant" interactions when used together with this drug. We have also included potentially serious interactions listed in the drug's FDA-approved professional product labeling or package insert. New scientific techniques have allowed researchers to predict some drug interactions before they have been documented in people. There may be other drugs, especially those in the families of drugs listed below, that also will react with this drug to cause severe adverse effects. The number of new drugs approved for marketing increases the chance of drug interactions, and new drug interactions are being identified with old drugs. Be vigilant. Make sure to tell your doctor and pharmacist the drugs you are taking and tell your doctor if you are taking any of these interacting drugs:

BENEMID, colistimethate sodium, COLYMYCIN M PARENTERAL, COUMADIN,

GARAMYCIN, gentamicin, probenecid, warfarin.

Adverse Effects

Call your doctor immediately if you experience:

- **signs of severe allergic reaction (anaphylactic shock):** severe asthma (wheezing), extreme weakness, abdominal pain, nausea or vomiting, diarrhea, rash

Call your doctor immediately, even if it has been a month since you stopped taking cephradine, if you experience:

- pain, cramps, or bloating in the abdomen or stomach
- severe, watery diarrhea (may contain blood)
- fever
- increased thirst
- abnormal tiredness
- abnormal weight loss or loss of appetite
- dizziness or headache
- joint pain
- skin rash, hives, itching, blistering, peeling or loosening
- swelling at place of injection
- unusual bleeding or bruising
- seizures
- urine decrease
- yellowing of eyes and skin

Call your doctor if these symptoms continue:

- mild diarrhea
- sore mouth or tongue
- mild stomach pain
- itching of the genital or rectal area

Periodic Tests

Ask your doctor which of these tests should be done periodically while you are taking this drug:

- bleeding time
- prothrombin time
- stool exam

Do Not Use
(Except in the hospital)

ALTERNATIVE TREATMENT:
If needed (outside the hospital), a less toxic antibiotic.

Chloramphenicol
CHLOROMYCETIN (Parke-Davis)

FAMILY: Antibiotics (see p. 468)

Although chloramphenicol (klor am *fen* i kole) **is effective in treating many conditions, it should be used only in a very limited number of situations because it is so dangerous.** It can cause an irreversible depression of the bone marrow (where blood cells and platelets are produced), which usually results in death.

Chloramphenicol should be used to treat serious diseases for which there is no better antibiotic available. Most of these diseases require hospital treatment, so there is rarely any reason to take chloramphenicol at home. The only exception is that you may need to take it at home to finish treatment that was begun in the hospital.

Oral chloramphenicol (taken by mouth) is usually prescribed inappropriately to treat trivial infections.[56] **Chloramphenicol should not be used for minor infections, and it will not help a cold or the flu.**

Limited Use

Ciprofloxacin
CIPRO (Bayer)
CILOXAN Eye Drops (Alcon)

GENERIC: not available

FAMILY: Antibiotics (see p. 468)
Fluoroquinolones (see p. 472)

Ciprofloxacin (sip row *flocks* a sin) is used to treat infections, such as urinary tract infections, osteomyelitis, infectious diarrhea, and gonorrhea. Ciprofloxacin eye drops are used to treat eye infections. (See p. 622 for the proper use of eye drops.) **Since older people tend to have reduced kidney function, they are usually prescribed low doses of ciprofloxacin.**

Ciprofloxacin belongs to a family of drugs called fluoroquinolones. These drugs are alternatives for individuals allergic to, or with infections resistant to, other antibiotics. A seven-day course of ciprofloxacin costs 5 to 10 times more than drugs such as amoxicillin (see p. 476) or trimethoprim-sulfamethoxazole (see p. 478), which are equally effective for most infections. Both resistance and allergy to one drug in this family usually cross to the rest of the fluoroquinolones and sometimes even occur during therapy.[57,58] Overgrowth of normal bacteria may cause yeast infections, especially when antibiotics are used for long periods. The fluoroquinolones can cause central nervous system problems and psychosis.[59] Severe, even fatal, allergic reactions have happened after just one dose. Collapse of the circulatory system has occurred. As a group fluoroquinolones are expensive, resistance is increasing, and effective alternatives are available.[60]

The Journal of the American Medical Association reports widespread misuse of ciprofloxacin. Ciprofloxacin is inappropriate for common sinus and ear infections and community-acquired pneumonias. For most pneumonias and streptococcal infections penicillin or a cephalosporin remain drugs of choice.[61,62,63] **Ciprofloxacin will not help a cold.**

Practice measures to prevent urinary tract infections. Drink plenty of fluids, especially water. While cranberry juice is unreliable as a cure for urinary tract infections, the juice may reduce odor from incontinence.[64] Practice meticulous hygiene. After using the toilet, wipe backward, not forward, then wash your hands. Prepare and store foods properly, especially when traveling, to prevent diarrhea. Restrict caffeine, which widens the urethra. Indwelling catheters invite urinary tract infections. However, unless there are symptoms of urinary infection, it is not always necessary to take medication just because bacteria are found in a urine test.[65] Women are particularly prone to repeated urinary tract infections. If urinary tract symptoms occur often, ask your doctor about keeping a supply of medication on hand. Ideally, the antibiotic you use should be the most effective, least toxic, and least costly.[66,67]

WARNING

Extreme caution should be used when fluoroquinolones such as ciprofloxacin are to be prescribed in conjunction with aminophylline or theophylline, particularly in elderly patients. Aminophylline or theophylline doses should be adjusted, perhaps reduced by 30% to 50% at the start of fluoroquinolone therapy. The reduction in dose must be guided by the clinical conditions of the patient, the use of other medications, and the baseline level of the aminophylline or theophylline in the blood. In addition, aminophylline or theophylline levels in the blood should be obtained following the start of a fluoroquinolone no later than two days into therapy.[68]

Before You Use This Drug

Tell your doctor if you have or have had:

- allergies to drugs
- epilepsy or seizures
- kidney problems alone
- kidney and liver problems
- myasthenia gravis[69]
- an implanted metal device[70]
- brain or spinal cord disease

Tell your doctor about any other drugs you take, including aspirin, herbs, vitamins, and other nonprescription products. It is especially important you tell your doctor if you take any theophylline drug (see p. 426).

When You Use This Drug

- **Take all the ciprofloxacin your doctor prescribed, even if you feel better before you run out. If you stop too soon, your symptoms could come back.**
- Do not drive or perform other activities that require alertness because this drug may make you drowsy, dizzy, or lightheaded.
- Drink plenty of fluids.
- Protect yourself from sunburn. Do not use a sunlamp.
- If you plan to have any surgery, including dental, tell your doctor that you take this drug.

How to Use This Drug

- Swallow tablet whole with **a full glass (eight ounces) of water.**
- If you miss a dose, take it as soon as you remember, but skip it if it is almost time for the next dose. **Do not take double doses.**
- Do not store in the bathroom. Do not expose to heat, moisture, or strong light.
- Do not take antacids, sucralfate (CARA-FATE), or products containing iron or zinc within two hours of taking ciprofloxacin.

Interactions with Other Drugs

The following drugs are listed in the *Evaluations of Drug Interactions* 1997 as causing "highly clinically significant" or "clinically significant" interactions when used together with this drug. We have also included potentially serious interactions listed in the drug's FDA-approved professional product labeling or package insert. New scientific techniques have allowed researchers to predict some drug interactions before they have been documented in people. There may be other drugs, especially those in the families of drugs listed below, that also will react with this drug to cause severe adverse effects. The number of new drugs approved for marketing increases the chance of drug interactions, and new drug interactions are being identified with old drugs. Be vigilant. Make sure to tell your doctor and pharmacist the drugs you are taking and tell your doctor if you are taking any of these interacting drugs:

aluminum hydroxide, AMPHOJEL, caffeine (beverages or drugs), calcium carbonate, CALTRATE, CARAFATE, COUMADIN, cyclosporine, FEOSOL, ferrous sulfate, MAALOX, magnesium hydroxide, NEORAL, OS-CAL 500, PHILLIPS' MILK OF MAGNESIA, SANDIMMUNE, SLOW FE, sucralfate, warfarin.

Caution should be taken when the following drugs are used with this one (see warning box): amino-phylline, ELIXOPHYLLIN, SLOBID, SOMOPHYLLIN, SOMOPHYLLIN DF, THEO-24, theophylline.

Adverse Effects

Call your doctor immediately if you experience:

- agitation
- difficulty breathing
- confusion, hallucinations
- fever

- skin rash, itching, redness, peeling
- seizure
- swelling of face, neck, calves or lower legs
- tremors
- blurred vision
- pain at site of injection
- pain in calves radiating to heels

Call your doctor if these symptoms continue:

- dizziness, lightheadedness
- drowsiness
- headache
- insomnia, restlessness
- nausea, vomiting, diarrhea
- pain in abdomen, stomach, joints
- increased sensitivity of skin to sunlight

PREGNANCY WARNING

This drug caused harm to developing fetuses in animal studies, or such studies were not done. Use during pregnancy only for clear medical reasons. Tell your doctor if you are pregnant or thinking of becoming pregnant before you take this drug.

WARNING

INCREASED RISK OF TENDINITIS AND TENDON RUPTURE WITH ALL FLUO-ROQUINOLONE ANTIBIOTICS

Public Citizen's Health Research Group petitioned the Food and Drug Administration (FDA) to add a warning for doctors to the labeling, or package, for all fluoroquinolone antibiotics about the risk of tendinitis, including the possibility of complete tendon rupture.

This adverse reaction most frequently involves the Achilles tendon, the tendon that runs from the back of the heel to the calf. Rupture of the Achilles tendon may require surgical repair. Tendons in the rotator cuff (the shoulder), the hand, the biceps, and the thumb have also been involved. This reaction appears to be more common in those taking steroid drugs, in older patients, and in kidney transplant recipients but cases have occurred in people without any of these risk factors. The onset of symptoms is sudden and has occurred as soon as 24 hours after starting treatment with a fluoroquinolone. Most people have recovered completely after one to two months.

If you experience unexpected tendon pain while taking a fluoroquinolone antibiotic, stop the drug immediately, call your doctor, and rest.

Limited Use

Clindamycin
CLEOCIN (Pharmacia & Upjohn)

GENERIC: available
FAMILY: Antibiotics (see p. 468)

Clindamycin (klin da *mye* sin) is used to treat life-threatening infections that do not respond to penicillin or other antibiotics, such as bone or abdominal infections. **Clindamycin will not help a cold or the flu, and it is too dangerous to use for sore throats and other upper respiratory infections.**

Clindamycin can have serious adverse effects. It can cause serious inflammation of the large intestine, abdominal cramps, and severe diarrhea, sometimes with passage of blood and mucus. These adverse effects can happen up to several weeks after you stop using the drug. Because of the possibility of these serious adverse effects, your doctor should prescribe a drug less toxic than clindamycin if at all possible. If you are taking clindamycin, watch closely for the serious adverse effects listed. If any occur, call your doctor immediately, stop taking clindamycin, and **do not take any other medication to treat your adverse effects**. When you take antidiarrheal drugs to treat diarrhea caused by clindamycin, they can prolong or worsen the diarrhea instead of helping.

If you have combined liver and kidney disease, you should take less than the usual adult dose of clindamycin.

Before You Use This Drug

Tell your doctor if you have or have had:

- allergies to drugs
- an unusual reaction to clindamycin or lincomycin (see p. 513)
- kidney or liver problems
- stomach or intestinal disease
- allergies to tartrazine (a food dye) or aspirin
- diarrhea

Tell your doctor about any other drugs you take, including aspirin, herbs, vitamins, and other nonprescription products.

When You Use This Drug

- Call your doctor if your symptoms do not improve in two or three days or if you get diarrhea.
- **Take all the clindamycin your doctor prescribed, even if you feel better before you run out. If you stop too soon, your symptoms could come back.**
- Do not give this drug to anyone else. Throw away outdated drugs.
- If you plan to have any surgery, including dental, tell your doctor that you take this drug.

How to Use This Drug

- **Take capsules with a full glass (eight ounces) of water or with food to avoid irritation or ulcers in the esophagus** (the tube that carries food from your mouth to your stomach).
- Do not refrigerate the liquid form. Shake well before using.

- If you miss a dose, take it as soon as you remember. If it is almost time for your next dose, space missed dose and next dose two to four hours apart. **Do not take double doses.**

Interactions with Other Drugs

The following drugs are listed in the *Evaluations of Drug Interactions* 1997 as causing "highly clinically significant" or "clinically significant" interactions when used together with this drug. We have also included potentially serious interactions listed in the drug's FDA-approved professional product labeling or package insert. New scientific techniques have allowed researchers to predict some drug interactions before they have been documented in people. There may be other drugs, especially those in the families of drugs listed below, that also will react with this drug to cause severe adverse effects. The number of new drugs approved for marketing increases the chance of drug interactions, and new drug interactions are being identified with old drugs. Be vigilant. Make sure to tell your doctor and pharmacist the drugs you are taking and tell your doctor if you are taking any of these interacting drugs:

ether, pancuronium, PAVULON.

Adverse Effects

Call your doctor immediately, even if these symptoms occur up to a month after you stop taking clindamycin:

- stomach cramps or abdominal pain
- severe, watery diarrhea (may contain blood)
- fever and sore throat
- increased thirst
- abnormal weakness or tiredness
- abnormal weight loss
- skin rash, redness and itching
- unusual bleeding or bruising

Call your doctor if these symptoms continue:

- mild diarrhea
- nausea or vomiting
- itching in the genital or rectal area
- sore mouth or tongue

Periodic Tests

Ask your doctor which of these tests should be done periodically while you are taking this drug:

- endoscopy, large bowel

Cloxacillin

Dicloxacillin
DYCILL (SmithKline Beecham)
DYNAPEN (Bristol-Myers Squibb)

GENERIC: available
FAMILY: Antibiotics (see p. 468)
Penicillins (see p. 470)

Cloxacillin (klox a *sill* in) and dicloxacillin (dye *klox* a sill in) are used to treat bacterial infections that are resistant to penicillin, such as certain infections of the skin, soft tissue (such as puncture wounds or deep cuts), and joints, and to prevent infection after hip surgery. Your doctor should usually do lab tests before prescribing either of these drugs, and should prescribe one of them only if tests show that the bacteria causing your infection are resistant to penicillin. If the bacteria are not resistant to penicillin, your doctor should prescribe penicillin instead. **These drugs will not help a cold or the flu.**

Cloxacillin and dicloxacillin should be used with caution in people who are over age 70, or people with impaired kidney function.[71]

Before You Use This Drug

Tell your doctor if you have or have had:

- allergies to drugs
- a reaction to any penicillin or cephalosporin (see p. 471 for examples)
- other allergies
- stomach or intestinal disease
- kidney disease
- congestive heart failure

Tell your doctor about any other drugs you take, including aspirin, herbs, vitamins, and other nonprescription products.

When You Use This Drug

- Call your doctor if your symptoms do not improve in two or three days or if you get diarrhea. Do not treat the diarrhea yourself.
- **Take all the cloxacillin or dicloxacillin your doctor prescribed, even if you feel better before you run out. If you stop too soon, your symptoms could come back.**
- **Caution diabetics:** see p. 550.
- If you plan to have any surgery, including dental, tell your doctor that you take this drug.

How to Use This Drug

- Take on an empty stomach (at least one hour before or two hours after meals) with **a full glass (eight ounces) of water.** Capsules may be opened and mixed with water.
- Store liquid form in the refrigerator but do not freeze. Shake well before using.
- Do not store capsules in the bathroom. Do not expose to heat, moisture, or strong light.
- If you miss a dose, take it as soon as you remember, but skip it if it is almost time for the next dose. **Do not take double doses.**

Interactions with Other Drugs

The following drugs are listed in the *Evaluations of Drug Interactions* 1997 as causing "highly clinically significant" or "clinically significant" interactions when used together with this drug. We have also included potentially serious interactions listed in the drug's FDA-approved professional product labeling or package insert. New scientific techniques have allowed researchers to predict some drug interactions before they have been documented in people. There may be other drugs, especially those in the families of drugs listed below, that also will react with this drug to cause severe adverse effects. The number of new drugs approved for marketing increases the chance of drug interactions, and new drug interactions are being identified with old drugs. Be vigilant. Make sure to tell your doctor and pharmacist the drugs you are taking and tell your doctor if you are taking any of these interacting drugs:

AUREOMYCIN, chlortetracycline, COUMADIN, GARAMYCIN, gentamicin, heparin, warfarin.

Adverse Effects

Call your doctor immediately if you experience:

- **signs of severe allergic reaction (anaphylactic shock):** severe asthma (wheezing), extreme weakness, abdominal pain, nausea or vomiting, diarrhea, rash

Call your doctor immediately, even if it has been a month since you stopped taking this drug, if you experience:

- pain, cramps, or bloating in the abdomen or stomach
- severe, watery diarrhea (may contain blood)
- fever
- nausea or vomiting
- increased thirst
- abnormal weakness or tiredness
- abnormal weight loss
- skin rash, hives, or itching

- sore throat
- seizure
- decreased urine
- depression
- pain at site of injection
- unusual bleeding or bruising
- yellow eyes or skin
- lightheadedness or fainting
- puffiness or swelling around face
- decrease in blood pressure
- red or scaly skin
- joint pain

Call your doctor if these symptoms continue:

- mild diarrhea
- sore mouth or tongue
- darkened or discolored mouth or tongue
- vaginal itching or discharge
- headache

Periodic Tests

Ask your doctor which of these tests should be done periodically while you are taking this drug:

- stool cytotoxin assays

 Do Not Use

ALTERNATIVE TREATMENT:
An antibiotic alone, if necessary.

Neomycin, Polymyxin B, and Hydrocortisone
CORTISPORIN Ear Drops (Otic)
(Monarch)

FAMILY: Antibiotics (see p. 468)
         Corticosteroids (see p. 651)

This combination of the drugs neomycin (nee oh *mye* sin), polymyxin (pol i *mix* in) B, and hydrocortisone (see p. 660) is used to treat ear infections caused by bacteria and allergies. **There is no persuasive proof that it is beneficial for this purpose.**

One of the drugs in this product, hydrocortisone, generally should not be used for treating infections at all, because it can hide the signs of an infection or make it spread. The other two drugs in this product, neomycin and polymyxin B, are antibiotics and are unnecessary, unless your ear problem is caused by a bacterial infection. If it is caused by a bacterial infection, you should be taking an antibiotic alone rather than this combination with hydrocortisone.

Neomycin commonly causes skin rashes in 8% of the people who use it.[72] Using neomycin can also make it hard for you to use other drugs in its family (aminoglycoside antibiotics, such as gentamicin and tobramycin, see p. 635) that may be needed later for serious infections.

Fluconazole
DIFLUCAN (Pfizer)

GENERIC: not available
FAMILY: Antifungals

WARNING
Fluconazole has been associated with serious liver toxicity, including deaths.

Fluconazole (flu *con* as ol) is used to treat severe fungal infections, such as meningitis and infections of the mouth or esophagus.[73,74] Often these infections occur when another condition, such as cancer, organ transplant, or HIV infection, reduces your immunity to infections. You may also be more prone to these fungal infections if you have been exposed to contaminated air conditioners, or certain animals or geographic areas. Outbreaks have occurred during remodeling of hospitals.[75] The drug should not be used to treat trivial fungal skin infections.

Fluconazole is also approved by the FDA to treat vaginal yeast infections (vaginal Candidiasis) in a single dose of 150 milligrams.

Before You Use This Drug

Tell your doctor if you have or have had:

- allergies to drugs
- cancer
- diabetes
- kidney or liver problems
- seizures
- tuberculosis
- alcohol abuse

Tell your doctor about any other drugs you take, including aspirin, herbs, vitamins, and other nonprescription products.

When You Use This Drug

- **Take all the fluconazole your doctor prescribed, even if you feel better before you run out. If you stop too soon, your symptoms could come back.**

How to Use This Drug

- If you miss a dose, take it as soon as you remember, but skip it if it is almost time for the next dose. **Do not take double doses.**
- Do not store capsules in the bathroom. Do not expose to heat, moisture, or strong light.

Interactions with Other Drugs

The following drugs are listed in the *Evaluations of Drug Interactions* 1997 as causing "highly clinically significant" or "clinically significant" interactions when used together with this drug. We have also included potentially serious interactions listed in the drug's FDA-approved professional product labeling or package insert. New scientific techniques have allowed researchers to predict some drug interactions before they have been documented in people. There may be other drugs, especially those in the families of drugs listed below, that also will react with this drug to cause severe adverse effects. The number of new drugs approved for marketing increases the chance of drug interactions, and new drug interactions are being identified with old drugs. Be vigilant. Make sure to tell your doctor and pharmacist the drugs you are taking and tell your doctor if you are taking any of these interacting drugs:

cisapride, COUMADIN, cyclosporine, DECADRON, dexamethasone, DILANTIN, DURAQUIN, glipizide, GLUCOTROL, HEXADROL, NEORAL, phenytoin, PROPULSID, QUINAGLUTE DURA-TABS, QUINIDEX, quinidine, RIFADIN, rifampin, RIMACTANE, SANDIMMUNE, SELDANE, terfenadine, warfarin.

Adverse Effects

Call your doctor immediately if you experience:

- unusual bleeding or bruising
- abdominal pain, especially on right side under ribs
- fever, chills and sore throat
- seizures
- yellowing of eyes or skin
- reddened, blistering, itching or peeling skin or mucous membranes
- dark, amber urine
- redness, swelling or pain at site of injection
- loss of appetite
- pale stools
- unusual tiredness or weakness
- stomach pain

Call your doctor if these symptoms continue:

- abdominal discomfort

- dizziness
- fatigue
- headache
- nausea, vomiting, diarrhea, constipation

Periodic Tests

Ask your doctor which of these tests should be done periodically while you are taking this drug:

- blood creatinine
- blood urea nitrogen (BUN)
- liver function tests
- potassium serum tests

PREGNANCY WARNING

This drug caused harm to developing fetuses in animal studies, or such studies were not done. Use during pregnancy only for clear medical reasons. Tell your doctor if you are pregnant or thinking of becoming pregnant before you take this drug.

Cefadroxil
DURICEF (Bristol-Myers Squibb)

GENERIC: available
FAMILY: Antibiotics (see p. 468)
Cephalosporins (see p. 470)

Cefadroxil (sef a *drox* ill) is used to treat some infections caused by bacteria, such as infections of the bladder or soft tissues (puncture wounds or deep cuts). For most of these infections, though, you could take an antibiotic from a different family that would be just as effective as cefadroxil and much less expensive.[76] For example, if you have an ordinary urinary tract infection and take cefadroxil, your treatment could cost 25 times as much as if you took another drug, generic sulfisoxazole (see p. 505), which works just as well.[77] **Cefadroxil will not help a cold or the flu.**

Sometimes doctors prescribe cefadroxil or another drug in its family because the person taking the drug is allergic to penicillin. However, there is a chance that someone allergic to penicillin will also be allergic to drugs in this family (cephalosporins).

If you have kidney disease, you may need to take less than the usual adult dose of cefadroxil.

Practice measures to prevent urinary tract infections. Drink plenty of fluids, especially water. While cranberry juice is unreliable as a cure for urinary tract infections, the juice may reduce odor from incontinence.[78] Practice meticulous hygiene. After using the toilet, wipe backward, not forward, then wash your hands. Prepare and store foods properly, especially when traveling, to prevent diarrhea. Restrict caffeine, which widens the urethra. Indwelling catheters invite urinary tract infections. However, unless there are symptoms of urinary tract infection, it is not always necessary to take medication just because bacteria are found in a urine test.[79] Women are particularly prone to repeated urinary tract infections. If urinary tract symptoms occur often, ask your doctor about keeping a supply of medication on hand. Ideally, the antibiotic you use should be the most effective, least toxic, and least costly.[80,81]

Before You Use This Drug

Tell your doctor if you have or have had:

- allergies to drugs
- a reaction to any penicillin or cephalosporin (see p. 471 for examples)
- stomach or intestinal disease
- kidney or liver problems
- a salt (sodium)-restricted diet (injected form of cefadroxil contains sodium)

Tell your doctor about any other drugs you take, including aspirin, herbs, vitamins, and other nonprescription products.

When You Use This Drug

- Call your doctor if your symptoms do not improve in two or three days or if you get diarrhea. Do not treat the diarrhea yourself.
- **Take all the cefadroxil your doctor prescribed, even if you feel better before you run out. If you stop too soon, your symptoms could come back.**
- **Caution diabetics:** see p. 550.
- Do not give this drug to anyone else. Throw away outdated drugs.
- If you plan to have any surgery, including dental, tell your doctor that you take this drug.

How to Use This Drug

- Taking cefadroxil with food may help prevent stomach upset. Capsules may be opened and mixed with food or water.
- Store liquid form in the refrigerator but do not freeze. Shake well before using.
- Do not store capsules in the bathroom. Do not expose to heat, moisture, or strong light.
- If you miss a dose, take it as soon as you remember, but skip it if it is almost time for the next dose. **Do not take double doses.**

Interactions with Other Drugs

The following drugs are listed in the *Evaluations of Drug Interactions* 1997 as causing "highly clinically significant" or "clinically significant" interactions when used together with this drug. We have also included potentially serious interactions listed in the drug's FDA-approved professional product labeling or package insert. New scientific techniques have allowed researchers to predict some drug interactions before they have been documented in people. There may be other drugs, especially those in the families of drugs listed below, that also will react with this drug to cause severe adverse effects. The number of new drugs approved for marketing increases the chance of drug interactions, and new drug interactions are being identified with old drugs. Be vigilant. Make sure to tell your doctor and pharmacist the drugs you are taking and tell your doctor if you are taking any of these interacting drugs:

BENEMID, COUMADIN, GARAMYCIN, gentamicin, probenecid, warfarin.

Adverse Effects

Call your doctor immediately if you experience:

• **signs of severe allergic reaction (anaphylactic shock):** severe asthma (wheezing), extreme weakness, abdominal pain, nausea or vomiting, diarrhea, rash

Call your doctor immediately, even if it has been a month since you stopped taking cefadroxil, if you experience:

- pain, cramps, or bloating in abdomen or stomach
- severe, watery diarrhea (may contain blood)
- fever
- increased thirst
- abnormal tiredness
- abnormal weight loss or loss of appetite
- dizziness or headache
- joint pain
- skin rash, hives, itching, blistering, peeling or loosening
- swelling at place of injection
- unusual bleeding or bruising
- seizures
- decreased urine
- yellowing of eyes and skin

Call your doctor if these symptoms continue:

- mild diarrhea
- sore mouth or tongue
- mild stomach pain
- muscle or joint pain
- itching in the genital or rectal area

Periodic Tests

Ask your doctor which of these tests should be done periodically while you are taking this drug:

- bleeding time
- prothrombin time
- stool exam

Erythromycin
ERYTHROCIN (Abbott)
EES (Abbott)

GENERIC: available
FAMILY: Antibiotics (see p. 468)

Erythromycin (eh rith roe *mye* sin) is used to treat infections such as diphtheria and some kinds of pneumonia. Your doctor may also prescribe erythromycin for other infections if you are allergic to penicillin. **Erythromycin will not help a cold or the flu.**

Erythromycin is one of the safest antibiotics available. However, people who use a particular type of erythromycin called erythromycin estolate (ILOSONE) are about 20 times more likely to suffer liver damage (toxicity) from the drug than people who use other forms.[82] Therefore, you should not take erythromycin estolate (ILOSONE, see p. 507).[83] **If you have liver disease, you should be taking less than the usual adult dose of erythromycin.**

Before You Use This Drug

Tell your doctor if you have or have had:

- allergies to drugs
- an unusual reaction to erythromycin
- heart or liver problems
- hearing loss

Tell your doctor about any other drugs you take, including aspirin, herbs, vitamins, and other nonprescription products.

When You Use This Drug

- Call your doctor if your symptoms do not improve in two or three days or if you get diarrhea. Do not treat the diarrhea yourself.
- **Take all the erythromycin your doctor prescribed, even if you feel better before you run out. If you stop too soon, your symptoms could come back.**
- Do not give this drug to anyone else. Throw away outdated drugs.
- If you plan to have any surgery, including dental, tell your doctor that you take this drug.

How to Use This Drug

Erythromycin taken by mouth:

- Most types must be taken on an empty stomach (at least one hour before or two hours after meals) with **a full glass (eight ounces) of water**.
- Some brands of enteric-coated erythromycin and erythromycin ethyl succinate can be taken on either a full or an empty stomach. Ask your doctor if you are taking one of these types.
- Chewable tablets should be chewed or crushed, not swallowed whole. Enteric-coated tablets (coated so they won't dissolve in your stomach) or capsules should be swallowed whole.
- Do not store in the bathroom. Do not expose to heat, moisture, or strong light. Store liquid erythromycin in the refrigerator (do not freeze) and shake well before using.
- If you miss a dose, take it as soon as you remember. If you are on a twice-a-day schedule, take the dose you missed and then wait six hours before taking the next one. If you are on a schedule of three doses or more a day, you can take the dose you missed and the next one at the same time.

Erythromycin eye ointment:

- If you are using eye ointment, see instructions on p. 622.
- If you miss an application, do it as soon as you remember, but skip it if it is almost time for the next application.

Interactions with Other Drugs

The following drugs are listed in the *Evaluations of Drug Interactions* 1997 as causing "highly clinically significant" or "clinically significant" interactions when used together with this drug. We have also included potentially serious interactions listed in the drug's FDA-approved professional product labeling or package insert. New scientific techniques have allowed researchers to predict some drug interactions before they have been documented in people. There may be other drugs, especially those in the families of drugs listed below, that also will react with this drug to cause severe adverse effects. The number of new drugs approved for marketing increases the chance of drug interactions, and new drug interactions are being identified with old drugs. Be vigilant. Make sure to tell your doctor and pharmacist the drugs you are taking and tell your doctor if you are taking any of these interacting drugs:

ALFENTA, alfentanil, carbamazepine, COUMADIN, cyclosporine, DEPAKENE/DEPAKOTE, digoxin, disopyramide, ELIXOPHYLLIN, ERGOMAR, ERGOSTAT, ergotamine, LANOXICAPS, LANOXIN, MEDROL, methylprednisolone, midazolam, NEORAL, NORPACE, ORAP, pimozide, PROGRAF, SANDIMMUNE, SLO-BID, tacrolimus, TEGRETOL, THEO-24, theophylline, TUBARINE, tubocurarine, valproic acid, VERSED, warfarin.

The following drugs should not be taken with erythromycin (see warning box): astemizole, cisapride, HISMANAL, PROPULSID, SELDANE, terfenadine.

Adverse Effects

Call your doctor immediately if you experience:

- severe, watery diarrhea (may contain blood)
- dark or colored urine
- light-colored stools
- severe stomach pain
- abnormal tiredness or weakness
- yellow eyes or skin
- temporary hearing loss (rare)
- fever
- nausea or vomiting
- skin rash, redness or itching
- pain, swelling or redness at site of injection

Call your doctor if these symptoms continue:

- sore mouth or tongue
- mild abdominal or stomach pain
- vaginal itching and discharge
- diarrhea

Periodic Tests

Ask your doctor which of these tests should be done periodically while you are taking this drug:

- electrocardiogram (ECG, EKG)
- liver function determinations

Limited Use

Metronidazole
FLAGYL (Searle)

GENERIC: available
FAMILY: Antibiotics (see p. 468)

Metronidazole (me troe *ni* da zole) is used to treat some serious infections caused by bacteria or protozoa, including trichomonas, amoebiasis, and giardiasis. **This drug will not help a cold or the flu.**

Metronidazole has been shown to cause cancer in mice and rats. Because of this connection, you should only be using metronidazole if you have a serious infection. Doctors sometimes prescribe metronidazole for a vaginal infection called trichomonas ("trich"), but you should not be using this drug for this kind of infection until you have tried other treatments such as taking a tub bath twice a day, wearing cotton underwear, and not wearing panty hose. If you have tried these treatments and you still have symptoms of a trichomonas infection, then metronidazole may be prescribed.[85]

If you are taking metronidazole for a vaginal trichomonas infection, it is best to use the form that must be taken for one day only. **If you are taking metronidazole for any reason and you have kidney or severe liver impairment, you may need to take less than the usual adult dose.**[86]

The information in this profile deals mostly with the forms of metronidazole taken by mouth—tablets and capsules.

Before You Use This Drug

Tell your doctor if you have or have had:

- allergies to drugs
- an unusual reaction to metronidazole
- disease of the central nervous system
- epilepsy
- severe liver disease
- blood problems
- heart problems

Tell your doctor about any other drugs you take, especially an anticoagulant such as warfarin or heparin, and including aspirin, herbs, vitamins, and other nonprescription products.

When You Use This Drug

- Do not drink alcohol. If you do, you may get abdominal cramps, nausea, vomiting, headaches, flushing, or low blood sugar.
- Call your doctor if your symptoms do not get better in two or three days.
- **Take all the metronidazole your doctor prescribed, even if you feel better before you finish. If you stop too soon, your symptoms could come back.**
- Do not give this drug to anyone else. Throw away outdated drugs.
- If you are going to have any medical tests done, first tell your doctor that you are taking metronidazole.
- Until you know how you react to this drug, do not drive or perform other activities requiring alertness.
- Metronidazole may cause your urine to get darker. This is normal and not dangerous.

How to Use This Drug

- If you are taking metronidazole by mouth, eat something at the same time to prevent stomach irritation.

- Always take your doses of metronidazole the same number of hours apart, even at night, to keep the amount of the drug in your body constant.
- Do not store in the bathroom. Do not expose to heat, moisture, or strong light.
- If you miss a dose, take it as soon as you remember, but skip it if it is almost time for the next dose. **Do not take double doses.**

Interactions with Other Drugs

The following drugs are listed in the *Evaluations of Drug Interactions* 1997 as causing "highly clinically significant" or "clinically significant" interactions when used together with this drug. We have also included potentially serious interactions listed in the drug's FDA-approved professional product labeling or package insert. New scientific techniques have allowed researchers to predict some drug interactions before they have been documented in people. There may be other drugs, especially those in the families of drugs listed below, that also will react with this drug to cause severe adverse effects. The number of new drugs approved for marketing increases the chance of drug interactions, and new drug interactions are being identified with old drugs. Be vigilant. Make sure to tell your doctor and pharmacist the drugs you are taking and tell your doctor if you are taking any of these interacting drugs:

alcohol, ANTABUSE, ARALEN, carbamazepine, chloroquine, COUMADIN, disulfiram, lithium, LITHOBID, LITHONATE, LUMINAL, phenobarbital, SOLFOTON, TEGRETOL, warfarin.

Adverse Effects

Call your doctor immediately if you experience:

- numbness, tingling, pain, or weakness in hands or feet

- clumsiness or unsteadiness
- seizures
- confusion, irritability, depression, weakness, or trouble sleeping
- mood or mental changes
- skin rash, redness, hives, or itching
- sore throat or fever
- vaginal dryness, discharge, or irritation
- pain, tenderness, redness or swelling over skin after injection

Call your doctor if these symptoms continue:

- nausea or vomiting
- diarrhea (even if you stopped taking the drug a month ago)
- dizziness or lightheadedness
- headache
- loss of appetite
- stomach cramps or pain
- sore mouth or tongue
- problems urinating
- dry mouth
- bad taste in mouth
- abnormal tiredness or weakness
- joint pain

Periodic Tests

Ask your doctor which of these tests should be done periodically while you are taking this drug:

- total and differential white blood cell counts (before and after long-term treatment)
- stool examinations

Limited Use

Ofloxacin
FLOXIN (Ortho/McNeil)
OCUFLOX Eye Drops (Allergan)

GENERIC: not available
FAMILY: Antibiotics (see p. 468)
Fluoroquinolones (see p. 472)

Ofloxacin (oh *flocks* a sin) kills a broad spectrum of bacteria and can cure infections caused by susceptible bacteria. Ofloxacin is primarily used to treat complicated infections of the urinary tract and prostate. Ofloxacin drops are used to treat eye infections. (See p. 622 for information about using eye drops.) It is also used for chronic bronchitis, pneumonia, soft skin infections, and uncomplicated gonorrhea. Ofloxacin is not a drug of choice for community-acquired pneumonias. Length of therapy varies from a few days to several weeks or months. Treatment of other conditions, or to prevent urinary tract infections is still under study.

Ofloxacin belongs to a family of drugs called fluoroquinolones. These drugs are alternatives for individuals allergic to, or with infections resistant to, other antibiotics. A seven-day course of ofloxacin costs 5 to 10 times more than drugs such as amoxicillin (see p. 476) or trimethoprim and sulfamethoxazole (see p. 478), which are equally effective for most infections. Both resistance and allergy to one drug in this family usually cross to the rest of the fluoroquinolones and sometimes even occur during therapy.[87,88] Overgrowth of normal bacteria may cause yeast infections, especially when antibiotics are used for long periods. The fluoroquinolones can cause central nervous system problems and psychosis.[89] Severe, even fatal, allergic reactions have happened after just one dose. Collapse of the circulatory system has occurred. As a group fluoroquinolones are expensive, resistance is increasing, and effective alternatives are available.[90]

In people over age 65, ofloxacin is excreted more slowly, so a lower dose is usually used.[91] One-dose therapies with ofloxacin are often followed by a recurrence of the infection.[92] Ofloxacin should not be used for minor infections. Ofloxacin is interchangeable with ciprofloxacin for most uses.

Practice measures to prevent urinary tract infections. Drink plenty of fluids, especially water. While cranberry juice is unreliable as a cure for urinary tract infections, the juice may reduce odor from incontinence.[93] Practice meticulous hygiene. After using the toilet, wipe backward, not forward, then wash your hands. Prepare and store foods properly, especially when traveling, to prevent diarrhea. Restrict caffeine, which widens the urethra. Indwelling catheters invite urinary tract infections. However, unless there are symptoms of urinary infection, it is not always necessary to take medication just because bacteria are found in a urine test.[94] Women are particularly prone to repeated urinary tract infections. If urinary tract symptoms occur often, ask your doctor about keeping a supply of medication on hand. Ideally, the antibiotic you use should be the most effective, least toxic, and least costly.[95,96]

WARNING

Extreme caution should be used when fluoroquinolones such as ofloxacin are to be prescribed in conjunction with aminophylline or theophylline, particularly in elderly patients. Aminophylline or theophylline doses should be adjusted, perhaps reduced by 30% to 50% at the start of fluoroquinolone therapy. The reduction in dose must be guided by the clinical conditions of the patient, the use of other medications, and the baseline level of the aminophylline or theophylline in the blood. In addition, aminophylline or theophylline levels in the blood should be obtained following the start of a fluoroquinolone no later than two days into therapy.[97]

Before You Use This Drug

Tell your doctor if you have or have had:

- allergies to any drugs
- kidney problems alone
- kidney and liver problems
- epilepsy or seizures
- brain or spinal cord disease

Tell your doctor about any other drugs you take, including aspirin, herbs, vitamins, and other nonprescription products.

When You Use This Drug

- Do not drive or perform other activities that require alertness because this drug may make you drowsy, dizzy, or lightheaded.
- Drink plenty of fluids (water, fruit and vegetable juices) to prevent crystals of ofloxacin forming in your urine.
- **Take all the ofloxacin your doctor prescribed, even if you feel better before you run out. If you stop too soon, your symptoms could come back.**
- Protect yourself from sunburn. Wear protective clothing, headgear, sunglasses, and use a sunscreen.

How to Use This Drug

- Swallow whole tablet. Take with **a full (eight ounces) glass of water.** Do not take with food.
- If you miss a dose, take it as soon as you remember, but skip it if it is almost time for the next dose. **Do not take double doses.**
- Do not store tablets in the bathroom. Do not expose to heat, moisture, or strong light.

Interactions with Other Drugs

The following drugs are listed in the *Evaluations of Drug Interactions* 1997 as causing "highly clinically significant" or "clinically significant" interactions when used together with

this drug. We have also included potentially serious interactions listed in the drug's FDA-approved professional product labeling or package insert. New scientific techniques have allowed researchers to predict some drug interactions before they have been documented in people. There may be other drugs, especially those in the families of drugs listed below, that also will react with this drug to cause severe adverse effects. The number of new drugs approved for marketing increases the chance of drug interactions, and new drug interactions are being identified with old drugs. Be vigilant. Make sure to tell your doctor and pharmacist the drugs you are taking and tell your doctor if you are taking any of these interacting drugs:

aluminum hydroxide, AMPHOJEL, caffeine (beverages, drugs), CARAFATE, COUMADIN, cyclosporine, DURAQUIN, MAALOX, magnesium hydroxide, NEORAL, PHILLIPS' MILK OF MAGNESIA, QUINAGLUTE DURA-TABS, QUINIDEX, quinidine, SANDIMMUNE, sucralfate, warfarin.

Caution should be taken when the following drugs are used with this one (see warning box): aminophylline, ELIXOPHYLLIN, SLO-BID, SOMOPHYLLIN, SOMO-PHYLLIN-DF, THEO-24, theophylline.

Adverse Effects

Call your doctor immediately if you experience:

- difficulty breathing or swallowing
- chest pain
- confusion, disorientation
- convulsions
- severe diarrhea

- dizziness, fainting
- fever
- hallucinations
- rapid heartbeat[98]
- itching
- muscle pain
- numbness or tingling sensation
- skin rash, hives, peeling
- swelling of face, throat, calves or lower legs
- tremors[99]
- agitation
- pain at site of injection
- pain in calves radiating to heels

Call your doctor if these symptoms continue:

- abdominal pain
- diarrhea
- dry mouth
- fatigue
- gas
- headache
- hearing loss, or ringing in ears
- insomnia
- loss of appetite
- nausea and vomiting
- nervousness
- taste changes
- vaginal discharge or itching
- vision change, inability to see red, blue[100]

Sulfisoxazole
GANTRISIN (Roche)

GENERIC: available
FAMILY: Antibiotics (see p. 468)
Sulfonamides

Sulfisoxazole (sul fi *sox* a zole) is used to treat urinary tract infections and some other infections. **If you have kidney or liver damage, you should take less than the usual adult dose. Sulfisoxazole will not help a cold or the flu.**

Sulfisoxazole is available in several forms. It is often taken by mouth. Another form is a vaginal cream that is used to treat vaginitis, but there is no evidence that this is an effective treatment. For eye infections, there is an eye ointment and eye solution, which are similar to sulfacetamide (see p. 641).

Practice measures to prevent urinary tract infections. Drink plenty of fluids, especially water. While cranberry juice is unreliable as a cure for urinary tract infections, the juice may reduce odor from incontinence.[101] Practice meticulous hygiene. After using the toilet, wipe backward, not forward, then wash your hands. Prepare and store foods properly, especially when traveling, to prevent diarrhea. Restrict caffeine, which widens the urethra. Indwelling catheters invite urinary tract infections. However, unless there are symptoms of urinary infection, it is not always necessary to take medication just because bacteria are found in a urine test.[102] Women are particularly prone to repeated urinary tract infections. If urinary tract symptoms occur often, ask your doctor about keeping a supply of medication on hand. Ideally, the antibiotic you use should be the most effective, least toxic, and least costly.[103,104]

Before You Use This Drug

Tell your doctor if you have or have had:

- allergies to drugs

• an unusual reaction to other sulfonamides (sulfa drugs), furosemide, thiazide diuretics, or diabetes or glaucoma drugs taken by mouth
• glucose-6-phosphate dehydrogenase deficiency
• kidney or liver disease
• porphyria
• anemia or other blood problems

Tell your doctor about any other drugs you take, including aspirin, herbs, vitamins, and other nonprescription products.

When You Use This Drug

• **Take each dose with a full glass (eight ounces) of water, and drink a few more glasses of water every day, unless your doctor tells you differently.**
• Call your doctor if your symptoms do not improve in two or three days.
• **Take all the sulfisoxazole your doctor prescribed, even if you feel better before you finish. If you stop too soon, your symptoms could come back.**
• Do not give the drug to anyone else. Throw away outdated drugs.
• **Caution diabetics:** see p. 550.
• Stay out of the sun as much as possible, and call your doctor if you get a rash, hives, or any other skin reaction. Sulfisoxazole makes you more sensitive to the sun.
• While taking this drug, you may need more vitamin K than usual. Ask your doctor.
• If you plan to have any surgery, including dental, tell your doctor that you take this drug.
• Until you know how you react to this drug, do not drive or perform other activities requiring alertness.

How to Use This Drug

• Take with **a full glass of water (eight ounces) on an empty stomach** (at least one hour before or two hours after meals). Tablets can be crushed and mixed with the water. Shake liquid form before using.
• If you are using sulfisoxazole eye drops or ointment, see instructions on p. 622.
• Do not store in the bathroom. Do not expose to heat, moisture, or strong light. Do not allow liquid form to freeze.
• If you miss an oral dose, take it as soon as you remember. If you are on a twice-a-day schedule for taking sulfisoxazole, take the dose you missed and then wait at least five or six hours before taking the next one. If you are taking sulfisoxazole three times a day or more, you can take the missed dose and the next one at the same time.
• If you miss an application of eye ointment or eye drops, do it as soon as you remember, but skip it if it is almost time for the next application.

Interactions with Other Drugs

The following drugs are listed in the *Evaluations of Drug Interactions* 1997 as causing "highly clinically significant" or "clinically significant" interactions when used together with this drug. We have also included potentially serious interactions listed in the drug's FDA-approved professional product labeling or package insert. New scientific techniques have allowed researchers to predict some drug interactions before they have been documented in people. There may be other drugs, especially those in the families of drugs listed below, that also will react with this drug to cause severe adverse effects. The number of new drugs approved for marketing increases the chance of drug interactions, and new drug interactions are being identified with old drugs. Be vigilant. Make sure to tell your doctor and pharmacist the drugs you are taking and tell your doctor if you are taking any of these interacting drugs:

COUMADIN, DILANTIN, methotrexate, ORINASE, phenytoin, RHEUMATREX DOSE PACK, tolbutamide, warfarin.

Adverse Effects

Call your doctor immediately if you experience:

- increased sensitivity of skin to sun (increased sunburn)
- skin rash, itching, blistering or peeling
- aching joints or muscles
- difficulty swallowing
- fever, pale skin, or sore throat
- abnormal bleeding or bruising
- abnormal tiredness or weakness
- yellow eyes or skin
- lower back pain
- increase in thirst
- difficulty urinating
- severe abdominal or stomach cramps
- watery and severe diarrhea (may be bloody)
- mood or mental changes
- swelling of neck

Call your doctor if these symptoms continue:

- diarrhea
- dizziness or headache
- loss of appetite
- nausea or vomiting

Periodic Tests

Ask your doctor which of these tests should be done periodically while you are taking this drug:

- complete blood count, if you take the drug for a long time
- urinalysis

PREGNANCY WARNING

This drug caused harm to developing fetuses in animal studies, or such studies were not done. Use during pregnancy only for clear medical reasons. Tell your doctor if you are pregnant or thinking of becoming pregnant before you take this drug.

 Do Not Use

ALTERNATIVE TREATMENT:
See erythromycin, p. 498.

Erythromycin Estolate
ILOSONE (Dista)

FAMILY: Antibiotics (see p. 468)

Erythromycin is one of the safest antibiotics available. However, people who use a particular type of erythromycin called erythromycin estolate (ILOSONE) are about 20 times more likely to suffer liver damage (toxicity) from the drug than people who use other forms.[105] Therefore, you should not take erythromycin estolate (ILOSONE).[106] **If you have liver disease, you should be taking less than the usual adult dose of erythromycin.**

WARNING

If you are using erythromycin do not use Propulsid, Seldane, Seldane-D or Hismanal. These drugs, when used in combination with erythromycin, can accumulate to dangerous levels in the body and can cause life-threatening, sometimes fatal heart arrhythmias.[107]

Isoniazid
INH

GENERIC: available
FAMILY: Antibiotics (see p. 468)
(for tuberculosis)

Isoniazid (eye soe *nye* a zid) is used to treat and prevent tuberculosis (TB). If you are an older adult who has had a positive TB skin test, you do not necessarily need preventive treatment for TB. You should be treated *only* if you are at special risk, for example if you have cancer, if you are taking high doses of corti-costeroid drugs on a long-term basis, or if you had a negative TB skin test until recently. If you have sudden, serious liver disease, you should not get preventive TB treatment. If you have confirmed tuberculosis, you should always get a second drug, rifampin (see p. 530), along with isoniazid, rather than taking only one. If you take only one, you may develop bacteria that are resistant to one of these drugs.[108]

Isoniazid can cause serious damage to your liver. Some people who have taken this drug, especially people over age 50, have developed severe and even fatal hepatitis (a liver disease). You are more likely to get hepatitis if you drink alcohol daily, so do not drink while taking this drug. Call your doctor immediately if you have any of the symptoms of hepatitis: fatigue, weakness, malaise (vague feeling of being unwell), loss of appetite, nausea, vomiting, or yellow eyes or skin. **Schedule monthly visits with your doctor while taking this drug. If you have impaired liver function or severe kidney failure, you should probably be taking less than the usual adult dose of isoniazid.**

A small number of people using isoniazid develop nerve pain and tenderness in their hands and feet. Taking 15 to 50 milligrams of vitamin B_6 every day can prevent this problem. If necessary, your doctor can give you a prescription for vitamin B_6 along with the isoniazid prescription.

WARNING

If you have nausea, vomiting, yellow eyes, dark urine, unexplained fatigue, or abdominal pain, stop taking this medication and call your doctor immediately.[109]

WARNING

There have been a number of case reports of liver damage involving a possible drug interaction between isoniazid, a medication used to prevent and treat tuberculosis, and acetaminophen, an over-the-counter painkiller and the active ingredient in Tylenol. Isoniazid alone, especially as people get older, has been documented to cause liver damage. Acetaminophen, alone in large doses or probably in combination with alcohol, also increases the risk of liver damage. The combination of acetaminophen with isoniazid, according to the authors of these case reports, may also be dangerous.

If you are taking isoniazid for tuberculosis or have a positive TB skin test and are using the drug, consult your physician before using acetaminophen or any combination product containing acetaminophen. Discuss alternatives to acetaminophen with your physician.[110,111]

Before You Use This Drug

Tell your doctor if you have or have had:

- allergies to drugs
- an unusual reaction to isoniazid, ethionamide, pyrazinamide, or niacin
- liver problems
- alcohol dependence
- epilepsy or seizures
- severe kidney disease

Tell your doctor about any other drugs you take, including aspirin, herbs, vitamins, and other nonprescription products.

When You Use This Drug

- Do not drink alcohol.
- Call your doctor if your symptoms do not get better in two or three weeks or if they get worse.

• You may need more vitamin B$_6$ and niacin than usual. Ask your doctor.

• Call your doctor if you get symptoms of a food reaction (see Adverse Effects).

• **Caution diabetics:** see p. 550.

• **Take all the isoniazid your doctor prescribed, even if you feel better in a few weeks. You might have to take it every day for a year or more. Do not miss doses. If you stop too soon, your symptoms could come back.**

• Do not give this drug to anyone else. Throw away outdated drugs.

• If you plan to have any surgery, including dental, tell your doctor that you take this drug.

How to Use This Drug

• Take with **a full glass (eight ounces) of water** on an empty stomach (at least one hour before or two hours after meals). If isoniazid upsets your stomach, try taking it with food. Tablets may be crushed and mixed with water.

• If you take antacids, take them at least one hour before or after you take your isoniazid.

• Do not store in the bathroom. Do not expose to heat, moisture, or direct light. Do not let the liquid form freeze.

• If you miss a dose, take it as soon as you remember, but skip it if it is almost time for the next dose. **Do not take double doses.**

Interactions with Other Drugs

The following drugs are listed in the *Evaluations of Drug Interactions* 1997 as causing "highly clinically significant" or "clinically significant" interactions when used together with this drug. We have also included potentially serious interactions listed in the drug's FDA-approved professional product labeling or package insert. New scientific techniques have allowed researchers to predict some drug interactions before they have been documented in people. There may be other drugs, especially those in the families of drugs listed below, that also will react with this drug to cause severe adverse effects. The number of new drugs approved for marketing increases the chance of drug interactions, and new drug interactions are being identified with old drugs. Be vigilant. Make sure to tell your doctor and pharmacist the drugs you are taking and tell your doctor if you are taking any of these interacting drugs:

carbamazepine, DILANTIN, phenytoin, RIFADIN, rifampin, RIMACTANE, TEGRETOL.

The following acetaminophen-containing drugs should not be taken with isoniazid (see warning box): acetaminophen, ESGIC, FIORICET, PERCOCET, TYLENOL, TYLENOL NO. 3, TYLOX, VICODIN.

Adverse Effects

Call your doctor immediately if you experience:

• **signs of overdose:** *early signs* are nausea, vomiting, dizziness, slurred speech, blurred vision, and hallucinations, including bright colors and strange designs; *late signs* are seizures, trouble breathing, stupor and coma
  • numbness, tingling, pain, or weakness of hands or feet
  • clumsiness or unsteadiness
  • dark urine
  • yellow eyes or skin
  • loss of appetite
  • light colored stools
  • headache
  • pain in stomach or abdomen
  • unexplained fatigue
  • nausea or vomiting
  • abnormal tiredness or weakness
  • blurring or changes in vision
  • seizures

- fever and sore throat
- joint pain
- depression, mood or other mental changes
- skin rash
- unusual bleeding or bruising
- **signs of food reaction:** red or itching skin, fast or pounding heartbeat, sweating, chills, or headache after eating certain foods such as cheese, fermented sausages, fish, herring, or sauerkraut. If you have such a reaction, you may have to avoid these foods while you are using isoniazid.

Call your doctor if these symptoms continue:

- dizziness or upset stomach
- breast enlargement in men
- diarrhea
- irritation at place of injection

Periodic Tests

Ask your doctor which of these tests should be done periodically while you are taking this drug:

- liver function tests, before treatment and regularly thereafter. (During nine months of treatment, you should have them at the end of months one, three, six, and nine.)
- ophthalmologic exams

Cephalexin
KEFLEX (Dista)

GENERIC: available

FAMILY: Antibiotics (see p. 468)
Cephalosporins (see p. 470)

Cephalexin (sef a *lex* in) is used to treat some infections caused by bacteria, such as infections of the bladder or soft tissues (puncture wounds or deep cuts). For most of these infections, though, you could take an antibiotic from a different family that would be just as effective as cephalexin and much less expensive.[112] **Cephalexin will not help a cold or the flu.**

Sometimes doctors prescribe cephalexin or another drug in its family because the person taking the drug is allergic to penicillin. However, there is a chance that someone allergic to penicillin will also be allergic to drugs in this family (cephalosporins).

If you have kidney disease, you may need to take less than the usual adult dose of cephalexin.

Practice measures to prevent urinary tract infections. Drink plenty of fluids, especially water. While cranberry juice is unreliable as a cure for urinary tract infections, the juice may reduce odor from incontinence.[113] Practice meticulous hygiene. After using the toilet, wipe backward, not forward, then wash your hands. Prepare and store foods properly, especially when traveling, to prevent diarrhea. Restrict caffeine, which widens the urethra. Indwelling catheters invite urinary tract infections. However, unless there are symptoms of urinary infection, it is not always necessary to take medication just because bacteria are found in a urine test.[114] Women are particularly prone to repeated urinary tract infections. If urinary tract symptoms occur often, ask your doctor about keeping a supply of medication on hand. Ideally, the antibiotic you use should be the most effective, least toxic, and least costly.[115,116]

Before You Use This Drug

Tell your doctor if you have or have had:

- allergies to drugs
- a reaction to any penicillin or cephalosporin (see p. 471 for examples)
- stomach or intestinal disease
- kidney or liver problems
- a salt (sodium)-restricted diet (the injected form of cephalexin contains sodium)

Tell your doctor about any other drugs you take, including aspirin, herbs, vitamins, and other nonprescription products.

When You Use This Drug

• Call your doctor if your symptoms do not improve in two or three days or if you get diarrhea. Do not treat the diarrhea yourself.

• **Take all the cephalexin your doctor prescribed, even if you feel better before you run out. If you stop too soon, your symptoms could come back.**

• **Caution diabetics:** see p. 550.

• Do not give this drug to anyone else. Throw away all outdated drugs.

• If you plan to have any surgery, including dental, tell your doctor that you take this drug.

How to Use This Drug

• Taking cephalexin with food may help prevent stomach upset.

• Store liquid form in the refrigerator but do not freeze. Shake well before using.

• Do not store capsules in the bathroom. Do not expose to heat, moisture, or strong light. Capsules may be opened and mixed with food or water.

• If you miss a dose, take it as soon as you remember, but skip it if it is almost time for the next dose. **Do not take double doses.**

Interactions with Other Drugs

The following drugs are listed in the *Evaluations of Drug Interactions* 1997 as causing "highly clinically significant" or "clinically significant" interactions when used together with this drug. We have also included potentially serious interactions listed in the drug's FDA-approved professional product labeling or package insert. New scientific techniques have allowed researchers to predict some drug interactions before they have been documented in people. There may be other drugs, especially those in the families of drugs listed below, that also will react with this drug to cause severe adverse effects. The number of new drugs approved for marketing increases the chance of drug interactions, and new drug interactions are being identified with old drugs. Be vigilant. Make sure to tell your doctor and pharmacist the drugs you are taking and tell your doctor if you are taking any of these interacting drugs:

BENEMID, colistimethate sodium, COLY-MYCIN M PARENTERAL, COUMADIN, GARAMYCIN, gentamicin, probenecid, warfarin.

Adverse Effects

Call your doctor immediately if you experience:

• **signs of severe allergic reaction (anaphylactic shock):** severe asthma (wheezing), extreme weakness, abdominal pain, nausea or vomiting, diarrhea, rash

Call your doctor immediately, even if it has been a month since you stopped taking cephalexin, if you experience:

• pain, cramps, or bloating in the abdomen or stomach
• severe, watery diarrhea (may contain blood)
• fever
• increased thirst
• abnormal tiredness
• abnormal weight loss or loss of appetite
• dizziness or headache
• joint pain
• skin rash, hives, itching, blistering, peeling or loosening
• swelling at place of injection
• unusual bleeding or bruising
• seizures
• urine decrease
• yellowing of eyes and skin

Call your doctor if these symptoms continue:

- mild diarrhea
- sore mouth or tongue
- mild stomach pain
- itching in the genital or rectal area

Periodic Tests

Ask your doctor which of these tests should be done periodically while you are taking this drug:

- bleeding time
- prothrombin time
- stool exam

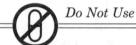

Do Not Use

ALTERNATIVE TREATMENT:
Nonprescription permethrin (Nix).

Lindane (gamma benzene hexachloride)
KWELL (Reedco)

FAMILY: Pediculicide, Scabicide

Lindane *(lynn* dane) shampoo is available to treat head lice, while lindane cream and lotion are available to treat scabies. Outbreaks of head lice are commonplace in day care centers, schools, and nursing homes. Scabies is epidemic in nursing homes, homeless shelters, and among people with AIDS.

Treatment of lice or scabies with lindane is neither safe nor effective. Lindane is a pesticide of the type called an organochlorine, in the same group as DDT. Although the Environmental Protection Agency drastically cut the amount of lindane used in industry and agriculture, this toxin is still available. Workers exposed to lindane for a long time may eventually develop damage to their bone marrow, kidneys, liver, and reproductive organs.[117] Lindane is classified as a carcinogen. Even individuals who use lindane briefly for lice or scabies, as well as people whose work exposes them to lindane, can experience rashes, dizziness, or convulsions. Vomiting, muscle cramps, nervousness, unsteadiness, and fast heartbeat have also been reported.

Lindane is readily absorbed through the skin, particularly skin that is broken or has residues of oils on it. Crusts formed in Norwegian scabies increase absorption of lindane even more.[118] The Centers for Disease Control and Prevention recommends that bathing prior to applying lindane lotion be avoided since toxicity is increased.[119] Lindane is contraindicated for premature infants. Children and the elderly are particularly prone to convulsions from lindane.[120] A further tragedy associated with lindane is misuse in infants and children. Lindane has been left on the skin 12 hours or longer without being washed off.[121] Such misuse has been fatal to some children.

A review of clinical tests of head lice products found that in the few well-designed studies lindane proved so ineffective that continued use could not be justified.[122] While no pediculicide is 100% effective, failure was at least eight times more likely with lindane than with permethrin (NIX). Lack of effectiveness encourages repeat applications. Prolonged use of lindane has lowered production of red blood cells. Concern also exists since some mites are now resistant to lindane and lice are suspected of developing resistance to lindane, as well as to alternative medications.

In 1995 Public Citizen filed a petition with the Food and Drug Administration to ban lindane.[123] The FDA later changed labeling requirements for lindane. Although repulsive, lice are not life-threatening.

Do Not Use

ALTERNATIVE TREATMENT:
See Clindamycin, p. 491.

Lincomycin
LINCOCIN (Pharmacia & Upjohn)

FAMILY: Antibiotics (see p. 468)

Lincomycin (lin koe *mye* sin) is similar to another antibiotic called clindamycin (see p. 491) and is also used to treat infections. Lincomycin does *not* have any advantage over clindamycin.[124] It is hard for your body to absorb, and it has more unwanted adverse effects than clindamycin. It should not be used.

Do Not Use

ALTERNATIVE TREATMENT:
See Ampicillin, p. 522, Trimethoprim, p. 528, and Trimethoprim and Sulfamethoxazole, p. 478.

Nitrofurantoin
MACRODANTIN (Proctor & Gamble)
FURADANTIN (Dura)
MACROBID (Proctor & Gamble)

FAMILY: Antibiotics (see p. 468)

Nitrofurantoin (nye troe fyoor *an* toyn) is used to treat certain urinary tract infections. **It is a dangerous drug and should not be used.** People over 60 who take this drug have such a high risk of harmful adverse effects that the World Health Organization has said older adults should not use it.[125]

Because your kidneys normally work less effectively as you grow older, they do not eliminate this drug from your body fast enough. Because of this, nitrofurantoin accumulates to dangerously high levels in your bloodstream, causing adverse effects. Two of the possible adverse effects, a nerve disease called peripheral neuropathy and scarring of the lungs, may be irreversible, and deaths from these adverse effects have been reported.[126] You can almost always take another drug that will be just as effective as nitrofurantoin and much safer. **If you are taking this drug, ask your doctor to change your prescription.**

Practice measures to prevent urinary tract infections. Drink plenty of fluids, especially water. While cranberry juice is unreliable as a cure for urinary tract infections, the juice may reduce odor from incontinence.[127] Practice meticulous hygiene. After using the toilet, wipe backward, not forward, then wash your hands. Prepare and store foods properly, especially when traveling, to prevent diarrhea. Restrict caffeine, which widens the urethra. Indwelling catheters invite urinary tract infections. However, unless there are symptoms of urinary infection, it is not always necessary to take medication just because bacteria are found in a urine test.[128] Women are particularly prone to repeated urinary tract infections. If urinary tract symptoms occur often, ask your doctor about keeping a supply of medication on hand. Ideally, the antibiotic you use should be the most effective, least toxic, and least costly.[129,130]

Miconazole
MONISTAT-DERM (Ortho)
MONISTAT 7 (Ortho)

GENERIC: available
FAMILY: Antifungals

Miconazole (mi *kon* a zole) is used to treat fungal infections and is available in several forms, including a cream, a lotion, and tablets. Since miconazole is most often used for skin and vaginal infections, the information here deals mostly with these forms of the drug.

Mild vaginal infections are often self-limiting.[131] For some women a bland cream (without drugs) relieves symptoms until infection spontaneously goes away.[132] Preventive measures include less sugar in the diet, and avoiding tight-fitting pants and panty hose. Cotton is preferable to synthetics.[133] Dry the vaginal area thoroughly after bathing or swimming.

Before You Use This Drug

Tell your doctor if you have or have had:

- allergies to drugs
- an unusual reaction to miconazole
- other allergies
- kidney or liver problems
- alcohol abuse

Tell your doctor about any other drugs you take, including aspirin, herbs, vitamins, and other nonprescription products.

When You Use This Drug

- **Take all the miconazole your doctor prescribed, even if you feel better before you finish. If you stop too soon, your symptoms could come back.**
- Do not give this drug to anyone else. Throw away outdated drugs.
- Do not store in the bathroom. Do not expose to heat, moisture, or strong light.

Using miconazole lotion, skin cream, liquid, or aerosol powder:

- Call your doctor if your skin problem does not improve within four to six weeks. (It will usually improve in the first week.)
- Call your doctor immediately if new symptoms appear—skin rash, itching, swelling, or other signs of skin irritation. This is rare.

Using miconazole vaginal cream or tablets:

- Call your doctor immediately if you develop new symptoms of vaginal burning, a skin rash, or abdominal cramps, or if your sex part-

ner feels burning or irritation of his penis after you start this treatment.
- Wear freshly washed cotton underwear. Wearing a sanitary napkin will protect your clothes from fluids draining from your vagina.
- Ask your doctor if you have questions about douching or having sex during treatment.

How to Use This Drug

Using miconazole lotion, skin cream, liquid, or aerosol powder:

- Apply enough to cover the affected area of skin and the surrounding area, and rub in gently.
- Do not apply an airtight dressing unless your doctor recommends it.
- Shake lotion and aerosol powder well before using.
- If you miss a dose, apply it as soon as you remember, but skip it if it is almost time for the next dose.
- Avoid getting this drug in your eyes.

Using miconazole vaginal cream or tablets:

- If you miss a dose, insert it as soon as you remember, but skip it if you don't remember until the next day.

Interactions with Other Drugs

Some other drugs that you may be taking (either over-the-counter or prescription drugs) can interact with this one, causing adverse effects. Ask your doctor what these drugs are and let him or her know if you are taking any of them.

When using topical products it is advisable not to apply other topical preparations, including cosmetics, to the same site. This prevents interactions that could irritate your skin.

Adverse Effects

Call your doctor immediately if you experience:

- redness, swelling or pain at site of injection
- fever and chills

- skin rash or itching
- dark or amber urine
- sore throat
- loss of appetite
- pale stools
- reddening, blistering, peeling of skin and mucous membranes
- stomach pain
- abnormal bleeding or bruising
- unusual tiredness or weakness
- yellow eyes or skin

Call your doctor if these symptoms continue:

- constipation
- diarrhea
- dizziness
- drowsiness
- flushing or redness of face or skin
- headache
- nausea or vomiting

Periodic Tests

Ask your doctor which of these tests should be done periodically while you are taking this drug:

- blood urea nitrogen tests
- liver function tests
- potassium serum levels

Clotrimazole
MYCELEX (Bayer)
LOTRIMIN (Schering)
GYNE-LOTRIMIN (Schering)

GENERIC: available
FAMILY: Antifungals

Clotrimazole (kloe *trim* a zole) is used to treat fungal infections in different parts of the body. For skin infections, you may be given clotrima-zole cream, lotion, or liquid to apply externally; for vaginal infections, vaginal cream or tablets placed in the vagina; and for mouth and throat infections, lozenges placed in the mouth. Since most often use of clotrimazole is for skin and vaginal infections, the information here deals mostly with these forms of the drug.

Mild vaginal infections are often self-limiting.[134] For some women a bland cream (without drugs) relieves symptoms until infection spontaneously goes away.[135] Preventive measures include less sugar in the diet, and avoiding tight-fitting pants and panty hose. Cotton is preferable to synthetics.[136] Dry the vaginal area thoroughly after bathing or swimming.

Before You Use This Drug

Tell your doctor if you have or have had:

- allergies to drugs
- an unusual reaction to clotrimazole
- other allergies

Tell your doctor about any other drugs you take, including aspirin, herbs, vitamins, and other nonprescription products.

When You Use This Drug

- **Take all the clotrimazole your doctor prescribed, even if you feel better before you finish. If you stop too soon, your symptoms could come back.**
- Do not give this drug to anyone else. Throw away outdated drugs.

How to Use This Drug

- Do not store in the bathroom. Do not expose to heat, moisture, or strong light.

Using clotrimazole skin cream, lotion, and liquid:

- Apply enough to cover the affected skin and the surrounding area, and rub in gently.
- Do not use an airtight bandage unless your doctor recommends it.

• If you miss a dose, apply it as soon as you remember, but skip it if it is almost time for the next dose.

• Avoid getting this drug in your eyes.

• Call your doctor if your skin problem does not improve within four weeks. (Usually it will improve in the first week.)

• Call your doctor immediately if new symptoms appear—skin rash, itching, swelling, or other signs of skin irritation. This is rare.

Using clotrimazole vaginal cream or tablets:

• If you miss a dose, insert it as soon as you remember, but skip it if you don't remember until the next day.

• Call your doctor immediately if you get new symptoms of vaginal burning, a skin rash, or abdominal cramps, or if your sex partner feels burning or irritation of his penis after you start this treatment.

• Wear freshly washed cotton underwear. Wearing a sanitary napkin will protect your clothes from fluid draining from your vagina.

• Ask your doctor if you have questions about douching or having sex during treatment.

Interactions with Other Drugs

Some other drugs that you may be taking (either over-the-counter or prescription drugs) can interact with this one, causing adverse effects. Ask your doctor what these drugs are and let him or her know if you are taking any of them.

When using topical products it is advisable not to apply other topical preparations, including cosmetics, to the same site. This prevents interactions that could irritate your skin.

Adverse Effects

Call your doctor immediately if you experience:

• vaginal burning, itching discharge or other irritation
• skin rash or hives

Call your doctor if these symptoms continue:

• abdominal or stomach cramps
• burning or irritation of penis of sexual partner
• headache

PREGNANCY WARNING

This drug caused harm to developing fetuses in animal studies, or such studies were not done. Use during pregnancy only for clear medical reasons. Tell your doctor if you are pregnant or thinking of becoming pregnant before you take this drug.

 Do Not Use

ALTERNATIVE TREATMENT:
Separate antifungal and corticosteroid ointments or creams.

Nystatin and Triamcinolone
MYCOBIOTIC II (Moore)
MYCOLOG II (Apothecon)

FAMILY: Antifungals
          Corticosteroids (see p. 651)

This combination of nystatin (see p. 517) and triamcinolone (see p. 656) is commonly prescribed by dermatologists (skin doctors) to treat fungal skin infections, such as the yeast infection called candidiasis. However, *one* of its ingredients, triamcinolone, may actually be dangerous to an infection because drugs in its family can hide the signs of an infection or make it spread. Therefore, this drug product is an irrational combination for treating an infection. Instead, your doctor should prescribe nystatin alone.

If you have a fungal skin infection that is inflamed, itching, or scaly, it may be appropriate to use hydrocortisone (see p. 660) in addition to an antifungal ointment such as nystatin for a few days. Each drug should be applied *separately* in a ratio determined by your doctor.

This drug, sold under the brand name Mycolog II, also has an older form which is called Mycolog cream. Mycolog cream is a combination of neomycin and gramacidin, and it should not be used either. Neomycin commonly causes skin rashes in 8% of the people who use it.[137] Using neomycin can also make it hard for you to use other drugs in its family (aminoglycoside antibiotics, such as gentamicin and tobramycin, see p. 635) that may be needed later for serious infections.[138]

Nystatin
MYCOSTATIN (Bristol-Myers Squibb)

GENERIC: available
FAMILY: Antifungals

Nystatin (nye *stat* in) is used to treat fungal infections in different parts of the body. For infections in your mouth, you may be given a liquid or powder form of nystatin, for intestinal infections, tablets that are swallowed, for a vaginal infection, tablets that are inserted in the vagina, and for skin infections, a powder that you apply to your skin.

Before You Use This Drug

Tell your doctor if you have or have had:

- allergies to drugs
- an unusual reaction to nystatin

Tell your doctor about any other drugs you take, including aspirin, herbs, vitamins, and other nonprescription products.

When You Use This Drug

- **Take all the nystatin your doctor prescribed, even if you feel better before you finish. If you stop too soon, your symptoms could come back.**
- Do not give this drug to anyone else. Throw away outdated drugs.

How to Use This Drug

- Do not store in the bathroom. Do not expose to heat, moisture, or strong light. Do not let the liquid form freeze.
- If you miss a dose, take it as soon as you remember, but skip it if it is almost time for the next dose. **Do not take double doses.**

Taking nystatin by mouth:

- *Dry powder:* When it is time to take a dose, add about ⅛ teaspoon of dry powder to a glass of water and stir well. Take one mouthful of this mixture and hold it in your mouth, swishing it around for as long as you can before swallowing. Continue, one mouthful at a time, until the whole glass is gone.
- *Liquid (suspension):* Shake well. Measure out the dose and put half of it in each side of your mouth. Hold it in your mouth or swish it around as long as you can before swallowing.

Using nystatin skin cream, ointment, or powder:

- Apply enough to cover the affected area.
- Do not use an airtight bandage unless your doctor recommends it.
- For fungal infection of the feet, dust powder onto feet, socks, and shoes.
- Call your doctor immediately if new symptoms appear—skin rash, itching, swelling, or other signs of skin irritation. This is rare.
- Do not let cream or ointment freeze.

Using nystatin vaginal tablets:

- If you miss a dose, insert it as soon as you remember, but skip it if you don't remember until the next day.

• Call your doctor immediately if you get new vaginal burning, a skin rash, or abdominal cramps.

• Wear freshly washed cotton underwear. Wearing a sanitary napkin will protect your clothes from fluid draining from your vagina.

• Ask your doctor if you have questions about douching or having sex during treatment.

Interactions with Other Drugs

Some other drugs that you may be taking (either over-the-counter or prescription drugs) can interact with this one, causing adverse effects. Ask your doctor what these drugs are and let him or her know if you are taking any of them.

When using topical products it is advisable not to apply other topical preparations, including cosmetics, to the same site. This prevents interactions that could irritate your skin.

Adverse Reactions

Call your doctor immediately if you experience:

- diarrhea
- nausea or vomiting
- stomach pain
- skin or vaginal irritation

PREGNANCY WARNING

This drug caused harm to developing fetuses in animal studies, or such studies were not done. Use during pregnancy only for clear medical reasons. Tell your doctor if you are pregnant or thinking of becoming pregnant before you take this drug.

 Do Not Use

ALTERNATIVE TREATMENT:
Cleaning the infected area well and taking antibiotics by mouth or as injections, if necessary.

Neomycin, Polymyxin B, and Bacitracin
NEOSPORIN MAXIMUM STRENGTH OINTMENT (Warner-Lambert)
MYCITRACIN (Pharmacia & Upjohn)

FAMILY: Antibiotics (see p. 468)

This combination of three antibiotics—neomycin (nee oh *mye* sin), polymyxin (pol i *mix* in) B, and bacitracin (bass i *tray* sin)—is used to treat a wide variety of skin infections. It is also used to prevent infection in burns or broken skin. It is available as an aerosol spray, powder, and ointment.

There is no satisfactory evidence that antibiotics applied directly to the skin (as opposed to injected or swallowed) help healing or prevent infection. Uninfected, well-cleaned wounds usually heal by themselves. If a wound is infected and antibiotics are needed, they should be given by mouth or by injection.

Despite the controversy over external use of antibiotics, dermatologists (skin doctors) often prescribe this combination drug to treat some superficial skin infections, such as inflammation of hair follicles (folliculitis) and impetigo.

Neomycin commonly causes skin rashes in 8% of the people who use it.[139] Using neomycin can also make it hard for you to use other drugs in its family (aminoglycoside antibiotics, such as gentamicin and tobramycin, see p. 635) that may be needed later for serious infections.

Norfloxacin
NOROXIN Tablets (Merck)
CHIBROXIN Eye Drops (Merck)

GENERIC: available
FAMILY: Antibiotics (see p. 468)
Fluoroquinolones (see p. 472)

Norfloxacin (nor *flocks* a sin) kills bacteria and can cure infections caused by susceptible organisms. Oral norfloxacin is used only to treat infections in the urinary tract, prostate gland, and sexually transmitted diseases. Drops of norfloxacin are used to treat eye infections.

Elderly people have suffered more severe adverse effects, fatalities, and harmful interactions from norfloxacin.[140,141] **Since in people over age 65 norfloxacin is excreted more slowly, a lower dose is usually used.**

Norfloxacin belongs to a family of drugs called fluoroquinolones. These drugs are alternatives for individuals allergic to, or with infections resistant to, other antibiotics. A seven-day course of norfloxacin costs 5 to 10 times more than drugs such as amoxicillin (see p. 476) or trimethoprim and sulfamethoxazole (see p. 478), which are equally effective for most infections. Both resistance and allergy to one drug in this family usually cross to the rest of the fluoroquinolones and sometimes even occur during therapy.[142,143] Overgrowth of normal bacteria may cause yeast infections, especially when antibiotics are used for long periods. The fluoroquinolones can cause central nervous system reactions and psychosis.[144] Severe, even fatal, allergic reactions have happened after just one dose. Collapse of the circulatory system has occurred. As a group fluoroquinolones are expensive, resistance is increasing, and effective alternatives are available.[145]

The same adverse effects of norfloxacin can result from either oral tablets or eye drops.

Practice measures to prevent urinary tract infections. Drink plenty of fluids, especially water. While cranberry juice is unreliable as a cure for urinary tract infections, the juice may reduce odor from incontinence.[146] Practice meticulous hygiene. After using the toilet, wipe backward, not forward, then wash your hands. Prepare and store foods properly, especially when traveling, to prevent diarrhea. Restrict caffeine, which widens the urethra. Indwelling catheters invite urinary tract infections. However, unless there are symptoms of urinary infection, it is not always necessary to take medication just because bacteria are found in a urine test.[147] Women are particularly prone to repeated urinary tract infections. If urinary tract symptoms occur often, ask your doctor about keeping a supply of medication on hand. Ideally, the antibiotic you use should be the most effective, least toxic, and least costly.[148,149]

WARNING

Extreme caution should be used when fluoroquinolones such as norfloxacin are to be prescribed in conjunction with aminophylline or theophylline, particularly in elderly patients. Aminophylline or theophylline doses should be adjusted, perhaps reduced by 30% to 50% at the initiation of fluoroquinolone therapy. The reduction in dose must be guided by the clinical conditions of the patient, the use of other medications, and the baseline level of the aminophylline or theophylline in the blood. In addition, aminophylline or theophylline levels in the blood should be obtained following the start of a fluoroquinolone no later than two days into therapy.[150]

Before You Use This Drug

Tell your doctor if you have or have had:

- allergies to drugs
- epilepsy
- kidney or liver problems
- seizures
- brain or spinal cord disease

Tell your doctor about any other drugs you take, including aspirin, herbs, vitamins, and other nonprescription products.

When You Use This Drug

- Do not drive or perform other activities that require alertness because this drug may make you drowsy, dizzy, or lightheaded.
- **Take all the norfloxacin your doctor prescribed, even if you feel better before you run out. If you stop too soon, your symptoms could come back.**
- Drink several glasses of fluids (water, fruit, and vegetable juices) each day. This flushes bacteria out of your bladder and prevents crystals of norfloxacin from forming.
- Restrict your use of caffeine.
- Limit exposure to bright light. Protect yourself from sunburn by wearing protective clothing, headgear, and sunglasses, and using a sunblock.
- If you plan to have any surgery, including dental, tell your doctor that you take this drug.

How to Use This Drug

- Swallow tablet whole. Take with **a full glass (eight ounces) of water,** one hour before or two hours after meals. Space doses evenly apart.
- Instill eyedrops according to instructions on p. 622.
- Avoid touching the tip of the container in or around your eye.

- Do not take antacids, sucralfate (CARAFATE), or products containing iron or zinc within two hours of taking norfloxacin.
- Do not store in the bathroom. Do not expose to heat, moisture, or strong light.
- If you miss a dose, take it as soon as you remember, but skip it if it is almost time for the next dose. **Do not take double doses.**

Interactions with Other Drugs

The following drugs are listed in the *Evaluations of Drug Interactions* 1997 as causing "highly clinically significant" or "clinically significant" interactions when used together with this drug. We have also included potentially serious interactions listed in the drug's FDA-approved professional product labeling or package insert. New scientific techniques have allowed researchers to predict some drug interactions before they have been documented in people. There may be other drugs, especially those in the families of drugs listed below, that also will react with this drug to cause severe adverse effects. The number of new drugs approved for marketing increases the chance of drug interactions, and new drug interactions are being identified with old drugs. Be vigilant. Make sure to tell your doctor and pharmacist the drugs you are taking and tell your doctor if you are taking any of these interacting drugs:

aluminum hydroxide, AMPHOJEL, caffeine (beverages, drugs), CARAFATE, cyclosporine, FEOSOL, FERGON, ferrous gluconate, ferrous sulfate, MAALOX, magnesium hydroxide, NEORAL, PHILLIPS' MILK OF MAGNESIA, SANDIMMUNE, SLOW FE, sucralfate.

A report in the *Archives of Internal Medicine* adds interaction with COUMADIN, warfarin as one most frequently reported in older people.[151]

Caution should be taken when the following drugs are used with this one (see warning box): aminophylline, ELIXOPHYLLIN, SLO-BID, SOMOPHYLLIN, SOMO-PHYLLIN–DF, THEO-24, theophylline.

Adverse Effects

Call your doctor immediately if you experience:

- agitation
- difficulty breathing or swallowing
- confusion, disorientation
- depression
- fainting
- fever
- hallucinations
- numbness
- seizures
- skin rash, itching or redness
- swelling of face, neck, tongue, fingers, joints, calves or lower legs
- tremors
- blurred vision
- pain at site of injection
- pain in calves radiating to heels

Call your doctor if these symptoms continue:

- abdominal pain
- anxiety, irritability, restlessness
- constipation, diarrhea
- dizziness, lightheadedness
- drowsiness, fatigue
- dry mouth
- headache
- indigestion
- insomnia, unusual dreams
- loss of appetite
- nausea or vomiting
- sensitivity to light, sunburn
- stomach pain
- bitter taste

WARNING

INCREASED RISK OF TENDINITIS AND TENDON RUPTURE WITH ALL FLUOROQUINOLONE ANTIBIOTICS

Public Citizen's Health Research Group petitioned the Food and Drug Administration (FDA) to add a warning for doctors to the labeling, or package, for all fluoroquinolone antibiotics about the risk of tendinitis, including the possibility of complete tendon rupture.

This adverse reaction most frequently involves the Achilles tendon, the tendon that runs from the back of the heel to the calf. Rupture of the Achilles tendon may require surgical repair. Tendons in the rotator cuff (the shoulder), the hand, the biceps, and the thumb have also been involved. This reaction appears to be more common in those taking steroid drugs, in older patients, and in kidney transplant recipients, but cases have occurred in people without any of these risk factors. The onset of symptoms is sudden and has occurred as soon as 24 hours after starting treatment with a fluoroquinolone. Most people have recovered completely after one to two months.

If you experience unexpected tendon pain while taking a fluoroquinolone antibiotic, stop the drug immediately, call your doctor, and rest.

PREGNANCY WARNING

This drug caused harm to developing fetuses in animal studies, or such studies were not done. Use during pregnancy only for clear medical reasons. Tell your doctor if you are pregnant or thinking of becoming pregnant before you take this drug.

Ampicillin
OMNIPEN (Wyeth-Ayerst)
POLYCILLIN (Apothecon)

GENERIC: available

FAMILY: Antibiotics (see p. 468)
         Penicillins (see p. 470)

Ampicillin (am pi *sill* in) is used to treat some bacterial infections such as ear, sinus, bladder, and intestinal infections, and to treat people with chronic lung disease who have acute bronchitis. **Ampicillin will not help if you have a cold or the flu. If you have kidney disease, you may need to take less than the usual adult dose of ampicillin.**

Many people who take ampicillin develop a slight skin rash. This may or may not be a sign that you are allergic to the drug. If you get a skin rash, call your doctor. Some of ampicillin's adverse effects can appear as much as a month after you stop taking it (see Adverse Effects).

Practice measures to prevent urinary tract infections. Drink plenty of fluids, especially water. While cranberry juice is unreliable as a cure for urinary tract infections, the juice may reduce odor from incontinence.[152] Practice meticulous hygiene. After using the toilet, wipe backward, not forward, then wash your hands. Prepare and store foods properly, especially when traveling, to prevent diarrhea. Restrict caffeine, which widens the urethra. Indwelling catheters invite urinary tract infections. However, unless there are symptoms of urinary infection, it is not always necessary to take medication just because bacteria are found in a urine test.[153] Women are particularly prone to repeated urinary tract infections. If urinary tract symptoms occur often, ask your doctor about keeping a supply of medication on hand. Ideally, the antibiotic you use should be the most effective, least toxic, and least costly.[154,155]

Before You Use This Drug

Tell your doctor if you have or have had:

- allergies to drugs
- a reaction to any penicillin or cephalosporin (see p. 471 for examples)
- other allergies
- stomach or intestinal disease
- kidney problems
- infectious mononucleosis
- a salt (sodium)-restricted diet (the injected form of ampicillin contains sodium)

Tell your doctor about any other drugs you take, including aspirin, herbs, vitamins, and other nonprescription products.

When You Use This Drug

- Call your doctor if your symptoms do not improve in two or three days or if you get diarrhea. Do not treat the diarrhea yourself.
- **Take all the ampicillin your doctor prescribed, even if you feel better before you run out. If you stop too soon, your symptoms could come back.**
- Do not give the drug to anyone else. Throw away outdated drugs.
- **Caution diabetics:** see p. 550.
- If you plan to have any surgery, including dental, tell your doctor that you take this drug.

How to Use This Drug

- Take ampicillin on an empty stomach (at least one hour before or two hours after meals) with **a full glass (eight ounces) of water.** Capsules may be opened and mixed with water.
- Store liquid form in the refrigerator but do not freeze. Shake well before using.
- Do not store capsules in the bathroom. Do not expose to heat, moisture, or strong light.
- If you miss a dose, take it as soon as you remember, but skip it if it is almost time for the next dose. **Do not take double doses.**

Interactions with Other Drugs

The following drugs are listed in the *Evaluations of Drug Interactions* 1997 as causing "highly clinically significant" or "clinically significant" interactions when used together with this drug. We have also included potentially serious interactions listed in the drug's FDA-approved professional product labeling or package insert. New scientific techniques have allowed researchers to predict some drug interactions before they have been documented in people. There may be other drugs, especially those in the families of drugs listed below, that also will react with this drug to cause severe adverse effects. The number of new drugs approved for marketing increases the chance of drug interactions, and new drug interactions are being identified with old drugs. Be vigilant. Make sure to tell your doctor and pharmacist the drugs you are taking and tell your doctor if you are taking any of these interacting drugs:

AUREOMYCIN, chlortetracycline, COUMADIN, GARAMYCIN, gentamicin, heparin, oral contraceptives, warfarin.

Adverse Effects

Call your doctor immediately if you experience:

- **signs of severe allergic reaction (anaphylactic shock):** severe asthma (wheezing), extreme weakness, puffiness or swelling around face, abdominal pain, nausea or vomiting, diarrhea, skin rash

Call your doctor immediately, even if it has been a month since you stopped taking ampicillin, if you experience:

- pain, cramps, or bloating in the abdomen or stomach
- severe, watery diarrhea (may contain blood)
- fever and sore throat

- nausea or vomiting
- increased thirst
- abnormal weakness or tiredness
- abnormal weight loss
- seizures
- difficulty urinating
- depression
- unusual bleeding or bruising
- yellow eyes or skin
- pain at site of injection

Call your doctor if these symptoms continue:

- mild diarrhea
- sore mouth or tongue
- darkened or discolored tongue
- vaginal itching and discharge

Periodic Tests

Ask your doctor which of these tests should be done periodically while you are taking this drug:

- stool cytotoxin assays

Limited Use

Enoxacin (en *ox* a sin)
PENETREX (Rhone-Poulenc Rorer)

Lomefloxacin (loe me *flox* a sin)
MAXAQUIN (Searle)

 Do Not Use

Sparfloxacin (spar *flox* a sin)
ZAGAM (Rhone-Poulenc Rorer)

Grepafloxacin (grep a *flox* a sin)
RAXAR (Glaxo Wellcome)

Do Not Use Until Five Years After Release (Except for Community-acquired Bacterial Pneumonia)

Levofloxacin (Do Not Use Until 2003)
LEVAQUIN (Ortho-McNeil)

Do Not Use Until Five Years After Release

Trovafloxacin (Do Not Use Until 2004)
TORVAN (Pfizer)

GENERIC: not available

FAMILY: Antibiotics (see p. 468)
Fluoroquinolones (see p. 472)

Trovafloxacin (trov a *flox* a sin) is the newest member of the fluoroquinolone family and because of this it is the one we know the least about. Grepafloxacin is also new and is being promoted for community-acquired pneumonia and a number of other types of infections. Levofloxacin (levo *flox* a sin), is listed as do not use until five years after release except for community-acquired bacterial pneumonia. We have made this designation because many of the bacteria that cause pneumonia have become resistant to older antibiotics and this drug may be your only future option for this very serious infection.[156]

Enoxacin is used for urinary tract infections and uncomplicated gonorrhea. It is similar to norfloxacin and lomefloxacin. It offers no advantage over ciprofloxacin, ofloxacin, or many other drugs that can be used to treat urinary tract infections or gonorrhea.[157] Each of the fluoroquinolones differs in its likelihood of causing harmful adverse effects.

Practice measures to prevent urinary tract infections. Drink plenty of fluids, especially water. While cranberry juice is unreliable as a cure for urinary tract infections, the juice may reduce odor from incontinence.[158] Practice meticulous hygiene. After using the toilet, wipe backward, not forward, then wash your hands. Prepare and store foods properly, especially when traveling, to prevent diarrhea. Restrict caffeine, which widens the urethra. Indwelling catheters invite urinary tract infections. However, unless there are symptoms of urinary infection, it is not always necessary to take medication just because bacteria are found in a urine test.[159] Women are particularly prone to repeated urinary tract infections. If urinary tract symptoms occur often, ask your doctor about keeping a supply of medication on hand. Ideally, the antibiotic you use should be the most effective, least toxic, and least costly.[160,161]

WARNING

Extreme caution should be used when fluoroquinolones are to be prescribed in conjunction with aminophylline or theophylline, particularly in elderly patients. Aminophylline or theophylline doses should be adjusted, perhaps reduced by 30% to 50% at the initiation of fluoroquinolone therapy. The reduction in dose must be guided by the clinical conditions of the patient, the use of other medications, and the baseline level of the aminophylline or theophylline in the blood. In addition, aminophylline or theophylline levels in the blood should be obtained following the start of a fluoroquinolone no later than two days into therapy.[162]

WARNING

GREPAFLOXACIN (RAXAR) AND SPARFLOXACIN (ZAGAM)

DRUG INTERACTIONS THAT CAN LEAD TO HEART RHYTHM DISTURBANCES

The FDA-approved package inserts for grepafloxacin and sparfloxacin warn that these fluoroquinolone antibiotics should not be used with other drugs that can potentially cause heart rhythm disturbances. These drugs include: amiodarone (Cordarone), astemizole (Hismanal), bepridil (Vascor), cisapride (Propulsid), disopyramide (Norpace and generics), erythromycin (EES, Erythrocin and generics), flecainide (Tambocor), mexiletine (Mexitil and generics), moricizine (Ethmozine), pentamidine (Pentam 300, Nebupent), phenothiazine antipsychotics, procainamide (Procanbid and generics), propafenone (Rythmol), quinidine (Duraquin, Quinaglute Duratabs, Quinidex, and generics), sotalol (Betapace), terfenadine (Seldane was removed from the market February 27, 1998), tocainide (Tonocard), and tricyclic antidepressants.

Tell your doctor if you have or have had:

- allergies to drugs
- brain or spinal cord disease
- epilepsy or seizures
- kidney and liver problems
- kidney problems alone

Tell your doctor about any other drugs you take, including aspirin, herbs, vitamins, and other nonprescription products. It is especially important you tell your doctor if you take any theophylline drug (See p. 426).

When You Use This Drug

- **Take all the antibiotic your doctor prescribed, even if you feel better before you run out. If you stop too soon, your symptoms could come back.**
- Do not drive or perform other activities that require alertness because these drugs may make you drowsy, dizzy, or lightheaded.
- Drink plenty of fluids.
- Protect yourself from sunburn. Do not use a sunlamp.
- If you plan to have any surgery, including dental, tell your doctor that you take these drugs.

How to Use This Drug

- Swallow tablet whole with **a full glass (eight ounces) of water.**
- If you miss a dose, take it as soon as you remember, but skip it if it is almost time for the next dose. **Do not take double doses.**
- Do not store in the bathroom. Do not expose to heat, moisture, or strong light.
- Do not take antacids, sucralfate (CARAFATE), or products containing iron or zinc within two hours of taking these drugs.

Interactions with Other Drugs

The following drugs are listed in the *Evaluations of Drug Interactions* 1997 as causing "highly clinically significant" or "clinically significant" interactions when used together with these drugs. We have also included potentially serious interactions listed in the drug's FDA-approved professional product labeling or package insert. New scientific techniques have allowed researchers to predict some drug interactions before they have been documented in people. There may be other drugs, especially those in the families of drugs listed below, that also will react with these drugs to cause severe adverse effects. The number of new drugs approved for marketing increases the chance of drug interactions, and new drug interactions are being identified with old drugs. Be vigilant. Make sure to tell your doctor and pharmacist the drugs you are taking and tell your doctor if you are taking any of these interacting drugs:

> aluminum hydroxide, AMPHOJEL, caffeine (beverages or drugs), calcium carbonate, CALTRATE, CARAFATE, COUMADIN, cyclosporine, FEOSOL, ferrous sulfate, MAALOX, magnesium hydroxide, NEORAL, OS–CAL 500, PHILLIPS' MILK OF MAGNESIA, SANDIMMUNE, SLOW FE, sucralfate, warfarin.

> *Caution should be taken when the following drugs are used with this one (see warning box):* aminophylline, ELIXOPHYLLIN, SLO-BID, SOMOPHYLLIN, SOMO-PHYLLIN–DF, THEO-24, theophylline.

Adverse Effects

Call your doctor immediately if you experience:

- agitation
- difficulty breathing
- confusion, hallucinations
- fever
- skin rash, itching, redness, peeling
- seizure
- swelling of face, neck, calves or lower legs
- tremors
- blurred vision
- pain at site of injection
- pain in calves radiating to heels

Call your doctor if these symptoms continue:

- dizziness, lightheadedness
- drowsiness
- headache
- insomnia, restlessness
- nausea, vomiting, diarrhea
- pain in abdomen, stomach, joints
- increased sensitivity of skin to sunlight

WARNING

INCREASED RISK OF TENDINITIS AND TENDON RUPTURE WITH ALL FLUO-ROQUINOLONE ANTIBIOTICS

Public Citizen's Health Research Group petitioned the Food and Drug Administration (FDA) to add a warning for doctors to the labeling, or package, for all fluoroquinolone antibiotics about the risk of tendinitis, including the possibility of complete tendon rupture.

This adverse reaction most frequently involves the Achilles tendon, the tendon that runs from the back of the heel to the calf. Rupture of the Achilles tendon may require surgical repair. Tendons in the rotator cuff (the shoulder), the hand, the biceps, and the thumb have also been involved. This reaction appears to be more common in those taking steroid drugs, in older patients, and in kidney transplant recipients, but cases have occurred in people without any of these risk factors. The onset of symptoms is sudden and has occurred as soon as 24 hours after starting treatment with a fluoroquinolone. Most people have recovered completely after one to two months.

If you experience unexpected tendon pain while taking a fluoroquinolone antibiotic, stop the drug immediately, call your doctor, and rest.

PREGNANCY WARNING

Maxaquin and Zagam caused harm to developing fetuses in animal studies, or such studies were not done. Use during pregnancy only for clear medical reasons. Tell your doctor if you are pregnant or thinking of becoming pregnant before you take these drugs.

Penicillin G

Penicillin V
PEN VEE K (Wyeth)

GENERIC: available

FAMILY: Antibiotics (see p. 468)
Penicillins (see p. 470)

These two forms of penicillin (pen i *sill* in) are taken by mouth (orally). They are used to treat some infections caused by bacteria, including strep throat, some other oral (mouth) infections, and skin infections. Your doctor may also prescribe oral penicillin for you to take at home if you are just getting out of the hospital and were getting antibiotic shots while you were in the hospital. **Penicillin will not help if you have a cold or the flu.**

If you are taking penicillin by mouth, penicillin V is the better form to take because your body absorbs it better. If you have kidney damage, you may need to take less than the usual adult dose.

Before You Use This Drug

Tell your doctor if you have or have had:

- allergies to drugs
- reaction to any penicillin or cephalosporin (see p. 471 for examples)
- other allergies
- stomach or intestinal disease
- kidney disease

Tell your doctor about any other drugs you take, including aspirin, herbs, vitamins, and other nonprescription products.

When You Use This Drug

- Call your doctor if your symptoms do not improve in two or three days or if you get diarrhea. Do not treat the diarrhea yourself.
- **Take all the penicillin your doctor prescribed, even if you feel better before you run out. If you stop too soon, your symptoms could come back.**
- Do not give the drug to anyone else. Throw away outdated drugs.
- If you plan to have any surgery, including dental, tell your doctor that you take penicillin.

How to Use This Drug

- Taking penicillin with food may help prevent stomach upset.
- Store liquid form of penicillin in the refrigerator but do not freeze. Shake well before using.
- Do not store capsules in the bathroom. Do not expose to heat, moisture, or strong light. Capsules may be opened and mixed with water or food.
- If you miss a dose, take it as soon as you remember, but skip it if it is almost time for the next dose. **Do not take double doses.**

Interactions with Other Drugs

The following drugs are listed in the *Evaluations of Drug Interactions* 1997 as causing "highly clinically significant" or "clinically significant" interactions when used together with this drug. We have also included potentially serious interactions listed in the drug's FDA-approved professional product labeling or package insert. New scientific techniques have allowed researchers to predict some drug interactions before they have been documented in people. There may be other drugs, especially those in the families of drugs listed below, that also will react with this drug to cause severe adverse effects. The number of new drugs approved for marketing increases the chance of drug interactions, and new drug interactions are being identified with old drugs. Be vigilant. Make sure to tell your doctor and pharmacist the drugs you are taking and tell your doctor if you are taking any of these interacting drugs:

AUREOMYCIN, chlortetracycline, COUMADIN, GARAMYCIN, gentamicin, heparin, warfarin.

Adverse Effects

Call your doctor immediately if you experience:

• **signs of severe allergic reaction (anaphylactic shock):** severe asthma (wheezing), extreme weakness, abdominal pain, nausea or vomiting, diarrhea, rash

Call your doctor immediately, even if it has been a month since you stopped taking penicillin:

• pain, cramps, or bloating in the abdomen or stomach
• severe, watery diarrhea (may contain blood)
• fever
• increased thirst
• abnormal tiredness
• abnormal weight loss or loss of appetite
• dizziness or headache
• joint pain
• skin rash, hives, itching, blistering, peeling or loosening
• swelling at place of injection
• seizures
• unusual bleeding or bruising
• yellowing of eyes and skin
• agitation, combativeness
• anxiety
• confusion
• fear of impending death
• feeling, hearing or seeing things not there

Call your doctor if these symptoms continue:

• mild diarrhea
• darkened or discolored tongue
• sore mouth or tongue
• mild stomach pain
• itching of the genital or rectal area

Periodic Tests

Ask your doctor which of these tests should be done periodically while you are taking this drug:

• bleeding time
• prothrombin time
• stool cytotoxin assays
• potassium and sodium levels

Trimethoprim
PROLOPRIM (Glaxo Wellcome)
TRIMPEX (Roche)

GENERIC: available
FAMILY: Antibiotics (see p. 468)
Urinary anti-infectives

Trimethoprim (trye *meth* oh prim) is used mainly to treat some urinary tract infections. **It will not help a cold or the flu.**

If you have severe kidney impairment, you should use caution in taking trimethoprim.[163] **If you have impaired kidney function, you may need to take less than the usual adult dose.** While taking trimethoprim, you may suffer a rash or itching.

Practice measures to prevent urinary tract infections. Drink plenty of fluids, especially water. While cranberry juice is unreliable as a cure for urinary tract infections, the juice may reduce odor from incontinence.[164] Practice meticulous hygiene. After using the toilet, wipe backward, not forward, then wash your hands. Prepare and store foods properly, especially when traveling, to prevent diarrhea. Restrict caffeine, which widens the urethra. Indwelling catheters invite urinary tract infections. However, unless there are symptoms of urinary infection, it is not always necessary to take medication just because bacteria are found in a urine test.[165] Women are particularly prone to repeated urinary tract infections. If urinary tract symptoms occur often, ask your doctor about keeping a supply of medication on hand. Ideally, the antibiotic you use should be the most effective, least toxic, and least costly.[166,167]

Before You Use This Drug

Tell your doctor if you have or have had:

- allergies to drugs
- an unusual reaction to trimethoprim
- folic acid (folate) deficiency
- kidney or liver problems
- anemia

Tell your doctor about any other drugs you take, including aspirin, herbs, vitamins, and other nonprescription products.

When You Use This Drug

- Call your doctor if your symptoms do not get better in two or three days.
- **Take all the trimethoprim your doctor prescribed, even if you feel better before you run out. If you stop too soon, your symptoms could come back.**
- Do not give this drug to anyone else. Throw away outdated drugs.
- Schedule regular doctor's visits to check your progress.
- If you take trimethoprim for a long time, ask your doctor if you need a folic acid supplement.
- If you plan to have any surgery, including dental, tell your doctor that you take this drug.

How to Use This Drug

- If the drug irritates your stomach, try taking it with food.

- Tablets may be crushed and mixed with food or water.
- Do not store in the bathroom. Do not expose to heat, moisture, or strong light.
- If you miss a dose, take it as soon as you remember. If you are taking trimethoprim only once a day, take the dose you missed and wait about 12 hours before taking the next one. If you are taking trimethoprim twice a day, take the dose you missed and wait about six hours before taking the next one.

Interactions with Other Drugs

The following drugs are listed in the *Evaluations of Drug Interactions* 1997 as causing "highly clinically significant" or "clinically significant" interactions when used together with this drug. We have also included potentially serious interactions listed in the drug's FDA-approved professional product labeling or package insert. New scientific techniques have allowed researchers to predict some drug interactions before they have been documented in people. There may be other drugs, especially those in the families of drugs listed below, that also will react with this drug to cause severe adverse effects. The number of new drugs approved for marketing increases the chance of drug interactions, and new drug interactions are being identified with old drugs. Be vigilant. Make sure to tell your doctor and pharmacist the drugs you are taking and tell your doctor if you are taking any of these interacting drugs:

COUMADIN, DILANTIN, methotrexate, phenytoin, RHEUMATREX DOSE PACK, warfarin.

Adverse Effects

Call your doctor immediately if you experience:

- fever or sore throat
- abnormal bleeding or bruising

- abnormal paleness, tiredness, or weakness
- bluish fingernails, lips, or skin
- trouble breathing
- headache
- nausea
- neck stiffness
- pale skin
- skin rash or itching
- joint and muscle ache
- skin red, blistering or peeling

Call your doctor if these symptoms continue:

- unusual taste in mouth
- diarrhea
- loss of appetite
- vomiting
- sore mouth or tongue
- stomach cramps or pain

Periodic Tests

Ask your doctor which of these tests should be done periodically while you are taking this drug:

- complete blood count (monthly, if you are on long-term therapy)

PREGNANCY WARNING

This drug caused harm to developing fetuses in animal studies, or such studies were not done. Use during pregnancy only for clear medical reasons. Tell your doctor if you are pregnant or thinking of becoming pregnant before you take this drug.

Rifampin
RIMACTANE (Novartis)
RIFADIN (Hoechst Marion Roussel)

GENERIC: not available

FAMILY: Antibiotics (see p. 468)
             (for tuberculosis)

Rifampin (rif *am* pin) is often used together with other drugs, such as isoniazid (see p. 507), to treat tuberculosis (TB). Rifampin and isoniazid are the most effective drugs to fight TB. If you test positive for TB in a skin test but do not have a confirmed case of the disease, and your doctor decides you need preventive treatment, your treatment will probably be isoniazid alone. If you are carrying a type of bacteria called meningitis but you have no symptoms, you may be prescribed a short course of rifampin alone. However, if you have confirmed tuberculosis, you should always take both of these drugs together. If you take only one, you may develop bacteria that are resistant to one of these drugs.[168]

Some people have developed severe and even fatal liver disease while taking rifampin. You increase your risk of liver disease if you drink alcohol daily, so do not drink while taking this drug. Call your doctor immediately if you have any symptoms of liver disease: fatigue, weakness, malaise (vague feeling of being unwell), loss of appetite, nausea, vomiting, or yellow eyes or skin. If you have impaired liver function, you will probably need to take less than the usual adult dose of rifampin.

Before You Use This Drug

Tell your doctor if you have or have had:

- allergies to drugs
- an unusual reaction to rifampin
- alcohol dependence
- liver problems

Tell your doctor about any other drugs you take, including aspirin, herbs, vitamins, and other nonprescription products.

When You Use This Drug

- Do not drink alcohol.
- Call your doctor if your symptoms don't get better in two or three weeks or if they get worse.
- **Take all the rifampin your doctor prescribed, even if you feel better in a few weeks. You may have to take rifampin every day for a year or more. If you stop too soon, your symptoms might come back.**
- Do not miss doses. If you do not keep to your schedule for taking rifampin, you are more likely to have serious adverse effects. Stopping and starting the drug can cause kidney failure, although this is rare.
- Do not give this drug to anyone else. Throw away outdated drugs.
- Your urine, stools, saliva, sweat, and tears might turn red or orange. This is no cause for alarm, but let your doctor know that it has happened and watch for signs of overdose (see Adverse Effects). If you wear soft contact lenses, they may be permanently discolored.
- If you plan to have any surgery, including dental, tell your doctor that you take this drug.

How to Use This Drug

- Take with **a full glass (eight ounces) of water** on an empty stomach (at least one hour before or two hours after meals). If it upsets your stomach, try taking it with food.
- Capsules may be opened and mixed with food such as applesauce or jelly.
- Do not store in the bathroom. Do not expose to heat or direct light.
- If you miss a dose, take it as soon as you remember, but skip it if it is almost time for the next dose. **Do not take double doses.**

Interactions with Other Drugs

The following drugs are listed in the *Evaluations of Drug Interactions* 1997 as causing "highly clinically significant" or "clinically significant" interactions when used together with this drug. We have also included potentially serious interactions listed in the drug's FDA-approved professional product labeling or package insert. New scientific techniques have allowed researchers to predict some drug interactions before they have been documented in people. There may be other drugs, especially those in the families of drugs listed below, that also will react with this drug to cause severe adverse effects. The number of new drugs approved for marketing increases the chance of drug interactions, and new drug interactions are being identified with old drugs. Be vigilant. Make sure to tell your doctor and pharmacist the drugs you are taking and tell your doctor if you are taking any of these interacting drugs:

CALAN SR, CATAPRES, chloramphenicol, CHLOROMYCETIN, clonidine, COUMADIN, COVERA–HS, CRIXIVAN, CRYSTODIGIN, cyclosporine, digitoxin, digoxin, DILANTIN, DOLOPHINE, DURAQUIN, ELIXOPHYLLIN, FLUOTHANE, FORTOVASE, halothane, indinavir, INH, INVIRASE, isoniazid, ISOPTIN SR, ketoconazole, LANOXICAPS, LANOXIN, LOPRESSOR, methadone, METHADOSE, metoprolol, METRETON, NEORAL, NIZORAL, oral contraceptives, phenytoin, PRED FORTE, prednisolone, QUINAGLUTE DURA-TABS, QUINIDEX, quinidine, RETROVIR, SANDIMMUNE, saquinavir, SLO–BID, THEO–24, theophylline, TOPROL XL, verapamil, VERELAN, warfarin, zidovudine (AZT).

Adverse Effects

Call your doctor immediately if you experience:

• **signs of overdose:** nausea, vomiting, extreme tiredness, malaise, abdominal pain, reddish color of skin, mouth, and eyeballs, swelling of eyes or face, itching, mental changes

• **flu-like symptoms:** fever, chills, trouble breathing, dizziness, headache, muscle or joint aches, shivering, skin rash, itching
  • confusion or inability to concentrate
  • loss of appetite
  • nausea or vomiting
  • abnormal tiredness or weakness
  • bloody or cloudy urine
  • noticeable decrease in frequency of urinating or amount of urine
  • sore throat
  • abnormal bruising or bleeding
  • yellow eyes or skin

Call your doctor if these symptoms continue:
  • diarrhea
  • stomach cramps or heartburn
  • sore mouth or tongue
  • blurring or any change in vision

Periodic Tests

Ask your doctor which of these tests should be done periodically while you are taking this drug:
  • liver function tests

PREGNANCY WARNING

This drug caused harm to developing fetuses in animal studies, or such studies were not done. Use during pregnancy only for clear medical reasons. Tell your doctor if you are pregnant or thinking of becoming pregnant before you take this drug.

Silver Sulfadiazine
SILVADENE (Hoechst Marion Roussel)

GENERIC: available

FAMILY: Antibiotics (see p. 468)
Sulfonamides

Silver sulfadiazine (sul fa *dye* a zeen) is a cream that is used on burns, to prevent and treat infection. **If you have decreased kidney and liver function, you may need to use less than the usual adult dose to prevent dangerous levels of this drug from accumulating in your body.** When you use this cream on burns over large areas of your body, your doctor should be carefully watching your kidney function and the levels of the drug in your body, and your urine should be tested for sulfa crystals.

Before You Use This Drug

Tell your doctor if you have or have had:

  • allergies to drugs
  • an unusual reaction to silver sulfadiazine
  • glucose-6-phosphate dehydrogenase deficiency
  • kidney or liver problems
  • blood problems
  • porphyria

Tell your doctor about any other drugs you take, including aspirin, herbs, vitamins, and other nonprescription products.

How to Use This Drug

• Do not store in the bathroom. Do not expose to heat, moisture or strong light.

• If you miss a dose, take it as soon as you remember, but skip it if it is almost time for the next dose. **Do not take double doses.**

Interactions with Other Drugs

Some other drugs that you may be taking (either over-the-counter or prescription drugs) can interact with this one, causing adverse effects. Ask your doctor what these drugs are and let him or her know if you are taking any of them.

Adverse Effects

Call your doctor immediately if you experience:

- burning, itching, or rash (rare)
- worsening of condition, or no improvement
- increased sensitivity to sun

Call your doctor if these symptoms continue:

- burning feeling on treated areas
- skin discoloration
- skin rash or itching

Because silver sulfadiazine is absorbed into the body, you may have other adverse effects like those that occur with the sulfonamides (sulfa drugs). See sulfisoxazole, p. 505, for examples.

Periodic Tests

Ask your doctor which of these tests should be done periodically while you are taking this drug:

- complete blood count
- serum sulfadiazine concentrations
- urinalysis

Do Not Use
(Except for serious fungal infection)

ALTERNATIVE TREATMENT:
This is a cosmetic,
not a medical problem;
no treatment recommended.

Itraconazole
SPORANOX (Janssen)

Terbinafine
LAMISIL (Novartis)

FAMILY: Antifungals

Itraconazole (i tra *koe* na zole) was first approved to treat serious fungal infections in people with compromised immune systems such as AIDS patients, and terbinafine (ter *bin* a feen) was previously available only for topical use. Both drugs are now being heavily promoted directly to consumers for the treatment of toenail fungus, with or without involvement of the fingernails. Fungal infections of the nails are generally resistant to topical treatment.

Serious adverse effects have been reported with terbinafine. These include liver and bone marrow toxicity, and changes in the lens and retina of the eye.[169] The relapse of toenail fungus with terbinafine is reported to be about 15%.[170] Nausea and vomiting are the most common adverse effects reported with itraconazole.[171]

The editors of *The Medical Letter on Drugs and Therapeutics,* the internationally respected, independent source of drug information, written for doctors and pharmacists said: *"The advisability of taking either of these expensive drugs [itraconazole or terbinafine] for months to treat an infection that is mainly cosmetic and may relapse is unclear."*[172] Our warning to consumers is stronger: Using these drugs for a cosmetic condition is risky.

```
┌─────────────────────────────────────────┐
│               WARNING                     │
│                                           │
│        LIFE-THREATENING DRUG              │
│     INTERACTIONS WITH ITRACONAZOLE        │
│                                           │
│    Serious heart rhythm disturbances have │
│  occurred when itraconazole is taken with │
│  terfenadine (Seldane), astemizole        │
│  (Hismanal) or cisapride (Propulsid).     │
│  Deaths have resulted when itraconazole   │
│  was taken with terfenadine or cis-       │
│  apride.                                  │
└─────────────────────────────────────────┘
```

Limited Use

Cefixime
SUPRAX (Lederle)

GENERIC: not available

FAMILY: Antibiotics (see p. 468)
Cephalosporins (see p. 470)

Cefixime (sef *ix* ime) is an antibiotic used for certain infections, such as uncomplicated urinary tract infections, gonorrhea, respiratory, sinus, or ear infections. Cefixime has no demonstrated clinical advantage over other antibiotics, some of which cost much less and **does not help a cold, or staph infections.** Gastrointestinal toxicity, mainly diarrhea, appears to be more frequent with cefixime than with some other drugs, such as amoxicillin (see p. 476) or cefaclor (see p. 482).[173]

Practice measures to prevent urinary tract infections. Drink plenty of fluids, especially water. While cranberry juice is unreliable as a cure for urinary tract infections, the juice may reduce odor from incontinence.[174] Practice meticulous hygiene. After using the toilet, wipe backward, not forward, then wash your hands. Prepare and store foods properly, especially when traveling, to prevent diarrhea. Restrict caffeine, which widens the urethra. Indwelling catheters invite urinary tract infections. However, unless there are symptoms of urinary infection, it is not always necessary to take medication just because bacteria are found in a urine test.[175] Women are particularly prone to repeated urinary tract infections. If urinary tract symptoms occur often, ask your doctor about keeping a supply of medication on hand. Ideally, the antibiotic you use should be the most effective, least toxic, and least costly.[176,177]

Before You Use This Drug

Tell your doctor if you have or have had:

- allergies to drugs
- colitis
- diabetes
- kidney problems
- other stomach or intestinal disorders
- a salt (sodium)-restricted diet (injected form of cefixime contains sodium)

Tell your doctor about any other drugs you take, including aspirin, herbs, vitamins, and other nonprescription products.

When You Use This Drug

- Call your doctor if your symptoms do not improve in two or three days or if you get diarrhea. Do not treat the diarrhea yourself.
- **Take all the cefixime your doctor prescribed, even if you feel better before you run out. If you stop too soon, your symptoms could come back.**
- **Caution diabetics:** see p. 550
- Do not give the drug to anyone else. Throw away outdated drugs.

- If you plan to have any surgery, including dental, tell your doctor that you take this drug.

How to Use This Drug

- Swallow tablet whole. If you take the liquid form, shake it well before measuring. Since the liquid contains sugar, rinse your mouth after swallowing a dose.
- If you miss a dose, take it as soon as you remember, but skip it if it is almost time for the next dose. **Do not take double doses.**
- Do not store tablets in the bathroom. Do not expose to heat, moisture, or strong light. The oral liquid may be refrigerated, but avoid freezing. Discard liquid after two weeks.

Interactions with Other Drugs

The following drugs are listed in the *Evaluations of Drug Interactions* 1997 as causing "highly clinically significant" or "clinically significant" interactions when used together with this drug. We have also included potentially serious interactions listed in the drug's FDA-approved professional product labeling or package insert. New scientific techniques have allowed researchers to predict some drug interactions before they have been documented in people. There may be other drugs, especially those in the families of drugs listed below, that also will react with this drug to cause severe adverse effects. The number of new drugs approved for marketing increases the chance of drug interactions, and new drug interactions are being identified with old drugs. Be vigilant. Make sure to tell your doctor and pharmacist the drugs you are taking and tell your doctor if you are taking any of these interacting drugs:

BENEMID, carbamazepine, probenecid, TEGRETOL.

Adverse Effects

Call your doctor immediately, even if it has been a month since you stopped taking cefixime, if you experience:

- pain, cramps or bloating in the abdomen or stomach
- abnormal bleeding or bruising
- difficulty breathing
- severe, watery diarrhea (may contain blood)
- dizziness
- fever
- headache
- seizures
- skin rash, hives, blistering, itching
- decrease in amount of urine
- increased thirst
- abnormal tiredness
- joint pain
- swelling at place of injection
- yellowing of eyes or skin

Call your doctor if these symptoms continue:

- loss of appetite
- mild diarrhea
- dry mouth
- gas, heartburn
- insomnia
- nausea, vomiting, mild diarrhea
- sore mouth or tongue
- mild stomach pain
- itching of the genital or rectal area

Periodic Tests

Ask your doctor which of these tests should be done periodically while you are taking this drug:

- bleeding time or prothrombin time
- stool exam

Amantadine
SYMMETREL (Endo)

GENERIC: available

FAMILY: Antivirals
         Antiparkinsonians

Amantadine (a *man* ta deen) is used to treat two different problems: diseases caused by a virus, such as flu, and Parkinson's disease. If you are over 60, you will probably need to take less than the usual adult dose. For use against flu, a lower dose of no more than 100 mg is recommended for older people, even less if your kidney function is impaired, or you are underweight.[178,179]

For the flu (influenza), it is best to get a flu shot early in the season. However, if you cannot get a flu shot because it is unavailable, or you have a medical condition that prevents it, you can use amantadine. During outbreaks of the flu, amantadine may be prescribed in addition to earlier flu shots. For amantadine to be effective against the flu, you must take it within 48 hours of your first flu symptoms.[180]

Your doctor may also prescribe amantadine if you have Parkinson's disease, usually as a supplement to another drug. A combination of two drugs called levodopa and carbidopa (see p. 582) is the best treatment for Parkinson's disease. Amantadine is often effective only for a limited time (less than six months), and it often produces adverse effects such as confusion, lightheadedness, hallucinations, and anxiety, which reduce its usefulness.[181] When you are taking amantadine, especially if you are a woman, the skin of your legs may become mottled (this is known as livedo reticularis). This will go away when you stop taking the drug.

If you have symptoms of parkinsonism, you should know that they might be caused by a drug that you are taking for another problem. As many as half of older adults with these symptoms may have developed them as an adverse effect of one of their drugs. A list of drugs that can cause symptoms of parkinsonism appears on p. 193. If you are taking any of the drugs on this list, discuss the possibility of drug-induced parkinsonism with your doctor, and ask to have your prescription changed or stopped.

Before You Use This Drug

Tell your doctor if you have or have had:

- allergies to drugs
- blood vessel disease of the brain
- congestive heart failure
- eczema (recurring)
- heart disease, swelling of feet and ankles
- kidney disease
- mental illness
- seizures, epilepsy
- stomach ulcers

Tell your doctor about any other drugs you take, including aspirin, herbs, vitamins, and other nonprescription products.

When You Use This Drug

- Keep to the schedule and dose your doctor prescribed for you. Do not use more or less often, or in a higher or lower dose, than was prescribed.
- Until you know how you react to this drug, do not drive or perform other activities requiring alertness. Amantadine can cause fainting and confusion.
- You may feel dizzy when rising from a lying or sitting position. If you are lying down, hang your legs over the side of the bed for a few minutes, then get up slowly. When getting up from a chair, stay by the chair until you are sure that you are not dizzy. (See p. 16.)
- Do not drink alcohol.
- Take measures to prevent falls. Hold on to handrails or steps, avoid using throw rugs.

How to Use This Drug

- Do not store in the bathroom. Do not expose to heat, moisture, or strong light. Do not let the liquid form freeze.

- If you miss a dose, take it as soon as you remember, but skip it if it is less than four hours until the next dose. **Do not take double doses.**

Interactions with Other Drugs

Some other drugs that you may be taking (either over-the-counter or prescription drugs) can interact with this one, causing adverse effects. Ask your doctor what these drugs are and let him or her know if you are taking any of them.

Adverse Effects

Call your doctor immediately if you experience:

- **signs of overdose**: severe confusion or other mental changes, seizures, severe nightmares, trouble sleeping
  - confusion or hallucinations
  - depression, mood or mental changes
  - difficulty urinating
  - fainting
  - slurred speech
  - uncontrolled rolling of eyes
  - sore throat and fever
  - swelling of feet or lower legs
  - shortness of breath
  - rapid weight gain
  - skin rash
  - vision changes
  - lack of coordination
  - irritation and swelling of the eye

Call your doctor if these symptoms continue:

- difficulty concentrating
- dizziness, lightheadedness
- irritability
- loss of appetite
- nausea, vomiting
- nervousness
- red, blotchy spots on skin

- nightmares, trouble sleeping
- constipation
- dry mouth, nose, and throat
- headache

Periodic Tests

Ask your doctor which of these tests should be done periodically while you are taking this drug:

- blood pressure

PREGNANCY WARNING

This drug caused harm to developing fetuses in animal studies, or such studies were not done. Use during pregnancy only for clear medical reasons. Tell your doctor if you are pregnant or thinking of becoming pregnant before you take this drug.

 Do Not Use

ALTERNATIVE TREATMENT:
See Clotrimazole (p. 515) and Miconazole (p. 513).

Terconazole
TERAZOL 3 Vaginal Cream or Suppositories (Ortho-McNeil)
TERAZOL 7 Vaginal Cream (Ortho-McNeil)

FAMILY: Antifungals

Terconazole (ter *kone* a zole) is used to treat vaginal fungal infections. It is equally as effective as some other antifungal creams (for example clotrimazole and miconazole), but it is absorbed into the body much more than these drugs, and can cause flu-like symptoms of headache, chills, fever, and a drop in blood pressure.[182,183] If you are using this drug, or if your doctor recommends it, ask your doctor to change your prescription.

Mild vaginal infections are often self-limiting.[184] For some women a bland cream (without drugs) relieves symptoms until infection spontaneously goes away.[185] Preventive measures include less sugar in the diet, and avoiding tight-fitting pants and panty hose. Cotton is preferable to synthetics.[186] Dry the vaginal area thoroughly after bathing or swimming.

 Do Not Use

ALTERNATIVE TREATMENT:
See Ampicillin, p. 522, Trimethoprim, p. 528, and Trimethoprim and Sulfamethoxazole, p. 478.

Atropine, Hyoscyamine, Methenamine, Methylene Blue, Phenyl Salicylate, and Benzoic Acid
URISED (PolyMedica)

FAMILY: Antibiotics (see p. 468)
         Antispasmodics
         Painkillers

This combination of six drugs, atropine (see p. 361), hyoscyamine (hye oh *sye* a meen), methenamine (meth *en* a meen), methylene (*meth* i leen) blue, phenyl salicylate (*fen* ill sa *li* si late), and benzoic (ben *zoe* ik) acid is used to treat symptoms of urinary tract infections. This combination of drugs is irrational and too complex, and it should not be used. Part of the problem is that because the dosage of each individual drug is fixed, your doctor cannot adjust dosages to ensure that the product will be safe and effective. And one drug in this combination, atropine, causes adverse effects so severe that people over 60 should not take it at all.

Some of the ingredients in this product may cause excitement, agitation, drowsiness, or confusion in older adults, even at the usual dose. Call your doctor if you have any of these symptoms. Also, in people over 40, this drug may cause glaucoma, an eye disease that often remains hidden.

WARNING: SPECIAL MENTAL AND PHYSICAL ADVERSE EFFECTS

Older adults are especially sensitive to the harmful anticholinergic (see Glossary, p. 768) effects of a family of drugs known as belladonna alkaloids. Atropine and hyoscyamine are both in this family. Drugs in this family should not be used unless absolutely necessary.

Mental Effects: confusion, delirium, short-term memory problems, disorientation, and impaired attention.

Physical Effects: dry mouth, constipation, difficulty urinating (especially for a man with an enlarged prostate), blurred vision, decreased sweating with increased body temperature, sexual dysfunction, and worsening of glaucoma.

Practice measures to prevent urinary tract infections. Drink plenty of fluids, especially water. While cranberry juice is unreliable as a cure for urinary tract infections, the juice may reduce odor from incontinence.[187] Practice meticulous hygiene. After using the toilet, wipe backward, not forward, then wash your hands. Prepare and store foods properly, especially when traveling, to prevent diarrhea. Restrict caffeine, which widens the urethra. Indwelling catheters invite urinary tract infections. However, unless there are symptoms of urinary infection, it is not always necessary to take medication just because bacteria are found in a urine test.[188] Women are particularly prone to repeated urinary tract infections. If urinary tract symptoms occur often, ask your doctor about keeping a supply of medication on hand. Ideally, the antibiotic you use should be the most effective, least toxic, and least costly.[189,190]

Mebendazole
VERMOX (Janssen)

GENERIC: not available
FAMILY: Antiparasites

Mebendazole (meb *n* dah zoll) is a drug of choice for hookworms, lungworm, pinworms, porkworms, roundworms, threadworms, and whipworms, as well as filiarsis caused by xmansonella perstans, and gnathomiasis. It is an alternative drug to treat creeping eruption. Mebendazole is also preferred for mixed infestations of two or more parasites. It deprives the invaders of sugar needed for energy, thereby killing or immobilizing the eggs, larvae, or adult form, depending on the parasite.

It is very important that these conditions be treated since if worms escape from the intestines, they can be quite disturbing under the skin, and dangerous in the heart, mouth, liver, or joints.[191,192] Masses of roundworms have blocked the intestines or bile duct during therapy.[193] In high doses mebendazole has suppressed the bone marrow. Mebendazole is not approved in the U.S. for tapeworm or hydatid diseases. Effectiveness of mebendazole depends on whether the infestation is minor or severe, how long it takes worms to pass through your digestive tract, whether or not you have diarrhea, and the susceptibility of the worms. It may take a few days for the body to expel dead forms in the stool.

Length of therapy varies from three days to several months, according to the type and number of parasites. At times treatment needs to be repeated at least once. In severe infections, use of mebendazole may prevent the need for a blood transfusion or surgery. Compared to some other pinworm medicine, mebendazole has an advantage of not staining clothing or bedding.

At times individuals recover spontaneously from lungworm.[194] However, it can persist in the body for decades.[195] You may be more susceptible to parasites if you take immunosuppressant drugs or corticosteroids.[196] Several measures can prevent infestation. Wear shoes. Do not go barefoot where human or animal feces may be on the ground, including beaches, children's sandboxes, and fertilized gardens. Wash fruits and vegetables thoroughly. Eat meat that is completely cooked. Wash your hands before preparing food, eating, and after going to the toilet. Use sanitary conditions to dispose of human feces. Be cautious when traveling to areas with dense shade, high humidity, and sandy soil, coupled with poor sanitation.

Before You Use This Drug

Tell your doctor if you have or have had:

- allergies to drugs
- AIDS[197]
- anemia
- Crohn's ileitis or colitis
- persistent or bloody diarrhea
- "ground itch" of feet or hands
- inflammatory bowel disease
- itching of anal area
- liver disease
- organ transplant[198]
- peptic ulcer
- stomach surgery[199]
- ulcerative colitis

Inform your doctor of activities, places, or work that may have exposed you to parasites, especially if you have:

- lived or traveled in tropical or subtropical areas, especially the Southeastern United

States, the Caribbean, Central and South America, the Philippines, Africa, Thailand, Vietnam, Burma, Turkey, and Eastern Europe.

• worked in agriculture, mining, plumbing, tunneling, or with foreign missions, immigrants, refugees, foreign visitors.

• been duck hunting.

Tell your doctor about any other drugs you take, including aspirin, herbs, vitamins, and other nonprescription products.

When You Use This Drug

• **Take all the mebendazole your doctor prescribed, even if you feel better before you run out. If you stop too soon, your symptoms could come back.**

• Disinfect toilets.

• Wash your hands often, especially before eating and after using the toilet. Use soap and water and clean under your fingernails.

• Change undergarments, bedding, towels, and nightclothes daily.

• Launder bedding, towels, and nightclothes to prevent reinfection of pinworms. Merely shaking bedding and clothes is not sufficient.

• Observe stools for signs of parasites. If you think there is reinfection, take a stool sample to your doctor.

• Ask your doctor about any diet changes, especially if you are on a low-fat diet.

• Ask your doctor if you need to take iron or folic acid supplements.

• Do not fast or use enemas or laxatives unless your doctor advises you to do so.

• Check with your doctor if there is no improvement within a few days.

How to Use This Drug

• Chew tablets, or swallow whole. If desired you may crush the tablets and mix with food. For severe whipworm infections, doctors sometimes order an enema of mebendazole for the pharma-cist to prepare.[200] If your doctor orders this, follow the instructions on your prescription label.

• If your dose is high, or your course of therapy long, then mebendazole should be taken with a fatty meal which allows your system to absorb the drug more efficiently.

• If you miss a dose, take it as soon as you remember. If it is almost time for the next dose: space according to the number of doses you take each day. For two doses a day: space the missed dose and the next dose at least four hours apart. If you take eight doses a day: space the missed dose and the next dose at least one and one-half hours apart.

• Do not store in the bathroom. Do not expose to heat, moisture, or strong light.

Interactions with Other Drugs

Some other drugs that you may be taking (either over-the-counter or prescription drugs) can interact with this one, causing adverse effects. Ask your doctor what these drugs are and let him or her know if you are taking any of them.

Adverse Effects

Call your doctor immediately if you experience:

• fever
• skin rash or itching
• sore throat
• unusual tiredness or weakness

Call your doctor if these symptoms continue:

• abdominal pain
• diarrhea
• dizziness
• hair loss
• headache
• nausea and vomiting
• numbness
• ringing in the ears

Periodic Tests

Ask your doctor which of these tests should be done periodically while you are taking this drug:

- complete blood count
- perianal exam
- stool exam

PREGNANCY WARNING

This drug caused harm to developing fetuses in animal studies, or such studies were not done. Use during pregnancy only for clear medical reasons. Tell your doctor if you are pregnant or thinking of becoming pregnant before you take this drug.

Doxycycline
VIBRAMYCIN (Pfizer)

GENERIC: available
FAMILY: Antibiotics (see p. 468)
Tetracyclines (see p. 474)

WARNING

The use of tetracyclines during tooth development (last half of pregnancy, infancy, and childhood to the age of eight years) may cause permanent discoloration (yellow-gray-brown) of the teeth.

Doxycycline (dox i *sye* kleen) is used to treat chronic infections of the prostate gland, urinary tract infections, pelvic inflammatory disease, and acute bronchitis (in people with chronic lung disease). **Doxycycline will not help a cold or the flu.**

Doxycycline is sometimes used to treat bacterial infections that are common in older adults, but it is rarely the best antibiotic for this purpose.[201] Penicillin would be a better choice. People with kidney damage who need to take a tetracycline drug are better off taking doxycycline than any other, but they should have their kidney function monitored carefully by their doctor while they are taking this drug. People with liver failure might need to take less than the usual adult dose of doxycycline.

When you take doxycycline, make sure that you either drink at least one full glass of water or take it with food. **Some people who have taken doxycycline at bedtime, without sufficient water to wash it down, have gotten esophageal ulcers (irritation of the esophagus, the tube leading from the throat to the stomach).**[202] Doxycycline is more likely than other pills to lead to this problem.

Practice measures to prevent urinary tract infections. Drink plenty of fluids, especially water. While cranberry juice is unreliable as a cure for urinary tract infections, the juice may reduce odor from incontinence.[203] Practice meticulous hygiene. After using the toilet, wipe backward, not forward, then wash your hands. Prepare and store foods properly, especially when traveling, to prevent diarrhea. Restrict caffeine, which widens the urethra. Indwelling catheters invite urinary tract infections. However, unless there are symptoms of urinary infection, it is not always necessary to take medication just because bacteria are found in a urine test.[204] Women are particularly prone to repeated urinary tract infections. If urinary tract symptoms occur often, ask your doctor about keeping a supply of medication on hand. Ideally, the antibiotic you use should be the most effective, least toxic, and least costly.[205,206]

Before You Use This Drug

Tell your doctor if you have or have had:

- allergies to drugs
- an unusual reaction to doxycycline, tetracycline or other drugs in this family
- liver problems

Tell your doctor about any other drugs you take, including aspirin, herbs, vitamins, and other nonprescription products.

When You Use This Drug

- Stay out of the sun as much as possible, and call your doctor if you get a rash, hives, or any other skin reaction. Doxycycline makes you more sensitive to the sun.
- Do not eat or drink milk or other dairy products, and do not take antacids or iron, vitamin, or mineral supplements for a few hours before and after you take each dose of doxycycline. These substances can stop your body from absorbing the drug, which makes it less effective.
- Call your doctor if your symptoms do not improve in two or three days or if you get diarrhea. Do not treat the diarrhea yourself.
- **Take all the doxycycline your doctor prescribed, even if you feel better before you run out. If you stop too soon, your symptoms could come back.**
- Do not give this drug to anyone else. Throw away outdated drugs.
- If you plan to have any surgery, including dental, tell your doctor that you take this drug.

How to Use This Drug

- Take on an empty stomach (at least one hour before or two hours after meals) with **a full glass (eight ounces) of water.** Take your last dose of the day with a full glass of water at least an hour before bedtime. If your stomach gets irritated when you take this drug, you can take it with food to help prevent that.
- Keep the container closed tightly and in a dry place. Do not store in the bathroom. Do not expose to heat, moisture, or strong light. Do not use if the appearance or taste has changed.
- Take doxycycline at least two hours apart from any other drug you are taking.
- If you miss a dose, take it as soon as you remember, but skip it if it is almost time for your next dose. **Do not take double doses** unless you are taking it three or more times a day (see p. 474).

Interactions with Other Drugs

The following drugs are listed in the *Evaluations of Drug Interactions* 1997 as causing "highly clinically significant" or "clinically significant" interactions when used together with this drug. We have also included potentially serious interactions listed in the drug's FDA-approved professional product labeling or package insert. New scientific techniques have allowed researchers to predict some drug interactions before they have been documented in people. There may be other drugs, especially those in the families of drugs listed below, that also will react with this drug to cause severe adverse effects. The number of new drugs approved for marketing increases the chance of drug interactions, and new drug interactions are being identified with old drugs. Be vigilant. Make sure to tell your doctor and pharmacist the drugs you are taking and tell your doctor if you are taking any of these interacting drugs:

aluminum hydroxide, AMPHOJEL, calcium carbonate, carbamazepine, CALTRATE, COUMADIN, DILANTIN, FEOSOL, FERGON, ferrous gluconate, ferrous sulfate, LUMINAL, MAALOX, magnesium hydroxide, oral contraceptives, OS-CAL 500, phenobarbital, phenytoin, PHILLIPS' MILK OF MAGNESIA, SLOW FE, SOLFOTON, TEGRETOL, warfarin.

Adverse Effects

Call your doctor immediately if you experience:

- skin rash or increased sensitivity of skin to sun
- changes in vision
- difficulty urinating
- increased thirst
- abnormal tiredness or weakness
- yellowing of skin
- abdominal pain
- change in soft spot on head (infants)
- headache
- loss of appetite

Call your doctor if these symptoms continue:

- stomach irritation or cramps
- diarrhea
- sore or discolored mouth or tongue
- itching in the genital or rectal area

```
PREGNANCY WARNING

This drug caused harm to developing fetuses in
animal studies, or such studies were not done. Use
during pregnancy only for clear medical reasons.
Tell your doctor if you are pregnant or thinking of
becoming pregnant before you take this drug.
```

Limited Use

Azithromycin
ZITHROMAX (Pfizer)

GENERIC: not available
FAMILY: Antibiotics (see p. 468)

Azithromycin (a *zyth* row my sin) is approved to treat infections, such as chlamydia, urethritis, and pneumonia. Your doctor may prescribe azithromycin for other infections if you are allergic to penicillin. **Azithromycin will not help a cold, but may be effective in the treatment of bronchitis and sinusitis.**[207]

Azithromycin belongs to the same family of antibiotics as erythromycin (see p. 498). For many infections azithromycin is similar in effectiveness to amoxicillin (see p. 476) and erythromycin. However, azithromycin costs much more than these alternative antibiotics. Some experts recommend that it be reserved, in most instances, to treat AIDS-related infections.

```
WARNING

If you are using azithromycin do not use Sel-
dane, Seldane-D or Hismanal. These drugs, when
used in combination with azithromycin can accu-
mulate to dangerous levels in the body and can
cause life-threatening, sometimes fatal heart
arrhythmias.[208]
```

Before You Use This Drug

Tell your doctor if you have or have had:

- allergies to drugs
- chronic bronchitis
- kidney or liver problems

Tell your doctor about any other drugs you take, including aspirin, herbs, vitamins, and other nonprescription products.

When You Use This Drug

- Call your doctor if your symptoms do not improve in two or three days or if you get diarrhea. Do not treat the diarrhea yourself.
- **Take all the azithromycin your doctor prescribed, even if you feel better before you run out. If you stop too soon, your symptoms could come back.**

• Do not give this drug to anyone else. Throw away outdated drugs.

• If you plan to have any surgery, including dental, tell your doctor that you take this drug.

How to Use This Drug

• Take with **a full glass (eight ounces) of water** on an empty stomach, at least one hour before or two hours after meals. Do not take with food, or at the same time as antacids containing aluminum or magnesium.[209,210,211]

• If you miss a dose, take it as soon as you remember, but skip it if it is almost time for the next dose. **Do not take double doses**.

• Do not store in the bathroom. Do not expose to heat, moisture, or strong light.

Interactions with Other Drugs

The following drugs are listed in the *Evaluations of Drug Interactions* 1997 as causing "highly clinically significant" or "clinically significant" interactions when used together with this drug. We have also included potentially serious interactions listed in the drug's FDA-approved professional product labeling or package insert. New scientific techniques have allowed researchers to predict some drug interactions before they have been documented in people. There may be other drugs, especially those in the families of drugs listed below, that also will react with this drug to cause severe adverse effects. The number of new drugs approved for marketing increases the chance of drug interactions, and new drug interactions are being identified with old drugs. Be vigilant. Make sure to tell your doctor and pharmacist the drugs you are taking and tell your doctor if you are taking any of these interacting drugs:

ALFENTA, alfentanil, carbamazepine, COUMADIN, cyclosporine, digoxin, disopyramide, ELIXOPHYLLIN, ERGOMAR, ERGOSTAT, ergotamine,

LANOXICAPS, LANOXIN, MEDROL, methylprednisolone, NEORAL, NORPACE, ORAP, pimozide, SANDIMMUNE, SLO-BID, TEGRETOL, THEO-24, theophylline, warfarin.

The following drugs should not be taken with azithromycin (see warning box): astemizole, HISMANAL, SELDANE, terfenadine.

Adverse Effects

Call your doctor immediately if you experience:

• severe, watery diarrhea
• skin rash
• difficulty breathing
• fever
• joint pain
• swelling of face, mouth, neck, hands and feet

Call your doctor if these symptoms continue:

• abdominal or stomach discomfort or pain
• dizziness
• headache
• nausea or vomiting
• taste change
• vaginal itching

Acyclovir
ZOVIRAX (Glaxo Wellcome)

GENERIC: not available
FAMILY: Antivirals

Acyclovir (ay *sye* kloe veer) is used mostly to treat genital herpes infections the first time they appear, and to prevent them from coming back. It is also used to treat chicken pox.

The benefits and risks of using acyclovir to prevent recurrence of genital herpes have not been precisely determined. If you have genital herpes, you should discuss this issue with your doctor. Adverse effects from this drug are rare, but are more common in people with kidney disease. You should use acyclovir as soon as herpes symptoms appear. The earlier you use it, the better it works. When you have a herpes outbreak, avoid irritating the sores, wear loose clothing, and keep the infected area dry and clean. To protect your sex partner from infection, do not have sex during an outbreak, and use condoms at all other times. Using condoms for sex during an outbreak can lower the risk that you will infect your partner, but it is not foolproof. Women with genital herpes may be more likely to get cancer of the cervix (the opening of the uterus) and should have an annual Pap smear to check for this.

Before You Use This Drug

Tell your doctor if you have or have had:

- allergies to drugs
- kidney or liver problems
- nerve disease

Tell your doctor about any other drugs you take, including aspirin, herbs, vitamins, and other nonprescription products.

When You Use This Drug

- Keep to the schedule and dose your doctor prescribed for you. Do not use more or less often, or in a higher or lower dose, than was prescribed.
- Until you know how you react to this drug, do not drive or perform other activities requiring alertness. Acyclovir can cause confusion and dizziness.

How to Use This Drug

- Capsules may be taken with food.

- Do not store in the bathroom or expose to heat, moisture, or strong light.
- If you miss a dose, take it as soon as you remember, but skip it if it is almost time for the next dose. **Do not take double doses.**

Interactions with Other Drugs

Some other drugs that you may be taking (either over-the-counter or prescription drugs) can interact with this one, causing adverse effects. Ask your doctor what these drugs are and let him or her know if you are taking any of them.

Adverse Effects

Call your doctor immediately if you experience:

If you take acyclovir by mouth:

- skin rash

If you get acyclovir injections:

- rash or hives
- blood in urine
- confusion or hallucinations
- trembling
- abdominal pain
- trouble breathing
- decreased urination
- nausea, vomiting, loss of appetite
- unusual thirst
- seizures
- unusual tiredness or weakness
- pain, swelling or redness at place of injection

Call your doctor if these symptoms continue:

If you take acyclovir by mouth:

- diarrhea
- dizziness
- headache
- joint pain
- nausea, vomiting

- acne
- trouble sleeping

If you get acyclovir injections

- lightheadedness
- headache
- unusual sweating

Periodic Tests

Ask your doctor which of these tests should be done periodically while you are taking this drug:

- pap smears

- kidney function tests (during long-term, continuous treatment)
- blood urea nitrogen and creatinine serum tests

PREGNANCY WARNING

This drug caused harm to developing fetuses in animal studies, or such studies were not done. Use during pregnancy only for clear medical reasons. Tell your doctor if you are pregnant or thinking of becoming pregnant before you take this drug.

NOTES FOR DRUGS FOR INFECTIONS

1. Nyquist A-C, Gonzales R, Steiner JF, Sande MA. Antibiotic prescribing for children with colds, upper respiratory tract infections, and bronchitis. *Journal of the American Medical Association* 1998; 279:875–7.

2. Gonzales R, Steiner JF, Sande MA. Antibiotic prescribing for adults with colds, upper respiratory tract infections, and bronchitis by ambulatory care physicians. *Journal of the American Medical Association* 1997; 278:901–4.

3. *National Disease and Therapeutic Index.* I.M.S., Ambler, PA, 1983.

4. *The Medical Letter on Drugs and Therapeutics.* New York: The Medical Letter Inc., 1992; 34:63–4.

5. Gleckman R, Esposito A. Antibiotics in the elderly: skating on therapeutic thin ice. *Geriatrics* 1980; 35:26–8,33–7.

6. James PR. Untoward effects of antimicrobial drugs. *Post-Graduate Medicine* 1971; 50:193–200.

7. Moellering RC. Factors influencing the clinical use of antimicrobial agents in elderly patients. *Geriatrics* 1978; 33:83–91.

8. Ibid.

9. Beam TR. The third generation of cephalosporins, Part II. *Rational Drug Therapy* 1982; 16:1–5.

10. DiPiro JT, Bowden TA, Hooks VH. Prophylactic parenteral cephalosporins in surgery: Are the newer agents better? *Journal of the American Medical Association* 1984; 252:3277.

11. *The Medical Letter on Drugs and Therapeutics.* New York: The Medical Letter Inc., 1985; 27:107.

12. *The Medical Letter on Drugs and Therapeutics,* 1992, op. cit. p. 87–8.

13. Ibid, p. 63–4.

14. *The Medical Letter on Drugs and Therapeutics.* New York: The Medical Letter Inc., 1986; 28:33–40.

15. American Society of Hospital Pharmacists. *American Hospital Formulary Service Drug Information,* Bethesda, MD, 1992: 2352–63.

16. Todd A, Faulds D. Ofloxacin: a reappraisal of its antimicrobial activity, pharmacology and therapeutic use. *Drugs* 1991; 42:825–76.

17. *The Medical Letter on Drugs and Therapeutics.* New York: The Medical Letter Inc., 1991; 33:71–3.

18. *The Medical Letter on Drugs and Therapeutics.* New York: The Medical Letter Inc., 1998; 40:33–42.

19. Orland MJ, Saltman RJ, eds. *Manual of Medical Therapeutics.* 25th ed. Boston: Little, Brown and Company, 1986:205.

20. AMA Department of Drugs. *AMA Drug Evaluations.* 5th ed. Chicago: American Medical Association, 1983:1674.

21. Kastrup EK, ed. *Facts and Comparisons.* St. Louis: J.B. Lippincott Co., July 1987:341.

22. American Society of Hospital Pharmacists. *American Hospital Formulary Service Drug Information,* Bethesda, MD, 1996: 355–65.

23. Gleckman, op. cit.

24. Moellering, op. cit.

25. Marderosian AD, Liberti L. *Natural Product Medicine.* Philadelphia, PA: George F. Stickley Co., 1988:282.

26. AMA Department of Drugs. *AMA Drug Evaluations.* Chicago: American Medical Association, 1992:1182.

27. Sarma PSA, Durairaj P. Randomized treatment of patients with typhoid and paratyphoid fevers using norfloxacin or chloramphenicol. *Transactions of the Royal Society of Tropical Medicine and Hygiene* 1991; 85:670–1.

28. Schubert ML, Sanyal AJ, Wong ES. Antibiotic prophylaxis for prevention of spontaneous bacterial peritonitis? *Gastroenterology* 1991; 101:550–1.

29. Larrey D, Vial T, Micaleff A, Babany B, Morichan-Beauchant M, Michel H, et al. Hepatitis associated with amoxicillin-clavulanic acid combination report of 15 cases. *Gut* 1992; 33:368–71.

30. Reddy KR, Brilliant P, Schiff ER. Amoxicillin-clavulanate potassium-associated cholestasis. *Gastroenterology* 1989; 96:1135–41.

31. Keisu M, Wiholm BE, Palmblad J. Trimethoprim-sulfamethoxazole-associated blood dyscrasias. Ten years' experience of the Swedish spontaneous reporting system. *Journal of Internal Medicine* 1990; 228:353–60.

32. Marderosian, op. cit.

33. AMA, 1992, op. cit.

34. Sarma, op. cit.

35. Schubert, op. cit.

36. Feder HM, Abrahamian LM, Grant-Kels JM. Is penicillin still the drug of choice for non-bullous impetigo? *Lancet* 1991; 338:803–5.

37. AMA Department of Drugs. *AMA Drug Evaluations.* Chicago: American Medical Association, 1991:1409–10.

38. Slocombe B, Perry C. The antimicrobial activity of mupirocin—an update on resistance. *Journal of Hospital Infection* 1991; 19 (Supplement B):19–25.

39. *USP DI, Drug Information for the Health Care Professional.* 12th ed. Rockville, MD: The United States Pharmacopeial Convention, Inc., 1992:1963–4.

40. Anderson G. Clarithromycin in the treatment of community-acquired lower respiratory tract infections. *Journal of Hospital Infection* 1991; 19 (Supplement A):21–7.

41. Gu JW, Scully BE, Neu HC. Bactericidal activity of clarithromycin and its 14-hydroxy metabolite against Haemophilus influenzae and streptococcal pathogens. *Journal of Clinical Pharmacology* 1991; 31:1146–50.

42. Warning Letters from Manufacturers.

43. AMA, 1983, op. cit., p. 1620.

44. *The Medical Letter on Drugs and Therapeutics.* New York: The Medical Letter Inc. 1979, 21:85–7.

45. *The Medical Letter on Drugs and Therapeutics,* 1998, op. cit.

46. Marderosian, op. cit.

47. AMA, 1992, op. cit.

48. Sarma, op. cit.

49. Schubert, op. cit.

50. AMA, 1983, op. cit., p. 1620.

51. *The Medical Letter on Drugs and Therapeutics,* 1985, op. cit.

52. Marderosian, op. cit.

53. AMA, 1992, op. cit.

54. Sarma, op. cit.

55. Schubert, op. cit.

56. Ray W, Federspiel C, Schaffner W. Prescribing of chloramphenicol in ambulatory practice. *Annals of Internal Medicine* 1976; 84:266.

57. American Society of Hospital Pharmacists, 1992, op. cit.

58. Todd, op. cit.

59. *The Medical Letter on Drugs and Therapeutics* 1991, op. cit..

60. *The Medical Letter on Drugs and Therapeutics* 1992, op. cit., p. 58–60.

61. Frieden T, Mangi R. Inappropriate use of oral ciprofloxacin. *Journal of the American Medical Association* 1990; 264:1438–40.

62. *The Medical Letter on Drugs and Therapeutics* 1991, op. cit., p. 53.

63. Ibid, p. 75–6.

64. Marderosian, op. cit.

65. AMA, 1992, op. cit.

66. Sarma, op. cit.

67. Schubert, op. cit.

68. Grasela TH, Dreis MW. An evaluation of quinolone-theophylline using the Food and Drug Administration spontaneous reporting system. *Archives of Internal Medicine* 1992; 152:617–21.

69. Mumford CJ, Ginsberg L. Ciprofloxacin and myasthenia gravis. *British Medical Journal* 1990; 301:818.

70. American Society of Hospital Pharmacists, 1992, op. cit., p. 417–26.

71. Hedstrom SA, Hybbinette CH. Nephrotoxicity in isoxazolypenicillin prophylaxis in hip surgery. *Acta Orthopedic Scandinavia* 1988; 59:44–7.

72. Dukes MNG, Beeley L. *Side Effects of Drugs Annual 15*, Amsterdam: Elsevier 1991:436.

73. Brown AE. Overview of fungal infections in cancer patients. *Seminars in Oncology* 1990; 17(Suppl. 6):2–5.

74. Evans TG, Mayer J, Cohen S, Classen D, Carroll K. Fluconazole failure in the treatment of invasive mycoses. *The Journal of Infectious Diseases* 1991; 164:1232–5.

75. Brown, op. cit.

76. AMA, 1983, op. cit., p. 1620.

77. *The Medical Letter on Drugs and Therapeutics,* 1979, op. cit.

78. Marderosian, op. cit.

79. AMA, 1992, op. cit.

80. Sarma, op. cit.

81. Schubert, op. cit.

82. 46 *Federal Register* 14355, February 27, 1981.

83. Orland, op. cit.

84. Warning Letters from Manufacturers.

85. *The Medical Letter on Drugs and Therapeutics.* New York: The Medical Letter Inc., 1975;17:53.

86. AMA, 1983, op. cit., p. 1717.

87. American Society of Hospital Pharmacists, op. cit., p. 2352–63.

88. Todd, op. cit.

89. *The Medical Letter on Drugs and Therapeutics,* 1991, op. cit., p. 71–3.

90. *The Medical Letter on Drugs and Therapeutics,* 1992, op. cit., p. 58–60.

91. Todd, op. cit.

92. Hooton TM, Johnson C, Winter C, Kuwamura L, Rogers ME, Roberts PL, et al. Single-dose and three-day regimens of ofloxacin versus trimethoprim-sulfamethoxazole for acute cystitis in women. *Antimicrobial Agents and Chemotherapy* 1991; 35:1479–83.

93. Marderosian, op. cit.

94. AMA, 1992, op. cit.

95. Sarma, op. cit.

96. Schubert, op. cit.

97. Grasela, op. cit.

98. American Society of Hospital Pharmacists, 1992, op. cit., p. 2352–63.

99. Sanders WE, Morris JF, Alessi L, Makris AT, McClosky RV, Trenholme GM, et al. Oral ofloxacin for the treatment of acute bacterial pneumonia: use of a nontraditional protocol to compare experimental therapy with 'Usual Care' in a multicenter clinical trial. *The American Journal of Medicine* 1991; 91:261–6.

100. Dukes, op. cit.

101. Marderosian, op. cit.

102. AMA, 1992, op. cit.

103. Sarma, op. cit.

104. Schubert, op. cit.

105. 46 *Federal Register,* op. cit.

106. Orland, op. cit.

107. Warning Letters from Manufacturers.

108. Gilman AG, Goodman LS, Rall TW, Murad F, eds. *The Pharmacological Basis of Therapeutics.* 7th ed. New York: Macmillan, 1985:1203–5.

109. Moulding TS, Redeker AG, Kanel GC. Twenty isoniazid-associated deaths in one state. *American Review of Respiratory Disease* 1989; 140:700–5.

110. Murphy R, Swartz R, Watkins PB. Severe acetaminophen toxicity in a patient receiving isoniazid. *Annals of Internal Medicine* 1990; 113:799–800.

111. Moulding TS, Redeker AG, Kanel GC. Acetaminophen, isoniazid, and hepatic toxicity. *Annals of Internal Medicine* 1991; 114:431.

112. AMA, 1983, op. cit., p. 1620.

113. Marderosian, op. cit.

114. AMA, 1992, op. cit.

115. Sarma, op. cit.

116. Schubert, op. cit.

117. Hart J, Holdren C, Schneider R, Shirley C. *Toxics A to Z.* Berkeley, CA: University of California Press, 1991:336–8.

118. *Physicians' Desk Reference.* 50th ed. Montvale, NY: Medical Economics, 1996:582–4.

119. Tenenbein M. Seizures after lindane therapy. *Journal of the American Geriatrics Society* 1991; 39:394–5.

120. Ibid.

121. Public Citizen Petition to FDA to immediately ban Lindane. Washington, DC, June 15, 1995.

122. Vander Stichele RH, Dezeure EM, Bogart MG. Systematic review of clinical efficacy of topical treatments for head lice. *British Medical Journal* 1995; 311:604–8.

123. Public Citizen Petition, op. cit.

124. AMA, 1983, op. cit, p. 1663.

125. *Drug Treatment in the Elderly.* 2nd ed. Copenhagen, Denmark: World Health Organization, 1997.

126. *Physicians' Desk Reference.* 40th ed. Oradell, NJ: Medical Economics, 1986:1278.

127. Marderosian, op. cit.

128. AMA, 1992, op. cit.

129. Sarma, op. cit.

130. Schubert, op. cit.

131. Thomason JL. Clinical evaluation of terconazole United States experience. *Journal of Reproductive Medicine* 1989; 34:597–601.

132. Doering PL, Santiago TM. Drugs for treatment of vulvovaginal candidiasis: comparative efficacy of agents and regimens. *DICP, The Annals of Pharmacotherapy* 1990; 24:1078–83.

133. *USP DI,* op. cit., p. 1558–62.

134. Thomason, op. cit.

135. Doering, op. cit.

136. *USP DI,* op. cit., p. 1558–62.

137. Patrick J, Panzer JD. Neomycin sensitivity in the normal (nonatopic) individual. *Archives of Dermatology* 1970; 102:532.

138. Ibid.

139. Ibid.

140. Jolson M, Tanner LA, Green L, Grasela TH. Adverse reaction reporting of interaction between warfarin and fluoroquinolones. *Archives of Internal Medicine* 1991; 151:1003–4.

141. Dukes, op. cit., p. 312–3.

142. American Society of Hospital Pharmacists, 1992, op. cit., 2352–63.

143. Todd, op. cit.

144. *The Medical Letter on Drugs and Therapeutics,* 1991, op. cit., p. 71–3.

145. *The Medical Letter on Drugs and Therapeutics,* 1992, op. cit., p. 58–60.

146. Marderosian, op. cit.

147. AMA, 1992, op. cit.

148. Sarma, op. cit.

149. Schubert, op. cit.

150. Grasela, op. cit.

151. Jolson, op. cit.

152. Marderosian, op. cit.

153. AMA, 1992, op. cit.

154. Sarma, op. cit.

155. Schubert, op. cit.

156. *The Medical Letter on Drugs and Therapeutics,* 1998, op. cit., p. 17–8.

157. *The Medical Letter on Drugs and Therapeutics,* 1992, op. cit., p. 103–4.

158. Marderosian, op. cit.

159. AMA, 1992, op. cit.

160. Sarma, op. cit.

161. Schubert, op. cit.

162. Grasela, op. cit.

163. *Physicians' Desk Reference,* 1986, op. cit., p. 759.

164. Marderosian, op. cit.

165. AMA, 1992, op. cit.

166. Sarma, op. cit.

167. Schubert, op. cit.

168. Gilman, op. cit.

169. *The Medical Letter on Drugs and Therapeutics.* New York: The Medical Letter Inc.: 1996; 38:72–4.

170. *Physician's Desk Reference,* 52nd ed. Montvale, NJ: Medical Economics Company, 1998:1861.

171. *The Medical Letter on Drugs and Therapeutics,* 1996, op. cit, p. 5–6.

172. *The Medical Letter on Drugs and Therapeutics,* 1996, op. cit, p. 72–4.

173. *The Medical Letter on Drugs and Therapeutics.* New York: The Medical Letter Inc., 1989; 31:73–5.

174. Marderosian, op. cit.

175. AMA, 1992, op. cit.

176. Sarma, op. cit.

177. Schubert, op. cit.

178. Degelau J, Somani S, Cooper SL, Irvine PW. Occurrence of adverse effects and high amantadine concentrations with influenza prophylaxis in the nursing home. *Journal of American Geriatric Society* 1990; 38:428–32.

179. Stange KC, Little DW, Blatnik B. Adverse reactions to amantadine prophylaxis of influenza in a retirement home. *Journal of American Geriatric Society* 1991; 33:700–5.

180. AMA, 1983, op. cit., p. 1457.

181. Vestal RE, ed. *Drug Treatment in the Elderly.* Sydney, Australia: ADIS Health Science Press, 1984:311.

182. Hirsch HA. Clinical evaluation of terconazole: European experience. *Journal of Reproductive Medicine* 1989; 34:594–6.

183. Moebius UM. Influenza-like syndrome after terconazole. *Lancet* 1988; ii:966–7.

184. Thomason, op. cit.

185. Doering, op. cit.

186. *USP DI,* op. cit., p. 1558–62.

187. Marderosian, op. cit.

188. AMA, 1992, op. cit.

189. Sarma, op. cit.

190. Schubert, op. cit.

191. Chippaux J. Mebendazole treatment of dracunculiasis. *Transactions of the Royal Society of Tropical Medicine* 1991; 85:280.

192. Walden J. Other roundworms trichuris, hookworm, and strongyloides. *Primary Care* 1991; 18:53–74.

193. Gilman AG, Rall TW, Nies AS, Taylor P, eds. *The Pharmacological Basis of Therapeutics.* 8th ed. New York: Pergamon Press, 1990:971.

194. *The Medical Letter on Drugs and Therapeutics,* 1992, op. cit., p. 17–26.

195. Walden, op. cit.

196. Ibid.

197. Ibid.

198. Ibid.

199. Ibid.

200. Ibid.

201. Gleckman, op. cit.

202. Amendola M, Spera TD. Doxycycline-induced esophagitis. *Journal of the American Medical Association* 1985; 253: 1009–11.

203. Marderosian, op. cit.

204. AMA, 1992, op. cit.

205. Sarma, op. cit.

206. Schubert, op. cit.

207. Bahal N, Nahata MC. The new macrolide antibiotics: azithromycin, clarithromycin, dirithromycin, and roxithromycin. *The Annals of Pharmacology* 1992; 26:46–55.

208. Warning Letters from Manufacturers.

209. Drew RH, Gallis HA. Azithromycin spectrum of activity, pharmacokinetics, and clinical applications. *Pharmacotherapy* 1992; 12:161–73.

210. Foulds G, Hilligoss DM, Henry EB, Gerber N. The effects of an antacid or cimetidine on the serum concentrations of azithromycin. *Journal of Clinical Pharmacology* 1991; 31:164–7.

211. Whitman MS, Tunkel AR. Azithromycin and clarithromycin: overview and comparison with erythromycin. *Infection Control and Hospital Epidemiology* 1992; 13:357–68.

Drugs for Diabetes

Diabetes and Its Treatment		**550**

DRUG LISTINGS

acarbose	Do Not Use Until Five Years After Release	564
acetohexamide	Ⓧ Do Not Use	555
AMARYL	Do Not Use Until Five Years After Release	555
chlorpropamide	Ⓧ Do Not Use	555
DIABETA	Limited Use	555
DIABINESE	Ⓧ Do Not Use	555
DYMELOR	Ⓧ Do Not Use	555
glimepiride	Do Not Use Until Five Years After Release	555
glipizide	Limited Use	555
GLUCOPHAGE	Ⓧ Do Not Use	558
GLUCOTROL	Limited Use	555
glyburide	Limited Use	555
HUMALOG	Limited Use	559
HUMULIN	Limited Use	559
ILETIN	Limited Use	559
INSULATARD	Limited Use	559
insulin (beef, pork)	Limited Use	559
insulin (human)	Limited Use	559
metformin	Ⓧ Do Not Use	558
MICRONASE	Limited Use	555
MIXTARD	Limited Use	559
NOVOLIN	Limited Use	559
ORINASE	Limited Use	555
PRECOSE	Do Not Use Until Five Years After Release	564
REZULIN	Ⓧ Do Not Use	565
tolazamide	Limited Use	555
tolbutamide	Limited Use	555
TOLINASE	Limited Use	555
troglitazone	Ⓧ Do Not Use	565
VELOSULIN	Limited Use	559

DIABETES AND ITS TREATMENT

What Is Diabetes?

Diabetes (diabetes mellitus) is a malfunction of the body's system that regulates glucose. Normally, sweets and starches (carbohydrates) are broken down in the intestines to simple sugars, mostly glucose. Glucose then circulates in the blood and enters cells all over the body where it is either stored or burned to produce energy. Insulin is a hormone made in the pancreas and released into the bloodstream. It enables some of the body's organs to take sugar from the bloodstream and use it for energy. When there isn't enough insulin, or when cells have too few receptors that recognize insulin, sugar is not removed from the bloodstream and high levels accumulate. High blood sugar stems from a defect in insulin production or a defect in insulin action or both.

Diabetes can lead to kidney disease, damage to the retina leading to blindness, nerve damage, foot ulcers, hardening of the arteries, heart disease, and bacterial or fungal infections. Three out of four diabetics die of cardiovascular (heart and blood vessel) disease related to their diabetes, and two of those three deaths are from heart disease.

Insulin-dependent Diabetes Mellitus (IDDM, Type-1)

A small fraction of all diabetics have IDDM and require insulin to live. With insulin, many live to an old age. Although this type of diabetes most commonly appears in childhood or adolescence, the term "juvenile-onset" is misleading. IDDM can first occur in much older patients as well. Therefore, physicians often refer to this type of diabetes in non-age-restricted terms as IDDM, or type-1 diabetes.

In type-1 diabetes, the pancreas cannot produce insulin. When a diabetic eats carbohydrates, their blood sugar rises sharply. This is because without insulin, glucose moves into the cells very slowly. Therefore, while a diabetic's blood contains concentrations of sugar, the cells are not able to absorb the glucose properly. Deprived of glucose, the cells may be forced to burn fat at an abnormally fast rate, a process that in turn floods the body with substances called ketones. This can lead to a condition known as ketoacidosis. Symptoms of ketoacidosis include vomiting, weakness, stomach pain, dehydration, and very low blood pressure. Untreated, it may even lead to coma and death.

Treatment

To prevent toxic levels of ketones from accumulating in the blood, a type-1 diabetic needs insulin injections daily. By adhering strictly to the American Diabetes Association's diet, a type-1 diabetic can regulate the amount and type of sugar taken into the body at various times throughout the day. The type-1 diabetic needs both insulin injections and a regimented diet to live.

Non-insulin-dependent Diabetes Mellitus (NIDDM, Type-2)

Of the millions of older Americans who have diabetes, 85 to 90% have type-2 diabetes. The vast majority of these people are obese, averaging about 50% over their ideal body weight. Type-2 diabetics have a hereditary tendency toward diabetes which is magnified when they become overweight. The symptoms of adult-onset diabetes involve, at the worst, increased urination, excessive eating and drinking, and perhaps occasional dizziness. Because of the vagueness of the symptoms, type-2 diabetes can often only be diagnosed with blood tests. The many long-term complications of diabetes make this disease the sixth leading cause of death in this country.

Like their type-1 counterparts, type-2 diabetics cannot remove sugar from the blood at a normal rate, but partly for a different reason. Type-2 diabetics do not respond normally to insulin (this is called "insulin resistance"); they require much larger amounts of insulin than do non-diabetics in order to control blood glucose. This resistance to insulin appears to be hereditary. Type-2 diabetics can make insulin, but not as much as can non-diabetics. This combination of increased insulin requirements and limited insulin secretion leads to the loss of control of blood glucose.

Obesity itself causes insulin resistance. Thus, type-2 diabetics who are overweight have even higher needs for insulin than do those who are not. Weight loss is the cornerstone of treatment for type-2 diabetics who are overweight: losing the excess weight makes the body more sensitive to insulin, and the amount of insulin produced will have much greater effects. Physically and psychologically, the benefits of a low calorie diet are achieved early (often within days) when patients are still overweight.[1]

Treatment

There are three kinds of treatment of type-2 diabetes: diet, oral hypoglycemic pills (anti-diabetes drugs taken by mouth), or insulin injections, alone or in combination. Below is a ranking of treatments from most hazardous to safest.

Diabetes pills, although the easiest therapy to follow, actually undermine the purpose of treating diabetes because they may increase your chances of dying from cardiovascular disease. The University Group Diabetes Program (UGDP) study, a study done on insulin and the antidiabetes drugs tolbutamide—a member of the sulfonylurea group of drugs—and phenformin (banned from the market)—a biguanide drug, and a first cousin to metformin (GLUCOPHAGE)—failed to prove that diabetes pills prevent the long-term complications of diabetes, such as heart disease, kidney disease, and blindness.[2] Moreover, it is probable that these drugs cause premature deaths from cardiovascular disease.[3]

Unlike insulin, oral hypoglycemics are only somewhat effective in lowering blood sugar. They fail to adequately control blood sugar in 20 to 40% of patients. But even if they work at first, they may fail later in as many as 30% of patients per year.[4]

After the UGDP report was released, two clinics that stopped using the sulfonylurea oral hypoglycemics found no change in blood sugar in about one-third to one-half of patients after stopping the drug, indicating that these people did not need to be on the drug in the first place.[5] The remaining patients were able to lower their blood sugar with diet alone or diet plus insulin. These results suggest that a majority of the people who take the sulfonylurea oral hypoglycemics could get along with mild dietary changes and not risk premature cardiovascular death.

Two oral hypoglycemics pose additional problems for older people. Chlorpropamide (DIABINESE) may cause *life-threatening*, long-lasting periods of low blood sugar. It may also cause difficulty breathing, drowsiness, muscle cramps, seizures, swelling of face, hands, or ankles, and unconsciousness, water retention, or weakness that could be life-threatening to people who have congestive heart failure or cirrhosis of the liver.[6] For these reasons, the World

Health Organization recommends that chlorpropamide not be used by people 60 years and older. Acetohexamide (DYMELOR) is eliminated from the body predominantly by the kidneys. Since kidney function decreases steadily with age, there is a possiblity that toxic amounts of this drug may accumulate in older people.

Chlorpropamide and acetohexamide should not be used in older people **and probably should be avoided at any age.** Other diabetes pills should only be used by people whose diabetes is not controlled by diet and who cannot inject insulin. Below is an informed consent statement containing information that Public Citizen's Health Research Group believes all patients should receive and sign before they are prescribed diabetes pills.

INFORMED CONSENT FOR USE OF ORAL DIABETES DRUGS

1. I have participated in a program of dietary control and physical exercise including at least 25 hours of instruction.

2. This program did not succeed in weight reduction or control of blood sugar. Dr. _____ told me that insulin was the preferred drug if one had to be used.

3. I refuse (or am physically unable) to take insulin.

4. I am aware of the increased risk of cardiovascular death from taking oral diabetes drugs and of the animal study showing that one of them (tolbutamide) causes a significant increase in coronary artery disease and that therapeutic efficacy has not been proven.

In light of the above, I agree to take

_____ (oral diabetes drug).

_____ Date

_____ Patient's signature

Insulin, like the diabetes pills, alters only the symptoms of the disease without treating the cause. In too large a dose, it may cause trembling, hunger, weakness, and irritability—symptoms of low blood sugar that can progress to insulin shock. Unlike the diabetes pills, however, insulin has not been shown to increase your chance of cardiovascular disease, **but does carry a risk of severe hypoglycemia (low blood sugar).**

It is very important that you understand the correct use of the needle and syringe and instructions that come in the insulin package. Ask for help if you are not sure about any part of your treatment. *Your doctor or the diabetes nurse-educator at your hospital can help you.* Improper cleansing or injection technique may cause skin problems. Tell your doctor if you are having skin problems or difficulty injecting insulin. Disposable syringes and needles are meant to be used only once. United States Pharmacopeia medical panels do not recommend reusing them. However, if you do reuse them, the syringe and needle must be used for only one person. After each use, wipe the needle with alcohol and replace the cap. These needles should definitely not be used more than a few times. Glass syringes need to be sterilized each time they are used.

Insulin should be refrigerated but not frozen. It can be kept at room temperature for a month, but it is better to keep it in the refrigerator. Do not expose it to hot temperatures or sunlight.

Insulin is available in a wide variety of preparations. Some last longer than others. Local allergy is more common with the less pure, older insulins and may be recognized by a hard, red, itching area at the injection site. **You should be using a human insulin rather than the older animal insulins.** Some people experience more serious allergic reactions (skin rash, swelling, stomach upset, difficulty breathing, and very rarely, low blood pressure or even death).[7] Call your doctor immediately if you think you may be experiencing an allergic reaction.

Diet is the safest, most effective treatment available for the vast majority of adult-onset diabetics. More than 90% of type-2 diabetics are overweight. In *many* cases, blood sugar levels return to normal and symptoms go away when the diabetic loses *enough* weight.

Since a large proportion of diabetics can be treated by diet alone, why are so many people taking pills? There are three reasons: drug companies, doctors, and patients. When the oral hypoglycemic agents became available, they were intended to serve as substitutes for insulin in the few adult-onset diabetics who needed diet plus insulin to control their diabetes. Instead, the pills became substitutes for the diet. With the availability of oral drugs, experts stopped stressing the role of diet in controlling the disease, mostly in those very people whose diabetes could have been controlled by an appropriate diet.

Doctors find it easier to prescribe a pill than to prod and nag patients into losing weight. Some assume that older people won't change their diet or lose weight. Doctors may not even suggest a trial weight loss period, but simply begin treatment by prescribing an oral hypoglycemic pill. Patients, who receive complex diet instructions from their physician and are referred to a dietitian for instructions on weighing food portions and memorizing food choices, often find it easier to take a pill than to change eating habits.

However, it is foolhardy to increase the already present risk of heart and blood vessel disease for the convenience of popping a pill, when proper instruction, limited dietary changes, and a little encouragement can help you to reach optimal weight, better health, and improved control of blood sugar. Below are some suggestions for successful weight loss, guidelines for developing a healthier diet, and details of some of the common pitfalls that cause people to become discouraged and discontinue dietary therapy for diabetes.

Diets that are very complicated or very different from what you are used to are hard to follow. The American Diabetes Association (ADA) diet is a highly structured plan based on exchange lists. Although it serves its purpose of regulating calorie and sugar intake quite well, the ADA diet may be difficult for older people to use. Successful use of this diet requires considerable time spent planning meal patterns and food portions. Older people often have trouble with this diet because the food lists are long and complicated and require considerable memorization. The amount of patience and manual dexterity necessary to properly weigh and measure foods may prove difficult, especially for older people. Furthermore, rigid control, such as that provided by the ADA diet, is not always necessary in type-2 diabetics. Often more gradual dietary change will reduce weight and lower blood sugar. See if your doctor or a dietitian can help you plan an easy-to-follow diet that will help to control your diabetes. The diet for a type-2 diabetic is based on the same nutritional principles as for a nondiabetic. Special foods ("dietetic") and imbalanced fad diets are unnecessary and sometimes dangerous. **The basic plan should be to avoid sugar and instead eat a diet high in starch and fiber.**

Many people are already eating a diet that is partly appropriate for diabetics. Only small changes may be needed. Eat fewer simple sugars. Instead of soft drinks, snack foods, and cookies, substitute sugar-free drinks, graham crackers, or bread sticks. To reduce your risk of atherosclerosis (hardening of the blood vessels) ask your doctor for a list of foods to avoid to reduce your intake of cholesterol and saturated fat. Start by cutting back meals that contain red meat (beef, pork, lamb) to three or fewer per week. These can be replaced with fish, chicken, turkey, or vegetable dishes.

A regular exercise program is recommended for people who have diabetes. Exercise helps to lower blood sugar and to reduce weight. It does not have to be strenuous; walking is often the best form of exercise. *Some complications of diabetes can limit your ability to exercise. Make sure your doctor thinks you have picked a form of exercise that is safe for you.*

Health Care for Diabetics

Because diabetes is such a complex disease, your overall health and your response to treatment need to be checked periodically. Schedule regular appointments with your doctor.

Most diabetics, even those treated by diet alone, should use one of the many machines currently available to test blood glucose at home at least once a day. This will let you know how well controlled your blood sugar is and will tell you if it is getting out of control. You should rotate the time of measurement (before breakfast one day, before lunch the next day, before supper the next, at bedtime the next, and then back to breakfast); this way you will know what happens to your blood sugar throughout the day. Write down your measurements and show them to your doctor at each visit (your doctor should make a copy for your medical record).

Also, at least two or three times a year your doctor should order a blood test called "hemoglobin A1c" or "glycosylated hemoglobin." This will tell your doctor how well your blood sugar has been controlled during the previous two to three months. If this test indicates that your blood sugar has been more than just slightly elevated, your doctor should consider changes in your treatment.

Foot care is a particular problem for diabetics. Between appointments be sure to check your feet regularly for sores, infections, and ulcers. These need prompt medical attention. Use cotton socks and wear well-fitted shoes.

Diabetic eye disease is one of the major causes of blindness in our country. Schedule an appointment with an ophthalmologist, (an eye doctor with an MD degree), at least every 12 months.

A number of drugs may raise blood sugar as an adverse effect. The most common are clonidine, corticosteroids, diuretics, gemfibrozil, narcotics, progesterone, and theophylline. If you are taking one of these drugs, ask your doctor whether you still need the medicine or if there is an alternative. Older people should not use chlorpropamide or acetohexamide.

DRUG PROFILES

 Do Not Use

Acetohexamide (a set oh *hex* a mide)
DYMELOR (Lilly)

Chlorpropamide (klor *proe* pa mide)
DIABINESE (Pfizer)

Limited Use

Glipizide (*glip* i zide)
GLUCOTROL (Pfizer)

Glyburide (*glye* byoo ride)
DIABETA (Hoechst Marion Roussel)

Tolazamide (tole *az* a mide)
TOLINASE (Upjohn)

Tolbutamide (tole *byoo* ta mide)
ORINASE (Upjohn)
MICRONASE (Pharmacia & Upjohn)

Do Not Use Until Five Years After Release

Glimepiride (gli *mip* ear ride)
(Do Not Use Until 2002)
AMARYL (Hoechst Marion Roussel)

GENERIC: available except for glimepiride
FAMILY: Antidiabetic Drugs (see p. 550)
Sulfonylurea Hypoglycemics

These drugs are taken by mouth (orally) to lower high blood sugar levels caused by NIDDM (type-2) diabetes (see p. 550). Most type-2 diabetics can control their disease by following a prescribed diet, or, if diet alone does not work, by following a diet and injecting insulin (see p. 550). The main reason to use these drugs is if diet alone fails to control your diabetes and you cannot inject insulin. If you do use these drugs, it is best to use them temporarily, while losing weight, not permanently.

If you have type-2 diabetes, before taking any of these pills, you should try following a prescribed diet to reduce your blood sugar levels and, if you are overweight, to lose weight. If this does not work and you need to take a drug, insulin is a better choice than any of these pills. Although taking these pills is easier and more convenient than injecting insulin, they have significant risks, including an increased risk of death from heart attacks and blood vessel disease.

If you do take a diabetes pill, you should make sure that you are taking the safest possible one. Tolbutamide is less likely than the other diabetes pills to cause low blood sugar (see Adverse Effects) and takes less time to be

> You should wait at least five years from the date of release to take any new drug unless it is one of those rare "breakthrough" drugs that offers you a documented therapeutic advantage over older proven drugs. New drugs are tested in a relatively small number of people before being approved, and serious adverse effects or life-threatening drug interactions may not be detected until the new drug has been taken by hundreds of thousands of people. A number of new drugs have been withdrawn within their first five years after release. Also, serious new adverse reaction warnings have been added to the labeling of a number of drugs, or new drug interactions have been detected, usually within five years after a drug's release.

eliminated from your body. It is also available in an inexpensive generic form.

Acetohexamide should *not* be used by people who have impaired kidney function.[8] Since many older adults do have impaired kidney function, *even though they have normal kidney function tests,* we do not recommend this drug for people over 60. We also strongly recommend that you do not use chlorpropamide because it takes a long time to be eliminated from the body and is more likely than other diabetes pills to cause serious adverse effects associated with low blood sugar (see Adverse Effects). Chlorpropamide appears on a World Health Organization list of drugs that older adults should not use.[9]

If you are over 60 and you use a diabetes pill, your doctor should start you off at no more than half the usual adult dose.

Before You Use This Drug

Do not use if you have or have had recent:

- severe burns or injuries
- severe infection
- major surgery or trauma
- high ketone levels
- acidosis
- diabetic coma or ketoacidosis

Tell your doctor if you have or have had:

- allergies to drugs
- adrenal gland disease
- kidney or liver problems
- thyroid disease
- pituitary gland disease
- recent nausea, vomiting, or high fever
- an unusual reaction to another diabetes drug, a sulfonamide (sulfa) antibiotic, or a thiazide diuretic (water pill)
- continuing diarrhea
- female hormone changes
- severe mental stress
- heart disease and water retention *(for chlorpropamide)*

Tell your doctor about any other drugs you take, including aspirin, herbs, vitamins, and other nonprescription products.

When You Use This Drug

- Call your doctor immediately and eat or drink something with sugar in it if you experience symptoms of low blood sugar (see Adverse Effects, below).
- Do not stop taking your drug without talking to your doctor.
- If you have a high fever, nausea and vomiting, severe infection, or any severe injury, tell your doctor. Your treatment may have to be changed.
- Do not drink alcohol. The combination of alcohol and diabetes pills may cause abdominal cramps, nausea, vomiting, headaches, flushing, and low blood sugar.
- If you plan to have any surgery, including dental, tell your doctor that you take an oral hypoglycemic.

For chlorpropamide only: Someone should check on you regularly for at least three to five days after you experience symptoms of low blood sugar.

HEAT STRESS ALERT

These drugs can affect your body's ability to adjust to heat, putting you at risk of "heat stress." If you live alone, ask a friend to check on you several times during the day. Early signs of heat stress are dizziness, lightheadedness, faintness, and slightly high temperature. Call your doctor if you have any of these signs.

Drink more fluids (water, fruit and vegetable juices) than usual—even if you're not thirsty—unless your doctor has told you otherwise. Do not drink alcohol.

How to Use This Drug

• If you miss a dose, take it as soon as you remember, but skip it if it is almost time for the next dose. **Do not take double doses.**

• Do not store in the bathroom. Do not expose to heat, moisture, or strong light.

Interactions with Other Drugs

The following drugs are listed in the *Evaluations of Drug Interactions* 1997 as causing "highly clinically significant" or "clinically significant" interactions when used together with this drug. We have also included potentially serious interactions listed in the drug's FDA-approved professional product labeling or package insert. New scientific techniques have allowed researchers to predict some drug interactions before they have been documented in people. There may be other drugs, especially those in the families of drugs listed below, that also will react with this drug to cause severe adverse effects. The number of new drugs approved for marketing increases the chance of drug interactions, and new drug interactions are being identified with old drugs. Be vigilant. Make sure to tell your doctor and pharmacist the drugs you are taking and tell your doctor if you are taking any of these interacting drugs:

alcohol, aspirin, ATROMID-S, GENUINE BAYER ASPIRIN, BUTAZOLIDIN, charcoal, chloramphenicol, CHLOROMYCETIN, cholestyramine, cimetidine, clofibrate, cortisone, CORTONE, dicumarol, doxepin, ECOTRIN, ESIDRIX, fenfluramine, gemfibrozil, hydrochlorothiazide, HYDRODIURIL, INDERAL, INDERAL LA, LEVOTHROID, levothyroxine, LOCHOLEST, LOPID, NARDIL, oxytetracycline, phenelzine, phenylbutazone, PONDIMIN, propranolol, QUESTRAN, SINEQUAN, sulfamethizole, SYNTHROID, TAGAMET, TERRAMYCIN, THIOSULFIL, URIOBIOTIC-250.

Adverse Effects

Call your doctor immediately if you experience:

• **signs of low blood sugar**: anxiety, blurred vision, cold sweats or cool, pale skin, confusion, difficulty concentrating, drowsiness, increased hunger, headache, nausea, nervousness, nightmares and restless sleep, rapid heartbeat, shakiness, slurred speech, unsteady walk, abnormal tiredness or weakness, unusual weight gain. *(This adverse effect may take several days to subside and require hospitalization.)*

• **signs of high blood sugar**: blurred vision, drowsiness, dry, flushed skin, breath smells of fruit, increased urination, loss of appetite, tiredness, abnormal thirst, deep rapid breathing, dizziness, dry mouth, headache, stomachache, nausea, vomiting, swelling of feet, legs
  • dark urine or pale stools
  • itching skin
  • yellow eyes and skin
  • sore throat and fever
  • unusual bleeding or bruising
  • weakness, fever
  • fainting or unconsciousness
  • seizures
  • chest pain
  • chills
  • coughing up blood or increased amount of phlegm
  • skin blisters
  • sweating
  • pale skin
  • sensitivity to the sun
  • difficulty breathing

For chlorpropamide only: difficulty breathing, shortness of breath, muscle cramps, swollen or puffy face, hands, or ankles, water retention

RISK OF LOW BLOOD SUGAR (HYPOGLYCEMIA) WITH INDIVIDUAL SULFONYLUREAS IN OLDER PEOPLE

A study has been published assessing the risk of serious hypoglycemia in diabetics over age 65 taking one of the sulfonylurea drugs.[10] The new sulfonylurea drug glimepiride was not included in the study.

Serious hypoglycemia was more than four times more frequent in those using glyburide or chlorpropamide than in users of tolbutamine. Serious hypoglycemia occurred twice as often among users of glyburide compared to those taking glipizide. Compared to tolbutamide, those taking glipizide experienced serious hypoglycemia 2.5 times more often in the study.

The table below lists the drugs taken by diabetics in the study, from glyburide, which caused the most reactions, to tolbutamide, which caused the fewest.

FREQUENCY OF SERIOUS HYPOGLYCEMIC REACTIONS WITH SULFONYLUREAS

1. glyburide
2. chlorpropamide
3. acetohexamide
4. tolazamide
5. glipizide
6. tolbutamide

Call your doctor if these symptoms continue:

- diarrhea
- dizziness
- headache
- heartburn
- nausea, vomiting, loss of appetite
- stomach pain
- skin rash

- taste changes
- constipation
- difficulty urinating

Periodic Tests

Ask your doctor which of these tests should be done periodically done while you are taking this drug:

- complete blood count
- blood sugar levels
- urine levels of sugar and ketones
- chronic high blood sugar levels
- potassium and sodium serum concentrations

PREGNANCY WARNING

Diabinese, Glucotrol, DiaBeta, Tolinase, Orinase and Micronase caused harm to developing fetuses in animal studies, or such studies were not done. Use during pregnancy only for clear medical reasons. Tell your doctor if you are pregnant or thinking of becoming pregnant before you take any of these drugs.

 Do Not Use

ALTERNATIVE TREATMENT:
Tolbutamide, glipizide, tolazamide, see p. 555.

Metformin
GLUCOPHAGE (Bristol-Meyers-Squibb)

FAMILY: Antidiabetic Drugs (see p. 550)
Biguanides

Metformin (met *for* min) is an oral treatment for diabetes in people who do not require insulin and whose blood sugar is not controlled by diet and exercise. This drug is a biguanide, the same family as phenformin (DBI), which was withdrawn from the market in 1977 because of hundreds of deaths from lactic acidosis, a serious disease—in this case an adverse drug reaction—caused by a buildup of lactic acid in the blood. Metformin also causes lactic acidosis, though to a lesser extent than phenformin. Lactic acidosis is estimated to be fatal about 50% of the time.

Metformin works by decreasing glucose production in the liver and inhibiting the metabolism of lactate, thus reducing high blood sugar. Improved blood sugar control is known to prevent or delay complications of diabetes in both type-1 and type-2 diabetes. Metformin by itself *can* cause too low a blood sugar (hypoglycemia). The elderly, debilitated or malnourished patients, and those with certain disorders of the adrenal or pituitary glands or alcohol intoxication are particularly susceptible to the hypoglycemic effects of metformin. When metformin is used in combination with a sulfonylurea, hypoglycemia is especially likely to occur. The effectiveness of metformin tends to decline over time.[11]

Metformin can reduce the absorption of folic acid and vitamin B_{12}, causing a deficiency. Metformin also tends to cause watery diarrhea and a metallic taste. It should not be used in people with kidney dysfunction, heart failure, lung, or liver disease, sepsis, hypoxia, and/or high blood sugar of 300 mg/dl or greater. Kidney function tends to decline with age, putting the elderly at greater risk of lactic acidosis. Severe infection, heart problems, or dehydration can also trigger lactic acidosis. In older people the test known as creatinine clearance overestimates kidney function.[12] Metformin is also costly.

The Food and Drug Administration approved metformin on the condition that Bristol-Myers-Squibb conduct a postmarketing safety study to determine risk of lactic acidosis with this drug. FDA policy allows drug companies to withhold the design of postmarketing safety studies from public scrutiny, claiming that this type of safety information is confidential. Public Citizen's Health Research Group filed a lawsuit in federal district court to obtain a copy of the metformin safety study design and won an important legal battle for consumers. A panel of outside scientific experts reviewed the metformin study design and found that the design was inadequate to answer the important question about the risk of lactic acidosis with metformin.

Limited Use

Insulins

Beef Insulin, Pork Insulin,
Human Insulin
HUMALOG (Lilly)
HUMULIN, ILETIN (Lilly)
**INSULATARD, MIXTARD, NOVOLIN,
VELOSULIN** (Novo Nordisk)

GENERIC: available
FAMILY: Antidiabetic Drugs (see p. 550)

Insulin (*in sull in*), a drug that is injected under the skin, controls diabetes that cannot be controlled by diet alone. The dose of insulin requires frequent adjustment if good blood sugar control is to be achieved and maintained. For a more thorough discussion of the two types of diabetes and their treatment, see p. 550.

Early insulin came from the pancreas of cows or pigs. Human insulin does not come from the human pancreas, but is prepared from bacteria with DNA technology. Lispro insulin (Humalog) is a synthetic derivative of insulin. It is also prepared with DNA technology but differs in chemical structure from human insulin. Lispro insulin has similar effects to human insulin, but is absorbed more rapidly after injection under the skin.

There are two types of diabetes, type-1 (also called insulin dependent diabetes mellitus or IDDM) and type-2 (also called non-insulin dependent diabetes mellitus or NIDDM). People with type-1 diabetes need to take insulin. People with type-2 diabetes need to take insulin only if their disease cannot be controlled by diet alone. Most diabetics with adult-onset disease can control their diabetes without drugs if they follow their prescribed diet (see p. 550). Only about 10–15% cannot control the disease by diet and must use a blood-sugar-lowering medicine. No absolute criteria exist for diagnosing diabetes in the elderly, and many studies on diabetes have not involved the elderly.[13, 14] Even if you follow a prescribed diet, unacceptable levels of blood sugar may occur after a number of years. In type-2 diabetes the ability of the pancreas to secrete insulin gradually decreases with time, while insulin resistance remains constant or even increases.[15] In a study done on more than 21,000 doctors, increased physical exercise showed promise as an approach to preventing non-insulin-dependent diabetes mellitus.[16] For a more thorough discussion of the two types of diabetes and their treatment see p. 550.

Insulin works by regulating the amount of sugar (glucose) in the blood and the speed at which sugar moves into cells. In diabetics, instead of moving into the cells, the sugar accumulates in the blood, resulting in very high blood sugar levels.

Your diet affects your cells' need for insulin and the insulin's ability to lower blood sugar when necessary. Therefore, for insulin to work, you must also follow a prescribed diet: **Insulin is not a replacement for such a diet.**

Too much insulin may cause low blood sugar (hypoglycemia). This happens most often in people who are over 60, especially if they have reduced kidney function, and also occurs frequently in young diabetics with type-1 diabetes. You may be more likely to suffer hypoglycemia if you skip or delay eating meals, exercise more than usual, or drink a significant amount of alcohol.

To prevent or delay severe consequences of diabetes, such as blindness, cataracts, gangrene, heart, circulatory, and kidney problems, lowering high blood sugar (hyperglycemia) is standard medical practice. Although there is a new emphasis on stricter glucose control than before, there are still concerns about the hazards of low blood sugar (hypoglycemia) if control is too strict.[17,18,19,20,21,22,23] Overly strict glucose control also resulted in more auto accidents for diabetics, due to sudden episodes of hypoglycemia.[24,25] Studies conflict on whether severe and frequent episodes of low blood sugar hasten decline in intellectual ability.[26,27,28] Prior objections to frequent testing centered on making people too preoccupied with being ill.

Diabetic therapy must be individualized.

Before You Use This Drug

Tell your doctor if you have or have had:

- allergies to drugs, beef, or pork
- adrenal or pituitary gland problems[29]
- eating disorders
- kidney or liver problems
- loss of consciousness
- nausea, vomiting, or diarrhea
- severe infections
- severe injuries or surgery
- thyroid problems
- changes in female hormones
- high fever
- psychological stress

Tell your doctor about any other drugs you take, including aspirin, herbs, vitamins, and other nonprescription products.

When You Use This Drug

- Know the warning signs of low blood sugar, high blood sugar and ketoacidosis (see Adverse Effects).
- Keep sugar on hand. Tubes or tablets of glucose, a piece of fruit, pure orange juice,

cheese, soda crackers, or one or two cups of milk will suffice. Honey, sugar candy, or syrup can also be used. Carry some with you at all times.

• Monitor your blood glucose. All diabetics should be using a machine to monitor blood glucose. Be sure you receive adequate instruction. Do not hesitate to ask or repeat questions until you feel comfortable using the device.

• Eat a diet high in complex carbohydrates and fiber, but low in saturated fats. Avoid sugar, alcohol, and smoking. Distribute your calories over several small meals, or meals and snacks to prevent low blood sugar. While these general diet guidelines should help, older diabetics should be aware that little information is available on the effect of diets in the elderly.[30]

• Whenever you cannot eat properly due to illness (fever, nausea, vomiting), continue your insulin, but realize your insulin requirements may change. Close medical supervision and hospitalization may be required.

• If you plan to have any surgery, including dental, tell your doctor that you are diabetic, and take insulin.

• Carry identification stating your condition and the type of insulin(s) you use.

• When you travel, pack an extra supply of insulin, syringes, glucose and ketone testing materials, snacks, and a prescription. Carry your supplies instead of checking them.

• Exercise regularly. Inconsistent exercise risks low blood sugar on days you exert more.

• Keep your feet clean, warm, and dry. If you cannot cut your toenails, find a community group that provides the service. Call your doctor if signs of infection appear.

• Wear well-fitting shoes, and break them in gradually. Avoid thongs, chemical corn and callous removers, and hot soaks or pads.

• Be cautious driving. Do not drive when your glucose levels are unstable.

• Choose nonprescription drugs and vitamins without sugar and alcohol. Lists of acceptable products are generally available from diabetes associations, your doctor and pharmacy. Check with your doctor if you have any doubts.

How to Use This Drug

• Insulin syringes come in 100- 50- and 25- or 30-unit sizes. For accuracy of dosing, you should use the smallest insulin syringe that will hold the dose to be given. Always use the same brand of syringes. Switching brands may result in using a different amount of insulin, due to differences in the unmeasured volume between the needle point and bottom calibration. Although it is not recommended, if you do reuse disposable syringes wipe the needle with alcohol, then recap. Reuse only for a limited number of injections.[31] Reusable glass syringes and metal needles can still be ordered. Before each use, the syringe, plunger, and needle must be boiled in water for five minutes, or immersed in 91% isopropyl alcohol for at least five minutes, then air dried. Insulin pen cartridges with replaceable needles are another alternative. Do not use conventional insulin syringes in those devices. Needleless jet injectors are available, but are limited by lack of predictability.[32] If you use an insulin pump, obtain instructions on how to fill the pump, check the tubing, and maintain the infusion site. Pumps have no well-documented advantage over insulin given by syringe.[33,34]

• If you cannot see well enough to measure insulin, contact community agencies to find someone to predraw your insulin.

• Insulin is stable for two weeks, in plastic syringes; in glass, it is stable for one week when refrigerated.[35]

• Verify the label on your insulin and examine the appearance of the insulin. Do not use regular insulin if it is cloudy or thick. Other insulins should appear uniformly milky, but not lumpy, grainy, stuck on the bottle, or unable to shake into suspension. Return questionable, unopened vials to your pharmacy.

• Wash your hands. Swab the top of the vial with alcohol.

• Except for regular (short-acting) insulin, roll the vial slowly between the palms of the hands until the insulin is uniformly mixed.

• Do not shake vigorously, or bubbles may interfere with a correct measurement of insulin.

• Draw air into the syringe equal to your insulin dose. Insert needle into the vial, then expel the air. Draw insulin into the syringe, check for air bubbles. Double check your dose.

• If you use more than one type of insulin, always draw in the same order. Draw regular (short-acting) insulin first. Before injecting, roll the syringe to remix. Several premixed insulins are now available. Do not mix buffered insulins with lente (longer-acting) insulins. Store prefilled syringes of mixtures vertically with the needle upwards to avoid plugging the needle.

• Select a site to inject insulin in the abdomen, buttocks, front thigh, or back of the arm. Stick to one area, then rotate sites within that area to prevent breakdown of fat tissue.[36] Maintain the same posture each time you inject. Avoid inflamed or infected sites.

• Clean the site before injecting. Inject needle at a 90 degree angle just under the skin (subcutaneously). Pull back on the plunger. If blood appears, try again. Inject in less than five seconds. Massaging the site after injection may speed absorption of the insulin.[37]

• Insulin comes in a variety of forms with different lengths of action. Do not change brands, strength, or type of insulin without checking with your doctor. Switches may call for a change in your insulin dose. If you use a less common form of insulin, deal with a pharmacy that promises to keep some in stock.

• Refrigeration prolongs stability, and prevents contamination of insulin. According to the International Diabetes Institute, unopened insulin, properly stored, loses 5% potency in 10 years.[38] Insulin (even old style) may be stored at room temperature. Once assembled, NovolinPen or PenFill must be stored at room temperature and must not be refrigerated.

Today, at home, most people with diabetes refrigerate insulin vials until opened, then store the vial being used at room temperature. Do not expose to high temperatures, or sunlight. Never freeze insulin or warm it in a microwave. Once opened, vials should be discarded after several weeks.[39] Policies for storing insulin in congregate living and institutions may differ from home practices.

• Dispose of your syringes according to local waste disposal regulations.

Interactions with Other Drugs

The following drugs are listed in the *Evaluations of Drug Interactions* 1997 as causing "highly clinically significant" or "clinically significant" interactions when used together with this drug. We have also included potentially serious interactions listed in the drug's FDA-approved professional product labeling or package insert. New scientific techniques have allowed researchers to predict some drug interactions before they have been documented in people. There may be other drugs, especially those in the families of drugs listed below, that also will react with this drug to cause severe adverse effects. The number of new drugs approved for marketing increases the chance of drug interactions, and new drug interactions are being identified with old drugs. Be vigilant. Make sure to tell your doctor and pharmacist the drugs you are taking and tell your doctor if you are taking any of these interacting drugs:

alcohol, ATROMID-S, clofibrate, fenfluramine, guanethidine, INDERAL, INDERAL LA, ISMELIN, LEVOTHROID, levothyroxine, NARDIL, oxytetracycline, phenelzine, PONDIMIN, propranolol, SYNTHROID, TERRAMYCIN, timolol, TIMOPTIC, UROBIOTIC-250.

Additionally, the *United States Pharmacopeia Drug Information,* 1998 lists these drugs as having interactions of major significance: DELTASONE, METICORTEN, NEBUPENT, pentamidine, PENTAM 300, prednisone.

Adverse Effects

Any insulin may cause allergies in a few individuals.[40,41] Skin cleansers and preservatives in the insulin also can cause local allergic reactions.[42]

Call your doctor immediately if you experience:

- **allergic reactions:** itching, rapid heartbeat, shortness of breath, swelling at injection site
  - out of control blood sugar
  - severe vomiting
  - severe symptoms of low or high blood sugar
  - seizures
  - faintness or unconsciousness
  - depressed or thickened skin at injection site
  - swelling of face, fingers, feet or ankles
- **signs of low blood sugar**: anxiety, blurred vision, cold sweats or cool, pale skin, confusion, difficulty concentrating, drowsiness, increased hunger, headache, nausea, nervousness, numbness,[43] nightmares and restless sleep, rapid heartbeat, shakiness, slurred speech, unsteady walk, abnormal tiredness or weakness, unusual weight gain.

Low blood sugar

- Low blood sugar can be caused by missed meals, increased exercise, consuming alcohol, changes in insulin dose, use of long-acting insulins, use of continuous infusion pumps[44,45] and certain illnesses.[46] An increase of even one unit of insulin can cause low blood sugar.[47]
- Hunger, sweating, and trembling are signs most diabetics rely on as a warning.[48,49] However, warnings vary with the individual, and whether or not an insulin pump is used. Warning signs may change if low blood sugar occurs often.[50] There is debate as to whether animal and human insulins differ in warnings each provide.[51,52,53,54,55,56,57,58,59,60]

- Every instance of these symptoms does not mean you have low blood sugar. Do not rely only on warning signs, but also test your blood sugar to see if it actually is low, if time permits.[61]
- More than half of episodes of low blood sugar happen during the night.[62] Testing blood glucose at bedtime is advisable.[63] So is keeping a source of sugar by your bed. However, you may not always be aware of low blood sugar that happened during the night. Clues on waking up are:[64] morning headaches, night sweats, symptoms of hypothermia (see glossary, p. 768)
- If you have low blood sugar often, call your doctor.

High blood sugar

- Symptoms of high blood sugar in the elderly may vary[65] but they can include: blurred vision, drowsiness, dry, flushed skin, breath smells of fruit, increased urination, loss of appetite, tiredness, abnormal thirst, deep rapid breathing, dizziness, dry mouth, headache, stomachache, nausea, vomiting, swelling of feet and legs.[66]
- High blood sugar is often due to severe lack of insulin or infection.

Periodic Tests

Ask your doctor which of these tests should be done periodically while you are taking this drug and how often they should be done:

- blood levels of glucose, ketones and potassium
- blood pH
- blood pressure
- glycosylated hemoglobin test
- urine ketone

Do Not Use Until Five Years After Release

Acarbose (Do Not Use Until 2001)
PRECOSE (Bayer)

GENERIC: not available

FAMILY: Antidiabetic Drugs (see p. 550)

> You should wait at least five years from the date of release to take any new drug unless it is one of those rare "breakthrough" drugs that offers you a documented therapeutic advantage over older proven drugs. New drugs are tested in a relatively small number of people before being approved, and serious adverse effects or life-threatening drug interactions may not be detected until the new drug has been taken by hundreds of thousands of people. A number of new drugs have been withdrawn within their first five years after release. Also, serious new adverse reaction warnings have been added to the labeling of a number of drugs, or new drug interactions have been detected, usually within the first five years after a drug's release.

Acarbose (*ak* ar bose) is used to treat people with diabetes who do not require insulin and whose diabetes is not controlled by diet alone. Acarbose slows digestion of sugars and complex carbohydrates by blocking digestive enzymes in the intestines. It is sometimes called a starch blocker. Acarbose decreases blood sugar, *to a relatively small degree,* usually without causing hypoglycemia (too low blood sugar).

Acarbose is not a substitute for a diet, and does not necessarily cause weight loss. The first dose is 25 mg three times daily. It may take two weeks to notice the effect of acarbose. Thereafter, dosage is adjusted at four to eight week intervals until the maximum dose of 50 mg three times daily for people weighing under 130 lbs. or 100 mg three times daily for people weighing over 130 lbs. is reached. Acarbose causes more carbohydrates to ferment in your colon, and you may experience rumbling noises in the bowels, gas, and diarrhea. These symptoms may subside. Acarbose may also inhibit absorption of iron. People who take high doses of acarbose and weigh less than 130 lbs. are at greater risk for liver complications. Acarbose is not recommended for people with kidney dysfunction. There is little available information on use of acarbose in the elderly.[67]

Before You Use This Drug

Tell your doctor if you have or have had:

- allergies
- anemia
- cirrhosis or other liver problems
- diabetic ketoacidosis
- hernia
- ongoing indigestion, intestinal blockage, or other gastrointestinal problems
- inflammatory bowel disease
- kidney problems
- ulceration of colon

Tell your doctor about any other drugs you take, including aspirin, herbs, vitamins, and other nonprescription products.

When You Use This Drug

- To limit adverse effects of gas, follow your diet, including high intake of complex carbohydrates and low intake of simple sugars, as sucrose.[68] Older people generally are at risk of malnutrition due to problems with food shopping, food preparation, and chewing and swallowing difficulties. Arrangements may be needed for timely access to daily meals.
- Maintain adequate iron intake.
- Continue to monitor your blood sugar and/or urine sugar.

• If your blood sugar becomes too low take glucose (dextrose), or lactose (glass of milk).[69] Do not take candy, Classic Coke, Life Savers, orange juice, (which contains sucrose, cane sugar) or starch to treat low blood sugar. Acarbose prevents these from working quickly enough.

• Maintain adequate exercise.

• Maintain proper foot care.

• Take precautions to avoid infections.

• If you plan to have any surgery, including dental, tell your doctor that you take this drug.

• If you miss a dose skip it, then take the next dose. **Do not take double doses.**

How to Use This Drug

• If your dose is half a tablet, split tablets at time you will take, not in advance. Exposure to moisture will cause discoloration of split tablets.

• Swallow or chew half or whole tablets according to your dose, with first bite of each meal.

• Store tablets at room temperature, not above 77°F. Do not store in the bathroom. Do not expose to heat, moisture, or strong light.

Interactions with Other Drugs

The following drugs are listed in the *Evaluations of Drug Interactions* 1997 as causing "highly clinically significant" or "clinically significant" interactions when used together with this drug. We have also included potentially serious interactions listed in the drug's FDA-approved professional product labeling or package insert. New scientific techniques have allowed researchers to predict some drug interactions before they have been documented in people. There may be other drugs, especially those in the families of drugs listed below, that also will react with this drug to cause severe adverse effects. The number of new drugs approved for marketing increases the chance of drug interactions, and new drug interactions are being identified with old drugs. Be vigilant. Make sure to tell your doctor and pharmacist

the drugs you are taking and tell your doctor if you are taking any of these interacting drugs:

charcoal, CREON, DONNAZYME, pancreatin.

Acarbose does not interact with alcohol, but if taken with beer, adverse effects of gas may increase.

Adverse Effects

Call your doctor immediately if you experience:

• dark stools

• high blood sugar

• weakness

• yellowing of skin or eyes, or pale skin

Call your doctor if these symptoms continue:

• abdominal swelling

• diarrhea or soft stools

• gas or other gastrointestinal problems

• sweating[70]

Periodic Tests

Ask your doctor which of these tests should be done periodically while you are taking this drug and how often they should be done:

• Have liver function (transaminase levels) tested every three months.

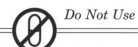 *Do Not Use*

ALTERNATIVE TREATMENT:
Tolbutamide, glipizide, tolazamide, p. 555.

Troglitazone
REZULIN (Parke-Davis)

FAMILY: Antidiabetic Drugs (see p. 550)

Troglitazone (*troe* glit a zone) is an expensive first entry to a new class of drugs for the treatment of type-2 diabetes. On December 1, 1997 the FDA announced additional warnings for troglitazone based on approximately 150 adverse reaction reports, including three deaths from liver failure linked to the use of the drug in Japan. Troglitazone remains on the market in the U.S. with the FDA saying that the benefits of this drug outweigh its risks, while in the United Kingdom the drug has been removed from the market based on the British authorities finding that troglitazone's risks outweigh its benefits.[71]

Why is there this discrepancy between the actions of the FDA and those of British regulatory authorities? To answer this question we first must examine the benefits of the antidiabetic drugs. There are four important facts to remember:

1. All of the antidiabetic drugs lower blood sugar.

2. These drugs are given not just to lower blood sugar, but to reduce the complications and prolong the lives of people with type-2 diabetes.

3. Diet and exercise should be tried as a method of controlling blood sugar before any of the antidiabetic drugs are prescribed.

4. Tolbutamide (ORINASE and generics), a member of the sulfonylurea family, and phenformin (the first cousin to metformin) banned from the market in 1977, are the only antidiabetic drugs that have ever been tested in a clinical study to see if the complications of type-2 diabetes could be prevented or delayed.

The study was called the University Group Diabetes Program (UGDP) and was stopped prematurely in 1970[72] because the death rate from heart problems was 2.5 times greater with tolbutamide and phenformin than in those treated with diet alone.

For the other antidiabetic drugs, metformin (GLUCOPHAGE), acarbose (PRECOSE), and

troglitazone that are not sulfonylureas, no studies have shown that these drugs can be taken safely for a long enough period of time to reduce the complications and prolong the lives of people with type-2 diabetes.

The British decision to withdraw troglitazone from the market was absolutely correct. Given that no antidiabetic drug has been shown to reduce the long term cardiovascular complications of type-2 diabetes and that the sulfonylureas, in fact, may cause harm, the risk of liver toxicity with troglitizone simply outweighs any known benefits of this drug. The FDA's action allowing troglitazone to remain on the market instead of banning the drug was irresponsible.

By June 1998, there were at least 21 deaths from liver failure in patients using troglitazone and three patients with liver damage so severe they required liver transplants. In July 1998, Public Citizen's Health Research Group petitioned the FDA to ban the drug.

NOTES FOR DRUGS FOR DIABETES

1. *Diabetes,* 1970; 19 (Suppl 2): 813.

2. Ibid.

3. Chalmers T. Settling the UGDP controversy. *Journal of the American Medical Association* 1975; 231:624.

4. Vestal RE, ed. *Drug Treatment in the Elderly.* Sydney, Australia: ADIS Health Science Press, 1984:231.

5. Chalmers, op. cit.

6. AMA Department of Drugs. *AMA Drug Evaluations.* 5th ed. Chicago: American Medical Association, 1983:1045.

7. Ibid, p. 1036.

8. Peden N, Newton RW, Feely J. Oral hypoglycaemic agents. *British Medical Journal* 1983; 286:1566.

9. *Drugs for the Elderly.* 2nd ed. Copenhagen, Denmark: World Health Organization, 1997:46.

10. Shorr RI, Ray WA, Daugherty JR, Griffin MR. Individual sulfonylureas and serious hypoglycemia in older people. *Journal of the American Geriatrics Society* 1996; 44:751–5.

11. American Diabetes Association Consensus Statement. The pharmacological treatment of hyperglycemia in NIDDM. *Diabetes Care* 1995; 18:1510–8.

12. Sambol NC, Chiang J, Lin ET, Goodman AM, Liu CY, Benet LZ, et al. Kidney function and age are both predictors of pharmacokinetics of metformin. *Journal of Clinical Pharmacology* 1995; 35:1094–102.

13. Lorenz RA, Santiago JV, Siebert C, Cleary PA, Heyse S, DCCT Research Group. Epidemiology of severe hypoglycemia in the Diabetes Control and Complications Trial. *The American Journal of Medicine* 1991; 90:450–9.

14. Porte D, Kahn SE. What geriatricians should know about diabetes mellitus. *Diabetes Care* 1990; 13 (Suppl. 2):47–54.

15. Expert Committee on the Diagnosis and Classification of Diabetes Mellitus. Report of the Expert Committee on the Diagnosis and Classification of Diabetes Mellitus. *Diabetes Care* 1997; 20:1183–97.

16. Manson JE, Nathan DM, Krolewski AS, Stampfer MJ, Willett WC, Hennekens CH. A prospective study of exercise and incidence of diabetes among U.S. male physicians. *Journal of the American Medical Association* 1992; 268:63–7.

17. Feingold KR. Hypoglycemia—a major risk of insulin therapy. *The Western Journal of Medicine* 1991; 154:469–71.

18. Lorenz, op. cit.

19. Porte, op. cit.

20. Ratner RE, Whitehouse FW. Motor vehicles, hypoglycemia, and diabetic drivers. *Diabetes Care* 1989; 12:217–22.

21. Reichard P, Berglund A, Britz A, Levander S, Rosenqvist U. Hypoglycaemic episodes during intensified insulin treatment: increased frequency but no effect on cognitive function. *Journal of Internal Medicine* 1991; 229:9–16.

22. Dukes MNG, Beeley L. *Side Effects of Drugs Annual* 15, Amsterdam: Elsevier, 1991:451.

23. Wolff SP. Is hyperglycemia risky enough to justify the increased risk of hypoglycemia linked with tight diabetes control? *Biochemical Medicine and Metabolic Biology* 1991; 46:129–39.

24. Lorenz, op. cit.

25. Ratner, op. cit.

26. Kerr D, Reza M, Smith N, Leatherdale BA. Importance of insulin in subjective, cognitive, and hormonal responses to hypoglycemia in patients with IDDM. *Diabetes* 1991; 40:1057–62.

27. Langan SJ, Deary IJ, Hepburn DA, Frier BM. Cumulative cognitive impairment following recurrent severe hypoglycemia in adult patients with insulin-treated diabetes mellitus. *Diabetologia* 1991; 34:337–44.

28. Reichard, op. cit.

29. Feingold, op. cit.

30. Porte, op. cit.

31. *USP DI, Drug Information for the Health Care Professional.* 12th ed. Rockville MD: The United States Pharmacopeial Convention, Inc., 1992:1580–6.

32. *Manual of Medical Therapeutics.* 26th ed. St. Louis: Washington University, 1989:381.

33. AMA Department of Drugs. *AMA Drug Evaluations.* Chicago: American Medical Association, 1992:943–4.

34. Gilman AG, Rall TW, Nies AS, Taylor P, eds. *The Pharmacological Basis of Therapeutics.* 8th ed. New York: Pergamon Press, 1990:1463–95.

35. Olin BR, ed. *Facts and Comparisons.* St. Louis: J.B. Lippincott Co., September 1992:129f-130d.

36. Gilman, op. cit.

37. *Manual of Medical Therapeutics,* op. cit.

38. Raab RS. Letter from the International Diabetes Institute, May 4, 1990.

39. American Society of Hospital Pharmacists. *American Hospital Formulary Service Drug Information.* Bethesda, MD, 1992:1883–8.

40. Balcells MC, Corcoy RM, Lleonart RB, Pujol RV, Mauricio DP, Garcia AP, et al. Primary allergy to human insulin in patients with gestational diabetes. *Diabetes Care* 1991; 14:423–4.

41. Dukes MNG, Beeley L. *Side Effects of Drugs Annual* 14, Amsterdam: Elsevier, 1990:372–3.

42. Olin, op. cit.

43. Kern W, Lieb K, Kerner W, Born J, Fehm HL. Differential effects of human and pork insulin-induced hypoglycemia on neuronal functions in humans. *Diabetes* 1990; 39:1091–8.

44. Dukes, 1990, op. cit.

45. Lorenz, op. cit.

46. Feingold, op. cit.

47. Gin H, Aparicio M, Potaux L, Merville P, Combe CH, de Precigout V, et al. Low-protein, low-phosphorus diet and tissue insulin sensitivity in insulin-dependent diabetic patients with chronic renal failure. *Nephron* 1991; 57:411–5.

48. Egger M, Smith GD, Teuscher AU, Teuscher A. Influence of human insulin on symptoms and awareness of hypoglycaemia: a randomised double blind crossover trial. *British Medical Journal* 1991; 303:622–6.

49. Muhlhauser I, Heinemann L, Fritsche E, von Lennep K, Berger M. Hypoglycemic symptoms and frequency of severe hypoglycemia in patients treated with human and animal insulin preparations. *Diabetes Care* 1991; 14:745–9.

50. Reichard, op. cit.

51. Bendtson I, Binder C. Counterregulatory hormonal response to insulin-induced hypoglycaemia in insulin-dependent diabetic patients: a comparison of equimolar amounts of porcine and semisynthetic human insulin. *Journal of Internal Medicine* 1991; 229:293–6.

52. Cherfas J. UK diabetics plan insulin suit. *Science* 1991; 253:1090.

53. Egger M, Smith GD, Imhoof H, Teuscher A. Risk of severe hypoglycaemia in insulin treated diabetic patients transferred to human insulin: a case control study. *British Medical Journal* 1991; 303:617–21.

54. Egger, Influence of Human Insulin, op. cit.

55. Human insulin. *British Medical Journal* 1991; 303:1265–8 [letters].

56. Jick SS, Derby LE, Gross KM, Jick H. Hospitalizations because of hypoglycemia in users of animal and human insulins. 2. Experience in the United States. *Pharmacotherapy* 1990; 1:398–9.

57. Lorenz, op. cit.

58. Muhlhauser, op. cit.

59. Dukes, 1990, op. cit.

60. Confusion over human insulin. *Lancet* 1991; 338:1213–4 [letters].

61. Feingold, op. cit.

62. Lorenz, op. cit.

63. Reichard, op. cit.

64. Gilman, op. cit.

65. Porte, op. cit.

66. Gilman, op. cit.

67. Mooradian AD. Drug therapy of non-insulin-dependent diabetes mellitus in the elderly. *Drugs* 1996; 51:931–41.

68. Ibid.

69. Yee HS, Fong NT. A review of the safety and efficacy of acarbose in diabetes mellitus. *Pharmacotherapy* 1996; 16:792–805.

70. Ibid.

71. Troglitazone (Romozin) withdrawn. *Current Problems in Pharmacovigilance* 1997; 23:13.

72. *Diabetes,* op. cit.

Drugs for Neurological Disorders

DRUG LISTINGS

ANTIPARKINSONIAN DRUGS

ARTANE	Ø Do Not Use	569
benztropine	Ø Do Not Use	570
bromocriptine		586
COGENTIN	Ø Do Not Use	570
deprenyl	Limited Use	576
ELDEPRYL	Limited Use	576
LARODOPA		582
levodopa		582
levodopa and carbidopa		582
PARLODEL		586
selegiline	Limited Use	576
SINEMET		582
trihexyphenidyl	Ø Do Not Use	569

ANTICONVULSANTS

carbamazepine		588
clonazepam		579
DEPAKENE		572
DEPAKOTE		572
DILANTIN		574
divalproex		572
KLONOPIN		579
LUMINAL	Limited Use	584
phenobarbital	Limited Use	584
phenytoin		574

SOLFOTON	Limited Use	584
TEGRETOL		588
valproate		572
valproic acid		572

DRUGS USED IN ALZHEIMER'S DISEASE

ARICEPT	Ø Do Not Use	571
COGNEX	Ø Do Not Use	571
donepezil	Ø Do Not Use	571
ergoloid mesylates	Ø Do Not Use	578
HYDERGINE	Ø Do Not Use	578
HYDERGINE LC	Ø Do Not Use	578
tacrine	Ø Do Not Use	571

DRUG PROFILES

Ø *Do Not Use*

ALTERNATIVE TREATMENT:
An antihistamine, see below.

Trihexyphenidyl
ARTANE (Lederle)

FAMILY: Antiparkinsonians

Trihexyphenidyl (try hex ee *fen* i dill) **should not be used to treat Parkinson's disease** because it can cause several serious adverse effects—more frequently in older adults. These effects include memory impairment, confusion, hallucinations, and retention of urine. If you use trihexyphenidyl, ask your doctor to change your prescription to an antihistamine such as diphenhydramine (BENADRYL, see p. 424). Antihistamines work in the same way as trihexyphenidyl, yet have milder adverse effects in older adults.[1,2] They are usually used either alone, to treat people with mild symptoms of Parkinson's disease, or in combination with another antiparkinsonian drug such as levodopa with carbidopa (see p. 582).

If you have symptoms of parkinsonism (tremor, rigid muscles, and disturbances in posture, walking, balance, speech, swallowing and muscle strength), there is a good chance that they are caused by a drug you are taking. As many as half of older adults with symptoms of parkinsonism may have developed them as adverse effects of a drug. A list of drugs that can cause symptoms of parkinsonism appears on p. 25. If you take any of the drugs on this list, discuss the possibility of drug-induced parkinsonism with your doctor, and ask to have your prescription changed or stopped.

WARNING: SPECIAL MENTAL AND PHYSICAL ADVERSE EFFECTS

Older adults are especially sensitive to the harmful anticholinergic (see Glossary, p. 768) effects of antiparkinsonian drugs such as trihexyphenidyl. Drugs in this family should not be used unless absolutely necessary.

Mental Effects: confusion, delirium, short-term memory problems, disorientation, and impaired attention.

Physical Effects: dry mouth, constipation, difficulty urinating (especially for a man with an enlarged prostate), blurred vision, decreased sweating with increased body temperature, sexual dysfunction, and worsening of glaucoma.

Do Not Use

ALTERNATIVE TREATMENT:
An antihistamine, see below.

Benztropine
COGENTIN (Merck)

FAMILY: Antiparkinsonians

Benztropine (*benz* troe peen) **should not be used to treat Parkinson's disease** because it can cause several serious adverse effects—more frequently in older adults. These effects include memory impairment, confusion, hallucinations, and retention of urine. If you use benztropine, ask your doctor to change your prescription to an antihistamine such as diphenhydramine (BENADRYL, see p. 424). Antihistamines work in the same way as benztropine, yet have milder adverse effects in older adults.[3,4] They are usually used either alone, to treat people with mild symptoms of Parkinson's disease, or in combination with another anti parkinsonian drug such as levodopa with carbidopa (see p. 582).

If you have symptoms of parkinsonism (tremor, rigid muscles, and disturbances in posture, walking, balance, speech, swallowing, and muscle strength), there is a good chance that they are caused by a drug you are taking. As many as half of older adults with symptoms of parkinsonism may have developed them as adverse effects of a drug. A list of drugs that can cause symptoms of parkinsonism appears on p. 25. If you take any of the drugs on this list, discuss the possibility of drug-induced parkinsonism with your doctor, and ask to have your prescription changed or stopped.

WARNING: SPECIAL MENTAL AND PHYSICAL ADVERSE EFFECTS

Older adults are especially sensitive to the harmful anticholinergic (see Glossary, p. 768) effects of antiparkinsonian drugs such as benztropine. Drugs in this family should not be used unless absolutely necessary.

Mental Effects: confusion, delirium, short-term memory problems, disorientation, and impaired attention.

Physical Effects: dry mouth, constipation, difficulty urinating (especially for a man with an enlarged prostate), blurred vision, decreased sweating with increased body temperature, sexual dysfunction, and worsening of glaucoma.

Do Not Use

ALTERNATIVE TREATMENT:
At this time there are no safe and effective treatments that improve cognition in Alzheimer's disease.

Tacrine
COGNEX (Parke-Davis)

Donepezil
ARICEPT (Pfizer)

FAMILY: Drugs Used in Alzheimer's Disease

Tacrine (*ta* crin) was the first drug approved by the Food and Drug Administration (FDA) for Alzheimer's disease and donepezil (doe *nep* pe zil) the second. The action of both drugs is to inhibit the enzyme that breaks down acetylcholine, a brain transmitter, a deficiency of which has been thought to play a role in Alzheimer's disease.

The major clinical trial evaluating tacrine found a statistically significant reduction in the decline of cognitive function in patients taking the drug compared to those taking a placebo (inactive sugar pill).[5] The editorial accompanying this clinical trial stated that the differences between the placebo and tacrine groups, although statistically significant, were "clinically trivial."[6] The editors of the internationally respected *Medical Letter on Drugs and Therapeutics,* an independent source of drug information, said: "Tacrine appears to improve or slow the decline in various test scores in a minority of patients with mild to moderate Alzheimer's disease, but there is no evidence from controlled trials that its use leads to substantial functional improvement. The drug can cause hepatic [liver] injury and may inhibit the metabolism of other drugs."[7]

Tacrine is still produced, although sales have slumped to the point where the drug's maker, Parke-Davis, has suspended promoting the drug to doctors and discontinued patient support programs. Parke-Davis will continue to produce tacrine, however.

The effectiveness of donepezil, the newest Alzheimer's disease drug, has not been compared with tacrine. Donepezil, like tacrine, has shown a modest effect of improvement compared with a placebo, and the differences between the donepezil and placebo groups were statistically significant. The most common adverse effects of donepezil have been nausea, diarrhea and vomiting. Insomnia, fatigue, muscle cramps and loss of appetite have also been reported by donepezil users. So far, the effect of serious liver injury that is present with tacrine has not been seen with donepezil. *The Medical Letter* editors in their 1997 review of donepezil said: "There is no evidence that use of either donepezil or tacrine leads to substantial functional improvement or prevents the progression of the disease."[8]

Divalproex/Valproate/Valproic Acid
DEPAKENE/DEPAKOTE (Abbott)

GENERIC: available
FAMILY: Anticonvulsants

WARNING: LIVER TOXICITY

Liver failure resulting in death has occurred in people receiving valproic acid and its derivatives. Experience has indicated that children under the age of two years are at a particular risk of developing fatal liver toxicity.

WARNING: BIRTH DEFECTS

Valproate can produce birth defects such as spina bifida. The use of valproate products in women of childbearing potential requires that the benefits of its use be weighed against the risk of injury to the baby.

Valproic acid (val *pro* ic acid) and its derivatives are approved to treat recurrent seizures and mania and to prevent migraine headaches. These drugs are also used for several other conditions not approved by the FDA, including other seizure disorders, aggression[9] and anxiety.

Doses vary with age, weight, the reason for taking valproic acid, and the nature of your response. It is best for older people to start with a low dose. Adverse effects may be decreased by increasing dosage incrementally and by taking enteric-coated tablets. Doses more than 250 mg are usually divided throughout the day. Long-term use of Valproic acid can lead to weight gain. Valproic acid and its derivatives can cause serious or fatal liver damage. Children under two years of age are particularly at risk. Persons with liver disease should not take valproic acid. Valproic acid can also adversely affect your blood by increasing blood platelets.

Most, but not all, of these serious reactions happen within the first six months. Valproic acid can cause neural tube defects in the fetus, so women who are pregnant should avoid this drug. Valproic acid also passes into breast milk and should be used with caution in women who are breastfeeding their infants, as the effects on the infant are unknown.

Valproic acid is sometimes taken in combination with other drugs for seizures.

Before You Use This Drug

Tell your doctor if you have or have had:

- allergies
- diabetes
- head injuries
- kidney or liver problems
- blood disease
- brain disease

Tell your doctor about any other drugs you take, including aspirin, herbs, vitamins, and other nonprescription products.

When You Use This Drug

- **Do not stop taking valproic acid abruptly.** Ask your doctor how to discontinue taking this drug.
- Do not drink alcohol or use other drugs that can cause drowsiness.
- Until you know how you react to this drug, do not drive or perform other activities that require alertness.
- If you plan to have any surgery, including dental, tell your doctor that you take this drug.

How to Use This Drug

- Measure dose of liquid with calibrated teaspoon. Swallow whole oral capsules or tablets according to dose. Take with food if it upsets your stomach or empty the contents of capsules and sprinkle onto a small amount of soft food, such as pudding or applesauce. Do not chew.

- Take at bedtime to minimize effects such as drowsiness.
- Store at room temperature. Do not store in the bathroom. Do not expose to heat, moisture, or strong light.

Interactions with Other Drugs

The following drugs are listed in the *Evaluations of Drug Interactions* 1997 as causing "highly clinically significant" or "clinically significant" interactions when used together with this drug. We have also included potentially serious interactions listed in the drug's FDA-approved professional product labeling or package insert. New scientific techniques have allowed researchers to predict some drug interactions before they have been documented in people. There may be other drugs, especially those in the families of drugs listed below, that also will react with this drug to cause severe adverse effects. The number of new drugs approved for marketing increases the chance of drug interactions, and new drug interactions are being identified with old drugs. Be vigilant. Make sure to tell your doctor and pharmacist the drugs you are taking and tell your doctor if you are taking any of these interacting drugs:

aspirin, GENUINE BAYER ASPIRIN, carbamazepine, COUMADIN, diazepam, DILANTIN, ECOTRIN, EES, ERYTHROCIN, erythromycin, ethosuximide, felbamate, FELBATOL, LAMICTAL, lamotrigene, LUMINAL, MYSOLINE, ORINASE, phenobarbital, phenytoin, primidone, RETROVIR, RIFADIN, rifampin, RIMACTANE, SOLFOTON, TEGRETOL, tolbutamide, VALIUM, warfarin, ZARONTIN, zidovudine (AZT).

Clonazepam (KLONOPIN) with divalproex/ valproic acid (DEPAKENE/DEPAKOTE)

may induce absence status (which may resemble a moment of absent-mindedness or daydreaming) in people who have had absence-type seizures (previously called petit-mal seizures).[10]

Adverse Effects

Call your doctor immediately if you experience:

- seizures
- increase or decrease in blood pressure
- dizziness
- difficulty breathing
- mood, mental or behavior changes
- fever
- increased heartbeat
- lack of muscle coordination
- pain in abdomen, stomach or joints
- rash
- swelling of face or legs
- suicidal thoughts
- tiredness, weakness
- tremor of hands and arms
- changes in vision
- vomiting
- weight loss
- yellowing of eyes or skin
- uncontrolled eye movements
- unusual bleeding or bruising

Call your doctor if these symptoms continue:

- diarrhea
- drowsiness
- dry skin or eyes
- hair loss
- nausea
- difficulty sleeping
- weight gain
- menstrual changes
- indigestion
- clumsiness or unsteadiness
- constipation
- headache
- unusual excitement, restlessness, irritability

Periodic Tests

Ask your doctor which of these tests should be done periodically while you are taking this drug:

- blood levels of ammonia
- bleeding time determinations
- complete blood count
- kidney function determination
- liver function tests, especially during the first six months of taking this drug.
- blood levels of valproate

Phenytoin
DILANTIN (Parke-Davis)

GENERIC: available

FAMILY: Anticonvulsants

Phenytoin (*fen* i toyn) is used to treat most forms of epilepsy, except a form called absence (petit mal) seizures. It is also used to treat a form of excruciating facial pain, called trigeminal neuralgia or tic douloureux, if the preferred drug, carbamazepine (see p. 588), does not work or causes an adverse reaction. **If you are over 60, you generally need to take less than the usual adult dose of phenytoin.** Many adverse effects can be controlled with a lower dose.

Phenytoin has caused serious, often permanent, and sometimes fatal, blood cell abnormalities in a few people. These disorders can occasionally be treated if detected early. If you are taking phenytoin and have any of the following symptoms, call your doctor immediately: fever and sore throat, ulcers in the mouth, easy bruising, or skin rashes. It is very important that your doctor check the level of phenytoin in your bloodstream frequently and adjust your dosage as needed.

Before You Use This Drug
Do not use if you have or have had:

- heart disease

Tell your doctor if you have or have had:

- allergies to drugs
- alcohol dependence
- blood cell abnormalities
- kidney or liver problems
- diabetes
- thyroid problems
- fever above 101°F. for longer than 24 hours
- porphyria
- systemic lupus erythematosus

Tell your doctor about any other drugs you take, including aspirin, herbs, vitamins, and other nonprescription products.

When You Use This Drug

- Until you know how you react to this drug, do not drive or perform other activities requiring alertness. Phenytoin can cause dizziness, blurred vision, drowsiness, and lack of muscle coordination.
- Schedule regular visits with your doctor to check your progress and test for adverse effects.
- Do not drink alcohol.
- Schedule frequent visits with your dentist to have your teeth cleaned, to prevent enlarged, tender, and bleeding gums.
- Wear a medical identification bracelet or carry a card stating that you take phenytoin.
- **Do not stop taking this drug suddenly. This may cause severe convulsions. Check with your doctor before stopping this drug, changing brands or dosage forms, or taking any other drugs (prescription or nonprescription).**
- If you plan to have any surgery, including dental, tell your doctor that you take this drug.

How to Use This Drug

- Take with food to decrease stomach upset.
- For epilepsy, you can take the total daily dose at one time, preferably at the same time each day (in the morning or at bedtime).

- Before using the liquid form, shake vigorously.
- Do not store in the bathroom. Do not expose to heat, moisture, or strong light.
- *If you miss a dose, use the following guidelines:* **If you take phenytoin only once a day,** take the missed dose as soon as you remember, but skip it if you don't remember until the next day.

If you take phenytoin more than once a day, take the missed dose as soon as possible, but skip it if it is less than four hours until your next scheduled dose.

Do not take double doses. Call your doctor immediately if you miss doses for two days in a row.

Interactions with Other Drugs

The following drugs are listed in the *Evaluations of Drug Interactions* 1997 as causing "highly clinically significant" or "clinically significant" interactions when used together with this drug. We have also included potentially serious interactions listed in the drug's FDA-approved professional product labeling or package insert. New scientific techniques have allowed researchers to predict some drug interactions before they have been documented in people. There may be other drugs, especially those in the families of drugs listed below, that also will react with this drug to cause severe adverse effects. The number of new drugs approved for marketing increases the chance of drug interactions, and new drug interactions are being identified with old drugs. Be vigilant. Make sure to tell your doctor and pharmacist the drugs you are taking and tell your doctor if you are taking any of these interacting drugs:

ADALAT, ADALAT CC, ADVIL, alcohol, ALERMINE, allopurinol, amiodarone, ANTABUSE, BiCNU, BUTAZOLIDIN, CALCIFEROL, CARAFATE, carmustine, charcoal, chloramphenicol, CHLOROMYCETIN, chlorpheniramine, CHLOR-TRIMETON, cimetidine, CORDARONE, cyclosporine, DECADRON, DEPAKENE/DEPAKOTE, dexamethasone, diazoxide, dicumarol, DIFLUCAN, digoxin, disopyramide, disulfiram, divalproex/valproic acid, dopamine, doxycycline, DURAQUIN, ELIXOPHYLLIN, ergocalciferol, felbamate, FELBATOL, fluconazole, fluoxetine, folic acid, FOLVITE, GANTANOL, HEXADROL, ibuprofen, INH, isoniazid, LANOXICAPS, LANOXIN, methotrexate, methoxsalen, metocurine, METUBINE, miconazole, MONISTAT-DERM, MONISTAT 7, MOTRIN, MYSOLINE, NEORAL, nifedipine, NORPACE, omeprazole, oral contraceptives, OXSORALEN, phenylbutazone, PRILOSEC, primidone, PROCARDIA, PROCARDIA XL, PROGLYCEM, PROLOPRIM, PROZAC, QUINAGLUTE DURA-TABS, QUINIDEX, quinidine, RHEUMATREX DOSE PACK, RIFADIN, rifampin, RIMACTANE, SANDIMMUNE, SLO-BID, sucralfate, sulfamethizole, sulfamethoxazole, TAGAMET, THEO-24, theophylline, THIOSULFIL, trimethoprim, TRIMPEX, VELBAN, VIBRAMYCIN, vinblastine, vitamin D, ZYLOPRIM.

Adverse Effects

Call your doctor immediately if you experience:

- **signs of overdose:** blurred vision, clumsiness or unsteadiness, confusion, severe dizziness or drowsiness, hallucinations, nausea or vomiting, slurred speech, staggering walk, uncontrolled eye movements
  - behavior, mood, or mental changes
  - clumsiness or unsteadiness
  - confusion

- seizures
- weakness or numbness of feet or legs
- enlarged, bleeding, or tender gums
- fever, sore throat, or enlarged lymph nodes in neck or underarms
- skin rash
- unusual bleeding or bruising
- dark urine, pale stools, yellow skin or eyes, loss of appetite, or stomach pain
- muscle pain
- trembling
- burning pain at site of injection
- chest discomfort
- joint pain
- painful erections
- unusual excitement, restlessness, agitation
- uncontrolled movement of lips, tongue, or cheeks
- unusual tiredness or weakness
- weight loss
- swelling around eyes and face[11]

Call your doctor if these symptoms continue:

- constipation
- dizziness, lightheadedness
- drowsiness
- nausea or vomiting
- excess hair growth on body and face
- headache
- muscle twitching
- enlargement of jaw or widening of nose tip
- insomnia
- swelling of breasts
- thickening of lips

Periodic Tests

Ask your doctor which of these tests should be done periodically while you are taking this drug:

- blood levels of phenytoin
- electroencephalogram (EEG)
- complete blood count
- thyroid function tests

- dental exam, every three months
- liver function tests
- blood levels of calcium
- cardiac respiratory function tests
- blood pressure
- blood levels of folate and phosphorus

Limited Use

Selegiline (Deprenyl)
ELDEPRYL (Somerset)

GENERIC: not available
FAMILY: Antiparkinsonians

Selegiline (sell *edge* ell lean) is sometimes used in the treatment of Parkinson's disease along with levodopa or carbidopa. While taking selegiline, less levodopa/carbidopa is required. Originally selegiline was thought to be most useful in the early stages of Parkinson's disease to slow the advance of the disease and to delay the need to institute levodopa. This practice has not proved to be effective.[12] Now selegiline is used only as adjunctive treatment in some patients. Selegiline is not recommended for those in the advanced stages of Parkinson's disease or with dementia.[13,14] Mental adverse effects are of special concern in the elderly.[15] Selegiline is also very expensive in the United States.[16,17]

If you have symptoms of parkinsonism (tremor, rigid muscles, and disturbances in posture, walking, balance, speech, swallowing and muscle strength), there is a good chance that they are caused by a drug you are taking. As many as half of older adults with symptoms of parkinsonism may have developed them as adverse effects of a drug. A list of drugs that can cause symptoms of parkinsonism appears on p. 25. If you take any of the drugs on this list, discuss the possibility of drug-induced parkinsonism with your doctor, and ask to have your prescription changed or stopped.

Selegiline belongs to a group of drugs called monoamine oxidase (MAO) inhibitors. Serious adverse effects and the severe dietary restrictions required when taking type A MAO inhibitors curtailed use of these drugs for depression. Selegiline is a type B MAO inhibitor purported to have fewer adverse effects. However, the same adverse effects can occur, especially at high doses.[18] In order to reduce adverse effects, it is a good practice to start with a low dose of selegiline, then increase the dose gradually.[19,20]

Before You Use This Drug

Tell your doctor if you have or have had:

- allergies to drugs
- stomach ulcers

Tell your doctor about any other drugs you take, including aspirin, herbs, vitamins, and other nonprescription products.

When You Use This Drug

- Do not eat highly fermented foods, which contain tyramine: aged cheese, beer and wines (including "alcohol-free" ones), sherry, liqueurs, fava and broad beans, smoked and pickled meats/fish, sausages, caviar, chicken livers, overripe fruit, yeast extracts (Marmite, packet soups).
- Avoid or eat only in moderation: sour cream, yogurt, soy sauce, chocolate, and caffeine. These dietary restrictions extend up to two weeks after you stop taking any MAO inhibitor, such as selegiline.
- You may feel dizzy when rising from a lying or sitting position. If you are lying down, hang your legs over the side of the bed for a few minutes, then get up slowly. When getting up from a chair, stay by the chair until you are sure that you are not dizzy. (See p. 16.)
- Protect yourself from sunburn.
- If you take levodopa, your dose will be reduced gradually.

- Take only cold, cough and diet pills recommended by your doctor.
- If you plan to have any surgery, including dental, tell your doctor that you take this drug.

How to Use This Drug

- Swallow tablet whole or break up. Time doses for morning or noontime. Do not take in late afternoon or bedtime. Take with meals.
- Do not store in the bathroom. Do not expose to heat, moisture, or strong light.
- If you miss a dose, take it as soon as you remember but skip it if it is almost time for the next dose. **Do not take double doses.**

Interactions with Other Drugs

The following drugs are listed in the *Evaluations of Drug Interactions* 1997 as causing "highly clinically significant" or "clinically significant" interactions when used together with this drug. We have also included potentially serious interactions listed in the drug's FDA-approved professional product labeling or package insert. New scientific techniques have allowed researchers to predict some drug interactions before they have been documented in people. There may be other drugs, especially those in the families of drugs listed below, that also will react with this drug to cause severe adverse effects. The number of new drugs approved for marketing increases the chance of drug interactions, and new drug interactions are being identified with old drugs. Be vigilant. Make sure to tell your doctor and pharmacist the drugs you are taking and tell your doctor if you are taking any of these interacting drugs:

DELSYM, DEMEROL, dextromethorphan, fluoxetine, imipramine, IMITREX, meperidine, nefazodone, PROZAC, SERZONE, sumatriptan, TOFRANIL.

Additionally, the *United States Pharmacopeia Drug Information,* 1998 lists this drug as having interactions of major significance: LARODOPA, levodopa (if you already take levodopa your dose should be lowered two to three days before starting selegiline).

Adverse Effects

Call your doctor immediately if you experience:

- agitation or irritability
- mood changes
- difficulty urinating
- dizziness, lightheadness, fainting or loss of balance
- chest pain or irregular heartbeat
- severe nausea or vomiting
- unusual or uncontrolled movements of the body, face or tongue
- enlarged pupils, sensitivity to light
- severe stomach pain
- difficulty breathing or speaking
- convulsions
- fever or chills
- hallucinations
- severe headache
- bloody or black, tarry stools
- increased sweating
- swelling of feet or legs
- stiff or sore neck
- vomiting of blood or material that looks like coffee grounds
- restlessness
- lip smacking or puckering
- puffing of cheeks
- irregular pulse
- severe spasm where head and heels are bent backward and the body arched forward

Call your doctor if these symptoms continue:

- dry mouth, burning of lips or throat, grinding of teeth
- insomnia
- numbness in feet or toes

- ringing in ears
- unusual tiredness or weakness
- blurred vision
- weight change or loss of appetite
- body ache or back or leg pain
- constipation or diarrhea
- burning of lips, mouth or throat
- heartburn
- memory problems
- red, raised or itchy skin
- taste changes
- clenching, gnashing or grinding teeth

PREGNANCY WARNING

This drug caused harm to developing fetuses in animal studies, or such studies were not done. Use during pregnancy only for clear medical reasons. Tell your doctor if you are pregnant or thinking of becoming pregnant before you take this drug.

 Do Not Use

ALTERNATIVE TREATMENT:
At this time there are no safe and effective treatments that improve cognition in Alzheimer's disease.

Ergoloid Mesylates
HYDERGINE, HYDERGINE LC (Novartis)

FAMILY: Drugs Used in Alzheimer's Disease

Ergoloid mesylates (*er* goe loid *mess* i lates) has been misleadingly promoted and advertised as effective therapy for "those who would be considered to suffer from some ill-defined process related to aging" and as "the only product for Alzheimer's dementia."[21] The truth is quite the opposite.

According to a review on geriatric medicine in the *Journal of the American Medical Association,* "One widely used treatment [for Alzheimer's] (ergoloid mesylates) has been convincingly demonstrated to be of no value. This trial [referring to the study discussed below], along with the absence of a convincing pathophysiologic basis for its use, indicates that this treatment should be abandoned."[22]

Hydergine (ergoloid mesylates) is the only drug approved by the Food and Drug Administration (FDA) for the treatment of mental deterioration in the elderly (in addition to Alzheimer's), and has been on the market for more than 30 years. A study, published in *The New England Journal of Medicine,*[23] shows ergoloid mesylates to be totally ineffective for mild to moderate Alzheimer's, and to actually accelerate patients' mental deterioration. This study was more carefully designed than previous research showing ergoloid mesylates to be effective. Potential participants underwent a rigorous evaluation at the start of the study to screen out those patients whose dementia was due to a medical or psychiatric problem other than Alzheimer's. More patients were studied (39 took ergoloid mesylates, and 41 took placebo), and the trial was continued for longer (24 weeks) than most previous studies.

Subjects taking Hydergine-LC, at the recommended dose of 1 mg three times daily, did worse than the control group on one measure of appropriate behavior and one measure of IQ. The authors said that the drug may either be directly toxic to the brain, or may somehow accelerate the progression of Alzheimer's.

The term "dementia" describes a collection of symptoms including confusion, disorientation, apathy, and memory loss. More than 60 disorders can cause dementia.[24] Alzheimer's dementia, which is not reversible, accounts for about 50 to 60% of the cases of dementia.[25] A smaller percentage of dementias are reversible.

A person showing signs of dementia should be completely tested to see whether he or she is suffering from one of the dementias that can be cured. These tests include complete physical, neurological, and psychiatric examinations as well as a chest X-ray, CT scan, and blood tests.[26] In addition, many cases of dementia are caused or worsened by prescription drugs such as tranquilizers and sleeping pills (see p. 178). If you are taking one of these drugs, ask your doctor about stopping or changing your prescription.

If, after testing, a physician determines that a person has Alzheimer's dementia, a health care team—including a doctor, a nurse, and a social worker experienced in working with dementia—can offer practical suggestions to increase the person's safety and comfort at home and can discuss alternative care options. Efforts to improve the mental and physical state of older or senile adults are most beneficial if they address social, physical, nutritional, psychological, occupational, and recreational needs.[27]

Clonazepam
KLONOPIN (Roche)

GENERIC: not available

FAMILY: Anticonvulsants
Benzodiazepines (see p. 178)

Clonazepam (clawn *az* ah pam) is approved for the control of several types of seizures in which myoclonus is a major element. Myoclonus refers to brusque, lightning-like movements of a muscle or part of a muscle, sometimes sufficiently strong enough to move an entire limb, and characterizes benign absence attacks, atypical petit mal, and the prodromal period of grand mal. Usually, other anticonvulsants are needed as well, to control the non-myoclonic elements of the seizure. Clonazepam is also useful in the control of myoclonus that sometimes follows recovery from anoxic brain damage and in the control of restless movements of the legs during sleep. Though unapproved for the purpose, clonazepam is also used to treat insomnia and a variety of psychiatric problems, such as anxiety and panic attacks. These latter disorders are treated far more effectively by drugs other than clonazepam.

Clonazepam is one of the benzodiazepine drugs (see p. 178), the best known of which are Valium, Xanax, Librium and Halcion. Elderly people are usually more sensitive to the central nervous system effects of these drugs.

Because clonazepam has been prescribed to treat panic attacks, anxiety and sleeplessness, it is important to rule out preventable causes of these problems. The cause of panic attacks may be thyroid disease, low blood sugar, overuse of caffeine and aspirin, or withdrawal from addictive drugs.[28] Before using drugs for panic disorders try controlled breathing, distraction, and relaxation.[29] Anxiety and sleeplessness may be aggravated by alcohol, caffeine, and a number of other drugs.

One hazard of taking clonazepam continuously for longer than several weeks is drug-induced dependence. **Do not stop taking your drug suddenly.** With the help of your doctor, work out a schedule for slowly decreasing the amount of the drug you take by about 5 to 10% each day. Keep a written record of the dosage reduction schedule with you. These steps will make it much easier to become drug free without developing distressing symptoms of drug withdrawal.

Before You Use This Drug

Do not use if you have or have had:

- alcohol dependence or drug addiction
- cirrhosis or other liver disease
- glaucoma (narrow angle)

Tell your doctor if you have or have had:

- allergies to drugs
- asthma
- mental depression
- seizures, epilepsy
- glaucoma, any type
- hepatitis
- hyperactivity

- kidney or liver problems
- low albumin
- low blood pressure
- lung problems
- myasthenia gravis
- porphyria
- smoked
- snore
- difficulty swallowing
- sleep apnea
- alcohol or drug abuse
- coma, shock
- brain disorders

Tell your doctor about any other drugs you take, including aspirin, herbs, vitamins, and other nonprescription products.

When You Use This Drug

- Do not drink alcohol or use other drugs that can cause drowsiness.
- Until you know how you react to this drug, do not drive or perform other activities requiring alertness.
- You may feel dizzy when rising from a lying or sitting position. If you are lying down, hang your legs over the side of the bed for a few minutes, then get up slowly. When getting up from a chair, stay by the chair until you are sure that you are not dizzy. (See p. 16.)
- Carry medical identification stating your condition and that you are taking clonazepam.
- If you plan to have any surgery, including dental, tell your doctor that you take this drug.

How to Use This Drug

- Swallow tablets whole or break apart. Some experts find taking clonazepam with food lessens adverse effects.[30]
- If you take different doses at different times of the day, take the largest dose at night.[31]

- If you miss a dose, take it if you remember within an hour. Otherwise, wait until time for the next dose. **Do not increase your dose or take double doses.**
- Do not store in the bathroom. Do not expose to heat, moisture, or strong light.
- Check with your doctor before you stop taking this drug. A gradual lowering of the dose is required to prevent seizures and other signs of withdrawal.
- If you need a refill, contact your pharmacy well ahead of time, to allow time for the pharmacist to contact your doctor before refilling.

Interactions with Other Drugs

The following drugs are listed in the *Evaluations of Drug Interactions* 1997 as causing "highly clinically significant" or "clinically significant" interactions when used together with this drug. We have also included potentially serious interactions listed in the drug's FDA-approved professional product labeling or package insert. New scientific techniques have allowed researchers to predict some drug interactions before they have been documented in people. There may be other drugs, especially those in the families of drugs listed below, that also will react with this drug to cause severe adverse effects. The number of new drugs approved for marketing increases the chance of drug interactions, and new drug interactions are being identified with old drugs. Be vigilant. Make sure to tell your doctor and pharmacist the drugs you are taking and tell your doctor if you are taking any of these interacting drugs:

BENADRYL, carbamazepine, cimetidine, digoxin, DILANTIN, diphenhydramine, itraconazole, KETALAR, ketamine, ketoconazole, LANOXICAPS, LANOXIN, LUMINAL, NIZORAL, phenobarbital, phenytoin, SOLFOTON, SOMINEX FORMULA, SPORANOX, TAGAMET, TEGRETOL.

Additionally, the *United States Pharmacopeia Drug Information,* 1998 lists Central nervous system depressant (CNS) drugs including alcohol, antidepressants, antihistamines, antipsychotics, some blood pressure medications (reserpine, methyldopa, beta-blockers), motion sickness medications, muscle relaxants, narcotics, sedatives, sleeping pills and tranquilizers, as well as M S CONTIN, morphine, ROXANOL as having interactions of major significance.

Adverse Effects

Call your doctor immediately if you experience:

- **signs of overdose:** confusion, unusual weakness, severe drowsiness, difficulty breathing, slurred speech, staggering, slow heartbeat, slowed reflexes, shakiness
  - difficulty concentrating, impaired memory, angry outbursts
  - depression
  - seizures
  - hallucinations
  - low blood pressure
  - muscle weakness
  - skin rash or itching
  - sore throat fever and chills
  - insomnia
  - ulcers or sores in mouth or throat
  - uncontrolled movements of body, including eyes
  - abnormal bleeding or bruising
  - unusual excitement, nervousness, irritability
  - severe and unusual tiredness or weakness
  - yellow eyes or skin

Call your doctor if these symptoms continue:
- clumsiness or unsteadiness
- dizziness or lightheadedness
- abdominal or stomach cramps or pain
- vision changes
- changes in sex drive or performance

- constipation or diarrhea
- dry mouth, increased saliva, increased thirst
- headache
- rapid heartbeat
- increased sensitivity to light, noise
- increased sweating
- loss of bladder control
- nausea or vomiting
- runny nose
- skin rash
- swelling of ankles, face, lymph glands
- twitching
- unusual eye movements
- muscle spasm
- difficulty urinating
- trembling

Call your doctor if these symptoms continue after you stop taking this drug:

When you stop taking clonazepam, symptoms of withdrawal may occur, even several days after cessation of the medication. In older people this time may be longer.[32] Tapering off the drug helps prevent these symptoms:

- irritability
- nervousness
- insomnia
- confusion
- irregular heartbeat
- increased sense of hearing
- increased sensitivity to touch and pain
- sweating
- loss of reality
- muscle cramps
- sensitivity of eyes to light
- tingling, burning or prickly sensations
- feelings of suspicion or distrust
- depression
- hallucinations
- seizures
- abdominal or stomach cramps
- excessive sweating
- tremors
- nausea or vomiting

Periodic Tests

Ask your doctor which of these tests should be done periodically while you are taking this drug:

- reassessment of the need for clonazepam
- blood levels

Levodopa
LARODOPA (Roche)

Levodopa and Carbidopa
SINEMET (Dupont)

GENERIC: available only for levodopa in capsule form
FAMILY: Antiparkinsonians

Levodopa (*lee* voe doe pa) and the combination of levodopa and carbidopa (*kar* bi doe pa) are both used to treat Parkinson's disease, a condition that produces tremor (shaking), rigid muscles, and disturbances in posture, walking, balance, speech, swallowing, and muscle strength. The combination drug is often a better choice for treating Parkinson's disease than levodopa alone, because carbidopa enhances the desired effects of levodopa and reduces its adverse effects. If you are taking levodopa alone, ask your doctor to switch you to a levodopa-carbidopa combination.

If you take levodopa alone, you should avoid foods and vitamins that contain vitamin B_6 (pyridoxine), since this vitamin can destroy the drug's effectiveness. To keep your intake of vitamin B_6 down, you should avoid: multiple vitamins, avocados, beans, peas, sweet potatoes, dry skim milk, oatmeal, pork, bacon, beef liver, tuna, and cereals fortified with vitamin B_6. If you take carbidopa with levodopa you do not need to worry about this.

If you have symptoms of parkinsonism (tremor, rigid muscles, and disturbances in posture, walking, balance, speech, swallowing and muscle strength), there is a good chance that they are caused by a drug you are taking. As many as half of older adults with symptoms of parkinsonism may have developed them as adverse effects of a drug. A list of drugs that can cause symptoms of parkinsonism appears on p. 25. If you take any of the drugs on this list, discuss the possibility of drug-induced parkinsonism with your doctor, and ask to have your prescription changed or stopped.

Before You Use This Drug

Tell your doctor if you have or have had:

- allergies to drugs
- bronchial emphyzema, asthma or other chronic lung disease
- heart or blood vessel disease
- diabetes
- hormone problems
- skin cancer
- glaucoma
- stomach ulcer
- seizure disorder, epilepsy
- kidney or liver problems
- mental illness

Tell your doctor about any other drugs you take, including aspirin, herbs, vitamins, and other nonprescription products.

When You Use This Drug

- **Use only as prescribed.**
- Until you know how you react to this drug, do not drive or perform other activities requiring alertness. This drug can cause faintness and lightheadedness.
- You may feel dizzy when rising from a lying or sitting position. When getting out of bed, hang your legs over the side of the bed for a few minutes, then get up slowly. When getting up from a chair, stay by the chair until you are sure that you are not dizzy. (See p. 16.)
- **Caution diabetics:** Levodopa may interfere with urine tests for sugar and ketones.
- Urine or sweat may get darker. This is no cause for alarm.
- If you plan to have any surgery, including dental, tell your doctor that you take this drug.

HEAT STRESS ALERT

These drugs can affect your body's ability to adjust to heat, putting you at risk of "heat stress." If you live alone, ask a friend to check on you several times during the day. Early signs of heat stress are dizziness, lightheadedness, faintness, and slightly high temperature. Call your doctor if you have any of these signs.

Drink more fluids (water, fruit and vegetable juices) than usual—even if you're not thirsty—unless your doctor has told you otherwise. Do not drink alcohol.

How to Use This Drug

- Take on an empty stomach, at least one hour before or two hours after meals. This drug will not work as well if you take it with or immediately after food. If the drug causes an upset stomach, eat something about 15 minutes after taking it.
- Do not store in the bathroom. Do not expose to heat, moisture, or strong light.
- If you miss a dose, take it as soon as you remember, but skip it if it is less than two hours until your next scheduled dose. **Do not take double doses.**

Interactions with Other Drugs

The following drugs are listed in the *Evaluations of Drug Interactions* 1997 as causing "highly clinically significant" or "clinically significant" interactions when used together with this drug. We have also included potentially serious interactions listed in the drug's FDA-approved professional product labeling or package insert. New scientific techniques have allowed researchers to predict some drug interactions before they have been documented in people. There may be other drugs, especially those in the families of drugs listed below, that also will react with this drug to cause severe adverse effects. The number of

new drugs approved for marketing increases the chance of drug interactions, and new drug interactions are being identified with old drugs. Be vigilant. Make sure to tell your doctor and pharmacist the drugs you are taking and tell your doctor if you are taking any of these interacting drugs:

FEOSOL, ferrous sulfate, NARDIL, phenelzine, RODEX, SLOW FE, vitamin B_6.

Adverse Effects

Call your doctor immediately if you experience:

- depression
- mood changes, aggressive behavior
- difficulty urinating
- dizziness or lightheadedness
- irregular heartbeat
- severe nausea or vomiting
- unusual or uncontrolled movements of the body
- spasm or closing of eyelids
- high blood pressure
- stomach pain
- unusual tiredness or weakness

Call your doctor if these symptoms continue:

- anxiety, confusion, nervousness
- constipation or diarrhea
- nightmares or trouble sleeping
- dry mouth
- flushed skin
- headache
- loss of appetite
- muscle twitching

Periodic Tests

Ask your doctor which of these tests should be done periodically while you are taking this drug:

- complete blood count
- liver function tests
- kidney function tests
- eye pressure tests
- cardiovascular monitoring
- creatinine phosphokinase concentrations

Limited Use

Phenobarbital
LUMINAL (Sanofi Winthrop)
SOLFOTON (ECR)

GENERIC: available
FAMILY: Barbiturates
Anticonvulsants

Phenobarbital (fee noe *bar* bi tal) is of limited benefit to older adults because it is addictive and has potentially serious adverse effects. You should not be taking it to promote sleep, relieve nervousness or anxiety, lower blood pressure, or reduce pain. Like other barbiturates, it is commonly misused as a painkiller, despite the fact that it can actually increase your sensation of, and reaction to, pain. **You should only be taking phenobarbital to control convulsions (seizures).** For this purpose, you can take it at doses well below those that cause you to go to sleep.

If your kidney or liver function is impaired, you need to take less than the usual adult dose of phenobarbital. Phenobarbital causes liver cancer in mice and rats.

One hazard of taking phenobarbital continuously for longer than several weeks is drug-induced dependence. **Do not stop taking your drug suddenly.** With the help of your doctor, work out a schedule for slowly decreasing the amount of the drug you take by about 5 to 10% each day. Keep a written record of the dosage reduction schedule with you. These steps will make it much easier to become drug free without developing distressing symptoms of drug withdrawal.

Before You Use This Drug

Do not use if you have or have had:

- porphyria

Tell your doctor if you have or have had:

- allergies to drugs
- alcohol or drug abuse
- mental depression
- asthma or other breathing difficulties
- diabetes
- kidney or liver problems
- anemia
- long-term pain
- adrenal gland problems
- overactive thyroid

Tell your doctor about any other drugs you take, including aspirin, herbs, vitamins, and other nonprescription products.

When You Use This Drug

- Until you know how you react to this drug, do not drive or perform other activities requiring alertness. Phenobarbital may cause drowsiness, dizziness, and lightheadedness.
- Do not drink alcohol or use other drugs that can cause drowsiness.
- Phenobarbital can worsen symptoms of Parkinson's disease.
- **Do not stop taking this drug suddenly. Your doctor must lower your dose gradually to prevent withdrawal symptoms.**
- If you plan to have any surgery, including dental, tell your doctor that you take this drug.

How to Use This Drug

- Do not store in the bathroom. Do not expose to heat, moisture, or strong light.
- If you miss a dose, take it as soon as you remember, but skip it if it is almost time for the next dose. **Do not take double doses.**

Interactions with Other Drugs

The following drugs are listed in the *Evaluations of Drug Interactions* 1997 as causing "highly clinically significant" or "clinically significant" interactions when used together with this drug. We have also included potentially serious interactions listed in the drug's FDA-approved professional product labeling or package insert. New scientific techniques have allowed researchers to predict some drug interactions before they have been documented in people. There may be other drugs, especially those in the families of drugs listed below, that also will react with this drug to cause severe adverse effects. The number of new drugs approved for marketing increases the chance of drug interactions, and new drug interactions are being identified with old drugs. Be vigilant. Make sure to tell your doctor and pharmacist the drugs you are taking and tell your doctor if you are taking any of these interacting drugs:

alcohol, chlorpromazine, COUMADIN, CRYSTODIGIN, cyclosporine, DECADRON, DEPAKENE/DEPAKOTE, dexamethasone, digitoxin, divalproex/valproic acid, doxycycline, DURAQUIN, ELIXOPHYLLIN, FLAGYL, HEXADROL, LOPRESSOR, methoxyflurane, metoprolol, metronidazole, NEORAL, oral contraceptives, PENTHRANE, QUINAGLUTE DURA-TABS, QUINIDEX, quinidine, SANDIMMUNE, SLO-BID, THEO-24, theophylline, THORAZINE, TOPROL XL, VIBRAMYCIN, warfarin.

Adverse Effects

Call your doctor immediately if you experience:

- **signs of overdose:** confusion, severe drowsiness, weakness, difficulty breathing, slurred speech, staggering, slow heartbeat, unusual eye movements, trouble sleeping, unusual irritability, decrease or loss of reflexes, low fever
- confusion
- hallucinations
- depression

- skin rash, hives, scaling
- swelling of eyelids, face, lips
- sore throat, fever
- unusual bleeding or bruising
- unusual excitement
- unusual tiredness or weakness
- yellow eyes or skin
- chest pain
- difficulty breathing
- sores, ulcers or white spots in mouth

Call your doctor if these symptoms continue:

- clumsiness, unsteadiness
- dizziness, lightheadedness
- drowsiness
- anxiety, nervousness
- constipation
- faintness
- headache
- nausea or vomiting
- nightmares, difficulty sleeping
- unusual irritability

Call your doctor if these symptoms continue after you stop taking this drug:

- anxiety or restlessness
- seizures
- dizziness or lightheadedness
- fainting
- hallucinations
- muscle twitching
- nausea or vomiting
- trembling of hands
- insomnia or increased dreaming or night-mares
- vision problems
- weakness

Periodic Tests

Ask your doctor which of these tests should be done periodically while you are taking this drug:

- complete blood count
- liver function tests
- kidney function tests

- blood levels of phenobarbital (when used as an anticonvulsant)
- folate concentrations
- hematopoetic function

PREGNANCY WARNING

This drug caused harm to developing fetuses in animal studies, or such studies were not done. Use during pregnancy only for clear medical reasons. Tell your doctor if you are pregnant or thinking of becoming pregnant before you take this drug.

Bromocriptine
PARLODEL (Novartis)

GENERIC: not available
FAMILY: Antiparkinsonians

Bromocriptine (broe moe *krip* teen) has several uses. This profile discusses its use for Parkinson's disease, for which it is the second-choice drug, after a combination of levodopa and carbidopa (see p. 582). If you have Parkinson's disease, your doctor should first try levodopa with carbidopa, and should prescribe bromocriptine only if the combination drug does not decrease your symptoms or if it causes too many adverse effects. Bromocriptine often works best when given with levodopa. **If you are over 60, you should generally be taking less than the usual adult dose.**

In older adults, bromocriptine often causes dizziness, nausea, constipation, and tingling in fingers or toes when exposed to the cold. It can also cause more serious adverse effects called choreiform movements—unusual and uncontrolled movements in the body, face, tongue, arms, hands, and upper body. About 25% of bromocriptine users in all age groups experience this adverse effect. If you have any of these symptoms, especially if they are severe or persistent, call your doctor and ask if your dose of bromocriptine should be reduced. Do not take less bromocriptine than your doctor prescribed unless he or she instructs you to do so.

If you have symptoms of parkinsonism (tremor, rigid muscles, and disturbances in posture, walking, balance, speech, swallowing, and muscle strength), there is a good chance that they are caused by a drug you are taking. As many as half of older adults with symptoms of parkinsonism may have developed them as adverse effects of a drug. A list of drugs that can cause symptoms of parkinsonism appears on p. 25. If you take any of the drugs on this list, discuss the possibility of drug-induced parkinsonism with your doctor, and ask to have your prescription changed or stopped.

DO NOT USE BROMOCRIPTINE FOR LACTATION SUPPRESSION

Following a petition and a lawsuit by Public Citizen's Health Research Group, there was a ban on the use of bromocriptine for suppressing lactation in women who had delivered a baby but did not want to breastfeed. The basis for this was a large number of strokes and heart attacks in women shortly after beginning to use bromocriptine. Since the effectiveness of the drug for this purpose is only temporary, the risks were unacceptable in view of the limited benefits.

Before You Use This Drug

Tell your doctor if you have or have had:

- allergies to drugs
- liver problems
- mental illness
- high blood pressure

Tell your doctor about any other drugs you take, including aspirin, herbs, vitamins, and other nonprescription products.

When You Use This Drug

- **Do not use more or less often or in a higher or lower dose than prescribed.** Higher doses increase the risk of adverse effects, while lower doses may worsen symptoms of parkinsonism.
- Until you know how you react to this drug, do not drive or perform other activities requiring alertness. Bromocriptine can cause drowsiness and lightheadedness.
- You may feel dizzy when rising from a lying or sitting position. When getting out of bed, hang your legs over the side of the bed for a few minutes, then get up slowly. When getting up from a chair, stay by the chair until you are sure that you are not dizzy. (See p. 16.)
- Try to stop smoking to lessen the chance of adverse effects from this drug.[33]

HEAT STRESS ALERT

This drug can affect your body's ability to adjust to heat, putting you at risk of "heat stress." If you live alone, ask a friend to check on you several times during the day. Early signs of heat stress are dizziness, lightheadedness, faintness, and slightly high temperature. Call your doctor if you have any of these signs.

Drink more fluids (water, fruit and vegetable juices) than usual—even if you're not thirsty—unless your doctor has told you otherwise. Do not drink alcohol.

How to Use This Drug

- Take with food to decrease stomach upset.
- Do not store in the bathroom. Do not expose to heat, moisture, or strong light.
- If you miss a dose, take it as soon as you remember, but skip it if it is less than four hours until your next scheduled dose. **Do not take double doses.**

Interactions with Other Drugs

The following drugs are listed in the *Evaluations of Drug Interactions* 1997 as causing "highly clinically significant" or "clinically significant" interactions when used together with this drug. We have also included potentially serious interactions listed in the drug's FDA-approved professional product labeling or package insert. New scientific techniques have allowed researchers to predict some drug interactions before they have been documented in people. There may be other drugs, especially those in the families of drugs listed below, that also will react with this drug to cause severe adverse effects. The number of new drugs approved for marketing increases the chance of drug interactions, and new drug interactions are being identified with old drugs. Be vigilant. Make sure to tell your doctor and pharmacist the drugs you are taking and tell your doctor if you are taking any of these interacting drugs:

MELLARIL, thioridazine.

Adverse Effects

Call your doctor immediately if you experience:

- dizziness or lightheadedness
- confusion or hallucinations
- unusual and uncontrolled movements of the body
- black, tarry stools or bloody vomit
- seizures
- sudden weakness
- vision changes
- shortness of breath
- nervousness
- severe chest pain
- fainting
- fast heartbeat
- headache
- sweating
- nausea and vomiting
- abdominal or stomach pain
- frequent urination
- loss of appetite
- lower back pain
- runny nose

Call your doctor if these symptoms continue:

- drowsiness
- depression
- headache
- constipation or diarrhea
- dry mouth
- leg cramps at night
- loss of appetite
- stuffy nose
- tingling in fingers or toes when exposed to cold

Periodic Tests

Ask your doctor which of these tests should be done periodically while you are taking this drug:

- blood pressure
- prolactin, serum
- pregnancy test
- visual field assessment

Carbamazepine
TEGRETOL (Novartis)

GENERIC: available

FAMILY: Anticonvulsants

Carbamazepine (kar ba *maz* e peen) is used to treat some forms of epilepsy that have not responded to other drugs and to treat a form of excruciating facial pain called trigeminal neuralgia or tic douloureux. This drug is *not* a simple painkiller and should *not* be used to treat general aches or pains.

If you are over 60, you will generally need to take less than the usual adult dose. Ask your doctor about starting with a daily dose of 50 milligrams to prevent harmful adverse effects, especially mental confusion and slowed pulse. Call your doctor if either of these adverse effects occurs. If you are taking carbamazepine for neuralgia, your doctor should try reducing your dose every few months to see if a smaller dose will relieve your symptoms.

Carbamazepine can cause serious and sometimes fatal, blood cell abnormalities in some people. These disorders can usually be treated if detected early. If you are taking carbamazepine and have any of the following symptoms, call your doctor immediately: fever and sore throat, ulcers in the mouth, easy bruising, or skin rashes.[34] Before you start using carbamazepine, you should have a complete blood count, to be certain that you don't have any potential blood abnormalities that could be worsened by the drug.

Carbamazepine causes malignant liver tumors in female rats and benign tumors of the testicles in male rats.[35]

Before You Use This Drug

Do not use if you have or have had:

- heart block
- blood disorders
- bone marrow depression

Tell your doctor if you have or have had:

- allergies to drugs
- heart, kidney, or liver problems
- diabetes
- glaucoma
- alcohol dependence
- retention of urine
- anemia
- behavioral problems
- a reaction to tricyclic antidepressant drugs (see p. 177)

Tell your doctor about any other drugs you take, including aspirin, herbs, vitamins, and other nonprescription products.

When You Use This Drug

- Until you know how you react to this drug, do not drive or perform other activities requiring alertness. Carbamazepine can cause dizziness, drowsiness, and lack of muscle coordination.
- **Schedule regular visits with your doctor to check your progress and test for adverse effects.**
- Wear a medical identification bracelet or carry a card stating that you take carbamazepine.
- **Do not stop taking this drug suddenly. This may cause convulsions.**
- If you plan to have any surgery, including dental, tell your doctor that you take this drug.

How to Use This Drug

- Take with food to decrease stomach upset.
- Do not store in the bathroom. Do not expose to heat, moisture, or strong light.
- If you miss a dose, take it as soon as you remember, but skip it if it is almost time for the next dose. **Do not take double doses.** Call your doctor immediately if you miss more than one dose in a day.

Interactions with Other Drugs

The following drugs are listed in the *Evaluations of Drug Interactions* 1997 as causing "highly clinically significant" or "clinically significant" interactions when used together with this drug. We have also included potentially serious interactions listed in the drug's FDA-approved professional product labeling or package insert. New scientific techniques have allowed researchers to predict some drug interactions before they have been documented in people. There may be other drugs, especially those in the families of drugs listed below, that also will react with this drug to cause severe adverse effects. The number of new drugs approved for marketing increases the chance of drug interactions, and new drug interactions are being identified with old drugs. Be vigilant. Make sure to tell your doctor and pharmacist the drugs you are taking and tell your doctor if you are taking any of these interacting drugs:

alcohol, CALAN SR, charcoal, cimetidine, COVERA-HS, cyclosporine, danazol, DANOCRINE, DARVON, DARVON-N, DECADRON, DEPAKENE/DEPAKOTE, dexamethasone, dicumarol, divalproex/valproic acid, doxycycline, EES, ELIXOPHYLLIN, ERYTHROCIN, erythromycin, erythromycin estolate, felbamate, FELBATOL, FLAGYL, HALDOL, haloperidol, HEXADROL, ILOSONE, INH, isoniazid, ISOPTIN SR, lithium, LITHOBID, LITHONATE, metronidazole, NEORAL, oral contraceptives, propoxyphene, SANDIMMUNE, SLO-BID, TAGAMET, THEO-24, theophylline, verapamil, VERELAN, VIBRAMYCIN.

Adverse Effects

Call your doctor immediately if you experience:

- **signs of overdose:** seizures, severe dizziness or drowsiness, irregular, slow, or shallow breathing, trembling, irregular heartbeat, poor control of body movements, clumsiness or unsteadiness, high or low blood pressure, decrease in urine, enlarged pupils, nausea or vomiting
  - blurred vision
  - confusion, slurred speech, or hallucinations
  - depression or other mood, mental or behavioral change
  - ringing or buzzing in the ears
  - dark urine, yellow skin and eyes, or pale stools
  - fainting
  - irregular or slow pulse
  - sudden increase or decrease in urine production
  - numbness, tingling, pain, or weakness in hands or feet
  - chest pain
  - pain, tenderness, bluish color, or swelling of legs, feet or hands
  - unusual tiredness or weakness
  - severe diarrhea

- continuing headache
- muscle or stomach cramps
- weight gain
- nausea and vomiting
- increased sensitivity of the skin to the sun

Call your doctor if these symptoms continue:

- aching joints or muscles
- constipation
- dry mouth
- increased sensitivity to sunlight
- irritation or inflammation of tongue or mouth
- appetite loss
- hair loss
- sexual problems
- skin rash
- stomach pain or discomfort
- increased sweating

Periodic Tests

Ask your doctor which of these tests should be done periodically while you are taking this drug:

- blood levels of carbamazepine
- complete blood count: before using the drug, weekly during the first three months of treatment, and monthly thereafter for at least two to three years
- kidney function tests
- liver function tests
- eye pressure tests
- complete urinalysis
- calcium and iron concentrations

PREGNANCY WARNING

This drug caused harm to developing fetuses in animal studies, or such studies were not done. Use during pregnancy only for clear medical reasons. Tell your doctor if you are pregnant or thinking of becoming pregnant before you take this drug.

NOTES FOR DRUGS FOR NEUROLOGICAL DISORDERS

1. AMA Department of Drugs. *AMA Drug Evaluations.* 5th ed. Chicago: American Medical Association, 1983:333.

2. Vestal RE, ed. *Drug Treatment in the Elderly.* Sydney, Australia: ADIS Health Science Press, 1984:310.

3. AMA, op. cit.

4. Vestal, op. cit.

5. Davis KL, Thal LJ, Gamzu ER, Davis CS, Woolson RF, Gracon SI, et al. A double-blind, placebo-controlled multicenter study of tacrine for Alzheimer's disease. *New England Journal of Medicine* 1992; 327:1253–9.

6. Growdon JH. Treatment for Alzheimer's disease. *New England Journal of Medicine* 1992; 327:1306–8[editorial].

7. *The Medical Letter on Drugs and Therapeutics.* New York: The Medical Letter Inc., 1993; 35:87–8.

8. *The Medical Letter on Drugs and Therapeutics.* New York: The Medical Letter Inc., 1997; 39:53–4.

9. Pabis DJ, Stanislav SW. Pharmacotherapy of aggressive behavior. *The Annals of Pharmacotherapy* 1996; 30:278–87.

10. Levien T, Baker DE. Valproate sodium injectable and bupropion hydrochloride. *Hospital Pharmacy* 1998; 33:213–27.

11. Grillone G, Myssiorek D. Otolaryngologic manifestations of phenytoin toxicity. *Clinical Otolaryngology* 1992; 17:185–91.

12. Parkinson Study Group. Impact of deprenyl and tocopherol treatment on Parkinson's disease in DATATOP patients requiring levodopa. *Annals of Neurology* 1996; 39:37–45.

13. Boyson SJ. Psychiatric effects of selegiline. *Archives of Neurology* 1991; 48:902.

14. Gilman AG, Rall TW, Nies AS, Taylor P, eds. *The Pharmacological Basis of Therapeutics.* 8th ed. New York: Pergamon Press, 1990:475.

15. Marsden CD. Parkinson's disease. *Lancet* 1990; 335:948–52.

16. Cotton P. Many researchers, few clinicians, using drug that may slow, even prevent, Parkinson's. *Journal of the American Medical Association* 1990; 264:1083–4.

17. Riley D, Devereaux M, Grossman G, Chandar K, Bahntge M. Deprenyl for the treatment of early Parkinson's disease. *New England Journal of Medicine* 1990; 322:1526–8 [letter].

18. Dukes MNG, Beeley L. *Side Effects of Drugs Annual* 14, Amsterdam: Elsevier, 1990:11–2.

19. Boyson, op. cit.

20. Saint-Hilaire M, Feldman RG, Durso R, Goldstein M, Lew JH. Deprenyl for the treatment of Parkinson's disease. *New England Journal of Medicine* 1990; 322:1526–8[letters].

21. Advertisement for Hydergine. *Journal of the American Medical Association* 1985; 254:2233.

22. Larson EB. Geriatric medicine. *Journal of the American Medical Association* 1991; 265:1325–6.

23. Thompson TL, Filley CR, Mitchell WD, Culig KM, LoVerde M, Byyny RL. Lack of efficacy of Hydergine in patients with Alzheimer's disease. *New England Journal of Medicine* 1990; 323:445–8.

24. Haase GR. Disease presenting as dementia. In *Dementia* 2nd ed., edited by CE Wells. Philadelphia: FA Davis, 1977:27–67.

25. Smith JS, Kiloh LF. The investigation of dementia: results in 200 consecutive admissions. *Lancet* 1981; 1:824–7.

26. Weatherall DJ, Ledingham JGG, Warrel DA, eds. In *Oxford Textbook of Medicine,* 1st ed. New York: Oxford University Press, Inc., 1983; 24:14.

27. *The Medical Letter on Drugs and Therapeutics.* New York: The Medical Letter Inc., 1974; 16:21.

28. Raj A, Sheehan DV. Medical evaluation of panic attacks. *Journal of Clinical Psychiatry* 1987; 48:309–13.

29. DeRubeis R, Beck A. Cognitive Therapy. In *Handbook of Cognitive-Behavioral Therapies.* New York: The Guilford Press, 1988.

30. Davidson JRT. Continuation treatment of panic disorder with high-potency benzodiazepines. *Journal of Clinical Psychiatry* 1990; 51 (12 Supplement A):31–7.

31. American Society of Hospital Pharmacists. *American Hospital Formulary Service Drug Information.* Bethesda, MD, 1992:1196–8.

32. *USP DI, Drug Information for the Health Care Professional.* 12th ed. Rockville MD: The United States Pharmacopeial Convention, Inc., 1992:601–10.

33. Melmed S, Braunstein GD. Bromocriptine and pleuropulmonary disease. *Archives of Internal Medicine* 1989; 149:258–9.

34. *Physicians' Desk Reference.* 40th ed. Oradell, N.J.: Medical Economics Company, 1986:900.

35. *USP DI, Drug Information for the Health Care Provider.* 6th ed. Rockville MD.: The United States Pharmacopeial Convention, Inc., 1986:441.

Nutritional Supplements   **592**

SUPPLEMENT LISTINGS

AQUASOL A	Limited Use	611
ARCO-CEE	Limited Use	614
CALCIFEROL	Limited Use	616
calcium carbonate		600
calcium citrate		600
calcium gluconate		600
calcium lactate		600
CALTRATE		600
CENTRUM		606
CEVI-BID	Limited Use	614
CITRACAL		600
FEOSOL		604
FEOSTAT		604
FERGON		604
ferrous fumarate (iron)		604
ferrous gluconate (iron)		604
ferrous sulfate (iron)		604
folic acid (folate)		602
FOLVITE		602
multivitamins		606
niacin (nicotinic acid, vitamin B$_3$)		607
niacin (sustained-release dosage)	Ⓧ Do Not Use	609
NICOBID	Ⓧ Do Not Use	609
NICOLAR		607
OS-CAL 500		600
SLO-NIACIN	Ⓧ Do Not Use	609
SLOW FE		604
THERAGRAN-M		606
thiamine (vitamin B$_1$)		610
vitamin A	Limited Use	611
vitamin B$_{12}$ (cyanocobalamin)	Limited Use	613
vitamin C (ascorbic acid)	Limited Use	614
vitamin D	Limited Use	616
vitamin E (alpha-tocopherol)	Ⓧ Do Not Use	618

NUTRITIONAL SUPPLEMENTS

Nutritional supplements are used by an estimated 40% of the U.S. population. Current sales approach $6 billion annually and this industry is expected to see sales in excess of $12 billion a year by 2001.[1] Nutritional supplements include vitamins, minerals, and combinations of the two, as well as supplements for which there are no known daily requirements for the human body, such as carnitine, lecithin, and inositol.

The promotion of nutritional supplements is now reminiscent of the "snake oil" sales seen at the beginning of the 20th century. The Dietary Supplement Health and Education Act, or DSHEA, enacted by Congress in 1994 allows supplement suppliers to sell almost anything as being beneficial without any evidence that it works as long as they do not make a medical claim. This ill-advised law has tied the hands of the Food and Drug Administration (FDA) and created an unregulated industry that has opened the floodgates and deluged the market with products that are falsely promoted, or unsafe, or both.

In addition, DSHEA does not require supplement suppliers to show proof of safety. Instead, DSHEA requires that the FDA must first show a supplement causes harm before any regulatory action can be taken. This is a particularly dangerous aspect of DSHEA because the FDA does not have a system in place that can accurately identify the number of people killed or injured from prescription drugs each year, let alone those killed or injured from nutritional supplements. If a large number of people are harmed in a short period of time in a unique way, then the FDA might recognize that a dangerous supplement is on the market.

Furthermore, because DSHEA ties the hands of the FDA, supplement manufacturing facilities are not inspected. In other words, what is listed on the label of some nutritional supplements may not be in the bottle.

One promotional strategy of supplement suppliers is to make people worry about whether they are getting enough nutrients. But do most people really need to take vitamins and minerals to supplement their diets? Or are they a waste of money? Are there better alternatives to taking supplements to ensure adequate nutrition? This section will attempt to answer these questions and help you sort through the fact and fantasy surrounding nutritional supplements.

Causes of Nutritional Deficiencies

It is a fact that some people do have nutritional deficiencies, usually older adults. They fall into three categories:

1. People who do not eat enough food–fewer than 1,500 calories a day.

2. People who eat enough food but have an unbalanced, low-quality diet, often deficient in fruits and vegetables.

3. People who have medical problems or take drugs that contribute to nutritional deficiencies.

Too Few Calories

The most common cause of inadequate nutrition is eating too few calories. A diet that provides less than 1,500 calories a day does not ensure an adequate intake of all necessary nutrients. This can occur at all ages but is a particular problem in older adults. There are special reasons why this can happen.

Physical changes occur with aging. A decrease in the sensitivity of smell and taste results in food not tasting as good, and a subsequent loss of appetite. Dental problems may make eating more difficult, especially raw vegetables and meat. Physical handicaps can hinder food preparation and eating.

Economic factors also play a role in preventing people from eating enough. **One out of every six older adults lives in poverty, which makes buying sufficient, wholesome food a difficult task.**

An Unbalanced, Low-quality Diet

Another group of adults at risk for nutritional deficiencies are those who eat enough food to feel full but eat an inadequate supply of necessary nutrients (vitamins and minerals which ensure your body's good health). Certain changes make a deficiency more likely to happen.

As a person ages, his or her daily requirement for calories decreases because of a reduction in basal metabolic rate and physical activity. In order to maintain a weight of 140 pounds, a 70-year-old must eat fewer calories than he or she did as a 40-year-old. The basal metabolic rate, which determines how many calories your body burns off while resting, can decrease as much as 15 to 20% between the ages of 30 and 75. As a result, older adults require fewer calories. Less exercise results in a loss of lean body weight with a decrease in muscle and an increase in fat.

Regular exercise is the only way to slow down or reverse this age-related process. Exercise can increase both your basal metabolic rate and the amount of muscle in your body. It can also quicken the rate at which your food is digested and used. These effects from exercise allow you to eat more food without gaining weight.

Although the number of calories needed decreases with age, nutrient needs remain about the same (unless there is a special situation, such as a physical condition or a drug, that creates a need for more). As a result, a high-quality diet becomes more essential.

One obstacle to this goal of adequate nutrition and high-quality diet is that older adults often do not shop for or prepare their own food. Eating out often makes it harder to choose a healthy diet. Being immobile or in long-term institutional care reduces control over dietary choices. Living alone is also a barrier because preparing meals for one and eating alone is not always that appealing.

Medical Problems and Drugs

Nutritional deficiencies can also be caused by medical problems, including alcohol dependence and drugs. For example, diseases of the intestine, pancreas, and liver cause decreased absorption of certain nutrients, and some chronic diseases reduce the appetite.

Certain prescription and nonprescription drugs and alcohol also cause increased requirements of certain nutrients. These are the most common drugs (see the individual drug listings for more details):

* Drugs that affect the stomach or intestines such as mineral oil and laxatives;
* Cholesterol-reducing drugs such as clofibrate and cholestyramine;
* Antibiotics such as the cephalosporins and isoniazid;
* Cytotoxic drugs (drugs that cause damage to cells) such as methotrexate, colchicine and many anticancer drugs;
* Anticonvulsants such as phenytoin and phenobarbital;

* Blood pressure drugs such as hydrochlorothiazide and hydralazine;
* Alcohol.

If you have any medical problems or use any drugs that increase the demand for certain vitamins and minerals, talk to your doctor about the best ways to increase your nutrient intake.

How to Prevent and Treat a Nutritional Deficiency

Should people who have nutritional deficiencies take vitamins or minerals? There is no simple answer to this question because of the various causes of nutritional deficiencies. Sometimes, taking a supplement will help. But supplements are never the complete answer to anyone's nutritional problems. It is far better to address the situation that could cause nutritional deficiency than to take a supplement and do nothing more.

Steps Toward a Better Diet

Eating a well-balanced diet with plenty of variety and high-quality food is the most important way to ensure good nutrition. Here are some healthy suggestions for doing that. If you decide to make changes in your diet, make them one at a time; you will have a better chance of succeeding.

1. *Decrease the amount of fat in your diet, particularly saturated fats.* Most Americans eat too much fat, which contributes to heart disease, the nation's number one killer. Fat should contribute only 30% of your total daily caloric intake. You can decrease the amount of fat by:
   * trimming fat off meat
   * eating more fish and chicken (without the skin) instead of red meat
   * drinking skim milk instead of whole milk and cutting down on your consumption of whole-milk dairy products

- eating fewer fried foods
- steaming or baking food instead of cooking with oils and butter

2. *Decrease the amount of salt in your diet.* Eating a high-salt diet contributes to high blood pressure, thereby increasing your risk of heart disease and stroke. Foods that are high in salt include processed food, condiments, and salted meats. It is possible to buy low-salt crackers, no-salt pretzels, unsalted nuts, and low-sodium canned goods and breakfast cereals.

3. *Eat more fruits, vegetables, and whole grains.* These are the best sources of complex carbohydrates (starches that provide fiber and essential nutrients) and are also good sources of vitamins and minerals. Carbohydrates should contribute 55% of your total daily caloric intake, with the majority of them being fruits, vegetables, and whole grains. They also provide the best source of natural fiber, which comes from nonprocessed foods that are often more difficult to chew—raw cauliflower, broccoli, carrots, and whole-grain breads, for example. Fiber also promotes regularity (see Psyllium, p. 380), and may help to significantly reduce your cholesterol level and/or blood pressure.[2]

4. *Decrease the amount of simple sugars in your diet.* Replace foods sweetened with refined sugar (sucrose), such as candy, ice cream, pastry, jam, with naturally sweet foods, such as oranges and apples.

5. *Decrease your alcohol intake.* Drink no more than three to five alcoholic drinks a week, if not fewer.

6. *Increase your fluid intake to six to eight glasses of fluids a day, especially water.* Kidney function is often reduced in older adults. Drinking more fluids helps the kidneys function better and also promotes regularity. However, first ask your doctor if you need to restrict your fluid intake.

7. *Eat a wide variety of foods.* A wide variety of wholesome foods will provide all the nutrients you need. It's not too late to try new foods and get into new habits if your diet has been limited. Change your eating habits a little bit at a time and soon you will notice a difference. If you want to change your diet to get more of a specific nutrient, there is a list of good dietary sources of the individual vitamins and minerals at the end of this section.

Who Needs Vitamin and Mineral Supplements?

Having said that eating good food is the best, and only sure way to improve your nutritional health, it should be added that for particular groups of older adults, taking nutritional supplements is entirely reasonable and, at times, necessary:

1. People who eat fewer than 1,500 calories a day.

2. People who are institutionalized.

3. People with certain chronic diseases, including alcoholism, as well as liver, kidney, and intestinal diseases.

4. People who take drugs that interfere with absorption of nutrients.

5. People with a specific diagnosed nutritional deficiency or those who are in a high-risk group for developing a deficiency. For example, postmenopausal women should take calcium to prevent osteoporosis and strict vegetarians who do not eat eggs or milk products should take vitamin B_{12}.

People who fit into these categories may require either a supplement of a specific nutrient or a multivitamin supplement with or without minerals. Either way, supplementation should be started only after discussion with and approval by your doctor.

Taking Vitamin and Mineral Supplements as "Insurance"

What about people who do not fall into these categories? For example, what if you eat an inadequate diet and find it hard to make changes toward a healthy diet? Many people in this situation take a vitamin and mineral supplement to provide adequate "insurance" for their diets. Is this a good idea? One needs to look at both sides of the issue. Supplements cannot provide "insurance" from a poor diet because vitamin and mineral deficiencies are not the only problems resulting from eating an unbalanced diet, and may not even be the most important ones.

A diet high in fat, cholesterol, and salt, for example, contributes to heart disease. A diet low in fiber causes constipation and irregularity of bowel movements, and contributes to development of diverticulitis, a disease of the intestine that can result in bleeding of the intestine. A vitamin and mineral supplement will not insure against any of these problems. Only changes in your diet can help you to prevent such diseases. Relying on supplements for insurance can give you a false sense of security about your diet. We all have met people who eat a poor diet and justify it by saying, "Well, at least I'm taking vitamins." This false sense of security may remove any incentive to improve diet.

What if you want to take a supplement anyway? There is no strong medical evidence of benefit from supplements when a specific deficiency does not exist, although it is a fact that people take them for peace of mind.

There is, however, one very well-controlled study, done in people 65 and older, some of whom had established deficiencies in one or more vitamins or minerals in which a multiple-vitamin pill with minerals was given to half of the people, and a placebo to the other half. At the end of one year, those who took the balanced supplement had significantly fewer days of illness due to infections than those who took the placebo. Other indicators of immune function were also improved in the vitamin group, suggesting that in people with deficiencies of one or more vitamins or minerals correction by multiple vitamin supplementation may improve immune function. The authors stressed that no large doses of any vitamin or mineral were used since they might actually impair immunity.[3]

On the other hand, there is no evidence that a regular multivitamin supplement, with or without minerals, taken in a dose less than or equal to the recommended dietary allowance (RDA) is detrimental to your health. This does not hold true, however, for doses that far exceed the RDA (megadoses) of vitamins and minerals. If you decide to use a supplement, there are a few things that you should know.

Guidelines for Selecting Supplements

Be rational about selecting a supplement. If you are not at risk for a specific vitamin or mineral deficiency, choose a basic multivitamin plus mineral supplement. Taking specific pills for specific vitamins is a marketing tactic designed to make supplements more expensive. The average multivitamin pill with close to 100% of the RDA of each of the vitamins is less expensive.

Read the mineral contents on the label if you are concerned about increasing your intake of minerals. Most multivitamin supplements with minerals contain close to 100% of the RDA for vitamins but not for minerals. Mineral deficiency is actually more common than vitamin deficiency, despite what advertising might say. In older postmenopausal women, for example, calcium deficiency is a major health problem. We concur with the National Institutes of Health's recommendation of 1,000 to 1,500 milligrams of calcium a day. If you cannot get this amount through your diet, take a calcium supplement (see p. 600), either alone or in combination with a vitamin supplement.

Do not buy a supplement that contains nutrients for which there are no known requirements or "new" vitamins, such as lecithin, carnitine, and inositol. Supporters of these supplements argue that we do not know all of what the human body really needs. Within the last 15 years, however, people with intestinal problems have been living successfully on injected solutions of protein, carbohydrates, fats, and established vitamins. If there were any unknown nutrients needed, this information would be known by now.

Buy the least expensive supplements. Many products are horrendously overpriced, being marked up to 1,000% over cost! Money that you overspend on supplements is money taken away from buying wholesome food. There is no benefit to be gained from a "natural" supplement versus a synthetic supplement. Brand name vitamins are no better than generic versions. Buy the generics, which will work exactly the same as the more expensive name brands.

Recommended Dietary Allowances (RDA)—What They Really Mean

There is no need to take vitamin or mineral doses above the recommended dietary allowances. The National Academy of Sciences is the organization that sets the recommended dietary allowance (RDA) for each vitamin and mineral, and this allowance varies for males, females, and different age groups. Because they are designed to account for differences between older and younger adults, the RDAs are the most appropriate ones for an older adult to use.

There is a prevailing myth that the RDA is no more than the amount of a vitamin or mineral that is needed to prevent deficiencies. This is not the case. When an RDA is set, the committee first decides how much of a vitamin or mineral the average person needs, and then raises this number to cover the needs of 98% of the healthy population. **This number is set at a level that is often two to three times higher than people's needs, resulting in a significant safety margin—the government's own "insurance" for your health.**

Because of this built-in safety margin, the vast majority of people do not even need to get 100% of the RDA, as it is defined by the RDA committee. Thus, there is no need to take supplements that go beyond the RDA.

You may be familiar with two other guidelines, the U.S. Recommended Daily Allowance (USRDA) and the Minimum Daily Requirement (MDR). Neither of these guidelines is as appropriate as the RDA, especially for older adults. The Food and Drug Administration sets a single USRDA, which is largely based on the RDA for teenage boys. This allowance is not appropriate for older adults, since it does not account for age differences. Most vitamin supplements will state on the label what percent of the USRDA they provide. The MDR was a forerunner of the USRDA and is now out of date.

The Myth of Megadose

There is a great deal of advertising that promotes the unproven benefits of taking "megadoses" of vitamins and minerals—supplements well beyond the RDA. Sensational claims of health and well-being are made for megadoses—they will "add vitality to your health," "restore the luster to your skin," and "perk up your sex life." When looked at critically, these claims just don't stand up.

To understand what vitamins or minerals can or cannot do, one must first understand their function in the human body. For the most part, a vitamin is a part of an enzyme (protein) which helps the enzyme perform certain chemical functions in the body. For example, many B vitamins help enzymes convert food into energy. Minerals act similarly. Calcium builds bones and also helps enzymes perform their functions. Iron is an essential element of red blood cells and helps them carry oxygen from the lungs to the tissues.

Vitamin functions were originally determined through vitamin deficiency diseases in people who were deprived of certain kinds of food for long periods of time. For instance, sailors often developed scurvy, a disease with such symptoms as bleeding into joints, poor healing of wounds, and emotional changes. It was determined that scurvy resulted from vitamin C deficiency when it was discovered that the sailors' symptoms dramatically disappeared once they ate citrus fruits.

The vitamin manufacturers take the process of deficiency diseases and vitamins one step further. For example, claims are made that vitamin C will help cure skin or emotional problems, colds, or cancer. The overwhelming majority of these problems are not caused by vitamin C deficiency, so they will not improve in the average person taking vitamin C.

The flaw in this logic can be demonstrated by substituting "food" for "vitamin" in an example of a deficiency. If you fast for a long time you will begin to develop certain symptoms, such as muscle aches, headaches, nausea, and dizziness. These symptoms of "food" deficiency will disappear dramatically once you begin to eat again. It does not follow from this that if you have symptoms of nausea, headaches, and dizziness while eating normally, that more food will cause them to go away. But this is the kind of logic most manufacturers use to make claims for the benefits of megadoses of supplements: If some is good, then more must be better.

The only way to determine a beneficial effect of a supplement is through controlled scientific experiments, in which a supplement's effects are compared with those of a placebo (dummy medication). No extravagant claims made by manufacturers for megadoses of any vitamins have stood up to these tests.

There are a few instances where vitamins have been determined to have specific additional benefits that have been demonstrated by rigorous scientific studies. Most of these therapeutic uses occur at doses not much greater than the RDA. They are discussed in the individual drug profiles which follow this section.

There are serious dangers associated with taking megadoses of many vitamins. People who take a multivitamin supplement in low doses have few risks; however, people who take high doses of certain vitamins have a risk of developing serious medical problems. Dangerous, toxic, and occasionally fatal effects have been associated with high doses of the fat-soluble vitamins A, D, E, and K. Even the water-soluble vitamin C and the B vitamins, which normally pass out of the body in your urine, can have adverse effects at high doses. Vitamin B_6 has been associated with nerve damage,[4] for example. Too much vitamin C can cause stomach cramps or diarrhea.

Some vitamins should not be taken—even in normal doses—if you use certain drugs or have certain medical problems. If you use warfarin (Coumadin) to prevent blood clots, you should not take vitamin K; it will inhibit warfarin's ability to work. If you are B_{12} deficient and take folic acid (folate) without taking B_{12} as well, neurological symptoms can be worsened. If you are going to take any type of supplement, be sure to discuss it with your doctor before you start.

Nutritional supplements are a booming business in this country. Many people are misled by advertising into thinking that taking a supplement will help get rid of many of their health problems. But this is not the case. The most important step that you can take to maintain your nutritional well-being is to eat a healthy and well-balanced diet.

Certain older adults may need specific vitamin and mineral supplementation and should talk to their doctors about this. If you do not fall into one of these categories and still wish to take a supplement, you should follow a few rules of thumb.

First, realize that supplements are by no means the complete answer to good nutrition. Taking a supplement is not an adequate replacement for eating healthy food. If you do buy supplements there is no need to buy anything more than a regular multivitamin or a mineral supplement. Take supplements less than or equal to the recommended dietary allowance for older adults. Try to buy the generic brands, not the expensive name brands and "natural" supplements. Finally, avoid megadoses of any supplement. They will give you no additional benefits from the supplement, but will greatly increase your chances of toxic adverse effects.

DIETARY SOURCES OF VITAMINS AND MINERALS

VITAMINS

A Beef liver*, carrots, sweet potatoes, tomatoes, green leafy vegetables, broccoli, watermelon, cantaloupe, apricots, peaches, butter*, margarine*, whole milk*, fortified skim milk

D Some fatty fishes* and fish-liver oils*, vitamin D-fortified milk* and bread, eggs*, chicken livers*

E Vegetable oils* (corn, cottonseed, soybean, safflower), wheat germ, whole-grain cereals, egg yolk*

K Green leafy vegetables, beef*, pork*

C Citrus fruits (oranges, grapefruit, lemons, limes), tomatoes, strawberries, cantaloupe, cabbage, broccoli, cauliflower, potatoes, raw peppers

B₁ (thiamine) Dried beans, peas, whole-grain or enriched breads and cereals, enriched or brown rice, enriched pasta, noodles, and other flour products, potatoes, pork*, beef liver*, nuts*

B₂ (riboflavin) Milk*, enriched and whole-grain products, green leafy vegetables, meat*, fish, poultry*, eggs*, liver*, cheese*

B₃ (niacin) Beans, peas, potatoes, enriched grain products, beef*, poultry*, pork*, liver*, nuts*

B₆ (pyridoxine) Wheat and corn products, soybeans, lima beans, yeast, beef*, poultry*, pork*, organ meats*

B₁₂ (cyanocobalamin) Shellfish*, tongue*, fish, milk*, eggs*, cheese*, peas, beans, lentils, tofu, nuts*, beef*, poultry*, pork*, organ meats*

Folic Acid (folate) Dried beans and nuts*, fruits, green leafy vegetables, organ meats*, whole grains, yeast

MINERALS

Calcium Milk*, cheese*, yogurt*, ice cream*—low-fat and nonfat dairy products can be used—canned salmon and sardines, shellfish*, broccoli, green leafy vegetables, including collards, bok choy, mustard and turnip greens

Iron Organ meats*, red meat*, fish, green leafy vegetables, peas, wheat germ, brewer's yeast, oysters*, dried beans and fruits

High in fat and/or cholesterol. Keep servings of these foods to a minimum. Ideally, the calories in all of these foods together should be less than 30% of your diet.

RECOMMENDED DIETARY ALLOWANCES FOR OLDER ADULTS

(National Academy of Sciences Recommendations for Adults over 50 Years) (1989)[5]

	Amount	
	Males	Females
VITAMINS		
A		
Retinol	1,000 mcg	800 mcg
Beta-carotene	6,000 mcg	4,800 mcg
International Units	3,300 i.u.	2,640 i.u.
D	400 i.u.	200 i.u.
E	10 mg	8 mg
C	60 mg	60 mg
Thiamine (B₁)	1.2 mg	1.0 mg
Riboflavin (B₂)	1.4 mg	1.2 mg
Niacin (B₃)	15 mg	13 mg
B₆	2.0 mg	1.6 mg
B₁₂	2.0 mcg	2.0 mcg
Folic Acid (folate)	200 mcg	180 mcg
MINERALS		
Calcium	800 mg	1,000–1,500 mg*
Phosphorus	800 mg	800 mg
Magnesium	350 mg	280 mg
Iron	10 mg	10 mg
Zinc	15 mg	12 mg
Iodine	150 mcg	150 mcg

i.u.= International Units
mcg = micrograms
mg = milligrams

This is not the official calcium RDA for women, which is 800 mg. Many experts consider this too low, including the National Institutes of Health which recommends an intake of 1,000–1,500 mg a day for women after menopause (we agree). See Calcium Supplements (p. 600) for further details.

SUPPLEMENT PROFILES

Calcium Supplements

Calcium Carbonate
OS-CAL 500 (SmithKline Beecham)
CALTRATE (Lederle Consumer)

Calcium Gluconate

Calcium Citrate
CITRACAL (Mission)

Calcium Lactate

GENERIC: available
FAMILY: Nutritional Supplements (see p. 592)

Calcium (*kal* see um) is a mineral that is stored in the bones and is necessary for bone growth and strength. It also benefits the nervous system, muscles, and heart. As your body ages, its ability to absorb calcium decreases, even though its need for calcium does not diminish. If you are older and also have a diet that lacks adequate calcium, both factors limit the amount of the mineral available for your body to use.

Calcium deficiency in older adults causes changes in the bones (osteomalacia) and diseases that increase the risk of falls, fractures, and deformity (osteoporosis). Osteomalacia is an overall decrease in bone density. Osteoporosis, which occurs most frequently in thin, small-boned, and white women, is a condition in which the bones become weak, so that they are more likely to break or become deformed.

How much calcium do you need? The recommended dietary allowance (RDA) for calcium is 800 to 1,200 milligrams per day, but many experts consider that too low for the population as a whole. In 1984, the National Institutes of Health recommended a calcium intake of 1,000 to 1,500 milligrams per day for women after menopause.[6] We think that this is a safe and desirable intake for all adults. It will not necessarily protect you against the fractures and deformity of osteoporosis, but it may help and it is unlikely to do you any harm. We do not recommend taking more than 1,500 milligrams per day, since the greater amount has no advantages and can cause some dangerous adverse effects (see Adverse Effects).

The best way to get calcium is to eat foods that are rich in it (see food sources, below). In particular, you can increase your calcium intake by drinking milk and adding liquid or powdered milk to almost any cooked food (you can use low-fat or nonfat milk if you want to keep your fat intake down). If you cannot get enough calcium from your diet, take a calcium supplement. However, if you have a history of kidney stones, do not increase your calcium intake without talking to your doctor first.

Many people, particularly women, take calcium supplements in the hope that it will decrease their risk of getting osteoporosis. While it has been shown that a diet containing adequate calcium can prevent high blood pressure, taking supplements to prevent osteoporosis is controversial. If you want to reduce your risk of osteoporosis, try quitting smoking, drinking alcohol in moderation if at all, and doing weight-bearing exercise such as walking, aerobics, jogging, dancing, tennis, and biking (although biking is less beneficial than the others).

If you decide to take a calcium supplement, some cautions are in order. You should not take calcium supplements that contain bonemeal and dolomite. The Food and Drug Administration reported that they might contain lead in amounts that could present a risk to older adults.[7] Furthermore, your body does not absorb all calcium supplements with equal ease. Unfortunately, it has not been determined which supplement is absorbed the best. One study showed that calcium citrate was best absorbed, but another showed that there was no significant difference in absorption among various types of supplements.[8,9] Ask your pharmacist or other health professional for suggestions.

When comparing calcium supplements, you should always check how much elemental (pure) calcium they contain. Because calcium supplements contain other ingredients in addition to calcium, a 100-milligram calcium supplement tablet does not contain 100 milligrams of calcium, and a 100-milligram tablet of one supplement does not necessarily have the same amount of calcium as a 100-milligram tablet of another. Calcium carbonate is 40% calcium, calcium gluconate is 9% calcium, and calcium citrate is 24% calcium. Read the label on the container to find out the amount of elemental calcium. This is the only measurement that counts as far as your body is concerned.

FOODS HIGH IN CALCIUM

Milk, liquid or powdered, including low-fat and nonfat milk, low-fat yogurt, ice cream, cheese (some are high in fat and/or cholesterol), canned salmon and sardines, shellfish, broccoli, green leafy vegetables.

1 cup plain low-fat yogurt	415 milligrams calcium
1 cup milk	300 milligrams calcium
3 1/2 ounces canned salmon with bones	198 milligrams calcium

Before You Use This Drug

Do not use if you have or have had:

- high level of calcium in your blood
- increased parathyroid gland function
- reduced parathyroid gland function (*only for calcium phosphate*)
- kidney stones
- irregular heartbeat

Tell your doctor if you have or have had:

- allergies to drugs
- symptoms of appendicitis (severe abdominal pain)

- blood in stool
- heart disease
- hemorrhoids
- high blood pressure
- peptic ulcer
- intestinal blockage
- kidney disease
- sarcoidosis

Tell your doctor about any other drugs you take, including aspirin, herbs, vitamins, and other nonprescription products.

When You Use This Drug

- **Call your doctor immediately if you have black, tarry stools or vomit material that looks like coffee grounds.**
- After taking a calcium supplement, wait one to two hours before taking any other drug by mouth.
- Do not drink milk or eat milk products, spinach, rhubarb, bran, or whole-grain cereals at the same time that you take calcium supplements. They decrease its absorption.

How to Use This Drug

- Do not store in the bathroom. Do not expose to heat, moisture, or strong light. Do not let liquid form freeze.
- If you are taking calcium supplements on a fixed schedule and you miss a dose, take it as soon as you remember, but skip it if it is almost time for the next dose. **Do not take double doses.**

Interactions with Other Drugs

The following drugs are listed in the *Evaluations of Drug Interactions* 1997 as causing "highly clinically significant" or "clinically significant" interactions when used together with this drug. We have also included potentially serious interactions listed in the drug's FDA-approved professional product labeling or package insert. New scientific techniques have allowed researchers to predict some drug interactions before they have been documented in people. There may be other drugs, especially those in the families of drugs listed below, that also will react with this drug to cause severe adverse effects. The number of new drugs approved for marketing increases the chance of drug interactions, and new drug interactions are being identified with old drugs. Be vigilant. Make sure to tell your doctor and pharmacist the drugs you are taking and tell your doctor if you are taking any of these interacting drugs:

ACHROMYCIN, aspirin, GENUINE BAYER ASPIRIN, CALAN SR, CHIBROXIN, chlorothiazide, CILOXAN, CIPRO, ciprofloxacin, COVERA–HS, DIURIL, ECOTRIN, enoxacin, FLOXIN, grepafloxacin, ISOPTIN SR, LEVAQUIN, levofloxacin, lomefloxacin, MAXAQUIN, norfloxacin, NOROXIN, OCUFLOX, ofloxacin, PANMYCIN, PENETREX, RAXAR, sparfloxacin, SUMYCIN, tetracycline, TORVAN, trovafloxacin, verapamil, VERELAN, ZAGAM.

Adverse Effects

Call your doctor immediately if you experience:

- severe constipation
- severe abdominal pain or cramping
- difficult or painful urination
- irregular heartbeat
- mood or mental changes
- nervousness or restlessness
- unpleasant taste in mouth
- unusual tiredness or weakness

Call your doctor if these symptoms continue:

- bloated stomach, belching
- chalky taste in mouth

Folic Acid (Folate)
FOLVITE (Lederle)

GENERIC: available

FAMILY: Nutritional Supplements (see p. 592)

Folic (*foe* lik) acid, also called folate or vitamin B_9, is essential for cell formation and growth, particularly of blood cells. It is found in several foods (see food sources, below). A well-balanced diet with a variety of healthful foods should supply all the folic acid your body needs. The recommended dietary allowance (RDA) of folic acid for older adults is 200 micrograms per day for men, 180 for women.

It is unlikely that you would have a diet-related folic acid deficiency. Rather, certain medical conditions or the long-term use of several drugs can lead to a folic acid deficiency. Alcoholism is perhaps the most common cause because alcoholics often eat an inadequate diet. Some diseases of the small intestine can also interfere with your body's absorption of folic acid, so there is less available for the body to use. Long-term treatment with drugs such as methotrexate, trimethoprim, triamterene, corticosteroids, certain painkillers, sulfasalazine, and some anticonvulsants (phenobarbital, phenytoin, and primidone) can also cause a folic acid deficiency.

If you have to increase your intake of folic acid in order to prevent or treat a deficiency, eat folate-rich foods rather than taking a vitamin supplement. You should only take a supplement when you have a clear need for more folic acid and when you cannot get enough from your diet. You should not take a supplement until your doctor has made sure that you do not have pernicious anemia, a disease resulting in vitamin B_{12} deficiency. Folic acid supplements can hide the easily detected symptoms of pernicious anemia while allowing irreversible nervous system damage to occur undetected.

Folic acid has been shown to prevent neural tube defects, a serious type of birth defect, and as of January 1998, all grains sold in the U.S. contain 140 micrograms of folic acid per 100 grams (about 3 ounces). Even this amount, however, may be inadequate for prevention of neural tube defects, which occur early in pregnancy, before most women know that they are pregnant. The current recommendation is that women of childbearing age should receive 400 micrograms of folic acid per day.[10]

If you take folic acid without a doctor's supervision, do not exceed the RDA.

FOODS HIGH IN FOLIC ACID (FOLATE)

Organ meats and nuts (both are high in cholesterol and/or fat), green vegetables, dried beans, fruits, yeast, whole grains. Cooking may destroy some folic acid.

1/2 cup spinach	110 micrograms folic acid
1 ounce chicken liver	108 micrograms folic acid
1/2 cup peanuts	60 micrograms folic acid
1 ounce shredded wheat	30 micrograms folic acid

Before You Use This Drug

Tell your doctor if you have or have had:

- allergies to drugs
- pernicious anemia

Tell your doctor about any other drugs you take, including aspirin, herbs, vitamins, and other nonprescription products.

How to Use This Drug

- Do not store in the bathroom. Do not expose to heat, moisture, or strong light. Do not let liquid form freeze.

- As with all drugs, it is important to take this one regularly. However, because of the length of time required for a folic acid deficiency to occur, there is no cause for concern if a dose is missed. If you miss a dose, take it when you remember.

Interactions with Other Drugs

The following drugs are listed in the *Evaluations of Drug Interactions* 1997 as causing "highly clinically significant" or "clinically significant" interactions when used together with this drug. We have also included potentially serious interactions listed in the drug's FDA-approved professional product labeling or package insert. New scientific techniques have allowed researchers to predict some drug interactions before they have been documented in people. There may be other drugs, especially those in the families of drugs listed below, that also will react with this drug to cause severe adverse effects. The number of new drugs approved for marketing increases the chance of drug interactions, and new drug interactions are being identified with old drugs. Be vigilant. Make sure to tell your doctor and pharmacist the drugs you are taking and tell your doctor if you are taking any of these interacting drugs:

cholestyramine, DILANTIN, LOCHOLEST, phenytoin, QUESTRAN.

Adverse Effects

Folic acid and other water-soluble vitamins seldom cause adverse effects in people whose kidneys function normally. If you have decreased kidney function or are taking large doses of this vitamin, you should *call your doctor immediately* if you experience any of these adverse effects:

- skin rash or itching
- fever

Iron Supplements

Ferrous Sulfate
FEOSOL (SmithKline Beecham)
SLOW FE (Novartis)

Ferrous Gluconate
FERGON (Bayer Consumer)

Ferrous Fumarate
FEOSTAT (Forest)

GENERIC: available

FAMILY: Nutritional Supplements (see p. 592)

Iron is a mineral that your body needs to man-ufacture hemoglobin, a substance in red blood cells that carries oxygen throughout the body. A lack of iron causes anemia, a condition in which the body has too few red blood cells, too little hemoglobin, or too little blood. Iron is found in many foods (see food sources below), and a well-balanced diet with a variety of foods should supply all the iron that your body needs. There is no reason to take an iron supplement unless you have a low iron count or iron defi-ciency anemia. The recommended dietary allowance (RDA) for older adults is 10 mil-ligrams per day.

Adults generally become iron-deficient from blood loss, rather than from a lack of iron in their diet. If your doctor says that you have iron deficiency anemia, she or he must deter-mine the site of the blood loss.

If you have iron deficiency anemia due to blood loss, you should add iron-rich foods to your diet as well as take an iron supplement. When comparing iron supplements, you should always check how much elemental (pure) iron they con-tain. For example, a 324 milligram ferrous sul-fate tablet contains 65 milligrams of elemental iron, while a 320 milligram ferrous gluconate tablet contains 37 milligrams of elemental iron, and a 100 milligram ferrous fumarate tablet contains 33 milligrams of elemental iron. You should start out with a supplement containing

ferrous sulfate, rather than one made of ferrous gluconate or ferrous fumarate.[11]

Do not use iron supplements that also con-tain other minerals such as calcium and mag-nesium, which can interfere with your body's absorption of iron. Also, do not use enteric-coat-ed tablets (tablets coated so they do not dis-solve in your stomach) or timed-release products because your body does not absorb them evenly. Do not take an iron supplement at the same time as eating foods high in fiber or calcium.

Within two weeks from when you begin to take an iron supplement, your red blood cell count should improve. If there is no improvement after three to four weeks, ask your doctor to reevaluate your situation. If you are anemic, you might need to take iron supplements for six months or longer to replenish the body's supply. If the cause of your iron deficiency is poor absorption of iron, a rare problem, you may have to take an iron sup-plement for longer than six months.

If you do not have a low iron count or iron deficiency anemia, there is no reason for you to take an iron supplement. Your body saves iron and cannot get rid of extra iron except by bleed-ing. Taking too much iron can cause an iron overload in the body and damage to your liver, heart, or kidneys.[12]

FOODS HIGH IN IRON

Organ meats, red meat, oysters (all are also high in cholesterol and/or fat), fish, green leafy vegetables, peas, brewer's yeast, wheat germ, certain dried beans and fruits. Iron from meats is absorbed an average of five times better than iron from vegetables.

3 1/2 ounces calves' liver	14 milligrams iron
1 lean hamburger	3.9 milligrams iron
3 1/2 ounces chickpeas	3 milligrams iron
1/2 cup cooked lima beans	3 milligrams iron

Before You Use This Drug

Do not use if you have or have had:

- diseases of iron overload (hemochromatosis, hemosiderosis)
- thalassemia (a hereditary anemia)

Tell your doctor if you have or have had:

- allergies to drugs
- alcohol dependence
- liver disease (hepatitis)
- active infections
- inflammation of the pancreas
- peptic ulcer
- disease of the intestines
- recent blood transfusion

Tell your doctor about any other drugs you take, including aspirin, herbs, vitamins, and other nonprescription products.

When You Use This Drug

- Do not use calcium carbonate antacids or calcium supplements, drink coffee, tea, or milk, or eat whole-grain breads or cereals, eggs or milk products within two hours of taking an iron supplement. They can decrease iron absorption.
- Your stools will probably turn black. This is a normal side effect and no cause for concern.

How to Use This Drug

- Take on an empty stomach, at least one hour before, or two hours after, meals. If the iron upsets your stomach, try taking it with food instead. If you can, drink a glass of fruit juice with your iron as this will improve its absorption.
- Liquid form or contents of capsules can be taken alone or can be mixed with juice, cereal, or other food.
- Do not store in the bathroom. Do not expose to heat, moisture, or strong light. Do not let the liquid form freeze.

- If you miss a dose, take it as soon as you remember, but skip it if it is almost time for the next dose. **Do not take double doses.**

Interactions with Other Drugs

The following drugs are listed in the *Evaluations of Drug Interactions* 1997 as causing "highly clinically significant" or "clinically significant" interactions when used together with this drug. We have also included potentially serious interactions listed in the drug's FDA-approved professional product labeling or package insert. New scientific techniques have allowed researchers to predict some drug interactions before they have been documented in people. There may be other drugs, especially those in the families of drugs listed below, that also will react with this drug to cause severe adverse effects. The number of new drugs approved for marketing increases the chance of drug interactions, and new drug interactions are being identified with old drugs. Be vigilant. Make sure to tell your doctor and pharmacist the drugs you are taking and tell your doctor if you are taking any of these interacting drugs:

ACHROMYCIN, ALDOMET, CHIBROXIN, CILOXAN, CIPRO, ciprofloxacin, CUPRIMINE, DEPEN, enoxacin, grepafloxacin, LARODOPA, LEVAQUIN, levodopa, levofloxacin, lomefloxacin, MAXAQUIN, methyldopa, norfloxacin, NOROXIN, PANMYCIN, PENETREX, penicillamine, RAXAR, sparfloxacin, SUMYCIN, tetracycline, TORVAN, trovafloxacin, ZAGAM.

Adverse Effects

Call your doctor immediately if you experience:

- stomach pain, cramping, soreness
- fresh red blood in stools

• **If you know that you or someone else has taken an overdose of an iron supplement, particularly if that person is a child, seek emergency room treatment immediately. Do not wait for symptoms, which may not appear for one hour.**

• **early signs of overdose:** diarrhea, nausea or vomiting, sharp stomach pain or cramping

• **late signs of overdose:** bluish lips, fingernails, and palms, drowsiness, pale, clammy skin, unusual tiredness, weak, fast heartbeat

Call your doctor if these symptoms continue:

- constipation or diarrhea
- dark urine
- heartburn
- nausea or vomiting

Periodic Tests

Ask your doctor which of these tests should be done periodically while you are taking this drug:

- hemoglobin tests
- reticulocyte (young red blood cell) counts
- total iron binding capacity (TIBC)
- iron concentration in the blood
- ferritin concentration in the blood

———

Multivitamins (with and without minerals)
THERAGRAN-M (Mead Johnson)
CENTRUM (Lederle)

GENERIC: available
FAMILY: Nutritional Supplements (see p. 592)

It is estimated that 40% of adults in the United States take nutritional supplements daily.[13] Is this necessary?

Vitamin deficiencies are rare in this country. Mineral deficiencies are more common, but taking a multivitamin supplement with minerals is often not the best way to get minerals. These products either do not supply enough of the mineral you lack, or they contain other minerals which reduce your body's ability to absorb the specific mineral you need. Instead of taking such supplements, try changing your diet so that you get more of just the mineral you need, or take a specific mineral supplement. For example, if you have iron deficiency anemia, you should be taking an iron supplement. Calcium deficiency is another example. Most multivitamin supplements with minerals do not supply enough calcium to meet the recommended dietary allowance (RDA), so taking these supplements may give you a false sense of security about your calcium intake. Changes in your diet, combined with a calcium supplement, may be the best way to increase your calcium intake. See the listings for individual minerals and vitamins for more details.

Who needs a multivitamin and mineral supplement? The following groups of older adults are at risk of vitamin deficiency and may need a supplement:

• those who eat fewer than 1,500 calories a day and may have a barely adequate vitamin intake;

• those who live alone, are institutionalized, have recently been discharged from the hospital, or cannot shop for their food;

• those who have certain medical problems (such as some intestinal disorders) or take certain drugs that interfere with their body's ability to absorb nutrients;

• those who drink too much alcohol, which can reduce the body's supply of certain vitamins (thiamine, riboflavin, folic acid, vitamins C and B_6).

The more of these groups you belong to, the greater your risk of having a low-calorie, unbalanced, and nutritionally deficient diet. If you have one or more of these factors, you should discuss the need for a multivitamin supplement with your doctor. Remember that a supplement will not completely make up for deficiencies in your diet, since vitamins are only a very small part of proper nutrition. Getting a good balance of protein, fat, carbohydrates, and fiber is also important, and you can only do this through a well-balanced diet.

If you don't fit into the risk categories above, should you take a supplement for "insurance"? If you are eating a well-balanced diet, there is no reason why you need one.

There is, however, one very well-controlled study, done in people 65 and older, some of whom had established deficiencies in one or more vitamins or minerals in which a multiple-vitamin pill with minerals was given to half of the people, and a placebo to the other half. At the end of one year, those who took the balanced supplement had significantly fewer days of illness due to infections than those who took the placebo. Other indicators of immune function were also improved in the vitamin group, suggesting that in people with deficiencies of one or more vitamins or minerals correction by multiple vitamin supplementation may improve immune function. The authors stressed that no large doses of any vitamin or mineral were used since they might actually impair immunity.[14]

If you take a multivitamin supplement, don't take doses significantly higher than the recommended dietary allowance (RDA). Doses higher than the RDA will either be eliminated from your body in your urine (in the case of water-soluble vitamins such as the B vitamins and vitamin C) or will accumulate in the body tissues and cause harmful adverse effects (in the case of the fat-soluble vitamins A, D, E, and K).

When choosing a multivitamin, keep in mind that many manufacturers use the same general trademark for several products that have different formulas. Some make drastic changes in the formula of a product and keep the same name. Read the labels and compare the contents of several products. Compare the label with the Recommended Dietary Allowances for Older Adults

(p. 597). There is not much logic in a formula that contains less than 50% of the RDA for some vitamins and more than 500% for others. Choose a supplement that comes as close as possible to 100% of the RDA for each ingredient.

Buy the least expensive supplement that meets your needs, and buy a generic version if you can. Generic products are cheaper and are just as effective as the brand name products.

———

Niacin (Vitamin B$_3$)
NICOLAR (Rhone-Poulenc Rorer)

GENERIC: available

FAMILY: Nutritional Supplements (see p. 592)
Cholesterol-lowering drugs (see p. 54)

Niacin (*nye* a sin), also called nicotinic acid or vitamin B$_3$, and its derivative niacinamide (nye a *sin* a mide), also called nicotinamide, are used by the body to help convert food to energy. Niacin is available in many types of foods (see food sources, below), and a well-balanced diet with a variety of healthful foods should supply all the niacin that your body needs. The recommended dietary allowance (RDA) is 15 milligrams for older men and 13 milligrams for older women.

Dietary deficiency of niacin, called pellagra, is rare. If you need to get more niacin, it is better to eat niacin-rich foods than to take a vitamin supplement. You should take niacin supplements to prevent and treat niacin deficiency only when your diet does not provide an adequate amount.

Niacin (nicotinic acid), but not niacinamide, has another use. It can be prescribed as part of a program to lower blood cholesterol or fat, which also includes a modified diet and exercise. The dose for this purpose, 300 milligrams or more, is much higher than the dose as a dietary supplement (10 to 20 milligrams). Taking niacin for this purpose is only an adjunct to weight reduction and exercise, not a substitute.

The adverse effects of niacin, such as blood vessel dilation which produces intense flushing and itching of the face and upper part of the body, may limit the usefulness of this treatment. **One aspirin taken 30 minutes before a dose of niacin may reduce this adverse effect.**[15]

Niacin is *not* useful in treating schizophrenia and other mental disorders unrelated to niacin deficiency. It has not been proven effective in treating any blood vessel diseases nor in treating acne, leprosy, or motion sickness.

If you use niacin without a doctor's supervision, do not exceed the RDA. Excess niacin, beyond what is needed each day, simply passes through you and is eliminated in the urine without being used by your body. **Avoid taking extended-release forms of niacin, since these may damage your liver (see p. 609).**

FOODS HIGH IN NIACIN (VITAMIN B$_3$)

Beef, pork, liver, eggs, nuts, poultry, milk and dairy products (all are high in cholesterol and/or fat), fish, whole-grain and enriched breads and cereals, beans, peas, potatoes. Cooking destroys some niacin.

3 1/2 ounces calves' liver	16.5 milligrams niacin
1 cup wheat flakes	14.7 milligrams niacin
4 ounces halibut	10.4 milligrams niacin
1/4 cup peanuts	10.0 milligrams niacin
3 1/2 ounces roast turkey	7.7 milligrams niacin
1 slice whole wheat bread	6 milligrams niacin

Before You Use This Drug

Tell your doctor if you have or have had:

- allergies to drugs
- arterial bleeding or hemorrhage
- liver disease
- diabetes
- gout
- glaucoma
- ulcer
- low blood pressure

Tell your doctor about any other drugs you take, including aspirin, herbs, vitamins, and other nonprescription products.

When You Use This Drug

- Until you know how you react to this drug, do not drive or perform other activities requiring alertness. Niacin may cause dizziness or fainting.

How to Use This Drug

- Take with food to reduce stomach upset.
- Do not store in the bathroom. Do not expose to heat, moisture, or strong light. Do not let liquid form freeze.
- If you take a high dose of niacin and want to stop using the drug, reduce the dose gradually. If you plan to take a high dose, work up to it gradually.
- As with all drugs, it is important to take niacin regularly. However, because of the length of time required for niacin deficiency to occur, there is no cause for concern if you are taking niacin to supplement your diet and you miss a dose. Take it when you remember.
- If you are taking niacin as a cholesterol-lowering agent and you miss a dose, take it as soon as you remember, but skip it if it is almost time for the next dose. **Do not take double doses.**

Interactions with Other Drugs

The following drugs are listed in the *Evaluations of Drug Interactions* 1997 as causing "highly clinically significant" or "clinically significant" interactions when used together with

this drug. We have also included potentially serious interactions listed in the drug's FDA-approved professional product labeling or package insert. New scientific techniques have allowed researchers to predict some drug interactions before they have been documented in people. There may be other drugs, especially those in the families of drugs listed below, that also will react with this drug to cause severe adverse effects. The number of new drugs approved for marketing increases the chance of drug interactions, and new drug interactions are being identified with old drugs. Be vigilant. Make sure to tell your doctor and pharmacist the drugs you are taking and tell your doctor if you are taking any of these interacting drugs:

When niacin is used in doses to lower cholesterol: atorvastatin, BAYCOL, cerivastatin, fluvastatin, LESCOL, LIPITOR, lovastatin, MEVACOR, PRAVACHOL, pravastatin, simvastatin, ZOCOR.

Adverse Effects

Niacin and other water-soluble vitamins seldom cause adverse effects in people whose kidneys function normally. If you have decreased kidney function or are taking large doses of niacin, you should ***call your doctor immediately*** if you experience any of these adverse effects:

- skin rash or itching
- wheezing, an allergic reaction

With prolonged use of extended-release niacin:

- darkening of urine
- light gray-colored stools
- loss of appetite
- severe stomach pain
- yellow eyes or skin

Call your doctor if these symptoms continue:

- flushing or warmth of skin
- headache
- diarrhea
- lightheadedness or dizziness
- dry skin
- nausea or vomiting
- stomach pain
- joint pain

Periodic Tests

Ask your doctor which of these tests should be done periodically while you are taking this drug:

For high-dose therapy:

- cholesterol levels
- blood sugar levels
- liver function tests
- blood levels of uric acid

━━━━━━━━━

 Do Not Use

ALTERNATIVE TREATMENT:
See Nonsustained-release Niacin (p. 607).

Niacin (Vitamin B₃) (All sustained-release dosage forms of niacin)
NICOBID (Rhone-Poulenc Rorer)
SLO-NIACIN (Upsher-Smith)

FAMILY: Nutritional Supplements (see p. 592)
Cholesterol-lowering Drugs (see p. 54)

Although niacin is useful and effective as a cholesterol-lowering drug (see p. 54), the extended dose/sustained-release forms can cause liver damage. In the past several years, a number of studies have documented that liver toxicity, sometimes quite serious, is much more commonly associated with the sustained-release form than with the crystalline or regular form.[16,17]

If you are taking niacin for its lipid-lowering effects, ask your doctor if it is the crystalline (regular) type (see p. 607). Be sure that the prescription is not changed to a slow-release preparation by a pharmacist and do not purchase slow-release pills over the counter. The doses used to lower blood lipids are much higher than the amount needed for normal metabolism, and the slow-release formulas probably promote excessive accumulation of the drug in the liver.

Thiamine (Vitamin B$_1$)

GENERIC: available

FAMILY: Nutritional Supplements (see p. 592)

Thiamine (*thye* a min), or vitamin B$_1$, helps the body use sugars and starches (carbohydrates) effectively. It is available in several kinds of foods (see food sources, below), and a well-balanced diet with a variety of healthful foods should supply all the thiamine that your body needs. The recommended dietary allowance (RDA) of thiamine is 1.2 milligrams per day for older men and 1.0 milligrams per day for older women.

The signs of thiamine deficiency include loss of feeling on areas of the hands and feet, decreased muscle strength, personality disturbances, depression, lack of initiative, and poor memory. Thiamine deficiency is most commonly seen in alcoholics (the condition caused by a severe deficiency is called beri-beri). Alcoholics can become thiamine deficient because their diets often do not provide enough thiamine and because alcohol hinders the absorption of what thiamine they have. Chronic diarrhea can also lead to a need for more thiamine.

Thiamine is effective for treating conditions resulting from a thiamine deficiency, as in alcoholism. It has not been proven effective for treating skin problems, persistent diarrhea, fatigue, mental disorders, multiple sclerosis, ulcerative colitis, or for use as an insect repellant or appetite stimulant.[18]

If you have to increase your intake of thiamine, eat more thiamine-rich foods rather than taking a vitamin supplement. You should take a supplement only when dietary changes are inadequate to treat a deficiency.

If you take thiamine supplements without a doctor's supervision, do not take more than the RDA. Excess thiamine, beyond what is needed each day, simply passes through you and is eliminated in the urine without being used by your body.

FOODS HIGH IN THIAMINE (VITAMIN B$_1$)

Meats (especially pork), organ meats, and nuts (all of which are high in cholesterol and/or fat), dried beans, peas, whole-grain or enriched breads and cereals, enriched or brown rice, enriched pasta, noodles, and other flour products, potatoes. Cooking destroys some thiamine.

1 loin chop	1.18 milligrams thiamine
1 ounce wheat germ	.56 milligrams thiamine
3 1/2 ounces roast pork	.39 milligrams thiamine

Before You Use This Drug

Tell your doctor if you have or have had:

- allergies to drugs

Tell your doctor about any other drugs you take, including aspirin, herbs, vitamins, and other nonprescription products.

When You Use This Drug

- Do not drink alcohol. It interferes with your body's absorption of thiamine.

How to Use This Drug

• Do not store in the bathroom. Do not expose to heat, moisture, or strong light. Do not let the liquid form freeze.

• As with all drugs, it is important to take this one regularly. However, because of the length of time required for thiamine deficiency to occur, there is no cause for concern if you miss a dose. Take it when you remember.

Interactions with Other Drugs

Some other drugs that you may be taking (either over-the-counter or prescription drugs) can interact with this one, causing adverse effects. Ask your doctor what these drugs are and let him or her know if you are taking any of them.

Adverse Effects

Thiamine and other water-soluble vitamins seldom cause adverse effects in people whose kidneys function normally. If you have decreased kidney function or are taking large doses of thiamine, you should *call your doctor immediately* if you experience any of these adverse effects:

• skin rash or itching
• wheezing, an allergic reaction

Limited Use

===

Vitamin A
AQUASOL A (Astra)

GENERIC: available
FAMILY: Nutritional Supplements (see p. 592)

Vitamin A is necessary for growth and bone development, vision, and healthy skin. It is

---

PREGNANCY WARNING

The following warning appears in the professional product labeling for vitamin A: Fetal abnormalities including urinary tract malformations, growth retardation, and bone changes have been reported in children whose mothers took more than 6,000 units of vitamin A (1,800 micrograms) per day during pregnancy.

---

found in many foods (see food sources, below), and a well-balanced diet with a variety of healthful foods should supply all the vitamin A that your body needs. The recommended dietary allowance (RDA) of vitamin A is 1,000 micrograms per day for men and 800 micrograms per day for women.

Vitamin A deficiency is rare, but older adults may develop this deficiency if they have certain intestinal and liver diseases, an overactive thyroid (hyperthyroidism), or diabetes. You may also develop vitamin A deficiency from an inadequate diet or if you take certain drugs such as cholestyramine, colestipol, mineral oil, neomycin, or sucralfate. The liver stores enough vitamin A to last several months, so symptoms of a deficiency may take a few months to develop. The symptoms include night blindness and dry, cracked skin.

If you have to increase your intake of vitamin A to prevent or treat a deficiency, eat more foods that are rich in the vitamin rather than taking a vitamin supplement. You should take a supplement only if your diet does not supply enough vitamin A.

You can get vitamin A from foods in two main forms. Animal sources such as liver, egg yolks, and butter provide a form of vitamin A called retinol. Plant sources such as carrots, squash, and some fruits provide a substance called beta-carotene, which your body converts into vitamin A in the body. Plant sources have several advantages over animal sources, the main one being that they are low in calories, fat, and cholesterol and high in fiber and other nutrients.

Some researchers claim that people who eat large amounts of foods containing beta-carotene have a lower risk of some types of cancer than those who eat less of these foods.[19] One large 12-year study found that beta-carotene supplements had no effect on the incidence of cardiovascular disease or malignancy. A second controlled clinical trial in Finnish smokers found an increased incidence of lung cancer by 18%, which was statistically significant.[20] No one should take beta-carotene supplements.

If you use vitamin A supplements without a doctor's supervision, do not exceed the RDA. Taking doses only a few times higher than the RDA can be risky. Unlike with some other vitamins, your body cannot eliminate excess vitamin A, so the vitamin can accumulate to dangerous, toxic levels in your body. The toxic effects of too much retinol include: liver damage, weakness, increased pressure in the brain, bone and joint pain and damage, and dry, rough skin. The effects from beta-carotene are not as serious.

FOODS HIGH IN RETINOL (ANIMAL SOURCES)

Beef liver, butter, egg yolks, fish-liver oils (all four are high in cholesterol and/or fat). Freezing may destroy some vitamin A in both types of food sources.

1 large carrot	11,000 International Units vitamin A
1 ounce calves' liver	9,340 International Units vitamin A
1/2 cup cooked spinach	7,300 International Units vitamin A
2/3 cup cooked broccoli	2,500 International Units vitamin A
1/4 cup cantaloupe	2,000 International Units vitamin A
1 cup milk	300–500 International Units vitamin A

FOODS HIGH IN BETA-CAROTENE (PLANT SOURCES)

Carrots, sweet potatoes, squash, broccoli, tomatoes, green leafy vegetables, cantaloupe, apricots, peaches, margarine.

Before You Use This Drug

Tell your doctor if you have or have had:

- allergies to drugs
- alcohol abuse
- viral hepatitis
- kidney or liver problems

Tell your doctor about any other drugs you take, including aspirin, herbs, vitamins, and other nonprescription products.

How to Use This Drug

- Take with food to reduce stomach upset.
- Swallow whole, or mix capsule contents with jam, applesauce or other foods.
- Liquid form can be taken alone or mixed with juice, cereal, or any other food.

- Do not store in the bathroom. Do not expose to heat, moisture, or strong light. Do not let the liquid form freeze.
- As with all drugs, it is important to take this one regularly. However, because of the length of time required for a vitamin A deficiency to occur, there is no cause for concern if you miss a dose. Take it when you remember.

Interactions with Other Drugs

Some other drugs that you may be taking (either over-the-counter or prescription drugs) can interact with this one, causing adverse effects. Ask your doctor what these drugs are and let him or her know if you are taking any of them.

Adverse Effects

Call your doctor immediately if you experience:

- pain in your bones or joints
- dizziness, weakness
- headaches, irritability
- dry, rough skin
- orange skin (*for beta-carotene*)
- vomiting, diarrhea
- tiredness
- loss of appetite
- increased sensitivity of skin to sunlight

Limited Use

Vitamin B$_{12}$

GENERIC: available
FAMILY: Nutritional Supplements (see p. 592)

Vitamin B$_{12}$, also called cyanocobalamin (sye an oh koe *bal* a min), is essential for cell growth and normal formation of blood cells. It is found in several kinds of foods (see food sources,

below), and a well-balanced diet with a variety of healthful foods should supply all the vitamin B$_{12}$ that your body needs. The recommended dietary allowance (RDA) of vitamin B$_{12}$ for older adults is 2–4 micrograms per day.

Even if you do not get enough vitamin B$_{12}$ in your diet, a vitamin B$_{12}$ deficiency may take years to develop because the liver stores a vast supply of this vitamin. You may develop a deficiency from certain physical conditions or from an inadequate diet. In adults, a vitamin B$_{12}$ deficiency usually comes from a defect in the digestive tract's absorption of the vitamin, a condition called pernicious anemia. You may also develop a deficiency if you have had parts of your stomach or small intestine removed, which prevents the digestive tract from adequately absorbing the vitamin. In both of these cases, you need vitamin B$_{12}$ injections. Since plants do not contain vitamin B$_{12}$, strict vegetarians who do not eat eggs or milk products also need a vitamin B$_{12}$ supplement, and can take one by mouth.

Vitamin B$_{12}$ deficiency can lead to anemia and to slow, progressive, irreversible damage to the nervous system. This damage will cause loss of feeling in the hands and feet, unsteadiness, loss of memory, confusion, and moodiness. To prevent these changes, people who require life-long treatment with monthly B$_{12}$ injections should be reevaluated at 6 to 12 month intervals by their doctor if they are otherwise well.[21]

Unless you have one of the conditions that requires B$_{12}$ injections, to prevent and treat a deficiency of vitamin B$_{12}$, you should eat more food that is rich in this vitamin rather than taking a vitamin supplement. You should take a supplement only if your diet does not provide an adequate amount.

The claims made for vitamin B$_{12}$ as a remedy for numerous conditions are unfounded. There is no evidence that supplements can provide more pep or counter depression or fatigue in people who do not have a deficiency.

FOODS HIGH IN VITAMIN B$_{12}$

Tongue, beef, pork, organ meats, eggs, nuts, milk, shellfish, poultry, cheese, (all may be high in cholesterol and/or fat), fish, peas, beans, lentils, tofu. Cooking is not likely to destroy vitamin B$_{12}$.

1 ounce beef liver	9–34 micrograms vitamin B$_{12}$
3 1/2 ounces round roast	4 micrograms vitamin B$_{12}$
3 1/2 ounces filet of sole	1.3 micrograms vitamin B$_{12}$
1 ounce swiss cheese	9 micrograms vitamin B$_{12}$
1 cup whole milk	5 micrograms vitamin B$_{12}$

Before You Use This Drug

Tell your doctor if you have or have had:

- allergies to drugs
- Leber's disease (an eye disease)

Tell your doctor about any other drugs you take, including aspirin, herbs, vitamins, and other nonprescription products.

How to Use This Drug

- Do not store in the bathroom. Do not expose to heat, moisture, or strong light. Do not let liquid form freeze.
- As with all drugs, it is important to take this one regularly. However, because of the length of time required for a vitamin B$_{12}$ deficiency to occur, there is no cause for concern if you miss a dose. Take it when you remember.

Interactions with Other Drugs

Some other drugs that you may be taking (either over-the-counter or prescription drugs) can interact with this one, causing adverse effects. Ask your doctor what these drugs are and let him or her know if you are taking any of them.

Adverse Effects

Vitamin B$_{12}$ and other water-soluble vitamins seldom cause adverse effects in people whose kidneys function normally. If you have decreased kidney function or are taking large doses of this vitamin, you should *call your doctor immediately* if you experience any of these adverse effects:

- skin rash or itching
- wheezing
- persistent diarrhea

Periodic Tests

Ask your doctor which of these tests should be done periodically while you are taking this drug:

- blood tests
- blood levels of folic acid, potassium, and vitamin B$_{12}$
- reticulocyte (young red blood cell) count

PREGNANCY WARNING

This drug caused damage to developing fetuses in animal studies, or such studies were not done. Use during pregnancy only for clear medical reasons. Tell your doctor if you are pregnant or thinking of becoming pregnant before you take this drug.

Limited Use

Vitamin C (Ascorbic Acid)
ARCO-CEE (Arco)
CEVI-BID (Geriatric)

GENERIC: available
FAMILY: Nutritional Supplements (see p. 592)

Ascorbic (a *skor* bic) acid, also called vitamin C, helps bind cells together and promotes healing. It is found in certain fruits and vegetables (see food sources, below), and a well-balanced diet with a variety of healthful foods should supply all the vitamin C that you need. The recommended dietary allowance (RDA) for older adults is 60 milligrams per day.

Vitamin C deficiency, known as scurvy, is rare. It is seen occasionally in people whose diet does not supply enough vitamin C—some older adults who live alone, alcoholics, and drug abusers, for example. Symptoms of scurvy include anemia, loose teeth, red and swollen gums, wounds that do not heal, and small broken blood vessels that cause tiny purplish-red spots in the skin. Scurvy is easily prevented and is treated by increasing the intake of vitamin C through diet and a supplement.

You should take a vitamin C supplement only if your diet does not supply enough to prevent and treat a vitamin C deficiency, or if your body has a special demand for more vitamin C due to surgery, smoking, or an infectious disease. Although doses that far exceed the RDA are touted as remedies for many conditions—from the common cold to cancer—research does not support such claims. There is no convincing evidence that taking supplements of vitamin C prevents any disease.[22]

If you use a vitamin C supplement without a doctor's supervision, do not take more than the RDA. Higher doses have few beneficial effects except in people with scurvy, and high-dose products are more expensive. Also, taking high doses of vitamin C is risky for people with a history of kidney stones and for people who use anticoagulants (drugs that prevent blood clots from forming in the blood vessels) such as warfarin (COUMADIN).[23] If you are taking high doses of vitamin C and want to stop, do not stop suddenly. Reduce your dose gradually because your body needs time to adjust to the reduction.

FOODS HIGH IN ASCORBIC ACID (VITAMIN C)

Citrus fruits and juices (oranges, lemons, limes, grapefruit), tomatoes, strawberries, cantaloupe, cabbage, broccoli, cauliflower, potatoes, and raw peppers. Vitamin C in foods is reduced by drying, salting, and ordinary cooking. Mincing fresh vegetables and mashing potatoes also reduces the vitamin C content.

6 or 7 brussels sprouts	87 milligrams vitamin C
1 cup cauliflower	62 milligrams vitamin C
1 medium orange or	60 milligrams vitamin C
1/2 cup orange juice	
1 cup shredded cabbage	47 milligrams vitamin C
1 slice watermelon	42 milligrams vitamin C
1/2 grapefruit or	40 milligrams vitamin C
2/3 cup grapefruit juice	
1 medium potato	30 milligrams vitamin C

Before You Use This Drug

Tell your doctor if you have or had:

- allergies to drugs
- kidney stones
- diabetes
- blood problems
- glucose-6-phosphate dehydrogenase deficiency

Tell your doctor about any other drugs you take, including aspirin, herbs, vitamins, and other nonprescription products.

How to Use This Drug

- Take with food to reduce stomach upset. Swallow with water.
- Do not crush, break, or chew extended-release capsules or tablets. Swallow them whole, or mix capsule contents with jam, applesauce or other food.

• Liquid form can be taken alone or can be mixed with juice, cereal, or any other food.

• Do not store in the bathroom. Do not expose to heat, moisture, or strong light. Do not let liquid form freeze.

• As with all drugs, it is important to take this one regularly. However, because of the length of time required for a vitamin C deficiency to occur, there is no cause for concern if you miss a dose. Take it when you remember.

Interactions with Other Drugs

The following drugs are listed in the *Evaluations of Drug Interactions* 1997 as causing "highly clinically significant" or "clinically significant" interactions when used together with this drug. We have also included potentially serious interactions listed in the drug's FDA-approved professional product labeling or package insert. New scientific techniques have allowed researchers to predict some drug interactions before they have been documented in people. There may be other drugs, especially those in the families of drugs listed below, that also will react with this drug to cause severe adverse effects. The number of new drugs approved for marketing increases the chance of drug interactions, and new drug interactions are being identified with old drugs. Be vigilant. Make sure to tell your doctor and pharmacist the drugs you are taking and tell your doctor if you are taking any of these interacting drugs:

flecainide, TAMBOCOR.

Adverse Effects

Call your doctor if these symptoms continue: (These can occur if you take more than 1 gram (1,000 milligrams) per day.)

• flushing or warmth of skin
• headache

• increased urination
• nausea, vomiting
• stomach cramps

Limited Use

Vitamin D
CALCIFEROL (Schwartz)

GENERIC: available
FAMILY: Nutritional Supplements (see p. 592)

Vitamin D maintains normal blood levels of calcium and phosphate, both of which are necessary for bone growth and strength. It is available in several foods (see food sources, below), and your body can also manufacture it (in the skin) if you are out in the sun. If you eat a well-balanced diet with a variety of healthful foods and spend some time in the sun, you should have all the vitamin D that your body needs. The recommended dietary allowance (RDA) is 400 International Units per day for men and 200 per day for women.

Vitamin D deficiency in older adults prevents your body from absorbing calcium and phosphate normally. This leads to an overall decrease in bone density and weakening of the bones, called osteomalacia. If you have to increase your intake of vitamin D, eat more foods rich in the vitamin rather than taking a vitamin pill. You should take a supplement only if your diet does not supply enough vitamin D to prevent and treat a deficiency or to treat a low blood level of calcium.

If you use vitamin D without a doctor's supervision, do not take more than the RDA. Unlike with some other vitamins, your body cannot eliminate excess vitamin D, so the vitamin can accumulate to dangerous, toxic levels. This is especially risky for people who take the heart medication digoxin (see p. 113), because vitamin D increases the adverse effects of digoxin. The signs of vitamin D poisoning are listed below. Vitamin D overdose may cause death as a result of heart, blood vessel, or kidney failure.

If your doctor has prescribed vitamin D to prevent low calcium levels, see him or her regularly to check your progress and reduce the risk of adverse effects. Tell your doctor if you are taking a calcium supplement and discuss how to best increase the amount of calcium in your diet.

FOODS HIGH IN VITAMIN D

Some fatty fishes and fish-liver oils, eggs, chicken livers, vitamin D-fortified milk (all are high in cholesterol and/or fat), and bread. Vitamin D is not affected by cooking.

½ ounce cod liver oil	1,400 International Units vitamin D
3 ½ ounces sardines	1,380 International Units vitamin D
3 ½ ounces salmon	300 International Units vitamin D
1 egg yolk	265 International Units vitamin D
1 cup vitamin D-fortified milk	100 International Units vitamin D

Before You Use This Drug

Do not use if you have or have had:

- high level of calcium in your blood

Tell your doctor if you have or have had:

- allergies to drugs
- heart or blood vessel disease
- kidney disease
- sarcoidosis

Tell your doctor about any other drugs you take, including aspirin, herbs, vitamins, and other nonprescription products.

How to Use This Drug

- Take with food to reduce stomach upset.
- Liquid form or contents of capsules can be taken alone or can be mixed with juice, cereal, or any other food.
- Do not store in the bathroom. Do not expose to heat, moisture, or strong light. Do not let the liquid form freeze.
- As with all drugs, it is important to take this one regularly. However, because of the length of time required for a vitamin D deficiency to occur, there is no cause for concern if a dose is missed. Take it when you remember. **Do not take double doses.**

Interactions with Other Drugs

The following drugs are listed in the *Evaluations of Drug Interactions* 1997 as causing "highly clinically significant" or "clinically significant" interactions when used together with this drug. We have also included potentially serious interactions listed in the drug's FDA-approved professional product labeling or package insert. New scientific techniques have allowed researchers to predict some drug interactions before they have been documented in people. There may be other drugs, especially those in the families of drugs listed below, that also will react with this drug to cause severe adverse effects. The number of new drugs approved for marketing increases the chance of drug interactions, and new drug interactions are being identified with old drugs. Be vigilant. Make sure to tell your doctor and pharmacist the drugs you are taking and tell your doctor if you are taking any of these interacting drugs:

aluminum hydroxide, AMPHOJEL, DILANTIN, phenytoin.

Adverse Effects

Call your doctor immediately if you experience:

• **early signs of vitamin D toxicity:** constipation, headache, loss of appetite, metallic taste in mouth, nausea or vomiting, dry mouth and increased thirst, tiredness and weakness, increased frequency of urination

• **late signs of vitamin D toxicity:** bone pain, cloudy urine, weight loss, convulsions, high blood pressure, eyes easily irritated by light, irregular heartbeat, itching, mood or mental changes, muscle pain, nausea or vomiting, severe stomach or flank pain

Periodic Tests

Ask your doctor which of these tests should be done periodically while you are taking this drug:

For high-dose therapy:

• kidney function tests
• blood calcium level (weekly, when therapy is started)

————

Do Not Use

ALTERNATIVE TREATMENT:
Eat a well-balanced diet with an adequate supply of vitamin E.

Vitamin E (alpha-tocopherol)

FAMILY: Nutritional Supplements (see p. 592)

Vitamin E is thought to work as an antioxidant, a substance that helps to protect cells from damage. It is found in many foods (see food sources, below), and a well-balanced diet with a variety of healthful foods should supply all the vitamin E that your body needs. The recommended dietary allowance (RDA) of vitamin E is 10 milligrams per day for older men and 8 milligrams per day for older women.

Vitamin E deficiency is rare and has not been known to occur solely from an inadequate diet. It has occurred mainly in people who have certain conditions of their intestines, pancreas, or liver that interfere with their body's ability to absorb this fat-soluble vitamin.

Vitamin E supplements have not been proven effective for treatment of beta-thalassemia, cancer, fibrocystic disease of the breast, inflammatory skin disorders, loss of hair, habitual abortion, leg cramps (intermittent claudication), menopausal syndrome, infertility, peptic ulcer, sickle cell disease, burns, porphyria, neuromuscular disorders, blood clots (thrombophlebitis), impotence, bee stings, liver spots on the hands, bursitis, diaper rash, lung toxicity from air pollution, or aging.

Taking vitamin E in doses that far exceed the RDA can be harmful. Some people who have taken more than 300 milligrams have suffered muscle weakness, fatigue, headaches, nausea, high blood pressure, and increased tendency toward blood clotting.[24]

A controlled clinical trial (the strongest type of scientific evidence) published in the journal *Lancet* in 1997 found that the number of heart attacks in men with a previous heart attack who smoked was not decreased with either alpha-tocopherol or beta-carotene (a natural product converted in the body to vitamin A) supplements. In fact, the risk of a fatal outcome increased in those men taking beta-carotene or the combination of alpha-tocopherol and beta-carotene. There was a decrease in non-fatal heart attacks in those taking alpha-tocopherol. The authors of this study did not recommend the use of these supplements in men who smoke and had a previous heart attack.[25]

Another clinical trial published in 1996 examined the effect of high doses of alpha-tocopherol in preventing a second heart attack in men and women with heart disease most of whom did not smoke. This study also found that the use of alpha-tocopherol reduced the rate of non-fatal heart attacks, but not fatal outcomes. The authors of this study recommended further reseach.[26]

There were differences in these two studies. In the first, the dose of alpha-tocopherol was much smaller and the first study used synthetic alpha-tocopherol while the second used a product derived from soya oil. At this time there is insufficient evidence to recommend the use of Vitamin E for the prevention of heart attacks.

FOODS HIGH IN VITAMIN E:

Vegetable oils (corn, cottonseed, soybean, safflower), egg yolk, (all of which are high in fat and/or cholesterol), wheat germ and whole-grain cereals. Some vitamin E may be lost in cooking.

1 ounce margarine	15 milligrams vitamin E
1/2 cup wheat germ	3 milligrams vitamin E
2 slices whole-wheat bread	2 milligrams vitamin E

NOTES FOR NUTRITIONAL SUPPLEMENTS

1. *F-D-C Reports—The Tan Sheet,* February 2, 1998, p. 14–15.

2. Schlamowitz P. Treatment of mild to moderate hypertension with dietary fibre. *Lancet* 1987; 8559:622.

3. Chandra RK. Effect of vitamin and trace-element supplementation on immune responses and infection in elderly subjects. *Lancet* 1992; 340:1124–7.

4. *The Medical Letter on Drugs and Therapeutics.* New York: The Medical Letter Inc., 1984; 25:73.

5. AMA Department of Drugs. *AMA Drug Evaluations Annual* 1992. Chicago: American Medical Association, 1992:2018–9.

6. Sheikh M. Gastrointestinal absorption of calcium from milk and calcium salts. *New England Journal of Medicine* 1987; 317:532–6.

7. Osteoporosis Part II: Prevention and Treatment. Public Citizen's Health Research Group *Health Letter* 1987; 3(6).

8. Sheikh, op. cit.

9. Osteoporosis Part II, op. cit.

10. *The Medical Letter on Drugs and Therapeutics.* New York: The Medical Letter Inc., 1998; 40:75–7.

11. AMA Department of Drugs. *AMA Drug Evaluations.* 5th ed. Chicago: American Medical Association, 1983:797.

12. Ibid, p. 1144.

13. *F-D-C Reports,* op. cit.

14. Chandra, op. cit.

15. Whelan AM, Price SO, Fowler SF, Hainer BL. The effect of aspirin on niacin-induced cutaneous reactions. *The Journal of Family Practice* 1992; 34:165–8.

16. Hodis HN. Acute hepatic failure associated with the use of low-dose sustained-release niacin. *Journal of the American Medical Association* 1990; 264:181.

17. Henkin Y, Oberman A, Hurst DC, Segrest JP. Niacin revisited: clinical observations on an important but underutilized drug. *American Journal of Medicine* 1991; 91:239–46.

18. *USP DI, Drug Information for the Health Care Professional.* 8th ed. Rockville MD: The United States Pharmacopeial Convention, Inc., 1988: 2077.

19. Colditz GA. Increased green and yellow vegetable intake and lowered cancer deaths in an elderly population. *American Journal of Clinical Nutrition* 1985; 41(32).

20. *The Medical Letter on Drugs and Therapeutics,* 1998, op. cit.

21. Gilman AG, Goodman LS, Rall TW, Murad F, eds. *The Pharmacological Basis of Therapeutics.* 7th ed. New York: Macmillan, 1985:1330.

22. *The Medical Letter on Drugs and Therapeutics,* 1998, op. cit.

23. Gilman, op. cit., p. 1570.

24. Roberts H. Perspective on vitamin E as therapy. *Journal of the American Medical Association* 1981; 246:129–30.

25. Rapola JM, Virtamo J, Ripatti S, Huttunen JK, Albanes D, Taylor PR, et al. Randomised trial of α-tocopherol and β-carotene supplements on incidence of major coronary events in men with previous myocardial infarction. *Lancet* 1997; 349:1715–20.

26. Stephens NG, Parsons A, Schofield PM, Kelly F, Cheeseman K, Mitchinson MJ, et al. Randomised controlled trial of vitamin E in patients with coronary disease: Cambridge Heart Antioxidant Study (CHAOS). *Lancet* 1996; 347:781–6.

Eye Drugs

General Instructions For Application of Eye Drops and Ointment   **622**

Glaucoma   **623**

DRUG LISTINGS

DRUGS FOR EYE DISEASES

acetazolamide		632
ADSORBOCARPINE		624
BETAGAN		626
betaxolol (eye drops)		629
BETOPTIC		629
BETOPTIC S		629
DIAMOX		632
dipivefrin		640
dorzolamide	Limited Use	645
ISOPTO CARPINE		624
levobunolol		626
methazolamide		638
NEPTAZANE		638
pilocarpine		624
PROPINE		640
timolol (eye drops)		643
TIMOPTIC		643
TRUSOPT	Limited Use	645

ANTI-INFECTIVES AND COMBINATIONS

BLEPHAMIDE	⊘ Do Not Use	632
GARAMYCIN	Limited Use	635
gentamicin	Limited Use	635
MAXITROL	⊘ Do Not Use Except After Intraocular Lens Surgery	636
NEODECADRON	⊘ Do Not Use Except After Intraocular Lens Surgery	638
neomycin and dexamethasone	⊘ Do Not Use Except After Intraocular Lens Surgery	638
neomycin, polymyxin B and dexamethasone	⊘ Do Not Use Except After Intraocular Lens Surgery	636
SULAMYD	Limited Use	641
sulfacetamide	Limited Use	641
sulfacetamide and prednisolone	⊘ Do Not Use	632
tobramycin	Limited Use	635
TOBREX	Limited Use	635
VASOCIDIN	⊘ Do Not Use	632

OTHER EYE DRUGS

AK-PENTOLATE	625
artificial tears	642
CYCLOGYL	625
cyclopentolate	625
fluorometholone	634
FML	634
HYPOTEARS	642
MYDRIACYL	637
TEARISOL	642
TEARS NATURALE	642
tropicamide	637

GENERAL INSTRUCTIONS FOR APPLICATION OF EYE DROPS AND OINTMENT

The normal eye can hold about 10 microliters (10 millionths of a quart) of liquid. A single drop formed by an eye dropper, however, ranges from 25 to 50 microliters. What happens to the excess 15 to 40 microliters when you apply eye drops? Two things occur:

1. Medicine overflows the eyelids and runs down your face, especially if you are upright when applying the drops. This is not a very efficient use of medicine but is relatively harmless.

2. Medicine drains from the eyes into a small opening located at the inside corner of the eye. This small opening is the entrance to a duct (the nasolacrimal duct) through which tears and moisture normally leave the eye and drain into the nose (which is why your nose usually runs when you cry). In the nose, the medicine is absorbed into the blood supply and carried throughout the body, where it can affect the brain, heart, digestive system, lungs and airways, and other areas of the body, causing adverse effects.

What can be done to maximize drug absorption in the eye and minimize drug absorption through the nasal blood vessels?

1. Do not apply more than one drop of medicine within a five minute period, regardless of whether the second drop is the same or a different drug. The eye cannot hold more than one drop at a time, so an extra drop both flushes out the first drop and is diluted by it. It also increases the amount that is absorbed through the nasal blood vessels. Therefore, always wait at least five minutes between drops to give adequate time for the drug to be absorbed by the eye.

2. Lie down when applying drops. This helps to prevent "tears" from rolling down your face

and through the nasolacrimal duct. As much as 10 times more drug is lost when you are in an upright position than when you are reclining.

3. Using your thumb and middle finger, apply gentle pressure to the inside corner of the eye for five minutes after applying each drop, to block the medicine from draining through the nasolacrimal duct.

This technique may be difficult for people who have arthritis, long fingernails, or tremors. An alternative method of decreasing nasolacrimal drainage is to stop "the pump." The nasolacrimal duct relies on the pumping action of the eyelids blinking. If you stop moving your eyelids, you stop the drainage of medicine from the eye. If you squeeze, blink, flutter, etc., the pump is activated. Simple, gentle, relaxed eyelid closure works best to stop the pump.

Either technique, compressing the duct or stopping the pump, if used for five minutes, allows enough time for the drug to be absorbed through the eye and decreases adverse effects.

To avoid contaminating the eye drops, **do not touch the applicator tip to any surface, including the eye.** Store the bottle tightly closed. To ensure sterility, periodically discard used bottles of medicine. Drops can be considered safe for four weeks and ointments for three months after they have been opened.

To apply drops, first wash your hands. To increase drug absorption, it is best to lie down while applying this medicine. With the middle finger of the hand on the same side as the eye (right eye, right hand, for example), apply pressure to the inside corner of your eye to block the drainage duct. After you have begun to apply pressure with your middle finger, tilt your head back. With the index finger of the same hand, pull the lower eyelid away from the eye to form a pouch. Place a drop of medicine into the pouch, remove the index finger and close your eyes gently, without blinking. Keep your eyes closed and continue to apply pressure for five minutes. Do not close your eyes tightly and do not blink.

To apply ointment, first wash your hands. Lie down or tilt your head back. Squeeze about 1/4 to 1/2 inch of ointment inside your lower lid without actually touching the tube to your lid. Close your eye gently and roll your eyeball in all directions while the eye is closed to evenly distribute the medicine. Wait at least 10 minutes before applying other medicines to your eyes. If you need to apply ointment and drops it is best to put the drops in prior to the ointment, as the ointment will all but prevent absorption of the drops because of its "Vaseline"-like character.

GLAUCOMA

Glaucoma is a slowly progressing disorder in which the pressure inside the eye gradually increases. If left untreated, this elevated pressure may lead to nerve damage, decreased vision, and blindness. In general, the higher the pressure inside the eye, the greater the chance of damaging the optic nerve (the nerve to the eye that allows us to see) and losing vision. Most people with glaucoma have no symptoms until extensive, irreversible damage to the optic nerve has occurred, so it is important to have regular eye exams as you grow older. It is also important to take your medicine regularly if you have glaucoma.

To understand what causes glaucoma, it helps to start by discussing how the eye normally works. The eye (shown below as it would appear when cut in half can be divided into three parts. The vitreous chamber is the large, round area behind the lens. The posterior chamber is the smaller area located behind the iris and in front and to the sides of the lens. The anterior chamber is located in front of the iris. Both the anterior and the posterior chambers are filled with a clear liquid called the aqueous humor. Normally, aqueous humor flows from the posterior chamber through the opening in the iris to the anterior chamber. It leaves the eye through a small opening, called the canal of Schlemm, at the outermost edges of the iris. In glaucoma, less aqueous humor drains from the eye, raising the pressure inside the eye. The disorder is similar to blowing up a balloon: If there is no opening for the air to flow out, the pressure in the balloon steadily increases as the balloon fills with air.

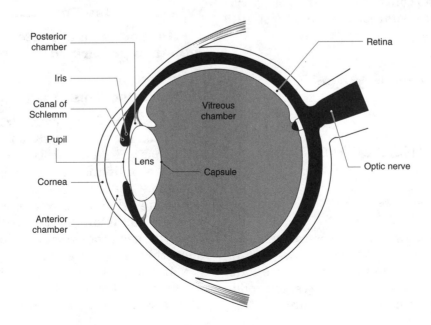

Posterior chamber · Iris · Canal of Schlemm · Pupil · Cornea · Anterior chamber · Lens · Capsule · Vitreous chamber · Retina · Optic nerve

Elevated pressure inside the eye can be treated in two ways:

• Increasing the amount of aqueous humor that leaves the eye through the canal of Schlemm; or

• Decreasing the amount of aqueous humor that is produced.

Drugs such as dipivefrin (PROPINE), pilocarpine (ADSORBOCARPINE, ISOPTO CARPINE), and physostigmine (ESERINE) increase aqueous humor outflow from the anterior chamber, whereas acetazolamide (DIAMOX), dorzolamide (TRUSOPT), and beta-blockers such as timolol (TIMOPTIC) decrease aqueous humor production. In either case, the total amount of aqueous humor is reduced and the pressure decreased. Timolol is often used for mild glaucoma, except for older adults who have congestive heart failure, abnormal heart rhythms, asthma, or emphysema. In these patients, pilocarpine or carbonic anhydase inhibitors like dorzolamide or acetazolamide can be an alternative choice. A combination of drugs may be necessary for more severe forms. Surgery is reserved for those people who continue to have optic nerve destruction and visual loss, in spite of multiple drug therapy.

DRUG PROFILES

Pilocarpine
ADSORBOCARPINE, ISOPTO CARPINE
(Alcon)

GENERIC: available

FAMILY: Antiglaucoma Drugs (see p. 623)

Pilocarpine (pye loe *kar* peen) is a drug used for treating most forms of glaucoma (see p. 623). Glaucoma is a condition in which the pressure of the fluid inside the eye increases, and pilocarpine lowers the increased pressure.

Pilocarpine makes the pupils of your eyes smaller and affects how quickly they react to light by enlarging or narrowing. Smaller pupils and their slower reaction allow less light to enter the eyes. This can hinder you from performing tasks such as driving at night. Be careful when performing such tasks. When used for a long time, the initial improvement may diminish.

Right after you use pilocarpine, your vision may be blurred, but it will clear. You might notice this more when viewing things at a distance.

Before You Use This Drug

Tell your doctor if you have or have had:

• allergies to drugs
• bronchial asthma
• eye infection or inflammation
• predisposition to, or retinal detachment

Tell your doctor about any other drugs you take, including aspirin, herbs, vitamins, and other nonprescription products.

When You Use This Drug

• **Do not use more often or in a higher dose than prescribed.**

How to Use This Drug

• Directions for applying drops appear on p. 622. If you use an eye system form, follow directions that accompany it. Do not use if system is damaged or if too much medication is being released.

• Store gel and eye system forms in refrigerator. Do not store in the bathroom. Do not expose to heat, moisture, or strong light. Do not allow this drug to freeze.

• If you miss a dose, apply it as soon as you remember, but skip it if it is almost time for the next dose. **Do not take double doses.**

Interactions with Other Drugs

Some other drugs that you may be taking (either over-the-counter or prescription drugs) can interact with this one, causing adverse effects. Ask your doctor what these drugs are and let him or her know if you are taking any of them.

Adverse Effects

Call your doctor immediately if you experience:

- muscle twitches or tremors
- nausea, vomiting, or diarrhea
- troubled breathing or wheezing
- increased sweating
- watering of mouth
- eye pain

Call your doctor if these symptoms continue:

- blurred vision
- brow ache
- headache
- irritation of eyes

Periodic Tests

Ask your doctor which of these tests should be done periodically while you are taking this drug:

- eye pressure tests at regular intervals

PREGNANCY WARNING

This drug caused harm to developing fetuses in animal studies, or such studies were not done. Use during pregnancy only for clear medical reasons. Tell your doctor if you are pregnant or thinking of becoming pregnant before you take this drug.

Cyclopentolate
AK-PENTOLATE (Akorn)
CYCLOGYL (Alcon)

GENERIC: available
FAMILY: Eye Drugs

Cyclopentolate (sye kloe *pen* toe late) is most commonly used to enlarge (dilate) the pupils of the eyes during an eye exam. It is also used to dilate the pupils before or after certain types of eye surgery, and to treat inflammation of the inner eye.

At first, cyclopentolate may cause a stinging sensation, blurred vision, and increased sensitivity to light. Check with your doctor if any of these effects lasts longer than 36 hours after the drug is applied.

Before You Use This Drug

Tell your doctor if you have or have had:

- allergies to drugs
- history of seizure
- glaucoma

Tell your doctor about any other drugs you take, including aspirin, herbs, vitamins, and other nonprescription products.

When You Use This Drug

- **Do not use more often or in a higher dose than prescribed.**

How to Use This Drug

- Directions for applying drops appear on p. 622.
- Do not store in the bathroom. Do not expose to heat, moisture, or strong light. Do not allow to freeze.
- If you miss a dose, apply it as soon as you remember, but skip it if it is almost time for the next dose. **Do not take double doses.**

Interactions with Other Drugs

Some other drugs that you may be taking (either over-the-counter or prescription drugs) can interact with this one, causing adverse effects. Ask your doctor what these drugs are and let him or her know if you are taking any of them.

Adverse Effects

Call your doctor immediately if you experience:

- clumsiness or unsteadiness
- confusion or unusual behavior
- fever
- flushed or red face
- hallucinations
- increased thirst, dry mouth
- skin rash
- slurred speech
- irregular heartbeat
- drowsiness, tiredness, weakness
- swollen stomach in infants

Call your doctor if these symptoms continue:

- blurred vision
- increased sensitivity to light
- stinging sensation in eyes
- headache
- irritation of eyes

PREGNANCY WARNING

This drug caused harm to developing fetuses in animal studies, or such studies were not done. Use during pregnancy only for clear medical reasons. Tell your doctor if you are pregnant or thinking of becoming pregnant before you take this drug.

Levobunolol
BETAGAN (Allergan)

GENERIC: available

FAMILY: Antiglaucoma Drugs (see p. 623)
Beta-blockers (see p. 52)

Levobunolol (levo *bewn* o lol) is available as an eye drop, specifically for treating glaucoma. It is well tolerated by most people, especially those who have cataracts or who have problems using another antiglaucoma drug called pilocarpine (see p. 624). Although levobunolol is an eye drop, some of it can be absorbed from the eyes into the bloodstream and the rest of the body, and if this happens you may experience some of the general adverse effects listed under Adverse Effects. (See p. 622 for directions on how to apply eye drops.)

Levobunolol belongs to the beta-blocker family of drugs and thus is similar in safety and efficacy to timolol (see p. 643).[1,2] Once in the eye, it takes levobunolol about an hour to begin working. If you use levobunolol in only one eye, it may also affect the other eye. Older people are especially sensitive to the harmful effects of levobunolol. Reduced kidney and liver function in the elderly may increase risk of adverse effects.

When used for a long time, the initial improvement may diminish. As with other beta-blockers, long-term use can exacerbate serious heart problems, even in people who did not previously have heart disease. Levobunolol, similarly to timolol, can decrease lung function by 30%, an adverse effect not seen in betaxolol, another beta-blocker.[3] Very rarely, serious harm, even fatalities have occurred, mostly to those with asthma or heart problems.[4] But according to *The Medical Letter,* betaxolol (see p. 629) may be less likely than timolol or levobunolol to have adverse effects on patients with asthma.[5]

At times levobunolol is used along with other medications for glaucoma, such as pilocarpine, dipivefrin, or acetazolamide. Use with epinephrine is controversial.

Before You Use This Drug

Levobunolol can be life-threatening to certain individuals.

Do not use if you have or have had:

- bronchial asthma
- congestive heart failure, slow heartbeat or heart block
- severe lung disease

Tell your doctor if you have or have had:

- allergies to drugs
- mental depression
- diabetes
- emphysema or chronic bronchitis
- heart problems
- myasthenia gravis
- smoked
- thyroid problems
- lung function impairment
- hypoglycemia
- impotence

Tell your doctor about any other drugs you take, including aspirin, herbs, vitamins, and other nonprescription products.

When You Use This Drug

- Restrict your use of caffeine, since it may add to the effect of levobunolol on the heart.[6]
- **Caution diabetics:** be aware that levobunolol may mask trembling and pulse rate used to signal low blood sugar.[7]
- If you plan to have any surgery, including dental, tell your doctor that you take this drug.

- Be cautious driving until the effect of the drug is complete (about two weeks),[8] and no blurred vision occurs.
- **Do not take other drugs without talking to your doctor first—especially nonprescription drugs for appetite control, asthma, colds, coughs, hay fever, or sinus problems.**

COLD STRESS ALERT

If levobunolol eye drops are absorbed into the body, older people have an increased risk of hypothermia.[9] Early signs are shivering, cold hands and feet, and memory lapse. Stay indoors, especially when it is cold and windy. Keep warm with extra clothes and blankets. If you must go outdoors, dress to protect yourself from the wind and cold. Avoid getting wet. Take along something to eat suitable to your diet such as trail mix.

How to Use This Drug

- Directions for applying drops appear on p. 622.
- If you use the compliance cap, whenever you start a new bottle click it until the number corresponding to the day of the week appears.
- After opening the cap, do not touch the tip of the applicator.
- Instill only one drop at a time, since the eye sac can only hold that amount (see p. 622 for directions on how to apply eye drops).
- Replace the cap. Hold the compliance cap between your thumb and forefinger, then rotate until it clicks.
- *If you miss a dose, use the following guidelines:* If you are using levobunolol only once a day, apply the missed dose as soon as you remember, but skip it if you don't remember until the next day.

If you are using levobunolol more than once a day, apply the missed dose as soon as you remember, but skip it if it is almost time for the next dose.

Do not apply double doses.

Interactions with Other Drugs

The following drugs are listed in the *Evaluations of Drug Interactions* 1997 as causing "highly clinically significant" or "clinically significant" interactions when used together with this drug. We have also included potentially serious interactions listed in the drug's FDA-approved professional product labeling or package insert. New scientific techniques have allowed researchers to predict some drug interactions before they have been documented in people. There may be other drugs, especially those in the families of drugs listed below, that also will react with this drug to cause severe adverse effects. The number of new drugs approved for marketing increases the chance of drug interactions, and new drug interactions are being identified with old drugs. Be vigilant. Make sure to tell your doctor and pharmacist the drugs you are taking and tell your doctor if you are taking any of these interacting drugs:

ADRENALIN (also in bee sting kits), ALDOMET, amiodarone, CALAN SR, CATAPRES, chlorpromazine, cimetidine, clonidine, cocaine, CORDARONE, COVERA–HS, DELTASONE, ELIXOPHYLLIN, epinephrine, FLUOTHANE, furosemide, halothane, HUMALOG, HUMULIN, INDOCIN, indomethacin, insulin, ISOPTIN SR, LASIX, levothyroxine, LEVOTHROID, lidocaine, lithium, LITHOBID, LITHONATE, methyldopa, METICORTEN, MINIPRESS, NEMBUTAL, NICODERM, NICORETTE, nicotine, pentobarbital, prazosin, prednisone, PRIMATENE MIST, RIFADIN, rifampin, RIMACTANE, SLO-BID, SYNTHROID, TAGAMET, THEO-24, theophylline, THORAZINE, tobacco

(inform your doctor if your smoking habits change while using levobunolol), TUBARINE, tubocurarine, verapamil, VERELAN, XYLOCAINE.

Adverse Effects

Levobunolol can be absorbed into the body through the eye. All adverse effects for oral beta-blockers are possible with levobunolol eyedrops.

Call your doctor immediately if you experience:

- cold hands and feet
- severe irritation or inflammation of the eye or eyelid
- vision change
- breathing difficulty, wheezing, coughing
- confusion or depression
- dizziness, or fainting
- headache
- slow or irregular heartbeat
- nausea or vomiting
- swelling of ankles, feet or legs
- unsteadiness, clumsiness
- unusual tiredness or weakness

Call your doctor if these symptoms continue:

- burning or stinging of the eye
- inflammation of eye or eyelids
- low blood pressure

Call your doctor if these symptoms continue after you stop taking the drug:

- chest pain
- irregular heartbeat
- weakness
- shortness of breath
- headache
- sweating
- trembling

Adverse effects to levobunolol can occur even a week after you stop using the drug.

More adverse effects information appears on p. 52.

Periodic Tests

Ask your doctor which of these tests should be done periodically while you are taking this drug:

- blood pressure and pulse rate
- heart function tests, such as electrocardiogram (ECG, EKG)
- blood glucose levels (for diabetics)
- eye pressure exams

PREGNANCY WARNING

This drug caused harm to developing fetuses in animal studies, or such studies were not done. Use during pregnancy only for clear medical reasons. Tell your doctor if you are pregnant or thinking of becoming pregnant before you take this drug.

Betaxolol (Eye Drops)
BETOPTIC (Alcon)
BETOPTIC S (Alcon)

GENERIC: not available

FAMILY: Antiglaucoma Drugs (see p. 623)
Beta-blockers (see p. 52)

Betaxolol (bait *ax* o loll) has two dosage forms for different uses: Kerlone tablets for the heart (see p. 154) and Betoptic drops for the eyes, specifically for treating glaucoma. This profile discusses betaxolol's use as an antiglaucoma drug.

Betaxolol drops are well tolerated by most people, especially those who have cataracts or who have problems using another antiglaucoma drug called pilocarpine (see p. 624). Although betaxolol is an eye drop, some of it can be absorbed from the eyes into the bloodstream and the rest of the body, and if this happens you may experience some of the general adverse effects listed under Adverse Effects. (See p. 622 for directions on how to apply eye drops.)

When used for a long time, the initial improvement may diminish. As with other beta-blockers, long-term use can exacerbate serious heart problems, even in people who did not previously have heart disease. Two other beta-blockers, levobunolol and timolol, can decrease lung function by 30%, an adverse effect not seen as much in betaxolol.[10] Very rarely, serious harm, even fatalities have occurred, mostly to those with asthma or heart problems.[11] But according to *The Medical Letter*, betaxolol may be less likely than timolol or levobunolol to have adverse effects on patients with asthma.[12] Older people are especially sensitive to the harmful effects of betaxolol.

At times betaxolol is used along with other eye drugs, such as pilocarpine. As the effect of betaxolol may diminish over time, it is sometimes necessary to supplement its use with other antiglaucoma medication.

Before You Use This Drug

Do not use if you have or have had:

- bronchial asthma
- congestive heart failure, slow heartbeat or heart block
- severe lung disease

Tell your doctor if you have or have had:

- allergies to drugs
- mental depression
- diabetes
- emphysema or chronic bronchitis
- heart problems
- myasthenia gravis
- smoked
- thyroid problems
- lung function impairment
- hypoglycemia
- impotence

Tell your doctor about any other drugs you take, including aspirin, herbs, vitamins, and other nonprescription products.

When You Use This Drug

• Restrict your use of caffeine, since it may add to the effect of betaxolol on the heart.[13]

• **Caution diabetics:** be aware that betaxolol may mask trembling and pulse rate used to signal low blood sugar.[14]

• If you plan to have any surgery, including dental, tell your doctor that you take this drug.

• Be cautious driving until the effect of the drug is complete (about two weeks),[15] and no blurred vision occurs.

• **Do not take other drugs without talking to your doctor first—especially nonprescription drugs for appetite control, asthma, colds, coughs, hay fever, or sinus problems.**

COLD STRESS ALERT

If betaxolol eye drops are absorbed into the body, older people have an increased risk of hypothermia.[16] Early signs are shivering, cold hands and feet, and memory lapse. Stay indoors, especially when it is cold and windy. Keep warm with extra clothes and blankets. If you must go outdoors, dress to protect yourself from the wind and cold. Avoid getting wet. Take along something to eat, suitable to your diet, such as trail mix.

How to Use This Drug

• Directions for applying drops appear on p. 622.

• If you use the suspension form, shake it well first.

• Wash your hands.

• After opening, avoid touching the tip against your eye or anything else.

• *If you miss a dose, use the following guidelines:* If you are using betaxolol only once a day, apply the missed dose as soon as you remember, but skip it if you don't remember until the next day.

If you are using betaxolol more than once a day, apply the missed dose as soon as you remember, but skip it if it is almost time for the next dose.

Do not apply double doses.

Interactions with Other Drugs

The following drugs are listed in the *Evaluations of Drug Interactions* 1997 as causing "highly clinically significant" or "clinically significant" interactions when used together with this drug. We have also included potentially serious interactions listed in the drug's FDA-approved professional product labeling or package insert. New scientific techniques have allowed researchers to predict some drug interactions before they have been documented in people. There may be other drugs, especially those in the families of drugs listed below, that also will react with this drug to cause severe adverse effects. The number of new drugs approved for marketing increases the chance of drug interactions, and new drug interactions are being identified with old drugs. Be vigilant. Make sure to tell your doctor and pharmacist the drugs you are taking and tell your doctor if you are taking any of these interacting drugs:

ADRENALIN (also in bee sting kits), ALDOMET, CALAN SR, CATAPRES, chlorpromazine, cimetidine, clonidine, cocaine, COVERA-HS, DELTASONE, ELIXOPHYLLIN, epinephrine, FLUOTHANE, furosemide, halothane,

HUMALOG, HUMULIN, INDOCIN, indomethacin, insulin, ISOPTIN SR, levothyroxine, LASIX, LEVOTHROID, lidocaine, lithium, LITHOBID, LITHONATE, methyldopa, METICORTEN, MINIPRESS, NEMBUTAL, NICODERM, NICORETTE, nicotine, pentobarbital, prazosin, prednisone, PRIMATENE MIST, RIFADIN, rifampin, RIMACTANE, SLO-BID, SYNTHROID, TAGAMET, THEO-24, theophylline, THORAZINE, tobacco (inform your doctor if your smoking habits change while using betaxolol), TUBARINE, tubocurarine, verapamil, VERELAN, XYLOCAINE.

Adverse Effects

Betaxolol can be absorbed into the body through the eye. All adverse effects for oral beta-blockers are possible with betaxolol eye-drops.

Call your doctor immediately if you experience:

- coughing, wheezing, difficulty breathing
- cold hands or feet
- depression, confusion
- dizziness, fainting
- headache
- slow or irregular heartbeat
- irritation, severe swelling or inflammation of eye or eyelids
- blurred vision or other visual changes
- difficulty swallowing, or painful tongue
- unusual tiredness or weakness
- insomnia
- hair loss
- eye pain
- raw or red areas of skin
- different size pupils or discoloration of eyeball
- skin rash, hives or itching
- swelling of feet, ankles or lower legs

Call your doctor if these symptoms continue:

- disturbed sleep, nightmares
- hallucinations[17]
- crusting of eyelashes
- diarrhea
- eye stinging or irritation when medicine is applied
- redness, itching or watering of eye
- dryness of eyes
- increased sensitivity to light

Call your doctor if these symptoms continue after you stop taking the drug:

- chest pain
- irregular heartbeat
- weakness
- shortness of breath
- headache
- sweating
- trembling

More adverse effects information appears on p. 52.

Periodic Tests

Ask your doctor which of these tests should be done periodically while you are taking this drug:

- blood pressure and pulse rate
- heart function tests, such as electrocardiogram (ECG, EKG)
- blood glucose levels (for diabetics)
- eye pressure exams

PREGNANCY WARNING

This drug caused harm to developing fetuses in animal studies, or such studies were not done. Use during pregnancy only for clear medical reasons. Tell your doctor if you are pregnant or thinking of becoming pregnant before you take this drug.

Do Not Use

ALTERNATIVE TREATMENT:
An antibiotic alone, if necessary.

Sulfacetamide and Prednisolone
BLEPHAMIDE (Allergan)
VASOCIDIN (Iolab)

FAMILY: Antibiotics (see p. 468)
Corticosteroids (see p. 651)

These are eye drops that contain two drugs, sulfacetamide (see p. 641) and prednisolone (see p. 711). The drops are used to treat some eye and eyelid infections caused by bacteria or allergies. **There is no persuasive proof that they are beneficial for this purpose.**

This combination is like several others that contain a drug from the corticosteroid family (in this case prednisolone) and one from the antibiotic family (in this case sulfacetamide). In general, combinations like this are not recommended for treating eye infections externally.[18] Corticosteroids like prednisolone may actually be dangerous because they can hide the signs of an infection or make it spread. For serious eye infections sulfacetamide may not be as effective as other antibiotics.

Acetazolamide
DIAMOX (Lederle)

GENERIC: available
FAMILY: Antiglaucoma Drugs (see p. 622)

Acetazolamide (a set a *zole* a mide) is most commonly used to treat glaucoma (see p. 623). It is also used to treat altitude sickness and to supplement other drugs used for seizure disorders such as epilepsy. In the past, acetazolamide was used as a diuretic (water pill) to treat high blood pressure, but it is outdated for this use because more effective drugs are now available.[19,20]

Acetazolamide belongs to the same family of drugs as methazolamide (NEPTAZANE). These drugs (carbonic anhydrase inhibitors) are cousins of sulfa drugs and thiazide diuretics, having the potential for the same adverse effects, but no action against bacteria. This family of drugs may cause kidney stones, gouty arthritis, and depress your bone marrow. Older people with decreased kidney function need to be cautious when taking these drugs. Many individuals cannot tolerate the adverse effects of this family of drugs for a prolonged time.[21]

Acetazolamide has caused a few cases of hives, fever, blood cell disorders, and kidney problems.[22] Stop taking the drug and call your doctor if you experience any of these reactions.

This drug may also reduce the amount of potassium in your body. To compensate for this loss, eat foods high in potassium (see p. 49).

Before You Use This Drug

Tell your doctor if you have or have had:

- allergies to drugs
- adrenal gland problem (Addison's disease)
- diabetes
- gout
- low blood levels of sodium or potassium
- kidney or liver problems
- emphysema or other chronic lung disease

Tell your doctor about any other drugs you take, including aspirin, herbs, vitamins, and other nonprescription products.

When You Use This Drug

• **Do not use more often or in a higher dose than prescribed. Do not stop taking** this drug suddenly. **Your doctor must lower your dose gradually.**

• Until you know how you react to this drug, do not drive or perform other activities requiring alertness. This drug may cause drowsiness, dizziness, lightheadedness, and tiredness.

• To help prevent kidney stones, **drink at least six to eight glasses (eight ounces each) of fluids each day.**

• **Caution diabetics:** This drug may elevate blood and urine sugar levels.

How to Use This Drug

• Directions for applying drops appear on p. 622.

• Take with food to decrease stomach upset.

• Do not store in the bathroom. Do not expose to heat, moisture, or strong light. Do not allow to freeze.

• If you miss a dose, take it as soon as you remember, but skip it if it is almost time for the next dose. **Do not take double doses.**

Interactions with Other Drugs

The following drugs are listed in the *Evaluations of Drug Interactions* 1997 as causing "highly clinically significant" or "clinically significant" interactions when used together with this drug. We have also included potentially serious interactions listed in the drug's FDA-approved professional product labeling or package insert. New scientific techniques have allowed researchers to predict some drug interactions before they have been documented in people. There may be other drugs, especially those in the families of drugs listed below, that also will react with this drug to cause severe adverse effects. The number of new drugs approved for marketing increases the chance of drug interactions, and new drug interactions are being identified with old

drugs. Be vigilant. Make sure to tell your doctor and pharmacist the drugs you are taking and tell your doctor if you are taking any of these interacting drugs:

aspirin, GENUINE BAYER ASPIRIN, cyclosporine, ECOTRIN, lithium, LITHOBID, LITHONATE, NEORAL, SANDIMMUNE.

Adverse Effects

Call your doctor immediately if you experience:

• blood in urine, difficulty urinating, pain in lower back, pain or burning during urination, or sudden decrease in amount of urine
  • bloody or black, tarry stools
  • clumsiness, unsteadiness
  • convulsions
  • dark urine, pale stools, or yellow eyes and skin
  • dry mouth or increased thirst
  • irregular heartbeat or weak pulse
  • mood or mental changes
  • muscle cramps, pain or weakness
  • nausea or vomiting
  • nearsightedness
  • unusual tiredness or weakness
  • fever and sore throat
  • unusual bruising or bleeding
  • hives, itching, or skin rash
  • mental confusion or depression
  • trouble breathing or shortness of breath
  • ringing or buzzing in ears

Call your doctor if these symptoms continue:

  • diarrhea
  • drowsiness
  • increased frequency of urination
  • loss of appetite, weight loss
  • metallic taste in mouth

- numbness, tingling, or burning sensation in hands, fingers, feet, toes, mouth, tongue, lips, or rectum
  - loss of taste and smell
  - headache
  - increased sensitivity to sunlight

Periodic Tests

Ask your doctor which of these tests should be done periodically while you are taking this drug:

- complete blood count
- blood electrolyte (sodium, potassium) tests
- platelet count
- tests of kidney function and kidney stone formation

Fluorometholone
FML (Allergan)

GENERIC: available
FAMILY: Corticosteroids (see p. 651)
         Eye Drugs

Fluorometholone (flure oh *meth* oh lone) is a steroid used to treat eye conditions that produce inflammation (swelling and redness), itching, or sensitivity. As with all drugs, you should always use the smallest dose of fluorometholone that works. You should also use it for as short a time as possible. **Check with your doctor if you do not notice improvement after five to seven days of taking the drug, or if your eye condition worsens.**

Corticosteroids (steroids) such as fluorometholone can cause *many* adverse effects, especially if you use them for a long time so that your entire body absorbs them. Steroids suppress your immune system, lowering your body's defense against disease. Because of this, if you use fluorometholone for a long time, you will be more likely to develop bacterial, fungal, parasitic, and viral infections.

Before You Use This Drug

Do not use if you have or have had:

- eye infections, such as herpes, tuberculosis, or others caused by a fungus or virus

Tell your doctor if you have or have had:

- allergies to drugs
- diabetes
- glaucoma
- cataracts
- other eye or ear infections

Tell your doctor about any other drugs you take, including aspirin, herbs, vitamins, and other nonprescription products.

When You Use This Drug

- **Do not use more often or in a higher dose than prescribed.**

How to Use This Drug

- Directions for applying drops appear on p. 622.
- If you miss a dose, take it as soon as you remember, but skip it if it is almost time for the next dose. **Do not take double doses.**

Interactions with Other Drugs

Some other drugs that you may be taking (either over-the-counter or prescription drugs) can interact with this one, causing adverse effects. Ask your doctor what these drugs are and let him or her know if you are taking any of them.

Adverse Effects

Call your doctor immediately if you experience:

- blurred or decreased vision
- eye pain
- headache

- seeing halos around lights
- drooping eyelids
- unusually large pupils
- eye infection
- nausea, vomiting

Call your doctor if these symptoms continue:

- burning, stinging, watering of the eyes

Periodic Tests

Ask your doctor which of these tests should be done periodically while you are taking this drug:

- eye exams

PREGNANCY WARNING

This drug caused harm to developing fetuses in animal studies, or such studies were not done. Use during pregnancy only for clear medical reasons. Tell your doctor if you are pregnant or thinking of becoming pregnant before you take this drug.

Limited Use

Gentamicin
GARAMYCIN (Schering)

Tobramycin
TOBREX (Alcon)

GENERIC: available
FAMILY: Antibiotics (see p. 468)
Aminoglycosides

Gentamicin (jen ta *mye* sin) and tobramycin (toe bra *mye* sin) are used in ointment, cream or liquid form to treat eye, ear, and skin infections. **Drugs in this family (aminoglycosides) are also given intravenously in the** hospital to treat serious infections, but the information on this page does *not* apply to this use.

Gentamicin is sometimes used on the skin to treat severe burns that are infected. This is not a recommended use. If you use gentamicin this way, you may develop bacteria that are resistant to the drug, and the injected form of gentamicin might then be ineffective if you ever received it.[23]

Before You Use This Drug

Tell your doctor if you have or have had:

- allergies to drugs
- an unusual reaction to any aminoglycoside (neomycin, for example)
- punctured eardrum or other ear problems (*if you are using the ear dosage form*)

Tell your doctor about any other drugs you take, including aspirin, herbs, vitamins, and other nonprescription products.

When You Use This Drug

- Your eyes may sting or burn just after using. Call your doctor if this problem does not go away in a few days.
- Call your doctor if your skin infection does not improve in a week or if it gets worse.
- **Use all the gentamicin or tobramycin your doctor prescribed, even if you feel better before you finish. If you stop too soon, your symptoms could come back.**

How to Use This Drug

- *For eye infections:* Follow the instructions on p. 622 for applying eye drops and ointment correctly, so that you won't absorb the drug into your body and possibly suffer serious adverse effects.
- *For skin infections:* Wash affected area with soap and water and dry completely, then apply a small amount of the medication to the skin.

• Do not store in the bathroom. Do not expose to heat, moisture, or strong light. Do not let liquid form freeze.

• If you miss an application, apply it as soon as you remember, but skip it if it is almost time for the next application. **Do not take double doses.**

Interactions with Other Drugs

Some other drugs that you may be taking (either over-the-counter or prescription drugs) can interact with this one, causing adverse effects. Ask your doctor what these drugs are and let him or her know if you are taking any of them.

Adverse Effects

Call your doctor immediately if you experience:

• itching, redness, swelling, or other irritation that has appeared since you started using the drug for a skin infection

---

PREGNANCY WARNING

Tobrex caused harm to developing fetuses in animal studies, or such studies were not done. Use during pregnancy only for clear medical reasons. Tell your doctor if you are pregnant or thinking of becoming pregnant before you take this drug.

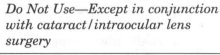

Do Not Use—Except in conjunction with cataract/intraocular lens surgery

ALTERNATIVE TREATMENT: *An antibiotic alone, if necessary.*

Neomycin, Polymyxin B, and Dexamethasone
MAXITROL (Alcon)

FAMILY: Antibiotics (see p. 468)
           Corticosteroids (see p. 651)

These are eye drops that contain three drugs, neomycin (nee oh *mye* sin), polymyxin (pol i *mix* in) B, and dexamethasone (see p. 665). The drops are used to treat some eye and eyelid infections caused by bacteria and allergies. **There is no persuasive proof that they are beneficial for this purpose.** However, ophthalmologists find this combination useful to prevent infections and reduce post-operative inflammation in the first few days after intraocular lens surgery.

One of the drugs in this combination, dexamethasone, belongs to a family called corticosteroids. Drugs in this family are not generally recommended for treating infections because they can hide the signs of an infection or make it spread. The other drugs in this combination, neomycin and polymyxin B, are antibiotics. If your eye problem is caused by a bacterial infection, an antibiotic might be needed. Otherwise, antibiotics are unnecessary and should not be used.[24]

Neomycin commonly causes skin rashes in 8% of the people who use it.[25] Using neomycin can also make it hard for you to use other drugs in its family (aminoglycoside antibiotics, such as gentamicin and tobramycin, see p. 635) that may be needed later to treat serious infections.

Tropicamide
MYDRIACYL (Alcon)

GENERIC: available

FAMILY: Eye Drugs

Tropicamide (troe *pik* a mide) is most commonly used to enlarge (dilate) the pupils of the eyes during an eye exam. It is also used to dilate the pupils before or after certain types of eye surgery.

At first this drug may cause a stinging sensation, blurred vision, and increased sensitivity to light. Check with your doctor if any of these effects lasts longer than 24 hours after you apply the drug.

WARNING: SPECIAL MENTAL AND PHYSICAL ADVERSE EFFECTS

Older adults are especially sensitive to the harmful anticholinergic (see Glossary, p. 768) effects of eye drugs such as tropicamide. Drugs in this family should not be used unless absolutely necessary.

Mental Effects: confusion, delirium, short-term memory problems, disorientation, and impaired attention.

Physical Effects: dry mouth, constipation, difficulty urinating (especially for a man with an enlarged prostate), blurred vision, decreased sweating with increased body temperature, sexual dysfunction, and worsening of glaucoma.

Before You Use This Drug

Tell your doctor if you have or have had:

- allergies to drugs
- glaucoma
- seizure disorder

Tell your doctor about any other drugs you take, including aspirin, herbs, vitamins, and other nonprescription products.

When You Use This Drug

- **Do not use more often or in a higher dose than prescribed.**

How to Use This Drug

- Directions for applying drops appear on p. 622.
- Do not store in the bathroom. Do not expose to heat, moisture, or strong light. Do not allow to freeze.
- If you miss a dose, apply it as soon as you remember, but skip it if it is almost time for the next dose. **Do not apply double doses.**

Interactions with Other Drugs

Some other drugs that you may be taking (either over-the-counter or prescription drugs) can interact with this one, causing adverse effects. Ask your doctor what these drugs are and let him or her know if you are taking any of them.

Adverse Effects

Call your doctor immediately if you experience:

- clumsiness or unsteadiness
- confusion or unusual behavior
- flushing or redness of face
- hallucinations
- increased thirst, dry mouth
- skin rash
- slurred speech
- fast heartbeat
- drowsiness, tiredness, weakness
- swollen stomach in infants

Call your doctor if these symptoms continue:

- blurred vision
- increased sensitivity to light
- stinging sensation in eyes

- headache
- irritation of eyes

Do Not Use—Except in conjunction with cataract/intraocular lens surgery.

ALTERNATIVE TREATMENT:
An antibiotic alone, if necessary.

Neomycin and Dexamethasone
NEODECADRON (Merck)

FAMILY: Antibiotics (see p. 468)
               Corticosteroids (see p. 651)

These are eye drops that contain two drugs, neomycin (nee oh *mye* sin) and dexamethasone (see p. 665). The drops are used to treat some eye and eyelid infections caused by bacteria and allergies. **There is no persuasive proof that they are beneficial for this purpose.** However, ophthalmologists find this combination useful to prevent infections and reduce post-operative inflammation in the first few days after intraocular lens surgery.

One of the drugs in this combination, dexamethasone, belongs to a family called corticosteroids. Drugs in this family are not recommended for treating infections because they can hide the signs of an infection or make it spread. The other drug in this combination, neomycin, is an antibiotic. If your eye problem is being caused by a bacterial infection, an antibiotic may be needed. Otherwise, antibiotics are unnecessary and should not be used.[26]

Neomycin commonly causes skin rashes in 8% of the people who use it.[27] Using neomycin can also make it hard for you to use other drugs in its family (aminoglycoside antibiotics such as gentamicin and tobramycin, see p. 635) that may be needed later to treat serious infections.

Methazolamide
NEPTAZANE (Lederle)

GENERIC: not available
FAMILY: Antiglaucoma Drugs (see p. 623)

Methazolamide (meth a *zoll* am ide) is an oral drug used to treat glaucoma. It lowers pressure in the eyes, and improves vision. Methazolamide is used long-term for open-angle glaucoma. It may be used temporarily before surgery for angle-closure (narrow angle) glaucoma. Studies of methazolamide to control essential tremor are not yet conclusive.[28]

Methazolamide belongs to the same family of drugs as acetazolamide (DIAMOX). These drugs are cousins of sulfa drugs and thiazide diuretics, having the potential for the same adverse effects, but no action against bacteria. This family of drugs may cause kidney stones, gouty arthritis, and depress your bone marrow. Older people with decreased kidney function need to be cautious when taking these drugs. Many individuals cannot tolerate the adverse effects of this family of drugs for a prolonged time.[29]

Methazolamide can upset the gastrointestinal tract, and severely deplete your calcium, potassium and other minerals. Unfortunately, stopping methazolamide does not always reverse the damage to bone marrow.[30] Anyone whose liver is impaired risks going into a coma while taking methazolamide.

Before You Use This Drug

Do not use if you have or have had:

- allergies to acetazolamide, sulfas, or thiazide diuretics
- acidosis, hyperchloremic type
- adrenal gland failure
- kidney or liver problems
- very low potassium or sodium levels
- diabetes

Tell your doctor if you have or have had:

- allergies to drugs

- adrenal gland problems (Addison's disease)
- diabetes
- gout
- low blood levels of sodium or potassium
- kidney or liver problems
- emphysema, or other chronic lung disease

Tell your doctor about any other drugs you take, including aspirin, herbs, vitamins, and other nonprescription products.

When You Use This Drug

- Until you know how you react to this drug, do not drive or perform other activities requiring alertness. This drug may cause drowsiness, dizziness, lightheadedness, and tiredness.
- To help prevent kidney stones, **drink at least six to eight glasses (eight ounces each) of fluids each day.**
- Eat foods rich in potassium to compensate for loss of potassium (see p. 49).
- If you plan to have any surgery, including dental, tell your doctor that you take this drug.

How to Use This Drug

- Swallow tablet whole or break in half. You may take methazolamide with food to decrease stomach upset.
- Do not store in the bathroom. Do not expose to heat, moisture, or strong light.
- If you miss a dose, take it as soon as you remember but skip it if it is almost time for the next dose. **Do not take double doses.**

Interactions with Other Drugs

The following drugs are listed in the *Evaluations of Drug Interactions* 1997 as causing "highly clinically significant" or "clinically significant" interactions when used together with this drug. We have also included potentially serious interactions listed in the drug's FDA-approved professional product labeling or package insert. New scientific techniques have allowed researchers to predict some drug interactions before they have been documented in people. There may be other drugs, especially those in the families of drugs listed below, that also will react with this drug to cause severe adverse effects. The number of new drugs approved for marketing increases the chance of drug interactions, and new drug interactions are being identified with old drugs. Be vigilant. Make sure to tell your doctor and pharmacist the drugs you are taking and tell your doctor if you are taking any of these interacting drugs:

aspirin, especially in large doses, GENUINE BAYER ASPIRIN, cyclosporine, ECOTRIN, lithium, LITHOBID, LITHONATE, NEORAL, SANDIMMUNE.

Additionally, the *United States Pharmacopeia Drug Interactions* 1998, lists these drugs as having interactions of major significance: amphetamines, DURAQUIN, HIPREX, INVERSINE, mecamylamine, methenamine, QUINAGLUTE DURATABS, QUINIDEX, quinidine, UREX.

Adverse Effects

Call your doctor immediately if you experience:

- blood in urine, difficulty urinating, pain or burning during urination, pain in lower back, or sudden decrease in amount of urine
  - bloody or black, tarry stools
  - clumsiness, unsteadiness
  - convulsions
  - dry mouth or increased thirst
  - irregular heartbeat, weak pulse
  - muscle cramps, weakness or pain
  - nausea or vomiting
  - unusual tiredness or weakness
  - fever and sore throat
  - unusual bruising or bleeding

- mental confusion or depression
- nearsightedness
- mood or mental changes
- trouble breathing or shortness of breath
- ringing or buzzing in ears
- hives, itching or skin rash
- tremors in hands or feet
- vision changes

Call your doctor if these symptoms continue:

- constipation or diarrhea
- dizziness, lightheadedness
- drowsiness
- increased amount or frequency of urination
- loss of appetite, weight loss
- metallic taste or loss of taste in mouth
- numbness or tingling of hands, fingers, feet, toes, mouth, tongue, lips or rectum
- hair loss
- headache
- impotence[31]
- increased sensitivity to sunlight

Periodic Tests

Ask your doctor which of these tests should be done periodically while you are taking this drug:

- complete blood count
- blood electrolyte (sodium, potassium) tests
- platelet count
- tests of kidney function and kidney stone formation

PREGNANCY WARNING

This drug caused harm to developing fetuses in animal studies, or such studies were not done. Use during pregnancy only for clear medical reasons. Tell your doctor if you are pregnant or thinking of becoming pregnant before you take this drug.

Dipivefrin
PROPINE (Allergan)

GENERIC: available
FAMILY: Antiglaucoma Drugs (see p. 623)

Dipivefrin (dye *pi* ve frin) is used to treat the most common form of glaucoma (see p. 623). In glaucoma, the pressure of the fluid inside the eye increases, and dipivefrin controls the pressure by reducing the amount of fluid that is produced and improving its circulation. It has not proven to be as effective in lowering intraocular pressure as pilocarpine (see p. 624) or beta-blockers such as timolol (see p. 643) or carbonic anhydrase inhibitors such as dorzolamide (see p. 645). When used for a long time, the initial improvement may diminish.

Before You Use This Drug

Tell your doctor if you have or have had:

- allergies to drugs
- the lens in your eye removed
- glaucoma

Tell your doctor about any other drugs you take, including aspirin, herbs, vitamins, and other nonprescription products.

When You Use This Drug

- **Do not use more often or in a higher dose than prescribed.**

How to Use This Drug

- Directions for applying drops appear on p. 622
- Do not store in the bathroom. Do not expose to heat, moisture, or strong light. Do not allow to freeze.
- If you miss a dose, apply it as soon as you remember, but skip it if it is almost time for the next dose. **Do not take double doses.**

Interactions with Other Drugs

Some other drugs that you may be taking (either over-the-counter or prescription drugs) can interact with this one, causing adverse effects. Ask your doctor what these drugs are and let him or her know if you are taking any of them.

Adverse Effects

Call your doctor immediately if you experience:

- rise in blood pressure
- fast or irregular heartbeat

Call your doctor if these symptoms continue:

- burning, stinging, or irritation of the eyes
- increased sensitivity to light

Periodic Tests

Ask your doctor which of these tests should be done periodically while you are taking this drug:

- eye pressure tests
- complete eye exam, including test for visual acuity

Limited Use

Sulfacetamide
SULAMYD (Schering)

GENERIC: available

FAMILY: Antibiotics (see p. 468)
Sulfonamides

Sulfacetamide (sul fa *see* ta mide) is used to treat some eye infections and is available as a liquid or an ointment. It can cause blurred vision, stinging, or burning after use. It also makes your eyes sensitive to bright light. Wearing sunglasses may help with this problem. For serious eye infections sulfacetamide may not be as effective as other antibiotics.

Before You Use This Drug

Tell your doctor if you have or have had:

- allergies to drugs
- an unusual reaction to other sulfa drugs, furosemide, thiazide diuretics (water pills), or diabetes or glaucoma drugs taken by mouth
- glucose-6-phosphate dehydrogenase deficiency

Tell your doctor about any other drugs you take, including aspirin, herbs, vitamins, and other nonprescription products.

When You Use This Drug

- Call your doctor if your symptoms do not improve in two or three days.
- If the liquid form of sulfacetamide gets dark, throw it away.
- **Use all the sulfacetamide your doctor prescribed, even if you feel better before you finish. If you stop too soon, your symptoms could come back.**
- Do not give this drug to anyone else. Throw away outdated drugs.

How to Use This Drug

- Directions for applying drops appear on p. 622
- Do not let the tip of the applicator touch your eye, your fingers, or anything else. It could become contaminated.
- Do not store in the bathroom. Do not expose to heat, moisture, or strong light. Do not allow this drug to freeze.
- If you miss a dose, apply it as soon as you remember, but skip it if it is almost time for the next dose. **Do not take double doses.**

Interactions with Other Drugs

Some other drugs that you may be taking (either over-the-counter or prescription drugs) can interact with this one, causing adverse effects. Ask your doctor what these drugs are and let him or her know if you are taking any of them.

Adverse Effects

Call your doctor immediately if you experience:

- itching, redness, or swelling not present before using this drug
- Because sulfacetamide is absorbed into the body, you may have other adverse effects like those that occur with the sulfonamides (sulfa drugs). See sulfisoxazole, p. 505, for examples.

Artificial Tears
TEARISOL (Iolab)
TEARS NATURALE (Alcon)
HYPOTEARS (Ciba Vision)

GENERIC: available
FAMILY: Eye Drugs

Artificial tears are used to treat people who do not produce tears normally. You can also use them on a temporary basis to moisten dry eyes. Do not use artificial tears for more than three days unless your doctor has prescribed them.

Most artificial tears preparations contain either polyvinyl alcohol or a methylcellulose solution for lubrication. Methylcellulose solutions stay in your eye longer, but they tend to form crusts on the eyelids. If you use artificial tears containing polyvinyl alcohol, do not also use an eye solution containing boric acid. The combination may form gummy deposits.[32]

To avoid eye infection, irritation, and other problems, take care to prevent contamination when applying eye drops. Do not allow the applicator tip to touch anything, including your eye. After applying drops, replace the cap tightly on the bottle.

Before You Use This Drug

Tell your doctor if you have or have had:

- allergies to drugs

Tell your doctor about any other drugs you take, including aspirin, herbs, vitamins, and other nonprescription products.

When You Use This Drug

- **Do not use more often or in a higher dose than prescribed.**
- Your eyes may sting or burn just after using. Call your doctor if this problem does not go away in a few days.

How to Use This Drug

- Directions for applying eye drops appear on p. 622.
- Do not store in the bathroom. Do not expose to heat, moisture, or strong light. Do not allow to freeze.

Interactions with Other Drugs

Some other drugs that you may be taking (either over-the-counter or prescription drugs) can interact with this one, causing adverse effects. Ask your doctor what these drugs are and let him or her know if you are taking any of them.

Adverse Effects

Call your doctor immediately if you experience:

- eye irritation that was not present before you started using artificial tears

Call your doctor if these symptoms continue:

- blurred vision
- matted or sticky eyelids

Timolol (Eye Drops)
TIMOPTIC (Merck)

GENERIC: available

FAMILY: Antiglaucoma Drugs (see p. 623)
Beta-blockers (see p. 52)

Timolol (*tim* oh lole) has two forms for different uses: Blocadren tablets for the heart (see p. 66) and Timoptic eye drops for the eyes, specifically for treating glaucoma (see p. 623). This profile discusses timolol's use as an antiglaucoma drug.

Timolol drops are well tolerated by most people, especially those who have cataracts or who have problems using another antiglaucoma drug called pilocarpine (see p. 624). Although timolol is an eye drop, some of it can be absorbed from the eyes into the bloodstream and the rest of the body, and if this happens you may experience some of the general adverse effects listed under Adverse Effects. (See p. 623 for directions on how to apply eye drops.)

When used for a long time, the initial improvement may diminish. As with other beta-blockers, long-term use can exacerbate serious heart problems, even in people who did not previously have heart disease. Timolol, similarly to levobunolol, can decrease lung function by 30%, an adverse effect not seen in betaxolol, another beta-blocker.[33] Very rarely, serious harm, even fatalities have occurred, mostly to those with asthma or heart problems.[34] But according to *The Medical Letter*, betaxolol (see p. 629) may be less likely than timolol or levobunolol to have adverse effects on patients with asthma.[35] Timolol taken by mouth has been shown to cause an increased number of adrenal, lung, uterine, and breast cancers in rats. This has not been shown for the eye drops.

Before You Use This Drug

Do not use if you have or have had:

- bronchial asthma
- congestive heart failure, slow heartbeat or heart block
- severe lung disease

Tell your doctor if you have or have had:

- allergies to drugs
- impotence
- mental depression
- diabetes
- emphysema or chronic bronchitis
- myasthenia gravis
- thyroid problems
- lung function impairment
- hypoglycemia

Tell your doctor about any other drugs you take, including aspirin, herbs, vitamins, and other nonprescription products.

When You Use This Drug

- Restrict your use of caffeine, since it may add to the effect of timolol on the heart.[36]
- **Caution diabetics:** be aware that timolol may mask trembling and pulse rate used to signal low blood sugar.[37]
- If you plan to have any surgery, including dental, tell your doctor that you take this drug.
- Be cautious driving until the effect of the drug is complete (about two weeks),[38] and no blurred vision occurs.
- **Do not take other drugs without talking to your doctor first—especially nonprescription drugs for appetite control, asthma, colds, coughs, hay fever, or sinus problems.**

COLD STRESS ALERT

If timolol eye drops are absorbed into the body, older people have an increased risk of hypothermia.[39] Early signs are shivering, cold hands and feet, and memory lapse. Stay indoors, especially when it is cold and windy. Keep warm with extra clothes and blankets. If you must go outdoors, dress to protect yourself from the wind and cold. Avoid getting wet. Take along something to eat, such as trail mix suitable to your diet.

How to Use This Drug

• Directions for applying drops appear on p. 622.

• Do not expose to heat or direct light.

• *If you miss a dose, use the following guidelines:* If you are using timolol only once a day, apply the missed dose as soon as you remember, but skip it if you don't remember until the next day.

If you are using timolol more than once a day, apply the missed dose as soon as you remember, but skip it if it is almost time for the next dose.

Do not apply double doses.

Interactions with Other Drugs

The following drugs are listed in the *Evaluations of Drug Interactions* 1997 as causing "highly clinically significant" or "clinically significant" interactions when used together with this drug. We have also included potentially serious interactions listed in the drug's FDA-approved professional product labeling or package insert. New scientific techniques have allowed researchers to predict some drug interactions before they have been documented in people. There may be other drugs, especially those in the families of drugs listed below, that also will react with this drug to cause severe adverse effects. The number of new drugs approved for marketing increases the chance of drug interactions, and new drug interactions are being identified with old drugs. Be vigilant. Make sure to tell your doctor and pharmacist the drugs you are taking and tell your doctor if you are taking any of these interacting drugs:

ADRENALIN (also in bee sting kits), ALEVE, ANAPROX, CALAN SR, CATAPRES, clonidine, cocaine, COVERA-HS, DELTASONE, ELIXOPHYLLIN, epinephrine, FLUOTHANE, halothane, HUMALOG, HUMULIN, insulin, ISOPTIN SR, LEVOTHROID, levothyroxine, lidocaine, lithium, LITHOBID, LITHONATE, METICORTEN, MINIPRESS, NAPROSYN, naproxen, prazosin, prednisone, PRIMATENE MIST, SLO-BID, SYNTHROID, THEO-24, theophylline, TUBARINE, tubocurarine, verapamil, VERELAN, XYLOCAINE.

Adverse Effects

Timolol can be absorbed into the body through the eye. All adverse effects for oral beta-blockers are possible with timolol eye-drops.

Call your doctor immediately if you experience:

• headache
• itching skin or rash
• nausea, vomiting, diarrhea
• decreased sexual ability
• numbness or tingling of limbs
• coughing, wheezing or difficulty breathing
• chest pain
• hallucinations
• cold hands or feet
• confusion, depression
• skin rash, hives or itching

- swelling of ankles, feet, or lower legs
- redness, itching, stinging, burning watering, irritation of eyes or eyelids
- blurred vision, seeing double or other vision changes
- droopy upper eyelid
- hair loss
- dizziness, faintness
- bloody, stuffy or runny nose
- heartbeat, fast or irregular

Call your doctor if these symptoms continue:

- anxiety, nervousness
- abnormal tiredness or weakness
- disturbed sleep, nightmares
- slow pulse
- burning or prickly feeling on body

Call your doctor if these symptoms continue after you stop taking the drug:

- chest pain
- irregular heartbeat
- weakness
- shortness of breath
- headache
- sweating
- trembling

More adverse effects information appears on p. 52.

Periodic Tests

Ask your doctor which of these tests should be done periodically while you are taking this drug:

- blood pressure and pulse rate
- heart function tests, such as electrocardiogram (ECG, EKG)
- blood glucose levels (*if diabetic*)
- eye pressure exams

Limited Use

Dorzolamide
TRUSOPT (Merck)

GENERIC: not available
FAMILY: Antiglaucoma Drugs (see p. 623)

Dorzolamide (dor *zole* a mide) is used to treat glaucoma, especially open-angle glaucoma, and to lower pressure in the eye. This medication is also used in certain eye surgeries. Excess pressure in the eye can damage the optic nerve and cause loss of vision. Dorzolamide blocks the enzyme carbonic anhydrase, as does the oral drug acetazolamide. Carbonic anhydrase is present in the eyes, kidney, lungs, and stomach. Dorzolamide belongs to the family of sulfa drugs.

The usual dose is one drop in the affected eye or eyes, three times daily. Some people may be able to use dorzolamide twice daily.[40] Drugs for glaucoma usually work more quickly in people with light colored eyes than in people with dark eyes.[41] Bitter taste is a common adverse effect to dorzolamide. If the container becomes contaminated it can damage your eye, even causing loss of vision. Dorzolamide does not lower pressure in the eye as much as acetazolamide or timolol.[42,43] When dorzolamide and timolol are both given, an additional lowering of pressure in the eye occurs. Adverse effects are generally less likely than with oral acetazolamide. However, dorzolamide, like other eye drops, is absorbed throughout your body. Potentially any adverse effect of sulfas or carbonic anhydrase inhibitors could occur with dorzolamide. These include rare, but sometimes fatal, severe allergic reactions, blood disorders, and bone marrow depression. If you stop taking dorzolamide, some of the drug may remain in your body for a few months.[44]

People who are allergic to sulfa drugs should not use dorzolamide. Dorzolamide has not been studied in people with liver problems. It is not recommended for people with narrow angle glaucoma, kidney disease, or people who wear soft contacts. Dorzolamide is also not recommended for children, or women who are pregnant or nursing. Information about dorzolamide, particularly effects after use for more than one year, remains limited.

Before You Use This Drug

Tell your doctor if you have or have had:

- allergies, including allergies to sulfa
- acidosis or electrolyte problems
- blood disorders
- other eye problems, especially cornea problems,[45] or acute-angle glaucoma
- kidney or liver problems
- pregnant or nursing
- respiratory problems
- wear contact lenses

Tell your doctor about any other drugs you take, including aspirin, herbs, vitamins, and other nonprescription products.

When You Use This Drug

- If you develop irritation or infection in your eye or have an injury to your eye, discontinue using dorzolamide and call your doctor.
- If you plan to have any surgery, including dental, tell your doctor that you take this drug.

How to Use This Drug

- Directions for applying drops appear on p. 622.
- Prevent the container from becoming contaminated. Avoid letting the tip of the container touch your eye, hands, or any other object.
- Recap the container immediately to prevent contamination and to prevent crystals from forming on the tip of the container.[46]
- If you use other eye medications, allow 10 minutes between the dose of that medication and dorzolamide.

- If you miss a dose, use it as soon as you remember but skip it if it is almost time for the next dose. **Do not take double doses**.
- Do not store in the bathroom. Do not expose to heat, moisture, or strong light.

Interactions with Other Drugs

The following drugs are listed in the *Evaluations of Drug Interactions* 1997 as causing "highly clinically significant" or "clinically significant" interactions when used together with this drug. We have also included potentially serious interactions listed in the drug's FDA-approved professional product labeling or package insert. New scientific techniques have allowed researchers to predict some drug interactions before they have been documented in people. There may be other drugs, especially those in the families of drugs listed below, that also will react with this drug to cause severe adverse effects. The number of new drugs approved for marketing increases the chance of drug interactions, and new drug interactions are being identified with old drugs. Be vigilant. Make sure to tell your doctor and pharmacist the drugs you are taking and tell your doctor if you are taking any of these interacting drugs:

acetazolamide, DIAMOX.

Other possible drug interactions are: cholinesterase inhibitors, such as ambenonium (MYTELASE), edrophonium (TENSILON), neostigmine (PROSTIGMIN), or pyridostigmine (MESTINON). The effect of these drugs (often used in myasthenia gravis) may be lowered by dorzolamide.[47] When taken with diuretics there can be a greater loss of potassium.[48] Use with phenytoin (DILANTIN) may aggravate osteoporosis.[49] Salicylic acid (SALSALATE) taken with dorzolamide can lead to acidosis.[50] Also, the preservative in dorzolamide drops (benzalkonium chloride) can interact with soft contact lenses.

Adverse Effects

Call your doctor immediately if you experience:

- abnormal bleeding[51]
- burning, itching, or stinging of eye or eyelid
- frequent infections[52]
- skin rash
- tiredness, fatigue[53]
- vision problems, including blurring, sensitivity to light
- blood in urine
- nausea or vomiting
- pain in side, back or abdomen

Call your doctor if these symptoms continue:

- bitter or metallic taste
- dry eyes
- headache
- excess tearing
- unusual tiredness or weakness

PREGNANCY WARNING

This drug caused harm to developing fetuses in animal studies, or such studies were not done. Use during pregnancy only for clear medical reasons. Tell your doctor if you are pregnant or thinking of becoming pregnant before you take this drug.

NOTES FOR EYE DRUGS

1. The Levobunolol Study Group. A four-year study of efficacy and safety in glaucoma treatment. *Ophthalmology* 1989; 96:642–5.

2. Silverstone D, Zimmerman T, Choplin N, Mundorf T, Rose A, Stoecker J, et al. Evaluation of once-daily levobunolol 0.25% and timolol 0.25% therapy for increased intraocular pressure. *American Journal of Ophthalmology* 1991; 112:56–60.

3. Dukes MNG, Beeley L. *Side Effects of Drugs Annual 15*, Amsterdam: Elsevier, 1991:510.

4. American Society of Hospital Pharmacists. *American Hospital Formulary Service Drug Information.* Bethesda, MD, 1992:1694–7.

5. *The Medical Letter on Drugs and Therapeutics.* New York: The Medical Letter Inc., 1986; 28:45–6.

6. *USP DI, Drug Information for the Health Care Professional.* 12th ed. Rockville MD: The United States Pharmacopeial Convention, Inc., 1992:1757–61.

7. Ibid, p. 656–9.

8. American Society of Hospital Pharmacists, op. cit.

9. *USP DI,* op. cit., p. 1757–61.

10. Dukes, op. cit.

11. American Society of Hospital Pharmacists, op. cit.

12. *The Medical Letter on Drugs and Therapeutics,* op. cit.

13. *USP DI,* op. cit., p. 1757–61.

14. Ibid, p. 656–9.

15. American Society of Hospital Pharmacists, op. cit.

16. *USP DI,* op. cit., p. 1751–61.

17. Allen RC, Hertzmark E, Walker AM, Epstein DL. A double-masked comparison of betaxolol vs. timolol in the treatment of open-angle glaucoma. *American Journal of Ophthalmology* 1986; 101:535–41.

18. AMA Department of Drugs. *AMA Drug Evaluations.* 1st ed. Chicago: American Medical Association, 1971:526.

19. *USP DI, Drug Information for the Health Care Provider.* 6th ed. Rockville MD: The United States Pharmacopeial Convention, Inc., 1986:448.

20. AMA Department of Drugs. *AMA Drug Evaluations.* 5th ed. Chicago: American Medical Association, 1983:763–4.

21. AMA Department of Drugs. *AMA Drug Evaluations.* Chicago: American Medical Association, 1992:1975–7.

22. AMA, 1983, op. cit.

23. Ibid, p. 1686.

24. AMA, 1971, op. cit.

25. Patrick J, Panzer JD. Neomycin sensitivity in the normal (nonatopic) individual. *Archives of Dermatology* 1970; 102:532–5.

26. AMA, 1971, op. cit.

27. Patrick, op. cit.

28. Koller WC. New drug for treatment of essential tremor? Time will tell. *Mayo Clinic Proceedings* 1991; 66:1085–7.

29. AMA, 1992, op. cit.

30. Moroi-Fetters SE, Metz EN, Chambers RB, Davidorf FH. Aplastic anemia with platelet autoantibodies in a patient after taking methazolamide. *American Journal of Ophthalmology* 1990; 110:570–1.

31. Dukes, op. cit., p. 513.

32. *Handbook of Nonprescription Drugs.* 7th ed. Washington, D.C.: American Pharmaceutical Association, 1982:425.

33. Dukes, op. cit., p. 510.

34. American Society of Hospital Pharmacists, op. cit.

35. *The Medical Letter on Drugs and Therapeutics,* op. cit.

36. *USP DI,* 1992, op. cit., p. 1757–61.

37. Ibid, p. 656–9.

38. American Society of Hospital Pharmacists, op. cit.

39. *USP DI,* 1992, op. cit., p. 1757–61.

40. Pfeiffer N. Dorzolamide: development and clinical application of a topical carbonic anhydrase inhibitor. *Survey of Ophthalmology* 1997; 42:137–51.

41. Ibid.

42. Heijl A, Strahlman E, Sverrisson T, Brinchman-Hansen O, Puustjarvi T, Tipping R. A comparison of dorzolamide and timolol in patients with pseudoexfoliation and glaucoma or ocular hypertension. *Ophthalmology* 1997; 104:137–42.

43. Mause TL, Larsson L, McLaren JW, Brubaker RF. Comparison of dorzolamide and acetazolamide as suppressors of aqueous humor flow in humans. *Archives of Ophthalmology* 1997; 115:45–9.

44. Pfeiffer, op. cit.

45. Ibid.

46. Zambarakji HJ, Spencer AF, Vernon SA. An unusual side effect of dorzolamide. *Eye* 1997; 11:418.

47. Pfeiffer, op. cit.

48. Ibid.

49. Ibid.

50. Ibid.

51. Ibid.

52. Ibid.

53. Ibid.

Drugs for Other Conditions

Corticosteroids		651

DRUG LISTINGS

CORTICOSTEROIDS

ACTHAR	Limited Use	654
AEROBID		703
ARISTOCORT		656
beclomethasone		736
BECLOVENT		736
betamethasone		675
CORTEF		660
corticotropin/ adrenocorticotropic hormone (ACTH)	Limited Use	654
CORTROPHIN-ZINC	Limited Use	654
DECADRON		665
DELTASONE		668
desoximetasone		733
dexamethasone		665
DIPROLENE		675
DIPROSONE		675
flunisolide		703
fluocinolone		730
fluocinonide		698
HEXADROL		665
hydrocortisone		660
KENALOG		656
LIDEX		698
LIDEX-E		698
MEDROL		700
methylprednisolone		700
METICORTEN		668
NASALIDE		703
PRED FORTE		711
prednisolone		711
prednisone		668
SYNALAR		730
SYNEMOL		730
TOPICORT		733
triamcinolone		656
VALISONE		675
VANCENASE		736
VANCERIL		736

HORMONES

AMEN	Limited Use	723
ANDROID	Limited Use	709
AYGESTIN	Limited Use	723
conjugated estrogens	Limited Use	714
DEMULEN		670
DES	Limited Use	714
DESOGEN	Ⓧ Do Not Use	673
desogestrel/ethinyl estradiol	Ⓧ Do Not Use	673
diethylstilbestrol	Limited Use	714
ESTRACE (cream)	Limited Use	714
ESTRADERM (patch)	Limited Use	680
estradiol (cream)	Limited Use	714
estradiol (patch)	Limited Use	680
estropipate	Limited Use	714
ethynodiol diacetate/ethinyl estradiol		670
EUTHROID		732
fluoxymesterone	Limited Use	709
GENORA 1/35		689

HALOTESTIN	Limited Use	709
LEVOTHROID		732
levothyroxine		732
liotrix		732
LO/OVRAL		689
LOESTRIN-FE 1.5/30		689
medroxyprogesterone	Limited Use	723
methyltestosterone	Limited Use	709
norethindrone acetate	Limited Use	723
norethindrone/ethinyl estradiol		689
norgestimate/ethinyl estradiol		689
norgestrel/ethinyl estradiol		689
OGEN	Limited Use	714
ORETON METHYL	Limited Use	709
ORTHO-CEPT	Ⓧ Do Not Use	673
ORTHO-CYCLEN		689
ORTHO-NOVUM 1/35		689
ORTHO-NOVUM 7/7/7		689
ORTHOTRI-CYCLEN		689
PREMARIN	Limited Use	714
PROVERA	Limited Use	723
SYNTHROID		732
thyroid		732
THYROLAR		732
TRI-LEVLEN		689
TRIPHASIL		689

MUSCLE RELAXANTS

carisoprodol	Ⓧ Do Not Use	730
chlorzoxazone	Ⓧ Do Not Use	711
cyclobenzaprine	Ⓧ Do Not Use	686
FLEXERIL	Ⓧ Do Not Use	686
methocarbamol	Ⓧ Do Not Use	728
NORFLEX	Ⓧ Do Not Use	708
orphenadrine	Ⓧ Do Not Use	708
PARAFON FORTE DSC	Ⓧ Do Not Use	711
ROBAXIN	Ⓧ Do Not Use	728
SOMA	Ⓧ Do Not Use	730

DRUGS FOR URINARY TRACT DISORDER

bethanechol		735
DITROPAN	Limited Use	677
oxybutynin	Limited Use	677
phenazopyridine	Ⓧ Do Not Use	725
PYRIDIUM	Ⓧ Do Not Use	725
URECHOLINE		735

DRUGS FOR TREATING CANCER

cyclophosphamide	Limited Use	663
CYTOXAN	Limited Use	663
EFUDEX		679
FLUOROPLEX		679
fluorouracil		679
NEOSAR	Limited Use	663
NOLVADEX	Limited Use	706
tamoxifen	Limited Use	706

SKIN & HAIR CARE DRUGS

minoxidil	Ⓧ Do Not Use	729
RENOVA	Ⓧ Do Not Use Except for Skin Cancer and Severe Acne	726
RETIN-A	Ⓧ Do Not Use Except for Skin Cancer and Severe Acne	726
ROGAINE	Ⓧ Do Not Use	729
tretinoin	Ⓧ Do Not Use Except for Skin Cancer and Severe Acne	726

DRUGS TO HELP STOP SMOKING

bupropion	Limited Use	739
HABITROL	Limited Use	692
NICODERM	Limited Use	692
NICORETTE	Limited Use	692
nicotine	Limited Use	692
NICOTROL	Limited Use	692
PROSTEP	Limited Use	692
ZYBAN	Limited Use	739

DRUGS FOR OSTEOPOROSIS

alendronate	Limited Use	687
CALCIMAR	Ⓧ Do Not Use	659
calcitonin	Ⓧ Do Not Use	659

EVISTA	Do Not Use Until Five Years After Release	683
FOSAMAX	Limited Use	687
MIACALCIN INJECTION	⊘ Do Not Use	659
MIACALCIN NASAL SPRAY	⊘ Do Not Use	659
raloxifene	Do Not Use Until Five Years After Release	683

DRUGS FOR MIGRAINE

IMITREX	Limited Use	695
sumatriptan	Limited Use	695
zolmitriptan	Do Not Use Until Five Years After Release	695
ZOMIG	Do Not Use Until Five Years After Release	695

DIET DRUGS

MERIDIA	⊘ Do Not Use	702
sibutramine	⊘ Do Not Use	702

PROSTATE DRUGS

finasteride	Limited Use	721
PROSCAR	Limited Use	721

DRUGS FOR ATTENTION DEFICIT DISORDER

methylphenidate	Limited Use	726
RITALIN	Limited Use	726

CORTICOSTEROIDS

Corticosteroids, commonly known as steroids or cortisone, are a class of hormones that regulate vital body functions. They affect carbohydrate, protein, and fat metabolism, maintain the body's water and electrolyte (salt and potassium, for example) balance, support normal heart and blood vessel function, influence mood and sleep patterns, and maintain normal muscle strength. Corticosteroids are produced by the adrenal glands, located just above the kidneys. Prescription corticosteroids are either identical to or a synthetic version of the adrenal hormones. They are given to either replace the body's corticosteroids when the adrenal glands are diseased or suppress inflammation in diseases such as arthritis or asthma.

Corticosteroids are taken in many different dosage forms. Nasal dosage, eye dosage, topical, and inhaler forms have been developed to deliver the corticosteroid directly to the affected area, which minimizes adverse effects. In this section you will find directions common to all corticosteroids, followed by specific information regarding the most common dosage forms.

General Directions

1. Do not allow corticosteroids to freeze.

2. Do not expose corticosteroids to heat or direct light.

3. Do not store in the bathroom. The moisture and heat will alter the structure of the drug, and it will no longer be effective.

4. Do not take more often or in higher doses than your doctor prescribed. **Do not stop taking this drug suddenly. Your doctor must lower your dose gradually to prevent withdrawal symptoms.** When your symptoms improve, ask your doctor about reducing your dosage. Higher doses and/or shorter intervals between doses can stop the body's production of its own corticosteroids. This leads to a lowered defense against disease (a depressed immune system) and can result in a greater likelihood of developing infections and tumors.

5. Do not use the drug to treat problems other than that for which it was prescribed without first checking with your doctor.

6. Corticosteroids should not be used for many bacterial, viral, and fungal infections.

Systemic Dosage Forms

The word *systemic* refers to something which affects the body as a whole. A drug, taken as tablets, capsules, or injections, is distributed throughout the body—to areas that require treatment as well as to those that do not. Because the entire body is exposed to the drug's action, there can be unnecessary adverse effects.

Adverse effects from systemic corticosteroids can be minimized by using alternate-day therapy. In this way, the body is only exposed to the drug's full effects every other day. If you will be taking systemic steroids on a long term basis, ask your doctor about switching to alternate-day therapy.

The body's own corticosteroids are released mostly in the early morning hours between 4:00 A.M. and 8:00 A.M., with very little being released in the evenings. The varying amounts of corticosteroids to which your body is exposed throughout the day help to set your body's clock and to establish sleep and waking cycles. Therefore, a single daily dose or an alternate-day dose should be taken in the morning prior to 8:00 a.m. for the least disruption of your body's natural rhythm.

Prednisone is the drug of choice for systemic steroids, because it is reliable, effective, less expensive, and available in a generic preparation that can be taken by mouth. Oral forms of prednisolone, methylprednisolone, and betamethasone should *not* be used.

Corticotropin (ACTH) has limited use—it should be used only for diagnostic testing of adrenal function. It should not be used for inflammation or disorders which respond to other more preferable corticosteroids.

Nasal Dosage Forms

There are two types of nasal dosage forms: the solution and the aerosol, both of which supply metered-dose sprays of corticosteroid. They are used to treat severe allergies, severe cases of hay fever, and sometimes nasal polyps.

If you have a very runny nose with a lot of secretions or swelling, most of the drug may not reach the nasal mucous membranes and therefore may not be absorbed. Blow your nose before using the spray or take a decongestant first if your nasal passages are blocked. You may require treatment with cortisone tablets or a cream to shrink the nasal blood vessels.

At recommended dosages, absorption of the drug into the body through the lining of the nose is minimal, and adverse effects are limited primarily to the nose. Nosebleeds, burning, irritation, and sneezing are common.

Eye Dosage Form

While taking this drug you should schedule regular appointments with an eye doctor to check your progress. For both drops and ointments, **call your doctor immediately if symptoms do not improve within five to seven days, if your condition worsens, or if you feel pain, itching or swelling.** Temporary blurring of sight may occur after you apply the medicine. This is normal and will clear shortly. The medicine may also cause sensitivity to bright light. Wearing sunglasses will help. See p. 622 for directions to safely and effectively apply drops and ointments.

Eye pressure should be rechecked approximately two weeks after you begin to use corticosteroid drops or ointment on your eye because these drugs can cause or worsen glaucoma.

Topical (Applied to Skin and Mouth) Dosage Form

There are two major categories of corticosteroid preparations that are applied to the skin: those that contain fluorine and those that do not. Neither should be used for prolonged periods on the face or around the eye. Systemic adverse effects are related to the amount of drug used, and can pose a problem when large areas of skin are treated. Unless you are using a weak nonfluorinated cream, thinning of skin may occur with prolonged use, particularly on the face, armpits and groin. If the area which you are treating becomes irritated, stop using the drug and call your doctor.

Fluorinated topical forms

Corticosteroids that contain fluorine are betamethasone (DIPROSONE, DIPROLENE, VALISONE), desoximetasone (TOPICORT), dexamethasone (DECADRON, HEXADROL), fluocinolone (SYNALAR, SYNEMOL), fluocinonide (LIDEX, LIDEX-E), and triamcinolone (KENALOG, ARISTOCORT). Fluorinated topical corticosteroids are generally more effective than those that do not contain fluorine. They are more likely, however, to cause adverse effects such as skin wasting, loss of pigment, and acne. Because of the potential adverse effects, high strength fluorine-containing steroids should be spread in a very thin layer, covering only the treatment area. Systemic effects are rare if these preparations are used correctly.

Some people find ointments too greasy, especially for hairy areas. In this case, a cream, lotion, or gel may come into better contact with the skin.

Nonfluorinated topical forms

Hydrocortisone (CORTAID) can now be purchased without a prescription in two strengths, 0.25% and 0.50%. The lowest concentration of this drug that is generally considered effective, however, is 0.50%. A soothing emollient, such as a lotion, cream, or ointment, that does not contain hydrocortisone is probably just as effective as the 0.25% hydrocortisone cream.

Inhalation Aerosol for Asthma

Corticosteroid inhalants, used with an inhaler that is placed in the mouth, primarily benefit those people with asthma who require regular, long-term use of corticosteroids to control their symptoms. Inhalants are rarely appropriate treatment for nonasthmatic bronchitis or emphysema. The inhalants should not be used when asthma responds to bronchodilators and other non-steroid drugs, or to systemic (tablets and capsules) steroids used infrequently.

Inhaled aerosol corticosteroids may be used instead of, or in addition to, systemic corticosteroids. They are preferable to the systemic forms because of the way they deliver the medication to where it is required. Inhaling the medication ensures that more of it is concentrated in the lungs where it is needed and less is available to the rest of the body through general absorption. This is better because it is the drug's actions on the rest of the body that causes most adverse effects.

Inhaled aerosol corticosteroids can take up to four weeks to produce improvement when used alone, and therefore are ineffective if taken on an intermittent basis. People who use corticosteriods infrequently cannot substitute an inhalation aerosol for the medication they use.

Continue to use the inhalant even if you do not notice immediate improvement. It often takes one to four weeks before seeing full benefit. To receive the most benefit from your inhaler, follow the directions on p. 408.

The inhalant predisposes you to fungal infections of the mouth and throat because some of the drug is absorbed when you inhale the dose. Therefore, **after each dose you should rinse out your mouth and gargle with water.** This flushes out the drug that did not go to your lungs and prevents it from being absorbed.

If you are switching from taking systemic medication to the inhalant, **it is important that you do not suddenly stop taking the tablets or injections.** Your body requires a few weeks or months to adjust to the loss of extra corticosteroids and to start making its own again. In the meantime, your doctor will give you a dosage schedule to slowly taper the amount of systemic steroids that you take each day. Failure to follow this schedule and gradually decrease your dosage can result in serious adverse effects, including death.

If you have a severe asthma attack, call your doctor immediately. Do *not* inhale an extra dose of the corticosteroid. The inhalant helps to prevent attacks, but it will not control an attack that has already started. You will need to resume taking systemic steroids if the attack occurs while you are changing from tablets or injections to the inhalant. You should carry a card stating that you may need supplementary steroids during periods of stress or illness. If you are only taking corticosteroids via an inhaler, you may still need stronger therapy to treat mucous plugs that may be present.

DRUG PROFILES

Limited Use

Corticotropin/Adrenocorticotropic Hormone (ACTH)
ACTHAR (Rhone-Poulenc Rorer)
CORTROPHIN-ZINC (Organon)

GENERIC: available

FAMILY: Corticosteroids (see p. 651)

Corticotropin (kor ti koe *troe* pin) and adrenocorticotropic hormone (ACTH) are two names for the same drug. Both of these drugs act in the same way as natural corticotropin, a hormone which is produced by the pituitary gland in your brain. Natural corticotropin signals your adrenal glands, located just above your kidneys, to produce a type of chemical called corticosteroids (see p. 651).

There are a number of conditions—conditions that produce inflammation, such as arthritis, asthma, and some skin and eye conditions, for example—that can be treated effectively with corticosteroids (also just called steroids). Doctors often prescribe the hormone corticotropin (ACTH) instead of steroids for these conditions, since corticotropin stimulates

your body's own production of steroids. However, **you should not take corticotropin for more than three consecutive days.** If you need long term treatment, it is better to take steroids. For treatment lasting three days or less, either corticotropin or steroids may be used, but steroids are much less expensive.

If you need steroids and can take them by mouth, prednisone (see p. 668) is the best drug because it is reliable, inexpensive, and available in a generic form.[1]

Corticotropin is also used to test how well the adrenal glands are functioning. For these tests, it is better to use the newer drug Cortrosyn, a synthetic hormone with fewer harmful adverse effects.

Corticotropin, which is derived from pork products, has caused allergic reactions in some people who have used it.

Before You Use This Drug

Do not use if you have or have had:

- congestive heart failure
- high blood pressure
- herpes simplex infection of the eye
- scleroderma
- osteoporosis
- recent surgery
- an allergy to pork

Tell your doctor if you have or have had:

- allergies to drugs
- AIDS
- heart, liver or kidney problems
- high blood pressure
- diabetes
- inflammation of throat, stomach, or intestines
- glaucoma
- fungal infections
- myasthenia gravis
- tuberculosis or positive TB test

Tell your doctor about any other drugs you take, including aspirin, herbs, vitamins, and other nonprescription products.

When You Use This Drug

• Do not drink alcohol. Drinking alcohol while taking this drug increases your chances of developing an ulcer.

• If you plan to have any surgery, including dental, tell your doctor that you take this drug.

• Eat a diet low in salt and rich in potassium, protein, and folic acid. Ask your doctor to tell you how you can get more potassium, protein, and folic acid in your diet.

How to Use This Drug

• **Do not take more than your doctor has prescribed.**

Interactions with Other Drugs

The following drugs are listed in the *Evaluations of Drug Interactions* 1997 as causing "highly clinically significant" or "clinically significant" interactions when used together with this drug. We have also included potentially serious interactions listed in the drug's FDA-approved professional product labeling or package insert. New scientific techniques have allowed researchers to predict some drug interactions before they have been documented in people. There may be other drugs, especially those in the families of drugs listed below, that also will react with this drug to cause severe adverse effects. The number of new drugs approved for marketing increases the chance of drug interactions, and new drug interactions are being identified with old drugs. Be vigilant. Make sure to tell your doctor and pharmacist the drugs you are taking and tell your doctor if you are taking any of these interacting drugs:

aspirin, GENUINE BAYER ASPIRIN, cyclosporine, dicumarol, DIFLUCAN, ECOTRIN, fluconazole, itraconazole, ketoconazole, NEORAL, NIZORAL, SANDIMMUNE, SPORANOX, timolol, TIMOPTIC.

Adverse Effects

Call your doctor immediately if you experience:

• decreased or blurred vision
• frequent urination
• increased thirst
• numbness, pain, tingling, redness, or swelling at site of injection
• hallucinations
• depression or mood changes
• skin rash or hives

For long-term corticotropin therapy:

• persistent abdominal or stomach pain
• acne or other skin problems
• bloody or black, tarry stools
• rounding out of the face
• hip pain
• increased blood pressure
• swelling of feet or lower legs
• unusual weight gain
• irregular heartbeats
• muscle cramps or pain
• unusual tiredness or weakness
• pain in back, ribs, arms, or legs
• muscle weakness
• nausea or vomiting
• pitting or depression of skin at place of injection
• thin, shiny skin
• unusual bruising
• wounds that will not heal

Call your doctor if these symptoms continue:

• indigestion
• increased appetite
• nervousness or restlessness

- trouble sleeping
- dizziness or lightheadedness
- flushed face
- headache
- increased joint pain
- nosebleeds
- increased body or facial hair

Periodic Tests

Ask your doctor which of these tests should be done periodically while you are taking this drug:

- skin testing for sensitivity to pork products
- blood or urine glucose concentration
- eye exams
- blood levels of potassium, sodium, and calcium
- stool tests for possible blood loss

Triamcinolone
ARISTOCORT (Fujisawa)
KENALOG (Westwood-Squibb)

GENERIC: available
FAMILY: Corticosteroids (see p. 651)

Triamcinolone (trye am *sin* oh lone), like other steroids (corticosteroids), has many uses. It is commonly used to treat inflammation (redness and swelling) and itching caused by certain skin conditions, arthritis and other bone and joint disorders that produce inflammation, and allergies and other breathing problems. In an inhaled form, triamcinolone is used to control asthma that requires regular, long-term use of steroids.

Triamcinolone is available in several forms for different uses. It can be injected into the muscle, joint, lesion, or soft tissue, applied to the skin and mouth (topical form), sprayed into the mouth and inhaled, or taken by mouth as tablets or syrup. You should not use triamcinolone tablets or syrup taken by mouth, because when taken in this form, the drug stays in the body for too long and causes adverse effects. If you need to take steroids by mouth, prednisone (see p. 668) is the best choice because it is reliable, inexpensive, and available in a generic form.[2]

Steroids suppress your immune system, lowering your defenses against disease and making you more vulnerable to infections. If you use triamcinolone for a long time, you increase your risk of getting bacterial, viral, parasitic, and fungal infections. Older adults using triamcinolone are more likely than younger users to develop the bone-weakening condition called osteoporosis. Older users are also more likely to develop high blood pressure and to retain fluid while taking this drug.

As with all drugs, you should use the smallest dose of triamcinolone that works. You should also use it for the shortest possible time. If you use systemic steroids (ones that are taken by mouth or injected so that your whole body is exposed to them) for a long time, you may suffer many adverse effects, and you may also suffer withdrawal symptoms if you stop abruptly.

Before You Use This Drug

Do not use if you have or have had:

For injections into the joint:

- blood clotting disorders
- fracture of the joint
- infection around the joint
- joint surgery
- osteoporosis
- unstable joint

Tell your doctor if you have or have had:

- allergies to drugs
- AIDS
- bone disease
- chicken pox
- measles
- colitis

- diverticulitis
- stomach ulcer
- diabetes
- fungus infection
- herpes eye infection
- recent surgery or serious injury
- tuberculosis
- glaucoma
- heart disease
- high blood pressure
- liver disease
- thyroid problems
- myasthenia gravis
- systemic lupus (SLE)

For skin preparations:

- infection or ulceration at place where you will be applying the drug

Tell your doctor about any other drugs you take, including aspirin, herbs, vitamins, and other nonprescription products.

When You Use This Drug

For long-term use, if you take the drug by mouth or injection:

- **Do not stop taking this drug suddenly.** Your doctor must lower your dose gradually to prevent withdrawal symptoms.
- If you plan to have any surgery, including dental, tell your doctor that you take this drug.

If you are using the inhaled aerosol spray:

- Wear a medical identification bracelet or carry a card stating that you may need additional steroids (tablets or injection) in times of unusual stress or sudden, severe asthma attack.

How to Use This Drug

- **Use only as prescribed.**
- If you miss a dose, take it as soon as you remember, but skip it if it is almost time for the next dose. **Do not take double doses.**

- Do not store in the bathroom. Do not expose to heat, moisture, or strong light.

On your skin:

- The preparation may sting when applied.
- Keep away from eyes.
- Apply cream or ointment with cotton applicator. Do not bandage or wrap the area being treated unless your doctor has told you to do so.
- If you use the drug correctly, there is no danger that it will be absorbed into your system.

In your mouth:

- Apply with cotton applicator by pressing (not rubbing) paste on the sore.
- Check with your doctor or dentist if your condition does not improve in one week or if it worsens.
- See p. 651 for information about the spray.

Interactions with Other Drugs

The following drugs are listed in the *Evaluations of Drug Interactions* 1997 as causing "highly clinically significant" or "clinically significant" interactions when used together with this drug. We have also included potentially serious interactions listed in the drug's FDA-approved professional product labeling or package insert. New scientific techniques have allowed researchers to predict some drug interactions before they have been documented in people. There may be other drugs, especially those in the families of drugs listed below, that also will react with this drug to cause severe adverse effects. The number of new drugs approved for marketing increases the chance of drug interactions, and new drug interactions are being identified with old drugs. Be vigilant. Make sure to tell your doctor and pharmacist the drugs you are taking and tell your doctor if you are taking any of these interacting drugs:

aspirin, GENUINE BAYER ASPIRIN, chlorpropamide, DIABINESE, dicumarol, DILANTIN, ECOTRIN, LUMINAL, phenobarbital, phenytoin, RIFADIN, rifampin, RIMACTANE, SOLFOTON, timolol, TIMOPTIC.

Adverse Effects

Call your doctor immediately if you experience:

- numbness, pain, tingling, redness, or swelling at place of injection
- hallucinations
- depression or mood changes
- skin rash or hives
- confusion
- excitement, restlessness, or nervousness
- vision changes
- frequent urination
- increased thirst

If using inhaled form:

- trouble breathing or pain or tightness in chest
- white patches in mouth or throat and/or pain when eating or swallowing

For long-term use:

- persistent abdominal or stomach pain
- acne or other skin problems
- bloody or black, tarry stools
- rounding out of the face
- hip or shoulder pain
- increased blood pressure
- swelling of feet or lower legs
- unusual weight gain
- irregular heartbeats
- muscle cramps or pain
- unusual tiredness or weakness
- pain in back, ribs, arms, or legs
- muscle weakness
- nausea or vomiting

- pitting or depression of skin at place of injection
- thin, shiny skin
- unusual bruising
- wounds that will not heal
- menstrual irregularities
- reddish, purplish lines on arms, face, legs, trunk or groin

Call your doctor if these symptoms continue:

- increased appetite
- nervousness or restlessness
- trouble sleeping
- dizziness or lightheadedness
- flushed face
- headache
- increased joint pain
- nosebleeds
- increase in hair on body or face
- indigestion
- loss of appetite
- darkening or lightening of skin color
- sweating

If using inhaled form:

- cough
- dry mouth or throat
- hoarseness
- unpleasant taste

Call your doctor immediately if these symptoms occur after you stop taking this drug:

- abdominal or back pain
- dizziness or fainting
- low grade fever
- persistent loss of appetite
- muscle or joint pain
- nausea or vomiting
- returning symptoms of the condition for which you were taking the drug
- shortness of breath
- frequent unexplained headaches
- unusual tiredness or weakness
- unusual weight loss

Periodic Tests

Ask your doctor which of these tests should be done periodically while you are taking this drug:

- blood or urine glucose concentration
- eye exams
- stool tests
- serum electrolyte determination
- growth and development determinations
- hypothalamus and pituitary secretion tests

PREGNANCY WARNING

This drug caused harm to developing fetuses in animal studies, or such studies were not done. Use during pregnancy only for clear medical reasons. Tell your doctor if you are pregnant or thinking of becoming pregnant before you take this drug.

 Do Not Use

ALTERNATIVE TREATMENT:
Estrogen plus medroxyprogesterone (see p. 714), alendronate (see p. 687).

Calcitonin (Calcitonin-Salmon, Calcitonin-Human)
CALCIMAR Injection (Rhone-Poulenc Rorer)
MIACALCIN Injection (Novartis)
MIACALCIN Nasal Spray (Novartis)

GENERIC: not available
FAMILY: Osteoporosis Drugs

Calcitonin (kal si *toe* nin) is a hormone produced by thyroid glands of mammals and fish. Synthetic forms have been made of the hormones from humans, pigs, salmon, and eels. Calcitonin is used to treat moderate to severe Paget's disease, high levels of calcium in the blood (such as occur with cancer), and osteoporosis in women five years or more after menopause. Calcitonin prevents further bone loss of the spine, and modestly increases bone density, when taken with adequate amounts of calcium and vitamin D.

Though calcitonin-salmon has a modest effect on bone loss and bone density, neither the nasal spray nor the injection has been shown to reduce the risk of fractures in postmenopausal women with osteoporosis. Calcitonin-salmon nasal spray was approved because it was shown in two studies—with a combined total of 325 women five years or more after menopause with severe osteoporosis—to increase bone mineral content or density (bone building effect) in the vertebrae of the back by 2% to 3% compared with women using an inactive placebo (nasal spray without calcitonin). This bone building effect was not seen in the forearms or hips of the women in the study.[3]

The goal of treating women with osteoporosis should be to reduce their risk of fracture—not just to build bone density. After being on the market for more than 20 years, we still do not know if the bone building effect of calcitonin-salmon reduces the risk of fracture. To gain FDA approval for calcitonin-salmon nasal spray, the manufacturer had to promise to conduct additional clinical trials to evaluate the drug's long-term effectiveness in preventing fractures. The manufacturer is conducting a five-year study designed to answer this question but the results have not been published.

WHAT YOU CAN DO TO PREVENT OSTEOPOROSIS

DIET AND EXERCISE

Many women are not at risk of developing hip or other types of fractures. Women who are thin or small-boned, particularly if they are Asian or white, and women who drink more than two alcoholic drinks per day are at higher risk of osteoporosis. Black women, heavy women and women who get lots of exercise are at a lower risk. There are steps women can take to prevent osteoporosis; for instance, a lot of calcium in the diet from early adulthood and "weight bearing" exercise such as jogging, walking, tennis and bicycling. You should be receiving from 800 to 1,200 milligrams of calcium per day in your diet depending on your age. Women who are postmenopausal require an average of 1,500 milligrams per day of calcium. These two steps are enough to prevent osteoporosis in many adults.

THINGS YOU CAN DO TO PREVENT FALLS

Falls, of course, will increase your chances of a fracture. Ask your doctor to review your continued need for and dose of any drug which causes you to be dizzy or drowsy. Check p. 27 for drugs that can cause falls. Check your home for situations that can lead to falls such as areas that are not well lighted or loose rugs on hardwood floors.

Hydrocortisone
CORTEF (Pharmacia & Upjohn)

GENERIC: available
FAMILY: Corticosteroids (see p. 651)

Hydrocortisone (hye droe *kor* ti sone), like other steroids (corticosteroids), has many uses. It is commonly used to treat skin conditions, eye infections, and arthritis and other disorders that produce inflammation. It is also used to treat allergies and other breathing problems.

Hydrocortisone is available in several forms for different uses. It can be taken by mouth (oral form). It can be injected into the muscle, joint, lesion, soft tissue, or bloodstream. It can be applied to the skin (topical form) in one of two strengths available without a prescription, 0.25% and 0.50%. It can be applied to the eye (ophthalmic form) or ear (otic form), although it is preferable to see your doctor rather than getting the over-the-counter eye preparation. It is also available as a dental paste and as a rectal suppository or ointment.

You should not use the form of hydrocortisone taken by mouth. If you need to take a steroid by mouth, prednisone (see p. 668) is the best choice because it is reliable, inexpensive, and available in a generic form.[4] You also should not use the weaker (0.25%) form of hydrocortisone applied to the skin, because it is ineffective.

Steroids suppress your immune system, lowering your defenses against disease and making you more vulnerable to infections. If you use hydrocortisone for a long time, you increase your risk of getting bacterial, viral, parasitic, and fungal infections. Older adults using hydrocortisone are more likely than younger users to develop the bone-weakening condition called osteoporosis. Older users are also more likely to develop high blood pressure and to retain fluid while taking this drug.

As with all drugs, you should use the smallest dose of hydrocortisone that works. You should also use it for the shortest possible time. If you use systemic steroids (ones that are taken by mouth or injected so that your whole body is exposed to them) for a long time, you may suffer many adverse effects, and you may also suffer withdrawal symptoms if you stop abruptly.

Before You Use This Drug

Do not use if you have or have had:

- bone disease
- colitis
- stomach ulcer
- fungus infection
- herpes eye infection
- recent surgery or serious injury

Tell your doctor if you have or have had:

- allergies to drugs, particularly other hydrocortisone-containing drugs[5]
- AIDS
- heart, liver, or kidney problems
- high blood pressure
- diabetes
- inflammation of throat, stomach, or intestines
- glaucoma
- fungal, viral, or bacterial infections
- myasthenia gravis
- herpes sores
- tuberculosis or positive TB skin test
- chicken pox or measles, present or recent
- systemic lupus (SLE)
- thyroid problems

For topical form:

- infection or ulceration at the place where you will be applying the drug

Tell your doctor about any other drugs you take, including aspirin, herbs, vitamins, and other nonprescription products.

When You Use This Drug

- If you plan to have any surgery, including dental, tell your doctor that you take this drug.

How to Use This Drug

- **Use only as prescribed.**
- If you miss a dose, take it as soon as you remember, but skip it if it is almost time for the next dose. **Do not take double doses.**
- Do not store in the bathroom. Do not expose to heat, moisture, or strong light.

On your skin:

- The preparation may sting when applied.
- Keep away from eyes.
- Do not bandage or wrap the area you are treating unless your doctor has told you to do so.
- If you use the drug correctly, there is no danger that it will be absorbed into your system.

In your mouth:

- Apply with cotton applicator by pressing (not rubbing) paste on the sore.
- Check with your doctor or dentist if your condition does not improve within one week or if it worsens.

Interactions with Other Drugs

The following drugs are listed in the *Evaluations of Drug Interactions* 1997 as causing "highly clinically significant" or "clinically significant" interactions when used together with this drug. We have also included potentially serious interactions listed in the drug's FDA-approved professional product labeling or package insert. New scientific techniques have allowed researchers to predict some drug interactions before they have been documented in people. There may be other drugs, especially those in the families of drugs listed below, that also will react with this drug to cause severe adverse effects. The number of new drugs approved for marketing increases the chance of drug interactions, and new drug interactions are being identified with old drugs. Be vigilant. Make sure to tell your doctor and pharmacist the drugs you are taking and tell your doctor if you are taking any of these interacting drugs:

aspirin, GENUINE BAYER ASPIRIN, chlorpropamide, cyclosporine, DIABINESE,

dicumarol, DILANTIN, ECOTRIN,
LUMINAL, NEORAL, phenobarbital,
phenytoin, SANDIMMUNE, SOLFOTON,
timolol, TIMOPTIC.

Adverse Effects

Call your doctor immediately if you experience:

- decreased or blurred vision or eye infection
- frequent urination
- increased thirst
- rectal bleeding, burning, itching
- numbness, pain, tingling, redness, or swelling at site of injection
- hallucinations
- depression or mood changes
- skin rash, hives, pain or blistering
- confusion
- excitement or restlessnes

For long-term use:

- persistent abdominal or stomach pain
- acne or other skin problems
- bloody or black, tarry stools
- rounding out of the face
- hip or shoulder pain
- increased blood pressure
- swelling of feet or lower legs
- unusual weight gain
- irregular heartbeats
- muscle cramps or pain
- unusual tiredness or weakness
- pain in back, ribs, arms, or legs
- muscle weakness
- nausea or vomiting
- pitting or depression of skin at place of injection
- thin, shiny skin
- unusual bruising
- wounds that will not heal
- menstrual irregularities
- reddish, purplish lines on arms, face, legs, trunk or groin

Call your doctor if these symptoms continue:

- indigestion
- increased appetite
- nervousness or restlessness
- trouble sleeping
- dizziness or lightheadedness
- flushed face
- headache
- increased joint pain
- nosebleeds
- increase in hair on body or face
- loss of appetite
- darkening or lightening of skin color
- sweating

Call your doctor immediately if these symptoms occur after you stop taking this drug:

- abdominal or back pain
- dizziness or fainting
- low grade fever
- persistent loss of appetite
- muscle or joint pain
- nausea or vomiting
- returning symptoms of the condition for which you were taking the drug
- shortness of breath
- frequent unexplained headaches
- unusual tiredness or weakness
- unusual weight loss

Periodic Tests

Ask your doctor which of these tests should be done periodically while you are taking this drug:

- blood or urine glucose concentration
- eye exams
- blood levels of potassium, sodium, and calcium
- stool tests
- hypothalamus and pituitary secretion tests
- growth and development determinations

```
┌─────────────────────────────────────────┐
│        PREGNANCY WARNING                  │
│  ─────────────────────────────────────   │
│   This drug caused harm to developing     │
│  fetuses in animal studies, or such       │
│  studies were not done. Use during        │
│  pregnancy only for clear medical rea-    │
│  sons. Tell your doctor if you are        │
│  pregnant or thinking of becoming         │
│  pregnant before you take this drug.      │
│                                           │
└─────────────────────────────────────────┘
```

Limited Use

Cyclophosphamide
CYTOXAN (Bristol-Meyers Squibb)
NEOSAR (Pharmacia & Upjohn)

GENERIC: available

FAMILY: Anticancer Drugs
Arthritis Drugs (see p. 265)

Cyclophosphamide (sye kloe *foss* fa mide) is used mainly to treat certain kinds of cancer. It is also used to treat some conditions that produce inflammation (redness, swelling, heat, or pain), such as rheumatoid arthritis (see p. 265) and systemic lupus erythematosus. This profile primarily discusses cyclophosphamide's use for conditions causing inflammation.

Cyclophosphamide should be used to treat only the most severe cases of rheumatoid arthritis that have not responded to the progressive use of other drugs for inflammation, such as aspirin, ibuprofen, gold salts (see p. 329), and penicillamine. Cyclophosphamide is the drug of last resort for rheumatoid arthritis because it has serious adverse effects, including nausea, vomiting, loss of appetite, blood problems, hair loss, and heart and lung problems. It can also cause other harmful effects such as leukemia and bladder cancer months or years after you stop taking it.

If you are taking cyclophosphamide and an adverse effect is disturbing you, ask your doctor or other health professional to suggest ways to avoid or decrease the problem. Be aware, however, that some adverse effects are unavoidable, and that some, in fact, are used to tell whether the drug is working.

Before You Use This Drug

Do not use if you have or have had:

- recent infection or exposure to chicken pox
- shingles (herpes zoster)

Tell your doctor if you have or have had:

- allergies to drugs
- loss of the adrenal glands
- bone marrow depression or tumor cell infiltration
- kidney stones
- kidney or liver problems
- recent infection
- gout

Tell your doctor about any other drugs you take, including aspirin, herbs, vitamins, and other nonprescription products.

When You Use This Drug

- **Do not use more or less often or in a higher or lower dose than prescribed.** Check with your doctor before you stop using this drug.
- **Check with your doctor to make certain your fluid intake is adequate and appropriate.**
- **Because this drug decreases the number of white blood cells, which fight infection, you are more likely to get an infection. Do not get immunizations without your doctor's approval.**
- Schedule regular visits with your doctor to check your progress.
- If you plan to have any surgery, including dental, tell your doctor that you take this drug.

How to Use This Drug

- To reduce stomach upset, your doctor may want you to take smaller doses throughout the day.
- Do not store in the bathroom. Do not expose to heat, moisture, or strong light. Do not allow liquid form to freeze.
- Call your doctor for instructions if you miss a dose or vomit shortly after taking the drug. **Do not take double doses.**

Interactions with Other Drugs

The following drugs are listed in the *Evaluations of Drug Interactions* 1997 as causing "highly clinically significant" or "clinically significant" interactions when used together with this drug. We have also included potentially serious interactions listed in the drug's FDA-approved professional product labeling or package insert. New scientific techniques have allowed researchers to predict some drug interactions before they have been documented in people. There may be other drugs, especially those in the families of drugs listed below, that also will react with this drug to cause severe adverse effects. The number of new drugs approved for marketing increases the chance of drug interactions, and new drug interactions are being identified with old drugs. Be vigilant. Make sure to tell your doctor and pharmacist the drugs you are taking and tell your doctor if you are taking any of these interacting drugs:

allopurinol, ANECTINE, chloramphenicol, CHLOROMYCETIN, COUMADIN, digoxin, LANOXICAPS, LANOXIN, succinylcholine, warfarin, ZYLOPRIM.

Adverse Effects

Call your doctor immediately if you experience:

- fever, chills, or sore throat
- confusion or agitation
- dizziness, tiredness, or weakness
- blood in urine
- painful or frequent urination
- cough or shortness of breath
- unusually fast heartbeat
- flank or stomach pain
- swelling of feet or lower legs
- joint pain
- unusual bleeding or bruising
- bloody or black, tarry stools
- sores in mouth or on lips
- unusual thirst
- yellow eyes and skin
- lower back or stomach pain
- pinpoint redspots on skin
- skipped menstrual period
- redness, swelling or pain at site of injection

Call your doctor if these symptoms continue:

- hair loss
- nausea, vomiting, appetite loss
- darkening of skin and fingernails
- flushed or red face
- headache
- rash, hives, or itching
- swollen lips
- increased sweating
- diarrhea

Call your doctor if these symptoms continue once you've stopped taking the drug:

- blood in urine

Periodic Tests

Ask your doctor which of these tests should be done periodically while you are taking this drug:

- kidney function tests
- liver function tests
- urine tests
- complete blood tests (including hematocrit, platelet count, white blood cell count)

PREGNANCY WARNING

This drug caused harm to developing fetuses in animal studies, or such studies were not done. Use during pregnancy only for clear medical reasons. Tell your doctor if you are pregnant or thinking of becoming pregnant before you take this drug.

Dexamethasone
DECADRON (Merck)
HEXADROL (Organon)

GENERIC: available
FAMILY: Corticosteroids (see p. 651)

Dexamethasone (dex a *meth* a sone), like other steroids (corticosteroids), has several uses and dosage forms. It can be taken by mouth to treat some types of cancer, to reduce swelling in the brain, and to help doctors diagnose a hormonal condition or depression. It can also be injected into the muscle, joint, lesion, soft tissue, and bloodstream, applied to the skin (topical form), eye (ophthalmic form), or ear (otic form), or sprayed into the nose or mouth. These forms are used to treat conditions that produce inflammation, such as arthritis and other joint and muscle disorders, allergies, hay fever, and other breathing problems, skin infections, and eye infections.

If you need to take a hormone by mouth, prednisone (see p. 668) is the best choice because it is reliable, inexpensive, and available in a generic form.[6]

Steroids suppress your immune system, lowering your defenses against disease and making you more vulnerable to infections. If you use dexamethasone for a long time, you increase your risk of getting bacterial, viral, parasitic, and fungal infections. Older adults using dexamethasone are more likely than younger users to develop the bone-weakening condition called osteoporosis. Older users are also more likely to develop high blood pressure and to retain fluid while taking this drug.

As with all drugs, you should use the smallest dose of dexamethasone that works. You should also use it for the shortest possible time. If you use systemic steroids (ones that are taken by mouth or injected so that your whole body is exposed to them) for a long time, you may suffer many adverse effects, and you may also suffer withdrawal symptoms if you stop abruptly.

Before You Use This Drug

Do not use if you have or have had:

For injections into the joint:

- joint surgery
- blood clotting disorders
- fracture of the joint
- osteoporosis
- infection around the joint
- unstable joint

For eye dosage form:

- eye infections such as tuberculosis, herpes simplex, or other fungal or viral diseases

Tell your doctor if you have or have had:

- allergies to drugs
- AIDS
- bone disease
- chicken pox
- measles
- colitis
- diverticulitis
- stomach ulcer
- diabetes
- fungus infection
- herpes eye infection
- recent surgery or serious injury
- tuberculosis
- glaucoma
- heart disease

- high blood pressure
- liver disease
- thyroid problems
- myasthenia gravis
- systemic lupus (SLE)

Tell your doctor about any other drugs you take, including aspirin, herbs, vitamins, and other nonprescription products.

When You Use This Drug

If taken by mouth or injection:

- **If you have been taking this drug for a long time, do not stop taking it suddenly.** Your doctor must lower your dose gradually to prevent withdrawal symptoms.
- Do not drink alcohol. Drinking alcohol when you are using this drug increases your chances of getting an ulcer.
- If you plan to have any surgery, including dental, tell your doctor that you take this drug.
- Avoid becoming constipated.[7] See ways to avoid constipation on p. 380.
- If you are taking this drug for a long time, eat a diet low in salt and rich in potassium, protein, and folic acid. Ask your doctor to tell you how you can get more potassium, protein and folic acid in your diet.

If you are using nose or mouth sprays:

- Wear a medical identification bracelet or carry a card stating that you may need additional steroids (tablets or injection) in times of unusual stress or sudden, severe asthma attack.

How to Use This Drug

- Crush tablet and mix with food or water, or swallow whole with water. Take with food to decrease stomach upset.
- **Use only as prescribed.**
- If you miss a dose, take it as soon as you remember, but skip it if it is almost time for the next dose. **Do not take double doses.**

- Do not store in the bathroom. Do not expose to heat, moisture, or strong light.
- See p. 651 for information on inhaled mouth and nose sprays.

For eye, ear, skin dosage forms:

- Check with your doctor if your condition does not improve in one week, or if it worsens.

Interactions with Other Drugs

The following drugs are listed in the *Evaluations of Drug Interactions* 1997 as causing "highly clinically significant" or "clinically significant" interactions when used together with this drug. We have also included potentially serious interactions listed in the drug's FDA-approved professional product labeling or package insert. New scientific techniques have allowed researchers to predict some drug interactions before they have been documented in people. There may be other drugs, especially those in the families of drugs listed below, that also will react with this drug to cause severe adverse effects. The number of new drugs approved for marketing increases the chance of drug interactions, and new drug interactions are being identified with old drugs. Be vigilant. Make sure to tell your doctor and pharmacist the drugs you are taking and tell your doctor if you are taking any of these interacting drugs:

aldesleukin/interleukin-2, aminoglutethimide, aspirin, GENUINE BAYER ASPIRIN, carbamazepine, chlorpropamide, cyclosporine, CYTADREN, DIABINESE, dicumarol, DILANTIN, ECOTRIN, ketoconazole, LUMINAL, NEORAL, NIZORAL, phenobarbital, phenytoin, PROLEUKIN, RIFADIN, rifampin, RIMACTANE, SANDIMMUNE, SOLFOTON, TAO, TEGRETOL, timolol, TIMOPTIC, troleandomycin.

Adverse Effects

Call your doctor immediately if you experience:

- decreased or blurred vision
- frequent urination
- increased thirst
- numbness, pain, tingling, redness, or swelling at site of injection
- hallucinations
- depression or mood changes
- skin rash, hives, pain or blistering
- muscle weakness
- confusion
- excitement or restlessness

If using eye dosage form:

- blurred vision
- eye pain
- headache
- seeing halos around lights
- drooping of the eyelids
- unusually large pupils

If using inhaled form:

- trouble breathing or pain or tightness in chest
- white patches in mouth or throat and/or pain when eating or swallowing

For long-term use:

- persistent abdominal or stomach pain
- acne or other skin problems
- bloody or black, tarry stools
- rounding out of the face
- hip or shoulder pain
- increased blood pressure
- swelling of feet or lower legs
- unusual weight gain
- irregular heartbeat
- muscle cramps or pain
- unusual tiredness or weakness
- pain in back, ribs, arms, or legs
- muscle weakness
- nausea or vomiting

- pitting or depression of skin at place of injection
- thin, shiny skin
- unusual bruising
- wounds that will not heal
- menstrual irregularities
- reddish, purplish lines on arms, face, legs, trunk or groin

Call your doctor if these symptoms continue:

- indigestion
- increased appetite
- nervousness or restlessness
- trouble sleeping
- dizziness or lightheadedness
- flushed face
- increased joint pain
- nosebleeds
- increase in hair on body or face
- loss of appetite
- darkening or lightening of skin color
- sweating

If using inhaled form:

- cough
- dry mouth or throat
- hoarseness
- unpleasant taste

Call your doctor immediately if these symptoms occur after you have stopped taking this drug:

- abdominal or back pain
- dizziness or fainting
- low grade fever
- persistent loss of appetite
- muscle or joint pain
- nausea or vomiting
- returning symptoms of the condition for which you were taking the drug
- shortness of breath
- frequent unexplained headaches
- unusual tiredness or weakness
- unusual weight loss

Periodic Tests

Ask your doctor which of these tests should be done periodically while you are taking this drug:

- blood or urine glucose concentration
- eye exams
- blood levels of potassium, sodium, and calcium
- stool tests for possible blood loss
- hypothalamus and pituitary secretion tests
- growth and development determinations

PREGNANCY WARNING

This drug caused harm to developing fetuses in animal studies, or such studies were not done. Use during pregnancy only for clear medical reasons. Tell your doctor if you are pregnant or thinking of becoming pregnant before you take this drug.

Prednisone
DELTASONE (Pharmacia & Upjohn)
METICORTEN (Schering)

GENERIC: available
FAMILY: Corticosteroids (see p. 651)

Prednisone (*pred* ni sone), like other steroids (corticosteroids), has many uses. It is used to treat asthma, bronchitis, allergies, and other breathing problems, conditions that produce inflammation, such as arthritis and other joint and muscle disorders, skin conditions, and certain kinds of cancer and infections. If you can take a steroid by mouth, prednisone is the drug of choice because it is reliable, inexpensive, and available in a generic form.[8]

Steroids suppress your immune system, lowering your defenses against disease and making you more vulnerable to infections. If you use prednisone for a long time, you increase your risk of getting bacterial, viral, parasitic, and fungal infections. Older adults using prednisone are more likely than younger users to develop the bone-weakening condition called osteoporosis even with short-term use or low doses.[9] Older users are also more likely to develop high blood pressure and to retain fluid while taking this drug.

As with all drugs, you should use the smallest dose of prednisone that works. You should also use it for the shortest possible time. If you use systemic steroids (ones that are taken by mouth or injected so that your whole body is exposed to them) for a long time, you may suffer many adverse effects, and you may also suffer withdrawal symptoms if you stop abruptly.

Before You Use This Drug

Tell your doctor if you have or have had:

- allergies to drugs
- AIDS
- bone disease
- chicken pox
- measles
- colitis
- diverticulitis
- stomach ulcer
- diabetes
- fungus infection
- herpes eye infection
- recent surgery or serious injury
- tuberculosis
- glaucoma
- heart disease
- high blood pressure
- liver disease
- thyroid problems
- myasthenia gravis
- systemic lupus (SLE)

Tell your doctor about any other drugs you take, including aspirin, herbs, vitamins, and other nonprescription products.

When You Use This Drug

- **If you have been using this drug for a long time, do not stop taking it suddenly.** Your doctor must lower your dose gradually, to prevent withdrawal symptoms.
- Do not drink alcohol. Drinking alcohol while taking this drug increases your risk of getting an ulcer.
- If you plan to have any surgery, including dental, tell your doctor that you take this drug.
- Eat a diet low in salt and rich in potassium, protein, and folic acid. Ask your doctor to tell you how you can get more potassium, protein, and folic acid in your diet.

How to Use This Drug

- Crush tablet and mix with food or water, or swallow whole with water. Take with food to decrease stomach upset.
- **Do not take more than prescribed.**
- If you miss a dose, take it as soon as you remember, but skip it if it is almost time for the next dose. **Do not take double doses.**
- Do not store in the bathroom. Do not expose to heat, moisture, or strong light.

Interactions with Other Drugs

The following drugs are listed in the *Evaluations of Drug Interactions* 1997 as causing "highly clinically significant" or "clinically significant" interactions when used together with this drug. We have also included potentially serious interactions listed in the drug's FDA-approved professional product labeling or package insert. New scientific techniques have allowed researchers to predict some drug interactions before they have been documented in people. There may be other drugs, especially those in the families of drugs listed below, that also will react with this drug to cause severe adverse effects. The number of new drugs approved for marketing increases the chance of drug interactions, and new drug interactions are being identified with old drugs. Be vigilant. Make sure to tell your doctor and pharmacist the drugs you are taking and tell your doctor if you are taking any of these interacting drugs:

aspirin, GENUINE BAYER ASPIRIN, chlorpropamide, cyclosporine, DIABINESE, dicumarol, digoxin, DILANTIN, ECOTRIN, ketoconazole, LANOXICAPS, LANOXIN, LUMINAL, NEORAL, NIZORAL, phenobarbital, phenytoin, RIFADIN, rifampin, RIMACTANE, SANDIMMUNE, SOLFOTON, TAO, timolol, TIMOPTIC, troleandomycin.

Adverse Effects

Call your doctor immediately if you experience:

- decreased or blurred vision
- frequent urination
- increased thirst
- hallucinations
- depression or mood changes
- skin rash or hives
- confusion
- excitement or restlessness

For long-term use:

- persistent abdominal or stomach pain
- acne or other skin problems
- bloody or black, tarry stools
- rounding out of the face
- hip or shoulder pain
- increased blood pressure
- swelling of feet or lower legs
- unusual weight gain
- irregular heartbeat
- muscle cramps or pain
- unusual tiredness or weakness
- pain in back, ribs, arms, or legs
- muscle weakness
- nausea or vomiting
- thin, shiny skin
- unusual bruising

- wounds that will not heal
- menstrual irregularities
- reddish, purplish lines on arms, face, legs, trunk or groin

Call your doctor if these symptoms continue:

- euphoria[10]
- depression[11]
- indigestion
- increased appetite
- nervousness or restlessness
- trouble sleeping
- dizziness or lightheadedness
- flushed face
- headache
- increased joint pain
- nosebleeds
- increase in hair on body or face
- loss of appetite
- darkening or lightening of skin color
- sweating

Call your doctor immediately if these symptoms occur after you stop taking this drug:

- abdominal or back pain
- dizziness or fainting
- low grade fever
- persistent loss of appetite
- muscle or joint pain
- nausea or vomiting
- returning symptoms of the condition for which you were taking the drug
- shortness of breath
- frequent unexplained headaches
- unusual tiredness or weakness
- unusual weight loss

Periodic Tests

Ask your doctor which of these tests should be done periodically while you are taking this drug:

- blood or urine glucose concentration
- eye exams

- blood levels of potassium, sodium, and calcium
- stool tests for possible blood loss
- hypothalamus and pituitary secretion test
- growth and development determinations

Ethynodiol diacetate/Ethinyl estradiol
DEMULEN (Searle)

GENERIC: not available
FAMILY: Oral contraceptives

Cigarette smoking increases the risk of serious cardiovascular adverse effects from oral contraceptive use. This risk increases with age and with heavy smoking (15 or more cigarettes per day) and is quite marked in women over 35 years of age. Women who use oral contraceptives are strongly advised not to smoke.

Are birth control pills the safest contraceptive option for you? There are many issues to consider, and like every other decision concerning your health, this is a highly individual one. Unfortunately, you will not be able to base your decision on assurances of absolute safety. In fact, even after 40 years of studying the pill, much about its long-term effect on human physiology is still unknown.

Although the convenience of the pill is obvious from the start, its problems are also evident. Many women suffer from headaches, bloating, nausea, irregular bleeding, breast tenderness, weight gain, or optical changes. Other unpleasant effects that can occur from a few months to a few years after starting oral contraceptive use include high blood pressure, gallbladder disease, liver tumors, depression, and metabolic disorders, such as diabetes. Temporary infertility has been associated with the period of time right after pill use is stopped.

But the long-term risks—which you should also consider—are still not fully known. True, oral contraceptives have come a long way since the early days—the 1960s and 1970s—when women were first given hormone doses so potent that heart attacks and strokes were not unusual among pill users. With hormone levels in the pill now much lower, the number of women suffering from heart attacks and strokes also appears to have dropped.

Today's pill is clearly safer in many respects. When used properly, it prevents pregnancy 98% of the time, and its unwanted clotting properties have been significantly reduced. But serious questions remain concerning the pill's relationship to breast cancer.[12]

Before You Use This Drug

Tell your doctor if you have or have had:

- known or suspected cancer of the breast
- cancer of the cervix or endometrium (the lining of the uterus)
- jaundice (yellowing of the skin or eyeballs) during pregnancy or with prior use of birth control pills
  - tumors or cancer of the liver
  - a pregnancy
  - a past history of blood clots
  - diabetes
  - elevated cholesterol or triglycerides
  - high blood pressure
  - migraine headache or epilepsy
  - mental depression
  - gallbladder problems
  - heart or kidney disease
  - history of irregular menstrual periods
  - fibroid tumors of the uterus

Tell your doctor about any other drugs you take, including aspirin, herbs, vitamins, and other nonprescription products.

When You Use This Drug

- You should receive regular check–ups by your doctor.
- If you miss taking a pill follow the directions in the FDA-approved patient information leaflet that you should receive from your pharmacist each time you get a prescription for birth control pills. This information will tell you what to do and when to use a back-up method of contraception.
- If you plan to have any surgery, including dental, tell your doctor that you take this drug.

How to Use This Drug

- Your pharmacist is required to dispense an FDA-approved patient information leaflet each time you receive a prescription for an oral contraceptive. Since the many different brands of oral contraceptives vary in the number of tablets taken per month and the colors of the pills, consult this information before starting to take your pills. Make sure you are receiving the FDA-approved information for the brand of birth control pills you are taking and not the printout from the pharmacist's computer system.
- Do not store in the bathroom. Do not expose to heat, moisture, or strong light.

Interactions with Other Drugs

The following drugs are listed in the *Evaluations of Drug Interactions* 1997 as causing "highly clinically significant" or "clinically significant" interactions when used together with this drug. We have also included potentially serious interactions listed in the drug's FDA-approved professional product labeling or package insert. New scientific techniques have allowed researchers to predict some drug interactions before they have been documented in people. There may be other drugs, especially those in the families of drugs listed below, that also will react with this drug to cause severe adverse effects. The number of new drugs approved for marketing increases the chance of drug interactions, and new drug interactions are being identified with old drugs. Be vigilant. Make sure to tell your doctor and pharmacist the drugs you are taking and tell your doctor if you are taking any of these interacting drugs:

> Certain drugs may interact with birth control pills to make them less effective in preventing pregnancy or cause an increase in breakthrough bleeding. Such drugs include rifampin (RIFADIN, RIMACTANE and generics), drugs used for seizures such as barbiturates (for example phenobarbital [LUMINAL, SOLFOTON]), anticonvulsants such as carbamazepine (TEGRETOL and generics), and phenytoin (DILANTIN and generics), and possibly other antibiotics. You may need to use additional contraception when you take these drugs.

Adverse Effects

Call your doctor immediately if you experience:

- chest pain
- coughing up blood
- sudden shortness of breath
- pain in the calf or groin
- severe and sudden headache
- vomiting
- dizziness or fainting
- slurring of speech
- weakness, or numbness in arms or legs
- partial or complete loss of vision.
- lumps in breast if you have a history of breast disease
- severe pain or tenderness in the stomach area
- insomnia
- abnormal weakness
- mood changes

- yellowing of the skin or eyeballs, accompanied frequently by fever, fatigue, loss of appetite, dark colored urine, or light brown colored bowel movements.
- loss of coordination
- changes in menstrual bleeding
- increased blood pressure
- vaginal infection
- fainting, nausea, pale skin or sweating if you have diabetes
- depression

Call your doctor if these symptoms continue:

- abdominal cramping or bloating
- acne
- breast pain, tenderness or swelling
- swelling of ankles or feet
- unusual tiredness or weakness
- vomiting
- brown, blotchy spots on skin
- gain or loss of body or facial hair
- weight gain or loss
- increased sensitivity to sun

Periodic Tests

Ask your doctor which of these tests should be done periodically while you are taking this drug:

- blood pressure
- liver function determinations
- pap smear
- glucose, lipid and lipoprotein serum levels
- FSH levels

PREGNANCY WARNING

This drug caused harm to developing fetuses in animal studies, or such studies were not done. Use during pregnancy only for clear medical reasons. Tell your doctor if you are pregnant or thinking of becoming pregnant before you take this drug.

Do Not Use

ALTERNATIVE TREATMENT:
Second generation oral contraceptives (see p. 689).

Desogestrel/Ethinyl Estradiol
DESOGEN (Organon)
ORTHO-CEPT (Ortho-McNeil Pharmaceutical)

FAMILY: Oral contraceptives (third generation)

Cigarette smoking increases the risk of serious cardiovascular adverse effects from oral contraceptive use. This risk increases with age and with heavy smoking (15 or more cigarettes per day) and is quite marked in women over 35 years of age. Women who use oral contraceptives are strongly advised not to smoke.

A bitter scientific debate has raged since late 1995 and early 1996 when four observational studies were published, showing that the risk of blood clots, or deep venous thrombosis, with "third generation" oral contraceptives is two times higher than with "second generation" birth control pills (see p. 689).

Combination oral contraceptives contain the hormones estrogen and progestin. These pills are classified as "second" or "third" generation based on their progestin component. Two third generation brands are available in the U.S., Ortho-Cept, produced by Ortho-McNeil Pharmaceuticals of Raritan NJ, and Desogen, sold by Organon Incorporated of West Orange NJ. Both drugs are exactly the same containing 0.15 milligrams of the progestin desogestrel and 0.03 milligrams of the estrogen ethinyl estradiol. "Second generation" contraceptives contain the progestins norgestrel, levonorgestrel and norethindrone.

A worldwide study conducted by the World Health Organization (WHO) and published in late 1995 found that the third generation oral contraceptives containing the progestins desogestrel and gestodene (this progestin is not available in the U.S.) were associated with an increased risk of blood clots.[13] Shortly thereafter, four more observational studies, published in rapid succession, confirmed that the risk of blood clots with the third generation pills was two times greater than with the older second generation contraceptives.[14,15,16,17]

In October 1995, the United Kingdom's equivalent of our Food and Drug Administration (FDA), the Committee on Safety of Medicines (CSM), warned the British public that third generation birth control pills containing the progestins desogestrel or gestodene could double the risk of blood clots compared to older second generation oral contraceptives containing the progestins norgestrel, levonorgestrel or norethindrone. British doctors were told that the third generation products should not be routinely prescribed and that women should be offered the choice to switch to the older, safer second generation pills. The CSM decided that the increased risk—estimated at 30 cases of blood clots for every 100,000 users of third generation pills a year, compared with 15 cases for every 100,000 women on second generation pills a year—was sufficient to warrant an urgent alert to women and their doctors.[18]

Proponents of the third generation pills maintained that any increase in the risks of blood clots may be offset by a reduced risk of heart attack.[19,20] The key phrase in the last sentence is "may be". The third generation pill proponents have not been able to produce any convincing evidence that there is any difference in the risk of heart attack between women using second or third generation pills.

While the British authorities took the responsible step in 1995 to inform women and their doctors about the risk of blood clots with the third generation pills, the FDA took no similar action in alerting the public. The action of the British authorities allowed "the user to be the chooser" by providing women with the information to make an informed decision about which contraceptive to use.

The professional product labeling, or package insert, and the patient labeling for Ortho-Cept now warn doctors and women about the risks of blood clots, but few doctors or pharmacists read the product labeling in detail and every woman may not receive the FDA-approved patient labeling from their pharmacist when Ortho-Cept is dispensed. Unlike the British authorities who used the news media to warn doctors and women, the FDA relied on the drug's labeling as the only warning. This is the statement contained in the Ortho-Cept professional package insert: *Data from case-control and cohort studies report that oral contraceptives containing desogestrel (ORTHO-CEPT contains desogestrel) are associated with a two-fold increase in the risk of venous thromboembolic disease as compared to other low-dose (containing less than 50 micrograms of estrogen) pills containing other progestins. According to these studies, this two-fold risk increases the yearly occurrence of venous thromboembolic disease by about 10–15 cases per 100,000 women.*[21]

The Ortho-Cept package insert also makes reference to the unsubstantiated theory that third generation birth control pills protect users from heart attacks. This is the statement, again directly from the Ortho-Cept package insert: *Desogestrel has minimum androgenic activity, and there is some evidence that the risk of myocardial infarction [heart attack] associated with oral contraceptives is lower when the progestogen has minimal androgenic activity.*[22]

Organon, the producer of Desogen, makes similar statements about the risks of blood clots and heart attacks in the Desogen professional package insert and the patient labeling for the drug.

To settle questions about the oral contraceptives the World Health Organization (WHO) convened an international meeting of experts in Switzerland in November 1997 with the overall objective of reviewing the current scientific data on the use of oral contraceptives and the risk of heart attack, stroke, and blood clots. Regarding blood clots and heart attack, the Scientific Group concluded that:

• Current users of combined oral contraceptives have a low absolute risk of venous thromboembolism which is nonetheless three-to six-fold higher than in nonusers. The risk is probably highest in the first year of use and declines thereafter, but persists until discontinuation.

• Combined oral contraceptive preparations containing desogestrel and gestodene probably carry a small risk of venous thromboembolism beyond that attributable to combined oral contraceptives containing levonorgestrel. There are insufficient data to draw conclusions with regard to combined oral contraceptives or combined oral contraceptives containing norgestimate.

• The available data do not allow a conclusion that the risk of myocardial infarction (heart attack) in users of low-dose combined oral contraceptives is related to progestogen type. The suggestion that gestodene- or desogestrel-containing low-dose combined oral contraceptives may carry a lower risk of myocardial infarction compared with low-dose formulations containing levonorgestrel remains to be substantiated.[23]

The risk of blood clots with combined oral contraceptives is small, but it is a real risk, and this risk is greater with the third generation pills than with the second generation oral contraceptives. There is no acceptable scientific evidence that a woman taking third generation pills reduces her risk of heart attack over a woman using the second generation products, and the second and third generation pills are equally effective in preventing pregnancy. In summary, there is no reason why women should be using third generation pills when equally effective and safer oral contraceptives are available.

Betamethasone
DIPROLENE, DIPROSONE, VALISONE
(Schering)

GENERIC: available

FAMILY: Corticosteroids (see p. 651)

Betamethasone (bay ta *meth* a sone), like other steroids (corticosteroids), is used in several different ways. It is commonly used to reduce inflammation (redness and swelling) and relieve itching caused by many kinds of skin conditions or by a type of mouth lesion. It is also used to treat other conditions which produce inflammation, such as arthritis and other joint problems, and allergies, hay fever, and other breathing problems.

Betamethasone has several forms. It can be injected into the muscle, joint, lesion, soft tissue, or bloodstream. It can be applied to the skin (topical form), to the eye (ophthalmic form), or to the ear (otic form). It also has a form that is taken by mouth, but this should not be used. If you need to take a steroid by mouth, prednisone (see p. 668) is the best choice because it is reliable, inexpensive, and available in a generic form.[24]

Steroids suppress your immune system, lowering your defenses against disease and making you more vulnerable to infections. If you use betamethasone for a long time, you increase your risk of getting bacterial, viral, parasitic, and fungal infections. Older adults using betamethasone are more likely than younger users to develop the bone-weakening condition called osteoporosis. Older users are also more likely to develop high blood pressure and to retain fluid while taking this drug.

As with all drugs, you should use the smallest dose of betamethasone that works. You should also use it for the shortest possible time. If you use systemic steroids (ones that are taken by mouth or injected so that your whole body is exposed to them) for a long time, you may suffer many adverse effects, and you may also suffer withdrawal symptoms if you stop abruptly.

Before You Use This Drug

Do not use if you have or have had:

For injections into the joint:

- blood clotting disorders
- fracture of the joint
- infection around the joint
- joint surgery
- osteoporosis
- unstable joint

Tell your doctor if you have or have had:

- bone disease
- chicken pox
- measles
- colitis
- diverticulitis
- stomach ulcer
- diabetes
- fungus infection
- herpes eye infection
- recent surgery or serious injury
- tuberculosis
- glaucoma
- heart disease
- high blood pressure
- liver disease
- thyroid problems
- myasthenia gravis
- systemic lupus (SLE)

For form applied to skin:

- infection or ulceration at place where you will be applying the drug

Tell your doctor about any other drugs you take, including aspirin, herbs, vitamins, and other nonprescription products.

When You Use This Drug

- If you plan to have any surgery, including dental, tell your doctor that you take this drug.

How to Use This Drug

- **Use only as prescribed.**
- If you miss a dose, take it as soon as you remember, but skip it if it is almost time for the next dose. **Do not take double doses.**
- Do not store in the bathroom. Do not expose to heat, moisture, or strong light.

On your skin:

- The preparation may sting when applied.
- Keep away from eyes.
- Do not bandage or wrap the area being treated unless your doctor has told you to do so.
- Check with your doctor if your condition does not improve in one week, or if it worsens.
- If you use the drug correctly, there is no danger that it will be absorbed into your system.

Interactions with Other Drugs

The following drugs are listed in the *Evaluations of Drug Interactions* 1997 as causing "highly clinically significant" or "clinically significant" interactions when used together with this drug. We have also included potentially serious interactions listed in the drug's FDA-approved professional product labeling or package insert. New scientific techniques have allowed researchers to predict some drug interactions before they have been documented in people. There may be other drugs, especially those in the families of drugs listed below, that also will react with this drug to cause severe adverse effects. The number of new drugs approved for marketing increases the chance of drug interactions, and new drug interactions are being identified with old drugs. Be vigilant. Make sure to tell your doctor and pharmacist the drugs you are taking and tell your doctor if you are taking any of these interacting drugs:

aldesleukin/interleukin-2, aminoglutethimide, aspirin, GENUINE BAYER ASPIRIN, chlorpropamide, cyclosporine, CYTADREN, DIABINESE, dicumarol, DILANTIN, ECOTRIN, ketoconazole, LUMINAL, NEORAL, NIZORAL, phenobarbital, phenytoin, PROLEUKIN, RIFADIN, rifampin, RIMACTANE, SANDIMMUNE, SOLFOTON, timolol, TIMOPTIC.

Adverse Effects

Call your doctor immediately if you experience:

- decreased or blurred vision
- frequent urination
- increased thirst
- numbness, pain, tingling, redness, or swelling at site of injection
- hallucinations
- depression or mood changes
- skin rash or hives
- confusion
- excitement or restlessness

For long-term use:

- persistent abdominal or stomach pain
- acne or other skin problems
- bloody or black, tarry stools
- rounding out of the face
- hip or shoulder pain
- increased blood pressure
- swelling of feet or lower legs
- unusual weight gain
- irregular heartbeat
- muscle cramps or pain
- unusual tiredness or weakness
- pain in back, ribs, arms, or legs
- muscle weakness
- nausea or vomiting
- pitting or depression of skin at place of injection
- thin, shiny skin
- unusual bruising
- wounds that will not heal

- menstrual irregularities
- reddish, purplish lines on arms, face, legs, trunk or groin

Call your doctor if these symptoms continue:

- indigestion
- increased appetite
- nervousness or restlessness
- trouble sleeping
- dizziness or lightheadedness
- flushed face
- headache
- increased joint pain
- nosebleeds
- increase in hair on body or face
- loss of appetite
- darkening or lightening of skin color
- sweating

Call your doctor immediately if these symptoms occur after you have stopped taking the drug:

- abdominal or back pain
- dizziness or fainting
- low grade fever
- persistent loss of appetite
- muscle or joint pain
- nausea or vomiting
- returning symptoms of the condition for which you were taking the drug
- shortness of breath
- frequent unexplained headaches
- unusual tiredness or weakness
- unusual weight loss

Periodic Tests

Ask your doctor which of these tests should be done periodically while you are taking this drug:

- blood or urine glucose concentration
- eye exams

- stool tests
- serum electrolyte determination
- growth and development determinations
- hypothalamus and pituitary secretion tests

PREGNANCY WARNING

This drug caused harm to developing fetuses in animal studies, or such studies were not done. Use during pregnancy only for clear medical reasons. Tell your doctor if you are pregnant or thinking of becoming pregnant before you take this drug.

Limited Use

Oxybutynin
DITROPAN (Hoechst Marion-Roussel)

GENERIC: available
FAMILY: Antispasmodics (urinary tract)
Anticholinergics

Oxybutynin (ox i *byoo* ti nin) is used to treat incontinence (loss of bladder control) and frequent urination. The drug decreases spasms in the bladder and increases its ability to hold urine. Oxybutynin has not been proven effective for treating disorders of the stomach and intestines.

This drug has adverse effects that severely limit its use in older adults. Potential adverse effects include severe memory impairment, difficulty swallowing, retention of urine, blurred vision, and constipation.[25,26] People over the age of 60 who are taking the usual dose of oxybutynin may experience excitement, restlessness, drowsiness, or confusion.[27]

WARNING: SPECIAL MENTAL AND PHYSICAL ADVERSE EFFECTS

Older adults are especially sensitive to the harmful anticholinergic (see Glossary, p. 768) effects of drugs such as oxybutynin. Drugs in this family should not be used unless absolutely necessary.

Mental Effects: confusion, delirium, short-term memory problems, disorientation, and impaired attention.

Physical Effects: dry mouth, constipation, difficulty urinating (especially for a man with an enlarged prostate), blurred vision, decreased sweating with increased body temperature, sexual dysfunction, and worsening of glaucoma.

Before You Use This Drug

Tell your doctor if you have or have had:

- allergies to drugs
- heart disease
- reflux esophagitis (a backward flow of stomach contents into the esophagus, which causes heartburn)
- abdominal obstruction or disease
- glaucoma
- kidney or liver problems
- high blood pressure
- lung disease
- myasthenia gravis
- enlarged prostate
- enlarged thyroid gland
- severe bleeding
- colitis
- severe and continuing dry mouth
- intestinal or urinary tract blockage or other problems
- toxemia of pregnancy

Tell your doctor about any other drugs you take, including aspirin, herbs, vitamins, and other nonprescription products.

When You Use This Drug

- Until you know how you react to this drug, do not drive or perform other activities requiring alertness. Oxybutynin may cause drowsiness, dizziness, and blurred vision.

How to Use This Drug

- Take with food or milk to decrease stomach upset.
- **Use only as prescribed.**
- Do not store in the bathroom. Do not expose to heat or direct light. Do not let liquid form freeze.
- If you miss a dose, take it as soon as you remember, but skip it if it is almost time for the next dose. **Do not take double doses.**

Interactions with Other Drugs

The following drugs are listed in the *Evaluations of Drug Interactions* 1997 as causing "highly clinically significant" or "clinically significant" interactions when used together with this drug. We have also included potentially serious interactions listed in the drug's FDA-approved professional product labeling or package insert. New scientific techniques have allowed researchers to predict some drug interactions before they have been documented in people. There may be other drugs, especially those in the families of drugs listed below, that also will react with this drug to cause severe adverse effects. The number of new drugs approved for marketing increases the chance of drug interactions, and new drug interactions are being identified with old drugs. Be vigilant. Make sure to tell your doctor and pharmacist the drugs you are taking and tell your doctor if you are taking any of these interacting drugs:

digoxin, LANOXICAPS, LANOXIN.

Central nervous system (CNS) depressant drugs including alcohol, antidepressants, antihistamines, antipsychotics, some blood pressure medications (reserpine, methyldopa, beta-blockers), motion sickness medications, muscle relaxants, narcotics, sedatives, sleeping pills and tranquilizers.

Adverse Effects

Call your doctor immediately if you experience:

- **signs of overdose:** clumsiness or unsteadiness, confusion, convulsions, dizziness, severe drowsiness, severe dry mouth, nose, or throat, fever, hallucinations, shortness of breath, slurred speech, unusual excitement, nervousness, or irritability, unusually fast heartbeat, unusual warmth or dryness of skin
  - eye pain
  - skin rash or hives

Call your doctor if these symptoms continue:

- blurred vision
- constipation
- decrease in sweating
- dry mouth, nose, throat, or skin
- difficulty urinating
- difficulty swallowing
- drowsiness, headache
- nausea or vomiting
- insomnia
- bloated feeling
- decreased flow of breast milk
- decreased sexual ability
- increased sensitivity to light
- unusual tiredness or weakness

Periodic Tests

Ask your doctor which of these tests should be done periodically while you are taking this drug:

- cystometry

Fluorouracil
EFUDEX (Roche)
FLUOROPLEX (Allergan)

GENERIC: available
FAMILY: Anticancer Drug

Fluorouracil (flure oh *yoor* a sill) is used to treat certain kinds of cancer, both inside the hospital in intravenous (IV) form and outside the hospital in a cream and a lotion. **This profile only discusses fluorouracil's use outside the hospital in cream or lotion form.**

Fluorouracil cream and lotion are used to treat certain cancers of the skin (basal cell cancers) and certain skin lesions which may lead to cancer. In most cases of cancer, it is better to remove the cancerous cells surgically than to treat them with fluorouracil.

When you apply fluorouracil to a lesion, it causes a sequence of redness, blistering, tenderness, and finally destruction and healing of the abnormal skin. This is a normal reaction. However, treatment may need to be stopped if an extreme reaction occurs in the normal skin around the lesion.

Treatment usually takes two to six weeks but may take up to 12 weeks. If you are using fluorouracil to treat cancer, or if you are using it to treat a lesion and the lesion comes back after treatment is stopped, you should have a biopsy to make sure that your condition is cured.

When you use fluorouracil on your skin, very little of the drug is absorbed into your system, so adverse effects such as those caused by intravenous fluorouracil are seldom seen.

Before You Use This Drug

Do not use if you have or have had:

- recent infection or exposure to chicken pox
- shingles (herpes zoster)

Tell your doctor if you have or have had:

- allergies to drugs
- bone marrow depression

- liver or kidney problems
- recent infection
- other skin problems

Tell your doctor about any other drugs you take, including aspirin, herbs, vitamins, and other nonprescription products.

When You Use This Drug

- Try to stay out of the sun as much as possible.
- Do not use a tight bandage over the area being treated unless your doctor has told you otherwise.
- Check with your doctor if the normal skin surrounding the area being treated becomes inflamed.
- **Check with your doctor immediately if you notice fever, chills, sore throat, or unusual bleeding or bruising during or after treatment.**
- **Because this drug, when absorbed into your body, decreases the number of white blood cells (which fight infection), you may be more likely to get an infection while taking it. Do not get immunizations without your doctor's approval.**
- If you plan to have any surgery, including dental, tell your doctor that you take this drug.

Interactions with Other Drugs

Some other drugs that you may be taking (either over-the-counter or prescription drugs) can interact with this one, causing adverse effects. Ask your doctor what these drugs are and let him or her know if you are taking any of them.

Adverse Effects

Call your doctor immediately if you experience:

- redness and swelling of normal skin

Call your doctor if these symptoms continue:

- hair loss
- nausea, vomiting, appetite loss
- rash, hives, itching or scaling of skin
- vaginal ulceration, discharge, itching[28]
- weakness
- burning where medicine was applied
- increased sensitivity to sunlight
- darkening of skin

Periodic Tests

Ask your doctor which of these tests should be done periodically while you are taking this drug:

- complete blood tests (including hematocrit, platelet count, white blood cell count)
- biopsy

PREGNANCY WARNING

This drug caused harm to developing fetuses in animal studies, or such studies were not done. Use during pregnancy only for clear medical reasons. Tell your doctor if you are pregnant or thinking of becoming pregnant before you take this drug.

Limited Use

Estradiol
ESTRADERM (Patch) (Novartis)

GENERIC: not available
FAMILY: Hormones

WARNING

Estrogen increases the risk of breast and endometrial (uterine) cancer in postmenopausal women.

For much more information on estrogens and the risk of breast cancer refer to p. 714.

Estradiol (est ra *dye* all) is an estrogen. In the patch form it is only approved for relief of symptoms of menopause, such as hot flashes, night sweats, and vaginal dryness, itching, or loss of elasticity and for prevention of osteoporosis (see p. 714). The patch form of estradiol may reduce adverse effects on the liver,[29] and be preferred for those who have had adverse effects from oral contraceptives.

Most women who are using estrogen for symptoms of menopause (such as hot flashes) do not need to take it forever. If you are using estrogen for this reason, you should begin by using it for no more than 6 to 12 months. There is no evidence for increased risk of breast cancer with such short-term use. Then your doctor should slowly take you off the drug, and watch to see if the symptoms return. You should start taking estrogen again only if the symptoms come back when you stop taking it. If you do keep using it, you should periodically try stopping it, under your doctor's guidance.

Estradiol will not relieve nervousness or depression,[30] nor keep you feeling "young" with soft skin. It is not for minor discomforts of menopause. A drawback for many women is return of monthly vaginal flow after menopause. Adverse effects increase with dose and length of time used.[31,32] Long-term effects, whether or not you continue to use the patch, are still unknown.[33,34] The lowest dose should be used for the shortest possible time.[35,36,37]

While risks of some diseases fall, other risks rise. Estradiol changes coagulation of blood, and can cause dangerous blood clots or inflame and enlarge veins. At times estrogens increase blood pressure, although the risk is less after menopause.[38]

To reduce the adverse effects of estrogens, a progesterone is often prescribed especially with the oral dosage form but also with the patch.[39] For more information on progesterone, see p. 723.

Menopause is a natural process. As with other changes in the body, disorders may happen. Reassurance should be a valid response from your doctor.

WARNING

Using estrogens increases your risk of endometrial cancer (cancer of the lining of the uterus) by six to eight times. This cancer can be cured by surgery only if it is detected early through a special examination called an endometrial biopsy, and such biopsies are usually done only when a woman is bleeding abnormally. Taking estrogen has also been linked to breast cancer in both men and women. The risk is higher for women who take higher doses or who have used estrogen longer. Experts from the National Cancer Institute and from other countries state that "the prolonged use of estrogens at the time of the menopause may increase the risk of breast cancer by 50% after a 5 to 10 year interval."

Before You Use This Drug

Do not use if you have or have had:

- history of blood clot formation
- abnormal or undiagnosed vaginal bleeding
- breast cancer or a strong family history of breast cancer

Tell your doctor if you have or have had:

- allergies to drugs
- asthma
- bone disease
- diabetes
- mental depression
- migraine headaches
- kidney or liver problems
- heart or circulatory disease
- pancreatitis
- high cholesterol or triglycerides
- colitis or diverticulitis

- chicken pox
- measles
- ulcers
- fungus infection or other infection
- recent surgery or serious injury
- tuberculosis
- glaucoma
- heart disease
- high blood pressure
- thyroid problems
- myasthenia gravis
- lupus

Tell your doctor about any other drugs you take, including aspirin, herbs, vitamins, and other nonprescription products.

When You Use This Drug

- Take with food to reduce nausea. Estrogen is most likely to cause nausea in the morning.
- **Do not use more or less often or in a higher or lower dose than prescribed by your doctor.**
- Do not smoke. Smoking increases your risk of serious adverse effects such as blood clots, heart attack, or stroke. The risk increases as you get older.
- Until you know how you react to this drug, do not drive or perform other activities requiring alertness. This drug can cause loss of coordination, blurred vision and drowsiness.
- If you plan to have any surgery, including dental, tell your doctor that you take this drug.
- Have your gums cleaned carefully by a dentist at least once a year, as estrogen can cause gum overgrowth.
- Stay out of the sun as much as possible and do not use sunlamps. Too much sun or sunlamp use while taking estrogen may produce brown, blotchy spots on your skin.

How to Use This Drug

- If you have been taking an oral estrogen, wait until a week after you stop before applying an estradiol patch.

- Wash and dry hands.
- Tear open new patch immediately before use. Do not use scissors to open. The device normally contains bubbles. Discard the liner.
- Remove old patch.
- Select an area on the abdomen or buttocks that is clean and dry, and free of hair, oil, breaks or cuts in the skin. Avoid applying to area where the patch is apt to rub loose, such as the waist. Rotate sites so no site is repeated during a week.
- Never apply patch to a breast.
- Press adhesive side of patch firmly on skin, using the palm of your hand and hold for about 10 seconds. Check that contact is good, especially around the edges.
- Apply the patch twice a week, the same two days each week, usually three weeks a month. A calendar is enclosed with the patch to aid scheduling.
- Reapply the same patch if it loosens or falls off. If necessary put on a new patch. Check patch after bathing, showering, or swimming.
- If you forget to change a patch, do so as soon as you remember, then adjust schedule.
- Store unopened patches at room temperature. Do not expose to heat. Do not store patches after protective liner has been removed.

Interactions with Other Drugs

Some other drugs that you may be taking (either over-the-counter or prescription drugs) can interact with this one, causing adverse effects. Ask your doctor what these drugs are and let him or her know if you are taking any of them.

Adverse Effects

Call your doctor immediately if you experience:

- persistent or abnormal vaginal bleeding
- drowsiness
- dribbling urination

- severe headache
- sudden loss of coordination
- pains in chest, groin, leg, or calf
- shortness of breath
- slurred speech
- vision changes
- weakness or numbness in arm or leg
- high blood pressure
- uncontrolled movements of body
- breast lumps or discharge
- depression
- pains in stomach or side
- yellowing of eyes or skin
- skin rash
- thick, white vaginal discharge
- swelling of ankles and feet
- breast swelling and tenderness

Call your doctor if these symptoms continue:

- bloating, cramping
- nausea, loss of appetite
- changes in weight
- changes in sexual desire
- changes in hair growth
- diarrhea
- dizziness, irritability
- decreased tolerance to wearing contact lenses
- skin irritation or redness where patch was worn
- vomiting
- headache

Periodic Tests

Ask your doctor which of these tests should be periodically done while you are taking this drug:

- blood pressure
- liver function test
- pap smear*
- yearly mammogram*
- physical examination at least every 6 to 12 months, with special attention to the breasts, and including a pelvic exam*

- endometrial biopsy
- bone age determination
- lipid profile determination

These should be a part of your normal health care routine.

PREGNANCY WARNING

This drug should not be used if you are pregnant or are thinking of becoming pregnant. The risk of use of this drug in pregnant women clearly outweighs any possible benefit.

Do Not Use Until Five Years After Release

Raloxifene (Do Not Use Until 2004)
EVISTA (Lilly)

GENERIC: not available
FAMILY: Osteoporosis Drugs

You should wait at least five years from the date of release to take any new drug unless it is one of those rare "breakthrough" drugs that offers you a documented therapeutic advantage over older proven drugs. New drugs are tested in a relatively small number of people before being approved, and serious adverse effects or life-threatening drug interactions may not be detected until the new drug has been taken by hundreds of thousands of people. A number of new drugs have been withdrawn within their first five years after release. Also, serious new adverse reaction warnings have been added to the labeling of a number of drugs, or new drug interactions have been detected, usually within the first five years after a drug's release.

The FDA approved raloxifene (ra lox i feen) for the prevention of osteoporosis, or thinning of the bones, in postmenopausal women. Raloxifene is the newest member of a family of drugs known as selective estrogen receptor modulators (SERMs) that act like estrogen in some tissues but not others. Whether this is important in terms of long-term adverse effects is unknown. Under FDA guidelines, drugs approved to prevent osteoporosis must be shown to preserve or increase bone density and maintain bone quality. Raloxifene does this, but not as well as conjugated estrogens (PREMARIN) (see p. 714) plus medroxyprogesterone (PROVERA and generics) (see p. 723) or alendronate (FOSAMAX) (see p. 687).

In a clinical study published in the *New England Journal of Medicine,* the effects of 30, 60, or 150 milligram doses of raloxifene per day were compared to a placebo (an inactive sugar pill) on bone density in different parts of the body.[40] In all, 601 women started, but only 452 finished the 24 month long study. The reason for the large number of "drop-outs", about 25%, was not clearly explained by the researchers.

All women in the study received between 400 and 600 mg of calcium daily in addition to raloxifene or placebo. At the end of the study the difference in bone density in the hip between women taking raloxifene and placebo ranged from 1.8% to 2.3% depending on the dose of raloxifene. This is less than the 3.3% change seen with both conjugated estrogens plus medroxyprogesterone and alendronate on bone density in the hip. The effect of raloxifene compared to placebo on bone density in the spine was between 2.1% and 3.0% depending again on raloxifene dosage. By comparison, a 5.2% change has been seen with conjugated estrogen plus medroxyprogesterone on the bone density of the spine and for alendronate a 5.8% change has been seen in the spine.

Raloxifene produced only a modest effect on bone density in this trial, less than that of either conjugated estrogen plus medroxyprogesterone or alendronate. More important than a drug's effect on bone density is its ability to reduce the risk of fracture, particularly hip fracture. The effect of raloxifene on fracture risk is not yet known but is being evaluated in ongoing trials.

At this time, only the conjugated estrogens and alendronate have been shown to reduce the risk of fractures. Observational studies have shown an approximately 60% reduction in hip and wrist fracture in women who began estrogen within a few years of menopause. Alendronate has been shown to produce a 48% reduction in the proportion of women experiencing one or more new vertebral fractures—a type of fracture of the spine that may go unnoticed by women—relative to those treated with placebo, but this is only a small 3% difference in the risk of vertebral fracture.

The most serious adverse effect associated with raloxifene was increased risk of venous thromboembolic events, or blood clots that form in the veins and may break off and travel to the lungs. The 2.5 fold increase in the risk for blood clots in women treated with raloxifene was similar to that reported for women on hormone replacement therapy. Other commonly reported adverse effects were hot flashes and leg cramps. Women with a history of blood clots in their veins should not use raloxifene, nor should women who are pregnant or may become pregnant, because of potential danger to the fetus. Abnormalities were observed in fetuses of rats given the drug.

Raloxifene produces only a modest effect on bone density compared to conjugated estrogens plus medroxyprogesterone or alendronate which have both been shown to reduce the risk of fracture unlike raloxifene. The long-term effects of raloxifene are unknown.

WHAT YOU CAN DO TO PREVENT OSTEOPOROSIS

DIET AND EXERCISE

Many women are not at risk of developing hip or other types of fractures. Women who are thin or small-boned, particularly if they are Asian or white, and women who drink more than two alcoholic drinks per day are at higher risk of osteoporosis. Black women, heavy women and women who get lots of exercise are at a lower risk. There are steps women can take to prevent osteoporosis; for instance, a lot of calcium in the diet from early adulthood and "weight bearing" exercise such as jogging, walking, tennis and bicycling. You should be receiving from 800 to 1,200 milligrams of calcium per day in your diet depending on your age. Women who are postmenopausal require an average of 1,500 milligrams per day of calcium. These two steps are enough to prevent osteoporosis in many adults.

THINGS YOU CAN DO TO PREVENT FALLS

Falls, of course, will increase your chances of a fracture. Ask your doctor to review your continued need for and dose of any drug which causes you to be dizzy or drowsy. Check p. 27 for drugs that can cause falls. Check your home for situations that can lead to falls such as areas that are not well lighted or loose rugs on hardwood floors.

Before You Use This Drug

Tell your doctor if you have or have had:

- a pregnancy
- breastfeeding
- congestive heart failure
- cancer
- blood clotting disorders
- liver disease

Tell your doctor about any other drugs you take, including aspirin, herbs vitamins, and other nonprescription products.

When You Use This Drug

- If you plan to have any surgery, including dental, tell your doctor that you take this drug.
- This drug can be taken without regard to meals.

How to Use This Drug

- Do not store in the bathroom. Do not expose to heat, moisture, or strong light.
- If you miss a dose, take it as soon as you remember, but skip it if it is almost time for the next dose. **Do not take double doses.**

Interactions with Other Drugs

The following drugs are listed in the *Evaluations of Drug Interactions* 1997 as causing "highly clinically significant" or "clinically significant" interactions when used together with this drug. We have also included potentially serious interactions listed in the drug's FDA-approved professional product labeling or package insert. New scientific techniques have allowed researchers to predict some drug interactions before they have been documented in people. There may be other drugs, especially those in the families of drugs listed below, that also will react with this drug to cause severe adverse effects. The number of new drugs approved for marketing increases the chance of drug interactions, and new drug interactions are being identified with old drugs. Be vigilant. Make sure to tell your doctor and pharmacist the drugs you are taking and tell your doctor if you are taking any of these interacting drugs:

cholestyramine, COUMADIN, estrogens, PREMARIN, LOCHOLEST, QUESTRAN, warfarin.

Call your doctor immediately if you experience:

- coughing up blood
- headache or migraine
- loss of or change in speech, coordination, or vision
- pain or numbness in chest, arm, or leg
- unexplained shortness of breath

Call your doctor if these symptoms continue:

- bloody or cloudy urine
- chest pain
- difficult, burning, or painful urination
- frequent urge to urinate
- fever
- infection, including body aches or pain, congestion in throat, cough, dryness or soreness of throat, and loss of voice
- runny nose
- leg cramping
- skin rash
- swelling of hands, ankles, or feet
- vaginal itching
- severe abdominal pain

Periodic Tests

Ask your doctor which of these tests should be done periodically while you are taking this drug:

- yearly physical examination with special attention give to the breast and pelvic organs

---

PREGNANCY WARNING

This drug should not be used if you are pregnant or are thinking of becoming pregnant. The risk of use of this drug in pregnant women clearly outweighs any possible benefit.

 Do Not Use

Cyclobenzaprine
FLEXERIL (Merck)

FAMILY: Muscle Relaxants

Cyclobenzaprine (sye kloe *ben* za preen) tablets are marketed for the relief of severe pain caused by muscle conditions such as sprains and back pain. However, they are not effective for these conditions. Instead of taking cyclobenzaprine, you should try rest, exercise, physical therapy, or other treatment recommended by your doctor.

The level of cyclobenzaprine in the tablets is not high enough to relax muscles, so this drug will not directly relax tense skeletal muscles. However, the drug is strong enough to have a sedative effect. **Cyclobenzaprine has not been shown to be any more effective than painkillers or anti-inflammatory drugs such as aspirin for relieving the pain of local muscle spasm,**[41] **yet it has a higher risk of adverse effects than these painkillers.**

Cyclobenzaprine is related to some drugs used to treat depression (tricyclic antidepressants such as amitriptyline, see p. 216, and imipramine, p. 203), and may cause some of the same adverse effects and dangerous drug interactions. Some people taking cyclobenzaprine have experienced drowsiness, dry mouth, dizziness, nausea, weakness, upset stomach, blurred vision, insomnia, and a fast heartbeat as adverse effects. If you take cyclobenzaprine for a long time, you can develop drug-induced dependence.[42] Cyclobenzaprine is particularly dangerous for people with glaucoma, an enlarged prostate, or heart problems.

Limited Use

Alendronate
FOSAMAX (Merck)

GENERIC: not available
FAMILY: Osteoporosis Drugs

Alendronate (a *len* dro nate) is approved to treat bone diseases such as osteoporosis and Paget's disease. It belongs to a class of drugs called bisphosphonates, which also includes etidronate (Didronel). Osteoporosis, a thinning of bones, is common in women after menopause, and may lead to fractures, curvature of the spine, and loss of height. About 16% of women have hip or wrist fractures. Some men also get osteoporosis.

Osteoporosis also develops in people who take corticosteroids for conditions such as asthma, skin disorders, or arthritis, for extended periods of time. This form of bone loss occurs by mechanisms very different from those in postmenopausal women and may not be expected to respond to the same types of drug treatment. At present corticosteroid osteoporosis is treated best by adequate intakes of dietary calcium and vitamin D.

Alendronate prevents loss of bone and even increases the amount of bone. This reduces new spinal fractures. Recent analysis suggesting alendronate also reduces hip fractures needs confirmation.[43] Since alendronate can irritate your esophagus (the tube that connects your mouth to your stomach), causing ulcers, and bleeding **it must be taken with water on an empty stomach and you must stay upright and fasting for at least half an hour** to ensure the tablet does not get stuck in your esophagus before reaching the stomach. Alendronate is not recommended in mild osteoporosis, to prevent osteoporosis, in people with severe kidney problems, or in women before menopause. Alendronate should not be given to people with dementia or who are otherwise unable to follow the recommendations on how to take the medication.

Alendronate is retained in bones for long periods of time, but long-term effects are still not known. Concern exists since some biphosphonates increase spontaneous fractures in animals.[44] Estrogen remains the treatment of choice for women able and willing to take it. Taking estrogen with alendronate is not currently recommended. Women over age 70 who have not had fractures may need only calcium and vitamin D supplements.[45] During clinical trials to approve alendronate, over 85% of women with osteoporosis who took the placebo for three years did not have a fracture of any type. Little information is available on the effect of alendronate in men.

Alendronate has also been shown to reduce the risk of hip fracture by 1.1% in women who had previously experienced at least one vertebral fracture. This is a 51% reduction relative to women who were taking a placebo. We are still waiting for the results of a study evaluating the effects of alendronate on hip fracture in postmenopausal women who have never experienced a vertebral fracture.

WHAT YOU CAN DO TO PREVENT OSTEOPOROSIS

DIET AND EXERCISE

Many women are not at risk of developing hip or other types of fractures. Women who are thin or small-boned, particularly if they are Asian or white, and women who drink more than two alcoholic drinks per day are at higher risk of osteoporosis. Black women, heavy women and women who get lots of exercise are at a lower risk. There are steps women can take to prevent osteoporosis; for instance, a lot of calcium in the diet from early adulthood and "weight bearing" exercise such as jogging, walking, tennis and bicycling. You should be receiving from 800 to 1,200 milligrams of calcium per day in your diet depending on your age. Women who are postmenopausal require an average of 1,500 milligrams per day of calcium. These two steps are enough to prevent osteoporosis in many adults.

THINGS YOU CAN DO TO PREVENT FALLS

Falls, of course, will increase your chances of a fracture. Ask your doctor to review your continued need for and dose of any drug which causes you to be dizzy or drowsy. Check p. 27 for drugs that can cause falls. Check your home for situations that can lead to falls such as areas that are not well lighted or loose rugs on hardwood floors.

Before You Use This Drug

Tell your doctor if you have or have had:

- allergies, including lactose
- Crohn's disease
- gastrointestinal problems
- hernia
- hypocalcemia or vitamin D deficiency
- kidney problems
- difficulty swallowing
- throat problems
- ulcers
- unable to sit or stand for 30 minutes

Tell your doctor about any other drugs you take, including aspirin, herbs, vitamins, and other nonprescription products.

When You Use This Drug

- Exercise regularly, preferably weight bearing exercise, such as bicycling, jogging, tennis, or walking.
- Eat a diet adequate in calcium. You may need to take a calcium supplement. If you do not live in a sunny climate you may need to take vitamin D, *particularly in the winter or if you do not go outdoors.*
- Prevent falls by using handrails on stairs, adequate lighting, and avoiding throw rugs and electric cords in your path. Use proper lifting techniques.
- Avoid alcohol and sedatives, which increase the risk of falls and fractures.
- Stop smoking, which increases the risk of osteoporosis.
- If a relative or friend takes alendronate at an institution, check that the timing and method for taking alendronate (as described below) is correct and followed closely.

How to Use This Drug

- On arising or soon after, sit or stand, then swallow tablet **with a full six to eight ounce glass of plain water.** Do not chew or suck on tablets. Take on an empty stomach. Wait at least 30 minutes before taking any food or beverage, including mineral water, coffee, tea, or juice. Do not take any other medications or dietary supplements during this time.
- Stay upright, standing or sitting, for at least 30 minutes, and until after your first food of the day.
- Take any calcium supplement one to four hours after alendronate, or with evening meal.

- Do not take at bedtime or before getting up for the day.
- Store tablets at room temperature.
- Do not store in the bathroom. Do not expose to heat, moisture, or strong light.
- If you miss a dose, skip it. **Do not take double doses.**

Interactions with Other Drugs

The following drugs are listed in the *Evaluations of Drug Interactions* 1997 as causing "highly clinically significant" or "clinically significant" interactions when used together with this drug. We have also included potentially serious interactions listed in the drug's FDA-approved professional product labeling or package insert. New scientific techniques have allowed researchers to predict some drug interactions before they have been documented in people. There may be other drugs, especially those in the families of drugs listed below, that also will react with this drug to cause severe adverse effects. The number of new drugs approved for marketing increases the chance of drug interactions, and new drug interactions are being identified with old drugs. Be vigilant. Make sure to tell your doctor and pharmacist the drugs you are taking and tell your doctor if you are taking any of these interacting drugs:

> aspirin, GENUINE BAYER ASPIRIN, ECOTRIN. Do not take calcium supplements or antacids at the same time of day as alendronate.

Adverse Effects

Call your doctor immediately if you experience:

- abdominal pain
- abnormal bleeding
- chest pain
- heartburn
- nausea or vomiting

- pain in bone, esophagus, or muscles
- skin rash
- swallowing difficulty

Call your doctor if these symptoms continue:

- constipation
- diarrhea
- gas or bloated feeling in stomach
- headache
- taste change

Periodic Tests

Ask your doctor which of these tests should be done periodically while you are taking this drug:

- bone mineral density
- alkaline phosphatase, calcium and creatinine serum levels
- urine tests

Norethindrone/Ethinyl Estradiol
GENORA 1/35 (Rugby)
ORTHO-NOVUM 1/35 (Ortho-McNeil Pharmaceutical)
LOESTRIN-FE 1.5/30 (Parke-Davis)
ORTHO-NOVUM 7/7/7 (Ortho-McNeil Pharmaceutical)

Norgestimate/Ethinyl Estradiol
ORTHO-CYCLEN (Ortho-McNeil Pharmaceutical)
ORTHOTRI-CYCLEN (Ortho-McNeil Pharmaceutical)

Norgestrel/Ethinyl Estradiol
TRIPHASIL (Wyeth-Ayerst)
LO/OVRAL (Wyeth-Ayerst)
TRI-LEVLEN (Berlex)

GENERIC: available
FAMILY: Oral Contraceptives (second generation)

> Cigarette smoking increases the risk of serious cardiovascular adverse effects from oral contraceptive use. This risk increases with age and with heavy smoking (15 or more cigarettes per day) and is quite marked in women over 35 years of age. Women who use oral contraceptives are strongly advised not to smoke.

Are birth control pills the safest contraceptive option for you? There are many issues to consider, and like every other decision concerning your health, this is a highly individual one. Unfortunately, you will not be able to base your decision on assurances of absolute safety. In fact, even after 40 years of studying the pill, much about its long-term effect on human physiology is still unknown.

Although the convenience of the pill is obvious from the start, soon its problems may also be evident. Many women suffer from headaches, bloating, nausea, irregular bleeding, breast tenderness, weight gain, or optical changes. Other unpleasant effects that can occur from a few months to a few years after starting oral contraceptive use include high blood pressure, gallbladder disease, liver tumors, depression, and metabolic disorders, such as diabetes. Temporary infertility has been associated with the period of time right after pill use is stopped.

But the long-term risks—which you should also consider—are still not fully known to medical science. True, oral contraceptives have come a long way since the early days—the 1960s and 1970s—when women were first given hormone doses so potent that heart attacks and strokes were not unusual among pills users. With hormone levels in the pill now much lower, the number of women suffering from heart attacks and strokes also appears to have dropped.

Today's pill is clearly safer in many respects. When used properly, it prevents pregnancy 98% of the time, and its unwanted clotting properties have been significantly reduced. But serious questions remain concerning the pill's relationship to breast cancer.[46]

Before You Use This Drug

Tell your doctor if you have or have had:

- known or suspected cancer of the breast
- cancer of the cervix or endometrium (the lining of the uterus)
- jaundice (yellowing of the skin or eyeballs) during pregnancy or with prior use of birth control pills
- tumors or cancer of the liver
- a pregnancy
- a past history of blood clots
- diabetes
- elevated cholesterol or triglycerides
- high blood pressure
- migraine headache or epilepsy
- mental depression
- gallbladder
- heart or kidney disease
- history of irregular menstrual periods
- fibroid tumors of the uterus

Tell your doctor about any other drugs you take, including aspirin, herbs, vitamins, and other nonprescription products.

When You Use This Drug

- You should receive regular check-ups by your doctor.
- If you miss taking a pill follow the directions in the FDA-approved patient information leaflet that you should receive from your pharmacist each time you get a prescription for birth control pills. This information will tell you what to do and when to use a back-up method of contraception.
- If you plan to have any surgery, including dental, tell your doctor that you take this drug.

How to Use This Drug

• Your pharmacist is required to dispense an FDA-approved patient information leaflet each time you receive a prescription for an oral contraceptive. Since the many different brands of oral contraceptives vary in the number of tablets taken per month and the colors of the pills, consult this information before starting to take your pills. Make sure you are receiving the FDA-approved information for the brand of birth control pills you are taking and not the printout from the pharmacist's computer system.

• Do not store in the bathroom. Do not expose to heat, moisture, or strong light.

Interactions with Other Drugs

The following drugs are listed in the *Evaluations of Drug Interactions* 1997 as causing "highly clinically significant" or "clinically significant" interactions when used together with this drug. We have also included potentially serious interactions listed in the drug's FDA-approved professional product labeling or package insert. New scientific techniques have allowed researchers to predict some drug interactions before they have been documented in people. There may be other drugs, especially those in the families of drugs listed below, that also will react with this drug to cause severe adverse effects. The number of new drugs approved for marketing increases the chance of drug interactions, and new drug interactions are being identified with old drugs. Be vigilant. Make sure to tell your doctor and pharmacist the drugs you are taking and tell your doctor if you are taking any of these interacting drugs:

Certain drugs may interact with birth control pills to make them less effective in preventing pregnancy or cause an increase in breakthrough bleeding. Such drugs include rifampin (RIFADIN, RIMACTANE and generics), drugs used for seizures such as barbiturates (for example phenobarbital [LUMINAL, SOLFOTON]), anticonvulsants such as carbamazepine (TEGRETOL and generics), and phenytoin (DILANTIN and generics), and possibly other antibiotics. You may need to use additional contraception when you take these drugs.

Adverse Effects

Call your doctor immediately if you experience:

• chest pain
• coughing up blood
• sudden shortness of breath
• pain in the calf or groin
• severe and sudden headache
• vomiting
• dizziness or fainting
• slurring of speech
• weakness, or numbness in arms or legs
• partial or complete loss of vision
• lumps in breast if you have a history of breast disease
• severe pain or tenderness in the stomach area
• insomnia
• abnormal weakness
• mood changes
• yellowing of the skin or eyeballs, accompanied frequently by fever, fatigue, loss of appetite, dark colored urine, or light brown colored bowel movements
• loss of coordination
• changes in menstrual bleeding
• increased blood pressure
• vaginal infection
• fainting, nausea, pale or sweating skin if you have diabetes
• depression

Call your doctor if these symptoms continue:

• abdominal cramping or bloating
• acne

- breast pain, tenderness or swelling
- swelling of ankles or feet
- unusual tiredness or weakness
- vomiting
- brown, blotchy spots on skin
- gain or loss of body or facial hair
- weight gain or loss
- increased sensitivity to sun

Periodic Tests

Ask your doctor which of these tests should be done periodically while you are taking this drug:

- blood pressure
- liver function determinations
- pap smear
- glucose, lipid and lipoprotein serum levels
- FSH levels

PREGNANCY WARNING

This drug should not be used if you are pregnant or are thinking of becoming pregnant. The risk of use of this drug in pregnant women clearly outweighs any possible benefit.

Limited Use

Nicotine
HABITROL (Novartis)
NICORETTE, NICODERM (SmithKline Beecham)
NICOTROL (McNeil)
PROSTEP (Lederle)

GENERIC: not available
FAMILY: Aids to Stop Smoking

WARNING

Nicotine has only been shown to be effective when used as an aid to a comprehensive smoking cessation program. Since the above products contain nicotine, **do not continue to smoke while using them**.

Nicotine (*nick* o teen), whether in a patch or gum, is used to assist quitting smoking. This is the same nicotine found in tobacco, pesticides, and some foods. In patches, gums, and several forms still being developed, nicotine serves as a temporary aid to giving up smoking, by reducing physical withdrawal symptoms. However, unless the nicotine gum or patch is accompanied by a smoking cessation program, the drug works no better than a placebo,[47] because it is treating only the physical, not the psychological addiction.

Withdrawal signs from smoking include fatigue, headache, slowed heart rate, hunger, difficulty concentrating, irritability, and dreams about smoking. These symptoms start about two hours after the last cigarette, increase for 24 hours, then decrease over several days or weeks.[48] Signs of withdrawal do not require medical attention. Even people who have severe withdrawal are able to be successful in quitting.[49,50]

Aids are simple to use and can lull you into unrealistic expectations. To be effective, nicotine patches and gum must be accompanied by changes in behavior. Set a quit date, learn ways to cope with urges to smoke (particularly in the morning, with company, and in response to advertising), and plan ways to cope with relapses.[51] Learn how to deal with anger, anxiety, depression, stress, and tension without smoking. People who smoke are more apt to have a history of being depressed.[52] In addition, those who are anxious or depressed tend to have severe withdrawal.[53,54] Without learning these coping skills, the patch does not work any better than a non-medicated band-aid. While these aids eliminate smoke, they still contain nicotine. **If you continue to smoke while using nicotine replacements, you risk serious heart disease.**[55] Success rates of stopping smoking by using nicotine replacements are low, especially after six months or a year.[56,57,58,59,60,61] However, smokers who try slow withdrawal are apt to smoke less if they do resume smoking.[62,63]

Nicotine gum continues to satisfy and reinforce oral habits, and may lessen weight gain.[64] The gum is harder and thicker than regular chewing gums and can loosen dental work. Not everyone masters the chewing technique. Patches are easier to use. The 16-hour patch mimics patterns of smoking, but the 24-hour patches may get you through the strong urge to smoke in the morning. Both types can irritate your skin. Overall, the various patches do not differ in the rate of people who quit smoking.[65]

You must also gradually stop using the gum or patches to prevent addiction to these nicotine products. Quitting smoking reduces your chances of bronchitis, cancers (especially of the lung, mouth, throat, and voicebox), emphysema, heart disease, duodenal ulcers, and dulled sense of smell and taste. People who smoke and take psychotropic drugs often require higher doses of the nicotine and are more apt to have serious adverse effects from the psychotropic drugs, such as akathisia (involuntary restlessness, such as rocking from foot to foot).[66,67] Typically, the amount of weight gain after stopping smoking is a minimal health risk compared to the risks of smoking.[68]

Although most people quit smoking without the aid of organized programs, we recommend such a program, especially if you are using these products. Nicotine replacement is not appropriate for light smokers. A number of nonprescription aids to smoking cessation are also available, including plain chewing gum.

According to one study, these work just as well as nicotine replacements for light smokers, in the absence of a comprehensive smoking cessation program.[69] These also are only temporary aids, and must be augmented by changes in behavior to be successful.

Before You Use This Drug

Do not use if you have or have had:

- myocardial infarction
- temporomandibular joint (TMJ) disorder *(for gum)*

Tell your doctor if you have or have had:

- allergies to drugs or substances such as adhesives or tapes
- angina, chest pain
- Buerger's disease
- dental work (bridges, crowns, dentures, fillings) *(for gum)*
- diabetes
- epilepsy[70]
- heart problems
- high blood pressure
- liver problems[71]
- pheochromocytoma
- skin problems
- throat inflammation or irritation *(for gum)*
- thyroid problems
- ulcers

Tell your doctor about any other drugs you take, including aspirin, herbs, vitamins, and other nonprescription products.

When You Use This Drug

- **Stop smoking, or using tobacco in any form. If you continue to smoke and use a nicotine aid, you could get an overdose of nicotine.**
- Build social support for your goal to stop smoking, bolstered by counseling and education programs.

• Learn skills to avoid giving in to the urge to smoke.

• Follow diet recommended by your doctor to avoid weight gain.

• Inform your dentist if you are using the gum form.

• If you plan to have any surgery, including dental, tell your doctor that you take this drug.

How to Use This Drug

For patches:

• Remove patch from outer pouch. A slight discoloration is normal.

• Select a site to apply the patch. The site should be clean and dry. The skin should not be broken, irritated, oily, or hairy. Do not use the same site more than once a week. Avoid areas where movement or clothing may dislodge the patch.

• Apply sticky side firmly, pressing about 10 seconds, checking that the edges are not loose.

• Wash hands after applying the patch.

• Leave patch on for the number of hours specified by your doctor.

• Replace a patch that falls off, but stay on schedule.

• Remove at the same time each day.

• Store unopened patches at room temperature. Do not expose to heat. Discard unused opened patches.

• Fold used patch with sticky sides together. Place in empty, opened pouch to discard.

For the gum:

• Carry the gum with you at all times.

• Chew one piece of nicotine gum when you feel the urge to smoke. Chew slowly until you can taste it, or you feel a tingling sensation in your mouth, about 15 chews. When the taste or sensation disappears, resume chewing. Repeat with the same piece of gum for 30 minutes. Avoid swallowing during this time. Do not drink carbonated beverages or coffee while chewing nicotine gum.[72]

• Do not chew the gum rapidly, or chew more than 24 pieces (60 mg) in one day. Reduce the number of pieces chewed each day over two to three months. After you are down to one or two pieces of gum a day, stop taking the nicotine gum.

• If you accidentally swallow one piece of nicotine gum be alert to gastrointestinal irritation and signs of overdose.

• Do not store in the bathroom. Do not expose to heat, moisture, or strong light.

Interactions with Other Drugs

The following drugs are listed in the *Evaluations of Drug Interactions* 1997 as causing "highly clinically significant" or "clinically significant" interactions when used together with this drug. We have also included potentially serious interactions listed in the drug's FDA-approved professional product labeling or package insert. New scientific techniques have allowed researchers to predict some drug interactions before they have been documented in people. There may be other drugs, especially those in the families of drugs listed below, that also will react with this drug to cause severe adverse effects. The number of new drugs approved for marketing increases the chance of drug interactions, and new drug interactions are being identified with old drugs. Be vigilant. Make sure to tell your doctor and pharmacist the drugs you are taking and tell your doctor if you are taking any of these interacting drugs:

DARVON, DARVON-N, ELIXOPHYLLIN, HUMALOG, HUMULIN, INDERAL, INDERAL LA, insulin, MINIPRESS, prazosin, propoxyphene, propranolol, SLO-BID, THEO-24, theophylline.

Adverse Effects

Most adverse effects of nicotine patches and gums are also potential adverse effects from smoking.

Call your doctor or dentist immediately if you experience:

- damage to dental work or teeth *(for gum)*
- involuntary movements of arms or legs[73]
- **signs of overdose:** abdominal pain, difficulty breathing, cold sweat, confusion, convulsions, severe diarrhea, dizziness, fainting, severe headache, hearing changes, nausea or vomiting, vision changes, severe watering of mouth, severe weakness, low blood pressure, irregular heartbeat

Call your doctor if these symptoms continue:

- belching, hiccups *(for gum)*
- body aches
- cough
- constipation
- dry mouth
- headache
- insomnia, disturbing dreams
- irritability
- itching, rash, redness of skin at site of application *(for patch)*
- aching jaw muscle *(for gum)*
- pain in joints or muscles
- sore mouth or throat *(for gum)*
- undesired weight gain
- drowsiness
- loss of appetite
- menstrual pain
- increased appetite
- indigestion
- sweating

Periodic Tests

Ask your doctor which of these tests should be done periodically while you are taking this drug:

- kidney function test
- liver function test

PREGNANCY WARNING

This drug caused harm to developing fetuses in animal studies, or such studies were not done. Use during pregnancy only for clear medical reasons. Tell your doctor if you are pregnant or thinking of becoming pregnant before you take this drug.

Limited Use

Sumatriptan
IMITREX (Glaxo Wellcome)

Do Not Use Until Five Years After Release

Zolmitriptan (Do Not Use Until 2004)
ZOMIG (Zeneca)

GENERIC: not available
FAMILY: Migraine Drugs

You should wait at least five years from the date of release to take any new drug unless it is one of those rare "breakthrough" drugs that offers you a documented therapeutic advantage over older proven drugs. New drugs are tested in a relatively small number of people before being approved, and serious adverse effects or life-threatening drug interactions may not be detected until the new drug has been taken by hundreds of thousands of people. A number of new drugs have been withdrawn within their first five years after release. Also, serious new adverse reaction warnings have been added to the labeling of a number of drugs, or new drug interactions have been detected, usually within five years after a drug's release.

Sumatriptan (soo ma *trip* tan) is used to relieve migraine headaches with or without aura. It narrows swollen blood vessels by the action of serotonin, a neurotransmitter. Sumatriptan belongs to the same family as zolmitriptan (zol ma *trip* tan). Sumatriptan may relieve nausea accompanying migraines. Only the injectable form is used to relieve cluster headaches. Sumatriptan should be used only after determining that acetaminophen or nonsteroidal anti-inflammatory drugs (NSAIDs) fail to work. Sumatriptan does not prevent or cure migraines, it does not reduce the frequency of migraines, and it is not recommended for migraines described as basilar artery or hemiplegic. Sumatriptan works for up to 65% of those who use it,[74] about 40% develop another migraine in one or two days.

Adverse effects occur more often with higher doses. Long-term use can lead to changes in eyesight. Older people are more likely to experience an increase in blood pressure. Older men with high blood pressure or family history of myocardial infarction are more likely to develop chest pain.[75] Sumatriptan can dangerously, even fatally, narrow arteries in the heart. Life-threatening allergic reactions are possible. Limited studies show that sumatriptan does not work as well in children.[76] People with angina or myocardial infarction and women who are pregnant or breastfeeding should not use sumatriptan.

WARNING
EFFECTS ON THE HEART

Sumatriptan has caused serious effects on the heart some of which have been fatal. This drug can cause the vessels of the heart to contract and should not be taken by people with heart disease including chest pain (angina), and a history of heart attack. Sumatriptan can also raise blood pressure.

Before You Use This Drug

Tell your doctor if you have or have had:

- allergies, including lactose
- high cholesterol
- diabetes
- heart problems, especially angina, heart attack, or family history of heart problems
- high blood pressure
- kidney or liver problems
- pain in abdomen[77]
- pregnant or nursing
- Raynaud's syndrome[78]
- seizures
- smoke

Tell your doctor about any other drugs you take, including aspirin, herbs, vitamins, and other nonprescription products.

When You Use This Drug

- Avoid triggers to your migraines, such as alcohol, certain foods, craning your neck forward, flickering lights, strong odors, overexertion, lack of sleep or oversleeping, and stress. Head injuries may induce migraines without aura.
- Avoid smoking while using sumatriptan.
- Use an ice pack on forehead and temples to lower intensity of pain. Massage or biofeedback may also be useful.
- If you have migraines more than twice a month, check with your doctor about preventive measures.
- Avoid medications that may trigger migraines, such as cimetidine, estrogen, fenfluramine, indomethacin, nifedipine, nitroglycerin, reserpine, and theophylline.[79] However, migraines during menstruation may be due to low estrogen levels, and may even be treated with estrogen.[80]
- Have your blood pressure checked after using sumatriptan.
- Avoid rebound headaches by not overusing any analgesics. Rebound headaches tend to occur daily, often on awakening.

• If you plan to have any surgery, including dental, tell your doctor that you take this drug.

How to Use This Drug

• It is advisable to have the first dose administered under medical care if you have diabetes, high cholesterol, are overweight, smoke, or, have a family history of coronary artery disease.

• Use sumatriptan after headache pain begins, preferably in a quiet, dark room.

• If you do not experience any relief, do not repeat the dose. If you experience some relief, but it is not sufficient or headache reoccurs, after two hours you may repeat the dose once. Do not use more than every five to seven days.

Oral:

• Swallow coated tablet(s), according to your dose. Do not break, crush, or chew tablets. Take with fluids. However, taking with food may delay relief.

• If you experience some, but inadequate relief, you may repeat the dose after two hours. Do not take more than 300 mg in one day. If you first used one injection, do not take more than 200 mg by mouth the same day.

• Store at room temperature below 86°F.

• Do not store in the bathroom. Do not expose to heat, moisture, or strong light.

Nasal Spray:

• Blow your nose to clear nasal passages.

• Hold head upright. Close one nostril with an index finger. Breathe through your mouth. Hold sumatriptan spray container with your other hand, using your thumb to support the bottle. Hold your other index and middle fingers on either side of the nozzle. Insert the nozzle into your open nostril about one-half inch. Tilt your head back slightly. Close your mouth while taking a breath through your nose, and press on the blue plunger to release your dose. Avoid contact with eyes.

• Remove nozzle for your nose. Hold head back for 10 to 20 seconds while breathing in through your nose and breathing out through your mouth.

• For doses of 10 mg you may spray 5 mg in each nostril.

• If your headache returns, after two hours you may repeat the dose. Do not use more than 40 mg in one day, nor use for more than four headaches in one month.

• Clean nozzle, then recap container.

• Store at room temperature below 86°F.

• Do not store in the bathroom. Do not expose to heat, moisture, or strong light.

Injection:

• Wash your hands. Cleanse the injection site.

• Inject just below the skin (subcutaneously) in the upper thigh, or outer upper arm. Do not inject into veins.

• If you experience some, but inadequate relief, or your headache returns, you may repeat the dose after one hour. Do not inject more than 12 mg in one day. Some doctors recommend not more than 12 mg in two days.

• Store injection at room temperature below 86°F. Protect from light and freezing.

• Discard used syringes securely.

Interactions with Other Drugs

The following drugs are listed in the *Evaluations of Drug Interactions* 1997 as causing "highly clinically significant" or "clinically significant" interactions when used together with this drug. We have also included potentially serious interactions listed in the drug's FDA-approved professional product labeling or package insert. New scientific techniques have allowed researchers to predict some drug interactions before they have been documented in people. There may be other drugs, especially those in the families of drugs listed below, that also will react with this drug to cause severe adverse effects. The number of new drugs approved for marketing increases the chance of drug interactions, and new drug interactions are being identified with old drugs. Be vigilant. Make sure to tell your doctor and pharmacist the drugs you are taking and tell your doctor if you are taking any of these interacting drugs:

ELDEPRYL, ergoloid mesylates, ERGOMAR, ERGOSTAT, ergotamine, fluoxetine, fluvoxamine, furazolidone, FUROXONE, GERIMAL, HYDERGINE, HYDERGINE LC, LUVOX, MATULANE, NARDIL, PARNATE, paroxetine, PAXIL, phenelzine, procarbazine, PROZAC, selegiline/deprenyl, sertraline, tranylcypromine, ZOLOFT.

Adverse Effects

Call your doctor immediately if you experience:

- bleeding from rectum
- breathing problems or wheezing
- chest pain, or feeling of heaviness, pressure, or tightness in chest or neck
- slower or more rapid heartbeat
- seizures
- skin rash, hives, or itching
- swallowing difficulty
- swelling of eyes, eyelids, face, or lips
- unwell feeling[81]
- no relief from sumatriptan

Call your doctor if these symptoms continue:

- anxiety
- discomfort in jaw, mouth, tongue, throat, nasal passages or sinuses
- dizziness or lightheadedness
- drowsiness
- flushed face
- hearing disturbance

- muscle aches, cramps, or stiffness
- nausea, or vomiting
- restlessness[82]
- sensation of burning, cold or heat, numbness, or tingling
- sweating
- tastes become bitter or changed
- thirst
- vision changes
- weakness
- bleeding, burning, pain, redness, or swelling at injection site
- discomfort or irritation of nasal passages or sinuses when nasal spray is used

---

PREGNANCY WARNING

This drug caused harm to developing fetuses in animal studies, or such studies were not done. Use during pregnancy only for clear medical reasons. Tell your doctor if you are pregnant or thinking of becoming pregnant before you take this drug.

Fluocinonide
LIDEX, LIDEX-E (Medicis)

GENERIC: available
FAMILY: Corticosteroids (see p. 651)

Fluocinonide (floo oh *sin* oh nide) is a steroid that is applied to the skin. It is used to reduce inflammation (redness and swelling) and relieve itching caused by many kinds of skin conditions, such as eczema and psoriasis.

Steroids suppress your immune system, lowering your defenses against disease and making you more vulnerable to infections. If you use fluocinonide for a long time, you increase your risk of getting bacterial, viral, parasitic, and fungal infections

As with all drugs, you should use the lowest possible dose of fluocinonide that works. You should also use it for as short a time as possible and limit the area of your body that you use it on, if possible. A steroid applied to the skin can cause many adverse effects, especially if you use it for a long time or over a large area so that your whole body absorbs the drug. **If you have used this drug for a long time do not stop suddenly. Your doctor must lower your dose gradually to prevent withdrawal symptoms.**

Before You Use This Drug

Tell your doctor if you have or have had:

- allergies to drugs
- herpes sores
- infection or ulceration at place where you will be applying the drug
- cataracts
- glaucoma
- diabetes
- tuberculosis

Tell your doctor about any other drugs you take, including aspirin, herbs, vitamins, and other nonprescription products.

When You Use This Drug

- **Use only as prescribed.**
- Check with your doctor if your condition does not improve in one week or if it worsens.

How to Use This Drug

- Spread a very thin layer over the area being treated to minimize absorption of the drug into your body. There is no danger of systemic absorption with correct use.
- The preparation may sting when applied.
- Do not bandage or wrap the area you are treating unless your doctor has told you to do so.
- Do not use around eyes for a long period.

Interactions with Other Drugs

Some other drugs that you may be taking (either over-the-counter or prescription drugs) can interact with this one, causing adverse effects. Ask your doctor what these drugs are and let him or her know if you are taking any of them.

Adverse Effects

Call your doctor immediately if you experience:

- pain, redness, or blisters containing pus
- burning, itching, or blistering that was not present before you began using this drug
- thinning of skin with easy bruising

For long term use:

- acne or other skin problem
- backache
- increased hair growth, especially on the face
- loss of hair, especially on scalp
- lack of healing of skin condition
- loss of top skin layer
- numbness in fingers
- blurred vision
- eye pain
- rounding out of face
- increased blood pressure
- irregular heartbeat
- irregular menstrual period
- irritability
- irritation of skin and mouth
- loss of appetite
- depression
- muscle cramps, pain or weakness
- nausea
- rapid weight gain or loss
- reddish, purplish lines on arms, face, legs, trunk or groin
- changes in skin color
- bloated or painful stomach

- softening of skin
- swelling of feet or lower legs
- decrease in sexual ability or desire
- tearing of the skin
- unusual increase or loss of hair growth
- unusual tiredness or weakness
- vomiting

Call your doctor if these symptoms continue:

- worsening of infections
- skin rash, irritation, burning or dryness

Periodic Tests

Ask your doctor which of these tests should be done periodically while you are taking this drug:

- blood or urine glucose concentration
- eye exams
- adrenal function assessment

Methylprednisolone
MEDROL (Pharmacia & Upjohn)

GENERIC: available
FAMILY: Corticosteroids (see p. 651)

Methylprednisolone (meth ill pred *niss* oh lone), like other steroids (corticosteroids), has many uses. It is used to treat conditions that produce inflammation, such as arthritis and other joint disorders, allergies, asthma (for which it is the drug of last resort) and other breathing problems, and skin infections. It is also used for acute spinal cord injuries.

Methylprednisolone has several forms for different uses. It can be injected into the muscle, joint, lesion, soft tissue or bloodstream, applied to the skin (topical form), or taken by mouth (oral form). The oral form has limited use. If you need to take a steroid by mouth, prednisone (see p. 668) is the best choice because it is reliable, inexpensive, and available in a generic form.[83]

Steroids suppress your immune system, lowering your defenses against disease and making you more vulnerable to infections. If you use methylprednisolone for a long time, you increase your risk of getting bacterial, viral, parasitic, and fungal infections. Older adults using methylprednisolone are more likely than younger users to develop the bone-weakening condition called osteoporosis. Older users are also more likely to develop high blood pressure and to retain fluid while taking this drug.

As with all drugs, you should use the smallest dose of methylprednisolone that works. You should also use it for the shortest possible time. If you use systemic steroids (ones that are taken by mouth or injected so that your whole body is exposed to them) for a long time, you may suffer many adverse effects, and you may also suffer withdrawal symptoms if you stop abruptly.

Before You Use This Drug

Do not use if you have or have had:

For injections into the joint:

- blood clotting disorders
- fracture of the joint
- infection around the joint
- joint surgery
- osteoporosis
- unstable joint

Tell your doctor if you have or have had:

- allergies to drugs
- AIDS
- bone disease
- chicken pox
- measles
- colitis
- diverticulitis
- stomach ulcer
- diabetes

- fungus infection
- herpes eye infection
- recent surgery or serious injury
- tuberculosis
- glaucoma
- heart disease
- high blood pressure
- liver disease
- thyroid problems
- myasthenia gravis
- systemic lupus (SLE)

Tell your doctor about any other drugs you take, including aspirin, herbs, vitamins, and other nonprescription products.

When You Use This Drug

If taken by mouth or injected:

- **If you have been taking this drug for a long time, do not stop taking it suddenly.** Your doctor must lower your dose gradually to prevent withdrawal symptoms.
- Do not drink alcohol. Drinking alcohol while taking this drug increases your risk of getting an ulcer.
- If you plan to have any surgery, including dental, tell your doctor that you take this drug.
- If you take this drug for a long time, eat a diet low in salt and rich in potassium, protein, and folic acid. Ask your doctor to tell you how you can get more potassium, protein and folic acid in your diet.

How to Use This Drug

- Crush tablet and mix with food or water, or swallow whole with water. Take with food to decrease stomach upset.
- **Use only as prescribed.**
- If you miss a dose, take it as soon as you remember, but skip it if it is almost time for the next dose. **Do not take double doses.**
- Do not store in the bathroom. Do not expose to heat, moisture, or strong light.

Interactions with Other Drugs

The following drugs are listed in the *Evaluations of Drug Interactions* 1997 as causing "highly clinically significant" or "clinically significant" interactions when used together with this drug. We have also included potentially serious interactions listed in the drug's FDA-approved professional product labeling or package insert. New scientific techniques have allowed researchers to predict some drug interactions before they have been documented in people. There may be other drugs, especially those in the families of drugs listed below, that also will react with this drug to cause severe adverse effects. The number of new drugs approved for marketing increases the chance of drug interactions, and new drug interactions are being identified with old drugs. Be vigilant. Make sure to tell your doctor and pharmacist the drugs you are taking and tell your doctor if you are taking any of these interacting drugs:

aspirin, GENUINE BAYER ASPIRIN, cyclosporine, dicumarol, DILANTIN, ECOTRIN, ketoconazole, LUMINAL, NEORAL, NIZORAL, phenobarbital, phenytoin, RIFADIN, rifampin, RIMACTANE, SANDIMMUNE, SOLFOTON, TAO, timolol, TIMOPTIC, troleandomycin.

Adverse Effects

Call your doctor immediately if you experience:

- decreased or blurred vision
- frequent urination
- increased thirst
- numbness, pain, tingling, redness, or swelling at site of injection
- hallucinations
- depression or mood changes
- skin rash or hives
- confusion
- excitement or restlessness

For long-term use:

- persistent abdominal or stomach pain
- acne or other skin problems
- bloody or black, tarry stools
- rounding out of the face
- hip or shoulder pain
- increased blood pressure
- swelling of feet or lower legs
- unusual weight gain
- irregular heartbeats
- muscle cramps or pain
- unusual tiredness or weakness
- pain in back, ribs, arms, or legs
- muscle weakness
- nausea or vomiting
- pitting or depression of skin at injection site
- thin, shiny skin
- unusual bruising
- wounds that will not heal
- menstrual irregularities
- reddish, purplish lines on arms, face, legs, trunk or groin

Call your doctor if these symptoms continue:

- indigestion
- increased appetite
- nervousness or restlessness
- trouble sleeping
- dizziness or lightheadedness
- flushed face
- headache
- increased joint pain
- nosebleeds
- increase in hair on body or face
- loss of appetite
- darkening or lightening of skin color
- sweating

Call your doctor immediately if these symptoms occur after you stop taking this drug:

- abdominal or back pain
- dizziness or fainting
- low grade fever

- persistent loss of appetite
- muscle or joint pain
- nausea or vomiting
- returning symptoms of the condition for which you were taking the drug
- shortness of breath
- frequent, unexplained headaches
- unusual tiredness or weakness
- unusual weight loss

Periodic Tests

Ask your doctor which of these tests should be done periodically while you are taking this drug:

- blood or urine glucose concentration
- eye exams
- blood levels of potassium, sodium, and calcium
- stool tests for possible blood loss
- hypothalamus and pituitary secretion tests
- growth and development determinations

 Do Not Use

ALTERNATIVE TREATMENT:
Lifestyle changes, diet and exercise.

Sibutramine
MERIDIA (Knoll)

FAMILY: Diet Drugs

Sibutramine (si *byoo* tra meen) received marketing approval from the Food and Drug Administration (FDA) in November 1997 for weight loss and weight maintenance when used with a reduced calorie diet in those who meet the medical definition of being overweight.

Sibutramine was evaluated at the September 1996 meeting of the FDA Endocrinologic and Metabolic Drugs Advisory Committee. This committee voted five to four against recommending approval on the grounds that the risks of this drug outweighed its benefits. Committee members were concerned about sibutramine's potential to raise blood pressure and increase heart rate.[84] These adverse effects could make this a dangerous drug for people with high blood pressure, heart disease, blood vessel disease, congestive heart failure, stroke, heart rhythm disturbances, and high thyroid hormone levels (hyperthyroidism). Less than two months later, in mid-November, the FDA, against the advice of the advisory committee, deemed that sibutramine could be approved.[85]

The FDA-approved professional product information, or package insert, for sibutramine contains a number of important warnings: "The long-term effects of MERIDIA on the morbidity and mortality associated with obesity have not been established. . . . The safety and effectiveness of MERIDIA, as demonstrated in double-blind, placebo-controlled trials, have not been determined beyond one year at this time. . . . MERIDIA is contraindicated in patients taking other centrally acting appetite suppressant drugs."

Sibutramine also carries the following warning in bold upper-case letters:

MERIDIA SUBSTANTIALLY INCREASES BLOOD PRESSURE IN SOME PATIENTS. REGULAR MONITORING OF BLOOD PRESSURE IS REQUIRED WHEN PRESCRIBING MERIDIA.[86]

Sibutramine inhibits the reuptake of the brain transmitter serotonin, as do the class of antidepressant drugs know as selective serotonin reuptake inhibitors (SSRIs). These antidepressants include: fluoxetine (PROZAC), fluvoxamine (LUVOX), paroxetine (PAXIL), and sertraline (ZOLOFT). A rare, but serious condition termed "serotonin syndrome" has been reported with the use of serotonin reuptake inhibitors including sibutramine in combination with drugs for migraine headache treatment, such as sumatriptan (IMITREX) and dihydroergotamine (D.H.E. 45), certain opioids, such as dextromethorphan (DELSYM), meperidine (DEMEROL), pentazocine (TALWIN), and fentanyl (DURAGESIC), lithium (LITHOBID, LITHONATE), or tryptophan. Serotonin syndrome has also been reported when two serotonin reuptake inhibitors are taken together.

Serotonin syndrome requires immediate medical attention and may include one or more of the following symptoms: excitement, restlessness, loss of consciousness, confusion, disorientation, anxiety, agitation, weakness, tremor, incoordination, shivering, sweating, vomiting, and rapid heartbeat.

Sibutramine is another in the long list of diet drugs that have never been shown that they can be taken safely for a long enough period of time to reduce the morbidity and mortality associated with obesity.

———

Flunisolide
NASALIDE (Nasal Solution Spray) (Dura)
AEROBID (Oral Aerosol Inhaler) (Forest)

GENERIC: not available
FAMILY: Corticosteroids (see p. 651)

Flunisolide (floo *niss* oh lide) is a steroid (corticosteroid) which is inhaled. It has two forms, a solution that is sprayed into the nose and an inhaler for the mouth. The nose spray is used to treat severe allergies and hay fever and sometimes smooth growths (polyps) in the nose. The inhaler for the mouth mainly benefits people with asthma who need regular, long-term treatment with steroids to control their symptoms. For these people, flunisolide is used after a drug from another family, albuterol or terbutaline (see p. 449) used alone, has not improved the severe chronic symptoms of asthma.[87]

Steroids suppress your immune system, lowering your defenses against disease and making you more vulnerable to infections. If you use flunisolide for a long time, you increase your risk of getting bacterial, viral, parasitic, and fungal infections, especially an infection called oral thrush.

As with all drugs, you should always use flunisolide in the lowest dose that works. You should also take it for the shortest possible time. **If you have used this drug for a long time do not stop suddenly. Your doctor must lower your dose gradually to prevent withdrawal symptoms.**

Before You Use This Drug

Do not use if you have or have had:

- an allergic reaction to fluorocarbon propellants *(the oral inhaler contains fluorocarbons)*

Tell your doctor if you have or have had:

- allergies to drugs
- amebiasis
- liver disease
- recent nose surgery
- glaucoma
- fungal, viral or bacterial infections
- herpes of the eye
- thyroid problems

For oral inhaler:

- current infection of the mouth
- osteoporosis
- tuberculosis or positive TB skin test

Tell your doctor about any other drugs you take, including aspirin, herbs, vitamins, and other nonprescription products.

When You Use This Drug

- If you plan to have any surgery, including dental, tell your doctor that you take this drug.
- **Do not use this drug to treat a sudden, severe asthma attack. This drug is not strong or fast enough for such an attack.**
- Wear a medical identification bracelet or carry a card stating that you may need additional steroids (tablets or injection) in times of unusual stress or sudden, severe asthma attack.

How to Use This Drug

- **Use only as prescribed.**
- If you miss a dose, take it if it is within an hour otherwise skip it. **Do not take double doses.**

Oral inhaler:

- Clean inhaler every day.
- Gargle and rinse your mouth after each time you use the drug, to wash out any of the drug that did not enter your lungs. If your mouth and throat absorb this drug, you may become more susceptible to an infection called thrush.
- See p. 408 for information on how to use an inhaler.
- See p. 402 for information about nasal dosage forms.

Interactions with Other Drugs

The following drugs are listed in the *Evaluations of Drug Interactions* 1997 as causing "highly clinically significant" or "clinically significant" interactions when used together with this drug. We have also included potentially serious interactions listed in the drug's FDA-approved professional product labeling or package insert. New scientific techniques have allowed researchers to predict some drug interactions before they have been documented in people. There may be other drugs, especially those in the families of drugs listed below, that also will react with this drug to cause severe adverse effects. The number of new drugs approved for marketing increases the chance of drug interactions, and new drug interactions are being identified with old drugs. Be vigilant. Make sure to tell your doctor and pharmacist the drugs you are taking and tell your doctor if you are taking any of these interacting drugs:

aldesleukin/interleukin-2, aspirin, GENUINE BAYER ASPIRIN, cyclosporine, dicumarol, ECOTRIN, ketoconazole, NEORAL, NIZORAL, PROLEUKIN, SANDIMMUNE, timolol, TIMOPTIC.

Adverse Effects

Call your doctor immediately if you experience:

For oral inhaler:

- chest pain, trouble breathing
- white patches in the nose or throat
- difficulty swallowing
- behavior changes
- depression
- restlessness

For nasal spray

- bloody mucus or unexplained nosebleeds
- burning or stinging in nose after use of spray
- white patches or sores in nose
- eye pain, loss of vision
- headache
- skin rash, hives
- lightheadedness, dizziness
- loss of sense of taste or smell
- nausea or vomiting
- breathing difficulty
- sore throat
- cough or hoarseness

- stomach pain
- watery eyes
- unusual tiredness or weakness
- acne
- rounding of the face
- menstrual irregularities

Call your doctor if these symptoms continue:

For oral inhaler:

- cough, dry mouth, hoarseness
- sore or dry throat
- headache
- nausea
- skin bruising or thinning
- unpleasant taste

For nasal spray:

- burning or irritation in nose
- sneezing
- irritation, itching or discomfort in throat

Periodic Tests

Ask your doctor which of these tests should be done periodically while you are taking this drug:

- blood or urine glucose concentration
- eye exams

PREGNANCY WARNING

This drug caused harm to developing fetuses in animal studies, or such studies were not done. Use during pregnancy only for clear medical reasons. Tell your doctor if you are pregnant or thinking of becoming pregnant before you take this drug.

Limited Use

Tamoxifen
NOLVADEX (Zeneca)

GENERIC: available

FAMILY: Cancer Drugs

On October 30, 1998, tamoxifen received FDA approval to be used for the reduction in breast cancer incidence in high risk women. High risk is defined as a five year predicted risk of breast cancer of at least 1.67%.

Confusion has erupted over whether the FDA approved tamoxifen for all women 60 years of age and older, without other risk factors for breast cancer. The news media was initially reporting that, regardless of other factors, all women 60 and older were at five year predicted risk of 1.67% (in the high risk category) for developing breast cancer and thus eligible to receive tamoxifen. This is not the case: **NOT ALL WOMEN OVER 60 ARE AT A HIGH RISK OF DEVELOPING BREAST CANCER AND NOT ALL WOMEN OVER 60 SHOULD BE RECEIVING TAMOXIFEN TO REDUCE THE RISK OF BREAST CANCER.**

This drug is a known human cancer causing agent. Before deciding to take tamoxifen to reduce the risk of breast cancer, you should have a careful individual consultation with a cancer specialist (oncologist) or a doctor knowledgeable about the benefits and risks of a drug such as tamoxifen for reducing the risk of breast cancer.

Tamoxifen (ta *mox* i fen) is used to treat breast cancer in women and men, including advanced stages of the disease. It is effective in more than half of women with tumors that are estrogen receptor positive, but in fewer than 15% of those with tumors that are estrogen receptor negative.[88] Tamoxifen therapy appears to reduce risk of cancer in the opposite breast. For those over age 70 risk of fatal myocardial infarction declines.[89] Higher doses are more apt to induce vomiting and adverse effects on the eyes.[90] Women who take tamoxifen may develop large endometrial (uterine) polyps.[91]

Due to the risk of endometrial cancer, tamoxifen is not recommended for prevention of breast cancer. Concern also exists that tamoxifen may induce cancer of the gastrointestinal tract.[92] In animals, tamoxifen has caused liver cancer. Serious blood disorders can develop while taking tamoxifen. There are conflicting reports on the effect of tamoxifen on osteoporosis.[93,94] Since tamoxifen stimulates ovulation, precautions should be taken not to become pregnant, as concern exists that tamoxifen could cause a DES-like syndrome in the fetus. People taking tamoxifen who have bone cancer with breast cancer can develop hypercalcemia (elevated levels of calcium in the blood), which can be life-threatening.

Tamoxifen may induce depression.[95] Sometimes white hair darkens during treatment with tamoxifen.[96] Tamoxifen may be used along with chemotherapy, radiation, and/or surgery.

Before You Use This Drug

Tell your doctor if you have or have had:

- allergies
- cancer
- cataracts or other visual problems
- high cholesterol

Tell your doctor about any other drugs you take, including aspirin, herbs, vitamins, and other nonprescription products.

Ask for exams of your eyes[97] and for a test to detect endometrial cancer before you start to take tamoxifen.[98]

When You Use This Drug

• Take analgesics if needed for pain, which often occurs when tamoxifen is started, but then subsides.

• Do not become pregnant. Use barrier or non-hormonal contraceptives.

How to Use This Drug

• Swallow whole tablet(s). If you obtain tamoxifen outside the U.S. it may be enteric-coated. When using this form do not crush or break these tablets, and do not take antacids or cimetidine, famotidine, nizatidine or ranitidine within one to two hours of taking tamoxifen. These drugs cause the enteric coating to dissolve too soon.

• If you miss a dose skip it. **Do not take double doses.**

• Do not store in the bathroom. Do not expose to heat, moisture, or strong light.

Interactions with Other Drugs

The following drugs are listed in the *Evaluations of Drug Interactions* 1997 as causing "highly clinically significant" or "clinically significant" interactions when used together with this drug. We have also included potentially serious interactions listed in the drug's FDA-approved professional product labeling or package insert. New scientific techniques have allowed researchers to predict some drug interactions before they have been documented in people. There may be other drugs, especially those in the family of drugs listed below, that also will react with this drug to cause severe adverse effects. The number of new drugs approved for marketing increases the chances of drug interactions, and new drug interactions are being identified with old drugs. Be vigilant. Make sure to tell your doctor and pharmacist the drugs you are taking and tell your doctor if you are taking any of these interacting drugs:

COUMADIN, ESTRADERM, estrogen, PREMARIN, warfarin.

The following drugs were also found to have a significant interaction: aminoglutethimide, CYTADREN[99].

Adverse Effects

Call your doctor immediately if you experience:

For both men and women:

• breathing difficulties
• confusion
• swelling or pain in legs
• vision changes
• weakness or sleepiness
• yellowing of skin or eyes

For women:

• pain or pressure in pelvis
• change in vaginal discharge or bleeding

Call your doctor if these symptoms continue:

For both men and women:

• decrease in appetite
• bone pain
• headache
• nausea or vomiting
• skin is dry or develops rash

For women:

• hot flashes
• itching in genital area
• menstrual changes
• vaginal discharge
• undesired weight gain

For men:

• impotence or decreased interest in sex

Periodic Tests

Ask your doctor which of these tests should be done periodically while you are taking this drug:

- blood levels of calcium, cholesterol and triglycerides
- complete blood count
- gynecologic exams
- hepatic function tests
- ophthalmic exams

PREGNANCY WARNING

This drug caused harm to developing fetuses in animal studies, or such studies were not done. Use during pregnancy only for clear medical reasons. Tell your doctor if you are pregnant or thinking of becoming pregnant before you take this drug.

 Do Not Use

ALTERNATIVE TREATMENT:
Rest, exercise, physical therapy, and an anti-inflammatory drug such as aspirin.

Orphenadrine
NORFLEX (3M)

FAMILY: Muscle Relaxants

Orphenadrine (or *fen* a dreen) is marketed for the relief of severe pain caused by muscle conditions such as sprains and back pain. However, neither the tablet nor the injected form of orphenadrine is effective for these conditions. Instead of taking orphenadrine, you should try rest, exercise, physical therapy, or other treatment recommended by your doctor.

The level of orphenadrine in this product is not high enough to relax muscles, so this drug will not directly relax tense skeletal muscles. However, the drug is strong enough to have a sedative effect. **Orphenadrine has not been shown to be any more effective than painkillers or anti-inflammatory drugs such as aspirin for relieving the pain of local muscle spasm,[100] yet it has a higher risk of adverse effects than these painkillers.**

Orphenadrine is similar to a family of drugs called antihistamines, which are used to relieve symptoms of hay fever and other allergies (see p. 402). It may cause some of the same adverse effects and dangerous drug interactions as antihistamines. Some people taking orphenadrine tablets have experienced blurred vision, dry mouth, mild excitement, temporary dizziness, and lightheadedness as adverse effects. Many of these effects occur more often in older adults, even at the usual adult dose. Orphenadrine is particularly dangerous for people who have glaucoma, myasthenia gravis, heart problems, or an enlarged prostate.

WARNING: SPECIAL MENTAL AND PHYSICAL ADVERSE EFFECTS

Older adults are especially sensitive to the harmful anticholinergic (see Glossary, p. 768) effects of orphenadrine because of its similarity to the antihistamines. Drugs in this family should not be used unless absolutely necessary.

Mental Effects: confusion, delirium, short-term memory problems, disorientation, and impaired attention.

Physical Effects: dry mouth, constipation, difficulty urinating (especially for a man with an enlarged prostate), blurred vision, decreased sweating with increased body temperature, sexual dysfunction, and worsening of glaucoma.

Methyltestosterone
ORETON METHYL (Schering)

Fluoxymesterone
HALOTESTIN (Pharmacia & Upjohn)
ANDROID (ICN)

GENERIC: available
FAMILY: Hormones (androgens)

Androgens (*an* droe jens) are male hormones. In older men, they are used to treat impotence, but they are only appropriate in a very limited number of cases. In older women, they are used as a second-choice therapy for advanced breast cancer that is spreading. They are also prescribed for adults with certain rare, hard-to-treat types of anemia.

Most of the prescriptions written for androgens in the United States are for conditions for which they are neither effective nor appropriate. Women have been prescribed androgens to treat a breast condition that most often occurs near or at menopause (fibrocystic disease) and a disorder of the uterine lining (endometriosis), but androgens should not be taken for these conditions. Men suffering from impotence should take androgens only if their condition is caused by abnormally low androgen levels, which is rare. Most cases of impotence can be more effectively treated by seeking and treating other possible medical causes for the problem, by eliminating medications that can cause impotence (see p. 28), and by counseling. Elderly, bedridden males may react adversely to overstimulation caused by androgens and should not take them.

Long-term, high-dose androgen treatment has been associated with life-threatening liver inflammation and cancer. For older men, taking androgens may increase the risk of developing an enlarged prostate or prostate cancer.

If you are taking androgens, avoid food and drugs containing salt, as they increase the amount of fluid that your body retains. Women who take androgens will notice changes in their body, such as a deeper voice and increased facial hair. Most of these changes are temporary. Women taking androgens for breast cancer should be monitored closely by their doctors because androgen therapy occasionally accelerates the disease.

Before You Use This Drug

Do not use if you have or have had:

- breast cancer
- prostate cancer

Tell your doctor if you have or have had:

- allergies to drugs
- diabetes
- kidney or liver problems
- heart or blood vessel disease
- heart attack
- swelling (edema)
- high levels of calcium in the blood
- enlarged prostate gland

Tell your doctor about any other drugs you take, including aspirin, herbs, vitamins, and other nonprescription products.

When You Use This Drug

- **Do not use more or less often or in a higher or lower dose than prescribed.**
- **Caution diabetics:** Check urine sugar levels regularly. This drug affects glucose tolerance.

How to Use This Drug

- *If you use the tablet that is to be swallowed,* take it with or after food to reduce stomach upset.
- *If you use the buccal tablet,* place it in the space between your cheek and gum and allow it

to dissolve slowly. Do not eat, drink, chew, or smoke while the tablet is dissolving. Do not swallow it. After the tablet is dissolved and you can no longer taste it, remove the remaining sugar residue by thoroughly brushing your teeth or rinsing your mouth.

• Do not store in the bathroom. Do not expose to heat, moisture, or strong light.

• If you miss a dose, take it as soon as you remember, but skip it if it is almost time for the next dose. **Do not take double doses.**

Interactions with Other Drugs

The following drugs are listed in the *Evaluations of Drug Interactions* 1997 as causing "highly clinically significant" or "clinically significant" interactions when used together with this drug. We have also included potentially serious interactions listed in the drug's FDA-approved professional product labeling or package insert. New scientific techniques have allowed researchers to predict some drug interactions before they have been documented in people. There may be other drugs, especially those in the families of drugs listed below, that also will react with this drug to cause severe adverse effects. The number of new drugs approved for marketing increases the chance of drug interactions, and new drug interactions are being identified with old drugs. Be vigilant. Make sure to tell your doctor and pharmacist the drugs you are taking and tell your doctor if you are taking any of these interacting drugs:

carbamazepine, cyclosporine, COUMADIN, NEORAL, SANDIMMUNE, TEGRETOL, warfarin.

Adverse Effects

Call your doctor immediately if you experience:

In women:

• acne or oily skin

• enlarged clitoris
• deepening or hoarseness of voice
• changes in hair growth
• decreased breast size
• irregular menstrual cycles
• blistering or itching of skin under patch

In men:

• frequent, painful, or continuing erection
• frequent or difficult urination
• breast swelling or tenderness
• unusual increase in sexual desire

In women and men:

• mental changes
• shortness of breath
• changes in skin color
• dizziness
• frequent or persistent headache
• unusual tiredness
• flushed or red skin
• nausea, vomiting, loss of appetite
• skin rash, hives, or itching
• swelling of feet or lower legs
• unusual bleeding
• yellow eyes or skin
• black, tarry or light colored stools
• vomiting blood
• dark urine
• abdominal pain or swelling
• sore throat and fever
• purple or red spots on body, nose, or inside of mouth
• rapid weight gain
• continuing bad breath odor

Call your doctor if these symptoms continue:

• changes in weight
• breast swelling and tenderness
• changes in sexual desire or drive
• changes in hair growth
• acne
• diarrhea
• insomnia

- infection, pain, redness or other irritation at site of injection
- decrease in testicle size

Periodic Tests

Ask your doctor which of these tests should be done periodically while you are taking this drug:

- physical exam, at least every 6 to 12 months
- liver function tests
- blood levels of calcium and cholesterol
- urine levels of calcium
- hemoglobin and hematocrit levels
- x rays of known or suspected metastases
- bone age determination

PREGNANCY WARNING

This drug should not be used if you are pregnant or are thinking of becoming pregnant. The risk of use of this drug in pregnant women clearly outweighs any possible benefit.

 Do Not Use

ALTERNATIVE TREATMENT: *Rest, exercise, physical therapy, and an anti-inflammatory drug such as aspirin.*

Chlorzoxazone
PARAFON FORTE DSC (Ortho-McNeil Pharmaceutical)

FAMILY: Muscle Relaxants

Chlorzoxazone (klor *zox* a zone) tablets are marketed for the relief of severe pain caused by muscle conditions such as sprains and back pain. However, the drug is not effective for these conditions. Instead of using chlorzoxa-

zone, you should try rest, exercise, physical therapy, or other treatment recommended by your doctor.

The level of chlorzoxazone in the tablets is not high enough to relax muscles, so this drug will not directly relax tense skeletal muscles. However, the drug is strong enough to have a sedative effect. **Chlorzoxazone has not been shown to be any more effective than painkillers or anti-inflammatory drugs such as aspirin for relieving the pain of local muscle spasm,[101] yet it has a higher risk of adverse effects than these painkillers.**

Some people taking chlorzoxazone have experienced drowsiness, headache, upset stomach, nausea, vomiting, heartburn, constipation, diarrhea, and loss of appetite as adverse effects. If you use this drug for a long time, you can develop drug-induced dependence.[102] Some people taking chlorzoxazone have developed liver problems,[103] and the drug is particularly dangerous for people with liver disease.

The brand name product containing chlorzoxazone was reformulated. The old version, PARAFON FORTE, contained chlorzoxazone and acetaminophen. The new product, PARAFON FORTE DSC, contains twice the amount of chlorzoxazone as the old version and no acetaminophen. Both products are equally ineffective.

Prednisolone
PRED FORTE (Allergan)

GENERIC: available
FAMILY: Corticosteroids (see p. 651)

Prednisolone (pred *niss* oh lone), like other corticosteroids (steroids), has many uses. It is most commonly used to treat eye infections that have produced inflammation. It is also used for other conditions in which there is inflammation, such as arthritis and other joint and muscle disorders, allergies, asthma, hay fever, and other breathing problems, and skin infections.

Prednisolone has several forms for different uses. It can be injected into the muscle, joint, lesion, soft tissue, or bloodstream, applied to the eye (ophthalmic form) or the ear (otic form), or taken by mouth. You should not use the form of prednisolone that is taken by mouth. If you need to take a steroid by mouth, prednisone (see p. 668) is the best choice because it is reliable, inexpensive, and available in a generic form.[104]

Steroids suppress your immune system, lowering your defenses against disease and making you more vulnerable to infections. If you use prednisolone for a long time, you increase your risk of getting bacterial, viral, parasitic, and fungal infections. Older adults using prednisolone are more likely than younger users to develop the bone-weakening condition called osteoporosis. Older users are also more likely to develop high blood pressure and to retain fluid while taking this drug.

As with all drugs, you should use the smallest dose of prednisolone that works. You should also use it for the shortest possible time. If you use systemic steroids (ones that are taken by mouth or injected so that your whole body is exposed to them) for a long time, you may suffer many adverse effects, and you may also suffer withdrawal symptoms if you stop abruptly.

Before You Use This Drug

Do not use if you have or have had:

For injections into the joint:

- joint surgery
- blood clotting disorders
- fracture of the joint
- osteoporosis

- infection around the joint
- unstable joint

For eye dosage form:

- eye infections such as herpes, tuberculosis, or others caused by a fungus or virus

Tell your doctor if you have or have had:

- allergies to drugs
- bone disease
- chicken pox
- measles
- colitis
- diverticulitis
- stomach ulcer
- diabetes
- fungus infection
- herpes eye infection
- recent surgery or serious injury
- tuberculosis
- glaucoma
- heart disease
- high blood pressure
- liver disease
- thyroid problems
- myasthenia gravis
- systemic lupus (SLE)

Tell your doctor about any other drugs you take, including aspirin, herbs, vitamins, and other nonprescription products.

When You Use This Drug

If taken by mouth or injected:

- **If you have been taking this drug for a long time, do not stop taking it suddenly.** Your doctor must lower your dose gradually, to prevent withdrawal symptoms.
- Do not drink alcohol. Drinking alcohol while taking this drug increases your risk of getting an ulcer.
- If you plan to have any surgery, including dental, tell your doctor that you take this drug.

- If you take this drug for a long time, eat a diet low in salt and rich in potassium, protein, and folic acid. Ask your doctor how you can get more potassium, protein, and folic acid in your diet.

How to Use This Drug

- **Use only as prescribed.**
- If you miss a dose, take it as soon as you remember, but skip it if it is almost time for the next dose. **Do not take double doses.**

Eye dosage form:

- Follow directions on p. 622 for applying eye drops.
- Check with your doctor if your condition does not improve in one week, or if it worsens.

Interactions with Other Drugs

The following drugs are listed in the *Evaluations of Drug Interactions* 1997 as causing "highly clinically significant" or "clinically significant" interactions when used together with this drug. We have also included potentially serious interactions listed in the drug's FDA-approved professional product labeling or package insert. New scientific techniques have allowed researchers to predict some drug interactions before they have been documented in people. There may be other drugs, especially those in the families of drugs listed below, that also will react with this drug to cause severe adverse effects. The number of new drugs approved for marketing increases the chance of drug interactions, and new drug interactions are being identified with old drugs. Be vigilant. Make sure to tell your doctor and pharmacist the drugs you are taking and tell your doctor if you are taking any of these interacting drugs:

aldesleukin/interleukin-2, aspirin, GENUINE BAYER ASPIRIN, chlorpropamide, cyclosporine, DIABINESE, dicumarol, digoxin, DILANTIN, ECOTRIN, ketoconazole, LANOXICAPS, LANOXIN, LUMINAL, NEORAL, NIZORAL, phenobarbital, phenytoin, PROLEUKIN, RIFADIN, rifampin, RIMACTANE, SANDIMMUNE, SOLFOTON, timolol, TIMOPTIC.

Adverse Effects

Call your doctor immediately if you experience:

- decreased or blurred vision
- frequent urination
- increased thirst
- numbness, pain, tingling, redness, or swelling at site of injection
- hallucinations
- depression or mood changes
- skin rash or hives
- confusion
- restlessness

If using eye dosage form:

- blurred vision
- eye pain
- headache
- seeing halos around lights
- drooping of the eyelids
- unusually large pupils

For long-term use:

- persistent abdominal or stomach pain
- acne or other skin problems
- bloody or black, tarry stools
- rounding out of the face
- hip or shoulder pain
- increased blood pressure
- swelling of feet or lower legs
- unusual weight gain
- irregular heartbeats
- muscle cramps or pain
- unusual tiredness or weakness

- pain in back, ribs, arms, or legs
- muscle weakness
- nausea or vomiting
- pitting or depression of skin at place of injection
- thin, shiny skin
- unusual bruising
- wounds that will not heal
- menstrual irregularities
- reddish, purplish lines on arms, face, legs, trunk or groin

Call your doctor if these symptoms continue:

- indigestion
- increased appetite
- nervousness or restlessness
- trouble sleeping
- dizziness or lightheadedness
- flushed face
- headache
- increased joint pain
- nosebleeds
- increase in hair on body or face
- loss of appetite
- darkening or lightening of skin color
- sweating

If using eye dosage form:

- burning, stinging, or watering of the eyes

Call your doctor immediately if these symptoms occur after you stop taking this drug:

- abdominal or back pain
- dizziness or fainting
- low grade fever
- persistent loss of appetite
- muscle or joint pain
- nausea or vomiting
- returning symptoms of the condition for which you were taking the drug
- shortness of breath
- frequent, unexplained headaches
- unusual tiredness or weakness
- unusual weight loss

Periodic Tests

Ask your doctor which of these tests should be done periodically while you are taking this drug:

- blood or urine glucose concentration
- eye exams
- blood levels of potassium, sodium, and calcium
- stool tests for possible blood loss
- hypothalamus and pituitary secretion tests
- growth and development determinations

PREGNANCY WARNING

This drug caused harm to developing fetuses in animal studies, or such studies were not done. Use during pregnancy only for clear medical reasons. Tell your doctor if you are pregnant or thinking of becoming pregnant before you take this drug.

Limited Use

Conjugated Estrogens
PREMARIN (Wyeth-Ayerst)

Estropipate
OGEN (Pharmacia & Upjohn)

Estradiol
ESTRACE (cream) (Mead Johnson)

Diethylstilbestrol
DES (Lilly)

GENERIC: available
FAMILY: Hormones (estrogens)

Estrogen (*ess* troe jen) is a hormone normally produced in women's bodies, mainly by the ovaries. When a woman reaches menopause, her body's production of estrogen declines noticeably. Doctors commonly prescribe estrogen for women at menopause to treat symptoms such as hot flashes and vaginal dryness. Doctors also prescribe estrogen to replace normal hormone production in women who have had their ovaries removed (usually as part of a hysterectomy, the removal of the uterus), to prevent a bone disease known as osteoporosis in older women, and to treat certain hormone-sensitive cancers in both men and women. Many women on estrogen pills have been told to take them for the rest of their lives. **Estrogens have several serious risks, and you should therefore take them only if absolutely necessary.**

Estrogens Cause Breast Cancer

The most thorough review of all valid epidemiological studies analyzing the relationship between menopausal estrogens and breast cancer was published in the *Journal of the American Medical Association.*[105] The authors, from the Centers for Disease Control and Prevention (CDC), found that there was a direct linear relationship between the duration of use of menopausal estrogens and the risk of breast cancer such that if a woman used the pills for 15 years, she had a 30% increased risk of breast cancer. If use were for 25 years, a "goal" toward which many doctors are pointing their patients, there would be a 50% increased risk of breast cancer. The authors divided up the studies according to the quality of the epidemiological research, such as how well the breast cancer cases were matched with the controls who did not have breast cancer to make the comparison more valid.

The results of this analysis showed that those studies which failed to show an increase in breast cancer associated with the use of menopausal estrogens were judged by the authors to be of significantly lower quality in terms of the validity of the research than the studies which found an increased risk of breast cancer.

The authors examined the increased risk of breast cancer in the five studies which were judged to be of high quality. When just the five high quality studies were analyzed, the 15-year risk was an increase of 60% in breast cancer and the 25-year risk would increase 100%, or a doubling in the amount of breast cancer.

The authors estimate that, based on an increased risk of 30% (the lower estimate, based on high and lower quality studies), the excess number of cases of breast cancer which would be caused by the use of estrogens by 3 million women for 15 years would be 4,708 new cases of breast cancer and 1,468 breast cancer deaths. If the excess risk is 60%, as found in the high quality studies, there would be about 10,000 excess cases of breast cancer and 3,000 deaths. For 25 years of use, these grim statistics would get even worse. National Cancer Institute epidemiologist Dr. Robert Hoover, director of NCI's Environmental Epidemiology Branch, who is a co-author of several of the studies reviewed by the CDC, has told us that: *"The fact that ovarian hormones might relate to increased risk of breast cancer is not on the bizarre fringe of biological reasoning. The biological plausibility was established 100 years ago, so new data which shows that women on replacement therapy have an increased risk is exactly what you would predict."*

Because of these risks, any older woman taking estrogen should have a yearly checkup that includes careful breast and pelvic examinations. It may also include an endometrial biopsy and mammography. All women should examine their own breasts monthly (your doctor can teach you how).

WARNING

Using estrogens increases your risk of endometrial cancer (cancer of the lining of the uterus) by six to eight times. This cancer can be cured by surgery only if it is detected early through a special examination called an endometrial biopsy, and such biopsies are usually done only when a woman is bleeding abnormally. Taking estrogen has also been linked to breast cancer in both men and women. The risk is higher for women who take higher doses or who have used estrogen longer. Experts from the National Cancer Institute and from other countries state that "the prolonged use of estrogens at the time of the menopause may increase the risk of breast cancer by 50% after a 5 to 10 year interval."[106]

Symptoms of Menopause

Most women who are taking estrogen for symptoms of menopause (such as hot flashes) do *not* need to take it forever. If you are taking estrogen for the symptoms of menopause, you should begin by taking it for no more than 6 to 12 months. Then your doctor should slowly take you off the drug and watch to see if the symptoms return. You should start taking estrogen again *only* if the symptoms come back when you stop taking it. If you do keep taking it, you should periodically try stopping it again, under your doctor's guidance.

Some women taking estrogen for symptoms of menopause should not be taking it at all. Estrogen should not be used to treat vague symptoms such as fatigue or sadness. For vaginal dryness, estrogen pills are effective, but there are equally effective alternatives which may be safer. If you need to treat vaginal dryness, you should start by trying lubricant creams without hormones, and if these fail, try a vaginal cream containing estrogen. Although the estrogen in vaginal creams is absorbed into your system, it is not yet clear whether this form has as high a risk as estrogen pills.

Osteoporosis

Estrogen is sometimes prescribed to prevent a bone disease called osteoporosis in older women. In osteoporosis, your bones become frail, placing you at greater risk of hip and other fractures. Many women will never develop this problem. Women who are thin or small-boned, particularly if they are Asian or white, and women who drink more than two alcoholic drinks a day are at higher risk of osteoporosis. Black women, heavy women, and women who get a lot of exercise have a lower risk.

Osteoporosis has no effective treatment, but you can take steps to prevent it. These include getting a lot of calcium in your diet from early adulthood on (see calcium, p. 600) and regularly doing "weight-bearing" exercise such as jogging, walking, tennis, and bicycling. These two steps are enough to prevent osteoporosis in many adults.

Ask your doctor to review your continued need and dose of any drug which causes you to be drowsy or dizzy. Certain diuretics (water pills) may prevent fractures by increasing minerals in the bone,[107] but cause fractures from falls due to dizziness. Paying attention to safety also prevents fractures. Use handrails going up or down stairs, and wear shoes with soles that grip. Use adequate light and vision correction, especially at night. Avoid using throw rugs.

Estrogen therapy, if begun within six years after menopause, will slow the weakening of bone in women's bodies. You should only be taking estrogen for this purpose if you are at high risk for osteoporosis. Only for women in the high-risk group may the benefits of estrogen in preventing osteoporosis outweigh the considerable risks of taking the drug. If you are taking estrogen for osteoporosis, you only need a low daily dose of 0.625 milligram.

Preventing Heart Disease?

Researchers are investigating the effect of estrogen therapy on women's risk of heart and blood vessel diseases such as heart attacks, stroke, and blood clots. In general, women are less likely to have heart attacks than men, but their risk increases after menopause. Some researchers have suggested that estrogen protects women from heart and blood vessel diseases and that their risk of these diseases rises after menopause because their bodies are producing less estrogen. This has led to research to see whether taking estrogen after menopause will protect women from heart disease. There is cause for concern, however, because estrogen in birth control pills used by younger women has been shown to increase the risk of heart and blood vessel disease.

Dr. Vandenbroucke of the Department of Clinical Epidemiology at Leiden University Hospital has seriously questioned the strength of the evidence that estrogens prevent heart disease. He pointed out that in the early 1960s several researchers argued that estrogens were the ultimate protection against all kinds of "senescence" [physical problems of aging] and that estrogens could "delay the 'natural' rise of cardiovascular disease with age." But in referring to studies published in the U.S. in the 1970s raising serious doubts about estrogen's cardioprotective effects,[108] Dr. Vandenbroucke says the main cardiovascular debate is just now beginning "after a lull caused by studies showing an *increased* risk of cardiovascular disease caused by estrogens."

One set of studies involved the use of higher-dose conjugated estrogens (such as in Premarin) in men with previous proven heart attacks.[109] The Coronary Drug Project, involving men, was randomized so that the drug and placebo groups were the same and the experiment had to be stopped because in the highest estrogen dose group (5 milligrams), men actually had an *increased* incidence of adverse events such as blood clots in the lungs and thrombophlebitis, with an increased incidence of heart attacks. In the lower (2.5 milligrams) dose group, there was also an increased amount of blood clots and thrombophlebitis. Not only did estrogens, at those doses, do more harm than good in men, but other estrogens, in the form of the birth control pill (estrogen plus progestagen—a combination of hormones now used by about ⅓ of women taking menopausal estrogens) also caused an increased cardiovascular risk in women. The current studies on women, with one exception, were not randomized so that the group getting estrogens was not necessarily the same as the control group.

In one widely-cited study on the beneficial cardiac effects of estrogens in women[110] the authors found a 50% reduction in coronary heart disease in nurses who used estrogen. But, when nurses who had cancer or coronary heart disease at the beginning of the study were excluded for the analysis, the risk reduction for total mortality, which Vandenbroucke correctly points out is more important than just cardiac deaths, was only 10% and was not statistically significant. In other nonrandomized studies, after adjusting for factors such as this, there was also a reduction in the apparent benefits of estrogens after the adjustments were made.

It is still entirely possible that a woman who receives a prescription for hormone replacement is, at the start, subtly healthier, or more determined to stay that way, than a woman who forgoes this therapy. A study on baseline risk factors in women who were part of a study on hormone replacement therapy found that almost twice as many women who did not take estrogens (28%) were in the top obesity group as women who took estrogens (15.4%). More nonestrogen takers also had diabetes and high blood pressure.[111] Vandenbroucke concludes that the current kind of studies on the benefit of estrogen therapy are unlikely to be useful because they "all have the same defect—i.e., lack of comparability between users and non-users. Perhaps we should demand some colossal well-controlled trials before we let the genie of universal preventive prescription escape from the bottle."[112]

A Food and Drug Administration hearing on estrogens and heart disease addressed the fact that if we would apply what is known about preventing heart disease in women without drugs—increases in exercise, weight loss, eating less cholesterol and harmful fats, stopping smoking and treating high blood pressure—we could reduce heart disease in women by 90%, without significantly increasing the risks of breast and uterine cancer as occurs with the estrogen approach.

To summarize, taking estrogen increases the risk of one serious disease (two kinds of cancer) and protects against another (osteoporosis). Researchers are still trying to define the risks and benefits of estrogen with regard to heart and blood vessel disease in older women. At this time, we do not have enough information to know whether long-term use of estrogen by most older women will, on balance, do more harm or more good.

Internist Dr. Paul Stolley, formerly President of the Society for Epidemiological Research, a Professor at the University of Maryland School of Medicine and an expert on estrogens, has said: *"The famous philosopher Bertrand Russell said that when the experts are not agreed, the non-expert does well to suspend judgement. That could apply to HRT (hormone replacement therapy). The woman with a predictably high risk of developing osteoporosis might wish to run the known and unknown risks of HRT (with careful monitoring for the fairly certain benefit in the prevention of osteoporo-*

sis). However, the woman with no special risk factors of osteoporosis would do well to consider waiting for a few years with the hope that new knowledge will permit a more informed choice."

After years of prescribing estrogens, hoping that they will protect women from heart disease, we finally have a partial answer to the question: Do estrogens protect women from heart disease? A randomized clinical trial published in 1998 has shown no overall benefit in protecting postmenopausal women who already had heart disease from subsequent heart disease. The authors of this study concluded that, based on the finding of no overall benefit and a pattern of early increase in the risk of heart disease, they do not recommend starting this treatment for the prevention of heart disease. They noted however, that because of a favorable pattern of heart disease after several years of treatment, it could be appropriate for women already receiving this treatment to continue. Nevertheless, answer to the question whether or not estrogen replacement protects women who do not have heart disease is years away.[113]

Doctors frequently prescribe estrogen together with a progestin (see p. 723), a synthetic version of another female hormone normally produced in a woman's body before menopause. It is hoped that a combination of estrogen and progestin will have a lower risk of cancer of the uterine lining than estrogen alone. Progestins carry their own risks of blood clots and breast cancer. It is not yet clear whether adding progestin to estrogen is more protective or more dangerous than taking estrogen alone.

If you are taking estrogen after menopause, you should usually be taking it on a cyclical schedule, such as three weeks on and one week off. For treatment of menopausal symptoms, estrogen is also available in a skin patch (see p. 680), which releases the drug into your body slowly.

Before You Use This Drug

Do not use if you have or have had:

- history of blood clot formation
- abnormal or undiagnosed vaginal bleeding
- breast cancer or a strong family history of breast cancer

Tell your doctor if you have or have had:

- allergies to drugs
- asthma
- cancer of the uterus, breast or bone
- diabetes
- endometriosis
- epilepsy, seizure disorder
- gallstones or gallbladder disease
- mental depression
- migraine headaches
- kidney disease
- bone disease
- breast disease or lumps
- heart or circulatory disease
- stroke
- high levels of calcium in the blood
- high blood pressure
- liver disease or jaundice
- non cancerous growths in uterus
- high cholesterol or triglycerides
- pancreatitis

Tell your doctor about any other drugs you take, including aspirin, herbs, vitamins, and other nonprescription products.

When You Use This Drug

- **Do not use more or less often or in a higher or lower dose than prescribed by your doctor.**
- Do not smoke. Smoking increases your risk of serious adverse effects such as blood clots, heart attack, or stroke. The risk increases as you get older.
- Until you know how you react to this drug, do not drive or perform other activities requiring alertness. This drug can cause loss of coordination, blurred vision and drowsiness.
- If you plan to have any surgery, including dental, tell your doctor that you take this drug.
- Have your gums cleaned carefully by a dentist at least once a year, as estrogen can cause gum overgrowth.
- Stay out of the sun as much as possible and do not use sunlamps. Too much sun or sunlamp use while taking estrogen may produce brown, blotchy spots on your skin.

How to Use This Drug

- Take with or right after food to decrease stomach upset. Estrogen is most likely to cause nausea in the morning.
- Do not store in the bathroom. Do not expose to heat, moisture, or strong light.
- If you miss a dose, take it as soon as you remember, but skip it if it is almost time for the next dose. **Do not take double doses.**
- **If you are using skin patches see p. 680.**

Interactions with Other Drugs

The following drugs are listed in the *Evaluations of Drug Interactions* 1997 as causing "highly clinically significant" or "clinically significant" interactions when used together with this drug. We have also included potentially serious interactions listed in the drug's FDA-approved professional product labeling or package insert. New scientific techniques have allowed researchers to predict some drug interactions before they have been documented in people. There may be other drugs, especially those in the families of drugs listed below, that also will react with this drug to cause severe adverse effects. The number of new drugs approved for marketing increases the chance of drug interactions, and new drug interactions are being identified with old drugs. Be vigilant. Make sure to tell your doctor and pharmacist the drugs you are taking and tell your doctor if you are taking any of these interacting drugs:

ANECTINE, DELTASONE, LUMINAL, METICORTEN, phenobarbital, prednisone, RIFADIN, rifampin, RIMACTANE, SOLFOTON, succinylcholine.

Additionally, the *United States Pharmacopeia Drug Information,* 1998 lists these drugs as having interactions of major significance: bromocriptine, cyclosporine, DANTRIUM, dantrolene, NEORAL, PARLODEL, SANDIMMUNE.

Adverse Effects

Call your doctor immediately if you experience:

- persistent or abnormal vaginal bleeding
- drowsiness
- dribbling urination
- breast pain or increase in breast size
- swelling of feet or lower legs
- weight gain
- high blood pressure
- uncontrolled movements of body
- breast lumps or discharge
- depression
- pains in stomach, side or abdomen
- yellowing of eyes or skin
- skin rash
- thick, white vaginal discharge

For men:

- severe headache
- sudden loss of coordination
- pains in chest, groin, leg, or calf
- shortness of breath
- slurred speech
- vision changes
- weakness or numbness in arm or leg

Call your doctor if these symptoms continue:

- bloating, cramping
- nausea, loss of appetite, vomiting
- changes in weight
- swelling of ankles and feet
- breast swelling and tenderness
- changes in sexual desire
- changes in hair growth
- diarrhea
- dizziness, irritability
- decreased tolerance to wearing contact lenses
- headache

Periodic Tests

Ask your doctor which of these tests should be done periodically while you are taking this drug:

- blood pressure
- liver function test
- pap smear*
- yearly mammogram*
- physical examination at least every 6 to 12 months, with special attention to the breasts, and including a pelvic exam*
- endometrial biopsy
- bone age determinations
- lipid profile determinations

These should be a part of your normal health care routine.

PREGNANCY WARNING

This drug caused harm to developing fetuses in animal studies, or such studies were not done. Use during pregnancy only for clear medical reasons. Tell your doctor if you are pregnant or thinking of becoming pregnant before you take this drug.

Finasteride
PROSCAR (Merck)

GENERIC: not Available
FAMILY: Prostate Drugs

Finasteride (fin *as* tur ide) is used to control symptoms of enlarged prostate called benign prostatic hyperplasia (BPH). It is used for mild to moderate BPH. Enlargement of the prostate gland blocks urination, causing a weak stream, double voiding, inability to empty the bladder completely, and urinary tract infections. Chronic obstruction can be life-threatening. BPH affects 50% of men over age 60 and 90% of men over age 80.

Finasteride blocks an enzyme that is necessary to convert the male sex hormone testosterone to another hormone that causes the prostate to grow. As a result, the size of the prostate gland is decreased. Other drugs that are used to treat BPH belong to a family of drugs that were originally developed to treat high blood pressure called alpha blockers. These drugs are doxazosin (CARDURA), tamsulosin (FLOMAX), and terazosin (HYTRIN). The alpha blockers work by relaxing the muscles around the neck of the bladder to improve urinary flow. A complete discussion of terazosin can be found on p. 105.

A large clinical trial compared the effect of finasteride with terazosin in more than 1,000 men with BPH. This study lasted one year. Overall, this study concluded that terazosin was effective therapy, finasteride was not, and the combination of terazosin and finasteride was not more effective than terazosin alone. However, the researchers did find that finasteride was effective in a group of men with very large glands, while terazosin was effective in men with both very large and smaller prostate glands.[114]

A recent study found that long-term use of finasteride reduces the probability of surgery for an enlarged prostate gland.[115] But, the editorial accompanying this study took a different view: ". . . treatment with finasteride to prevent these complications may be unwarranted for most men with symptoms of this disorder [BPH]." The editorial relates a hypothetical conversation between a man asking about finasteride and reducing the risk of prostate surgery and a very good doctor who explains the results of the study.

Patient: Doctor, my wife just read about this new drug for the prostate. She said it was like an insurance policy. You pay a little premium each day to avoid needing surgery later.

Physician: That is a good way to think about it. After four years, 13 of 100 men had complete urine blockage or needed surgery for their prostate. A drug called finasteride reduced the chances of these problems; instead of occurring in 13 of 100 men, they occurred in 7 of 100. In other words, about 6 out of 100 men benefited after four years of taking the drug.

Patient: So 100 men paid the premium for four years and 6 of them got the benefit?

Physician: You seem to have the basic point. Those men who kept taking the drug also said that their urinary symptoms were a little better—an improvement of 2 points on a 35-point scale. But a few men taking the drug had impotence, breast tenderness, and loss of energy.[116]

If your BPH symptoms are minimal, no treatment is necessary, no matter what the size of your prostate may be. If you have BPH symptoms and do not have a very enlarged gland, terazosin would be the best drug to use. If your prostate is very enlarged, treatment with either finasteride or terazosin would be reasonable. If your BPH symptoms are severe, surgery may be the best treatment.[117]

PERCENTAGES OF MEN
REPORTING SELECTED ADVERSE
REACTIONS WITH FINASTERIDE
(PROSCAR) AND TERAZOSIN
(HYTRIN)[118]

	Finasteride	Terazosin
Dizziness	8%	26%
Weakness	7%	14%
Impotence	9%	6%
Inflammation of Nasal Mucous Membranes	3%	7%
Ejaculatory Problems	2%	0.3%
Decreased Libido	5%	3%

Before You Use This Drug

Tell your doctor if you have or have had:

- allergies, including lactose
- heart problems
- liver problems
- difficulties urinating

Tell your doctor about any other drugs you take, including aspirin, herbs, vitamins, and other nonprescription products.

Before you start this drug have your doctor do a digital rectal exam, baseline PSA test, and check that you do not have conditions with similar symptoms, such as infection, prostate cancer, stricture disease, or hypotonic bladder.

When You Use This Drug

- Do not let any women who are pregnant or could become pregnant crush your tablets or touch your medication.
- Protect any women you have intercourse with from pregnancy, since finasteride in semen can harm the fetus.
- Do not drink alcohol or coffee in the evening.
- Read information about your prescription each time in case new information has become available.

How to Use This Drug

- Swallow tablets whole or crushed. Take without regard to food.
- If you miss a dose, take it as soon as you remember but skip it if it is almost time for the next dose. **Do not take double doses.**
- Do not store in the bathroom. Do not expose to heat, moisture, or strong light.
- Check with your doctor before discontinuing finasteride.

Interactions with Other Drugs

The following drugs are listed in the *Evaluations of Drug Interactions* 1997 as causing "highly clinically significant" or "clinically significant" interactions when used together with this drug. We have also included potentially serious interactions listed in the drug's FDA-approved professional product labeling or package insert. New scientific techniques have allowed researchers to predict some drug interactions before they have been documented in people. There may be other drugs, especially those in the families of drugs listed below, that also will react with this drug to cause severe adverse effects. The number of new drugs approved for marketing increases the chance of drug interactions, and new drug interactions are being identified with old drugs. Be vigilant. Make sure to tell your doctor and pharmacist the drugs you are taking and tell your doctor if you are taking any of these interacting drugs:

ADRENALIN (also in bee sting kits), AKINETON, aminophylline, ANTIVERT, ARTANE, atropine, belladonna, BENADRYL, BENTYL, benztropine, biperiden, clidinium, COGENTIN, cyclizine, DEXATRIM, dicyclomine, dimenhydrinate, diphenhydramine, DRAMAMINE, ECSTACY, ELIXOPHYLLIN, ephedrine, epinephrine, ethopropazine, glycopyrrolate, HOMAPIN, homatropine, KEMADRIN, MAREZINE, meclizine, methoscopolamine,

PAMINE, PARSIDOL, phenylpropanolamine, PRIMATENE MIST, PRO–BANTHINE, procyclidine, propantheline, pseudoephedrine, QUARZAN, ROBINUL, scopolamine, SLO-BID, SOMINEX FORMULA, SOMOPHYLLIN, SOMOPHYLLIN-DF, SUDAFED, THEO-24, theophylline, TIGAN, TRANSDERM-SCOP, trihexyphenidyl, trimethobenzamide.

Adverse Effects

Call your doctor immediately if you experience:

- pelvic or testicular pain
- skin rash
- swelling of lips
- vision changes
- breast enlargement or tenderness

Call your doctor if these symptoms continue:

- abdominal pain
- decreased amount of ejaculation
- dizziness
- gas
- headache
- impotence
- diarrhea

Periodic Tests

Ask your doctor which of these tests should be done periodically while you are taking this drug:

- digital rectal examination

PREGNANCY WARNING

Women who are pregnant or thinking of becoming pregnant should not handle finasteride tablets because of the possibility of harm to the developing fetus.

Limited Use

Medroxyprogesterone
PROVERA (Pharmacia & Upjohn)
AMEN (Carnrick)

Norethindrone Acetate
AYGESTIN (Wyeth-Ayerst)

GENERIC: available
FAMILY: Hormones (Progestins)

Progesterone is a hormone normally produced in women's bodies. Progestins (proe *jess* tins) are synthetic variations of progesterone. For younger women, doctors prescribe synthetic progesterone to treat irregular menstrual bleeding and endometriosis. Doctors are increasingly prescribing progestins to older women who are taking another hormone, estrogen, to treat symptoms of menopause (such as hot flashes) or to prevent osteoporosis (bone frailty). Progestins are also used in special circumstances to treat uterine, breast, and kidney cancer. If you are taking progestins, you may bleed every month even if you have passed menopause.

Because progestins have potentially significant risks, you should only use them (or progestin and estrogen combinations) to treat serious symptoms, and then for as short a time as possible. It is still unclear whether the benefits of long-term treatment with estrogen and progestins outweigh the risks.

When you take estrogen (for example, to treat symptoms of menopause), the lining of your uterus thickens. Many doctors are prescribing progestins along with estrogen to slow this thickening and to prevent the cancer of the lining of the uterus (endometrial cancer) that estrogen can cause.

Progestin use has been associated with blood clots, strokes, and blindness in women. The drug causes breast and uterine cancers when administered to laboratory mammals, and researchers are investigating whether it causes breast cancer in women by itself or further increases the risk of breast cancer when used with estrogen.

The combination of progestins and estrogen that many doctors are prescribing to older women is similar to that in birth control pills. In birth control pills, this combination has been known to cause serious adverse effects to the heart and blood vessels, such as heart attack and stroke. These adverse effects are more common in older women, especially older women who smoke. Using an estrogen-progestin combination later in life for purposes other than birth control may also increase the risk of such adverse effects (see p. 714).

Before You Use This Drug

Do not use if you have or have had:

- stroke
- varicose veins
- breast disease
- history of blood clot formation
- abnormal or undiagnosed uterine, vaginal or urinary tract bleeding
- liver disease
- pregnancy, known or suspected

Tell your doctor if you have or have had:

- allergies to drugs
- asthma
- cancer
- diabetes
- epilepsy, seizure disorder
- mental depression
- migraine headaches
- kidney or liver problems
- breast disease or lumps
- heart or circulatory disease
- high blood cholesterol
- osteoporosis risk

Tell your doctor about any other drugs you take, including aspirin, herbs, vitamins, and other nonprescription products.

When You Use This Drug

- **Do not use more or less often or in a higher or lower dose than your doctor has prescribed.**
- If you plan to have any surgery, including dental, tell your doctor that you take this drug.

How to Use This Drug

- Take with or right after food to decrease stomach upset.
- Do not store in the bathroom. Do not expose to heat, moisture, or strong light.
- If you miss a dose, take it as soon as you remember, but skip it if it is almost time for the next dose. **Do not take double doses.**

Interactions with Other Drugs

Some other drugs that you may be taking (either over-the-counter or prescription drugs) can interact with this one, causing adverse effects. Ask your doctor what these drugs are and let him or her know if you are taking any of them.

Adverse Effects

Call your doctor immediately if you experience:

- persistent or abnormal vaginal bleeding
- bulging eyes
- double vision, loss of vision
- skin rash, itching
- severe headache
- sudden loss of coordination
- pains in chest, groin, leg, calf
- sudden shortness of breath
- loss of or change in speech

- vision changes
- weakness or numbness in arm or leg
- breast lumps or discharge or unexpected or increased milk flow
- depression
- pains in stomach or side
- yellow eyes or skin
- dry mouth
- frequent urination
- loss of appetite
- unusual thirst

Call your doctor if these symptoms continue:

- nausea, loss of appetite
- changes in weight
- swelling of face, ankles or feet
- breast swelling and tenderness
- changes in sexual desire
- changes in hair growth
- acne
- abdominal pain or cramping
- increase in blood pressure
- headache
- mood changes
- brown spots on exposed skin
- hot flashes
- insomnia
- nervousness
- pain or irritation at injection site
- unusual tiredness or weakness

Periodic Tests

Ask your doctor which of these tests should be done periodically while you are taking this drug:

- physical exam, at least every 6 to 12 months*
- breast self-examination, monthly*
- pap smear*

*These should be a part of your normal health care routine.

PREGNANCY WARNING

This drug should not be used if you are pregnant or are thinking of becoming pregnant. The risk of use of this drug in pregnant women clearly outweighs any possible benefit.

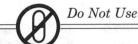 *Do Not Use*

ALTERNATIVE TREATMENT: *Drink plenty of fluids and treat the cause of the pain, such as the urinary tract infection.*

Phenazopyridine
PYRIDIUM (Warner-Chilcott)

FAMILY: Urinary Analgesics (Painkillers)

Phenazopyridine (fen az oh *peer* i deen) is used to treat pain, burning, and other symptoms when the lower part of the urinary tract (bladder) is irritated due to an infection or surgery. **Do not take this drug.** Because older people's bodies eliminate drugs less effectively than younger people's, this drug can stay in your system much longer than it should, and can build up until it reaches dangerously high levels in your bloodstream. This can lead to harmful adverse effects. Also, this drug can cause cancer, according to the World Health Organization's International Agency for Research on Cancer.[119]

Instead of prescribing this drug to relieve pain and irritation, a physician should find and treat the *cause* of the pain and irritation. See p. 484 for ways to avoid urinary tract infections.

Do Not Use (Except for treatment of certain types of skin cancer and severe acne)

ALTERNATIVE TREATMENT:
Protection from the sun.

Tretinoin
RETIN-A (Ortho)
RENOVA (Ortho Dermatological)

FAMILY: Wrinkle Remover

Tretinoin (*tret* in oyn) has been used for a long time to treat certain types of acne. It does not cure acne. Tretinoin cream has been used more recently, despite insufficient information about safety and effectiveness, to reverse skin damage from the sun, which increases with aging. Concern exists that since tretinoin causes increased sensitivity to sunburn, over a long time it could actually increase the risk of skin cancer.[120]

Cosmetically, tretinoin may smooth out fine wrinkles, but it is not yet known if wrinkles return. Deep, coarse wrinkles may not improve.[121] Even if tretinoin reduces wrinkles caused by sun damage, it is not known if it works on wrinkles from normal aging, or how older people react to the topical form of tretinoin. At times tretinoin causes a change in pigmentation, which may last months after discontinuing the drug.[122] Some patients cannot tolerate the irritating effect of the drug,[123] and the safety of long-term use on photo-(sun) damaged skin remains to be determined.

To prevent sun damage to the skin, avoid prolonged exposure to the sun, including at work, while driving, and from reflection off water and snow. Wear long sleeves, protective hats, dark sunglasses, and use a sunscreen. Avoid dry air and smoking to reduce premature wrinkling. Alcohol, either regularly taken as a beverage, or applied in cosmetics can aggravate wrinkles. Don't overdo activities that dry the skin, such as frequent bathing or swimming. To lessen dry, wrinkled skin, use a moisturizer, such as products containing lanolin, urea or lactic acid.

Limited Use

Methylphenidate
RITALIN (Novartis)

GENERIC: available
FAMILY: Central nervous system stimulants

> ### DRUG DEPENDENCE
>
> Methylphenidate can cause dependence. Chronic overuse of this drug can lead to varying degrees of abnormal behavior. Psychotic episodes can occur. Careful supervision is required during withdrawal from methylphenidate, since severe depression and other adverse effects can occur.

Methylphenidate (meth ill *fen* i date) is approved by the FDA for the treatment of attention deficit disorders and for the sudden uncontrollable need to sleep at irregular intervals called narcolepsy. More than four million prescriptions were sold for methylphenidate in 1997.[124]

There is no doubt that although this drug can be effective in helping children (or adults) who actually have attention deficit disorder (ADD), it is greatly overused and misused. Many children diagnosed with this condition actually have problems which are caused or worsened by inadequate teachers in the schools they attend or by problems with their parents. Similarly, many adults may have interpersonal problems which need to be dealt with by psychotherapy. Until these causes of what might appear to be ADD are searched for and ruled out in a systematic way, it is not appropriate to use Ritalin or similar drugs.

Methylphenidate should not be used in children under six years of age, since safety and efficacy in this age group have not been established. Little information is available on the long-term safety and effectiveness of this drug in children. Suppression of growth has been reported with the long-term use of stimulants in children.

Before You Use This Drug

Do not use if you have or have had:

- family history or diagnosis of Tourette's syndrome
- glaucoma
- anxiety, tension, agitation

Tell your doctor if you have or have had:

- allergies to drugs
- alcohol or drug dependence
- epilepsy
- high blood pressure
- psychosis
- mental depression
- tics other than Tourette's syndrome

Tell your doctor about any other drugs you take, including aspirin, herbs, vitamins, and other nonprescription products.

When You Use This Drug

- Methylphenidate should be taken after meals or with a snack.
- To prevent trouble sleeping, take the last dose of the short-acting tablets before 6 pm, unless you are told to do otherwise by your doctor.
- Do not crush or chew the long acting form of this drug. These tablets must be swallowed whole.

How to Use This Drug

- **Use only as prescribed.**
- If you miss a dose, take it as soon as possible. Then take any remaining doses for that day at regularly spaced intervals. **Do not take double doses.**
- Do not store in the bathroom. Do not expose to heat, moisture, or strong light.

Interactions with Other Drugs

The following drugs are listed in the *Evaluations of Drug Interactions* 1997 as causing "highly clinically significant" or "clinically significant" interactions when used together with this drug. We have also included potentially serious interactions listed in the drug's FDA-approved professional product labeling or package insert. New scientific techniques have allowed researchers to predict some drug interactions before they have been documented in people. There may be other drugs, especially those in the families of drugs listed below, that also will react with this drug to cause severe adverse effects. The number of new drugs approved for marketing increases the chance of drug interactions, and new drug interactions are being identified with old drugs. Be vigilant. Make sure to tell your doctor and pharmacist the drugs you are taking and tell your doctor if you are taking any of these interacting drugs:

Central nervous system (CNS) depressant drugs including alcohol, antidepressants, antihistamines, antipsychotics, some blood pressure medications (reserpine, methyldopa, beta-blockers), motion sickness medications, muscle relaxants, narcotics, sedatives, sleeping pills and tranquilizers.

Monoamine oxidase (MAO) inhibitors: deprenyl, ELDEPRYL, furazolidone,

FUROXONE, isocarboxazid, MARPLAN, MATULANE, NARDIL, PARNATE, phenelzine, procarbazine, selegiline, tranylcypromine should not be used at the same time or within two weeks of taking methylphenidate.

The following drug was also found to have a significant interaction: ORAP, pimozide.

Adverse Effects

Call your doctor immediately if you experience:

- agitation
- severe confusion
- seizures
- dryness of the mouth or mucous membranes
- false sense of well-being
- fast, pounding, or irregular heartbeat
- fever
- severe headache
- increased blood pressure
- increased sweating
- enlarged pupils
- muscle twitching
- seeing, hearing, or feeling things that are not there
- trembling
- vomiting

Call your doctor if these symptoms continue:

- loss of appetite
- nervousness
- trouble sleeping
- dizziness
- drowsiness
- headache
- nausea
- stomach pain
- black, tarry stools
- blood in urine or stools
- chest pain

- joint pain
- pinpoint red spots on skin
- skin rash or hives
- unusual bleeding or bruising
- blurred vision or any change in vision
- uncontrolled vocal outburst and tics
- mood or mental changes

Call your doctor immediately if these symptoms occur after you stop taking this drug:

- depression
- unusual behavior
- unusual tiredness or weakness

Periodic Tests

Ask your doctor which of these tests should be done periodically while you are taking this drug:

- blood pressure
- complete blood cell, differential, and platelet counts
- monitoring of growth, both height and weight gain, in children
- reassessment for the need for therapy in children

 Do Not Use

ALTERNATIVE TREATMENT: *Rest, exercise, physical therapy, and an anti-inflammatory drug such as aspirin.*

Methocarbamol
ROBAXIN (Robins)

FAMILY: Muscle Relaxants

Methocarbamol (meth oh *kar* ba mole) is marketed for the relief of severe pain caused by muscle conditions such as sprains and back pain. However, it is not effective for these conditions. Instead of taking methocarbamol, you should try rest, exercise, physical therapy, or other treatment recommended by your doctor.

The level of methocarbamol in this product is not high enough to relax muscles, so this drug will not directly relax tense skeletal muscles. However, the drug is strong enough to have a sedative effect. **Methocarbamol has not been shown to be any more effective than painkillers or anti-inflammatory drugs such as aspirin for relieving the pain of local muscle spasm,[125] yet it has a higher risk of adverse effects than these painkillers.**

Methocarbamol's adverse effects include drowsiness, lightheadedness, dizziness, nausea, vomiting, heartburn, abdominal distress, constipation, diarrhea, and loss of appetite. If you use this drug for a long time, you may develop drug-induced dependence.

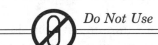 *Do Not Use*

ALTERNATIVE TREATMENT:
This is a cosmetic, not a medical problem. No treatment recommended.

Minoxidil
ROGAINE (Pharmacia & Upjohn)

FAMILY: Hair Growth Drugs

Minoxidil (min *ox* id ill) applied to the scalp is used to treat baldness, especially male-pattern baldness. It stimulates hair growth, or at least slows down the rate of hair loss, but does not cure baldness. The same drug in the form of an oral tablet (LONITEN) controls high blood pressure. Studies are underway to evaluate the use of topical minoxidil in women and some show effectiveness in women.[126,127,128] It takes four months to a year to promote hair growth, with results varying widely. **Minoxidil works best in men under age 40,** whose hair has been thinning less than two years, and when the bald area covers less than 50% of the scalp.

Hair is more apt to regrow on the crown, and less apt on temples and receding hair lines. The first hair growth is usually short and soft, resembling a newborn's. Subsequent growth matches your hair in color (which can be white) and thickness. About 25% of men obtain some regrowth of hair. Less than 1% experience thick regrowth.[129] Complete coverage of a bald area rarely occurs. Expectations often determine satisfaction with the results. At best, one-third rate the results good to excellent.[130] For smokers, a side benefit may be a distaste for smoking cigarettes.[131]

People over age 50 should weigh the risks and benefits carefully,[132] and as indicated above this is a Do Not Use drug for people over the age of 60. Minoxidil is less likely to work the older you are, if baldness has existed more than five years, or is primarily on the sides. Effectiveness in women past menopause has not been studied.

The alcohol in minoxidil solution sometimes irritates the scalp, or eyes if it accidentally gets into the eye. Adverse effects increase with higher strengths of minoxidil. Although absorption of minoxidil is low, when absorbed, all harmful effects of oral minoxidil (LONITEN) are possible. Topical minoxidil may cause changes in heart function, such as increased heart rate. Later development of a heart problem or other condition might require discontinuing the drug.

To be effective, treatment must continue. Once minoxidil is stopped, new hair growth disappears over a few months and hair growth returns to the previous pattern. Expenses associated with the use of minoxidil run about $400 a year.

Hair regrowth can occur spontaneously when baldness is due to disease, drugs, or radiation once the disease is cured or exposure stopped. Immune diseases, including seasonal allergies, can aggravate hair loss.[133] Options besides minoxidil include hair pieces, hair transplants, and accepting baldness as a natural process.

 Do Not Use

ALTERNATIVE TREATMENT:
*Rest, exercise, physical therapy, and
anti-inflammatory drugs such as aspirin.*

Carisoprodol
SOMA (Wallace)

FAMILY: Muscle Relaxants

Carisoprodol (kar eye soe *proe* dole) tablets are promoted for the relief of severe pain caused by muscle conditions such as sprains and back pain. However, this drug is not effective for these conditions. Instead of taking carisoprodol, you should try rest, exercise, physical therapy, or other treatment recommended by your doctor.

The level of carisoprodol in the tablets is not high enough to relax muscles, so this drug will not directly relax tense skeletal muscles. However, the drug is strong enough to have a sedative effect. **Carisoprodol has not been shown to be any more effective than painkillers or anti-inflammatory drugs such as aspirin for relieving the pain of local muscle spasm,[134] yet it has a higher risk of adverse effects than these painkillers.**

Some people taking carisoprodol have experienced drowsiness, lightheadedness, dizziness, nausea, vomiting, heartburn, abdominal distress, constipation, diarrhea, and loss of appetite as adverse effects. If you take cariso-

prodol for a long time, you may become addicted to it.[135] Carisoprodol is particularly dangerous for people with acute intermittent porphyria.

Carisoprodol occasionally causes a reaction within the first few minutes or hours after the first dose. Symptoms of a reaction are agitation, confusion, unsteadiness, disorientation, weakness, speech or vision problems, and temporary inability to move arms or legs.

Fluocinolone
SYNALAR, SYNEMOL (Medicis)

GENERIC: available
FAMILY: Corticosteroids (see p. 651)

Fluocinolone (floo oh *sin* oh lone) is used to reduce inflammation (redness and swelling) and relieve itching caused by many skin conditions, such as eczema and psoriasis. It is a topical solution and comes in cream and ointment form.

Steroids suppress your immune system, lowering your defenses against disease and making you more vulnerable to infections. If you use fluocinolone for a long time, you increase your risk of getting bacterial, viral, parasitic, and fungal infections.

As with all drugs, you should use the lowest possible dose of fluocinolone that works. You should also use it for as short a time as possible and limit the area of your body that you use it on, if possible. A steroid applied to the skin can cause many adverse effects, especially if you use it for a long time or over a large area so that your whole body absorbs the drug. **If you have used this drug for a long time do not stop suddenly. Your doctor must lower your dose gradually to prevent withdrawal symptoms.**

Before You Use This Drug

Tell your doctor if you have or have had:

- allergies to drugs
- herpes sores
- infection or ulceration at the place where you will be applying the drug
- cataracts
- glaucoma
- diabetes
- tuberculosis

Tell your doctor about any other drugs you take, including aspirin, herbs, vitamins, and other nonprescription products.

When You Use This Drug

- Check with your doctor if your condition does not improve in one week or if it worsens.

How to Use This Drug

- **Use only as prescribed.**
- Spread a very thin layer over the area being treated to minimize absorption of the drug into your body. (There is no danger of systemic absorption with correct use.)
- The preparation may sting when applied.
- Do not bandage or wrap the area you are treating unless your doctor has told you to do so.
- Do not use around eyes for a long period.

Interactions with Other Drugs

Some other drugs that you may be taking (either over-the-counter or prescription drugs) can interact with this one, causing adverse effects. Ask your doctor what these drugs are and let him or her know if you are taking any of them.

Adverse Effects

Call your doctor immediately if you experience:

- pain, redness, or blisters containing pus
- burning, itching, or blistering that was not present before you began using this drug
- acne or other skin problems
- thinning of skin
- bruising
- increased hair growth, especially on the face
- loss of hair, especially on scalp
- lack of healing of skin condition
- loss of top skin layer
- numbness in fingers

Call your doctor if these symptoms continue:

- acne or other skin problem
- backache
- blurred vision
- eye pain
- rounding out of face
- increased blood pressure
- irregular heartbeat
- irregular menstrual period
- irritability
- irritation of skin and mouth
- loss of appetite
- depression
- muscle cramps, pain or weakness
- nausea
- rapid weight gain or loss
- reddish, purplish lines on arms, face, legs, trunk or groin
- changes in skin color
- stomach bloating or pain
- softening of skin
- swelling of feet or lower legs
- decrease in sexual ability or desire
- tearing of the skin
- unusual increase or loss of hair growth
- unusual tiredness or weakness
- vomiting
- worsening of infections
- skin rash, irritation, burning or dryness

Periodic Tests

Ask your doctor which of these tests should be done periodically while you are taking this drug:

- blood or urine glucose concentration
- eye exams
- adrenal function assessment

Levothyroxine
SYNTHROID (Knoll)
LEVOTHROID (Forest)

Liotrix
EUTHROID (Parke-Davis)
THYROLAR (Forest)

Thyroid

GENERIC: available
FAMILY: Hormones (thyroid)

Thyroid (*thye* roid) hormone pills are prescribed for people whose thyroids do not produce a normal amount of these hormones. Most people, however, are unnecessarily prescribed thyroid hormone even though their own levels are in the normal range. Most people who actually *need* to be on thyroid replacement therapy need to take these hormones for the rest of their lives. **In general, if you are over 60, you need to take only about three-fourths of the usual adult dose.**

Levothyroxine (lee voe thye *rox* een) is the usual first-choice drug for thyroid replacement therapy. Older adults should start at a dose of just 25 micrograms (.025 milligram), with cautious increases every two to four weeks if necessary. Starting with a low dose will reduce the risk of heart failure or chest pain.[136] Whichever type of thyroid hormone you use, check with your doctor before switching brands. Brands can vary in

concentration, so switching brands can cause you to get too much or too little of the hormone.

Natural thyroid extract (thyroid) is an older drug that is now considered obsolete. It can produce hazardous adverse effects in older people. **You should not take this form of thyroid hormone unless you have already been taking it for years.**[137]

Before You Use This Drug

Tell your doctor if you have or have had:

- allergies to drugs
- heart or circulatory disease
- diabetes
- underactive adrenal or pituitary gland
- high blood pressure
- thyroid problems

Tell your doctor about any other drugs you take, including aspirin, herbs, vitamins, and other nonprescription products.

When You Use This Drug

- You may need to take this medicine for the rest of your life. Schedule regular checkups. Do not stop taking this drug without talking to your doctor first.
- **Talk to your doctor before taking any other prescription or nonprescription drugs. They may interfere with the effects of thyroid hormone.**
- **Caution diabetics:** see p. 550.
- If you plan to have any surgery, including dental, tell your doctor that you take this drug.

How to Use This Drug

- **Do not use more or less often or in a higher or lower dose than prescribed by your doctor.**
- Do not store in the bathroom. Do not expose to heat, moisture, or strong light.

- If you miss a dose, take it as soon as you remember, but skip it if it is almost time for the next dose. **Do not take double doses.** Check with your doctor if you miss more than two doses.

Interactions with Other Drugs

The following drugs are listed in the *Evaluations of Drug Interactions* 1997 as causing "highly clinically significant" or "clinically significant" interactions when used together with this drug. We have also included potentially serious interactions listed in the drug's FDA-approved professional product labeling or package insert. New scientific techniques have allowed researchers to predict some drug interactions before they have been documented in people. There may be other drugs, especially those in the families of drugs listed below, that also will react with this drug to cause severe adverse effects. The number of new drugs approved for marketing increases the chance of drug interactions, and new drug interactions are being identified with old drugs. Be vigilant. Make sure to tell your doctor and pharmacist the drugs you are taking and tell your doctor if you are taking any of these interacting drugs:

cholestyramine, COUMADIN, CRYSTODIGIN, digitoxin, digoxin, HUMALOG, HUMULIN, imipramine, INDERAL, INDERAL LA, insulin, LANOXICAPS, LANOXIN, LOCHOLEST, propranolol, QUESTRAN, TOFRANIL, warfarin.

Adverse Effects

Call your doctor immediately if you experience:

- **signs of overdose:** changes in appetite, changes in menstrual period, vomiting, weight loss, chest pain, diarrhea, fever, hand tremors, headache, irritability, leg cramps, nervousness, rapid or irregular heartbeat, sensitivity to heat, sweating, shortness of breath, trouble sleeping, skin rash, hives, or itching

Call your doctor if these symptoms continue:

- clumsiness
- feeling cold
- constipation
- dry, puffy skin
- headache
- unusual tiredness or weakness
- muscle aches
- weight gain
- change in appetite

Periodic Tests

Ask your doctor which of these tests should be done periodically while you are taking this drug:

- thyroid hormone levels
- examination for signs of irregular heart rhythm
- bone age and growth measurement

Desoximetasone
TOPICORT (Hoechst-Marion Roussel)

GENERIC: available

FAMILY: Corticosteroids (see p. 651)

Desoximetasone (des ox i *met* a sone) is a steroid that is applied to the skin. It is used to reduce inflammation (redness and swelling) and relieve itching of many kinds of skin conditions, such as psoriasis and eczema.

Steroids suppress your immune system, lowering your defenses against disease and making you more vulnerable to infections. If you use desoximetasone for a long time, you increase your risk of getting bacterial, viral, parasitic, and fungal infections.

As with all drugs, you should use the lowest possible dose of desoximetasone that works. You should also use it for as short a time as possible and limit the area of your body that you use it on, if possible. A steroid applied to the skin can cause many adverse effects, especially if you use it for a long time or over a large area so that your whole body absorbs the drug. **If you have used this drug for a long time do not stop suddenly. Your doctor must lower your dose gradually to prevent withdrawal symptoms.**

Before You Use This Drug

Tell your doctor if you have or have had:

- allergies to drugs
- herpes sores
- infection or ulceration at the place where you will be applying the drug

Tell your doctor about any other drugs you take, including aspirin, herbs, vitamins, and other nonprescription products.

How to Use This Drug

- **Use only as prescribed.**
- Spread a very thin layer over the area to be treated, to minimize absorption of the drug into your body. (There is no danger of systemic absorption with correct use.)
- The preparation may sting when applied.
- Do not bandage or wrap the area being treated unless your doctor has told you to do so.
- Do not use around eyes for a long period.
- Check with your doctor if your condition does not improve in one week, or if it worsens.

Interactions with Other Drugs

Some other drugs that you may be taking (either over-the-counter or prescription drugs) can interact with this one, causing adverse effects. Ask your doctor what these drugs are and let him or her know if you are taking any of them.

Adverse Effects

Call your doctor immediately if you experience:

- pain, redness, or blisters containing pus
- burning, itching, or blistering that was not present before you began using this drug
- thinning of skin with easy bruising

For long-term use:

- acne or other skin problems
- backache
- increased hair growth, especially on the face
- loss of hair, especially on scalp
- lack of healing of skin condition
- loss of top skin layer
- numbness in fingers
- blurred vision
- eye pain
- rounding out of face
- increased blood pressure
- irregular heartbeat
- irregular menstrual period
- irritability
- irritation of skin and mouth
- loss of appetite
- depression
- muscle cramps, pain or weakness
- nausea
- rapid weight gain or loss
- reddish, purplish lines on arms, face, legs, trunk or groin
- changes in skin color
- bloated or painful stomach
- softening of skin

- swelling of feet or lower legs
- decrease in sexual ability or desire
- tearing of the skin
- unusual increase or loss of hair growth
- unusual tiredness or weakness
- vomiting

Call your doctor if these symptoms continue:

- worsening of infections
- skin rash, irritation, burning or dryness

Periodic Tests

Ask your doctor which of these tests should be done periodically while you are taking this drug:

- blood or urine glucose concentration
- eye exams

PREGNANCY WARNING

This drug caused harm to developing fetuses in animal studies, or such studies were not done. Use during pregnancy only for clear medical reasons. Tell your doctor if you are pregnant or thinking of becoming pregnant before you take this drug.

Bethanechol
URECHOLINE (Merck)

GENERIC: available
FAMILY: Cholinergics

Bethanechol (be *than* e kole) helps stimulate the emptying of the bladder and is used to treat the retention of urine. Although the drug is also used to prevent the backward flow of stomach contents into the esophagus (reflux esophagitis), it is not effective or approved for this purpose.[138]

Before You Use This Drug

Tell your doctor if you have or have had:

- allergies to drugs
- asthma
- recent bladder or abdominal surgery
- slow pulse
- coronary artery disease
- epilepsy
- abdominal or stomach obstruction or problems
- urinary tract obstruction
- high or low blood pressure
- enlarged thyroid gland
- Parkinson's disease

Tell your doctor about any other drugs you take, including aspirin, herbs, vitamins, and other nonprescription products.

When You Use This Drug

- You may feel dizzy when rising from a lying or sitting position. When getting out of bed, hang your legs over the side of the bed for a few minutes, then get up slowly. When getting up from a chair, stay by the chair until you are sure that you are not dizzy. (See p. 16.)
- Until you know how you react to this drug, do not drive or perform other activities requiring alertness. Bethanechol may cause dizziness and blurred vision.

How to Use This Drug

- Take on an empty stomach to decrease nausea and vomiting.
- **Use only as prescribed.**
- Do not store in bathroom. Do not expose to heat or direct light. Do not let liquid form freeze.

• If you miss a dose, take it if it is within an hour otherwise skip it. **Do not take double doses.**

Interactions with Other Drugs

Some other drugs that you may be taking (either over-the-counter or prescription drugs) can interact with this one, causing adverse effects. Ask your doctor what these drugs are and let him or her know if you are taking any of them.

Adverse Effects

Call your doctor immediately if you experience:

• shortness of breath, wheezing or chest tightness

Call your doctor if these symptoms continue:

• nausea, vomiting, or diarrhea
• belching
• changes in vision
• dizziness or lightheadedness
• frequent urge to urinate
• increased watering of mouth
• sweating
• flushing of skin or feeling of warmth
• seizures
• insomnia
• nervousness
• stomach discomfort or pain

PREGNANCY WARNING

This drug caused harm to developing fetuses in animal studies, or such studies were not done. Use during pregnancy only for clear medical reasons. Tell your doctor if you are pregnant or thinking of becoming pregnant before you take this drug.

Beclomethasone
VANCENASE (Nasal Aerosol Spray) (Schering)
BECLOVENT (Glaxo Wellcome)
VANCERIL (Oral Aerosol Inhalers) (Schering)

GENERIC: not available
FAMILY: Corticosteroids (see p. 651)

Beclomethasone (be kloe *meth* a sone) is a steroid (corticosteroid) that is inhaled. It has one form that you spray into your nose and another form that you inhale into your mouth. The nose spray is used to treat severe allergies and hay fever and sometimes smooth growths (polyps) in the nose. The inhaler for the mouth mainly benefits people with asthma who need regular, long-term steroid treatment to control their symptoms. For these people, beclomethasone is used after a drug from another family, albuterol or terbutaline (see p. 449) used alone, has not improved the severe chronic symptoms of asthma.[139]

Steroids suppress your immune system, lowering your defenses against disease and making you more vulnerable to infections. If you use beclomethasone for a long time, you increase your risk of getting bacterial, viral, parasitic, and fungal infections, especially an infection called oral thrush.

As with all drugs, you should always use beclomethasone in the lowest dose that works. You should also take it for the shortest possible time. **If you have used this drug for a long time do not stop suddenly. Your doctor must lower your dose gradually to prevent withdrawal symptoms.**

Before You Use This Drug

Do not use if you have or have had:

• an allergic reaction to fluorocarbon propellants (found in aerosol sprays)

Tell your doctor if you have or have had:

- allergies to drugs
- AIDS
- heart, liver or kidney problems
- high blood pressure
- diabetes
- inflammation of throat, stomach, or intestines
- glaucoma
- fungal, viral or bacterial infections
- myasthenia gravis
- osteoporosis
- herpes sores of the eyes or mouth
- tuberculosis or positive TB skin test
- present or recent chicken pox or measles
- thyroid problems

For oral inhaler:

- current infection of the mouth, throat, or lungs

For nose spray:

- any eye infection
- recent nose surgery or injury
- ulcers of the nasal septum

Tell your doctor about any other drugs you take, including aspirin, herbs, vitamins, and other nonprescription products.

When You Use This Drug

- If you plan to have any surgery, including dental, tell your doctor that you take this drug.
- **Do not use to treat a sudden, severe asthma attack. This drug is not strong enough or fast enough for such an attack.**
- Wear a medical identification bracelet or carry a card stating that you may need additional steroids (tablets or injection) in times of unusual stress or sudden, severe asthma attack.

How to Use This Drug

- **Use only as prescribed.**

- If you miss a dose, take it as soon as you remember, but skip it if it is almost time for the next dose. **Do not take double doses.**
- Do not store in the bathroom. Do not expose to heat, moisture, or strong light.

Oral Inhaler:

- Clean inhaler every day.
- Gargle and rinse your mouth after each time you use the drug, to wash out any of the drug that did not enter your lungs. If your mouth and throat absorb the drug, you may become more susceptible to an infection called thrush.
- See p. 408 for instructions on using an inhaler.

Nose spray:

- See p. 402 for information about nasal dosage forms.

Interactions with Other Drugs

The following drugs are listed in the *Evaluations of Drug Interactions* 1997 as causing "highly clinically significant" or "clinically significant" interactions when used together with this drug. We have also included potentially serious interactions listed in the drug's FDA-approved professional product labeling or package insert. New scientific techniques have allowed researchers to predict some drug interactions before they have been documented in people. There may be other drugs, especially those in the families of drugs listed below, that also will react with this drug to cause severe adverse effects. The number of new drugs approved for marketing increases the chance of drug interactions, and new drug interactions are being identified with old drugs. Be vigilant. Make sure to tell your doctor and pharmacist the drugs you are taking and tell your doctor if you are taking any of these interacting drugs:

aldesleukin/interleukin-2, aspirin,
GENUINE BAYER ASPIRIN, cyclosporine,

DELTASONE, dicumarol, ECOTRIN, ketoconazole, LUMINAL, METICORTEN, NEORAL, NIZORAL, phenobarbital, prednisone, PROLEUKIN, SANDIMMUNE, SOLFOTON, TAO, troleandomycin.

Adverse Effects

Call your doctor immediately if you experience:

- decreased or blurred vision
- hallucinations
- depression or mood changes
- skin rash or hives
- confusion
- excitement or restlessness
- frequent urination
- increased thirst

For long-term use:

- persistent abdominal or stomach pain
- acne or other skin problems
- bloody or black, tarry stools
- rounding out of the face
- increased blood pressure
- swelling of feet or lower legs
- unusual weight gain
- irregular heartbeats
- muscle cramps or pain
- unusual tiredness or weakness
- pain in back, ribs, arms, or legs
- muscle weakness
- nausea or vomiting
- unusual bruising
- wounds that will not heal
- menstrual irregularities
- reddish, purplish lines on arms, face, legs trunk or groin

If using oral inhaler:

- chest pain
- chills, cough, fever, sneezing
- ear congestion
- hoarseness or other voice changes

- nose congestion or runny nose
- sore throat
- white patches inside mouth
- difficulty swallowing
- eye pain, redness, or tearing

Call your doctor if these symptoms continue:

- indigestion
- increased appetite
- nervousness or restlessness
- trouble sleeping
- dizziness or lightheadedness
- flushed face
- headache
- increased joint pain
- nosebleeds
- increase in hair on body or face
- loss of appetite
- darkening or lightening of skin color
- sweating

If using oral inhaler:

- mild abdominal pain, bloated feeling, or gas
- constipation or diarrhea
- decrease in appetite
- dry or irritated mouth, nose, tongue, or throat
- loss of sense of smell or taste

If using nose spray:

- bloody mucus or nosebleeds
- crusting inside nose
- sore throat
- difficulty breathing
- nausea or vomiting
- loss of sense of taste or smell
- persistent stuffy nose
- headache

Call your doctor immediately if these symptoms occur after you have stopped taking the drug:

- abdominal or back pain

- dizziness or fainting
- low grade fever
- persistent loss of appetite
- muscle or joint pain
- nausea or vomiting
- returning symptoms of the condition for which you were taking the drug
- shortness of breath
- frequent, unexplained headaches
- unusual tiredness or weakness
- unusual weight loss

Periodic Tests

Ask your doctor which of these tests should be done periodically while you are taking this drug:

- blood or urine glucose concentration
- eye exams
- blood levels of potassium, sodium, and calcium
- stool tests for possible blood loss
- hypothalamus and pituitary secretion tests
- growth and development determinations

Limited Use

Bupropion
ZYBAN (Glaxo Wellcome)

GENERIC: not available
FAMILY: Antidepressants (see p. 196 for a discussion of depression)
Aids to Stop Smoking

Bupropion (byu *pro* pee on) is used to treat severe depression that is not caused by other drugs, alcohol, or emotional losses (such as

EXTREME CAUTION

Bupropion has been approved by the Food and Drug Administration (FDA) for use in smoking cessation for people 18 years of age and older under the brand name Zyban. Zyban and Wellbutrin are exactly the same drug. Taking Zyban and Wellbutrin together will increase the risk of seizure. See the warning about bupropion-induced seizure below.

death in the family). It can take four weeks to be effective. Bupropion controls, but does not cure depression. Although it has been used for several years in some people,[140] the manufacturer does not recommend use beyond six weeks. Bupropion is related to amphetamines and diethylpropion (TENUATE), but purportedly is not habit-forming. Although bupropion is preferred for the elderly by some doctors,[141] it has not been studied much in older people.

Weight loss is a common adverse effect. A number of people also become restless when taking bupropion.

Higher doses increase likelihood of harmful effects. With doses of more than 450 milligrams per day the risk of seizures increases tenfold and no one should take more than 450 mg per day.[142] Because of the high incidence of seizures with doses over 450 milligrams, bupropion was temporarily banned in the United States. People age 60 and over are more likely to experience adverse effects, such as heart complications. Due to age-related decrease in kidney and liver function, the lowest effective dose should be used.

The length of time it takes an antidepressant to work can overlap with the time of spontaneous recovery especially if the depression is situational—caused by a death or other external circumstances. The majority of people lift themselves out of depression with friends, or activities such as exercise, work, reading, play, art, travel, and spiritual resources. If depression is not overcome by these measures, seek help from mental health professionals, such as therapists or psychiatrists. Antidepressant drugs should be reserved for depression that is major and does not respond to psychotherapy alone.

WARNING: SPECIAL MENTAL AND PHYSICAL ADVERSE EFFECTS

Older adults are especially sensitive to the harmful anticholinergic (see Glossary, p. 768) effects of antidepressants such as bupropion. Drugs in this family should not be used unless absolutely necessary.

Mental Effects: confusion, delirium, short-term memory problems, disorientation, and impaired attention.

Physical Effects: dry mouth, constipation, difficulty urinating (especially for a man with an enlarged prostate), blurred vision, decreased sweating with increased body temperature, sexual dysfunction, and worsening of glaucoma.

Before You Use This Drug

Do not use if you have or have had:

- eating disorders, such as anorexia or bulimia
- seizures

Tell your doctor if you have or have had:

- allergies to drugs
- bipolar disorder (manic depression)
- brain tumor

- drug abuse
- electroshock therapy[143]
- head injury
- heart, kidney, or liver problems
- myocardial infarction
- psychosis
- tumor of the central nervous system

Tell your doctor about any other drugs you take, including aspirin, herbs, vitamins, and other nonprescription products.

When You Use This Drug

- Until you know how you react to this drug, do not drive or perform other activities requiring alertness.
- Do not drink alcohol.

How to Use This Drug

- Swallow tablet whole. Take with food to lessen stomach upset.
- Space doses evenly apart during the day, but avoid taking at bedtime.
- If you miss a dose, take it as soon as you remember, but skip it if it is within four hours of the next dose. **Do not take double doses.**
- Do not store in the bathroom. Do not expose to heat, moisture, or strong light.

Interactions with Other Drugs

The following drugs are listed in the *Evaluations of Drug Interactions* 1997 as causing "highly clinically significant" or "clinically significant" interactions when used together with this drug. We have also included potentially serious interactions listed in the drug's FDA-approved professional product labeling or package insert. New scientific techniques have allowed researchers to predict some drug interactions before they have been documented in people. There may be other drugs, especially those in the families of drugs listed below, that also will react with this drug to cause severe adverse effects. The number of new drugs approved for marketing increases the chance of drug interactions, and new drug interactions are being identified with old drugs. Be vigilant. Make sure to tell your doctor and pharmacist the drugs you are taking and tell your doctor if you are taking any of these interacting drugs:

At least two weeks should elapse after you stop taking a monoamine oxidase (MAO) inhibitor and start taking bupropion. The same is true if you stop taking bupropion and then start one of these MAO inhibitors: deprenyl, ELDEPRYL, EUTONYL, furazolidone, FUROXONE, isocarboxazid, MARPLAN, MATULANE, NARDIL, PARNATE, phenelzine, procarbazine, selegiline, tranylcypromine.

Taking bupropion with other drugs that also affect the central nervous system adds to adverse effects, including risk of seizures: alcohol, amitriptyline, chlorpromazine, clozapine, CLOZARIL, DESYREL, ELAVIL, fluoxetine, HALDOL, haloperidol, lithium, LITHOBID, LITHONATE, loxapine, LOXITANE, LUDIOMIL, maprotiline, MOBAN, molindone, NAVANE, PROZAC, thiothixene, THORAZINE, trazodone.

Adverse Effects

Call your doctor immediately if you experience:

- agitation, anxiety
- confusion
- convulsions
- fainting
- hallucinations
- severe headache
- irregular or fast heartbeat
- insomnia, restlessness
- skin rash, itching
- seizures

Call your doctor if these symptoms continue:

- anger, hostility
- increase or decrease in blood pressure
- constipation, diarrhea
- dizziness
- drowsiness
- dry mouth or increased saliva
- fever, chills
- impotence
- uncoordination
- inflammation of the mouth
- decrease in appetite
- muscle spasms, tremor, twitching
- nausea or vomiting
- tinnitus, ringing in ears[144]
- increased sweating
- undesired weight change
- unusual tiredness
- increase in frequency of urination, especially at night, or difficulty urinating
- blurred vision
- difficulty concentrating

Periodic Tests

Ask your doctor which of these tests should be done periodically while you are taking this drug:

- kidney function tests
- liver function tests
- supervision for suicidal tendencies

NOTES FOR DRUGS FOR OTHER CONDITIONS

1. AMA Department of Drugs. *AMA Drug Evaluations.* 5th ed. Chicago: American Medical Association, 1983:893.

2. Ibid.

3. Miacalcin spray approved in U.S. *SCRIP* August 25, 1995; 2054: 17.

4. AMA, op. cit.

5. Wilkinson SM, Cartwright PH, English JSC. Hydrocortisone: an important cutaneous allergen. *Lancet* 1991; 337:761–2.

6. AMA, op. cit.

7. Fadul CE, Lemann W, Thaler HT, Posner JB. Perforation of GI tract in patients receiving steroids for neurologic disease. *Neurology* 1988; 38:348–52.

8. AMA, op. cit.

9. Laan RFJM, van Riel PLCM, van Erning LJTO, Lemmens JAM, Ruijs SHJ, van de Putte LBAR. Vertebral osteoporosis in rheumatoid patients. *British Journal of Rheumatology* 1992; 31:91–6.

10. Minden SL, Orav J, Schildkraut JJ. Hypomanic reactions to ACTH and prednisone treatment for multiple sclerosis. *Neurology* 1988; 38:1631–4.

11. Ibid.

12. Wolfe SM. *Women's Health Alert.* New York: Addison-Wesley, Inc., 1991:115–45.

13. World Health Organization Collaborative Study of Cardiovascular Disease and Steroid Hormone Contraception. Venous thromboembolic disease and combined oral contraceptives: results of international multicentre case-control study. *Lancet* 1995; 346:1575–82.

14. World Health Organization Collaborative Study of Cardiovascular Disease and Steroid Hormone Contraception. Effect of different progestagens in low oestrogen oral contraceptives on venous thromboembolic disease. *Lancet* 1995; 346:1582–8.

15. Jick H, Jick SS, Gurewich V, Myers MW, Vasilakis C. Risk of idiopathic cardiovascular death and nonfatal venous thromboembolism in women using oral contraceptives with differing progestagen components. *Lancet* 1995; 346:1589–93.

16. Bloemenkamp KWM, Rosendaal FR, Helmerhorst FM, Büller HR, Vandenbroucke JP. Enhancement by factor V Leiden mutation of risk of deep-vein thrombosis associated with oral contraceptives containing a third-generation progestagen. *Lancet* 1995; 346:1593–6.

17. Spitzer WO, Lewis MA, Heinemann LAJ, Thorogood M, MacRae KD on behalf of Transnational Research Group on Oral Contraceptives and the Health of Young Women. Third generation oral contraceptives and risk of venous thromboembolic disorders: an international case-control study. *British Medical Journal* 1996; 312:83–8.

18. Carnall D. Controversy rages over new contraceptive data. *British Medical Journal* 1995; 311:1117–8.

19. MacRae K, Kay C. Third generation oral contraceptive pills. *British Medical Journal* 1995; 311:1112.

20. Lewis MA, Spitzer WO, Heinemann LAJ, MacRae KD, Bruppacher R, Thorogood M on behalf of Transnational Research Group on Oral Contraceptives and the Health of Young Women. Third generation oral contraceptives and risk of myocardial infarction: an international case-control study. *British Medical Journal* 1996; 312:88–90.

21. Ortho-Cept Product Information. *Physician's Desk Reference* 1998. Montvale NJ: Medical Economics, p. 2013–20.

22. Ibid.

23. WHO scientific group meeting on cardiovascular disease and steroid hormone contraceptives. *WHO Weekly Epidemiological Record* 1997; 72:357–64.

24. AMA, op. cit.

25. *USP DI, Drug Information for the Health Care Provider.* 6th ed. Rockville MD: The United States Pharmacopeial Convention, Inc., 1986:1147.

26. Vestal RE, ed. *Drug Treatment in the Elderly.* Sydney, Australia: ADIS Health Science Press, 1984:250.

27. *USP DI,* op. cit.

28. Krebs H. Chronic ulcerations following topical therapy. *Obstetrics and Gynecology* 1991; 78:205–8.

29. Boschetti C, Cortellaro M, Nencioni T, Bertolli V, Della Volpe A, Zanussi C. Short- and long-term effects of hormone replacement therapy (transdermal estradiol vs oral conjugated equine estrogens, combined with medroxyprogesterone acetate) on blood coagulation factors in postmenopausal women. *Thrombosis Research* 1991; 62:1–8.

30. Studd J, Watson N, Henderson A. Oestrogen therapy for the menopause. *British Journal of Psychiatry* 1990; 157:931–2.

31. Sillero-Arenas M, Delgado-Rodriguez M, Rodrigues-Canteras R, Bueno-Cavanillas A, Galvez-Vargas R. Menopausal hormone replacement therapy and breast cancer: a meta-analysis. *Obstetrics and Gynecology* 1992; 79:286–94.

32. Steinberg KK, Thacker SB, Smith SJ, Stroup DF, Zack MM, Flanders WD, et al. A meta-analysis of the effect of estrogen replacement therapy on the risk of breast cancer. *Journal of the American Medical Association* 1991; 265:1985–90.

33. Hormone replacement therapy in general practice. *British Medical Journal* 1991; 302:1601–2 [letters].

34. Miller AB. Risk/benefit considerations of antiestrogen/estrogen therapy in healthy postmenopausal women. *Preventive Medicine* 1991; 20:79–85.

35. L'Hermite M. Sex hormones and cardiovascular risk. *Acta Cardiologica* 1991; 46:357–72.

36. Dukes MNG, Beeley L. *Side Effects of Drugs Annual* 15, Amsterdam: Elsevier, 1991:436

37. Steinberg, op. cit.

38. L'Hermite, op. cit.

39. Clisham R, Cedars MI, Greendale G, Fu S, Gambone J, Judd HL. Long-term transdermal estradiol therapy on endometrial histology and bleeding patterns. *Obstetrics and Gynecology* 1992; 79:196–201.

40. Delmas PD, Bjarnason ND, Mitlak BH, Ravoux A, Shah AS, Huster WJ, et al. Effects of raloxifene on bone mineral density, serum cholesterol concentrations, and uterine endometrium in postmenopausal women. *New England Journal of Medicine* 1997; 337:1641–7.

41. AMA Department of Drugs, *AMA Drug Evaluations.* 6th ed. Chicago: American Medical Association 1986: 232–3.

42. Ibid.

43. Karpf DB, Shapiro DR, Seeman E, Ensrud KE, Johnston CC, Adami S, et al. Prevention of nonvertebral fractures by alendronate. *Journal of the American Medical Association* 1997; 277: 1159–64.

44. Marcus R, Papapoulos SE, editors. Chapter 64 Bisphosphonates: Pharmacology and use in the treatment of osteoporosis. San Diego: Academic Press, 1996: 1209–30.

45. Hodsman A, Adachi J, Olszynski W. Use of bisphosphonates in the treatment of osteoporosis. *Canadian Medical Association Journal* 1996; 155: 945–8.

46. Wolfe, op. cit.

47. Wolfe S. Testimony at Food and Drug Administration advisory committee hearing on nicotine patches, July 14, 1992.

48. Gunther V, Gritsch S, Meise U. Smoking cessation—gradual or sudden stopping? *Drug and Alcohol Dependence* 1992; 29:231–6.

49. West R. The focus and conduct of clinical trials. *British Journal of Addiction* 1991; 86:663–6.

50. West R. The 'nicotine replacement paradox' in smoking cessation: how does nicotine gum really work? *British Journal of Addiction* 1992; 87:165–7.

51. Morgan GD, Villagra VG. The nicotine transdermal patch: a cautionary note. *Annals of Internal Medicine* 1992; 116:424.

52. Benowitz NL. Cigarette smoking and nicotine addiction. *Medical Clinics of North America* 1992; 76:415–37.

53. Breslau N, Kibley MM, Andreski P. Nicotine withdrawal symptoms and psychiatric disorders: findings from an epidemiologic study of young adults. *American Journal of Psychiatry* 1992; 149:464–9 [abstract].

54. West, 1991, op. cit.

55. Wolfe Testimony, op. cit.

56. American Society of Hospital Pharmacists. *American Hospital Formulary Service Drug Information.* Bethesda, MD, 1992:754–9.

57. *The Medical Letter on Drugs and Therapeutics.* New York: The Medical Letter Inc., 1992; 34:37–8.

58. Russell MAH, Jarvis MJ. Skin patches to prevent lung cancer. *European Journal of Cancer* 1991; 27:223–4.

59. Sawe U. From smoking behaviour to nicotine addiction: the history of research. *Journal of the Royal Society of Medicine* 1992; 85:184 [letter].

60. Tonnesen P, Norregaard J, Simonsen K, Sawe U. A double-blind trial of a 16-hour transdermal nicotine patch in smoking cessation. *New England Journal of Medicine* 1991; 325:311–5.

61. Transdermal Nicotine Study Group. Transdermal nicotine for smoking cessation: six-month results from two multicenter controlled clinical trials. *Journal of the American Medical Association* 1991; 266:3133–8.

62. Gunther, op. cit.

63. Transdermal Nicotine Study Group, op. cit.

64. Perkins KA. Metabolic effects of cigarette smoking. *Journal of Applied Psychology* 1992; 72:401–9.

65. Transdermal nicotine patch for smoking cessation *New England Journal of Medicine* 1992; 326:344–5 [letters].

66. Kirch DG. Where there's smoke . . . nicotine and psychiatric disorders. *Biological Psychiatry* 1991; 30:107–8.

67. Menza MA, Grossman N, Van Horn M, Cody R, Forman N. Smoking and movement disorders in psychiatric patients. *Biological Psychiatry* 1991; 30:109–15.

68. Perkins, op. cit.

69. Jensen EJ, Schmidt E, Pederson B, Dahl R. Effect on smoking cessation of silver acetate, nicotine and ordinary chewing gum. *Psychopharmacology* 1991; 104:470–4.

70. Yokota T, Kagamihara Y, Hayashi H, Tsukagoshi H, Tanabe H. Nicotine-sensitive paresis. *Neurology* 1992; 42:382–8.

71. Kyerematen G, Vesell E. Metabolism of nicotine. *Drug Metabolism Reviews* 1991; 23:3–41.

72. Gilman AG, Rall TW, Nies AS, Taylor P, eds. *The Pharmacological Basis of Therapeutics.* 8th ed. New York: Pergamon Press, 1990:545–9.

73. Yokota, op. cit.

74. Sumatriptan: does it have a place in the routine treatment of migraine? *WHO Drug Information* 1996; 10:26–7.

75. Ottervanger JP, Valkenburg HA, Grobbee DE, Stricker BH. Characteristics and determinants of sumatriptan-associated chest pain. *Archives of Neurology* 1997; 54:1387–92.

76. Hamalainen ML, Hoppu K, Santavuori P. Sumatriptan for migraine attacks in children: a randomized placebo-controlled study. *Neurology* 1997; 48: 1100–3.

77. Ottervanger, op. cit.

78. Ibid.

79. Moore KL, Noble SL. Drug treatment of migraine: part 1. acute therapy and drug-rebound headache. *American Family Physician* 1997; 56:2039–52.

80. Fettes I. Menstrual migraine. *Postgraduate Medicine* 1997; 101: 67–76.

81. Glaxo Wellcome, Package Insert, September, 1997

82. Lopez-Alemany M, Ferrer-Tuset C, Bernacer-Alpera B. Akathisia and acute dystonia induced by sumatriptan. *Journal of Neurology* 1997; 244:131–3.

83. AMA, 1983, op. cit.

84. U.S. FDA panel rejects Knoll's sibutramine. *SCRIP* 1996; 2169: 21.

85. Knoll Meridia "approvable": labeling discussions on use by diabetics. *F-D-C Reports* November 18, 1996, T&G 5–7.

86. Meridia (sibutramine) Professional Product Labeling. Knoll Pharmaceutical Company, 1997.

87. AMA, 1986, op. cit., p. 399.

88. *Goodman and Gilman's The Pharmacological Basis of Therapeutics.* 9th ed. New York: McGraw-Hill, 1996: 1275.

89. Jordan VC. An overview of considerations for the testing of tamoxifen as a preventative for breast cancer. *Annals of The New York Academy of Sciences* 1995; 768:141–7.

90. Goodman, op. cit.

91. Ismail SM. Pathology of endometrium treated with tamoxifen. *Journal of Clinical Pathology* 1994; 47:827–33.

92. Nightingale SL. From the Food and Drug Administration. *Journal of the American Medical Association* 1994; 271:1472.

93. Goodman, op. cit.

94. Aronson JK, VanBoxtel CJ. *Side Effects of Drugs Annual* 19, Amsterdam: Elsevier, 1995:400-3.

95. Shariff S, Cumming CE, Lees A, Handman M, Cumming DC. Mood disorder in women with early breast cancer taking tamoxifen, an estradiol receptor antagonist: An expected or unexpected effect? *Annals of the New York Academy of Sciences* 1995; 761:365–8.

96. Hampson JP, Donnelly A, Lewis-Jones MS, Pye JK. Tamoxifen-induced hair color change. *British Journal of Dermatology* 1995; 132:483.

97. Nayfield SG, Gorin MB. Tamoxifen-associated eye disease: a review. *Journal of Clinical Oncology* 1996; 14:1018–26.

98. Jordan, op. cit.

99. Hansten and Horn, *Drug Interactions,* Applied Therapeutics, 1997; 26.

100. AMA, 1986, op. cit., p. 232–3.

101. Ibid.

102. Ibid.

103. Ibid.

104. AMA, 1983, op. cit.

105. Steinberg, op. cit.

106. *International Journal of Cancer,* 1986; 37:173–7.

107. Forbes AP. Fuller Albright: his concept of postmenopausal osteoporosis and what came of it. *Clinical Orthopedics* 1991; 269:128–40.

108. Vandenbroucke JP. Postmenopausal oestrogen and cardioprotection. *Lancet* 1991; 337:833–4.

109. The Coronary Drug Project. Findings leading to discontinuation of the 2.5 mg day estrogen group. *Journal of the American Medical Association* 1973; 226:652–7.

110. Stampfer MJ, Willett WC, Colditz GA, Rosner B, Speizer FE, Hennekens CH. *New England Journal of Medicine* 1985; 313:1044–9.

111. Wolf PH, Madans JH, Finucane FF, Higgins M, Kleinman JC. Reduction of cardiovascular disease—related mortality among postmenopausal women who use hormones: evidence from a national cohort. *American Journal of Obstetrics and Gynecology* 1991; 161:489–94.

112. Vandenbroucke, op. cit.

113. Hulley S, Grady D, Bush T, Furberg C, Herrington D, Riggs B, et al. Randomized trial of estrogen plus progestin for secondary prevention of coronary heart disease in postmenopausal women. *Journal of the American Medical Association* 1998; 280:605–13.

114. Lepor H, Williford WO, Barry MJ, Brawer MK, Dixon CM, Gormley G, et al. The efficacy of terazosin, finasteride, or both in benign prostatic hyperplasia. *New England Journal of Medicine* 1996; 335:533–9.

115. McConnell JD, Bruskewitz R, Walsh P, Andriole G, Lieber M, Holtgrewe HL, et al. The effect of finasteride on the risk of acute urinary retention and the need for surgical treatment among men with benign prostatic hyperplasia. *New England Journal of Medicine* 1998; 338:557–63.

116. Wasson JH. Finasteride to prevent morbidity from benign prostatic hyperplasia. *New England Journal of Medicine* 1998; 338:612–3[editorial].

117. Walsh PC. Treatment of benign prostatic hyperplasia. *New England Journal of Medicine* 1996; 335:586–7[editorial].

118. Lepor, op. cit.

119. *International Agency for Research on Cancer Monographs on the Evaluation of the Carcinogenic Risk of Chemicals to Humans,* Vol. 24: Some Pharmaceutical Drugs. Lyon, France: International Agency for Research on Cancer, 1980:163.

120. Randall T. FDA scrutinizes 'off-label' promotions. *Journal of the American Medical Association* 1991; 266:11.

121. American Society of Hospital Pharmacists, op. cit., p. 2158–9.

122. *USP DI, Drug Information for the Health Care Professional.* 12th ed. Rockville MD: The United States Pharmacopeial Convention, Inc., 1992:2695–7.

123. *The Medical Letter on Drugs and Therapeutics,* 1992, op. cit., p. 28–9.

124. The top 200 drugs. *American Druggist* February 1998:46–53.

125. AMA, 1986, op. cit., p. 232–3.

126. Olsen EA. Topical minoxidil in the treatment of androgenetic alopecia in women. *CUTIS* 1991; 48:243–8.

127. Saxena U, Ramesh V, Misra RS. Topical minoxidil in monilethrix. *Dermatologica* 1991; 182:252–3.

128. Wilson C, Walkden V, Powell S, Shaw S, Wilkinson J, Dawber R. Contact dermatitis in reaction to 2% topical minoxidil solution. *Journal of the American Academy of Dermatology* 1991; 24:661–2.

129. Gilman, op. cit., p. 1587.

130. AMA Department of Drugs. *AMA Drug Evaluations Annual 1992.* Chicago: American Medical Association, 1992:1123.

131. Trattner A, Ingber A. Topical treatment with minoxidil 2% and smoking intolerance. *Annals of Pharmacotherapy* 1992; 26:198–9.

132. American Society of Hospital Pharmacists, op. cit., p. 2180–5.

133. Fiedler V. Alopecia areata: current therapy. *Journal of Investigative Dermatology* 1991; 96:69S-70S.

134. AMA, 1986, op. cit., p. 232–3.

135. Ibid.

136. *Drugs for the Elderly.* 2nd ed. Copenhagen, Denmark: World Health Organization, 1997, 85–6.

137. AMA, 1986, op. cit., p. 802.

138. *The Medical Letter on Drugs and Therapeutics.* New York: The Medical Letter Inc., 1980; 22:27.

139. AMA, 1986, op. cit., p. 399.

140. Harsch HH. Bupropion. *American Family Physician* 1991; 43:1789–90.

141. Gelenberg AJ. Imperfect drugs in an imperfect world. *Journal of Clinical Psychiatry* 1992; 53:39–40.

142. Davidson J. Seizures and bupropion: a review. *Journal of Clinical Psychiatry* 1989; 50:256–61.

143. Rudorfer MV, Manji HK, Potter WZ. Bupropion, ECT, and dopaminergic overdrive. *American Journal of Psychiatry* 1991; 148:1101–2 [letter].

144. Settle EC. Tinnitus related to bupropion treatment. *Journal of Clinical Psychiatry* 1991; 52:352.

4

PROTECTING YOURSELF AND YOUR FAMILY FROM PREVENTABLE DRUG-INDUCED INJURY

Doctors and pharmacists often "blame" the adverse effects of prescription drugs on patients for improperly taking their medications. The standard solution offered by some health professionals is to get patients to better "comply" with doctors' instructions by using what are called compliance programs or strategies. (Another word for *compliance* is, of course, *obedience.)* Occasionally, the blame is also put on doctors for misprescribing and overprescribing, on pharmacists for failing to detect serious drug interactions, and only rarely on the drug industry for overselling drugs to doctors and now directly to patients through direct-to-consumer advertising. Even when health professionals are portrayed as being partially responsible for adverse reactions, the proposed solution is a ritual of faith, hoping the system of professional education will do a better job so that doctors will better learn about the proper use of drugs and pharmacists will do a better job of learning about and detecting dangerous drug interactions.

While important changes need to be made in the way patients, doctors, and pharmacists do things, they are not likely to occur without other, more primary changes. First, improved **communication** with your doctor is necessary. Second, you must have access to comprehensive **objective information** about the risks and benefits of prescription drugs written in nontechnical language distributed to you by your pharmacist with each new and refill prescription.

Communication: Activating Yourself and Your Doctor

Patients, their families, and friends need to feel comfortable approaching the doctor, with the help of their pharmacist, and to begin working with the doctor to reduce the number of drugs and the dosage of drugs being used. In most cases, this will result not only in fewer adverse reactions, including life-threatening ones, but also in fewer drugs being used. Equally important, this process will improve patients' ability to properly take the drugs that are actually needed. Studies show that more drugs lead to poorer patient compliance with instructions, while fewer drugs lead to better compliance.[1]

This problem is most serious for older patients, who proportionately take a higher number of drugs than their younger counterparts, but it can be a significant problem for younger patients as well. This chapter assumes that most doctors who take care of older patients, and even many doctors who treat younger age groups, have not had adequate training in the problems of drug prescribing and rely too heavily on drug company promotion to make prescribing decisions. For example, too many doctors usually employ the same decision-making process (when to treat and what drug and dose to use) for older adults as for younger people. This too often results in their prescribing too many drugs at doses that are too high. In addition, many older people see multiple doctors—an internist, a gynecologist, and a heart specialist, for example.

Communication among physicians about what drugs are prescribed is often deficient. We assume that most doctors are quite willing to learn to prescribe fewer and safer drugs, but this is most likely to occur if you follow the Ten Rules for Safer Drug Use outlined in this chapter and have access to objective drug information written specifically for patients. Being shy with your doctors or pharmacists is not only inappropriate, but may be dangerous to your health. If you do not understand any of the sections on the Drug Worksheet, for Patient, Family, Doctor and Pharmacist (see p. 747) or any of the Ten Rules below, ask your doctor. Remember—the doctor is working for you, and with you.

Ten Rules for Safer Drug Use

Rule 1: Have "Brown Bag Sessions" with Your Primary Doctor. Fill out the Drug Worksheet enclosed with this book.

It is impossible to overemphasize the importance of this first and most crucial step in preventing adverse drug reactions. Whenever you go to a doctor you have not previously seen or to one with whom you have never had a brown-bag session, put all prescription and over-the-counter drugs you are using, have used in the last month, or are likely to use in a bag, and bring them to the doctor so a list can be made and you can start to fill out the Drug Worksheet enclosed. (See p. 747 for a sample of this worksheet that you can use.)

Doctors should never prescribe a drug or renew a prescription, nor should you be willing to get a new prescription, without full, up-to-date knowledge of all drugs already being taken or likely to be taken.

Before your brown bag session with the doctor, your neighborhood pharmacist may help you to fill out some of the blanks on your drug worksheet.

Once you have brought in all the drugs you are taking, ask your doctor to help you fill out the drug worksheet. You will probably be able to fill out more of the information concerning over-the-counter drugs yourself, since doctors often do not know that you are taking them or for what purpose. The doctor will be able to help you to fill out most of the information concerning prescription drugs, at least the ones that he or she has prescribed for you.

Explanation of Items on Drug Worksheet (p. 747)

a. Name of drug, of doctor who wrote the prescription, and date drug was started or the dosage changed: Drugs should be listed by both brand and generic names, since both are commonly used. All drugs prescribed by all doctors should be listed. Over-the-counter drugs and the amount of alcohol, tobacco, and caffeine used should also be indicated. There are many dangerous interactions between drugs and between drugs and alcohol, so this information is extremely important in avoiding adverse drug interactions.

b. Purpose of the drug: Identify the reason for which each drug is being taken. Often, because physicians are frustrated at not being able to do anything else for the patient, or sometimes because the doctor believes that the patient will not be satisfied unless a pill is recommended, prescriptions are written without a valid medical reason. In one study, patients reported that one out of every four times (25.4%) they received a prescription, they were not told the purpose of the drug being prescribed.[2]

c. Dose, frequency of use, and duration of use: It is important to know what the dose is, how often it is supposed to be taken, at what hours, and for how long.

d. When the drug should be stopped or the need for its use reevaluated. For any drug, new or old, you should assume that it should be used for as short a time as possible unless there is evidence that its continued use is necessary. Evaluation at least every three to six months for each drug being used will reduce

Sample Page of Drug Worksheet for Patients, Family, Doctor and Pharmacist

Name Beatrice Jones

Primary Doctor's Name Dr. Jackson

Page 1

Doctor's Telephone 555-1212

a. Generic Name of Drug / Brand Name of Drug	Doctor, date started & changes	b. Reason why prescribed or changed?	Dose? (Each time)	c. Times per day	What time of day?	d. How long should you take drug? days / weeks / months	e. Problems to watch out for which this drug can cause	f. Interactions of this drug with other drugs or food; diet recommendations	g. How are you actually taking the drug?	h. New problems or complaints since drug started (Date it began)	i. Is drug working?
Example: hydrochlorothiazide — HydroDiuril (This is an example only.)	Dr. Jackson 2/10/92	high blood pressure 180/100	12.5 mg 1/2 pill	once	morning	at least till next visit in 1 month	muscle weakness; cramps from low potassium; frequent urination common	1) Eat raisins, bananas, wheat germ & drink orange juice for potassium	most days 5-6/wk	No	No
	3/8/92	pressure still high 165/100	25 mg 1 pill	once	morning	till next visit, 2 months		2) Avoid salt	stopped 4/1— felt too weak	feeling tired 3/22/92	No
	4/15/92	pressure 165/95	12.5 mg 1/2 pill	once	morning	till next visit, 2 months		3) may lower effectiveness of diabetes drugs	every day	NONE	Yes
	Dr. Lewis 10/10/92	pressure 155/87	same	same	same	till next visit, 6 months			every day	NONE	Yes

Instructions:

1. Include all over-the-counter drugs you take as well as prescription drugs.
2. When you change doses draw a single line through the old dose.
3. Bring this with you every time you go to a doctor or pharmacist.
4. Be straightforward with your doctor and yourself about how often you take medicine and why.

the number of drugs being taken. For some drugs, such as tranquilizers, sleeping pills, antidepressants, and others, much more frequent reevaluation is necessary.

e. Important possible adverse effects of the drug: Because many of the most serious perceptible adverse effects of drugs are often wrongly attributed to such things as "growing old," it is important for patients to know about the adverse effects of the drugs they take so they can recognize them and report them to the doctor. In one study, researchers found that 37% of documented adverse drug reactions had not been recognized by patients and reported to their doctors, and that the majority of these patients had not been informed about possible adverse drug reactions by their doctors.[3]

f. Important possible drug and food interactions, especially with over-the-counter drugs, and diet recommendations: Ask your doctor which foods and other drugs taken along with your drug can interact and cause side effects, and ask for dietary recommendations.

g. How you are actually taking the drug: Always be straightforward with your doctor about whether or not you are taking your medicine and how often. Do this even if you had no defined reason for stopping. This is important because not giving your doctor this information can lead to mistaken conclusions about what dosage or drugs work.

h. New problems or complaints noticed by the patient, friends, or family since any of the drugs listed on the worksheet have been started: As mentioned above, patients themselves often do not notice a change, especially older adults who are inclined to blame many of their problems on aging. Friends and relatives are often the first to notice adverse drug reactions, especially ones that affect thinking or mood. An additional difficulty is that patients are often reluctant to tell their doctors that something the doctor did to try to make them better actually made them worse. The safest assumption is that any worsening of a patient's condition or any new symptoms that develop after a drug is started are an adverse drug reaction, until proven otherwise.

i. In the judgment of you, your family, and your doctor, is the drug working? Have the purposes for which the drug is being prescribed (as in *b*) been achieved?

Do Not Use Drugs

If a drug already being used or being considered for use is one of the 160 drugs that we list as **Do Not Use** (see Index of Drugs, p. xxv), **Do Not Use Until . . . ,** or **Last Choice Drug,** ask your doctor about alternative therapy, which could be either nondrug therapy or a safer drug. If the drug you are using is listed in this book as **Limited Use,** it may also be a good idea to discuss the drug with your doctor to see if a better alternative might be found.

> Talk to your doctor before deciding to make any changes in your prescription drugs based on information in this book.

Rule 2: Find Out If You Are Having Any Adverse Drug Reactions.

Even before you have a brown bag session with your doctor, if you develop any of the following reactions after beginning to use any drug, contact your doctor. Ask if you really need a drug in the first place and, if you do, whether a safer drug can be substituted or whether a lower dose could be used to reduce or eliminate the adverse effect. Look in Chapter 2, Adverse Drug Reactions, p. 9, for the lists of widely used drugs that can cause each of these adverse effects.

• Mental adverse drug reactions: depression, hallucinations, confusion, delirium, memory loss, impaired thinking, and insomnia

• Nervous system adverse drug reactions: parkinsonism, involuntary movements of the face, arms, and legs (tardive dyskinesia), dizziness on standing, falls (which can sometimes result in hip fractures), automobile accidents that result in injury because of sedation, and sexual dysfunction

• Gastrointestinal adverse drug reactions: loss of appetite, nausea, vomiting, abdominal pain, bleeding, constipation, and diarrhea

• Urinary tract adverse drug reactions: difficulty urinating or loss of bladder control (incontinence)

If you or a relative or friend have any of the above problems or develop other problems after starting a new drug and are taking any of the drugs listed under each problem in Chapter 2, notify your doctor or tell your friend or relative to notify his or hers.

Another way of identifying possible adverse drug reactions you may be having is to look in the Index of Drugs, p. xxv, for the name of the drug you are using. Then turn to the page in the drug profile with the details on any adverse reactions caused by the drug.

The remaining rules for safer drug use (or nonuse) were compiled from a number of lists, but particularly from the World Health Organization's *General Prescribing Principles for the Elderly.* These rules, however, apply to all age groups[4,5,6,7]—and all doctors and patients who are involved in drug therapy should know them.

Rule 3: Assume That Any New Symptom You Develop After Starting a New Drug Might Be Caused by the Drug.

If you have a new symptom, report it to your doctor.

Rule 4: Make Sure Drug Therapy Is Really Needed.

Often, drugs are prescribed to treat situational problems such as loneliness, isolation, and confusion. Whenever possible, nondrug approaches to these problems should be tried. These include hobbies, socializing with others, and getting out of the house. When a person is suffering from an understandable depression after losing a loved one, for example, support from friends, relatives, or a psychotherapist is preferable to drugs such as antidepressants. (See discussion on depression for proper use of antidepressant drugs, p. 196.)

Nondrug therapy such as weight loss and exercise is preferable to drugs for such problems as mild high blood pressure and adult-onset diabetes. (See discussions of these two problems on pp. 44, 550.) Increasing fiber and liquid in the diet is preferable to using laxatives (see p. 380). For swollen legs due to "bad" veins in the legs (not due to heart disease), wearing support hose is less expensive, safer, and probably more effective than taking heart pills or water pills.

Anxiety or difficulty sleeping are two situations for which drugs should rarely, if ever, be prescribed, particularly in older adults. See discussions of these problems and nondrug solutions on p. 178.

A last category of "disease" for which drug therapy is rarely, if ever, appropriate is drug-induced disease or adverse drug reactions. The proper treatment for drug-induced parkinsonism is not a second drug to treat the problem caused by the first drug, but stopping the first drug.

For any condition, always consider and discuss with the doctor whether the drug that is being selected may cause problems (adverse effects) worse than the disease being treated. A very common example of this is the extraordinary overtreatment of older people with slightly high blood pressure but without any symptoms of or problems caused by high blood pressure. (See guidelines for treatment of hypertension, p. 44.) In most cases, the person will feel worse because of the treatment, without any evidence of benefit. Always consider the seriousness of the condition that your doctor is considering treating, and try to make sure that the treatment is not worse than the disease.

The guiding principle is to use as few drugs as possible, in order to reduce adverse reactions and increase the odds of properly taking the ones that are really necessary.

Rule 5: If Drug Therapy Is Indicated, in Most Cases, Especially in Older Adults, It Is Safer to Start With a Dose That Is Lower Than the Usual Adult Dose.

"Start low, go slow." The lowest effective dose for any patient is always the best, because a lower dose will cause fewer adverse effects, which are almost always related to dose. In the elderly, some experts suggest starting with one third to one half of the usual adult dose for most drugs and watching for side effects, increasing the dose slowly and only if necessary to get the desired effect.

Rule 6: When Adding a New Drug, See If It Is Possible to Discontinue Another Drug.

If your doctor is considering the addition of a new drug, this should always be used as an opportunity to reevaluate existing drugs and eliminate those that are not absolutely essential. The possibility of an adverse drug interaction between the new drug and one of the old ones may force dropping or changing a drug.

Rule 7: Stopping a Drug Is As Important As Starting It.

Regularly review with your doctor, at least every three to six months, the need to continue each drug being taken. For many mind-affecting drugs, such as sleeping pills, tranquilizers, and antidepressants, and for antibiotics, this reevaluation should be more frequent and sooner. The prevailing principle for doctors and patients should be to discontinue any drug unless it is essential. Many adverse drug reactions are caused by drugs that were continued long after any rational duration of use ended. Many drugs such as antidepressants, sleeping pills, tranquilizers, digoxin, and others that are prescribed for an acute problem are not needed beyond a short period, and cause risks without providing benefits. Slow and careful weaning

off these drugs may significantly improve the user's health. In addition to considering whether to stop the drug, you and your doctor should discuss the possibility of lowering the dose.

Rule 8: Make Sure Your Drug-Using Instructions Are as Clear as Possible to You and at Least One Other Person.

Regardless of how old someone is, the chance of adverse reactions is high enough that at least one other person—a spouse, child, or friend—should know about these possibilities. In the presence of such adverse reactions as confusion and memory loss, this is especially critical. For older adults, the complexities of drug use may be greater, especially for people taking more than one drug and people with physical or mental disabilities. In these cases, it is even more important to inform another person about possible adverse drug reactions.

Ask your doctor to make sure that the label on the drug states, if at all possible, the purpose for which the drug is being used. This is especially important when you are using multiple drugs, but is always important as a way of increasing your and your family's or friend's participation. All information concerning the proper use of the drug should also be on the label. In addition to the label, you should get a separate instruction sheet and have it explained to you.

Rule 9: Discard All Old Drugs Carefully.

Many people are tempted to keep and reuse drugs obtained in the past, even though their condition has changed. Additional drugs used may make the earlier drugs much more dangerous. In addition, you may be tempted to give drugs to a friend or relative who you believe may benefit from them. Resist these temptations and avoid further problems caused by using outdated drugs by throwing them away when you are done with your course of therapy.

Rule 10: Ask Your Primary Doctor to Coordinate Your Care and Drugs.

If you see a specialist and he or she wants to start you on new medicines in addition to the ones you are on, check with your primary doctor first—usually an internist or general or family practitioner. It is equally important to use one pharmacist, if possible.

SPECIAL PROBLEMS IN NURSING HOMES

All of the problems of dangerous misprescribing of drugs for people living in the community are even worse in many nursing homes. For example, one study found that almost 40% of nursing home residents were being given antipsychotic drugs even though only a small fraction of them actually were psychotic. Another study found that one third of people in nursing homes were getting seven or more prescription drugs. (See p. 1 for more information on the extent of prescription drug use in nursing homes.) Most of the above rules for safer drug use apply in all situations, including the nursing home situation, but there are some differences. The main one is that for patients in nursing homes, the brown bag session and filling out the Drug Worksheet should be done by the nursing home staff, including the nurse, doctor, and pharmacist.

If you are the child, other relative, or friend of a nursing home resident, you have the right, with his or her permission, to demand and receive a completed Drug Worksheet for that person and an explanation of the reasons for each drug being used. The process of obtaining this information, with the help of your own pharmacist and possibly your own doctor, will very likely lead to a reduced number of drugs being given and, where appropriate, reduced doses of those still judged to be necessary. By taking care of these matters, you will have made a major contribution to the health and well-being of your loved one(s) in nursing homes.

What You Can Do: Finding Information About New Drugs

If you want information on 456 commonly used drugs, you can consult this book. For monthly updates on new drugs and newly reported adverse drug reactions, you can turn to the Public Citizen's Health Research Group newsletter, *Worst Pills, Best Pills News* (see back of book for more information). But what if you are prescribed one of the flood of new drugs that are now coming on the market? In 1994 and 1995, for example, 50 new drugs were marketed in the United States, while in the following two year period, 1996 and 1997, this number almost doubled to 92 new drugs. Where else can you go for objective drug information? Until the Food and Drug Administration (FDA) requires the distribution of objective information written in nontechnical language, placing the risks and benefits of prescription drugs in a context meaningful for patients with each new and refill prescription, you have two choices—the nearest pharmacy or the local library. You should *not* turn to most sites on the Internet. Drug companies and marketing firms working for drug companies maintain Internet sites that are nothing more than a new platform for drug advertising and, as with all advertising for drugs, the benefits are overemphasized and the risks are understated.

Packaged with every bottle of a prescription drug delivered to the pharmacy—these usually contain a very large number of pills—the FDA requires drug companies to attach detailed written information for doctors and pharmacists about the drug's uses, adverse effects, drug interactions, and dosage recommendations. This piece of paper goes by several names; the most common is simply the *package insert*. Only information that has first been approved by the FDA can be included in a package insert, and it is usually the best picture we have of the risks, at the time of approval, of a new drug. FDA-approved package inserts are not routinely given out by pharmacists, but it's easy for you to get one for either a new or an old drug—just ask your pharmacist. If your pharmacist tells you that she or he can't give you the package insert because it is against the law or regulation, get a new pharmacist.

The package insert is written in technical language, in very small print, and you may need some help with the jargon. Despite what some paternalistic doctors and pharmacists think, there is little in the package insert about a drug's risks that can't be understood by a motivated patient.

For the elderly or others with substandard vision, reading the small print may be a bigger problem than understanding the contents of the package insert. Help on this score is available in the form of the *PDR—Physicians' Desk Reference*—a dictionary-sized, annual compilation of FDA-approved package inserts that often can be found on public library reference shelves. Helped along by *Dorland's Illustrated Medical Dictionary* or some other medical dictionary (also available in many public libraries), the average reader can usually get a general idea of the drug's indications (approved uses), contraindications (no-no's), and other potential hazards. Even if you don't fully understand the complex medical language, the *PDR* will often flash a warning that tells the prudent reader to ask the doctor some pertinent questions. One big advantage of the book over the actual package inserts is that the print is a lot easier on the eyes. Because the *PDR* is published only once a year, however, information about the very newest drugs may be absent. Also, not all older drugs are included, and the main edition of the *PDR* does not include OTC (over-the-counter, or nonprescription) drugs although they do publish a separate book of this information.

The information in package inserts is divided into a number of sections. Those sections of greatest importance to patients include the following:

Indications and Usage

Indication is the term used for a drug's FDA-approved use. The FDA has approved the drug only for the specific uses, or indications, listed in the package insert. Clinical studies and a rigorous FDA review are required to establish a drug's safety and effectiveness for a particular use. Doctors are not bound by law or regulation to prescribe drugs only for FDA-approved uses, and there may or may not be adequate scientific evidence supporting the safety and effectiveness for a drug when it is prescribed for a use not approved by the FDA.

Contraindications

These include other drugs or medical conditions with which the drug should not be used because of serious safety concerns. For example, the use of the common antibiotic erythromycin is contraindicated in people taking cisapride, a drug for nighttime heartburn, or astemizole, an antihistamine, because of a drug interaction that is potentially life-threatening. Another example of a contraindication is the use of the fluoroquinolone antibiotic sparfloxacin in people whose lifestyle or employment brings them into direct exposure to the sun while they are taking the drug, because they could have a very serious adverse reaction known as phototoxicity.

Adverse Reactions

The adverse drug effects listed in this section of the package insert have usually come from the clinical studies that were done before the drug was approved for sale. This is a good source of information about the adverse effects of a new drug and may be as much as we know about these risks when a drug is first marketed.

However, this risk information must be placed in its proper context. The number of patients receiving a drug in clinical trials is relatively small—typically only a few thousand individuals at the most. Rare, but serious, adverse reactions to a drug may not be detected until years later, after large numbers of people have been exposed to the drug.

Consider this: If the average number of patients receiving a drug in clinical trials is 3,000, and the drug causes a serious adverse reaction in 1 in 5,000 patients, 15,000 patients would have to receive the drug in clinical trials to have a 95% chance of detecting the adverse reaction occurring only one time. This is why we recommend that you do not take a new drug until it has been released for at least five years, unless it is one of the rare "breakthrough" drugs that offer some important documented advantage over older proven drugs. Remember, most new drugs are not breakthrough drugs.

Precautions

The precautions section of the package insert contains information about other drugs and medical conditions for which the drug should be used only if its potential benefits outweigh the risks. These situations often require special monitoring for toxicity by the doctor. In addition, this section contains information about the known drug interactions when a new drug is approved. The drug interaction information in the package insert can be lifesaving.

Dosage and Administration

Not only are the specific uses for a drug approved by the FDA, but also the dosage range and sometimes even the duration of treatment. Dosages or durations of treatment not listed in this section may or may not be safe or effective. Frequently, most of the patients studied in clinical trials are younger or middle-aged men, and information may not be avail-able on the proper dosage of a drug for women, the elderly, or children. If special dosage information is known, it will appear in this section of the package insert.

You can ask your pharmacist for a package insert; in fact, you can do this even before you have a prescription filled. Read it over, and if you think it describes a drug you should not be taking or if you have questions about it, talk with your doctor.

You have a right to all of the information in the package insert and it can be lifesaving. Assert this right; it could save your life.

Beware of Patient Information Leaflets (PILs) Distributed by Pharmacists

Many pharmacists are distributing patient information leaflets (PILs). Do not confuse these with FDA-approved package inserts for the drugs you are taking. Pharmacists' PILs are produced by commercial information vendors and printed out on pharmacists' computer systems, but there is little or no evidence supporting the completeness or quality of information contained in these leaflets. In fact, guidelines for the quality of information contained in PILs distributed by pharmacists were not established until 1996.[8] However, these guidelines are only voluntary and patients have no way of knowing if a particular PIL meets them.

The FDA conducted a survey of PILs for alprazolam, amoxicillin, and enalapril produced by eight commercial vendors and found that these leaflets were inadequate and that substantial differences existed in the quality of information provided by the different vendors' PILs.[9] In a study to assess pharmacists' ability to detect the potentially life-threatening interaction between terfenadine and erythromycin, researchers found that some PILs distributed by pharmacists only suggested checking with a doctor if these drugs were prescribed together, while others only contained general advice to report any other drugs being taken to the prescribing doctor.[10]

We have also obtained PILs from pharmacists containing unapproved use information for short-acting nifedipine and bromocriptine. Not only were these uses unapproved, but they had also been disapproved by the FDA for safety reasons. The short-acting nifedipine PIL listed blood-pressure-lowering as a use. This form of nifedipine has never been approved for blood-pressure-lowering (see p. 56). Breast milk suppression was listed as a use on one commercial vendor's PIL for bromocriptine. The Public Citizen's Health Research Group was instrumental in having this use finally removed from the labeling of bromocriptine in 1994, because of heart attacks and strokes occurring in new mothers using this drug to stop milk production.[11]

In 1997, we reviewed the PILs for 15 non-steroidal anti-inflammatory drugs (NSAIDs) for sufficient risk information for NSAID users to reduce their likelihood of gastrointestinal bleeding, a life-threatening adverse effect of NSAIDs. None of the PILs surveyed contained all the information necessary for patients to understand the risks of this family of drugs, how to recognize the symptoms of gastroin-

testinal toxicity, and what steps to take should gastrointestinal toxicity develop (see p. 263).[12]

Recently, we have completed a study of the information content of the PILs for five fluoroquinolone antibiotics produced by four commercial information vendors. The information contained in these PILs was compared with the information contained in the professional product labeling or package inserts for the five antibiotics. Overall, depending on the vendor and the antibiotic, the PILs only included from 16% to 57% of the important information that was contained in the package inserts.[13] In other words, in some of these PILs 84% of the information you need to take the drug safely and effectively was missing.

The PILs currently being distributed by pharmacists are misleading and potentially dangerous because of the amount of important safety information that is omitted. In addition, some PILs have been found that contain indications, or uses for drugs, that are not FDA-approved and are also FDA-disapproved (because there is no evidence of a benefit for that particular use but there are serious safety concerns). Pharmacists' PILs should not be considered as a reliable source of information for the safe and effective use of prescription drugs.

NOTES

1. Hulka BS, Kupper LL, Cassel JC, Efird RL, Birdette JA. Medication use and misuse: Physician-patient discrepancies. *Journal of Chronic Diseases* 1975; 28:7–21.

2. German PS, Klein LE. Adverse drug experience among the elderly. In *Pharmaceuticals for the Elderly*. Pharmaceutical Manufacturers Association, November 1986.

3. Ibid.

4. *Drugs for the Elderly*. 2nd ed. Copenhagen, Denmark: World Health Organization: 1997.

5. Vestal RE, ed. *Drug Treatment in the Elderly*. Sydney, Australia: ADIS Health Science Press, 1984:24–6.

6. Carruthers SG. Clinical pharmacology of aging. In *Fundamentals of Geriatric Medicine*. New York: Raven Press, 1983.

7. Avorn JL, Lamy PP, Vestal RE. Prescribing for the elderly—safely. *Patient Care* June 1982:14–62.

8. Action Plan for the Provision of Useful Prescription Medicine Information, presented to Donna E. Shalala, Secretary of the Department of Health and Human Services by the Steering Committee for the Collaborative Development of a Long-Range Action Plan for the Provision of Useful Prescription Medicine Information, December 1996.

9. 60 *Federal Register* 44194. August 24, 1995.

10. Cavuto NJ, Woosley RL, Sale M. Pharmacies and prevention of potentially fatal drug interactions. *Journal of the American Medical Association* 1996; 275:1086 [letter].

11. Letter from Sidney M. Wolfe, MD, and Stephen G. Moore, MD, MPH, of Public Citizen's Health Research Group to David Kessler, MD, JD, Commissioner, Food and Drug Administration, dated September 2, 1993.

12. Sasich LD, Wolfe SM. Deficiencies in patient information leaflets concerning gastrointestinal complications of nonsteroidal anti-inflammatory drugs. *Journal of General Internal Medicine* 1997; 12(suppl 1):79 [abstract].

13. Bradley LR, Sasich LD. The information content of patient medication information leaflets: Examination of five fluoroquinolone antibiotics. *Journal of the American Pharmaceutical Association* 1998; 38:278–9 [abstract].

5

SAVING MONEY WHILE AVOIDING INJURY WHEN BUYING PRESCRIPTION DRUGS

There are at least three ways you can save money on the high cost of prescription drugs: (1) If appropriate, ask your doctor to help you try to manage your condition using a nondrug treatment first; (2) Avoid **"Do Not Use"** drugs, and wait at least five years to take any new drug unless it is one of the rare "breakthrough" drugs; and (3) When you can, buy generic drugs. By following this advice, you can also reduce your risk of preventable drug-induced injury.

Nondrug Treatments

For many conditions, such as mild to moderate high blood pressure, high cholesterol, type-2 diabetes, obesity, and insomnia, changes in lifestyle are just as effective, safer, and less expensive than prescription drugs for many people. In fact, in many instances, nondrug interventions are recommended as the first-line treatment for these conditions before drugs are tried.

It may be easier for you to take pills, but pills may not be the safest or best management for your condition, and they are certainly more expensive than nondrug treatments.

"Do Not Use" or "Do Not Use Until Five Years After Release"

Avoiding drugs listed as **"Do Not Use"** or **"Do Not Use Until Five Years After Release"** can both save you money and help you to avoid needless drug-induced injury. For example, in the treatment of high blood pressure, a 30-day supply of the diuretic hydrochlorothiazide from a generic company at a dosage of 25 milligrams per day (12.5 milligrams can be used by many people) will cost you $5.99 at a Washington, D.C., pharmacy chain, while the same 30-day supply of the new calcium channel blocker mibefradil (Posicor), at the same pharmacy, in the recommended dosage of 100 milligrams per day, was $79.99. Mibefradil was definitely not a breakthrough drug; in fact, we listed it as **"Do Not Use"** because shortly after it was released, serious adverse effects were discovered (see p. 146). It was subsequently banned from the market in June 1998. The savings on hydrochlorothiazide over mibefradil was almost $900 per year if you need to use 25 milligrams per day of hydrochlorothiazide, and even greater if your blood pressure can be controlled with the 12.5 milligram dosage. There are additional proven benefits with hydrochlorothiazide. It has been shown to reduce the risk of heart attack and stroke in people with high blood pressure, while mibefradil has killed and injured hundreds of people.

The release of mibefradil is an example of a strategy now being used by brand name manufacturers to combat competition from generic companies. This strategy is to flood the market with new drugs that are protected by patents. Until the patent expires, no generic alternative can be made available. This strategy increases drug costs and keeps profits high for the brand name companies.

In 1996 and 1997, a total of 92 drugs were approved for marketing by the FDA. This is almost double the 50 new drugs cleared in 1994 and 1995 combined. In 1993, a year in which only 25 new drugs were released, brand name products lost about $1 billion of sales when patents expired, with generic equivalents achieving about $400 million in sales. This was a net loss of a little under $600 million lost as drugs went off-patent. New drugs introduced that year only achieved $560 million in sales. In subsequent years, with more new drugs being released—drugs which only rarely offer an important advantage over older, proven, less expensive drugs—the rate of sales growth for newly released drugs has soared, from $563 million in 1993 to $3 billion in 1996 for brand name companies.[1]

According to the market research firm IMS America, total pharmaceutical sales for 1997 were $81.17 billion with drugs first cleared for marketing in 1997—39 in all—contributing $3.28 billion to the total. Seven of these 39 drugs accounted for almost $1.4 billion towards your drug bills.[2] We listed six of these drugs as either **"Do Not Use"** or **"Do Not Use Until Five Years After Release:"**

atorvastatin (LIPITOR, see p. 130)

This drug was the fifth member of the "statin" family of cholesterol-lowering drugs approved by the FDA. Atorvastatin was the leading drug launched in 1997, averaging $48.6 million per month in sales after hitting the market in January, or $582.7 million for the year. The older drugs in the "statin" family have only shown a modest effect in reducing the risk of a first or second heart attack, while atorvastatin has not been shown to reduce the risk of heart attack. We recommend that you **Do Not Use Until Five Years After Release** (2002) for atorvastatin. For most people, lifestyle changes remain the management of first choice for high cholesterol.

troglitazone (REZULIN, see p. 565)

We listed this new blood-sugar-lowering drug as **"Do Not Use"** because of reports of liver toxicity and liver failure. Troglitazone was removed from the market in the United Kingdom in 1997 because British drug regulatory authorities found that the drug's risks outweighed its benefits. U.S. sales averaged $32.4 million per month after troglitazone was released in March. This is a total of $324 million for 1997.

donepezil (ARICEPT, see p. 571)

We concur with the editors of the highly respected independent source of drug information, *The Medical Letter on Drugs and Therapeutics,* written for doctors and pharmacists, that there is no evidence that use of either donepezil or tacrine, an older drug in the same class, leads to substantial functional improvement or prevention of the progression of Alzheimer's disease. We recommend that you **"Do Not Use"**. Donepezil sold $166 million in 1997, averaging $13.9 million per month in sales.

bromfenac (DURACT, see p. 292)

NOTE: removed from the market on June 22, 1998. This was a new member of the nonsteroidal anti-inflammatory drug family, or NSAIDs, and is listed as **"Do Not Use"** because of the possibility of serious liver toxicity. We recommend that you do not use bromfenac because there are safer, less expensive alternatives, such as ibuprofen, available. After entering the market in July, bromfenac sales averaged $11.4 million per month, totaling $68.4 million for 1997.

mibefradil (POSICOR, see p. 146)

NOTE: removed from the market on June 8, 1998 for safety reasons. Mibefradil, the example used above, is the ninth member of the calcium channel blocker family, and is used for both high blood pressure and chest pain (angina). We listed this drug as **"Do Not Use"** because it was found to cause a serious slowing of the heart rate and to be associated with potentially fatal drug interactions. Even if a calcium channel blocker is your only treatment option, there is no medical reason why you should be using this drug rather than one of the older drugs in this family, many of which are less expensive. With sales averaging $4.3 million per month after its release in July, mibefradil sales totaled $25.8 million for 1997.

valsartan (DIOVAN, see p. 90)

This drug is a member of a new family of drugs for high blood pressure known as angiotensin antagonists that we list as **Do Not Use Until Five Years After Release** (2002). Valsartan is not a first choice drug for treating high blood pressure. Valsartan sold $3.4 million per month after it entered the market in February 1997 for a total of $37.4 million for that year.

levofloxacin (LEVAQUIN, see p. 523)

This antibiotic is a new member of the fluoroquinolone family that now contains nine drugs. There are many other drugs that can be used to treat the same infections as levofloxacin that are safer and less expensive. Levofloxacin averaged $12.9 million per month for total 1997 sales of $154.8 million. We categorize this drug as **"Limited Use."**

We find it troubling that these seven new drugs, six of which we have listed as **"Do Not Use"** or **"Do Not Use Until Five Years After Release"** made almost $1.4 billion in sales in 1997. All of them have unknown safety and effectiveness compared to older, proven alternatives or nondrug treatments. These figures are a condemnation of the way many doctors prescribe drugs and reflect the effectiveness of drug company advertising.

Saving Money by Buying Generic Drugs

Unless you want to waste a large amount of money—often hundreds of dollars a year—by using brand name instead of generic drugs, you should ask for the generic version, especially if you are starting on a drug for the first time. (See chart below.) One of the few bits of comparative information about prescription drugs readily accessible to consumers is the retail price of brand name versus generic drugs. You can get this information easily, by

Retail Price of Brand Name vs Generic Drugs at a Washington DC Pharmacy Chain

USE	BRAND NAME	PRICE	GENERIC DRUG	PRICE	DURATION OF TREATMENT
high blood pressure	Inderal 40 mg #60	$50.59	propranolol 40 mg #60	$10.59	1 month
antibiotic	Bactrim DS #20	$40.19	trimethoprim/ sulfamethoxazole #20	$11.69	10 days
antibiotic	Keflex 250 mg #40	$87.99	cephalexin 250 mg #40	$23.39	10 days
antidepressant	Tofranil 25 mg #30	$18.79	imipramine 25 mg #30	$6.39	1 month
NSAID*	Motrin 400 mg #120	$37.69	ibuprofen 400 mg #120	$15.49	1 month

*Nonsteroidal anti-inflammatory drug for pain and arthritis

asking your pharmacist. The chart below was prepared by simply phoning a local pharmacy.

Brand name drug manufacturers have gone to extraordinary lengths to mislead doctors, pharmacists, and the public into believing that their products are produced to higher standards, and thus are safer and more effective than the same drugs produced by generic companies. These strategies have included setting up sham patient groups to lobby state legislatures to protect their brand name drugs, and the suppression of scientific research by at least one brand name company that showed their brand name product was no better than those of generic companies.

Should You Use Generic Drugs?

The quality of prescription drugs, brand name or generic, does not solely depend on the manufacturer, but also on a strong and vigilant FDA. Both brand name and generic drug companies are regulated by the FDA using the same standards for manufacturing facilities, quality and purity, and content of prescription drugs.

The Question of Brand Name Quality

Many brand name drug companies such as Warner-Lambert, and its subsidiary, Parke-Davis denigrate the quality of generic drugs in an attempt to hold market share from generics and protect profits. However, the facts about this brand-name manufacturer bear examining.

From 1990 to the end of 1995, there were a total of 64 recalls of Warner-Lambert products as listed in Food and Drug Administration (FDA) recall reports. In 1990, there were 3 recalls, 1 in 1991, 3 in 1992, 24 in 1993, 13 in 1994, and 20 in 1995. For their brand of phenytoin (DILANTIN) alone—a drug used primarily for treating seizure disorders and one where the amount of drug in the blood is critical—there have been 12 recalls during this period. Nine of these involved problems with dissolv-

ing of the drug, which can result in an insufficient amount being absorbed by the body. More than 975,000 bottles (some of which contained 1,000 capsules) and more than 30,000 injectable doses of Dilantin were affected by these recalls.[3]

In this case, Warner-Lambert officials pleaded guilty to criminal charges for withholding important information about sloppy manufacturing practices from the FDA.

FDA Repels Attacks on Generic Drugs

If you worry about the health hazards of prescription drugs, should you be more worried about brand name drugs or about the less-expensive generic copies of those brand name drugs which are no longer on patent? In reviewing the major prescription drug disasters of the last two decades, in every case of death or serious injury, the cause was a brand name drug, never a generic one.

Examples of such disasters, which collectively have killed hundreds of Americans and injured thousands more, have involved the arthritis drugs or painkillers Oraflex, Suprol, and Zomax, the antidepressant Merital, the high blood pressure drug Selacryn, and the diet drugs Pondimin, one-half of the once popular "fen/phen" combination, and its close chemical cousin Redux, Posicor, a drug for high blood pressure and chest pain, and the painkiller Duract. Because of the serious dangers of these nine drugs, all were taken off the market.

In fact, all of these tragedies involved brand name drugs which had only recently come onto the market, except for Pondimin, which was only available from a brand name company, making it impossible in eight of these nine cases for there even to be a generic version, because the patent had not yet expired. In other words, once a drug has been on the market long enough for the patent to have expired and for there to be a generic equivalent, there is very little chance that some previously unde- tected danger will come to light unless the drug was misprescribed as with Pondimin. This is much more likely to happen with drugs on the market for only a short time.

But what about those drugs which have been on the market for a long enough time for the patents to have expired and which are avail- able in both brand name and generic versions? Which version is safer or more effective? It has always been our position that there is no dif- ference between generic and brand name drugs as far as the odds that there will be something found wrong with the amount of active ingredi- ent or the purity. Over the years, there have been recalls because of these kinds of problems with both generic and brand name drugs.

In the past, however, there has been some legitimate concern about generic drugs by doc- tors, pharmacists, and patients. The passage of legislation shortening the approval process for generic copies of brand name drugs once the brand name patent had expired inspired some generic companies to stoop to criminal activity— such as bribing FDA officials—to push their drug through the approval process and on the market more quickly. Both FDA and drug com- pany officials have been successfully prosecuted for these actions. As a result, the process of look- ing at data upon which to base a decision whether to approve a generic drug is probably tighter and more patient-protective than ever. Fortunately, even though these procedural irreg- ularities occurred, there is no evidence that any patients were harmed as a result of taking the generic drugs made by these companies.

A 1990 study by Food and Drug Administra- tion laboratories from all over the country, found that those classes of prescription drugs which theoretically could be most likely to pose safety or effectiveness problems if they were not manufactured properly, met the applicable standards in virtually all cases. The classes of drugs tested included contraceptives, antibi- otics, and medications prescribed for asthma,

epilepsy, high blood pressure, and abnormal heart rhythms. Of the 429 samples of 24 differ- ent drugs which were tested, including both brand name and generic drugs, there were no samples tested which posed a health hazard to patients when examined for potency and, where applicable, dissolution rate and content uniformity.

The reason that these 24 different drugs were chosen is that they all have a narrow therapeu- tic range. This means that, unlike most kinds of drugs, for which there is a relatively large range of dosages which are both effective and rela- tively safe, the amount of these drugs which gets into the body must be more tightly con- trolled. If it is not, the drug may too easily lose its effectiveness (if the dose is too low) or become toxic (if the dose is too high).

The drugs which were tested included six asthma drugs, four for treating epilepsy, four high blood pressure drugs, four drugs for treat- ing heart arrhythmias, a birth control pill, one antibiotic, a drug for treating depression, and a so-called blood-thinning drug. In six categories of drugs, both brand name and generic versions were tested. In the case of the birth control pill, all of the major brand names, but no generic version, were tested.

For 23 of the 24 different drugs, there was no difference between the brand name and the generic versions in the FDA laboratories tests for purity or quality. For aminophylline, an asthma drug which we do not recommend as a first line treatment, five batches from two man- ufacturers failed to meet the FDA standards. Although none of these five batches posed a health hazard, all were recalled.[4]

Listed below are the names, both brand and generic, by therapeutic class, of all the drugs studied except for the birth control pill (because no generic version was studied) and aminophylline (see p. 417). Many of these manufacturers have changed since the 1990 study because of mergers and acquisitions within the drug industry.

In an article reprinted in the World Health Organization's *Essential Drugs Monitor* in 1988, the FDA rebuts what it calls "10 charges or myths currently being raised, under the guise of independent dialogue, aimed at discouraging health professionals from prescribing or dispensing generic drugs":

Myth 1: The 1984 action by Congress has eliminated safety and effectiveness testing requirements for generic drugs and has thus reduced the confidence that physicians and patients can have in the safety and effectiveness of generic drugs.

Fact 1: What the law in fact does is eliminate the unnecessary requirement for duplicative testing to redemonstrate the safety and effectiveness of active drug ingredients that have already been shown to be safe and effective by adequate and well-controlled studies and that have been widely used and accepted by the medical community for many years.

Myth 2: FDA requires pioneer drug manufacturers to study their drugs in thousands of patients, but it requires generic firms to test their drug products in 20 or 30 healthy volunteers.

Fact 2: This statement is misleading. Testing in a large number of patients is required for the pioneer drug in order to establish the safety and effectiveness of the new active drug ingredient. Once this has been established, the FDA need ensure only that others wanting to market a copy of the innovator's product make their product correctly and that similar amounts of the drug enter the bloodstream.

Myth 3: Plasma level studies (measuring the amount of a drug in the blood) do not show how a drug acts at the site of action and therefore are not indicative of how well a drug will perform.

Fact 3: Once the active ingredient is shown to enter the bloodstream at the same rate and extent as the same active ingredient from another similar drug product, there is no currently recognized scientific basis to allege that the therapeutic effects or adverse effects of the two drugs will differ.

Myth 4: Bioequivalence studies which measure the absorption of a drug into the blood (drug products made by different companies having the same absorption characteristics are called bioequivalent) are performed in healthy volunteers, who are usually in their twenties. However, many of the drugs are used primarily in elderly patients. These elderly patients can be expected to absorb and metabolize the drug differently than do the healthy volunteers. Therefore bioequivalence testing is not an indicator of how the drug will perform in patients.

Fact 4: The testing in healthy volunteers, which shows an equivalent blood level between the generic and the brand name product, is a strong indicator that the two tested dosage forms will behave the same under the same conditions. No one has demonstrated that two products found by conventional tests to be bioequivalent perform inequivalently in different patients. It is also preferable to subject healthy people, rather than already weakened or disabled patients, to the blood sampling and other discomforts of bioequivalence testing.

Myth 5: The FDA applies lower standards for generic approval compared to those required for the brand name products.

Fact 5: The lesser standard that is usually implied in such a statement relates to the safety and efficacy testing mentioned earlier. The FDA in fact requires that the manufacturers in both instances follow good manufacturing practice, that they show that their drug is stable, that it is bioequivalent, and that it meets the same standards of identity, strength, quality and purity.

Myth 6: The FDA has no written rules or criteria for how it determines bioequivalence.

Fact 6: The FDA has required generic drugs to be bioequivalent to brand name products since the mid-1970s, and it published final regulations on bioequivalence in January 1977.

ASTHMA DRUGS

Brand Name	Generic Name	Manufacturers of Brand Name or Generic Drugs
Lufyllin	dyphylline	Altana Inc., Lemmon Company, Wallace Laboratories
	isoetharine mesylate	Reedco, Inc.
Medihaler, Isuprel	isoproterenol inhaler	Abbott Laboratories, Barre-National Inc., Sterling Drug Inc.
Alupent, Metaprel	metaproterenol	American Therapeutics, Inc., Boehringer Ingelheim Pharmacy, Pharmaceutical Basics Inc., Sandoz Pharmaceuticals
Choledyl	oxtriphylline	Bolar Pharmaceutical Co. Inc., Warner Lambert Company
Slo-Phyllin, Quibron-T-Sr	theophylline	Banner Gelatin Products, Bristol-Myers USPNG, Central Pharmaceuticals, Cord Laboratories, Graham, DM Laboratories I, Inwood Labs, KV Pharmaceutical Co., Paco PR, Inc., Riker Labs/3M Pharmaceuticals, Rorer Pharmaceutical Corp., Schering-Plough Products, Searle & Co., Inc.

EPILEPSY DRUGS

Tegretol	carbamazepine	Geigy Pharmaceuticals, Inwood Labs, Pharmaceutical Basics Inc., Purepac, Sidmark Laboratories, Teva Pharmaceuticals, Warner Chilcot
Dilantin	phenytoin	Bolar Pharmaceutical Co., Inc., Lannett Company, Inc., Mason Distributors, Inc., Warner Lambert, Inc., Zenith Labs Inc.
Mysoline	primidone	Bolar Pharmaceutical Co., Inc., Danbury Pharmacal., Inc., Lannett Company Inc., Wyeth-Ayerst Labs
Depakene	valproic acid	Abbott Laboratories, Chase Chemical Co., Pharmaceutical Basics Inc., Scherer, R.P., North America

HIGH BLOOD PRESSURE DRUGS

Catapres	clonidine	American Therapeutics Inc., Barr Labs Inc., Boehringer Ingelheim Pharm., Bolar Pharmaceutical Co. Inc., Cord Laboratories, Danbury Pharmacal. Inc., Duramed Pharmaceuticals, Interpharm Inc., Kalipharma Inc., Lederle Laboratories, Par Pharmaceutical, Warner Lambert
Esimil, Ismelin	guanethidine	Bolar Pharmaceutical Co. Inc., Ciba Geigy Corp.

HIGH BLOOD PRESSURE DRUGS *(Cont.)*

Brand Name	Generic Name	Manufacturers of Brand Name or Generic Drugs
Loniten	minoxidil	Danbury Pharmacal Inc., Par Pharmaceutical, Quantum Pharmics Ltd., Upjohn Company
Minipress	prazosin hydrochloride	Danbury Pharmacal Inc., Kalipharma Inc., Mylan Pharmaceuticals, Inc., Pfizer Inc., Zenith Labs Inc.

ANTIARRYTHMIC DRUGS

Norpace	disopyramide	Barr Labs Inc., Biocraft Labs Inc., Cord Laboratories, Danbury Pharmacal Inc., Interpharm Inc., KV Pharmaceutical Co., Searle & Co., Inc., Zenith Labs Inc.
Pronestyl	procainamide	Bolar Pharm Co. Inc., Chelsea Labs, Copley Pharmaceutical Inc., Cord Laboratories, Danbury Pharmacal Inc., Sidmak Laboratories, Squibb Corp., Warner Lambert, Zenith Labs Inc.
Quinaglute	quinidine gluconate	Berlex Labs, Bolar Pharmaceutical Co. Inc., Cord Laboratories, Halsey Drug Co. Inc.
	quinidine sulfate	American Cyanamid Co., Barr Labs Inc., Chelsea Labs, Cord Laboratories, Danbury Pharmacal., Inc., Halsey Drug Co. Inc., Kalipharma Inc., Lannett Company Inc., Lilly, Eli & Co., Mutual Pharmaceutical Co., Private Formulations Inc., Reid-Rowell Inc., Richlyn Labs Inc., Robins, A.H. Company, Inc., Roxane Laboratories Inc., Vitarine Pharmaceuticals, Warner Lambert

ANTIBIOTIC DRUGS

Cleocin	clindamycin	Upjohn Company, Vitarine Pharmaceuticals

ANTIDEPRESSANT DRUGS

Eskalith	lithium carbonate	Bolar Pharmaceutical Co. Inc., Pfizer Inc., Reid-Rowell Inc., Roxane Laboratories Inc., SmithKline & French

BLOOD-THINNER DRUGS

Coumadin	warfarin sodium	Abbott Laboratories, Bolar Pharmaceutical Co. Inc., DuPont Pharmaceuticals, Pharmaceutical Basics Inc.

Myth 7: Because the FDA allows a variation of +/− 20 or 30% in the blood levels between the brand name and the generic products, generics may differ by as much as 60% from each other.

Fact 7: The test that the FDA employs, and the standard that is applied, is a statistical one. It is virtually impossible for a generic product to pass if it in fact differs in its average plasma level by 20% from the standard product. Deviations of more than 10% between generic and brand name products are rare; usually the differences are much less than 10%.

Myth 8: Brand name drugs are made in modern facilities, while generics are often made in substandard facilities. Thus generics are of generally inferior quality.

Fact 8: No one has been able to demonstrate that the quality of generic drugs differs from that of the brand name counterparts. The rates of defects found by the FDA in both brand name and generic products are extremely low and speak well of the pharmaceutical industry's care in producing prescription drugs. In fact, the innovator drug firms themselves account for an estimated 70–80% of the generic drug market. Thus, to believe generics are inferior, one would have to accept the premise that the research-oriented drug firms can't adequately manufacture products other than the ones they pioneered. It is also true that many innovator drug firms distribute products made by smaller generic firms. It is unlikely they would continue such arrangements if they really doubted the ability of generic firms to manufacture quality products.

Myth 9: In calling drugs bioequivalent, the FDA overlooks documented cases of bioinequivalence.

Fact 9: While there have been a few well-known, documented cases of bioinequivalence, they are either examples from many years ago that have long since been corrected or problems resulting from drugs which had never gone through FDA's approval system. The FDA is not aware of a single documented bioinequivalence involving any generic drug product that has been approved by the FDA as bioequivalent.

Myth 10: Patients using generic products are more likely to suffer adverse reactions than those taking the brand name drug.

Fact 10: There is no evidence of a different rate of adverse drug reactions (ADRs) between brand name products and their generic equivalents. There have been some efforts recently by several brand name firms to stimulate reporting to FDA's voluntary ADR system of adverse reactions to the products of their generic competitors. The FDA has vigorously opposed any such attempts.

The FDA has a public obligation to investigate thoroughly all allegations of drug product defects or failures. The agency has not found any of the allegations raised thus far in the brand name versus generic drug controversy to be valid. The FDA also has an obligation to make known to health care professionals and to the public its conclusions that false or misleading reports are being generated.

New Attacks on Generic Drugs

Dupont Merck Pharmaceutical, formed in 1991 by the merger of two industry giants, has created a campaign for promoting disinformation about generic drugs to health professionals and the public. Dupont Merck produces the anti-coagulant (blood thinner) warfarin (COUMADIN), a drug whose patent protection expired years ago, but which ranked No.11 on the list of most frequently dispensed drugs, with more than 14 million prescriptions filled in 1996. Generic warfarin was a drug tested by the FDA in 1990 and found to meet all applicable standards. When a competitor, Barr Laboratories, sought FDA approval of its generic warfarin product in May 1995, Dupont Merck went to extraordinary lengths to protect its bottom line from competition. Barr Laboratories has recently been granted approval to market its warfarin.

With a $75,000 grant, Dupont Merck created the Health Alliance for Narrow Therapeutic Index Patient Safety, an organization claiming to be dedicated to the protection of the millions of Americans (read protection of market share) who take one or more drugs known as narrow therapeutic index (NTI) drugs. If you telephone this organization, Goodard Claussen Campaigns (a Washington, D.C. public relations firm) answers. Dupont Merck's misleading message, conveyed through its sham patient group, is that FDA testing requirements for generic drugs used since 1984 are not adequate to protect the public's safety when generic NTI drugs are substituted for brand name ones by pharmacists.

Dupont Merck knew it had no scientific basis for such a claim, so it hired lobbyists to influence changes in state pharmacy and medical laws to make generic substitution for NTI drugs more difficult. For example, in North Carolina, a state where the interests of prescription drug consumers were sacrificed, provisions of a new Prescription Refill Safety Act require that consumers taking an NTI drug who are seeking a prescription refill must receive the same drug, produced by the same manufacturer, as they are already taking, unless both consumer and prescribing physician approve substitution of a different manufacturer's product. The only beneficiary of this legislation will be Dupont Merck, by making it more difficult for consumers to switch to less costly generic warfarin meeting FDA standards.

In fact, there is no formal designation by the FDA of any compound as an "NTI" drug. Agency regulations do define drugs with what is called a "narrow therapeutic ratio." The list of narrow therapeutic ratio drugs given above was prepared by the agency to assist FDA District Offices in their testing after the generic drug scandal of the late 1980s. Warfarin was on this list, and the FDA found no difference between the brand name product and two generic competitors.

The FDA makes scientifically based judgments about generic drugs. It is the agency's position—and ours—that brand name drugs are no different than generic equivalents in meeting FDA standards, and that patients and doctors can expect the same response and benefit from approved generic products as from brand name drugs.

The Levothyroxine (SYNTHROID) Scandal

Boots Pharmaceuticals which became the Knoll Pharmaceutical Company of Mt. Olive, N.J., in March 1995, suppressed publication of scientific research for more than two years in order to perpetuate the incorrect public impression that their brand name version of levothyroxine (SYNTHROID) was more reliable than generic levothyroxine products from three competing companies. The cost to the American public in excessive charges for Synthroid over these two years has been estimated to be $800 million.

Research that contradicted the Boot's/Knoll's superiority claim was finally published in the April 16, 1997 issue of the *Journal of the American Medical Association*. It found four generic and brand name drugs—Synthroid and the three competing levothyroxines—to be bioequivalent by current FDA standards and interchangeable without loss of therapeutic efficacy in the majority of patients for treatment of hypothyroidism (low thyroid).[5]

The powerful lesson in this story is in the extraordinary deception that first Boots, then later Knoll, undertook to protect their business interests, including corrupting the ethical foundations on which objective scientific research is based and violating federal law to perpetuate the myth that Synthroid was better than generic brands.

Knoll's predecessor, Boots, contracted with a faculty member and researchers at the University of California at San Francisco (UCSF), in 1987 for a bioequivalence study comparing Synthroid with three competitors' levothyroxine products. The company paid the researchers $250,000 to do the study. In this case, a finding of bioequivalence would allow consumers the choice of Synthroid or less expensive, equally effective generic products. Boots' expectation was that the study would find Synthroid to be superior to the generics.

The contract contained a clause giving Boots veto power over publication of the study's results. The problems began in late 1990, when it became known that Synthroid and the other three levothyroxines were the same.

Over the next four years, Boots waged a calculated campaign to discredit the researchers and their work. Once it was clear that the study would not support the claim of Synthroid's superiority, Boots alleged scores of deficiencies and errors in the study. The university conducted an investigation of how the research was done and found only minor and easily correctable problems. Some members of the investigating panel found Boots' interactions with the researchers to be "harassment" and characterized the company's actions as "deceptive and self-serving." The university concluded that the study was carefully done and complied fully with terms of the contract.[6]

The results of the study were submitted to the *Journal of the American Medical Association* in April 1994. The study was sent to five experts for peer review and was accepted for publication in November 1994 with its publication scheduled in the January 25, 1995 issue of the *Journal*. On January 13, 1995, the researchers suddenly withdrew the study from publication, citing as the reason "impending legal action by Boots Pharmaceuticals, Inc. against UCSF and the investigators." Because of the clause in the contract giving the company veto power over publication, UCSF said it would not defend the researchers if the study was printed without the company's permission.[7]

Then, in a move striking at the very core of ethical scientific standards, the company's senior director for medical research took the study results and, without giving credit to the UCSF researchers, published a misleading version in an obscure journal of which he was also an associate editor. The new version was used to support the company's previous assertion of Synthroid's superior reliability.

In November 1996, more than a year after the Boots-Knoll changeover, Knoll was caught distributing misleading advertising about Synthroid to doctors, and was cited by the FDA's Division of Drug Marketing, Advertising and Communications for violating federal law. The company was passing out a study claiming Synthroid had better absorption characteristics compared with a competing generic company's levothyroxine, while knowing that the UCSF study showed no difference between the two products. This new study was co-authored by Knoll's own senior director for medical research and was done on normal volunteers without a low thyroid condition, and was tested on these subjects for only 48 hours.[8] The company's claim of Synthroid's superiority could not possibly have been supported by this type of study.

Six years after it was known that there was no difference between Synthroid and generic levothyroxine products, and more than two years after the UCSF research should have been published, the *Journal of the American Medical Association* published the research just as it would have appeared in January 1995 had it not been for Boots' interference.

To sum it all up, generic drugs are just as effective and safe as brand name drugs. Unless you want to waste quite a bit of money, ask your pharmacist to fill your prescription with a generic drug. If the brand name drug is not yet off-patent, your pharmacist will advise you of this.

NOTES

1. Managed Care Spurs Industry Growth. *Scrip* 1997; 2273:15.

2. Post-1990 launches represent 43% of Rx market, IMS says. *F-D-C Reports* 1998; 60(10):9–10.

3. Statement by Sidney M. Wolfe, MD, Public Citizen's Health Research Group Concerning Warner-Lambert's Criminal Conviction and Poor Manufacturing Practices, November 29, 1995.

4. Survey of Narrow Therapeutic Range Drug Quality. Food and Drug Administration, September 12, 1990.

5. Dong BJ, Hauck WW, Gambertoglio JG, Gee L, White JR, Bubp JL, et al. Bioequivalence of generic and brand-name levothyroxine products in the treatment of hypothyroidism. *Journal of the American Medical Association* 1997; 277:1205–13.

6. Rennie D. Thyroid storm. *Journal of the American Medical Association* 1997; 277:1238–43[editorial].

7. Ibid.

8. Letter to Robert Ashwood, Ph.D., Director, Regulatory Affairs, Knoll Pharmaceuticals from Minnie Baylor-Henry, R.Ph., JD, Director, Division of Drug Marketing, Advertising and Communications, Food and Drug Administration.

GLOSSARY

ACE inhibitor: Angiotensin-converting enzyme inhibitor. Drugs such as captopril, mainly used to treat high blood pressure or heart failure.

Akathisia: Restless leg syndrome. Can be drug-induced, involving an inability to remain in a sitting position, promoting restlessness and a feeling of muscular jitters.

Akinesia: Weakness and muscular fatigue. Can be drug-induced, involving nerve problems which make patient appear listless, disinterested and depressed. Additional problems can include infrequent blinking, slower swallowing of saliva with drooling, and a lack of facial expression.

Allergy: Hypersensitivity (overreaction) to substances such as drugs, food, and pollen.

Analgesic: A drug used to relieve pain.

Anemia: Decrease in red blood cells or in hemoglobin of the blood.

Angiotensin II modifiers: A family of high-blood-pressure-lowering drugs that includes losartan (COZAAR), valsartan (DIOVAN), and irbesartan (AVAPRO).

Antacid: A drug used to neutralize excess acid in the stomach.

Antiarrhythmic: A drug used to treat abnormal heart rhythms.

Antibiotic: A drug derived from molds or bacteria which is used to treat bacterial infections.

Anticholinergic: A drug that blocks the effects of acetylcholine, a substance produced by the body which is responsible for certain nervous system activities (parasympathetic). Drugs with anticholinergic effects (including antidepressants, antihistamines, antipsychotics, drugs for intestinal problems, antiparkinsonians) inhibit the secretion of acid in the stomach, slow the passage of food through the digestive system, inhibit the production of saliva, sweat, and bronchial secretions, and increase the heart rate and blood pressure. Adverse effects of these drugs include dry mouth, constipation, difficulty urinating, confusion, worsening of glaucoma, blurred vision, and short-term memory problems.

Anticoagulant: A drug that inhibits or slows down blood clotting.

Anticonvulsant: A drug that prevents or treats seizures (convulsions or fits).

Antidepressant: A drug used to treat mental depression.

Antiflatulent: A drug used to relieve "excess gas" in the stomach or intestines.

Antifungal: A drug used to treat infections caused by a fungus (such as ringworm, thrush, or athlete's foot).

Antihistamine: A drug used to prevent or relieve the symptoms of allergy (such as hay fever).

Antihypertensive: A drug used to lower high blood pressure.

Antiparkinsonian: A drug used to control the symptoms of Parkinson's disease.

Antiprotozoal: A drug used to treat infections caused by protozoa (tiny, one-celled animals).

Antipsychotic: A drug used to treat certain serious mental conditions such as schizophrenia.

Antispasmodic: A drug used to reduce smooth muscle spasms (for example, stomach, intestinal, or urinary tract spasms).

Antitubercular: A drug used to treat tuberculosis (TB).

Aortic stenosis: Narrowing of one of the valves (aortic valve) in the heart or of the aorta itself (one of the major blood vessels in the body).

Arthritis: A chronic disease marked by painful, stiff, swollen, and sometimes red joints.

Asthma: A chronic disorder characterized by wheezing, coughing, difficulty in breathing, and a suffocating feeling. Can be caused by allergies or infections.

Barbiturate: A drug used to produce drowsiness and/or a hypnotic state. It can become addictive if taken for a long period of time.

Benzodiazepines: A family of drugs that are prescribed for nervousness and sleeping problems and to relax muscles and control seizures. They can be addictive if taken for an extended period of time. Adverse effects include confusion, drowsiness, hallucinations, mental depression, and impaired coordination resulting in falls and hip fractures.

Beta-blocker: A drug used to treat high blood pressure, angina, and irregular heart rhythms and to prevent migraine headaches. They work to dilate (open) the blood vessels and to decrease the number of heartbeats per minute thereby lowering blood pressure.

Bone marrow depression: The body produces new red and white blood cells by making blood cells in the bone marrow, the core of the bones. Certain types of drugs reduce the ability of the marrow to produce new blood cells, leaving fewer blood cells to circulate in the body to carry oxygen or fight infection.

Bronchodilator: A drug used to open the bronchial tubes (air passages) of the lungs to increase the flow of air through them. Used by patients who have asthma, chronic bronchitis, or emphysema.

Bronchospasm: Temporary narrowing of the air passages in the lungs, decreasing the flow of air. This occurs in patients who have asthma, chronic bronchitis, or emphysema.

Calcium channel blocker: A drug used to control high blood pressure (hypertension) and heart rate and to improve blood flow to the heart. It works by lowering the calcium concentrations in certain smooth muscles in the blood vessels, causing blood vessels to dilate (open) and heart rate to decrease thereby lowering blood pressure.

Cardiovascular system: The system which allows circulation of oxygen and blood. It consists of the heart and blood vessels.

Carotid sinus: Location of a special receptor in the carotid artery, a major blood vessel in the body, which is sensitive to changes in blood pressure.

Cephalosporins: A family of antibiotics which has antibacterial activity similar to the penicillins, but which can work against a wider range of infections and kill some bacteria resistant to penicillins.

Cholesterol: A fat-like substance found in blood and most tissues. Too much cholesterol is associated with such health risks as hardening of the arteries and heart attacks.

Cholesterol-lowering drug: A drug which works— by various mechanisms including blocking cholesterol synthesis or increasing cholesterol breakdown—to lower blood cholesterol levels.

Colitis: Inflammation of the colon (large bowel).

Complete blood count (CBC): An examination of the blood to detect red cell and white cell counts.

Congestive heart failure: A medical condition in which the heart does not pump adequately and fluid accumulates in the lungs and in the legs. Body tissues also do not receive an adequate blood supply.

Corticosteroids: A family of drugs similar to the chemical cortisone, produced by the adrenal gland, which are used as anti-inflammatory agents and to control the body's salt/water balance if needed.

Dementia: Deterioration or loss of intellectual faculties, reasoning power, will, and memory due to organic brain disease; characterized by confusion, disorientation, and stupor of varying degrees.

Diabetes mellitus: Also known as sugar diabetes. A disorder in which the body cannot process sugars to produce energy, due to lack of a hormone called insulin. This leads to too much sugar in the blood (hyperglycemia), and an increased risk of coronary artery disease, kidney disease, and other problems.

Diuretic: Also known as a water pill. A drug that increases the amount of urine produced, by helping the kidneys get rid of water and salt.

Diverticulitis: Inflammation of small pocket (abnormal sac) protruding outward from the lining of the intestine.

Eczema: Inflammation of the skin marked by itching, redness, swelling, blistering, watery discharge, and scales.

Edema: Swelling in the body, most notably feet and legs, caused by accumulation of fluid. This may be due to diseases in the veins of the legs or heart problems.

Electrolytes: Important chemicals such as sodium, potassium, calcium, magnesium, chloride, and bicarbonate, found in the body tissues and fluids.

Emphysema: Condition of the lungs characterized by swelling of the alveoli (small air cells of the lungs) causing breathlessness and difficulty breathing.

Endogenous depression: Serious depression not precipitated by outside factors, such as death of spouse, job loss, etc.

Endometriosis: Condition in which material similar to the lining of the womb (uterus) is present at other sites outside of the womb (including the pelvic cavity, intestines, and lung). This condition may cause pain and bleeding.

Enzyme: A chemical which acts on other substances to speed up a chemical reaction. Enzymes in the intestines help to break down food.

Expectorant: A drug promoted to thin mucus in the airways, so that the mucus may be coughed up more easily. None of these drugs are effective.

Fecal impaction: A collection of stool in the rectum or colon which is difficult to pass.

Fixed-ratio combination drug: A combination of two or more ingredients, each ingredient in a set amount. This means that you cannot take more or less of one ingredient without also changing the amount of the other ingredient.

Fluoroquinolones: A family of antibiotics that includes ciprofloxacin (CIPRO, CILOXAN), ofloxacin (FLOXIN, OCUFLOX), lomefloxacin (MAXAQUIN), and others.

G6PD (glucose-6-phosphate dehydrogenase) deficiency: An inherited medical condition marked by a lack of or reduced amounts of an enzyme (glucose-6-phosphate dehydrogenase) that breaks down certain sugar compounds in the body.

Glaucoma: A condition in which partial or complete loss of vision occurs because of abnormally high pressure in the eye.

Gout: A form of arthritis caused by too much uric acid buildup in the blood which then becomes deposited around the joints.

Heart block: Failure of the electrical conduction tissue of the heart to conduct impulses normally from one part of the heart to another, causing altered rhythm of the heartbeat. There are varying degrees of severity. Slow heartbeat with fainting, seizure, or even death can result from this abnormality.

Heart failure: See congestive heart failure.

Herpes simplex: Also known as cold sores. Inflammation of the skin, caused by a virus, resulting in groups of small, painful blisters. They may occur either round the mouth or, in the case of genital herpes, around the genitals (sex organs).

Histamine: A chemical made by the body especially during an allergic reaction. It produces dilation of small blood vessels causing redness, localized swelling, and often itching; lowers the blood pressure; and increases secretions from the stomach, the salivary glands, and other organs.

Hormone: Substance produced in one part of the body (usually a gland) which then passes into the bloodstream and is carried to other organs or tissues, where it helps them to function.

Hypersensitivity: An exaggerated response to a foreign stimulus.

Hypertension: High blood pressure.

Hypoglycemia: A low blood sugar level.

Hypothermia: A condition resulting from overexposure to cold temperatures. The symptoms include shivering, cold hands and feet, and memory lapse.

Infection: Disease resulting from presence of certain microorganisms or matter in the body. *Viral:* flu or cold, for example; cannot be treated with drugs except for herpes, flu, or AIDS. *Bacterial:* often treated with antibiotics.

Laxative: A drug used to encourage bowel movements.

Leukotriene modifiers: A new family of asthma drugs that includes zafirlukast (ACCOLATE) and zileuton (ZYFLO).

Me-too drugs: Drugs which offer no significant benefit over drugs already on the market.

Myasthenia gravis: A chronic disease marked by abnormal weakness, and sometimes paralysis of certain muscles.

Narcotic: A drug used to relieve pain but which also may produce insensibility or stupor.

Nervous system: The brain, spinal cord, and nerves throughout the body.

Nonsteroidal anti-inflammatory drug (NSAID): A drug (such as aspirin or ibuprofen) used to treat pain, fever, and swelling. It does not contain corticosteroids.

Osteomalacia: Softening of the bones due to lack of vitamin D.

Osteoporosis: Loss of bone tissue which occurs most often in older women (thin, small-boned, white women in particular), resulting in bones that are brittle and easily broken.

Parkinson's disease: Disorder of the nervous system marked by tremor (shaking), muscular rigidity, slow movements, stooped posture, salivation, and an immobile facial expression.

Parkinsonism, drug-induced: A tremor often indistinguishable from Parkinson's disease caused by a drug.

Peptic ulcer: A localized loss of tissue, involving mainly the lining of areas of the digestive tract exposed to acid produced by the stomach. Usually involves the lower esophagus, the stomach, or the beginning of the small intestine (duodenum).

Pneumonia: Disease of the lungs in which the tissue becomes inflamed, hardened, and watery. Causes include bacteria, viruses, chemical inhalation, and trauma.

Polyps: Swollen or tumorous tissues which may or may not be cancerous. They may be found in various parts of the body such as the lining of the digestive tract, bladder, nose, or throat.

Porphyria: Rare, inherited blood disease.

Progestins: Synthetic variations of the naturally occurring hormone in women's bodies called progesterone.

Prostate: A walnut-sized gland found only in males, located deep inside the abdomen just below the bladder. The prostate gland surrounds the urethra, the canal which carries urine from the bladder. The prostate gland is responsible for producing semen, the liquid which carries sperm. It enlarges with age and can cause difficulty with starting and stopping urination.

Psoriasis: Chronic skin condition marked by itchy, scaly, dry, red skin patches.

Psychosis: Severe mental illness marked by loss of contact with reality, often involving delusions, hallucinations, and disordered thinking.

Raynaud's syndrome: Condition marked by paleness, numbness, redness, and discomfort in the toes and fingers when they are exposed to cold. It rarely occurs in males.

Salicylate: A drug used to treat rheumatism and relieve pain.

Sarcoidosis: A chronic disorder in which the lymph nodes in many parts of the body are enlarged, and small fleshy swellings develop in the lungs, liver, and spleen.

Serotonin: A clinical transmitter found in many areas of the body including the brain where it is found in relatively high concentrations.

Schizophrenia: Serious mental illness (the most common type of psychosis) marked by a breakdown of the thinking process, of contact with reality, and of normal emotional responses. People with schizophrenia often have hallucinations.

Scleroderma: Persistent hardening and shrinking of the body's connective tissue.

Selective serotonin reuptake inhibitors (SSRIs): Drugs such as fluoxetine (PROZAC), fluvoxamine (LUVOX), paroxetine (PAXIL), and sertraline (ZOLOFT) that increase levels of serotonin in the brain to treat depression.

Sick sinus syndrome: Abnormality in the wiring system of the heart marked by periods of rapid and/or extremely slow heartbeats which may cause fainting, chest pain, or palpitations.

Sjogren's syndrome: Condition marked by swollen glands, dryness of the mouth and often the eyes, and arthritis.

Spasm: A sudden contraction of a muscle which can cause pain and restrict movement.

Statins: This term refers to the family of cholesterol-lowering drugs that include lovastatin (MEVACOR), simvastatin (ZOCOR), fluvastatin (LESCOL), and others.

Stool: Bowel movement.

Sulfonamide: An antibiotic drug derived from sulfa compounds.

Sympathomimetic: A drug that increases blood pressure and heartbeat. They are related to the chemical produced naturally in the body, adrenaline. These drugs also relieve nasal congestion by causing constriction of blood vessels.

Systemic lupus erythematosus: Also known as lupus or SLE. A chronic disease affecting the skin, blood vessels, and various internal organs, often accompanied by arthritis.

Tardive dyskinesia: Slow, involuntary movements of the tongue, lips, arms, and other body parts often brought on by certain drugs, especially antipsychotic drugs.

Thalassemia: An inherited blood disorder which causes anemia that is most often seen in persons of Mediterranean descent.

Thyroid: A large gland in front and on either side of the trachea which secretes thyroxine, a hormone regulating the growth of the body. Malfunctioning of the gland (hyperthyroidism, hypothyroidism) can cause medical problems.

Toxic: Poisonous; potentially deadly.

Tuberculosis: Also known as TB. An infectious disease, usually of the lungs, marked by fever, night sweats, weight loss, and coughing up blood.

Ulcer: Localized loss of surface tissue of the skin or mucous membrane.

Uric acid: One of the products made when protein is broken down in the body. It is normally eliminated from the body by the kidneys. Too high levels of uric acid in the body cause gout.

Urinalysis: An examination of the urine to detect abnormalities such as sugar, protein, bacteria, or crystals, and to check the pH.

Ventricular fibrillation: A life-threatening rapid, irregular contraction of the heart.

Vertigo: Dizziness. A sensation of irregular or whirling motion, either of oneself or of external objects. Elderly people often experience "postural vertigo" when rising from a lying or sitting position.

Vitamin: A substance found in foods which does not provide energy, but is needed by the body in small amounts for normal functioning.

Wolff-Parkinson-White syndrome: Also known as WPW syndrome. An abnormality of the heart marked by periods when the heart rate is very fast and must be controlled with medication or electrical shock to the heart (defibrillation).

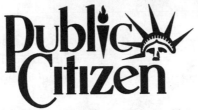

Public Citizen

Buyers Up • Congress Watch • Critical Mass • Global Trade Watch • Health Research Group • Litigation Group
Joan Claybrook, President

25+ Years of Consumer Activism

Dear Friend,

It has been over twenty-five years since a hardy group of enterprising young people came to the nation's capital to start an experiment in citizenship. The first "Nader's Raiders" showed special grit, integrity, and idealism that still serve us today. I am writing to ask all buyers of *Worst Pills, Best Pills* to please help us continue this record—and nurture those values—by joining Public Citizen today.

You hold in your hands an example of the important work we do every day. Public Citizen is the only organization with the courage to write *Worst Pills, Best Pills*. We name names and tell the real facts. When you join Public Citizen with a gift of $35 or more you'll get our monthly health publication, which will update you with new information on dangerous drugs and provide you with other information important to your health and safety. You'll also receive our bi-monthly member publication *Public Citizen News* which will keep you abreast of all the work that Public Citizen does on behalf of citizens across the country.

We've helped purge cancer-producing additives from dozens of food products. Workplaces have fewer safety and health hazards. Many ineffective, unsafe drugs and medical devices have been forced from the market as a result of our tireless efforts. We have helped to force government decision-making out of the smoke-filled back rooms, but there is so much left to do.

We need to remove the flood of soft money polluting our political system; stop federal give-aways to corporate fat cats; rewrite unfair trade legislation that hurts American workers and weakens our environmental laws; pass new and improved laws to protect our health and safety; and force federal agencies to enforce the laws we already have. *But we can't do it without you!*

To retain its independence, Public Citizen does not accept government or corporate funds. Our support comes from individual members who believe there should be full-time advocates of democratic principles working on their behalf, and from foundation grants and publication sales. To remain effective, Public Citizen needs you. Please join us. As Ralph Nader reminds us, "together we *can* make a difference."

Sincerely,

Joan Claybrook

Joan Claybrook
President

Ralph Nader, Founder

1600 20th Street NW • Washington, DC 20009-1001 • (202) 588-1000

Printed on Recycled Paper

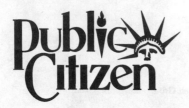

Corporations, trade associations, and other special interest groups send lobbyists to Washington, D.C., to advance their very particular agendas. Most speak for business or industry.

Public Citizen speaks for you—

> before Congress,
> in the courts,
> in the hallways of federal regulatory agencies.

Ralph Nader founded Public Citizen to empower ordinary citizens to protect the rights of consumers and give them a voice in the halls of power.

Public Citizen exposes threats to health and safety, and presses for freedom of information and public disclosure. We've won important victories for citizens and consumers on issues concerning health care, injury prevention, campaign finance reform, cutting corporate subsidies, and fair trade.

Join together with thousands of other like-minded citizens, and you can help transform many issues at the national level.

"There can be no daily democracy without daily citizenship."

> —Ralph Nader, founder of Public Citizen

1971
■ Public Citizen petitions the Food and Drug Administration (FDA) to ban the use of Red Dye #2 as food coloring.

1972
■ Public Citizen files a lawsuit that obligates airlines to pay damages to consumers bumped from flights.
■ Public Citizen asks courts to order increased disclosure of political campaign contributions.

1973
■ In response to Public Citizen's suit, President Nixon's firing of Special Prosecutor Archibald Cox is ruled illegal.

1974
■ Public Citizen convinces Congress to override President Ford's veto and pass major improvements to the Freedom of Information Act.

1975
■ Public Citizen successfully lobbies Congress for energy conservation laws, including fuel economy requirements for cars.

1976
■ FDA bans Red Dye #2 after Public Citizen's four-year campaign.
■ A Public Citizen petition leads to FDA ban on use of cancer-causing chloroform in cough medicines and toothpaste.

1977
■ Public Citizen challenges the airline industry's failure to provide adequate seating for nonsmokers.
■ Public Citizen mobilizes citizens who persuade President Carter to halt the construction of the Clinch River Breeder Reactor.

1978
■ Cyclamates are banned after Public Citizen raises safety concerns about the widely used artificial sweetener.
■ Congress passes Public Citizen's National Consumer Cooperative Bill, authorizing $300 million seed money for consumer cooperatives.

1979
■ Public Citizen helps defeat legislation that would have raised sugar price supports, saving consumers $300 million per year.
■ A Public Citizen petition leads the Environmental Protection Agency (EPA) to ban the use of DBCP, a pesticide proven to cause sterility in men.

1980
■ A Public Citizen lawsuit opens the Chrysler bailout board proceedings to the public.
■ Public Citizen plays a critical role in the passage of the Superfund law, requiring cleanup of toxic waste sites.

1981
■ Public Citizen secures Toxic Shock Syndrome warning labels on tampons.
■ Public Citizen helps thwart President Reagan's attempts to dismantle the Clean Air Act and diminish the authority of the Consumer Product Safety Commission.

1982
■ After an extensive Public Citizen campaign, cancer-causing urea formaldehyde is banned in home insulation.
■ The arthritis drug Oraflex is withdrawn from the market after Public Citizen exposes deaths and injuries caused by the drug.

1983
■ Public Citizen participates in a landmark Supreme Court decision overturning President

Reagan's revocation of auto safety standards for automatic restraints.

1984
■ Following the AT&T divestiture, Public Citizen mounts a nationwide "Campaign for Affordable Phones," successfully opposing rate hikes for residential customers.
■ Public Citizen wins a court order forcing the EPA to recall 700,000 GM cars with faulty emission controls.

1985
■ FDA requires a Reye's Syndrome warning label on aspirin after a four-year campaign by Public Citizen.
■ Public Citizen reveals the locations of more than 250 work sites nationwide where workers have been exposed to hazardous chemicals.

1986
■ Congress requires health warning labels on chewing tobacco and snuff, capping Public Citizen's two-year campaign.
■ A Public Citizen suit defeats a Bush administration plan to block low-income housing programs by refusing to spend appropriated funds.

1987
■ Public Citizen helps convince Congress to pass legislation restricting the time banks can hold checks after being deposited.
■ After eight years of litigation by Public Citizen, the Occupational Safety and Health

Administration (OSHA) imposes standards for exposure to cancer-causing ethylene oxide.

1988
■ Public Citizen publishes the best-selling *Worst Pills, Best Pills,* a consumer guide to dangerous and ineffective drugs and their safer alternatives, selling 2 million copies over the next 10 years.

1989
■ Public Citizen and Ralph Nader lead successful opposition to a $45,500 congressional pay raise.
■ Public Citizen helps persuade California voters to shut down the Rancho Seco nuclear plant.

1990
■ A Public Citizen court victory forces the Nuclear Regulatory Agency to require training for nuclear plant workers.

1991
■ OSHA imposes a standard to protect workers from cadmium, linked to lung cancer and kidney damage, after Public Citizen wins a court order.
■ Public Citizen wins a landmark ruling that the Federal Election Commission (FEC) cannot restrict the use of campaign finance data.

1992
■ Public Citizen's four-year campaign leads the FDA to severely restrict the use of silicone gel breast implants.

1993
■ Public Citizen plays a leading role in opposition to the North American Free Trade Agreement (NAFTA).
■ Public Citizen wins a landmark court victory that preserves the electronic records of the White House under Reagan, Bush, and Clinton.

1994
■ Public Citizen helps to enlist nearly 100 cosponsors for a single payer health care reform bill.
■ Public Citizen wins consumer protections against home equity scams.

1995
■ Public Citizen lawyers defend tobacco industry whistle blowers.
■ Congressional gift ban and lobbying registration reform passed after a major Public Citizen campaign.

1996
■ Public Citizen wins a Supreme Court decision upholding the right of people injured by federally regulated defective medical devices to sue for compensation.
■ Public Citizen wins a court ruling that class actions cannot be used to deprive future victims of their right to sue.
■ Public Citizen wins release of Nixon's White House tapes, after fifteen years of litigation.

1997
■ Public Citizen defends consumer interests as the electricity industry deregulates.

■ Public Citizen wins fights to prevent passage of damaging fast-track legislation, to ensure that global trade agreements do not sweep away health and safety standards.

1998
■ Public Citizen protests and helps force redesign of unethical AIDS research in Africa which would have denied known effective treatment to HIV-positive pregnant women.
■ Public Citizen again stops passage of undemocratic fast-track trade legislation.
■ Campaign Finance Reform passes House with continued pressure from Public Citizen. Senate leaders kill it with a filibuster.
■ Public Citizen helps stop two bills that would have limited the power of federal agencies to protect public health, safety, and the environment and taken away consumers' legal rights to hold accountable corporations that manufacture defective products that injure and kill.
■ Public Citizen played instrumental role in enactment of a new law to require reengineered airbags to protect small adults and children.

Public Citizen
Health Research Group Publications

Delivering a Better Childbirth Experience
A Consumer's Guide

Get the answers to the most common questions asked about nurse-midwives with this valuable consumer guide.

This report includes descriptions of 414 nurse-midwifery practices in 47 states that attend in-hospital births and details of 41 freestanding birth center practices.

1995, Item #F8018
$15.00

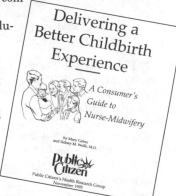

Medical Records: Getting Yours

If you needed your medical records to check an insurance policy or to check their accuracy, would you know how to go about getting them? Does your state allow full access?

This useful guide for consumers and professionals includes:
•Definitions of medical records •Step-by-step guide to getting your medical records •Glossary of terms to help you understand your own records •State-by-state access guide.

1995, Item #F8565
$10.00

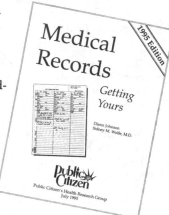

Questionable Doctors, Regional Editions

This is the only state-by-state listing of doctors who have been disciplined by state and federal agencies—doctors who may be continuing to treat unsuspecting patients.

When ordering *Questionable Doctors* regional editions, please specify the number of the region you are ordering. Regional editions are $20 each.

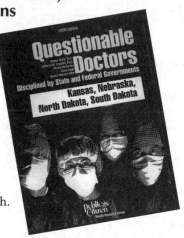

Region 1 (#FQ801): Arkansas, Louisiana, Mississippi
Region 2 (#FQ802): Alaska, Idaho, Montana, Oregon, Washington, Wyoming
Region 3 (#FQ803): Arizona, Colorado, Nevada, New Mexico, Utah
Region 4 (#FQ804): California, Hawaii
Region 5 (#FQ805): Connecticut, Maine, Massachusetts, New Hampshire, Rhode Island, Vermont
Region 6 (#FQ806): Delaware, New Jersey
Region 7 (#FQ807): District of Columbia, Maryland, Virginia
Region 8 (#FQ808): Florida

Region 9 (#FQ809): Alabama, Georgia
Region 10 (#FQ810): Illinois, Indiana
Region 11 (#FQ811): Iowa, Missouri
Region 12 (#FQ812): New York
Region 13 (#FQ813): Kentucky, North Carolina, South Carolina, Tennessee
Region 14 (#FQ814): Kansas, Nebraska, North Dakota, South Dakota
Region 15 (#FQ815): Oklahoma, Texas
Region 16 (#FQ816): Minnesota, Wisconsin
Region 17 (#FQ817): Michigan, Ohio
Region 18 (#FQ818): Pennsylvania, West Virginia

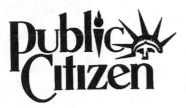

Public Citizen

1600 20th Street, NW, Washington, DC 20009-1001

Order Form

Public Citizen Membership/Newsletter Subscription

Qty	Item Description	Price	Subtotal
	Basic membership (includes PC News)	$20.00	
	Combination membership with *Health* Letter	$35.00	
	I want to help even more with an additional contribution of: $_____	$	
	Membership/Subscription subtotal		

Publications from Public Citizen

Qty	Item Description	Price	Subtotal
	F6672 *Worst Pills, Best Pills*	$16.00	
	FQ8 _____ *Questionable Doctors,* Regional Edition (write in region #)	$20.00	
	F8565 *Medical Records: Getting Yours*	$10.00	
	F8018 *Delivering a Better Childbirth Experience*	$15.00	
	Publications subtotal		
	Publications shipping (see chart)		
	TOTAL		

BWPBK3

CUT HERE

See over for ordering instructions

Name (please print)

Mailing address

City/State/Zip

Phone Number

Payment (all orders must be prepaid)

Charge to credit card: VISA   MC   AMEX   DISC

Charge will appear on statement as Public Citizen

Expiration Date: ———————————

Credit Card Number

Signature (as it appears on card)

Payment enclosed (make check or money order payable to Public Citizen)

Shipping and Handling

Publications Subtotal	S&H charge	Mail to: PUBLIC CITIZEN
$1.00–5.99	Add $1.00	1600 20th Street N.W.
$6.00–11.99	Add $2.50	Washington, D.C. 20009
$12.00–24.99	Add $3.50	
$25.00–99.99	Add $5.00	
$100.00–$150.00	Add $7.50	

Please allow 4–6 weeks for delivery of publications; 6–8 weeks for your first issue of subscriptions.

These titles represent only a portion of our current publications. For a complete brochure, to order publications by phone, get information on overnight delivery orders or orders outside the continental U.S., or for information on membership/subscriptions call (800) 289-3787 or (202) 588-1000, M–F 9AM–5PM EST, or check our web site at www.citizen.org.

Contributions to Public Citizen Foundation, which supports Public Citizen's education, litigation, research, and public information activities, are tax-deductible in excess of your annual $20 membership dues. Contributions to Public Citizen, Inc., a nonprofit membership organization that lobbies for strong citizen and consumer protection laws, are not tax-deductible.

A copy of our latest financial statement may be obtained by sending a large, self-addressed, stamped envelope to Public Citizen, 1600 20th Street N.W., Washington, D.C. 20009

Get monthly updates on dangerous pills in WORST PILLS/BEST PILLS NEWS!

Your copy of the new edition of WORST PILLS, BEST PILLS brings you up-to-date on the benefits and risks of hundreds of commonly used drugs.

Right now there are scores of *new drugs* in the pipeline that will soon be in pharmacies—available by prescription and over-the-counter.

America's drug companies will spend *billions* promoting these new drugs. And most doctors and pharmacists will be too busy to provide you with the information you need to protect yourself against dangerous reactions.

Which new drugs will be safe and effective? Which will be dangerous? Which will waste your money? Which should never be taken with other drugs?

You'll find the answers in monthly issues of WORST PILLS/BEST PILLS NEWS.

Edited by Dr. Sidney Wolfe, editor of WORST PILLS, BEST PILLS, and published by Public Citizen's Health Research Group, WORST PILLS/BEST PILLS NEWS brings you the *latest findings* about dangerous drugs and their safer alternatives. It also contains a wide range of information about health, health policy issues, evaluations of alternative medicine, vitamins and herbal products, and more.

(Continued on back)

This is potentially life-saving information you cannot get from any other single source. And it's *authoritative* information—provided by knowledgeable physicians and researchers as opposed to questionable information available from drug industry ads, on the Internet and from other sources.

In recent years, WORST PILLS/BEST PILLS NEWS has warned readers about several dangerous drugs and drug interactions and urged that they be banned—or warning labels issued—long before FDA action was taken. For example, our readers knew about the danger of the diet combination fen/phen many months before the lethal drugs were withdrawn from the market.

SAVE $10 . . . GET 3 FREE ISSUES IN THE BARGAIN!

To introduce readers of WORST PILLS, BEST PILLS who are not yet subscribers, we offer 15 monthly issues of WORST PILLS/BEST PILLS NEWS for only $10. The regular subscription price for 12 issues is $20, so you save $10 *plus you get 3 issues free!*

Your satisfaction is guaranteed! If you wish to cancel your subscription at any time, for any reason, your $10 payment will be refunded *in full!*

Use the coupon below to subscribe. Continue protecting your health—and the health of those you love—with a life-saving, money-saving subscription to WORST PILLS/BEST PILLS NEWS!

$10 SAVINGS . . . PLUS 3 FREE ISSUES!
SPECIAL OFFER FOR NEW SUBSCRIBERS ONLY

Yes, I want to be updated each month and avoid dangerous drugs. Please enter my introductory subscription to WORST PILLS/BEST PILLS NEWS for 15 months at only $10. That's 50% off the regular 12-month subscription price, plus I'll receive 3 issues free.

I understand I may cancel at any time and receive a full refund.

☐ Enclosed is my payment of $10 (Make check or money order payable to "Pills News")
Please charge my ☐ VISA ☐ MC ☐ DISC ☐ AMEX
Charge will appear on statement as Public Citizen

Credit Card # ————————————————————

Expiration Date ————————————————————

Signature ————————————————————

My Name ————————————————————

Address ————————————————————

City ———————————————— State ———————— Zip ————————

9P4PWP9

Look for your first issue in 6–8 weeks.
Offer expires December 31, 2000.

Mail to: WORST PILLS/BEST PILLS NEWS • P.O. Box 96978
Washington, DC 20090-6978